HIGH-DOSE CANCER THERAPY

HIGH-DOSE CANCER THERAPY

Pharmacology, Hematopoietins, Stem Cells

Edited by

James O. Armitage, M.D.
Professor of Medicine
University of Nebraska Medical Center
Omaha, Nebraska

Karen H. Antman, M.D.
Associate Professor of Medicine
Harvard Medical School
Dana-Farber Cancer Institute
Boston, Massachusetts

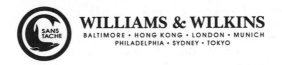

WILLIAMS & WILKINS
BALTIMORE · HONG KONG · LONDON · MUNICH
PHILADELPHIA · SYDNEY · TOKYO

Editor: Jonathan W. Pine, Jr.
Managing Editor: Carol Eckhart
Copy Editor: Rebecca Marnhout
Designer: Wilma E. Rosenberger
Illustration Planner: Wayne Hubbel
Production Coordinator: Barbara J. Felton
Cover Designer: Wilma E. Rosenberger

Copyright © 1992
Williams & Wilkins
428 East Preston Street
Baltimore, Maryland 21202, USA

Accurate indications, adverse reactions, and dosage schedules for drugs are provided in this book, but it is possible that they may change. The reader is urged to review the package information data of the manufacturers of the medications mentioned.

Printed in the United States of America

Library of Congress Cataloging-in-Publication Data

High-dose cancer therapy : pharmacology, hematopoietins, stem cells / edited by
  James O. Armitage, Karen H. Antman.
        p.   cm.
    Includes bibliographical references and index.
    ISBN 0-683-00254-6
    1. Cancer—Chemotherapy.   2. Cancer—Chemotherapy—Complications—
Prevention.   3. Drugs—Dosage.   4. Hematopoietic growth factors—Therapeutic
use.   5. Bone marrow—Effect of drugs on.   I. Armitage, James O., 1946–
II. Antman, Karen.   III. Title: High dose cancer therapy.
    [DNLM: 1. Antineoplastic Agents—administration & dosage.   2. Dose-Response
Relationship. Drug.   3. Hematopoietic Cell Growth Factors—therapeutic
use.   4. Neoplasms—drug therapy.   QZ 267 H638]
RC271.C5H54   1992
616.99'4061—dc20
DNLM/DLC
for Library of Congress   92-5759
                                                                     CIP

                                        92   93   94   95   96
                            1   2   3   4   5   6   7   8   9   10

Dedicated to our children in hopes of an effective treatment for cancer within their lifetimes

FOREWORD

Since the earliest trials of chemotherapy to treat cancer, evidence has accumulated that increased doses yield a higher cure rate in some tumors. The earliest and still dramatic example is the use of allogeneic marrow transplantation to treat leukemia. With allogeneic marrow transplantation the immunologic effects of the reinfused marrow also seem important in effecting cure in leukemias, demonstrating the importance of the immune system acting in concert with effective cytotoxic chemotherapy in the treatment of cancer.

Myelotoxicity of dose-intensive treatment can also be ameliorated with autologous marrow or peripheral blood stem cell support. Some patients who had not been cured with treatments at lower doses can be cured with high-dose therapy and hematopoietic stem cell support. The introduction of hematopoietic growth factors into the clinic raises the possibility that higher than conventional dose cytotoxic therapy might be repetitively administered without reinfusion of any hematopoietic stem cells.

These dramatic advances in the treatment of selected cancers have been paralleled by an increased understanding of the biology of hematopoiesis and the pharmacology of cancer chemotherapeutic agents. Some of these new insights will likely have application beyond the treatment of cancer.

This book is unique in that it integrates basic and clinical aspects of high-dose therapy of malignancy in one volume. It is divided into sections that deal first with the pharmacologic and biologic principles of high-dose cancer therapy and the varied strategies utilized for the application of these principles. Next is a series of up-to-date reviews of the various methods used to reestablish effective hematopoiesis after high-dose cancer therapy—including allogenic marrow, autologous marrow, or blood-derived stem cell transplantation, as well as very high-dose therapy utilizing hematopoietic growth factors without hematopoietic stem cell transplantation. The data from each of the hematopoietic growth factors now in clinical usage are reviewed. The extensive laboratory and clinical support necessary for effective high-dose therapy is detailed in the following section, including the controversial issues of tumor cell detection and marrow purging. Finally, the last section provides a clear and comprehensive review of the variety of malignancies currently treated with high-dose therapy regimens.

The issues addressed in this text will have increasing application in the treatment of patients with malignant diseases over the next decade. This volume will have wide interest and utility for all the scientists and clinicians who work in the broad field of cancer therapy.

—E. Donnall Thomas, M.D.
Professor of Medicine, Emeritus
University of Washington
Member, Fred Hutchinson Cancer Center
Nobel Laureate in Medicine, 1991

PREFACE

More than a century ago, in 1891, Brown-Sequard first attempted to orally "transplant" human bone marrow. Fifty years passed, during which administration of allogeneic marrow was attempted intramuscularly and by intramedullary injection, before the intravenous route was finally adopted in 1939 after animal experiments. Only after research in radiobiology and immunology between 1945 and 1965 defined the effects of total body radiotherapy and the necessary immunologic requirements for successful allogeneic engraftment was the first small series of patients transplanted for relapsed leukemia and aplastic anemia published in 1968.

In 1977, Thomas and colleagues in Seattle reported 100 patients with acute leukemia in relapse at the time of transplant. Thirteen were disease-free one to four and a half years after transplantation. Encouraged by these results in advanced leukemia, subsequent patients were transplanted in remission, a strategy that resulted in a substantial increase in the percentage of patients surviving disease-free. The availability of platelet transfusions, intensive supportive care, protected environments, and a wider variety of effective antibiotics have considerably decreased the risks of high-dose therapy. Simultaneously, moderate gains have been made in the treatment of graft-versus-host disease. The net result is that approximately 50% of acute myelogenous leukemia patients transplanted during first remission with HLA-matched sibling donor marrow are now cured.

However, allogeneic bone marrow transplantation (BMT) is intrinsically limited by the lack of an available matched sibling marrow for two-thirds of patients and a high incidence of lethal graft-versus-host disease in patients over age 35. To avoid these limitations, the use of autologous bone marrow reinfusion in the treatment of malignancy was first reported in 1959. Technical problems impeded the development of the technique. Initially, the harvested marrow was refrigerated or stored at room temperature. Reliable marrow cryopreservation (not required for sibling donor marrows) was subsequently developed, increasing the scope and duration of available drug therapy.

The preparative regimens developed for leukemia were next applied to lymphomas. Although the duration of follow-up of patients treated with BMT for lymphoma is considerably shorter than for transplanted leukemia, 10 to 50% of lymphoma patients failing conventional treatment have been long-term disease-free survivors.

The role of high-dose therapy in the treatment of common solid tumors has only recently come under the kind of scrutiny applied to leukemias and lymphomas a decade ago. Myelosuppression is the dose-limiting toxicity for many chemotherapy regimens for solid tumors. However, for many tumors, optimum response cannot be achieved without exceeding the dose of chemotherapeutic agents which causes unacceptable myelosuppression. The design of effective regimens is considerably more complex because of the diversity of solid tumors and the likelihood that different regimens will be required for the various tumors. Many patients with common solid tumors have a readily available source of tumor-free compatible bone marrow, thus obviating the risk of graft-versus-host disease. Lessons learned from the early leukemic transplantation experience, however, are clearly applicable to the current studies in solid tumors. Most important is the need to transplant patients relatively early in the disease course, before the development of resistance to available ablative chemotherapy regimens.

The current availability of effective recombinant hematopoietic growth factors has ensured that high-dose therapy for cancer will be applied more widely (with or without hematopoietic stem cell support) to an increasing number of diseases. Dose intensification offers the best currently available strategy to overcome the resistance to therapy. With the advent of clinical use of growth factors, it is likely that "standard" doses will increase substantially. This can be done expeditiously because many toxicity studies have already been done with bone marrow support.

Thus an opportunity exists for a comprehensive text to encompass this emerging field in the management of patients with cancer. This book is intended for hematologists and medical oncologists at levels from fellowship to faculty or practice. It is likely that this text also will be of interest to many practicing oncologists because the area of growth factors and dose-intensive treatment is evolving and expanding rapidly.

—*Karen Antman, M.D.*
—*James Armitage, M.D.*

CONTRIBUTORS

Kenneth C. Anderson, M.D.
Medical Director, Blood Component
Laboratory
Dana-Farber Cancer Institute
Associate Professor of Medicine
Harvard Medical School
Boston, Massachusetts

Karen H. Antman, M.D.
Associate Professor of Medicine
Harvard Medical School
Dana-Farber Cancer Institute
Boston, Massachusetts

James O. Armitage, M.D.
Professor and Chairman
Department of Internal Medicine
University of Nebraska Medical Center
Omaha, Nebraska

Lois J. Ayash, M.D.
Harvard Medical School
Dana-Farber Cancer Institute
Boston, Massachusetts

Giuseppe Bandini, M.D.
Institute of Hematology
L & A Seragnoli
St. Orsola University Hospital
Bologna, Italy

Bart Barlogie, M.D.
Professor and Director
Division of Hematology/Oncology
University of Arkansas for Medical
Sciences
Director of Research
Arkansas Cancer Research Center
Little Rock, Arkansas

Amy L. Billett, M.D.
Instructor in Pediatrics
Harvard Medical School
Clinical Associate Professor in Pediatrics
Dana-Farber Cancer Institute
Assistant Professor in Medicine
(Hematology/Oncology)
Children's Hospital
Boston, Massachusetts

Jean-Yves Blay, M.D.
Bone Marrow Transplantation Unit
Department of Immunology
Centre Léon Berard
Lyon, France

Karl G. Blume, M.D., F.A.C.P.
Professor of Medicine
Director, Bone Marrow Transplantation
Program
Stanford University Medical Center
Stanford, California

K. Bross, M.D.
Department of Hematology
University of Freiburg
Freiburg, Germany

E. Randolph Broun, M.D.
Assistant Professor of Medicine
Division of Hematology/Oncology
Department of Medicine
Indiana University School of Medicine
Indianapolis, Indiana

Sherri Brown
Amgen Inc.
Thousand Oaks, California

W. Brugger, M.D.
Department of Hematology
University of Freiburg
Freiburg, Germany

Anna Butturini, M.D.
Transplantation Biology Program
UCLA School of Medicine
Los Angeles, California

Nelson J. Chao, M.D.
Assistant Professor of Medicine
Assistant Director, Bone Marrow
   Transplantation Program
Stanford University Medical Center
Stanford, California

Bruce D. Cheson, M.D.
Head, Medicine Section
Clinical Investigations Branch
Cancer Therapy Evaluation Program
National Cancer Institute
Bethesda, Maryland

R. Chopra, M.D.
Department of Haematology
University of College Hospital
London, England

David A. Crouse, Ph.D.
Departments of Anatomy and Radiology
University of Nebraska Medical Center
Omaha, Nebraska

Christopher E. Desch, M.D.
Assistant Professor of Medicine
Virginia Commonwealth University
Medical College of Virginia
Richmond, Virginia

Frank R. Dunphy, M.D.
Division of Medical Oncology
St. Louis University Medical Center
St. Louis, Missouri

Connie J. Eaves, M.D.
Professor of Medical Genetics
University of British Columbia
Senior Scientist
Terry Fox Laboratory
British Columbia Cancer Centre
Vancouver, British Columbia, Canada

Stephen G. Emerson, M.D., Ph.D.
Associate Professor
Departments of Internal Medicine and
   Pediatrics
Associate Chief
Division of Hematology and Oncology
University of Michigan Medical Center
Ann Arbor, Michigan

Mary Ann Foote
Manager
Medical Writing
Amgen Inc.
Thousand Oaks, California

Theresa Franco, R.N., M.S.N.
University of Nebraska Medical Center
Omaha, Nebraska

Emil Frei III, M.D.
Physician-in-Chief, Emeritus
Chief, Division of Cancer Pharmacology
Dana-Farber Cancer Institute
Richard and Susan Smith Professor of
   Medicine
Harvard Medical School
Boston, Massachusetts

J. Frisch, M.D.
Department of Hematology
University of Freiburg
Freiburg, Germany

Zvi Y. Fuks, M.D.
Member and Chairman
Department of Radiation Oncology
Memorial Sloan-Kettering Cancer Center
New York, New York

Robert Peter Gale, M.D., Ph.D.
Department of Medicine
Division of Hematology/Oncology
UCLA School of Medicine
Los Angeles, California

L. Michael Glode, M.D.
Professor of Medicine
Division of Medical Oncology
University of Colorado Cancer Center
University of Colorado Health Sciences
   Center
Denver, Colorado

A. H. Goldstone, F.R.C.P., F.R.C.Path.
Department of Haematology
University of College Hospital
London, England

N. Claude Gorin, M.D.
Director of the Bone Marrow Transplant
Unit
Department of Hematology
Hôpital St. Antoine
Paris, France

John R. Graham-Pole, M.D.
Department of Pediatric Hematology/
Oncology
University of Florida
Gainesville, Florida

James D. Griffin, M.D.
Division of Tumor Immunology
Dana-Farber Cancer Institute
Boston, Massachusetts

William D. Haire, M.D.
Assistant Professor of Medicine
University of Nebraska Medical Center
Section of Oncology/Hematology
Omaha, Nebraska

Lisa S. Hami, B.S., M.T.(A.S.C.P.)
Bone Marrow Transplant Program
University of Colorado
Denver, Colorado

Roger H. Herzig, M.D.
Marion F. Beard Professor and Co-Chief
Division of Hematology-Medical
Oncology
Director, James Graham Brown Cancer
Center
University of Louisville
Louisville, Kentucky

Bruce E. Hillner, M.D.
Assistant Professor of Medicine
Division of General Internal Medicine
Richmond, Virginia

Thomas D. Horn, M.D.
Assistant Professor
Department of Dermatology
The Johns Hopkins University
Baltimore, Maryland

Sundar Jagannath, M.D.
Division of Hematology-Oncology
University of Arkansas Medical Sciences
Little Rock, Arkansas

Charles S. Johnston, M.T.(A.M.T.)
Bone Marrow Transplant Program
University of Colorado
Denver, Colorado

Roy B. Jones, M.D.
Director, Bone Marrow Transplant
Program
University of Colorado Health Sciences
Center
Denver, Colorado

Lothar Kanz, M.D.
Department of Medicine I, Hematology/
Oncology
Albert-Lûdwigs University Medical
Center
Freiburg, Germany

Armand Keating, M.D.
Director, University of Toronto
Autologous Bone Marrow Transplant
Program
Toronto Hospital
Toronto, Ontario, Canada

Anne Kessinger, M.D.
Chief, Section of Oncology/Hematology
University of Nebraska Medical Center
Omaha, Nebraska

Catherine E. Klein, M.D.
Associate Professor of Medicine
University of Colorado Health Sciences
Center
Denver Veteran's Affairs Medical Center
Denver, Colorado

Peter M. Lansdorp, M.D., Ph.D.
Terry Fox Laboratory
British Columbia Cancer Research
Center
Vancouver, British Columbia, Canada

Paul D. Lindower, M.D.
Cardiology Fellow
Division of Cardiovascular Diseases
Department of Internal Medicine
University of Iowa Hospitals and Clinics
Iowa City, Iowa

Robert B. Livingston, M.D.
Professor of Medicine
Head, Division of Oncology
University of Washington
Seattle, Washington

Dominique Maraninchi, M.D.
Professor of Medicine
Oncology-Hematology
Director, Regional Cancer Center
Marseilles, France

Steven Matthes, M.D.
University of Colorado Health Sciences
    Center
Denver, Colorado

Rosemary Mazanet, M.D., Ph.D.
Dana-Farber Cancer Institute
Boston, Massachusetts

A. K. McMillan, M.D.
Department of Haematology
University of College Hospital
London, England

Roland H. Mertelsmann, M.D., Ph.D.
Department of Medicine, Hematology/
    Oncology
University of Freiburg Medical Center
Freiburg, Germany

Mauricette Michallet, M.D.
Service d'Hematologie
Chu A. Michallon
Grenoble, France

Carole B. Miller, M.D.
Assistant Professor of Oncology
Bone Marrow Transplant Program
The Johns Hopkins Oncology Center
Baltimore, Maryland

George Morstyn, M.D., Ph.D.
Principal Research Fellow
Ludwig Institute for Cancer Research
Royal Melbourne Hospital
Victoria, Australia
Vice-President
Medical and Clinical Affairs
Amgen Inc.
Thousand Oaks, California

John Nemunaitis, M.D.
Director, Hematopoiesis Program
Western Pennsylvania Cancer Institute
West Penn Hospital
Pittsburgh, Pennsylvania

Craig R. Nichols, M.D.
Assistant Professor of Medicine
Division of Hematology/Oncology
Department of Medicine
Indiana University School of Medicine
Indianapolis, Indiana

Michael C. Perry, M.D., F.A.C.P.
Professor of Medicine and Senior
    Associate Dean
Medical Director, Ellis Fischer Cancer
    Center
University of Missouri Health Science
    Center
Columbia, Missouri

Thierry O. Philip, M.D.
Léon Berard Oncology Center
Lyon, France

Gordon L. Phillips, M.D.
Leukemia and Bone Transplantation of
    British Columbia
Vancouver, British Columbia, Canada

Syed M. Quadri, Ph.D.
Department of Medicine
University of Nebraska Medical Center
Omaha, Nebraska

Elizabeth C. Reed, M.D.
Assistant Professor of Medicine
Section of Oncology/Hematology
Department of Internal Medicine
University of Nebraska Medical Center
Omaha, Nebraska

Stephen I. Rennard, M.D.
Larsen Professor
Pulmonary and Critical Care Medicine
University of Nebraska Medical Center
Omaha, Nebraska

Ellen Beth Rest, M.D.
Assistant Professor
Department of Dermatology
University of Minnesota
Minneapolis, Minnesota

Richard A. Robbins, M.D.
Pulmonary and Critical Care Medicine
University of Nebraska Medical Center
Omaha, Nebraska

Rein Saral, M.D.
Professor of Medicine
Director, Bone Marrow Transplantation
    Program
Emory University School of Medicine
Atlanta, Georgia

Christian R. Schmitt, M.D.
CHU Pitié-Salpétrière
Laboratoire d'immunologie CNRS URA
Groupe d'Immuno-Hématologie
    Moléculaire
Paris, France

J. Graham Sharp, Ph.D.
Department of Anatomy
University of Nebraska Medical Center
Omaha, Nebraska

Elizabeth J. Shpall, M.D.
Associate Director
Bone Marrow Transplant Program
University of Colorado
Denver, Colorado

Jack W. Singer, M.D.
Professor of Medicine
University of Washington
Chief of Medical Oncology
Veterans Affairs Medical Center
Member, Fred Hutchinson Cancer
    Research Center
Seattle, Washington

Joseph H. Sisson, M.D.
Pulmonary and Critical Care Medicine
University of Nebraska Medical Center
Omaha, Nebraska

David J. Skorton, M.D.
Professor and Associate Chair for
    Clinical Programs
Department of Internal Medicine,
    College of Medicine
Professor, Department of Electrical and
    Computer Engineering
College of Engineering
The University of Iowa
Consulting Physician, Department of
    Veterans Affairs Medical Center
Iowa City, Iowa

Thomas J. Smith, M.D.
Director of Cancer Education
Massey Cancer Center
Medical College of Virginia
Richmond, Virginia

Verneeda Spencer, M.D.
Division of Medical Oncology
Bone Marrow Transplantation
St. Louis University Medical Center
St. Louis, Missouri

Gary Spitzer, M.D.
Division of Bone Marrow
    Transplantation, Oncology and
    Hematology
St. Louis University Medical Center
St. Louis, Missouri

John R. Spurzem, M.D.
Pulmonary and Critical Care Medicine
University of Nebraska Medical Center
Omaha, Nebraska

Michel Symann, M.D., Ph.D.
Professor of Medicine
Head, Laboratory of Experimental
    Hematology and Oncology and
Department of Clinical Oncology
Catholic University of Louvain Medical
    School
University Hospital Sainte Luc
Brussels, Belgium

Beverly A. Teicher, Ph.D.
Associate Professor of Pathology and
    Radiation Therapy
Dana-Farber Cancer Institute
Harvard Medical School
Boston, Massachusetts

Terry E. Thomas, Ph.D.
Terry Fox Laboratory
British Columbia Cancer Research
    Centre
Vancouver, British Columbia, Canada

William P. Vaughan, M.D.
University of Alabama
Birmingham, Alabama

David Vesole, M.D.
Division of Hematology-Oncology
University of Arkansas Medical Sciences
Little Rock, Arkansas

Patrice Viens, M.D.
Institut Paoli-Calmettes
Marseilles, France

Julie M. Vose, M.D.
Department of Internal Medicine
University of Nebraska Medical Center
Omaha, Nebraska

Huib M. Vriesendorp, M.D., Ph.D.
Radiation Therapy Department
M.D. Anderson Cancer Center
Houston, Texas

Jerry R. Williams, Sc.D.
Professor of Oncology
The Johns Hopkins Oncology Center
Baltimore, Maryland

Robert P. Witherspoon, M.D.
Director, Preadmission Department
Associate Member, Fred Hutchinson
    Cancer Research Center
Associate Professor of Medicine
University of Washington
Seattle, Washington

Steven N. Wolff, M.D.
Division of Medical Oncology
Vanderbilt University
Nashville, Tennessee

Joachim Yahalom, M.D.
Department of Radiation Oncology
Assistant Attending Memorial Sloan-
    Kettering Cancer Center
Assistant Professor
Cornell University Medical Center
New York, New York

CONTENTS

═══════════════════ Section II ═══════════════════
Reestablishing Hematopoiesis after Dose-Intensive Therapy

===================== Section III =====================
Laboratory and Clinical Support for Dose-Intensive Therapy

=========================== Section IV ===========================
Clinical Applications of High-Dose Therapy

Section I

Strategies for the Use of Agents at High Dose

1

PHARMACOLOGIC STRATEGIES FOR HIGH-DOSE CHEMOTHERAPY

Emil Frei III

The alkylating agents are primarily employed in intensification regimens for bone marrow transplantation because myelosuppression is dose limiting. For other classes of cancer chemotherapeutic agents, nonhematopoietic toxicity parallels myelosuppression as being dose limiting. Accordingly, this chapter will focus on alkylating agent dose intensity (1).

DOSE

Proportional Ratio

Assuming for the moment that dose-response curves for alkylating agents are steep, one basis for selecting alkylating agents for use in the intensification autologous bone marrow transplantation (ABMT) setting would relate to proportional dose escalation. By this is meant the maximum tolerated dose (MTD) for the transplant dose divided by this standard dose. These ratios are estimates primarily because of variation in what is considered to be the nontransplant dose. Using the criterion, thiotepa with a proportional ratio of 30 is particularly impressive. Most of the alkylating agents have ratios in the 4- to 10-fold range, with some agents, such as mitomycin C, at 2- to 3-fold. Nitrogen mustard and cisplatin are not candidates for major dose escalation since nonmyelosuppressive toxicity precludes dose escalation of more than 2-fold (2).

Pharmacology of Dose

The second issue that one would want to investigate about alkylating agents in the dose context is whether there are pharmacologic factors that might adversely affect biologic effect as dose is increased. For example, if a biotransformation process producing an active metabolic product were saturated shortly above the standard dose, the advantage of high-dose treatment in terms of biologic endpoints would not be realized. There is evidence for ifosfamide and for thiotepa that the P450 system, which produces 4-hydroxy ifosfamide and TEPA, respectively, becomes slightly to somewhat saturated with dose increase (3, 4). This is probably not important biologically for thiotepa, and its importance remains to be seen for ifosfamide. On the other hand, if the catabolic pathway were to become saturated with increasing doses, the biologic effect might increase disproportionately with higher doses. This is not known to occur for the alkylating agents.

Dose and Multi-Log Effect

Most important, in experimental systems, one would want to be assured that the steep dose-response curve for alkylating agents was maintained down through multiple logs of cell kill, given the need to destroy up to as many as 12 logs of cells to cure patients with clinically evident disease (5). This is dealt with in Figure 1.1, wherein the human MCF 7 breast cancer cell line in vitro is plotted with respect to log kill on the y axis and dose on the x axis. Dose is plotted as multiples of IC 90. This was done because an IC 90 represents a good partial or complete remission and normalizes all of the agents for the first log of cell kill. With the linear increase in dose, a log increase in cell kill (straight line) occurs for x-irradiation. The alkylating agents exhibit slightly curvilinear curves, whereas the nonalkylating agents, particularly the antimetabolites, lose effect very substantially after 1 or 2 logs of cell kill. Doxorubicin (Adriamycin) is intermediate. The optimal schedule was employed in Figure 1.1 in an attempt to rule out so-called cytokinetic resistance. It is our assumption that the degree of curvilinearity relates directly to the proportion and the degree of drug resistance in the original population (see below) (6–8).

Dose and Alkylating Agent Resistance

This is demonstrated directly in Figure 1.2, which is a summary of a large experience

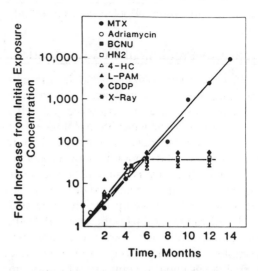

Figure 1.2.   Increase in resistance to antitumor agents (vertical axis) as a result of increasing selection pressure (horizontal axis). See text.

in producing resistance to the various alkylating agents by selection pressure in a number of human tumor cell lines (6). With representative nonalkylating agents such as methotrexate and doxorubicin, high levels of resistance can be produced with increasing selection pressure. For the alkylating agents, the concentration could be progressively increased to approximately 20-fold, at which point any increment resulted in total cell death. Thus we stabilized the cell lines at 20-fold resistance for a number of months. The colonies were then cloned, and resistance to the alkylating agents was found to vary between 3- and 15-fold. For x-irradiation, on the other hand, numerous investigators have failed to produce more than 2- to 3-fold resistance by multiple selection pressure. These data are consistent with those in Figure 1.1, suggesting that the probable lack of major curvilinearity for alkylating agents, at least down through 4 logs, relates to their relative "resistance to resistance development." Moreover, the fact that a maximum of 3- to 15-fold resistance can be achieved suggests that the 5- to 30-fold increase in dose achieved in the marrow transplant setting may be capable of

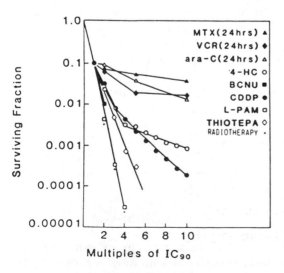

Figure 1.1.   MCF 7 (breast cancer) in vitro dose-response curves.

destroying the entire population of tumor cells (9).

Dose in Preclinical in Vivo Models

This in vitro situation may be misleading since the correlation between in vitro and in vivo resistance is controversial (10). Therefore, studies were done of dose response using the excision assay (Fig. 1.3). In this study, a solid tumor was developed to the point where it was palpable. The animals were treated with a single dose of agent across a dose-response curve up into the transplant or lethal range. At 24 hours, after all of the biochemical pharmacology presumably was complete, the tumor was excised and cloned. Lethal doses could be employed because antitumor agents produce deaths delayed beyond 3 days. These studies found that alkylating agents produced linear curves when log kill was plotted as a function of dose and therefore were similar to the in vitro studies (8).

Dose and Clinical Bone Marrow Transplantation Studies

The most compelling evidence for a steep dose-response curve for alkylating agents derives from clinical bone marrow transplantation studies. Thus cyclophosphamide plus total body radiotherapy in the bone marrow transplantation setting delivered to patients with acute myelogenous leukemia (AML) in complete remission produced a high cure rate. Either agent used alone at standard doses was ineffective. Moreover, the same can be achieved when busulfan is substituted for total body radiation (11). These data in patients receiving allogeneic bone marrow transplantation are not completely interpretable since there is evidence for a graft-versus-leukemia effect. However, that is factored out in autologous bone marrow transplantation. In this setting, a significant cure rate can also be achieved in patients with AML and acute lymphocytic leukemia (ALL), and importantly, a 40% cure rate can be achieved in selected patients with non-Hodgkin's lymphoma. Thus a 5- to 10-fold increase in dose can make the difference between response short of cure and a significant cure rate for the hematologic malignancies. Whether a substantial percentage of patients with solid tumors, particularly common solid tumors such as breast cancer and small cell lung cancer, can be cured is

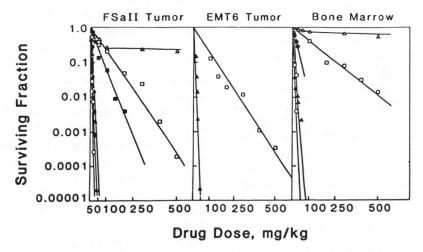

Figure 1.3. In vivo excision assay of antitumor agents in two mouse transplanted tumors, and the bone marrow. Cisplatin, ●; melphalan, ○; BCNU, ■; cyclophosphamide, □; thiotepa, ▲; or methotrexate △. The results are presented as the mean of three independent determinants.

the modern challenge and will be discussed below (11).

COMBINATION CHEMOTHERAPY RATIONALE

Dose is an established principle of cancer chemotherapy. The same is true for combination chemotherapy. Indeed, essentially all forms of curative chemotherapy for cancer involve combinations (12). Where single agents appear to have a cure rate (adjuvant breast cancer and early stage choriocarcinoma or Burkitt's lymphoma), combinations in the same setting produce a higher cure rate. Basic tumor biology provides a thoroughly compelling basis for combination chemotherapy. Thus while tumor cells are clonal in origin, they are plastic and dynamic in terms of frequency and magnitude of rearrangements, deletions, aneuploidy, and mutations—features that accelerate variation among daughter cells. Subsequently, selection is applied to those daughter cells that can survive in the cancerous milieu. This survival is dependent upon phenotypic characteristics that are good for the tumor and bad for the host, which include, particularly for our purposes, drug resistance. Thus the process of clonal evolution to heterogeneity is thoroughly Darwinian (13). Tumor cell heterogeneity implies a quantitative and perhaps qualitative range of targets and makes it extremely unlikely that an antitumor agent directed at one target that is absent or infrequent in, for example, 10^{-5} cells would be curative. On the other hand, multitargeted chemotherapy in the form of combination chemotherapy, both theoretically and in preclinical models and, as it turns out, in the clinic, will cure leukemias, pediatric solid tumors, lymphomas, testis cancer, and, in the adjuvant situation (micrometastatic disease), certain solid tumors (5, 12, 14).

Selection of Agents

How does one select agents for use in combination? First, it is important to realize that where a combination requires a reduction in dose because of additive toxicity, the advantage of the combination may be neutralized by the disadvantage of dose reduction. There are numerous clinical examples of this. The combinations that are effective are those wherein qualitatively different toxicity allows for little or no dose reduction. Under these circumstances, a major additive and sometimes synergistic effect with a cure rate can be achieved. The evidence for this in the hematologic malignancies is well known (12). In testis cancer, for example, actinomycin D, methotrexate, and chlorambucil were all individually substantially active but when employed in combination by M. C. Li many years ago, produced at best a 10%–20% cure rate. Examination of that experience indicates that all three agents were myelosuppressive, and substantial dose reduction was required. On the other hand, the modern combinations for testis cancer, which include cisplatin, bleomycin, and velban, have differing dose-limiting toxicities and therefore can be applied at full dose, with resulting cure rates in the 80%–90% range (15, 16).

Comparative Toxicity

The use of alkylating agents in combination in standard protocols has not been particularly successful since they are myelosuppressive agents, and substantial dose reduction is required for their use in combination. On the other hand, in the bone marrow transplant situation, nonmyelosuppressive toxicity becomes dose limiting, and such toxicity is qualitatively different for many of the alkylating agents. Thus the transplant dose-limiting toxicity for cyclophosphamide is cardiac; for melphalan and thiotepa, mucositis; for BCNU, liver and lung damage; for busulphan, venoocclusive disease; and for carboplatin, cholestatic liver damage. Thus there would appear to be many opportunities where these agents could be combined in the transplant setting without compromise in dose. However, many of the above manifestations, particularly mucositis and liver damage, occur at a lower dose when the alkylating agent is given with another alkylating agent, and toxicities not otherwise prominent may become manifest. Multiple organ system failure may occur with combinations, something that is not seen when they are employed separately at the same dose. In summary, it is often possible to give 60%–80% of the single-dose transplant MTD in combinations of three agents in the transplant setting.

Thus if toxicity were totally additive, the combination of three agents would yield a value of 1 MTD since the dose of each would have to be reduced to 0.33 of single-dose MTD if used in the combination. On the other hand, if toxicity were nonadditive a value of 3 would be achieved. If in practice the doses of each had to be reduced to 0.7, a score of 2.1 overall dose intensity would be achieved in the combination (2). This achievement is intermediate but nevertheless important considering the steep dose-response curve. Clearly, use of agents with nonadditive toxicity and supportive care methods that would allow the delivery of higher doses in combination are fertile and important areas for research.

The importance of maintaining dose in the transplant setting while employing agents in combination cannot be overemphasized. Thus alkylating agents with nonmyelosuppressive dose-limiting toxicity different from that of those already in common use would be of interest. In the schedule for the intensification regimen, how necessary is it that the drugs be given concurrently—that is, that the tumor cells see the two or three agents simultaneously? If that is not of critical importance, the alkylating agents can be scheduled within the context of the short intensification regimen in a way that might reduce toxicity. Other approaches to reducing toxicity through modulation and supportive care will be discussed below and elsewhere in this volume.

Cross-Resistance

The next and crucial issue for the use of agents in *combination* relates to *cross-resistance*. If the individual alkylating agents at transplant equivalent doses, as indicated in Figure 1.1, produce a 4–5 (or greater) log kill with reasonable linearity, then assuming there is no cross-resistance, three agents together should produce a 12 log kill (making certain assumptions), a potency sufficient to produce cytoeradication (cure) for patients with overt metastatic tumor. On the other hand, if there is absolute cross-resistance between all three agents, the effect of the three agents should be no greater than that of the single agent; that is, the log kill would be only in the range of 4–5.

In Figure 1.2, as indicated, we produced resistance for many different human tumor cells to a number of different alkylating agents. We then examined the issue of cross-resistance (Table 1.1). As indicated, lack of cross-resistance was the rule. Low levels of cross-resistance were common; high levels of cross-resistance, such as that for the Raji BCNU, were the exception. This led both Schabel and our group to conduct studies of in vitro and in vivo combinations of alkylating agents, the results of which are generally consistent with non-cross-resistance (8, 17, 18). These data, interpreted in light of the above kinetics, provide a powerful rationale for the use of alkylating agents in combination.

Summary

In summary, the choice of agent(s) for intensification should relate to

1. the effectiveness of that agent against the tumor in question
2. the steepness of the dose-response curve for that agent in experimental and clinical systems
3. the proportionality between the transplant dose and the standard dose
4. nonadditive toxicity when employed in combination
5. non-cross-resistance with other compounds to be employed in the combination

Table 1.1. Resistance Ratios to Various Alkylating Agents[a]

Cell Line	HN$_2$	L-PAM	CDDP	BCNU	4-HC	TSPA	MitoC
Breast (MCF7/CDDP)	1.6	2.0	6.5	1.4	1.1	3.1	1.3
Breast (MCF7/4HC)	2.0	1.0	1.3	1.1	*9.0*	2.0	1.0
H&N (SCC-25/CDDP)	1.8	5.0	*12.0*	2.0	2.8	1.7	1.0
Lymphoma (Raji/BCNU)	1.9	4.0	4.0	*5.3*	1.6		
Lymphoma (Raji/HN$_2$)	*6.6*	1.4	2.3	1.9	2.8	1.6	1.4

[a]Number = fold resistance.

Another important quality of alkylating agents and other agents chosen for intensification regimens is their ability to be modulated (see below).

CLINICAL EXPERIENCE WITH COMBINED ALKYLATING AGENTS IN THE AUTOLOGOUS BONE MARROW TRANSPLANTATION SETTING

These considerations led to the construction of the initial combined alkylating agent intensification regimens for the treatment of solid tumors. I will not review the clinical details of these studies here, as they will be covered elsewhere. Briefly, in breast cancer it has been found that combined alkylating agent regimens in patients with advanced refractory metastatic disease produce high partial response rates of relatively short duration and significant toxicity. When these programs were moved forward to newly diagnosed patients responding with metastatic breast cancer, we saw for the first time high complete response rates (40%–60%) with durable complete responses in perhaps 30% of patients. Toxicity was still considerable but less (19–21).

When these same programs were moved forward to the micrometastatic disease setting, that is, in patients with high-risk primary breast cancer (10 or more positive nodes), Peters has found in over 90 patients studied over a 5-year period that the actuarial disease-free survival at 4 years is 82% as compared to historical controls that range from 10%–30%. This important observation is now the subject of a comparative study in the Cancer and Leukemia Group B (CALGB) (Peters, personal communication).

FOCUS ON PATIENTS WITH MINIMAL PRIOR CHEMOTHERAPY AND MINIMAL TUMOR BURDEN

Thus another crucial principle of the application of high-dose alkylating agents in the autologous transplant setting is to focus on patients who have had no prior treatment, who ideally are currently responding to non-intensification treatment, and, finally and most important, who have micrometastatic disease. Whether the production of micrometastatic disease by producing complete remission with induction chemotherapy is comparable to the post-primary local treatment setting remains to be determined. The response to chemotherapy situation involves cells with a longer mitotic history and a selection process that might be somewhat adverse when compared to the unperturbed micrometastases existing following control of the primary with local therapy.

While it is clear that high response rates including complete response rates can be obtained through this approach in many patients with alkylating agent–sensitive tumors such as breast cancer, small cell lung cancer, childhood solid tumors, testis cancer, and perhaps others, it remains true that a substantial proportion of patients relapse, and further strategies for improving the intensification regimens are indicated. Quite obviously, improvement in induction regimens and local treatment approaches to sites of high risk for relapse are also important but will not be covered in this presentation.

MODULATION

The modulation approach has been employed experimentally in chemotherapy for a number of years, but only recently has come into its own as having an established place in clinical therapeutics. This relates to the modulation of fluorouracil by leucovorin wherein by stabilizing the ternary thymidylate complex, a markedly enhanced biochemical effect is achieved that translates into a better therapeutic effect in colorectal carcinoma, particularly, but also in head and neck cancer, breast cancer, and perhaps other forms of cancer (22–24). This realization provides major impetus to the studies of the clinical modulation of alkylating agents.

A modulator has not been carefully defined. For our purposes, a modulator is an agent that modifies the biochemical pharmacology of the parent antitumor agent in a way that improves the therapeutic index. A modulator ideally should not itself be toxic and should not compromise the dose of alkylating agent delivered.

The modulation potential for alkylating agents derives from our knowledge of the cellular and molecular pharmacology of the alkylating agents and from studies of alkylating agent resistance, as above.

Cellular Pharmacology of Alkylating Agents

The cellular and biochemical pharmacology of alkylating agents is presented in schematic form in Figure 1.4. Briefly, some alkylating agents pass the plasma membrane by active transport, a phenomenon that can be modulated but not, at least so far, in a therapeutically positive direction (25). The alkylating agent then enters the cytoplasm. As a free radical, it is subject to conjugation and inactivation by scavengers, particularly glu-tathione, which is present in millimolar concentrations. This conjugation is facilitated by the multienzyme system glutathione S-1 transferase. Other scavengers in the cytoplasm include metallothionein (26–28).

If they survive as alkylating agents through the cytoplasm, they enter the nucleus and produce DNA damage. It has been shown for several alkylating agents such as thiotepa (and it is known to be true for doxorubicin and bleomycin) that oxygen is essential for optimal DNA damage. It is inferred that this is true for other alkylating agents because correction of hypoxia in tumors increases their antitumor activity (29). In any event, hypoxia within tumors would appear to be a significant limitation in the capacity of the alkylating agents to produce DNA damage. Unrepaired DNA damage leads to arrest in G-2, a cascade of oncogene expression, nuclease release, disruption of internucleosomal DNA, and the so-called ladder effect on chromatograms, all of which constitute programmed cell death, or apoptosis.

However, the alkylating agent damage to DNA can be repaired, another mechanism of resistance. This can be accomplished by highly specific enzymes such as the alkyl transferase, which removes the nitrosourea monoligand from the O6 methyl group of guanine (30, 31). Other mechanisms of repair that may be accelerated in resistant cells have been described by alkaline elution–type techniques, the specific biochemical mechanisms for which have not been definitively described. Topoisomerase II, particularly, and topoisomerase I as well, modify the DNA topology, in the direction of providing an ideal setting for enzymatic DNA repair. Inhibition of topoisomerase II, for example, will favorably modulate alkylating agents, perhaps by indirect inhibition of the repair process (32).

Alkylating Agent Resistance Mechanisms

We have not discussed the mechanisms whereby the resistance and cross-resistance

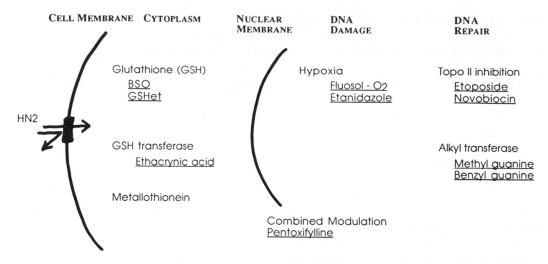

Figure 1.4.   Modulation of alkylating agents (schematic). Underlined agents have modulation potential.

patterns seen in Table 1.1 and Figure 1.4 are explained. Without going into this in detail, the generalization can be made that essentially all the above hurdles that the alkylating agent must go through to provide unrepaired DNA damage have been found to be modified in different alkylating agent–resistant cell types. Thus inhibition of transport, increase in glutathione (GSH), increase in GSH transferase, increase in metallothionein, hypoxia, and increase in DNA repair have been observed in alkylating agent–resistant tumors. The fact that there are so many potential mechanisms for resistance explains the fact that cross-resistance is the exception rather than the rule. Of importance is the fact that resistance within a given cell line is often multifactorial; that is, two or three mechanisms contribute to the overall degree of resistance. This is presumably responsible for the low level of cross-resistance, which is common. Finally, the fact that multiple mechanisms for resistance within a given cell line commonly apply means that to be effective, modulation may require combined modulators (33).

Specific Modulations (Figure 4.4.)

Fortunately, there are effective ways to modulate the aforementioned determinants of alkylating agent sensitivity and resistance. GSH levels can be lowered some 10-fold by the GSH synthesis inhibitor buthionine sulfoximine (BSO). BSO is currently under study in the clinic (34). Glutathione transferase activity can be reduced by ethacrynic acid and related compounds (28). Aldehyde dehydrogenase in the cytoplasm, which converts aldophosphamide, the active metabolite of cyclophosphamide, to carboxyphosphamide, which is inactive, can be inhibited by disulfiram.

Hypoxia can be corrected by Fluosol and oxygen (35), and oxygen can be mimicked by nitroimidazole compounds (36). The alkyl transferase repair mechanism can be inhibited by the administration of methyl or benzyl guanines, which saturate substrate sites on the alkyl transferase, precluding repair, and, finally, DNA repair mechanisms can be inhibited directly or indirectly by agents that inhibit topoisomerase II (novobiocin) or topoisomerase I (camptothecan) or effect transit through the G-2 portion of the cell cycle (pentoxifylline). Again, combinations of the above modulators have proven synergistic in preclinical systems (32, 37, 38).

All of the above mechanisms for modulation have been shown to reverse resistance or to increase sensitivity to the alkylating agents in in vitro systems, and many have proven effective in increasing the therapeutic index in preclinical in vivo systems. Many are in the early stages of clinical trials, including BSO, ethacrynic acid, pentoxifylline, novobiocin, Fluosol-oxygen, camptothecan analogues, and etanidazole.

Modulation—Protection of Host

The aforementioned modulation focuses on increasing the activity of the alkylating agent against the tumor. Protecting the host is also a critical approach to improving the therapeutic index. WR 2721 is an organic sulfhydryl compound that in experimental and clinical studies shows evidence of protecting the host and not the tumor. Similarly, GSH ethylester is sufficiently lipid soluble to enter cells. (GSH does not.) GSH ethylester is hydrolyzed within cells and provides selective protection for host tissues as compared to tumor tissues (39).

The aforementioned modulation approaches are designed to improve the cytoreduction capacity of intensification regimens with alkylating agents. The complexity of the above boggles the mind with respect to clinical trial strategy. The number of phase II and probably phase III studies that would have to be done is excessive, given particularly the limited numbers of patients. For this, surrogate endpoints are under development, such as tumor PO_2 measurements (for the Fluosol approach) and DNA damage assessment for some of the other modulation approaches.

Modulation of P450 System

Another approach to modulation requires manipulation of the microsomal drug-metabolizing P450 system. This system activates cyclophosphamide by ring hydroxylation, ring opening, and the production of active metabolites. Stimulation of the P450 system has been shown to increase the rate

but not the overall magnitude of active metabolite production, so that no significant change in the biologic effect occurs. On the other hand, for ifosfamide production of active metabolites is slow and particularly at high doses may be incomplete. The use of P450 inducers in this setting is under study in experimental systems (D Waxman, personal communication).

Thiotepa is converted to TEPA in a number of active metabolites by the P450 system. There is evidence, particularly at high doses, that this conversion may be relatively saturated. The issue as to the relative contribution to toxicity and therapeutic effect of thiotepa on the one hand and of TEPA and its metabolic products (many of which are active) on the other must be resolved. Studies of P450 manipulation may provide evidence as to the potential effectiveness of this approach on the therapeutic index (40).

PHARMACOKINETICS—VARIABILITY OF BIOAVAILABILITY AMONG THE ALKYLATING AGENTS

The dose of alkylating agents, including high doses, is based on body surface area. It has been demonstrated that body surface area correlates closely with lean body mass, which in turn correlates closely with pharmacokinetic parameters, such as total body clearance. Thus a given alkylating agent administered at a given dose should ideally produce a constant bioavailability, that is, area under the plasma curve—and such doses might be expected to produce relatively homogeneous toxicity, that is, a narrow range of toxicity, as well as a predictable therapeutic effect. Such is not the case for most of the alkylating agents. There is a 2- to 5-fold variation in area under the curve (AUC) per given dose. It might be expected that the higher the AUC per given dose, the greater the toxicity, and this has been demonstrated for venoocclusive disease in patients receiving busulfan (41). The AUC for

BCNU has been particularly hypervariable (10-fold range around the median AUC at 600 mg/m^2) (42). While the number of patients studied was limited, there is preliminary evidence that the higher AUCs of BCNU were associated with more frequent and more serious toxicity, such as lung and liver damage. Clearly, dosing based on achieving a constant AUC is more rational in the appropriate circumstances that dosing based on surface area. The development of practical techniques for evaluating alkylating agent blood levels in real time should provide for approaches to dose adjustment to achieve a given AUC. This should substantially improve the efficacy and safety of bone marrow transplantation. Obviously, the alkylating agents have to be approached individually in this regard. It must be demonstrated that the parent compound and/or active metabolites measured are active in the context of correlating with biologic effect, that is, toxicity, and antitumor effect.

CONCLUSION

Intensification regimens for bone marrow transplantation have been developed empirically with a focus on biologic, clinical, and toxicologic parameters. Major but limited progress has been achieved in that a major limitation to increasing cure rates with bone marrow transplantation for many tumors results from limitations of the intensification regimen. Molecular, cellular, preclinical in vivo pharmacologic, and pharmacokinetic studies provide important basic insights into drug action, including sensitivity, drug resistance, and toxicology, and such knowledge provides major leads in the direction of improving the therapeutic index of intensification regimens.

REFERENCES

1. Frei E III, Canellos G. Dose: a critical factor in cancer chemotherapy. AM J Med 1980;69:585–594.
2. Herzig G. Autologous marrow transplantation in cancer therapy. In: Brown, ed. Prog Hematol 1981;12:1–23.
3. Egorin M, Cohen B, Herzig R, et al. Human plasma pharmacokinetics and urinary excretion of thiotepa and its metabolites in patients receiving high-dose thiotepa therapy. In: Herzig G, ed. High-dose thiotepa and autologous marrow transplantation: advances in cancer chemotherapy. New York: Wiley & Sons, 1987:3–8.
4. Henner W, Shea T, Furlong E, et al. Pharmacokinetics of continuous-infusion high-dose thiotepa. Cancer Treat Rep 1987;71:1043–1047.
5. Frei E III, Freireich E. Progress and perspectives in the chemotherapy of acute leukemia. In: Goldin A, Hawking F, Schnitzer, eds. Advances in chemotherapy. Vol. 2. New York: Academic Press, 1965:269–298.
6. Frei E III, Cucchi C, Rosowsky A, et al. Alkylating agent resistance: in vitro studies with human cell lines. Proc Natl Acad Sci USA 1985;82:2158–2162.
7. Frei E III. Combined intensive alkylating agents with autologous bone marrow transplantation for metastatic solid tumors. In: Dicke K, Spitzer G, Zander A, eds. Autologous bone marrow transplantation: proceedings of the First International Symposium. Houston: The University of Texas M.D. Anderson Hospital and Tumor Institute at Houston, 1985:509–511.
8. Frei E III, Teicher B, Cucchi C, et al. Resistance to alkylating agents: basic studies and therapeutic implications. In: Woolley P III, Tew K, eds. Mechanisms of drug resistance in neoplastic cells. New York: Academic Press, 1988:69–87.
9. Frei E III, Antman K, Teicher B, et al. Bone marrow autotransplantation for solid tumors—prospects. J Clin Oncol 1989;7:515–526.
10. Teicher B, Herman T, Holden S, et al. Tumor resistance to alkylating agents conferred by mechanisms operative only in vivo. Science 1990;247:1457–1461.
11. Santos G, Tutschka P, Brookmeyer R, et al. Marrow transplantation for acute non lymphocytic leukemia after treatment with busulfan and cyclophosphamide. N Engl J Med 1983;309:1347–1353.
12. Frei E III. Curative cancer chemotherapy. Cancer Res 1985;45:6523–6537.
13. Frei E III. Pathobiology of cancer. In: Federman D, Rubenstein E, eds. Medicine. Vol. 12. New York: Scientific American, 1986:1–17.
14. Frei E III. Combination cancer therapy: presidential address. Cancer Res 1972;32:2593–2607.
15. Li M, Whitmore W, Golbey R, Grabstalb H. Effects of combined drug therapy on metastatic cancer of the testis. JAMA 1960;174:1291–1299.
16. Einhorn L, Donohue J. Cis-diamninedichloroplatinum, vinblastine and bleomycin: combination chemotherapy in disseminated testicular cancer. Ann Intern Med 1977;87:293–298.
17. Teicher B, Holden S, Kelley M, et al. Alkylating agents: in vitro studies of cross-resistance patterns. Cancer Res 1986;46:4379–4383.
18. Schabel F. Patterns of resistance and therapeutic syn-

ergism for alkylating agents. Antibiot Chemother 1978;23:200.

19. Peters W, Eder J, Henner W, et al. High-dose combination alkylating agents with autologous bone marrow support: a phase I trial. J Clin Oncol 1986;4:646–654.

20. Antman K, Gale P. High dose chemotherapy and autotransplants for breast cancer. Ann Intern Med 1988;108:570–574.

21. Antman K, Eder J, Frei E III. High-dose chemotherapy with bone marrow support for solid tumors. In: DeVita V Jr, Hellman S, Rosenberg S, eds. Important advances in oncology 1987. Philadelphia: JB Lippincott, 1987:221–235.

22. Rustum Y, Trave F, Zakrzewski SF, et al. Biochemical and pharmacologic basis for potentiation of fluorouracil action by leucovorin. NCI Monogr 1987;5:165.

23. Doroshow J, Multhauf P, Leong L, et al. Prospective randomized comparison of fluorouracil versus fluorouracil and high-dose continuous infusion leucovorin calcium for the treatment of advanced measurable colorectal cancer in patients previously unexposed to chemotherapy. J Clin Oncol 1990;3:491–501.

24. Dreyfuss A, Clark J, Wright J, et al. Continuous infusion high-dose leucovorin with 5-fluorouracil and cisplatin for untreated stage IV carcinoma of the head and neck. Ann Intern Med 1990;112:167–172.

25. Goldenberg G, Vanstone C, Israels L, et al. Evidence for a transport carrier of nitrogen mustard in nitrogen mustard sensitive and resistant L5178Y lymphoblasts. Cancer Res 1970;30:2285.

26. Meister A. Glutathione metabolism and its selective modification. J Biol Chem 1988;268:17205–17208.

27. Ozols R, Hamilton T, Masuda H, et al. Manipulation of cellular thiols to influence drug resistance. In: Woolley, P, Tew K, eds. Mechanisms of drug resistance in neoplastic cells. New York: Academic Press, 1988:289–306.

28. Tew K, Bomber A, Hoffman S. Ethacrynic acid and piriprost as enhancers of cytotoxicity in drug resistant and sensitive cell lines. Cancer Res 1988;48:3622–3625.

29. Teicher B, Holden S. A survey of the effect of adding Fluosol-DA 20%/O2 to treatment with various chemotherapeutic agents. Cancer Treat Rep 1987;71:173–177.

30. Sedgwick B, Lindahl T. A common mechanism for repair of O6-methylguanine and O6-ethylguanine in DNA. J Molec Biol 1982;154:169.

31. Scudiero D, Meyer S, Clatterbuck B, et al. Sensitivity of human cell strains having different abilities to repair O6-methylguanine in DNA to inactivation by alkylating agents including chloroethylnitrosureas. Cancer Res 1984;44:2467.

32. Eder J, Teicher B, Holden S, Cathcart K, Schnipper L. Novobiocin enhances alkylating agent cytotoxicity and DNA interstrand crosslinks in a murine model. J Clin Invest 1987;79:1524–1528.

33. Teicher B, Frei E III. Modulation of antitumor alkylating agents. In: Ozols R, ed. Molecular and clinical advances in anticancer drug resistance. Boston: Kluwer Academic Publishers, 1991:261–295.

34. Ozols R, Louie K, Plowman J, et al. Enhanced melphalan cytotoxicity in human ovarian cancer in vitro and in tumor-bearing nude mice by buthionine sulfoximine depletion of glutathione. Biochem Pharmacol 1987;36:147–153.

35. Hasegawa T, Rhee J, Levitt S, Song C. Increase in tumor pO2 by perfluorochemicals and carbogen. Int J Radiat Oncol Biol Phys 1987;13:569–574.

36. Brown J. Keynote address: hypoxic cell radiosensitizers: where next? Int J Radiat Oncol Biol Phys 1989;16:987–993.

37. Herman T, Teicher BA, Pfeffer M. Combined modulators (fluosol/DA/etanidazole) of alkylating agent activity. Proc Am Assoc Cancer Res 1990;31:407.

38. Fingert J, Chang J, Pardee A. Cytotoxic, cell cycle, and chromosomal effects of methylxanthines in human tumor cells treated with alkylating agents. Cancer Res 1986;46:2463–2467.

39. Teicher B, Crawfor J, Holden S, et al. Glutathione monoethyl ester can selectively protect liver from high dose BCNU or cyclophosphamide. Cancer 1988;62:1275–1281.

40. Ng SF, Waxman DJ. N,N',N'' Triethylenethiophosphoramide (Thio-TEPA) oxygenation by constitutive hepatic P450 enzymes and modulation of drug metabolism and clearance in vivo by P450-inducing agents. Cancer Res 1991;51:2340–2345.

41. Grochow L, Jones R, Brundrett R, et al. Pharmacokinetics of busulfan: correlation with veno-occlusive disease in patients undergoing bone marrow transplantation. Cancer Chemother Pharmacol 1989;25(1):55–61.

42. Henner W, Peters W, Eder J, et al. Pharmacokinetics and immediate effects of high-dose carmustine in man. Cancer Treat Rep 1986;70:877–880.

2

PRECLINICAL MODELS FOR HIGH-DOSE THERAPY

Beverly A. Teicher

The preclinical study of cancer therapy relevant to the high-dose setting has required the development of preclinical models that go beyond the standard endpoints of increase-in-life span and tumor growth delay. The ability to determine whether combination therapies, especially chemotherapy combinations, retain increasing efficacy in the high-dose setting is critical to the development of new treatment regimens. The ability to detect and effectively treat minimal residual disease is critical to the cure of both leukemias and solid tumors. This chapter will address these issues and discuss preclinical data describing alkylating agent/modulator combinations that may potentially be useful in the treatment of clinical disease.

ENDPOINTS

The earliest in vivo preclinical tumor models were leukemias grown as ascites tumors. The endpoint of experiments with these tumors was most often increase-in-life span. As solid tumor models were developed, the appropriate endpoints devised were tumor growth delay or tumor control of a primary implanted tumor. These assays require that drugs be administered at doses producing little normal tissue toxicity so that the response of the tumor to the treatment can be observed for a relatively long period of time.

These endpoints cannot be applied to the high-dose setting in which normally lethal doses of anticancer therapies can be administered with normal tissue support such as bone marrow transplantation. Response to high-dose therapies can be assessed by use of excision assays (1).

One important difference between excision assays and the in situ assays of increase in life span, tumor growth delay, or local tumor control is that excision assays require removal of the tumor from the environment in which it was treated. This difference and the nature of the assay procedure leads to a number of advantages and disadvantages in using excision assays rather than in situ assays. The ability to measure cell survival directly is important, because it gives basic information about what is perhaps the ultimate definitive cellular effect. Tumor excision assays also allow greater accuracy and finer resolution between various therapeutic regimens. Supralethal treatments can be tested. Perhaps the greatest disadvantage of excision assays is that extended treatment regimens cannot be used owing to tumor cell loss and tumor cell proliferation over the treatment time.

The survival of tumor cells from tumors treated in vivo and then excised is often determined by in vitro colony formation. This requires use of tumor models that grow well in vivo and also have a high plating efficiency in vitro (ideally on the order of 20%). However, in vivo colony formation such as spleen colony formation for leukemias is also often used as an excision assay endpoint.

In summary, the use of excision assays to determine survival curves for tumor cells treated in vivo can provide insights concerning both treatment efficacy and tumor biology.

THERAPEUTIC SYNERGY/ISOBOLOGRAM ANALYSIS

In the study of multimodality therapy or combined chemotherapy, it is of interest to determine whether the combined effects of two agents are additive or whether their combination is substantially different from the sum of their parts. Conceptual foundations for this form of data analysis are based on the construction of an envelope of additivity in an isoeffect plot (isobologram) (2). This approach provides a rigorous basis for defining regions of additivity, supraadditivity, subadditivity, and protection. This method of analysis is based on a clear formulation of the way that drugs or agents can be expected to show additivity. The first form of additivity is conceptually simple and is defined as mode I by Steel and Peckham (2). For a selected level of effect (for example, tumor cell survival) on a log scale, the dose of agent A to produce this effect is determined. A lower dose of agent A is then selected, the difference in effect from the isoeffect level is determined, and the dose of agent B needed to make up this difference is derived from the survival curve for agent B.

Mode II additivity is conceptually more complex but corresponds to the notions of additivity discussed by Berenbaum (3). For any given level of effect, the dose of agent A needed to produce the effect is determined from the survival relationship. The isoeffect dose of agent B is calculated as the amount of agent B needed to produce the given effect starting at the level of effect produced by

agent A. Graphically, on a linear dose scale, mode II additivity is defined as the straight line connecting the effective dose of agent A alone and the effective dose of agent B alone. This relationship is also described by the equation

$$\frac{\text{Dose of A}}{A_e} + \frac{\text{Dose of B}}{B_e} = 1$$

where A_e and B_e are the doses of agent A and agent B, respectively, needed to produce the selected effect.

Overall, combinations that produce the desired effect that are within the boundaries of mode I and mode II are considered additive. Those displaced to the left are supraadditive (synergistic), while those displaced to the right are subadditive. Combinations that produce effects outside the rectangle defined by the intersections of A_e and B_e are protective. This type of classical isobologram methodology is cumbersome to use experimentally as each combination must be carefully titrated to produce a constant level of effect. Dewey et al. (4) described an analogous form of analysis for the special case in which the dose of one agent was held constant. Using full survival curves of each agent alone, this method produces envelopes of additive effect for different levels of the variable agent. It is conceptually identical to generating a series of isoeffect curves and then plotting the survivals from a series of these at constant dose of agent A on a log effect by dose of agent B coordinate system (5). This approach can often be applied to the experimental situation in a more direct and efficient manner, and isobolograms can be derived describing the expected effect (mode I and mode II) for any level of the variable agent and constant agent combinations. This chapter will discuss several studies in which isobologram methodology has been used.

LEUKEMIAS

At the Southern Research Institute sublines of murine leukemia L1210 and P388 and several solid tumors have been selected for resistance to a variety of anticancer drugs and are maintained by serial passage in vivo (6–9). Using an in vivo/in vivo tumor excision assay that is treatment of a tumor-bearing animal followed by passage of known numbers of the treated tumor cells to fresh hosts, extensive quantitative studies on the resistance and cross-resistance of L1210 sublines selected for resistance to three alkylating agents were carried out. The L1210/CPA line selected by DeWys (10) is a stably resistant mutant. The L1210/BCNU subline is also stably resistant (11). The L1210/melphalan subline was maintained under treatment with melphalan in passage (6). Using as a criterion the ability of an optimal single-dose intraperitoneal (ip) treatment with each drug to kill up to 10^6 tumor cells, the L1210/CPA cell line is completely resistant in vivo to cyclophosphamide, and the L1210/BCNU and L1210/melphalan lines are about threefold resistant to BCNU and melphalan, respectively, compared to the parent L1210 line. These cell lines have been widely used in both in vivo and in vitro studies of alkylating agent resistance. One of the issues that these quantitative assessments of leukemic cell survival brought to the fore was that *undertreatment* with representatives of all of the chemical and functional classes of clinically useful anticancer agents is the most likely reason for the variable cure and/or regression rates among drug-sensitive tumors in man and grossly evident tumors in animals (8).

It has long been recognized that the schedule and sequence of drugs in combination can affect therapeutic outcome. Over the last 15 years the definition of additivity and therapeutic synergism has evolved with increasing stringency. In the work of Schabel et al. (6–8), therapeutic synergism between two drugs was defined to mean that "the effect of the two drugs in combination was significantly greater than that which could be obtained when either drug was used alone under identical conditions of treatment." Using this definition, the combination of cyclo-

phosphamide and melphalan has been reported to be therapeutically synergistic in L1210 and P388 leukemias (6). Cyclophosphamide plus a nitrosourea (BCNU, CCNU, or MeCCNU) have also been reported to be therapeutically synergistic in increase-in-life span and growth delay assays, using this definition (6).

More recently, the BN acute myelocytic leukemia (BNML) in the Brown Norway rat has proven to be a very useful model of human acute myelocytic leukemia for both analysis of disease progression and development of therapeutic regimens involving bone marrow transplantation (12, 13). Studies in the BNML model have added considerably to the understanding of various processes that occur during the development of leukemia—e.g., the interaction of leukemic cells and normal hematopoietic stem cells in relation to the microenvironment (14). Martens and Hagenbeek (15) showed that during the invasion of leukemic cells of the BNML model in the bone marrow, the number of normal bone marrow stem cells (CFU-S) decreased while simultaneously an increase of CFU-S in the leukemic spleen was observed. A small reduction in the tumor load by low-dose cyclophosphamide treatment (10 mg/kg) caused a temporary CFU-S recovery in the bone marrow. After a therapeutic dose of cyclophosphamide (100 mg/kg), the CFU-S numbers in femur and spleen decreased to low levels, but they rapidly increased immediately thereafter. In the spleen, however, the CFU-S increase halted when femoral CFU-S numbers reached normal levels. Splenectomy following cyclophosphamide treatment revealed that the splenic CFU-S population did not play a role in regeneration of hematopoiesis. During the subsequent leukemia relapse, CFU-S in the femur decreased again while spleen CFU-S tended to rise. They concluded that the bone marrow CFU-S, which survive both the leukemia and the remission-induction treatment and not the migrated, extramedullary localized stem cells, are the major source for the restoration of normal hematopoiesis (15).

The methodology developed in the BNML model allows the quantification of the relative effectiveness of any given treatment with regard to its antileukemic activity compared with its toxicity for normal host tissues. Furthermore, the cell kinetic studies performed in the BNML as a consequence of timed sequential chemotherapy have been helpful in designing an approach to take advantage of this phenomenon in the treatment of acute leukemia (16). The comparison of the various treatment modalities employed for conditioning prior to bone marrow transplantation allows determination of the relative effectiveness of the approaches. The fractionation of total body irradiation for conditioning purposes was thought to have a negligible effect with regard to a reduced antileukemic effect. Detailed studies that were conducted in the BNML model did not confirm this hypothesis, indicating that (hyper-)fraction of total body irradiation results in a reduced antileukemic effect (16). Recently, Nooter et al. (17) investigated the effects of low-dose cyclophosphamide pretreatment on daunorubicin concentrations in leukemic bone marrow in rats. At day 12 after transplantation of the leukemia, rats were injected intraperitoneally with cyclophosphamide (30 mg/kg). Two days later the leukemic rats received daunorubicin intravenously (7.5 mg/kg). Cyclophosphamide pretreatment led to a significant increase in daunorubicin concentration in the femoral bone marrow, by a factor of about 7. The log leukemic stem cell kill values, as estimated by a survival assay, were 1.8, 0.7, and 5.4 for the leukemic rats injected with cyclophosphamide (day 12), with daunorubicin (day 14), or with cyclophosphamide (day 12) plus daunorubicin (day 14), respectively. Low-dose cyclophosphamide pretreatment led to an increased daunorubicin accumulation in femoral bone marrow of leukemic rats and was synergistic with daunorubicin (17).

The in vitro purging studies in the BNML as well as in other model systems aimed at the elimination of residual leukemic cells in autologous bone marrow transplantation contributed to the introduction of this method in clinical practice (18–23). However, extended studies in the BNML model also indicated that the residual leukemia cell contributed more to relapse than did the residual cells in the autologous marrow graft. Hagenbeek and Martens (24) also examined the survival of pluripotent hematopoietic stem cells and in vivo clonogenic leukemic cells after cryopreservation in the BNML model. These stem cell populations can be selectively quantified with modified spleen colony assays (day 8 and day 12 CFU-S; LCFU-S). It appeared that the most primitive rat hematopoietic stem cell (day 12 CFU-S) was significantly less vulnerable to the freezing and thawing procedure as compared with the clonogenic leukemic cell (30% and 1.4% survival, respectively; $p = .0026$). Survival of the day 8 CFU-S population fell between those percentages (8.6%). In view of autologous bone marrow transplantation (ABMT), an attempt was made to extrapolate these and previously reported BNML rat data to man. Taking into account that (a) only 1% of the clonogenic leukemic cells survive cryopreservation, (b) the fraction of clonogenic leukemic cells in man is approximately 0.001, (c) leukemic cells reinfused with the autologous marrow graft may lodge at sites unfavorable for growth, and (d) supralethal high-dose chemoradiotherapy significantly hampers the regrowth of leukemia, it becomes rather unlikely that leukemic cells in the autologous marrow graft significantly contribute to a leukemia relapse after ABMT. Therefore, residual leukemia in the host surviving high-dose chemoradiotherapy is the most crucial factor as regards the final outcome of ABMT in acute leukemia (24).

A major contribution of the BNML model was achieved in a study of the area of so-called minimal residual disease (MRD) (14). A number of so-far unknown aspects of relapsing leukemia were identified and studied. A new concept of discriminating locally relapsing leukemia and a delayed occurrence of generalized spreading of leukemia formed the basis for the explanation of the observed heterogeneity in the distribution of leukemic cells during the remission and the subsequent relapse phase. Martens, Schultz, and Hagenbeek (25) investigated the distribution of leukemic cells in bone marrow samples from various sites using monoclonal antibodies and flow cytometry. Rats were studied before chemotherapy as well as thereafter—i.e., in the MRD phase. Bone marrow from different types of bones was analyzed from each animal. Before treatment, the ratio of the measured extreme values (i.e., highest/lowest value) for leukemic cell frequencies in bones from individual rats ranged from 3.7 to 11.7. During the MRD phase the ratios of the extremes ranged from a factor of 36 to a factor of more than 13,000 from one rat to another. The variability between bones of comparable size was estimated by studying the ribs from each individual animal. Within individuals the extremes differed by a factor of 1.2 to 4.0 before chemotherapy and from 2.4 to greater than 320 after chemotherapy. The variability within the marrow cavity of a single bone was determined by analyzing multiple samples from femoral bones cut into slices. The leukemic cell frequency appeared to vary considerably—i.e., before treatment from 1.7 to 7.3 and during MRD from 4 to 28,000. These data may contribute to understanding the sometimes conflicting observations in leukemic patients.

For complete elimination of MRD in the BNML, Hagenbeek and Martens (14) found that high doses of drugs have to be used even when the tumor load is as small as 1×10^4 cells. Cures could be obtained with various treatment protocols—e.g., cyclophosphamide only, cyclophosphamide combined with total body irradiation followed by bone marrow transplantation (BMT) (26), treatment with piperazinedione (27), or with 4-amino-N-(2-aminophenyl)benzyamide (NSC 328786) (28). Because treatment should result in a 5-log leukemic cell kill, BMT following the treatment was required except after 4-amino-

N-(2-aminophenyl)benzyamide (NSC 328786) treatment (28) and after cyclophosphamide treatment with a moderate dose (i.e., 100 mg/kg).

Leukemia relapses in man occasionally occur after remission periods of up to 5 years or more. These late relapses cannot be explained by the same growth kinetics that apply to regrowth of leukemia after short duration of remission. Leukemia relapses originating from very low numbers of leukemic cells develop much slower than expected. A similar break in the survival curve was observed in BNML rats that were known to carry very low (<10) levels of leukemic cells. These cells may have survived as "sleeper-cells" in protected "niches" (14).

It became apparent that other factors (e.g., immunologic processes) may also play a role in the eradication of small numbers of leukemic cells. This was indicated by experiments in which a specific immunostimulation with bacillus Calmette-Guérin (BCG) resulted in effective cure in 100% of the animals (29). This finding is of special significance since there is no evidence that the BNML is immunogenic.

The acute myelogenous leukemia model in the BN rat has contributed considerably to improved understanding of the various aspects of leukemia growth, responses to chemotherapy, application of BMT as therapy, and the possibilities and limitations for the detection of residual disease during the remission phase (14, 16). Obviously, there are restrictions with regard to the extrapolation of the rat data to the human situation. Leukemia growth in inbred rats is highly reproducible, while in humans there is a high degree of individual variation. However, some characteristics are shared, and the aim is to identify the similarities as well as the dissimilarities between human and rat leukemia. In that way progress may be envisaged with respect to reaching the final goal of curing human leukemia (14).

SOLID TUMORS

Several high-dose combination chemotherapy regimens with autologous bone marrow transplantation are under clinical study as therapy for solid tumors. Drug selection for these regimens was based on a knowledge of the mechanisms of action, the known dose-limiting toxicities, and some cross-resistance data from tissue culture and animal tumor studies (30–37). The relative success of these initial studies has inspired refined high-dose combination chemotherapy regimens directed toward specific malignancies. One of the strategies that will be used in several new high-dose chemotherapy regimens is to combine treatment with alkylating agents with the administration of "modulators" or "chemosensitizers," that is, drugs that have little toxicity or activity alone but that significantly increase the therapeutic efficacy of antitumor alkylating agents.

ETANIDAZOLE

The combination of cis-diamminedichloroplatinum(II) (CDDP) and cyclophosphamide has been well established in the treatment of ovarian carcinoma (38, 39). In recent years, several clinical trials have been conducted comparing (40) the efficacy of carboplatin with CDDP alone (41–44) and in combination with cyclophosphamide (38, 39) in ovarian carcinoma. The overall conclusion from many of these studies has been that, at doses that produce response rates equal to those achieved with CDDP, the spectrum of normal tissue toxicities seen with carboplatin is much more tolerable than that seen with CDDP (43). However, complete response rates in these clinical trials are still in the range of 20%–35%, indicating that there is much room for improvement.

The 2-nitroimidazole radiosensitizer, etanidazole (ETA), is also a hypoxic cellselective cytotoxic agent (45, 46) and a chemosensitizer or modulator of some antitumor drugs (47–49). The mechanisms by which ETA acts as a chemosensitizer are not known. The most important mechanisms appear to occur at the level of the cell and may involve interaction of a metabolite of the 2-nitroim-idazole with the alkylating agent in the vicinity of the DNA (49–54). Isobologram analysis (55) was used to examine the ability of etanidazole to potentiate the tumor cell killing and tumor growth delay of cyclophosphamide (CTX), CDDP, and carboplatin (Carbo) alone and in combination in the FSaIIC fibrosarcoma. Bone marrow CFU-GM survival was used to estimate the effects of the combinations on a representative normal tissue. The object in conducting these studies was to attempt to markedly improve the antitumor efficacy of these alkylating agents using the relatively nontoxic drug, ETA.

FSaIIC tumor cell survival curves and bone marrow CFU-GM survival curves for CTX, CDDP, and Carbo administered as single bolus injections with or without ETA are shown in Figure 2.1 (56). Treatment with ETA (1 g/kg) produced very little kill for the FSaIIC tumor cells (S.F. = 0.65) and no measurable kill of bone marrow CFU-GM from the same animals. However, when administration of ETA just preceded treatment with CTX, there was a 10-fold increase in tumor cell killing across the dosage range tested. In contrast, with the addition of ETA to treatment with CTX there was only a 1.5- to 2-fold increase in the killing of bone marrow CFU-GM from the same animals. ETA had a dose-modifying effect on tumor cell killing by CDDP; that is, the enhancement in the tumor cell killing produced by CDDP increased from about 4-fold to about 30-fold over the dosage range of CDDP examined. CDDP has only a limited cytotoxicity toward bone marrow CFU-GM, and this cytotoxicity was increased from about 1.2- to 2-fold over the CDDP dosage range with the addition of ETA (56). As with CDDP, ETA had a dose-modifying effect on the cytotoxicity of Carbo toward FSaIIC tumor cells. The enhancement in the tumor cell killing of Carbo by ETA increased from about 6-fold to more than 37-fold over the Carbo dosage range tested. Treatment with ETA did not increase the cytotoxicity of Carbo toward the bone marrow CFU-GM. Overall, therefore, if bone marrow CFU-GM is a representative sensitive

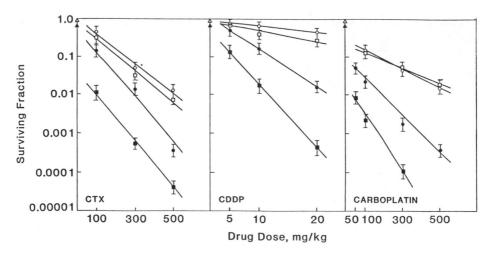

Figure 2.1. Survival of FSaIIC tumor cells (●, ■, ▲) and bone marrow CFU-GM (○, □, △) from animals treated in vivo with ETA (1 g/kg) administered immediately prior to a single dose of each alkylating agent (■, □) or with a single dose of the alkylating agent alone (●, ○). Shown on the axis is ETA (1 g/kg) (▲, △). (From Teicher BA, Herman TS, Shulman L, et al. Combinations of etanidazole with cyclophosphamide and platinum complexes. Cancer Chemother Pharmacol 1991;28:153–158.)

normal tissue, there was a marked increase in the therapeutic index of each of these three drugs when they were used in combination with ETA.

To examine the combination of CTX with CDDP, a dose of 150 mg/kg of CTX was selected (Fig. 2.2) (56). When CTX just preceded treatment with CDDP, the resulting tumor cell killing was greater than additive as determined by isobologram analysis. When the combination of ETA and CTX preceded treatment with CDDP, the complete treatment regimen produced greater than additive tumor cell killing with lower doses of CDDP and additive tumor cell killing with high dose CDDP. The bone marrow CFU-GM cytotoxicity of the combination of CTX (150 mg/kg) and CDDP appeared to be primarily additive. However, there was an additional approximately 3-fold enhancement in bone marrow CFU-GM cytotoxicity when ETA was added to treatment with CTX and CDDP.

Similar experiments were conducted to examine the effect of the combination of CTX (150 mg/kg) with a range of Carbo dosage levels on tumor cell killing in the FSaIIC fi-brosarcoma (Fig. 2.3) (56). The tumor cell killing achieved with CTX and Carbo was additive over the range of Carbo doses examined. When ETA and CTX were added to treatment with Carbo, the combination was most effective at lower Carbo doses, as with CDDP. At the lower doses of Carbo tumor cell killing was at the limits of the envelope of additivity and almost reached supraadditivity, but the combination with higher doses of Carbo was well within the envelope of additivity. The combination of CTX with Carbo produced killing of the bone marrow CFU-GM that was only equivalent to that of Carbo alone. However, adding ETA to treatment with CTX and Carbo increased the killing of the bone marrow CFU-GM about 8- to 10-fold over the Carbo dosage range examined.

These preclinical results suggest that ETA could significantly improve the therapeutic efficacy of these alkylating agents individually or in combination. Based on these findings, a high-dose chemotherapeutic regimen consisting of ETA/Carbo/CTX directed toward ovarian carcinoma is planned at Dana-Farber.

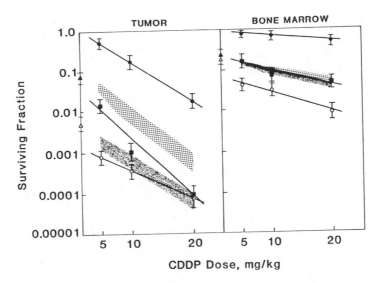

Figure 2.2. Survival of FSaIIC tumor cells and bone marrow CFU-GM from animals treated in vivo with single doses of CDDP alone (●) preceded by CTX (150 mg/kg) (■) or preceded by ETA (1 g/kg) with CTX (150 mg/kg) (○). Shown on the axis is CTX (150 mg/kg) (▲) and ETA (1 g/kg) with CTX (150 mg/kg) (△). Shaded areas indicate the envelopes of additivity determined by isobologram analysis of the survival curves for each drug combination. (From Teicher BA, Herman TS, Shulman L, et al. Combinations of etanidazole with cyclophosphamide and platinum complexes. Cancer Chemother Pharmacol 1991;28:153–158.)

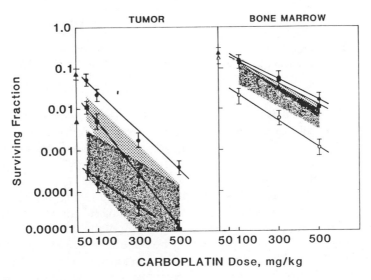

Figure 2.3 Survival of FSaIIC tumor cells and bone marrow CFU-GM from animals treated in vivo with single doses of carboplatin alone (●) preceded by CTX (150 mg/kg) (■) or preceded by ETA (1 g/kg) with CTX (150 mg/kg) (○). Shown on the axis is CTX (150 mg/kg) (▲) and ETA (1 g/kg) with CTX (150 mg/kg) (△). Shaded areas indicate the envelopes of additivity determined by isobologram analysis of the survival curves for each drug combination. (From Teicher BA, Herman TS, Shulman L, et al. Combinations of etanidazole with cyclophosphamide and platinum complexes. Cancer Chemother Pharmacol 1991;28:153–158.)

LONIDAMINE

Lonidamine,1-[(2,4-dichlorophenyl)methyl]-1H-indazole-3-carboxylic acid, affects the energy metabolism of cells (57–62). In both normal and neoplastic cells, oxygen consumption is strongly inhibited by this drug; furthermore, in tumor cells, aerobic and anaerobic glycolysis are additionally affected (57, 59–62). Based on these data, mitochondria have been considered the primary intracellular targets of the drug. As data have been accrued, it has become evident that lonidamine is not equally effective in all cell types and that the mitochondrial effects of lonidamine can be reversible if the drug is removed after short time exposure (63). Ultrastructural studies by DeMartino et al. (58) indicate that the inhibition of energy metabolism in cells by lonidamine is a consequence of damage to the inner and outer mitochondrial membranes, which leads to inhibition of respiration and glycolysis and finally loss of cell viability (58).

Lonidamine could be an important component of a combined modality regimen if repair of damage by a cytotoxic treatment is an energy-dependent process. Working with Chinese hamster HA-1 cells in culture, Hahn et al. (64) showed that at concentrations achievable in vivo lonidamine inhibited the repair of potentially lethal damage caused by x-rays, methyl methane sulfonate, bleomycin, and hyperthermia. Kim et al. (65–67) showed that lonidamine potentiated the effects of radiation and the effects of hyperthermia (66) in murine tumor models. Lonidamine has also been shown to enhance the cytotoxicity of several alkylating agents (88) as well as Adriamycin in culture (69).

Using the FSaIIC fibrosarcoma in vivo–in vitro tumor system, the response of tumors in vivo was examined to increasing single doses of alkylating agents in the presence or absence of lonidamine (Fig. 2.4) (70). Tumor cell kill was quantified by colony formation, and the survival of bone marrow from the same animals was measured by the CFU-

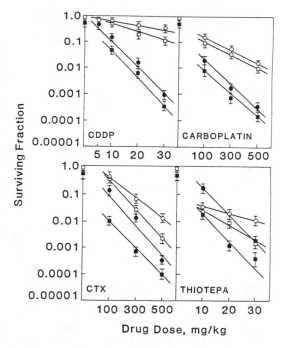

Figure 2.4. Survival of FSaIIC tumor cells (●, ■) and bone marrow CFU-GM (○, □) from animals treated in vivo with lonidamine (5 × 50 mg/kg) over 36 hours alone or with a single dose of an alkylating agent administered with the third dose of lonidamine (■, □) or with a single dose of the alkylating agent alone (●, ○). (From Teicher BA, Herman TS, Holden SA, et al. Lonidamine as a modulator of alkylating agent activity in vitro and in vivo. Cancer Res 1991;51:780–784.)

GM assay. The treatment schedule for lonidamine was five ip injections of 50 mg/kg given at 7–10 hour intervals over 36 hours, with the alkylating agent being administered as a single dose ip immediately following the third lonidamine injection. Lonidamine, on this treatment schedule, resulted in about a 50% killing of the tumor cells and no toxicity to the bone marrow CFU-GM. Each of the four alkylating agents produced log-linear increasing tumor cell killing with increasing dose of the drug. The addition of lonidamine prior to, during, and following treatment with CDDP resulted in a 2- to 3-fold increase in tumor cell killing and a smaller increase in bone marrow CFU-GM killing. A similar effect was observed with carbo in vivo where, in the presence of lonidamine treatment, there was a 2- to 2.5-fold increase in the killing of FSaIIC tumor cells and a smaller increase in the killing of bone marrow CFU-GM.

The addition of lonidamine to treatment with CTX in vivo resulted in 10-fold additional tumor cell killing in the normal therapeutic range of CTX doses (100–300 mg/kg) and a much smaller increase in the killing of bone marrow CFU-GM of 0- to 3-fold in that same dosage range (Fig. 2.4) (70). There was a similar 10-fold increase in the killing of tumor cells by thiotepa with the addition of lonidamine to treatment with that drug. The 10-fold increase in tumor cell killing by thiotepa persisted over the entire dosage range (10–30 mg/kg) examined. The killing of bone marrow CFU-GM by thiotepa with the addition of lonidamine increased to a lesser extent than did the tumor cell killing, so that there was equal or greater tumor cell than bone marrow CFU-GM killing by thiotepa over the dosage range examined.

These results indicate that lonidamine has the potential to increase the efficacy of antineoplastic alkylating agents without a reduction in the dosage of the alkylating agents and that a greater potentiation of the effect of the alkylating agents may occur in the tumor compared with the bone marrow. Clinical protocols utilizing lonidamine with antitumor alkylating agents are being considered.

PENTOXIFYLLINE

Pentoxifylline is a methylxanthine that is used to treat vascular occlusive disease in human beings (71–76). Like other methylxanthines (77–89), pentoxifylline has been shown to enhance the cytotoxicity of x-irradiation, alkylating agents, and other anticancer drugs in cell culture (89–91). Evidence indicates that methylxanthines enhance the lethality of alkylating agents in cell culture by preventing delays in the cell cycle transit through the G-2 phase, thus not allowing time for repair of DNA cross-links which augments formation of lethal chromosome aberrations

(81, 86, 87, 89). Enhancements in the cytotoxicity of nitrogen mustard and thiotepa by caffeine or pentoxifylline of up to 10-fold have been reported (89). However, to achieve these effects in cell culture requires several hours of exposure to relatively high (1–2 mM) concentrations of caffeine or pentoxifylline (77–89). Although it is not possible to achieve millimolar concentrations of caffeine or pentoxifylline in vivo, caffeine has been shown to increase antitumor activity of some chemotherapeutic agents in several model systems (92–95).

At doses readily achievable in man, pentoxifylline has significant hemorheologic effects upon red blood cells and platelets. Pentoxifylline increases red blood cell deformability, inhibits platelet aggregation, and inhibits fibrolytic activity so that red blood cells are better able to traverse narrowed arterioles and capillaries, thereby increasing tissue oxygenation (71–76, 91). These biologic effects of pentoxifylline have been attributed to enhanced vascular wall production of prostacyclin (PGI_2) and intracellular cyclic adenosine monophosphate (cAMP) in platelets, polymorphonuclear leukocytes, and monocytes (96, 97). At biologically achievable doses, pentoxifylline as well as other methylxanthines can suppress the production of both biologically active tumor necrosis factor (TNF) and TNF mRNA expression (98, 99). Since cAMP can function in intracellular signal transduction and regulate monokine production (100), this mechanism may be involved in pentoxifylline-induced inhibition of TNF production (99).

The survival of tumor cells from FSaIIC fibrosarcoma tumors and of bone marrow CFU-GM from the same animals after treatment was CDDP or Carbo in the presence or absence of pentoxifylline is shown in Figure 2.5 (101). Pentoxifylline itself was not toxic to the tumor or to the bone marrow (data not shown). CDDP killed increasing numbers of FSaIIC tumor cells with increasing doses of the drug in a log-linear manner. When a single dose of pentoxifylline (100 mg/kg)

Figure 2.5. Survival of FSaIIC tumor cells (●, ▲, ■) and bone marrow CFU-GM (○, △, □) from animals treated in vivo with single doses of CDDP, Carbo, thiotepa, or CTX (●, ○); single doses of CDDP or Carbo preceded by a single dose of pentoxifylline (100 mg/kg) (▲, △); or five doses of pentoxifylline (50 mg/kg) over 24 hours with CDDP, Carbo, thiotepa, or CTX administered immediately after the third dose of pentoxifylline (■, □). (From Teicher BA, Holden SA, Herman TS, et al. Effect of pentoxifylline as a modulator of alkylating agent activity in vitro and in vivo. Cancer Lett 1991, in press.)

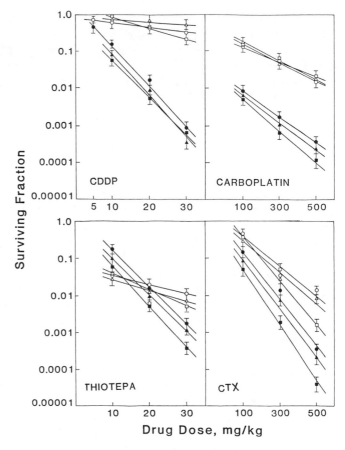

preceded CDDP administration or when five doses of pentoxifylline (50 mg/kg) were administered over a 24-hour period and CDDP was injected immediately after the third dose of pentoxifylline, no significant effect on cell killing resulted. Overall, pentoxifylline administered either on the single-dose or multiple-dose schedule did not alter the killing of bone marrow cells by CDDP. A very similar pattern was obtained with Carbo in vivo. As the dose of Carbo was increased, there was a log-linear increase in the killing of tumor cells by the drug. Administration of pentoxifylline (100 mg/kg) prior to Carbo resulted in a slight increase in tumor cell killing, while administering five doses of pentoxifylline (50 mg/kg) with Carbo given immediately after the third dose of pentoxifylline produced a two- to threefold increase in tumor cell kill-

ing compared to Carbo alone. Neither single-dose nor multiple-dose administration of pentoxifylline altered the killing of bone marrow CFU-GM produced by Carbo.

More positive results were obtained when pentoxifylline was added to the treatment of FSaIIC tumor-bearing animals with thiotepa or CTX (Fig. 2.5) (101). Thiotepa killed increasing numbers of FSaIIC tumor cells with increasing dosage of the drug in a log-linear manner. When a single dose of pentoxifylline (100 mg/kg) preceded the dose of thiotepa, only a slight increase in tumor cell killing resulted. However, when five doses of pentoxifylline were administered over a 24-hour period and thiotepa was given immediately after the third dose of pentoxifylline, tumor cell killing by thiotepa was increased by three-fold with 10 mg/kg of thiotepa and by 6-fold at the high dose of 30 mg/kg of thiotepa. The killing of bone marrow CFU-GM by thiotepa was increased to a much lesser extent than the killing of the tumor cells with the addition of pentoxifylline to treatment with drug. Overall, the increase in bone marrow CFU-GM killing by the combination of pentoxifylline and thiotepa was two- to three-fold compared to results with thiotepa alone. Interestingly, while at the lower end of the thiotepa dose range bone marrow killing actually exceeded tumor cell killing, at the high dose end this pattern was reversed.

The effect of tumor cell killing with CTX by pentoxifylline was similar to that seen with thiotepa (Fig. 2.5) (101). CTX killed increasing numbers of FSaIIC tumor cells with increasing dose of the drug in a log-linear manner. A single dose of pentoxifylline (100 mg/kg) immediately prior to treatment with CTX resulted in about a twofold increase in the killing of tumor cells by the drug. However, when five doses of pentoxifylline (50 mg/kg) were administered over 24 hours and CTX was given immediately after the third injection of pentoxifylline, a threefold increase in tumor cell killing was obtained with 100 mg/kg of CTX, which increased to ninefold with 500 mg/kg of CTX. In the lower dosage range of CTX (100–300 mg/kg) the enhancement in the killing of tumor cells was larger than the enhancement in the killing of bone marrow CFU-GM. However, at the highest dose of CTX of 500 mg/kg, there was a ninefold increase in the killing of bone marrow CFU-GM, which was equal to the increase in the killing of tumor cells by the drug combination.

A standard dose phase I clinical study of pentoxifylline in combination with thiotepa has been completed (102). The pentoxifylline was administered orally and dose-escalated. The recommended dose of pentoxifylline was 1600 mg three times daily. In three patients it was noted that pentoxifylline appeared to decrease levels of cachexia and TNF mRNA in circulating mononuclear cells (99). This decrease in TNF correlated with an improved feeling of well-being in these patients. A standard dose phase II study of pentoxifylline and chemotherapy is underway at Dana-Farber.

L-BUTHIONINE SULFOXIMINE

Glutathione is the major intracellular nonprotein sulfhydryl compound. One of its functions is to reduce the cytotoxic effects of endogenous or exogenous electrophiles, including chemotherapeutic alkylating agents (103, 104). L-buthionine sulfoximine (BSO) is a selective inhibitor of g-glutamylcysteine synthetase, effecting depletion of glutathione in vitro and in vivo (105–107). Calcutt and Connors (108) initially demonstrated the role of glutathione in mediating tumor cell sensitivity to the antitumor nitrogen mustard melphalan (L-PAM). Studies with L1210 leukemia cells and human ovarian carcinoma cell lines have demonstrated glutathione-mediated resistance to L-PAM and reversal of this resistance following glutathione depletion mediated by BSO (105–107), 109–111). Furthermore, L-PAM cytotoxicity was enhanced following glutathione depletion in both sensitive and resistant cells (112).

Although several studies have suggested that the combination of BSO with several alkylating agents does not increase toxic effects in the host (113, 114), carefully controlled studies of normal tissue toxicity have not yet been reported for many BSO/alkylating agent combinations. The recent description of hepatoxic effects and enhanced nephrotoxic effects following administration of BSO and semustine to Fischer 344 rats suggests that BSO and alkylating agents administered in combination can have toxicologic consequences (115). Attempts to selectively deplete tumor cells but not normal cells have been only partially successful in murine cells in vivo and human cells in vitro (114, 116). Timing of glutathione depletion to allow maximal enhancement of the therapeutic effect while minimizing the toxic effect will need to be identified for optimal use of BSO/

alkylating agent combination therapy, perhaps using glutathione monoethyl ester as a normal tissue protector (117). BSO-mediated glutathione depletion may offer a means of increasing the activity of certain alkylating agents as well as a means of reversing glutathione-mediated drug resistance. The observation that glutathione depletion may also serve as a radiosensitizer (118) offers another potential means to exploit BSO therapeutically in the treatment regimens without the concerns of enhanced systemic toxicity.

Early initial studies suggested that the central nervous system is relatively refractory to BSO, with minimal depletion of brain glutathione (105). However, studies by Skapek et al. (119) with the human glioma cell line D-54 MG growing intracranially in BSO-treated athymic mice clearly demonstrated the selective depletion of xenograft glutathione levels with minimal effects on contralateral normal brain (119). Studies of [^{35}S]BSO accumulation in xenograft and surrounding non-tumor-bearing brain suggested that this selectivity resulted from differential BSO transport between normal brain and tumor tissue. Skapek et al. (120) also demonstrated enhanced L-PAM cytotoxicity to human medulloblastoma xenografts (TE-671) grown subcutaneously in BSO-treated athymic mice (120). Recently, Friedman et al. (121) demonstrated enhanced L-PAM cytotoxicity with significant increases in median survival following treatment with BSO in human glioma and medulloblastoma xenografts growing intracranially. However, the marked permeability of intracranial D-54 MG and TE-671 xenografts (122, 123) may overestimate the tumor-induced disruption of the blood-brain barrier seen in patients, with consequent decreased delivery of water-soluble agents such as BSO. In those studies, Friedman et al. (121) treated xenograft-bearing mice with L-PAM alone or BSO followed by L-PAM. Administration of BSO depleted intracellular glutathione to 7.5% of the control level. BSO plus melphalan resulted in a significant increase in median survival over that produced by L-

PAM alone: 45.3% versus 26.4% in TE-671 and 69% versus 27.6% in D-54 MG.

Soble and Dorr (124) demonstrated that CTX treatment of CD-1 mice following BSO-mediated depletion of glutathione resulted in sudden death within hours of CTX administration. Friedman et al. (125) explored the mechanism of this effect and confirmed that administration of CTX at a dose lethal to 10% of control athymic nude mice resulted in sudden death within 3 hours in all mice that had been pretreated with BSO. In Fischer 344 rats pretreated with BSO, the CTX dose producing 100% acute toxicity was lowered from 500 to 150 mg/kg; cardiac monitoring revealed ventricular fibrillation to be the cause of death. These studies demonstrated that cytoplasmic glutathione is an important protectant against the cardiac and skeletal muscle toxicity of CTX and indicate that such toxicity may be substantially increased by glutathione depletion. Therefore, caution must be observed is using these combinations.

COMBINED MODULATORS

Fluosol-DA/Oxygen and Etanidazole

The perfluorochemical emulsion Fluosol-DA in combination with an intake of a 100% or 95% oxygen atmosphere has been shown to enhance the response of several solid rodent tumors to single-dose and fractionated radiation treatment (126–132). On the basis of these promising preclinical results, several clinical phase I/II studies and a phase III trial have been initiated with Fluosol-DA and oxygen breathing in conjunction with radiation treatment (133, 134).

The level of cellular oxygenation is also an important factor in the action of many antineoplastic agents, several of which have been classified in vitro (135) and in vivo (136) by their selective cytotoxicity toward oxygenated and hypoxic tumor cells. Fluosol-DA and carbogen (95% oxygen and 5% carbon dioxide) breathing have been shown to enhance the antitumor activity and cytocidal activity of each of the antitumor tumor alkylating agents described below: CDDP (136–138), CTX (136, 138, 139), Carbo (140), thiotepa (140), BCNU (141, 142), and L-PAM (138, 143–145).

However, because of the short diffusion distance and metabolic instability of oxygen, it is unlikely that Fluosol-DA and carbogen or oxygen breathing can be 100% efficient in oxygenating tumor masses (126, 128). Using microoxygen electrodes, Hasegawa et al. (126) and Song (128) showed substantially increased oxygenation of tumors in the presence of Fluosol-DA/carbogen, but some hypoxic regions remained. These regions of hypoxic cells may remain viable and contribute to tumor regrowth. Use of selective hypoxic cell cytotoxic agents in conjunction with Fluosol-DA plus oxygen breathing is, therefore, a logical combination approach. Teicher et al. (146) examined the ability of the 2-nitroimidazole ETA to act as a chemosensitizer of a series of antitumor alkylating agents in conjunction with Fluosol-DA and carbogen breathing.

The addition of ETA or Fluosol-DA/carbogen resulted in approximately 10-fold additional tumor cell killing compared with CDDP alone (Fig. 2.6) (146). The combination of modulators, ETA, and Fluosol-DA/carbogen resulted in an increase in tumor cell killing of only 2-fold compared with each modulator individually with CDDP. At the lowest Carbo dose there was about an 8-fold increase in tumor cell killing, and at the higher dosage level (300 and 500 mg/kg), this increased to more than 50-fold. Using the two modulators in combination again added little to the enhancement of tumor cell killing by Carbo obtained in conjunction with either modulator alone. The addition of ETA and Fluosol-DA/carbogen to CDDP resulted in only a 2- to 3-fold increase in the cytotoxicity of CDDP and a small (2- to 3-fold) decrease in cytotoxicity by Carbo to the bone marrow CFU-GM. The use of ETA and/or Fluosol-DA/carbogen in combination with CTX or thiotepa is shown in Figure 2.7. The addition of ETA

or Fluosol-DA/carbogen to treatment with CTX resulted in about a 10-fold increase in tumor cell killing across the dosage range examined. The combination of modulators ETA with Fluosol-DA/carbogen and CTX resulted in an additional 5- to 7-fold increase in tumor cell killing over that obtained with CTX and each single modulator. The addition of ETA to treatment with thiotepa resulted in about a 2- to 3-fold increase in tumor cell killing. The addition of Fluosol-DA/carbogen to treatment with the thiotepa resulted in about a 5- to 8-fold increase in tumor cell killing by the drug. The combination of modulators resulted in an additional 2- to 3-fold tumor cell killing over that achieved with Fluosol-DA/carbogen and thiotepa, so that over the dosage range of thiotepa examined, there was about an 8- to 10-fold increase in tumor cell killing compared with thiotepa alone. The addition of ETA and Fluosol-DA/carbogen to treatment with CTX did not alter the cytotoxicity of CTX to the bone marrow CFU-GM. The combination of modulators with thiotepa produced only about a 2-fold increase in the killing of bone marrow CFU-GM with the low dose of thiotepa (10 mg/kg), which increased to about 10-fold at the highest thiotepa dose level of 30 mg/kg.

ETA resulted in a 5- to 7-fold increase in tumor cell killing over the L-PAM dosage range examined (Fig. 2.8) (146). Fluosol-DA/carbogen was a more effective modulator of L-PAM than was ETA, resulting in about a 9- to 11-fold increase in tumor cell killing. The combination of ETA and Fluosol-DA/carbogen produced a larger increase in tumor cell killing than either single modulator alone, resulting in about a 10- to 50-fold increase in tumor cell killing compared with L-PAM alone. ETA produced about a 2- to 5-fold increase in tumor cell killing, and Fluosol-DA/carbogen produced about a 4- to 9-fold increase in tumor cell killing compared with BCNU alone. The combination of modulators was much more effective than either single modulator alone with BCNU in the killing of tumor cells and resulted in a 10- to 50-fold increase com-

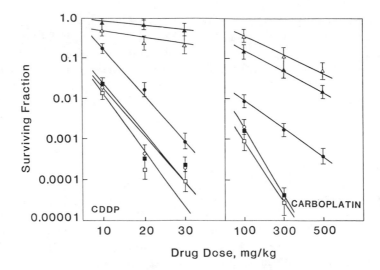

Figure 2.6. Survival of FSaIIC tumor cells and bone marrow CFU-GM from animals treated in vivo with single doses of CDDP or Carbo alone (●, tumor; △, bone marrow), preceded by a single dose of ETA (1g/kg) (○, tumor), preceded by a single dose of Fluosol-DA (0.3 ml, 12 ml/kg) and followed by carbogen breathing (6 hours) (■, tumor), or with the combination of the two modulators (□, tumor; △, bone marrow). (From Teicher BA, Herman TS, Tanaka J, et al. Modulation of alkylating agents by etanidazole and Fluosol-DA/carbogen in the FSaIIC fibrosarcoma and EMT6 mammary carcinoma. Cancer Res 1991;51:1086–1091.)

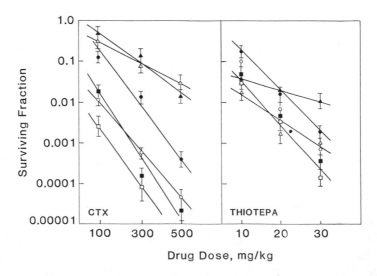

Figure 2.7. Survival of FSaIIC tumor cells and bone marrow CFU-GM from animals treated in vivo with single doses of CTX or thiotepa alone (●, tumor; △, bone marrow), preceded by a single dose of ETA (1 g/kg) (○, tumor), preceded by a single dose of Fluosol-DA (0.3 ml, 12 ml/kg) and followed by carbogen breathing (6 hours) (■, tumor), or with the combination of the two modulators (□, tumor; △, bone marrow). (From Teicher BA, Herman TS, Tanaka J, et al. Modulation of alkylating agents by etanidazole and Fluosol-DA/carbogen in the FSaIIC fibrosarcoma and EMT6 mammary carcinoma. Cancer Res 1991;51:1086–1091.)

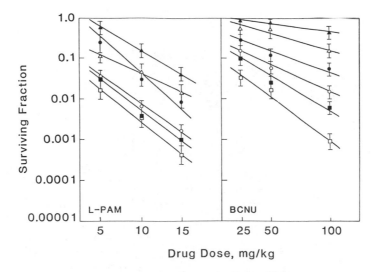

Figure 2.8. Survival of FSaIIC tumor cells and bone marrow CFU-GM from animals treated in vivo with single doses of L-PAM or BCNU alone (●, tumor; △, bone marrow), preceded by a single dose of ETA (1 g/kg) (○, tumor), preceded by a single dose of Fluosol-DA (0.3 ml, 12 ml/kg) and followed by carbogen breathing (6 hours) (■, tumor), or with the combination of the two modulators (□, tumor; △, bone marrow). (From Teicher BA, Herman TS, Tanaka J, et al. Modulation of alkylating agents by etanidazole and Fluosol-DA/carbogen in the FSaIIC fibrosarcoma and EMT6 mammary carcinoma. Cancer Res 1991;51:1086–1091.)

pared with BCNU alone. The modulator combination increased the killing of bone marrow CFU-GM 5- to 7-fold compared with L-PAM alone and produced a 3- to 5-fold increase in the killing of bone marrow CFU-GM by BCNU.

To determine the effectiveness of these various treatments on environmentally determined tumor subpopulations, tumors were treated as in the above tumor cell excision assays and then sorted into subpopulations by the Hoechst dye method (Figure 2.9) (146). In these experiments, Fluosol-DA/carbogen was nontoxic, whereas ETA killed about 5% of bright cells and about 40% of dim cells. The 10% brightest cells are believed to represent a population near the tumor vasculature (euoxic) and the 20% dimmest to represent a cellular population distal from the tumor vasculature (hypoxic). CDDP (10 mg/kg) was about 2-fold more toxic toward bright cells than toward dim cells. The combination of the two modulators with CDDP increased the killing of bright cells 23-fold and the killing of dim cells 51-fold compared with CDDP

alone. CTX (150 mg/kg) was about 6.3-fold more cytotoxic toward bright cells than toward dim cells. The combination of modulators was highly effective, increasing the killing of bright cells by about 9.5-fold and the killing of dim cells by about 55-fold.

L-PAM was about 2.2-fold more cytotoxic toward bright tumor cells than toward dim tumor cells. The combination of modulators was, again, highly effective, resulting in about a 25-fold increase in the killing of bright cells and about a 44-fold increase in the killing of bright cells compared with L-PAM alone. BCNU (50 mg/kg) was about 3.2-fold more cytotoxic toward bright cells than toward dim cells. The combination of modulators increased the killing of bright cells by about 45-fold and increased the killing of dim cells by about 23-fold.

Fluosol-DA/Oxygen and Lonidamine or Pentoxifylline

The combination of modulators, lonidamine and Fluosol-DA/carbogen (6 hours)

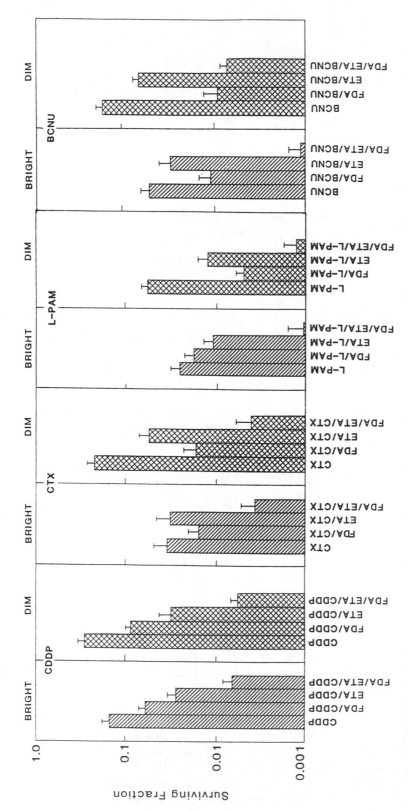

Figure 2.9. Survival of subpopulations based on Hoechst 33342 fluorescence intensity of FSaIIC cells from FSaIIC tumors treated with a single dose of CDDP (10 mg/kg), CTX (150 mg/kg), L-PAM (10 mg/kg), or BCNU (50 mg/kg) with or without ETA (1 g/kg), and/or Fluosol-DA (12 ml/kg) and carbogen breathing (6 hours). (From Teicher BA, Herman TS, Tanaka J, et al. Modulation of alkylating agents by etanidazole and Fluosol-DA/carbogen in the FSaIIC fibrosarcoma and EMT6 mammary carcinoma. Cancer Res 1991;51:1086–1091.)

administered ip to animals bearing the FSaIIC fibrosarcoma just prior to ip administration of a range of doses of CDDP resulted in an additional 10-fold increase in tumor cell killing compared with Fluosol-DA/carbogen/CDDP and a 100-fold increase in tumor cell killing compared with CDDP alone (Fig. 2.10) (147). The cytotoxicity of CDDP toward bone marrow CFU-GM was unaffected by the addition of lonidamine (100 mg/kg) or Fluosol-DA (0.3 ml, 12 ml/kg)/carbogen (6 hours). However, the combination of modulators resulted in about a 10-fold increase in the cytotoxicity of CDDP toward bone marrow CFU-GM.

Using the combination of modulators, lonidamine and Fluosol-DA/carbogen did not further increase the tumor cell killing compared with what was obtainable with Fluosol-DA/carbogen and L-PAM. Neither lonidamine nor Fluosol-DA/carbogen increased the toxicity of L-PAM to bone marrow as compared with the drug alone. However, as was the case with CDDP, the combination of modulators markedly increased the cytotoxicity of L-PAM to the bone marrow CFU-GM (by 10- to 50-fold over the L-PAM dosage range compared with L-PAM alone). The addition of lonidamine (100 mg/kg) to treatment with Fluosol-DA/carbogen and CTX did not alter the tumor cell killing produced by Fluosol-DA/carbogen with CTX. There was no significant difference in the toxicity of CTX to bone marrow CFU-GM when the drug was administered in combination with lonidamine or with Fluosol-DA/carbogen. The combination of modulators with CTX, however, resulted in about 10-fold additional killing of bone marrow CFU-GM compared with CTX alone. The combination of the two modulators, lonidamine and

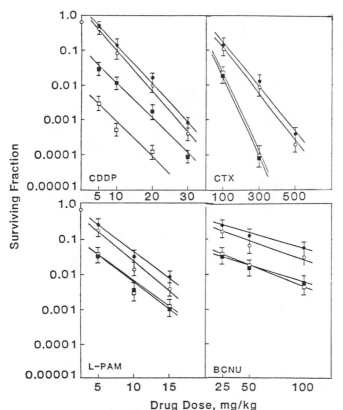

Figure 2.10. Survival of FSaIIC tumor cells from animals treated in vivo with single doses of CDDP, L-PAM, CTX, or BCNU alone (●), preceded by a single dose of lonidamine (100 mg/kg) (○), preceded by a single dose of Fluosol-DA (0.3 ml, 12 ml/kg) and followed by carbogen breathing (6 hours) (■), or with the combination of the two modulators (□). (From Teicher BA, Herman TS, Tanaka J, et al. Fluosol-DA/carbogen with lonidanine or pentoxifylline as modulators of alkylating agents in the FSaIIC fibrosarcoma. Cancer Chemother Pharmacol 1991;28:45–50.)

Fluosol-DA/carbogen, did not further increase tumor cell killing by BCNU compared
with Fluosol-DA/carbogen and BCNU. As with
the other three drugs, neither lonidamine nor
Fluosol-DA/carbogen alone increased the cytotoxicity of BCNU to bone marrow CFU-GM;
however, the combination of modulators increased the killing of bone marrow CFU-GM
by BCNU by about 5-fold.

In combination with Fluosol-DA/car-
bogen and CDDP, pentoxifylline increased
tumor cell killing by about 2-fold (Fig. 2.11)
(147). Pentoxifylline (100 mg/kg) alone and
in combination with Fluosol-DA/carbogen had
a dose-modifying effect on the cytotoxicity of
CDDP to the bone marrow CFU-GM. The cytotoxicity of CDDP to the bone marrow CFU-
GM was increased about 2-fold with 5 mg/
kg of CDDP (with or without Fluosol-DA/car-
bogen) and about 50-fold with 30 mg/kg of

CDDP (with or without Fluosol-DA/carbo-
gen). The combination of pentoxifylline and
Fluosol-DA/carbogen further increased the
killing of bone marrow CFU-GM by L-PAM, so
that the level of bone marrow CFU-GM killing by the combination was about 20-fold
greater than that of L-PAM alone.

Pentoxifylline (100 mg/kg) with or
without Fluosol-DA/carbogen when used with
CTX resulted in a 1.5- to 2-fold increase in
the killing of tumor cells compared with CTX
or Fluosol-DA/carbogen and CTX. Although
neither pentoxifylline nor Fluosol-DA/car-
bogen increased the cytotoxicity of CTX toward the bone marrow CFU-GM, the combination of modulators produced a dose-
modifying effect on the cytotoxicity of CTX
toward bone marrow CFU-GM. The enhancement in bone marrow CFU-GM cytotoxicity
increased from about 5-fold at 100 mg/kg of

Figure 2.11. Survival of FSaIIC tumor
cells from animals treated in vivo with
single doses of CDDP, L-PAM CTX, or
BCNU alone (●), preceded by a single
dose of pentoxifylline (100 mg/kg) (○),
preceded by a single dose of Fluosol-DA
(0.3 ml, 12 ml/kg) and followed by carbogen breathing (6 hours) (■), or with the
combination of the two modulators (□).
(From Teicher BA, Herman TS, Tanaka J,
et al. Fluosol-DA/carbogen with lonidanine or pentoxifylline as modulators of alkylating agents in the FSaIIC fibrosarcoma. Cancer Chemother Pharmacol
1991;28:45–50.)

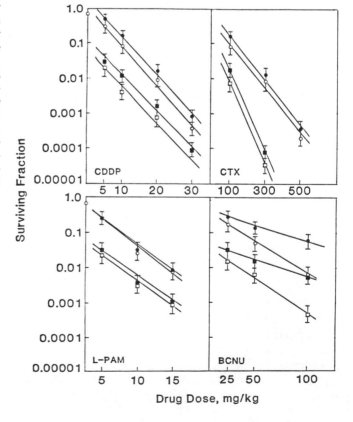

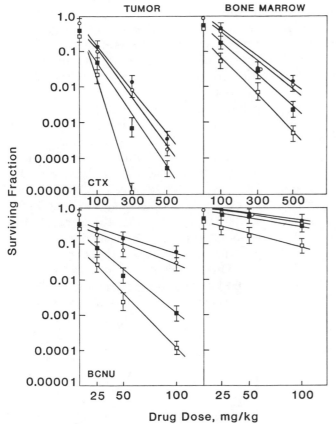

Figure 2.12. Survival of FSaIIC tumor cells and bone marrow CFU-GM from animals treated in vivo with single doses of CTX or BCNU alone (●), preceded by a single dose of lonidamine (100 mg/kg) (○) preceded by a single dose of etoposide (20 mg/kg), or with the combination of the two modulators (□). (From Tanaka J, Teicher BA, Herman TS, et al. Etoposide with lonidamine or pentoxifylline as modulators of alkylating agent activity in vivo. Int J Cancer 1991;48:631–637.)

CTX to about 100-fold at 500 mg/kg of CTX.

Dose modification of the killing of tumor cells was observed when pentoxifylline was used in combination with Fluosol-DA/carbogen and BCNU. The combination of modulators with BCNU resulted in about a 20-fold enhancement in tumor cell killing by 25 mg/kg of BCNU, which increased to about a 200-fold enhancement in tumor cell killing by 100 mg/kg of BCNU. Neither pentoxifylline nor Fluosol-DA/carbogen increased the cytotoxicity of BCNU to the bone marrow CFU-GM; however, the combination of the two modulators had a dose-modifying effect on the cytotoxicity of BCNU toward the bone marrow CFU-GM, such that there was about a 4-fold increase in cytotoxicity with 25 mg/kg of BCNU and about a 25-fold increase in cytotoxicity with 100 mg/kg BCNU.

ETOPOSIDE AND LONIDAMINE OR PENTOXIFYLLINE

DNA topoisomerase type II enzymes are proteins found in both prokaryotic and eukaryotic cells that control and modify the topological states of DNA. By transiently breaking a pair of complementary DNA strands and passing another double-stranded segment through the area, topoisomerase type II can catalyze many types of interconversions between DNA topological isomers (148, 149). DNA topoisomerases have been found to affect a number of vital biologic functions, including the replication and repair of DNA (149–152). DNA topoisomerase type II is a useful focus for cancer therapy on two levels, first as a target itself through the formation of the tertiary complex of drug-enzyme-DNA, which can lead directly to a cytotoxic event, and, second, since formation of the tertiary complex locks the DNA into a conformation that may be more susceptible to the actions of antitumor bifunctional alkylating agents or may inhibit repair of monoadducts (153, 154). Molecules from several chemical families have been shown to interact with DNA topoisomerase II; one type of these is the antitumor epipodophyllotoxins such as etoposide (VP-16-213) and VM-26 (148, 154, 155).

Etoposide (20 mg/kg) produced additive FSaIIC tumor cell killing with CTX (Fig. 2.12) (156). Addition of lonidamine to treatment with etoposide and CTX appeared to have a dose-modifying effect. At a dose of 300 mg/kg of CTX, lonidamine cotreatment increased tumor killing of FSaIIC cells by etoposide and CTX by about 1.5 logs. Although

lonidamine addition to treatment with etoposide and CTX increased the killing of bone marrow CFU-GM, the level of increase was only 3- to 4-fold. Etoposide (20 mg/kg) had a dose-modifying effect on BCNU that resulted in an increase in FSaIIC tumor cell killing of about 3-fold at 25 mg/kg of BCNU to about 50-fold at 100 mg/kg of BCNU. The addition of lonidamine to treatment with etoposide and BCNU resulted in an additional dose-modifying effect. There was about a 3-fold increase in tumor cell killing at 25 mg/kg of BCNU that increased to about 10-fold at 100 mg/kg of BCNU. There was a much lesser effect of the combination treatment on the cytotoxicity of BCNU to bone marrow CFU-GM, which resulted in about a 5-fold increase in the killing of bone marrow CFU-GM.

Pentoxifylline did not increase tumor cell

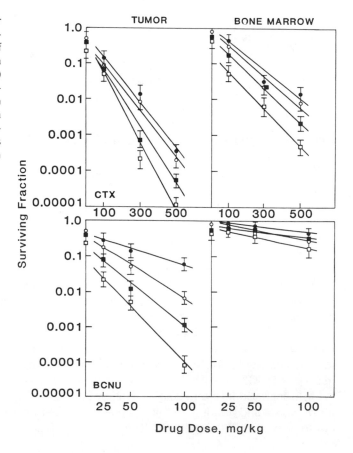

Figure 2.13. Survival of FSaIIC tumor cells and bone marrow CFU-GM from animals treated in vivo with single doses of CTX or BCNU alone (●), preceded by a single dose of pentoxifylline (100 mg/kg) (○), preceded by a single dose of etoposide (20 mg/kg), or with the combination of the two modulators (□). (From Tanaka J, Teicher BA, Herman TS, et al. Etoposide with lonidamine or pentoxifylline as modulators of alkylating agent activity in vivo. Int J Cancer 1991;48:631–637.)

killing by the combination of etoposide and CTX (100 mg/kg); however, there was about a 5-fold increase in tumor cell killing by the combination of etoposide and CTX (500 mg/kg) (Fig. 2.13) (156). Although pentoxifylline did not significantly increase the cytotoxicity of CTX toward bone marrow CFU-GM, the addition of pentoxifylline to the combination of etoposide and CTX increased the killing of bone marrow CFU-GM by 10- to 50-fold over the dosage range of CTX examined, compared with CTX alone. A similar dose-modifying effect was observed when pentoxifylline was added to treatment with the combination of etoposide and BCNU, so that overall there was about a 15- to 1000-fold increase in tumor cell killing with pentoxifylline/etoposide/BCNU compared with BCNU alone and about a 4- to 12-fold increase as compared with etoposide plus BCNU. Interestingly, there was little increase in the killing of bone marrow CFU-GM by the addition of pentoxifylline to treatment with BCNU and etoposide. Overall there was about a 2- to 3-fold increase in the killing of bone marrow

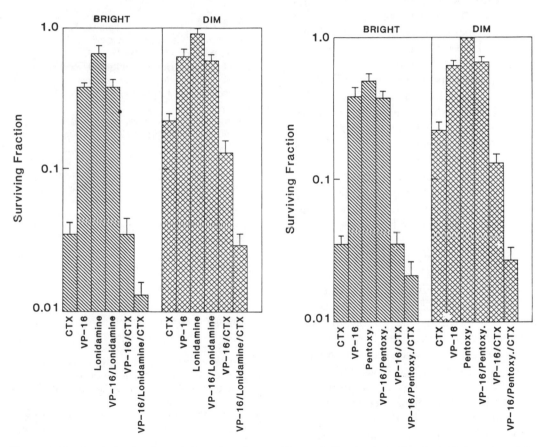

Figure 2.14. Survival of subpopulations based on Hoechst 33342 fluorescence intensity of FSaIIC cells from FSaIIC tumors treated with a single dose of CTX (150 mg/kg) with or without lonidamine (100 mg/kg) and/or etoposide (20 mg/kg). (From Tanaka J, Teicher BA, Herman TS, et al. Etoposide with lonidamine or pentoxifylline as modulators of alkylating agent activity in vivo. Int J Cancer 1991;48:631-637.)

Figure 2.15. Survival of subpopulations based on Hoechst 33342 fluorescence intensity of FSaIIC cells from FSaIIC tumors treated with a single dose of CTX (150 mg/kg) with or without pentoxifylline (100 mg/kg) and/or etoposide (20 mg/kg). (From Tanaka J, Teicher BA, Herman TS, et al. Etoposide with lonidamine or pentoxifylline as modulators of alkylating agent activity in vivo. In J Cancer 1991;48:631–637.)

CFU-GM with the combination of pentoxifyl-line/etoposide/BCNU compared with BCNU alone. For all the combinations tested, the greatest differential between tumor and bone marrow killing was seen with pentoxifylline and etoposide added to BCNU, especially at the highest BCNU dose tested.

CTX was about 7-fold more cytotoxic toward bright cells than toward dim cells (Fig. 2.14) (156). Etoposide (20 mg/kg) addition to treatment with CTX did not alter the kill-ing of bright cells but increased the killing of dim cells by about 1.7-fold compared to the drug alone. The combination of lonidamine with etoposide and CTX was more effective, producing increases in tumor cell killing of 2.7-fold in bright cells and 7.6-fold in dim cells compared with CTX alone.

Pentoxifylline added to treatment with etoposide and CTX resulted in a 1.7-fold in-crease in bright tumor cell killing compared with CTX alone or with etoposide/CTX (Fig. 2.15) (156). However, in the dim cells, ad-dition of pentoxifylline to treatment with eto-poside and CTX resulted in an 8.1-fold in-crease in tumor cell killing compared with CTX alone and in a 4.8-fold increase in tumor cell killing compared with etoposide/CTX.

Conclusion

Preclinical studies from the earliest mu-rine leukemia model systems to the present range of leukemia, solid tumor, and xeno-graft models have provided both cancer sci-entists and physicians with the awareness that tumor cure requires the eradication by ex-ogenous treatments of nearly all tumor cells to be curative. High-dose chemotherapy reg-imens are based on the premise that under-treatment is the reason for failure to achieve cure in many cases. Through the use of in vivo/in vivo and in vivo/in vitro excision as-says, preclinical models have reached to high-dose levels of chemotherapy and have been able to demonstrate continued tumor cell killing. The use of rigorous analytical tech-niques has allowed the determination of the effectiveness of drug combination in the high-dose setting.

Several clinical leads have developed from the preclinical results presented herein for both the treatment of leukemias and solid tumors. Through the use of modulators, it is hoped that the selectivity of current antican-cer agents can be further increased. Several high-dose clinical trials of modulators and al-kylating agents, including ETA/Carbo/CTX in ovarian carcinoma and pentoxifylline/eto-poside/BCNU/CTX in lymphoma, are planned.

REFERENCES

1. Hill RP. Excision assays. In: Kallman RF, ed. Rodent tumor models in experimental cancer therapy. New York: Pergamon Press, 1987:67–75.
2. Steel GG, Peckham MJ. Exploitable mechanisms in combined radiotherapy-chemotherapy: the concept of additivity. Int. J Radiat Oncol Biol Phys 1979;5:85–91.
3. Berenbaum MC. Synergy, additivism and antago-nism in immunosuppression. Clin Exp Immunol 1977;28:1–18.
4. Dewey WC, Stone LE, Miller HH, Giblak RE. Radi-osensitization with 5-bromodeoxyuridine of Chinese hamster cells X-irradiated during different phases of the cell cycle. Radiat Res 1971;47:672–688.
5. Deen DF, Williams MW. Isobologram analysis of X-ray-BCNU interactions *in vitro*. Radiat Res 1979; 79:483–491.
6. Schabel FM, Trader MW, Laster WR, Wheeler GP, Witt MH. Patterns of resistance and therapeutic syn-ergism among alkylating agents. Antibiot Chemo-ther 1978;23:200–215.
7. Schabel FM, Griswold DP, Corbett TH, Laster WR, Mayo JG, Lloyd HH. Testing therapeutic hypotheses in mice and man: observations on the therapeutic activity against advanced solid tumors of mice treated with anticancer drugs that have demonstrated or potential clinical utility for treatment of advanced solid tumors of man. Methods Cancer Res 1979;17:3–51.
8. Schabel FM, Griswold DP, Corbett TH, Laster WR. Increasing therapeutic response rates to anticancer drugs applying the basic principles of pharmacol-ogy. Pharmacol Ther 1983;20:283–305.
9. Schabel FM Jr, Skipper HE, Trader MW, Laster WR Jr, Griswold DP Jr, Corbett TH. Establishment of cross-resistance profiles for new agents. Cancer Treat Rep 1983;67:905.
10. DeWys DW. A dose-response study of resistance to leukemia L1210 to cyclophosphamide. J Natl Cancer Inst 1973;50:783.

11. Schabel FM Jr. Nitrosoureas: a review of experimental antitumor activity. Cancer Treat Rep 1976; 60:665.

12. Hagenbeek A, van Bekkum DW. Comparative evaluation of the L5222 and the BNML rat leukemia models and their relevance for human acute leukemia. Leuk Res 1977;1:75–255.

13. van Bekkum DW, Hagenbeek A. Relevance of the BN leukemia model as a model for human acute myeloid leukemia. Blood Cells 1977;3:565–579.

14. Martens AC, van Bekkum DW, Hagenbeek A. The BN acute myelocytic leukemia (BNML) (a rat model for studying human acute myelocytic leukemia [AML]). Leukemia 1990;4:241–257.

15. Martens AC, Hagenbeek A. Kinetics of normal hemopoietic stem cells during leukemia growth before and after induction of a complete remission. Studies in a rat model for acute myelocytic leukemia (BNML). Leuk Res 1987;11:453–459.

16. Martens ACM. Normal and leukemic stem cells during minimal residual disease. Studies in an experimental rat leukemia model (BNML) [Monograph]. Rijswijk: The Radiobiologic Institute TNO, 1988.

17. Nooter K, de Vries A, Martens AC, Hagenbeek A. Effect of cyclophosphamide pretreatment on daunorubicin in rat acute leukaemia model. Eur J Cancer 1990;26:729–732.

18. Sharkis SJ, Santos GW, Colvin M. Elimination of acute myelogenous leukemic cells from marrow and tumor suspensions in the rat with 4-hydroperoxycyclophosphamide. Blood 1980;55:521–532.

19. Hagenbeek A, Martens ACM. Toxicity of ASTA-Z-7557 to normal and leukemic stem cells: implications for autologous bone marrow transplantation. Invest New Drugs 1984;2:237–242.

20. Martens ACM, van Bekkum DW, Hagenbeek A. Heterogeneity within the speen colony forming cell population in rat bone marrow. Exp Hematol 1986;14:714–718.

21. Kaizer H, Stuart RK, Brookmeyer R, et al. Autologous bone marrow transplantation (BMT) in acute leukemia: a phase I study of in vitro treatment of marrow with 4-hydroperoxycyclophosphamide (4-HC) to purge tumor cells. Blood 1985;65:1504–1510.

22. Rowley SD, Colvin M, Stuart RK. Human multilineage progenitor cell sensitivity to 4-hydroperoxycyclophosphamide. Exp Hematol 1985;13:295–298.

23. Gordon MY, Goldman JM, Gordon-Smith EC. 4-Hydroxycyclophosphamide inhibits proliferation by human granulocyte-macrophage colony-forming cells but spares more primitive progenitor cells. Leuk Res 1985;9(8):1017–1021.

24. Hagenbeek A, Martens SC. Cryopreservation of autologous marrow grafts in acute leukemia: survival of in vivo clonogenic leukemic cells and normal hemopoietic stem cells. Leukemia 1989;3:535–537.

25. Martens AC, Schultz FW, Hagenbeek A. Nonhomogenous distribution of leukcmia in the bone marrow during minimal residual disease. Blood 1987;70:1073–1078.

26. Hagenbeek A, Martens ACM. The efficacy of high dose cyclophosphamide in combination with total body irradiation in the treatment of acute myelocytic leukemia. Studies in a relevant rat model (BNML). Cancer Res 1983;43:408–412.

27. Hagenbeek A, Martens ACM. The efficacy of piperazindeione (NSC135758) prior to bone marrow transplantation. Studies in a rat model for acute myelocytic leukemia. Cancer Treat Rep 1981;65:575–582.

28. Hagenbeek A, Weiershausen U, Martens ACM. Dinaline: a new oral drug against acute myelocytic leukemia? Leukemia 1988;2:226–230.

29. Hagenbeek A, Martens ACM. BCG treatment of residual disease in acute leukemia. Studies in a rat model for human acute myelocytic leukemia (BNML). Leuk Res 1983;7:547–555.

30. Frei E III. Curative cancer chemotherapy. Cancer Res 1985;45:6523–6537.

31. Frei E III, Canellos GP. Dose: a critical factor in cancer chemotherapy. Am J Med 1980;69:585–594.

32. Skipper HE, Schabel FM, Jay R, et al. Experimental evaluation of potential antitumor agents: on the criteria and kinetics associated with curability of experimental leukemia. Cancer Chemother Rep 1964;35:1–37.

33. Skipper HE. Combination therapy: some concepts and results. Cancer Chemother Rep 1974;4:137–145.

34. Blum R, Frei E III. Combination chemotherapy: methods in cancer research. Cancer Res 1979;17:215–257.

35. Frei E III. Combination cancer therapy: presidential address. Cancer Res 1972;32:2593–2607.

36. Frei E III, Karon M, Levin RH, et al. The effectiveness of combinations of antileukemic agents in inducing and maintaining remission in children with acute leukemia. Blood 1965;26:642–656.

37. Holland JR. Breaking the cure barrier. J Clin Oncol 1983;1:75–90.

38. Alberts DS, Green SJ, Hannigan EV, et al. Improved efficacy of carboplatin plus cyclophosphamide versus cisplatin plus cyclophosphamide: preliminary report by the Southeast Oncology Group of a phase III randomized trial in stages III and IV suboptimal ovarian cancer. Proc Am Soc Clin Oncol 1989;8:151.

39. Carney DN, Teeling M. Carboplatin plus cyclophosphamide for epithelial ovarian carcinoma. In: Bunn PA, Canetta R, Ozols RF, et al., eds. Carboplatin (JM-8): current perspectives and future directions. Philadelphia: Harcourt, Brace, Jovanovich, 1990;125–132.

40. Eisenhauer EA, Swenerton KD, Sturgeon JF, et al. Phase II study of carboplatin in patients with ovarian carcinoma: a National Cancer Institute of Can-

ada Clinical Trials Group study. Cancer Treat Rep 1986;70:1195–1198.

41. ten Bokkel Huinink WW, Rodenhuis S, Simonetti G, et al. Studies with carboplatin in ovarian cancer: experience of the Netherlands Cancer Institute and GCCG of the European Organization for Research and Treatment of Cancer. In: Bunn PA, Canetta R, Ozols RF, et al., eds. Carboplatin (JM-8): current perspectives and future directions. Philadelphia: Harcourt, Brace, Jovanovich, 1990:165–174.

42. Kavanagh JJ. Carboplatin in refractory epithelial ovarian cancer. In: Bunn PA, Canetta R, Ozols RF, et al., eds. Carboplatin (JM-8): current perspectives and future directions. Philadelphia: Harcourt, Brace, Jovanovich, 1990:141–146.

43. Rozencweig M, Martin A, Beltangady M, et al. In: Bunn PA, Canetta R, Ozols RF, et al., eds. Carboplatin (JM-8): current perspectives and future directions. Philadelphia: Harcourt, Brace, Jovanovich, 1990:175–186.

44. Speyer JL, Richards D, Beller U, et al. Trials of intraperitoneal carboplatin in patients with refractory ovarian cancer. In: Bunn PA, Canetta R, Ozols RF, et al., eds. Carboplatin (JM-8): current perspectives and future directions. Philadelphia: Harcourt, Brace, Jovanovich, 1990:153–162.

45. Coleman NC. Hypoxic cell radiosensitizers: expectations and progress in drug development. Int J Radiat Oncol Biol Phys 1985;11:323–329.

46. Teicher BA, Herman TS, Holden SA. Effect of pH oxygenation and temperature on the cytotoxicity and radiosensitization by etanidazole. Int J Radiat Onc Biol Phys 1991;20:723–731.

47. Herman TS, Teicher BA, Holden SA, Pfeffer MR, Jones SM. Addition of 2-nitroimidazole radiosensitizers to trimodality therapy (cis-diamminedichloroplatinum II/hyperthermia/radiation) in the murine FSaIIC fibrosarcoma. Cancer Res 1990;50:2734–2740.

48. Teicher BA, Herman TS, Holden SA, Jones SM. Addition of misonidazole, etanidazole, or hyperthermia to treatment with Fluosol-DA/carbogen/radiation. J Natl Cancer Inst 1989;12:929–934.

49. Siemann DW. Modification of chemotherapy by nitroimidazoles. Int J Radiat Oncol Biol Phys 1984;10:1585–1594.

50. Franko AJ. Misonidazole and other hypoxia markers: metabolism and applications. Int J Radiat Oncol Biol Phys 1986;12:1195–1202.

51. Laderoute KR, Eryzvec E, McClelland RA, Rauth AM. The production of strand breaks in DNA in the presence of the hydroxylamine of SR-2508 (1-[N-(2-hydroxyethyl)acetamido]-2-nitroimidazole) at neutral pH. Int J Radiat Oncol Biol Phys 1986;12:1215–1218.

52. McNally NJ. Enhancement of chemotherapy agents. Int J Radiat Oncol Biol Phys 1982;8:593–598.

53. Roizen-Towle L, Hall EJ, Piro JP. Oxygen dependence for chemosensitization by misonidazole. Br J Cancer 1986;54:919–924.

54. Teicher BA, Pfeffer MR, Alvarez Sotomayor E, Herman TS. DNA cross-linking and pharmacokinetic parameters in target tissues with cis-diamminedichloroplatinum (II) and etanidazole with or without hyperthermia. Int J Hyperthermia 1991;7:773–784.

55. Teicher BA, Holden SA, Jones SM, Eder JP, Herman TS. Influence of scheduling on two drug combinations of alkylating agents in vivo. Cancer Chemother Pharmacol 1989;25:161–166.

56. Teicher BA, Herman TS, Shulman L, Bubley G, Coleman CN, Frei E III. Combination of etanidazole with cyclophosphamide and platinum complexes. Cancer Chemother Pharmacol 1991;28:153–158.

57. DeMartino C, Battelli T, Paggi MG, et al. Effects of lonidamine on murine and human tumor cells in vitro. Oncology 1984;41(suppl):15–29.

58. DeMartino C, Malorni W, Accinni L, et al. Cell membrane changes induced by lonidamine in human erythrocytes and T lymphocytes, and Ehrlich ascites tumor cells. Exp Molec Pathol 1987;46:15–30.

59. Floridi A, Lehninger AL. Action of the antitumor and antispermatogenic agent lonidamine on electron transport in Ehrlich ascites tumor mitochondria. Arch Biochem Biophys 1983;226:73–83.

60. Floridi A, Paggi MG, D'Arti, et al. Effect of lonidamine on the energy metabolism of Ehrlich ascites tumor cells. Cancer Res 1981;41:4661–4666.

61. Floridi A, Paggi MG, Marcante ML, et al. Lonidamine, a selective inhibitor of aerobic glycolysis of murine tumor cells. J Natl Cancer Inst 1981;66:497–499.

62. Floridi A, Bahnato A, Bianchi C, et al. Kinetics of inhibition of mitochondrial respiration by antineoplastic agent lonidamine. J Exp Clin Cancer Res 1986;5:273–280.

63. Szekely JG, Lobreau AU, Delaney S, Raaphorst GP, Feeley M. Morphological effects of lonidamine on two human tumor cell culture lines. Scanning Microsc 1989;3:681–693.

64. Hahn GM, vanKersen I, Silvestrini B. Inhibition of the recovery from potentially lethal damage by lonidamine. Br J Cancer 1984;50:657–660.

65. Kim JH, Alfieri A, Kim SH, Young CW, Silvestrini B. Radiosensitization of Meth-A fibrosarcoma in mice by lonidamine. Oncology 1984;41(suppl 1):36–38.

66. Kim JH, Kim SH, Alfieri A, Young SW, Silvestrini B. Lonidamine: a hyperthermic sensitizer of HeLa cells in culture and of the Meth-A tumor in vivo. Oncology 1984;41(Suppl 1):30–35.

67. Kim JH, Alfieri AA, Kim SH, Young CW. Potentiation of radiation effects on two murine tumors by lonidamine. Cancer Res 1986;46:1120–1123.

68. Rosbe KW, Brann TW, Holden SA, Teicher BA, Frei E III. Effect of lonidamine on the cytotoxicity of four

alkylating agents *in vitro*. Cancer Chemother Pharmacol 1989;25:32–36.

69. Zupi G, Greco C, Laudino N, Benassi M, Silverstrini B, Caputo A. *In vitro* and *in vivo* potentiation by lonidamine of the antitumor effect of Adriamycin. Anticancer Res 1986;6:1245–1250.

70. Teicher BA, Herman TS, Holden SA, Epelbaum R, Liu S, Frei E III. Lonidamine as a modulator of alkylating agent activity *in vitro* and *in vivo*. Cancer Res 1991;51:780–784.

71. Ward A, Clissold SP. Pentoxifylline: a review of its pharmacodynamic and pharmacokinetic properties, and its therapeutic efficacy. Drugs 1987;34:50–97.

72. Ehrly AM. The effect of pentoxifylline on the flow properties of human blood. Curr Med Res Opin 1978;5:608–613.

73. Ehrly AM. The effect of pentoxifylline on the deformability of erythrocytes and on the muscular oxygen pressure in patients with chronic arterial disease. J Med 1979;10:331–338.

74. Aviado DM, Porter JM. Pentoxifylline: a new drug for the treatment of intermittent claudication. Pharmacotherapy 1984;6:297–307.

75. Perego MA, Sergio G, Artale F, Giunti P, Danese C. Haemorheological improvement by pentoxifylline in patients with peripheral arterial occlusive disease. Curr Med Res Opin 1986;10:135–138.

76. Poggesi L, Scarti L, Boddi M, Masotti G, Serneri GG. Pentoxifylline treatment in patients with occlusive peripheral vascular disease. Angiology 1985;36:628–637.

77. Waldren CA, Rasko I. Caffeine enhancement of x-ray killing in cultured human and rodent cells. Radiat Res 1978;73:95–110.

78. Busse PM, Bose SK, Jones RW, Tolmach LJ. The action of caffeine on x-irradiated HeLa cells. II: Synergistic lethality. Radiat Res 1977;71:666–677.

79. Tolmach LJ, Busse PM. The action of caffeine on x-irradiated HeLa cells. IV: Progression delays and enhanced cell killing at high caffeine concentrations. Radiat Res 1980;82:374–392.

80. Busse PM, Bose SK, Jones RW, Tolmach LJ. The action of caffeine on x-irradiated HeLa cells. III: Enhancement of x-ray-induced killing during G_2 arrest. Radiat Res 1978;76:292–307.

81. Painter RB, Young BR. Radiosensitivity in ataxia-telangiectasia: a new explanation. Proc Natl Acad Sci 1980;77:7315–7317.

82. Tolmach LJ, Duncan PG, Beetham KL. The action of caffeine on x-irradiated HeLa cells. IX: Hypothermic effects. Radiat Res 1990;122:280–287.

83. Fraval HNA, Roberts JJ. Effects of *cis*-platinum(II) diamine dichloride on survival and the rate of DNA synthesis in synchronously growing Chinese hamster V79-379A cells in the absence and presence of caffeine inhibited post replication repair: evidence for an inducible repair mechanism. Chem Biol Interact 1978;23:99.

84. Fraval HNA, Roberts JJ. Effects of *cis*-platinum(II) diamine dichloride on survival and the rate of DNA synthesis in synchronously growing HeLa cells in the absence and presence of caffeine. Chem Biol Interact 1978;23:111.

85. Evenson DP, Baer RK, Jost LK, Gesch RW. Toxicity of thiotepa on mouse spermatogenesis as determined by dual-parameter flow cytometry. Toxicol Appl Pharmacol 1986;82:151.

86. Lau CC, Pardee AB. Mechanism by which caffeine potentiates lethality of nitrogen mustard. Proc Natl Acad Sci 1982;79:2942–2946.

87. Hansson K, Kihlman BA, Tanzarella C, Palitti F. Influence of caffeine and 3-aminobenzamide in G_2 on the frequency of chromosomal aberrations induced by thiotepa, mitomycin C, and N-methyl-N-nitro-N'-nitrosoguanidine in human lymphocytes. Mutat Res 1984;126:251.

88. Kihlman BA, Anderson HC. Synergistic enhancement of the frequency of chromatid aberrations in cultured human lymphocytes by combinations of inhibitors of DNA repair. Mutat Res 1985;150:313.

89. Fingert HJ, Chang JD, Pardee AB. Cytotoxic, cell cycle, and chromosomal effects of methylxanthines in human tumor cells treated with alkylating agents. Cancer Res 1986;46:2463–2467.

90. Fingert HJ, Pu AT, Chen Z, Googe PB, Alley MC, Pardee AB. In vivo and in vitro enhanced antitumor effects by pentoxifylline in human cancer cells treated with thiotepa. Cancer Res 1988;48:4375–4381.

91. Dion MD, Hussey DH, Osborne JW. The effect of pentoxifylline on early and late radiation injury following fractionated irradiation in C3H mice. Int J Radiat Oncol Biol Phys 1989;17:101–107.

92. Rose WC, Trader MW, Dykes DJ, Laster WR Jr, Schabel FM Jr. Therapeutic potentiation of nitrosoureas using chlorpromazine and caffeine in the treatment of murine tumors. Cancer Treat Rep 1978;62:2085–2093.

93. Kyriazis AP, Kyriazis AA, Yagoda A. Enhanced therapeutic effect of *cis*-diamminedichloroplatinum(II) against nude mouse grown human pancreatic adenocarcinoma when combined with U-B-D-arabinofuranosylcytosine and caffeine. Cancer Res 1985;45:6083–6087.

94. Allen TE, Aliano NA, Cowan RJ, et al. Amplification of the antitumor activity of phleomycins and bleomycins in rats and mice by caffeine. Cancer Res 1985;45:2516–2521.

95. Osieka R, Glatte P, Pannenbacker R, Schmidt CG. Enhancement of semustine-induced cytotoxicity by chlorpromazine and caffeine in a human melanoma xenograft. Cancer Treat Rep 1986;70:1167–1171.

96. Schror RH. Antithrombotic potential of pentoxifylline—a hemorheologically active drug. Angiology 1985;36:387–398.

97. Bessler H, Gilgal R, Diadetti M, Zahavi I. Effect of pentoxifylline on the phagocytic activity, cAMP levels and superoxide anion production by monocytes and polymorphonuclear cells. J Leukocyte Biol 1986;40;747–754.

98. Strieter RM, Remick DG, Ward PA, Spengler RN, Lynch JP III, Kunkel SL. Cellular and molecular regulation of tumor necrosis factor-alpha production by pentoxifylline. Biochem Biophys Res Comm 1988;155:1230–1236.

99. Dezube BJ, Fridovich-Keil JL, Bouvard I, Lange RF, Pardee AB. Pentoxifylline and well-being in patients with cancer. Lancet 1990;335–662.

100. Knudsen PJ, Dinarello CA, Strom TB. Prostaglandins posttranscriptionally inhibit monocyte expression of interleukin 1 activity by increasing intracellular cyclic adenosine monophosphate. J Immunol 1986;137:3189–3194.

101. Teicher BA, Holden SA, Herman TS, Epelbaum R, Pardee AB, Dezube B. Effect of pentoxifylline as a modulator of alkylating agent activity *in vitro* and *in vivo*. Cancer Lett 1992, in press.

102. Dezube BJ, Eder JP, Pardee AB. Phase I trial of escalating pentoxifylline dose with constant dose thiotepa. Cancer Res 1990;50:6806–6810.

103. Meister A. Metabolism and transport of glutathione and other γ-glutamyl compounds. In: Larson A, Orrenius S, Holmgren A et al., eds. Functions of glutathione: biochemical, physiological, toxicological, and clinical aspects. New York: Raven Press, 1983:1–21.

104. Griffith OW. Glutathione and cell survival. In: Sebashi S, ed. Cellular regulation and malignant growth. Tokyo: Japanese Scientific Society Press, Springer-Verlag, 1985:292–300.

105. Griffith OW, Meister A. Potent and specific inhibition of glutathione synthesis by buthionine sulfoximine (S-n-butyl homocysteine sulfoximine). J Biol Chem 1979;254–7558;–7560.

106. Griffith OW. Mechanism of action, metabolism and toxicity of buthionine sulfoxinime and its higher homologs, potent inhibitors of glutathione synthesis. J Biol Chem 1982;257:13704–13712.

107. Somfai-Relle S, Suzukake K, Vistica BP, et al. Reduction in cellular glutathione by buthionine sulfoximine and sensitization of murine tumor cells resistant to L-phenylalanine mustard. Biochem Pharmacol 1984:33:485–490.

108. Calcutt G, Connors TA. Tumor sulfhydryl levels and sensitivity to the nitrogen mustard melphalan. Biochem Pharmacol 1963;12:839–845.

109. Green JA, Vistica DT, Young RC, et al. Potentiation of melphalan cytotoxicity in human ovarian cancer cell lines by glutathione depletion. Cancer Res 1984;44:5427–5431.

110. Kramer RA, Greene K, Ahmad S, et al. Chemosensitization of L-phenylalanine mustard by the thiol-modulating agent buthionine sulfoximine. Cancer Res 1987;47:1593–1597.

111. Ozols RF, Louis KG, Plowman J, et al. Enhanced melphalan cytotoxicity in human ovarian cancer in vitro and in tumor-bearing nude mice by buthionine sulfoximine depletion of glutathione. Biochem Pharmacol 1987;36:148–153.

112. Hamilton TC, Winker MA, Louie KG, et al. Augmentation of Adriamycin, melphalan, and cisplatin cytotoxicity in drug-resistant and -sensitive human ovarian carcinoma cell lines by buthionine sulfoximine mediated glutathione depletion. Biochem Pharmacol 1985;34:2583–2586.

113. Russo A, Tochner L, Phillips T, et al. In vivo modulation of glutathione by buthionine sulfoximine: effect on marrow response to melphalan. Int J Radiat Oncol Biol Phys 1986;12:1187–1189.

114. Lee FYF, Allalunis-Turner MJ, Siemann DW. Depletion of tumour versus normal tissue glutathione by buthionine sulfoximine. Br J Cancer 1987;50:33–38.

115. Kramer RA, Schuller HM, Smith AC, et al. Effects of buthionine sulfoximine on the nephrotoxicity of 1-(2-chloroethyl)-3-(trans-4-methylcyclohexyl)-1-nitrosourea (MeCCNU). J Pharmacol Exp Ther 1985;234:498–506.

116. Russo A, DeGraft W, Friedman N, et al. Selective modulation of glutathione levels in human normal versus tumor cells and subsequent differential response to chemotherapy drugs. Cancer Res 1986; 46:2845–2848.

117. Teicher BA, Crawford JM, Holden SA, et al. Glutathione monoethyl ester can selectively protect liver from high dose BCNU or cyclophosphamide. Cancer 1988;62:1275–1281.

118. Dethmers JK, Meister A. Glutathione export by human lymphoid cells: depletion of glutathione by inhibition of its synthesis decreases export and increases sensitivity to irradiation. Proc Natl Acad Sci USA 1981;78:7492–7496.

119. Skapek SX, Colvin OM, Griffith OW, et al. Buthionine sulfoximine-mediated depletion of glutathione in intracranical human glioma-derived xenografts. Biochem Pharmacol 1988;37(22):4313–4317.

120. Skapek SX, Colvin OM, Griffith OW, et al. Enhanced melphalan cytotoxicity following buthionine sulfoximine-mediated glutathione depletion in a human medulloblastoma xenograft in athymic mice. Cancer Res 1988;48(10):2764–2767.

121. Friedman HS, Colvin OM, Griffith OW, et al. Increased melphalan activity in intracranial human medulloblastoma and glioma xenografts following buthionine sulfoximine-mediated glutathione depletion. J Natl Cancer Inst 1989;81:524–527.

122. Groothiuis DR, Blasberg RG. Rational brain tumor chemotherapy: the interaction of drug and tumor. Neurol Clin 1985;3:810–816.

123. Warnke PC, Friedman HS, Bigner DD, Groothuis DR.

Simultaneous measurements of blood flow and blood-to-tissue transport in xenotransplanted medulloblastomas. Cancer Res 1987;47:1687–1690.

124. Soble MJ, Dorr RT. Lack of enhanced myelotoxicity with buthionine sulfoximine and sulfhydryl-dependent anticancer agents in mice. Res Commun Chem Pathol Pharmacol 1987;55:161–180.

125. Friedman, HS, Colvin OM, Aisaka K, et al. Glutathione protects cardiac and skeletal muscle from cyclophosphamide-induced toxicity. Cancer Res 1990; 50:2455–2462.

126. Hasegawa T, Rhee JG, Levitt SH, et al. Increase in tumor PO₂ by perfluorochemicals and carbogen. Int J Radiat Oncol Biol Phys 1987;13:569–574.

127. Rockwell S. Use of perfluorochemical emulsion to improve oxygenation in a solid tumor. Int J Radiat Oncol Biol Phys 1985;11:97–103.

128. Song CW. Increase in pO_2 and radiosensitivity of tumors by Fluosol-DA (20%) and carbogen. Cancer Res 1987;47:442–446.

129. Teicher BA, Rose CM. Perfluorochemical emulsion can increase tumor radiosensitivity. Science 1984; 223:934–936.

130. Teicher BA, Rose CM. Sensitization of solid mouse tumor to x-ray treatment by oxygen-carrying perfluorochemical emulsion. Cancer Res 1984;44:4285–4288.

131. Teicher BA, Rose CM. Effect of dose and scheduling on growth delay of the Lewis lung carcinoma produced by the perfluorochemical emulsion Fluosol-DA. Int J Radiat Oncol Biol Phys 1986;12:1311–1313.

132. Zhang WL, Pence D, Patten M, et al. Enhancement of tumor response to radiation by Fluosol-DA. Int J Radiat Oncol Biol Phys 1984,10.172 175.

133. Lustig R, McIntosh-Lowe NL, Rose C, et al. Phase I–II study of Fluosol-DA and 100% oxygen breathing as an adjuvant to radiation in the treatment of advanced squamous cell tumors of the head and neck. Int J Radiat Oncol Biol Phys 1989;16:1587–1593.

134. Rose C, Lustig R, McIntosh N, Teicher B. A clinical trial of Fluosol-DA in advanced squamous cell carcinoma of the head and neck. Int J Radiat Oncol Biol Phys 1986;12:1325–1327.

135. Teicher B, Lazo JS, Sartorelli AC. Classification of antineoplastic agents by their selective toxicities toward oxygenated and hypoxic tumor cells. Cancer Res 1981;41:73–81.

136. Teicher BA, Holden SA, Al-Achi A, Herman TS. Classification of antineoplastic treatments by their differential toxicity toward putative oxygenated and hypoxic tumor subpopulations in vivo in the FSaIIC murine fibrosarcoma. Cancer Res 1990;50:3339–3344.

137. Teicher BA, McIntosh-Lowe NL, Rose CM. Effect of various oxygenation conditions and Fluosol-DA on cancer chemotherapeutic agents. Biomater Artif Cells Artif Organs 1988;16:533–546.

138. Teicher BA, Holden SA. A survey of the effect of adding Fluosol-DA 20/O₂ to treatment with various chemotherapeutic agents. Cancer Treat Rep 1987; 71:173–177.

139. Teicher BA, Herman TS, Holden SA, Cathcart KNS. The effect of Fluosol-DA and oxygenation status on the activity of cyclophosphamide in vivo. Cancer Chemother Pharmacol 1988;21:286–291.

140. Teicher BA, Waxman DJ, Holden SA, et al. Evidence for enzymatic activation and oxygen involvement in cytotoxicity and antitumor activity of N,N′N″-triethylenethiophosphoramide. Cancer Res 1989;49: 4996–5001.

141. Teicher BA, Holden SA, Rose CM. Effect of Fluosol-DA/O₂ on tumor cell and bone marrow cytotoxicity of nitrosoureas in mice bearing FSaII fibrosarcoma. Int J Cancer 1986;38:285-288.

142. Teicher BA, Herman TS, Rose CM. Effect of Fluosol-DA on the response of intracranial 9L tumors to x-rays and BCNU. Int J Radiat Oncol Biol Phys 1988;15:1187–1192.

143. Teicher BA, Holden SA, Rose CM. Differential enhancement of melphalan cytotoxicity in tumor and normal tissue by Fluosol-DA and oxygen breathing. Int J Cancer 1985;36:585–589.

144. Teicher BA, Holden SA, Jacobs JL. Approaches to defining the mechanism of Fluosol-DA 20%/carbogen enhancement of melphalan antitumor activity. Cancer Res 1987;47:513–518.

145. Teicher BA, Crawford JM, Holden SA, Cathcart KNS. Effects of various oxygenation conditions on the enhancement by Fluosol-DA of melphalan antitumor activity. Cancer Res 1987;47:5036–5041.

146. Teicher BA, Herman TS, Tanaka J, et al. Modulation of alkylating agents by etanidazole and Fluosol-DA/carbogen in the FSaIIC fibrosarcoma and EMTG mammary carcinoma. Cancer Res 1991;51:1086–1091.

147. Teicher BA, Herman TS, Tanaka J, Dezube B, Pardee A, Frei E III. Fluosol-DA/carbogen with lonidamine or pentoxifylline as modulators of alkylating agents in the FSaIIC fibrosarcoma. Cancer Chemother Pharmacol 1991;28:45–50.

148. Catten M, Bresnahan D, Thompson S, Chalkly R. Novobiocin precipitates histones at concentrations normally used to inhibit eukaryotic type II topoisomerase. Nucleic Acid Res 1986;14:3671.

149. Wang JC. Recent studies of DNA topoisomerases. Biochem Biophys Acta 1987;909:1.

150. Holm CT, Gato T, Wang JC, Botstein D. DNA topoisomerase II is required at the time of mitosis in yeast. Cell 1985;41:553.

151. Prem veer Reddy G, Pardee A. Inhibitor evidence for allosteric interaction in the replicase complex. Nature 1983;304:86.

152. Ryaji M, Worcel A. Chromatin assembly in Xenopus oocytes: in vivo studies. Cell 1984;37:21.

153. Mattern MR, Scudiero DA. Characterization of the

inhibition of replicative and repair type DNA synthesis by novobiocin and nalidixic acid. Biochem Biophys Acta 1981;653:248.

154. Ross WE. DNA topoisomerases as targets for cancer therapy. Biochem Pharmacol 1985;34:4191.

155. Glisson B, Gupta R, Hodges P, Ross W. Cross resistance to intercalating agents in an epipodophyllo-toxic-resistant Chinese hamster ovary cell line: evidence for a common intracellular target. Cancer Res 1986;46:1939.

156. Tanaka J, Teicher BA, Herman TS, Holden SA, Dezube B, Frei E III. Etoposide with lonidamine or pentoxifylline as modulators of alkylating agent activity in vivo. Int J Cancer 1991;48:631–637.

3

PHARMACOKINETICS

Roy B. Jones and Steven Matthes

METHODS AND RATIONALE FOR PHARMACOKINETIC STUDIES

Pharmacokinetics can be defined as the study of the behavior of drugs in the blood, its components, other accessible body fluids, or tissues. Practically speaking, such studies usually involve repetitive sampling of blood and measurement of the changes in serum or plasma drug concentration over time. Such measurements can be used to construct a curve describing these changes. A typical curve describing the changes in plasma drug concentration following rapid intravenous injection is shown in Figure 3.1. Using mathematical modeling techniques such as nonlinear least squares regression analysis, a best-fit smooth curve can be matched to the data. Once the curve is generated, derived pharmacokinetic parameters such as maximal drug concentration (Cmax), elimination half-life ($t_{1/2}$elim), area under the curve (AUC), and clearance (Cl) can be derived. Readers are assumed to be familiar with these terms; further definitions as well as information on methods of curve fitting may be obtained from standard reference sources (1, 2).

While these analyses and values have important and intrinsic value for basic pharmacology research, their major value for clinicians lies in their application to rational drug dosing in patients. Examples of such use are described below.

Initial Design of Dosing Schemes

Antineoplastic agents with a short $t_{1/2}$elim are often rationally dosed using multiple divided doses or as a prolonged infusion. Drugs with a long $t_{1/2}$elim can usually be given as a single dose without major loss of therapeutic benefit.

Antineoplastic agents with known renal clearance significantly higher than the creatinine clearance are likely to undergo renal elimination by both filtration and secretion. Coadministration of other agents known to affect or utilize renal secretory pathways may alter the antineoplastic agent pharmacokinetics, with unpredictable effects on toxicity and therapeutic effect.

It is important to note at the outset that systematic pharmacokinetic measurements on populations treated with high-dose chemotherapy have not been frequently performed. Thus the thrust of this chapter will be not only to describe the available data in this area but also to discuss the rationale, design, assay development, analysis, and practical use of these studies and data.

Attempts to measure the nature of drug handling in individual patients for the purpose of providing uniform drug exposure are called *therapeutic drug monitoring*. Many are familiar with this concept when employed as "peak and trough" drug measurements. The peak measurement is designed to describe the Cmax, the trough is designed to describe

43

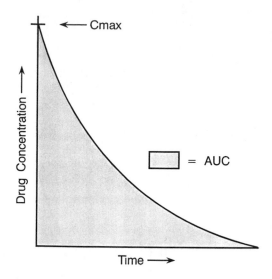

Figure 3.1. Typical mathematical model of drug disappearance from plasma following a bolus intravenous injection.

the elimination phase. Together, these measures can be used to estimate the AUC, or integral of drug exposure at the cell surface over time.

INTERPATIENT VARIABILITY OF DRUG HANDLING

Pharmacokinetic parameters have important utility for detecting differences in drug handling between patients. This is because these parameters describe the concentration-time aggregate of drug exposure at the cell surface. While differences in drug handling inside the cell clearly exist, the processes of drug absorption, distribution, and elimination are usually normally distributed continuous variables within common patient populations. For many classes of drugs, it has clearly been established that differences in the AUC, Cmax, or both are proportional to toxic or therapeutic effects (3, 4). The study of these phenomena is termed *pharmacodynamics.*

Such clear-cut proportionality between pharmacokinetic parameters and biologic effects has been reported less frequently for antineoplastic agents than for several other

classes of drugs. There are several reasons for this lack of data. Most other classes of drugs are administered as frequent intravenous or oral doses, and thus measurement is easier to accomplish. Frequent monitoring allows cruder estimates of pharmacokinetic parameters with each individual dose, because serial refinement of the estimates is possible as subsequent doses are given. Because antineoplastic drugs are given less frequently, more precise estimates of pharmacokinetic parameters (i.e., more frequent blood sampling) of each dose is required.

Ironically, the frequency and relative simplicity of measurement of adverse effects has also retarded the development of antineoplastic therapeutic drug monitoring. "See how sick the patient becomes and adjust the dose accordingly" is standard practice for conventional dose treatment. Implicit in this treatment guideline is that avoidance of toxicity, as opposed to therapeutic benefit, is the driving force for dosing. In the setting of high-dose chemotherapy with bone marrow support, the driving force is to maximize therapeutic benefit by maximizing dose. Unfortunately, the cost of excessive dosing in this setting can be fatal organ injury. Thus the more intensive the treatment regimen becomes, the more therapeutic drug monitoring may benefit the patient.

Despite the difficulties inherent in antineoplastic drug pharmacology, some reports of pharmacokinetic-pharmacodynamic relationships have appeared. A summary of some of these reports is shown in Table 3.1.

IDENTIFICATION OF THE TOXIC OR THERAPEUTIC SPECIES— WHAT SHOULD BE MEASURED?

Commonly, the "parent" drug that is administered is a prodrug that must be converted to other species to produce its effects. In fact, many drugs undergo complex metabolism producing multiple metabolites, each having different balances of toxic and therapeutic effects. How can one hope to perform

Table 3.1. Antineoplastic Pharmacodynamic Analysis: Selected Precedents[a]

Biologic Effect	Drug	Investigator
Leukopenia	Menogaril	Egorin et al. 1986 (74)
RR, colon cancer	5-FU	Hillcoat et al. 1978 (75)
Nephrotoxicity	cDDP	Campbell 1983 (76)
Thrombocytopenia	CBDCA	Egorin et al. 1985 (77)
Cardiotoxicity	Adriamycin	Legha et al. 1982 (78)
Neurotoxicity	Vincristine	Desai et al. 1982 (79)
RR, AML	Ara-C	Baguley, Faulkenberg, 1974 (69)
RR, AML	Adriamycin	Priesler et al. 1984 (80)
DFI, ALL	MTX	Evans et al. 1984 (81)

[a]Abbreviations: RR, relapse rate; DFI, disease-free interval; 5-FU, 5-fluorouracil; cDDP, cisplatin; CBDCA, carboplatin; Ara-C, (cytosine arabinoside); MTX, methotrexate.

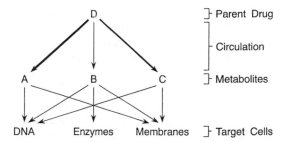

Figure 3.2. Schematic representation of one cancer drug (D) which, following administration, results in several circulating metabolites (A, B, C) in various proportions (represented by the thickness of the *arrows*). Each metabolite may have several cellular and subcellular targets.

effective therapeutic drug monitoring in this circumstance?

If this issue is viewed as a statistical problem, it is possible that over a population a rough proportionality exists between the aggregate of toxic and therapeutic effects of the sum of the metabolites and the amount of prodrug measured in the plasma. While such formulations are not particularly pleasing to the analytical pharmacologist or pharmacokineticist, the necessity for such an approach becomes more clear when it is recognized that pharmacokinetic-pharmacodynamic relationships of necessity reflect the effect of these metabolites on a variety of cellular targets. Unfortunately, a large majority of antineoplastic agents form reactive or tight-binding intermediates capable of affecting a multiplicity of cellular targets (Fig. 3.2). For example, methotrexate (MTX) is frequently believed to produce its effects solely by tight-binding to dihydrofolate reductase. In fact, MTX exerts additional important effects by interacting with membrane-associated folate uptake pathways (5), affecting regulation of purine biosynthetic enzymes (6), altering the dynamics of the folate polyglutamylation system (7), and affecting S-adenosyl methionine synthesis and regulation (8). Additionally, it has been shown that MTX is metabolized, and the metabolites have important therapeutic and toxic activity (9).

Despite this complexity, therapeutic drug monitoring of MTX has been useful in reducing high-dose MTX toxicity and directing folinic acid rescue techniques (10).

The utility of drug monitoring for a given drug species can only be estimated by the usual (incomplete) understanding of the drug's known metabolism and intracellular targets. Obviously, the more pharmacokinetic monitoring can be predicted to account for major toxic and therapeutic species, the more likely it will be valuable in pharmacodynamic analyses. The final and only acceptable definition of the utility of monitoring, however, comes from the performance of systematic pharmacokinetic measurements in a patient population and the use of statistical techniques, such as multivariate regression analysis (11), to evaluate the relationship of pharmacokinetics to a biologic outcome.

PRACTICAL ISSUES

How should one evaluate already existing pharmacokinetic studies and their usefulness? The basic goal of such evaluation should be to decide, within practical limitations, whether or not the proposed methods have taken into account predictable factors that might affect the outcome of later pharmacokinetic-pharmacodynamic analyses.

1. *What is the relevance of the assay target to knowledge of the drug's metabolism and known active species?* Is there reason to believe that the drug species to be measured is the toxic or therapeutic effector species, or that the assay target will be present in an amount proportional to known active species? Since the majority of agents used with intensive therapy function through reactive (therefore unstable) intermediates, surrogate measures such as measuring the parent compound of the reactive species are often required.
2. Is the assay scientifically sound? Does the proposed assay methodology measure the free (unbound) drug fraction, or another fraction proportional to it?
3. Are sufficient computing resources and pharmacokinetic expertise available to allow accurate design of blood sampling, determination of pharmacokinetic parameters, and database storage of pharmacokinetic parameters in a form that will allow statistical comparison to toxicity and therapeutic outcome?

ANTINEOPLASTIC DRUG MONITORING LABORATORY— DESIGN AND FUNCTION

Once the above issues have been evaluated, practical aspects of drug assay methodology and design must be addressed. While a detailed exposition of these issues is beyond the scope of this chapter, a condensed overview is presented here. Clinicians who contemplate establishment of such a laboratory or review results produced by one should have some understanding of the procedures required to generate pharmacokinetic data. Only through this understanding can feasi-

bility be assessed or frailties of results be understood.

An ultimate goal of a cancer drug monitoring laboratory is to direct the administration of the antineoplastic agents on a daily basis to achieve predictable and uniform plasma drug levels from patient to patient. It is important that the drug or metabolites (analytes) chosen for quantitation be biologically relevant (active) species or be directly and predictably related to active species. This choice must be made prior to the methods development stage to maximize the odds of accruing data that can be effectively utilized for pharmacodynamic analyses.

Once the relevant analyte has been determined, a clinical assay must be developed. A clinical assay imposes different and more extensive design requirements than those required by a valid research assay. Research assays are often used to analyze many samples saved over long periods and ultimately run in a "batch" mode. Since the assay is run at only a few points in time, interrun precision (the variability of the assay result when analyzing a specimen of standard composition at several different times) is a secondary objective of assay design. A clinical assay must place priority upon reliability, reproducibility, and delivery of results in a timely fashion to the clinician. The method must be reproducible on a day-to-day basis with acceptable and clearly defined quality control procedures for all phases of the analysis, from specimen accrual to end result. A clinical assay must be efficient, allowing rapid performance, minimal cost per analysis, and measurement of multiple analytes (if required) with each assay. (See Table 3.2.)

Analytical Equipment

The basic requirements for a quality, clinically useful pharmacokinetic laboratory demand analytical methodologies that are specific for the clinically significant species (including possible metabolite investigation) and sensitive enough to detect the analyte over

Table 3.2 Essential Features of a Well-Designed Clinical Assay

Low inter- and intrarun variability
Rapid analysis time
Low cost
Simultaneous measurement of multiple analytes
Backup instrumentation available
Sensitivity at relevant drug concentrations
Lack of interference by other drugs

the full range of concentrations relevant to clinical dosing. These requirements limit the value of assays dependent on radiolabeling, enzymatic pathways, or fluorescence polarization. Additionally, these latter methods require substantial development time, which is beyond the usual scope of such laboratories.

More appropriate assay methodologies for this laboratory include high-performance liquid chromatography (HPLC) with ultraviolet or fluorescence detectors and gas-liquid phase chromatography (GLPC) using a capillary column and either a flame ionization detector (FID) or, where applicable, a nitrogen-phosphorus detector (NPD) (12–14). Either chromatographic technique may also employ a mass spectrophotometric (MS) detector that will increase the sensitivity of detection and, in the case of HPLC, facilitate metabolite investigation. MS and the required interfaces markedly increase the price of the equipment, however, and the higher doses of chemotherapy administered with intensive therapy usually do not require the sensitivity of MS. If cisplatin, carboplatin, or other platinum analogues are to be used, atomic absorption spectrophotometry (AAS), used alone or after initial separation of platinum species by HPLC, is a useful analytical tool.

Selection of Assay Methodology

A search of the literature may often produce an analytical method for GLPC or HPLC for the desired drug. Often, however, this assay is a research methodology. Quality control data required for therapeutic drug monitoring may be limited or absent; the method may be too cumbersome for rapid, frequent analyses; and few or no data may exist on whether concomitantly administered drugs will interfere with the assay. Such methods provide useful starting points for further development, however.

Sample Preparation

Proper sample preparation is critical to the production of clinically valuable analyses. It is important to determine the extent of plasma protein binding of the analyte and its stability in plasma at room temperature, in ice, and frozen. If the analyte is unstable in plasma in vitro, the rapidity of decomposition must be determined and assay conditions adjusted to overcome this problem. While organic solvent extraction of blood or plasma is frequently used in sample work-up, this technique may extract drug that is tightly bound to proteins or cells and is unavailable to produce toxic or therapeutic effects in vivo. Such analysis may lose power for pharmacodynamic determinations.

If an important fraction of the analyte is protein bound, determination of the unbound drug fraction will likely be important for pharmacokinetic-pharmacodynamic analysis because only this fraction may be accessible to the intracellular space. This is most conveniently done by rapid centrifugation of plasma through a membrane that excludes any large molecular weight protein and assaying the protein-free fraction. Further work-up of plasma or protein-free plasma filtrate is usually required to eliminate contaminants that may interfere with the assay or damage the chromatographic column or detector. The most frequently used techniques involve solid phase extraction (SPE) and/or micro liquid/liquid extraction of the filtrate into an organic phase (15).

Assay Normalization and Quality Control

Once a proper sample preparation method is available, a known amount of analyte is added to pooled banked plasma or whole blood (a "standard sample") in a range of concentrations designed to encompass clinically important concentrations. These specimens are then processed by the designated method (Fig. 3.3). Following chromatography, the relationship between detector response and analyte concentration is determined by graphing the two variables on linear axes. Ideally, the relationships should be linear or, at a minimum, a predictable simple function of one another (such as exponential or logarithmic). In practice, most modern chromatographs are equipped with integrators that express the area under the curve of each detector peak. An internal standard compound is added to the patient sample or standard sample prior to any other manipulation in the laboratory. It should be a compound that extracts and chromatographs similarly to the analyte. In practice, this is usually accomplished by identifying a structurally similar chemical compound (for example, doxorubicin and daunorubicin). Expressing the detector response of analyte and internal standard as a ratio thus "corrects" for incompleteness or variability of recovery of analyte during the sample-processing phase (16).

A peak area-detector response ratio of the standard analyte to an internal standard is, in fact, more commonly compared to the known analyte concentration. Repeated measures of the linearity and coefficient of variation of this "standard curve" and its component samples can serve as quality control measures for the assay. The assay reliability is defined by the inter- and intrarun precision or coefficient of variation of standard sample analyses.

The sensitivity of the assay is determined by adding internal standards and decreasing concentrations of the analyte to pooled plasma or whole blood and then processing and analyzing the sample in a standard manner. The minimal concentration for which the detector response can be reliably quantitated defines the sensitivity limit. The specificity of the assay is determined by two methods: (a) adding any drugs to which the patient might be exposed to pooled plasma or blood and verifying that there is no detector response in the area of the analyte, or (b) analyzing patient blood or plasma immediately prior to drug administration to validate that the detector response in the area of the analyte is zero (the so-called 0 time point).

The array of standard samples is used to define a standard curve expressing the detector response ratio (patient sample:internal standard) as a function of known standard analyte concentration. When a patient sample with added internal standards is analyzed, the standard curve is used to relate the observed detector response ratio to analyte concentration in that sample. In practice, commercially available computer software packages such as Maxima (Millipore/Waters Assoc., New Milford, MA) are used to perform these analyses in an automated fashion.

Patient Sampling and Derivation of Pharmacokinetic Parameters

Selecting time points for patient blood sampling and methods of sample collection and storage is critical in achieving reliable results. Published data with half-life of elimination, clearance mechanisms, and protein binding are available for most antineoplastic agents. Relating this information to the type and length of administration is critical when selecting time points for samples since it is crucial to definitively describe the elimination curve for each drug. As a first approximation, a drug with a short half-life of elimination such as carmustine (BCNU) requires a concentration of time points during the infusion and immediately following it. Drugs with longer half-lives (e.g., mitoxantrone) require much more prolonged sampling to describe the elimination curve. As a first approximation, sampling for any drug should continue for at least three times the $t_{1/2}$elim beyond the end of the infusion to ensure reasonable analysis. The exact timing of individ-

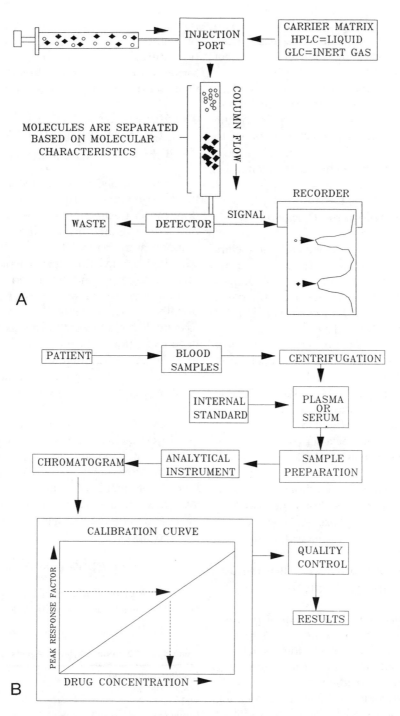

Figure 3.3. Schematic representation of a chromatograph. An idealized plasma extract containing a drug (black squares) and an internal standard (white circles) are injected through a column containing an inert stationary phase that has different affinity for each sample constituent. The drug and internal standard are separated and passed through a detector that produces an electronic signal proportional to the amount of material present.

ual samples should be discussed with investigators experienced in pharmacokinetic studies to maximize the information content obtained from them.

A major source of error for any pharmacokinetic analysis is improper timing and labeling of individual patient samples by the patient care staff. It is critically important to provide unambiguous instructions and a clear rationale for careful technique to them.

Modeling—Derivation of Pharmacokinetic Parameters

To derive pharmacokinetic parameters such as the AUC, $t_{1/2}$elim, clearance, and the like, the concentration/time specific samples must be analyzed as a data set and a smoothed curve fit to the data. This curve is employed for pharmacokinetic data derivation using standardized computer programs, several of which may be implemented on microcomputers (PC NONLIN, Statistical Consultants Inc., Lexington, KY; Minsq, MicroMath Scientific Software, Salt Lake City, UT). The shape of the curve may be defined by a best fit approximation of each data set (so-called stripping programs such as R-strip [MicroMath] may be used to refine this process) or predefined prior to the analysis. The choice and methodology of this analysis should be governed by individuals with pharmacokinetic expertise and is reviewed in standard texts (1).

Computerization and Automated Sample Analysis

It is imperative that a clinical pharmacokinetic laboratory for cancer treatment be automated with computer interfacing between autosampling analytical instruments, quality control instrumentation, and a dedicated pharmacokinetic analysis computing resource to accomplish the tasks described here. The laboratory will often be required to analyze 50–75 specimens overnight with acceptable quality control and provide pharmacokinetic parameter estimates to the cli-

nician early the next morning. Development of such power, however, offers extensive opportunities to utilize therapeutic drug monitoring to provide uniform drug dosing to patients receiving intensive anticancer therapies.

PHARMACOKINETICS OF AGENTS COMMONLY EMPLOYED IN HIGH-DOSE CANCER THERAPY

Historically, alkylating agents have been the most common drugs employed in high-dose cancer treatment regimens. This is in part due to the pioneering preclinical studies of Skipper and Shabel (17–19), who demonstrated that alkylating agents typically demonstrate a steep and linear dose:antitumor relationship over a wide dose range. Additionally, alkylating agents have predominant toxicity for marrow, allowing considerable dose escalation before extramedullary toxicity becomes dose limiting.

A list of the common alkylating agents used in high-dose therapy is shown in Table 3.3.

Other agents that have frequently been employed in high-dose therapy include etoposide, mitoxantrone, and cytosine arabinoside. In subsequent sections the pharmacokinetics of each agent will be discussed and available pharmacokinetic-pharmacodynamic data and potential organ toxicities commented upon.

Cyclophosphamide

Cyclophosphamide (CPA) is the most common agent used for high-dose therapy,

Table 3.3.   Common Alkylating Agents

Cyclophosphamide
Ifosfamide
Melphalan
Busulfan
Carmustine (BCNU)
Cisplatin
Carboplatin
Thiotepa

and its pharmacokinetic behavior and metabolism has been extensively studied. Important metabolic pathways are shown in Figure 3.4.

CPA is a prodrug that is hydroxylated by hepatic microsomal enzymes (20) or cooxidized via pathways involving prostaglandin synthase (21) to produce 4-hydroxycyclophosphamide (4-OHCPA). It is generally believed that the components of the aldophosphamide-4-OHCPA tautomeric equilibrium are responsible for transport of cytotoxic metabolites into cells (22). Phosphoramide mustard, primarily formed intracellularly, is the predominant antitumor metabolite (23). Acrolein, excreted in the urine, is the major cause of hemorrhagic cystitis (24) and also may play a role in organ toxicity produced by high doses of CPA, such as hemorrhagic myocarditis (25), hepatic venoocclusive disease (26), or pulmonary injury (27). Little intact CPA is excreted in the urine.

Measurement of both components of the aldophosphamide:4-OHCPA equilibrium process would be required to directly quantitate the delivery of cytotoxic species to cells. While this has been done in cell-free fluids, technical difficulties have to date prevented rapid, accurate measurement in patient blood or plasma (28). Fortunately, Sladek has shown that changes in plasma CPA dose are roughly proportional to changes in the reactive intermediate AUC in experimental systems, using an assay not suitable for routine clinical monitoring (29). Measurement of CPA may thus be a possible surrogate measure of reactive intermediate delivery to cells.

CPA is usually delivered in a divided total dose of 5–8 gm/m^2 over 2–4 days. The divided dose pattern arose from observations that single large doses of CPA produced important cardiotoxicity that was reduced when the dose was divided over several days (30, 31). Pharmacokinetic data from a cohort of 68 patients treated with 1875 mg/m^2 CPA daily for 3 days are shown in Table 3.4.

Of interest, the AUC declines and clearance increases over the 3 days, consistent with

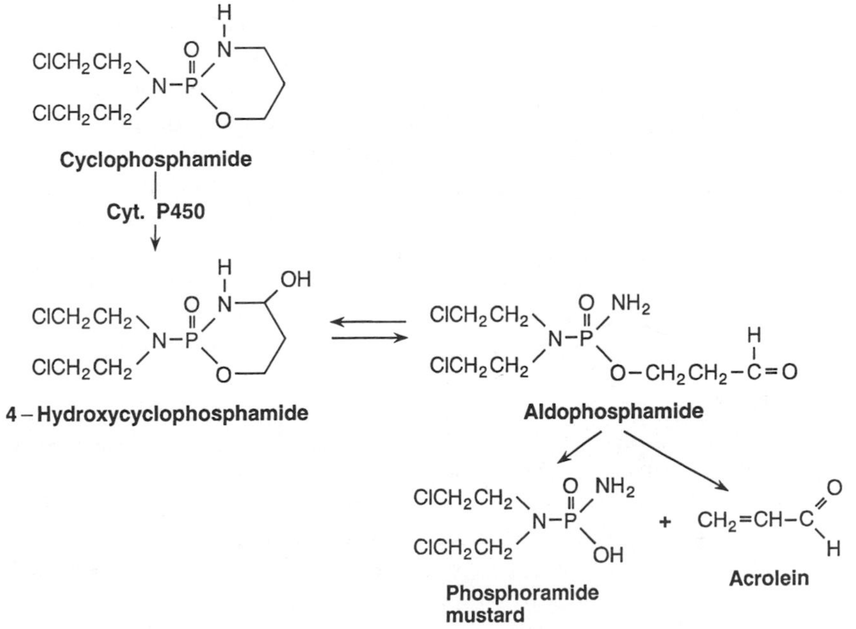

Figure 3.4. Abbreviated metabolic pathways for cyclophosphamide.

Table 3.4. Typical High-Dose Cyclophosphamide Pharmacokinetic Parameters

Parameter (units)	Mean	Std. Dev.
Day 1		
AUC, μg-min/ml	67000	74600
Cmax, μg/ml	141	82.2
T1/2elim, minutes	350	426
Vol. dist., liter/m^2	11.0	6.28
Cl(TB), ml/min/m^2	46.9	32.6
Day 2		
AUC	48100	83500
Cmax	142	95.6
$T_{1/2}$elim	224	215
Vol. dist.	16.4	14.2
Cl(TB)	82.1	72.6
Day 3		
AUC	34600	21400
Cmax	136	136
$T_{1/2}$elim	192	52.3
Vol. dist.	16.2	15.5
Cl(TB)	89.6	82.1

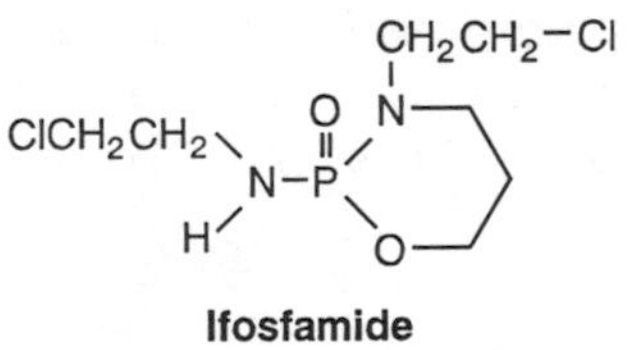

Ifosfamide

Figure 3.5. Structure of ifosfamide.

other reports (32). It has been hypothesized that CPA induces its own metabolism, even though the time course is relatively short for such phenomena. Considerable interpatient variation in the AUC is seen, consistent with the possibility that such variability could produce differences in pharmacodynamic outcome.

Ifosfamide

Ifosfamide (IPA), a structural isomer of CPA, is shown in Figure 3.5. It is also a prodrug, activated by 4-hydroxylation. The rate of ring hydroxylation is slower than for CPA, resulting in lower peak levels of 4-hydroxyifosfamide (4-OHIPA) and more prolonged production and excretion of mustard and ac-

rolein metabolites. For high-dose therapy, the drug is often given by continuous infusion in doses of 8–18 gm/m^2 over 4 days (33). The usual IPA $t_{1/2}$elim of 6–8 hours is prolonged to approximately 15 hours if more than 3.8 gm/m^2 is given as a single daily dose, and at this dose more than 50% of the drug is excreted intact in the urine. Since intact urinary excretion of drug implies lack of microsomal hydroxylation (drug activation), dose rates of >2.0 gm/m^2/8 h should probably be avoided in high-dose regimens. At these doses, no population data are currently available with respect to changes in clearance rate with time or interpatient AUC variability. Additionally, no data analyzing the proportionality of changes in 4-hydroxy IPA relative to changes in IPA AUC have been reported.

In spite of the relatively limited use of IPA in high-dose therapy, it is clear that bladder, mucosal, renal, and CNS toxicity can all be dose limiting (33).

IPA is usually given in conjunction with sodium mercaptoethane sulfonate (mesna), a sulfhydryl compound that chemically combines with acrolein to reduce the incidence of hemorrhagic cystitis. Mesna ($t_{1/2}$elim = 30 minutes) is usually given in a 60%–100% mg equivalent dose to IPA and rapidly dimerizes in the plasma to form dimesna ($t_{1/2}$elim = 70 minutes). Because of the short $t_{1/2}$elim of mesna and dimesna relative to IPA and its metabolites, the dose must be divided or administered by continuous infusion, with the last of the mesna given at least one IPA $t_{1/2}$elim after the last of the IPA is given.

Melphalan

Melphalan (L-PAM) is only available for noninvestigational use in the United States as an oral formulation, which is poorly suited for high-dose therapy. An intravenous formulation is available, however, and is used extensively in other countries. L-PAM alkylates target tissues after spontaneous formation of a mustard-type reactive intermediate in vivo and is hydrolyzed to a dihydroxy product as the major route of elimination (Fig. 3.6). Less than 15% of intact drug is renally excreted, but severe renal failure delays excretion of intravenously administered drug, with important pharmacokinetic-pharmacodynamic (34, 35). The plasma $t_{1/2}$elim is reportedly between 40 minutes and 2 hours (36, 37).

L-PAM is usually administered as a single rapid intravenous infusion in doses of 80–140 mg/m^2. Tranchand et al. have demonstrated that a small intravenous test dose of drug can be used to predict pharmacokinetic parameters for a larger therapeutic dose. This is particularly important in view of the three- to fourfold variability in the AUC that has been seen in such patients when identical doses of drug are given (36). Such test dosing represents an important mechanism to provide uniform pharmacokinetic dosing of drug when a single therapeutic dose is contemplated.

Gastrointestinal toxicity is usually dose limiting.

Busulfan

Busulfan (Bu) is frequently used in high-dose therapy but also is limited by the lack of an intravenous formulation. This bifunctional methane sulfonate is capable of spontaneous alkylation in vivo, as shown in Figure 3.7. It is eliminated through extensive but incompletely characterized metabolism and tissue alkylation (38). The plasma $t_{1/2}$elim is 2.5–3.5 hours in adults (39) but is 2 hours or less in children (40, 41), correlating with a decreased risk of Bu-associated neurotoxicity seen in children given equivalent doses of drug. The increased clearance of the drug in children obviously results in decreased exposure of the CNS to drug or toxic metabolite(s), but the mechanism of this increased clearance is unknown. Presumably, the increased clearance also produces an inferior antitumor effect, but this also is not proven.

Bu was the second drug for which a clear-cut pharmacodynamic organ toxicity relationship at high dose was established, namely, risk of hepatic venoocclusive disease (VOD) with increasing drug exposure, as shown by Groshow et al. (39). They described a seven- to eightfold variability in the AUC ascribed primarily to differences in absorption. VOD is known to be the dose-limiting organ toxicity of this agent (42).

Bu is commonly administered orally to adult patients in 1 mg/kg doses every 6 hours for 16 doses.

Carmustine

Carmustine (BCNU) is a poorly soluble nitrosourea that is frequently employed in high-dose therapy. It is formulated for intravenous use as a 10% ethanol solution and is generally administered as a 2-hour infusion through a central intravenous catheter. BCNU undergoes spontaneous hydrolysis in intravenous solutions or plasma. This process is accelerated by increasing temperature or light. Six percent of the compound undergoes hydrolysis within 3 hours of reconstitution and storage at room temperature; therefore, it must be used rapidly after formulation, and pharmacokinetic samples must be processed rapidly after phlebotomy. Because of its poor

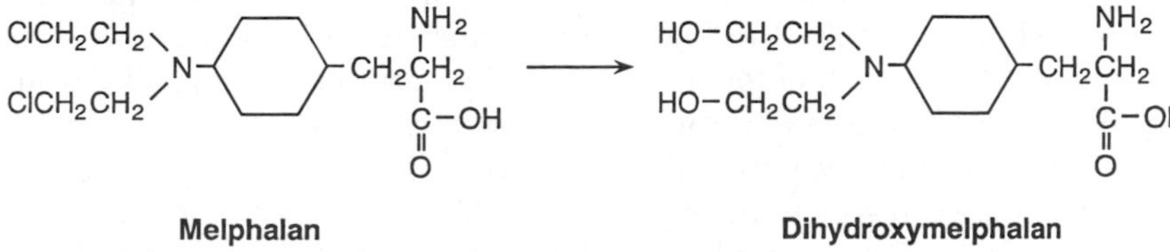

Figure 3.6 Melphalan and its hydrolysis product.

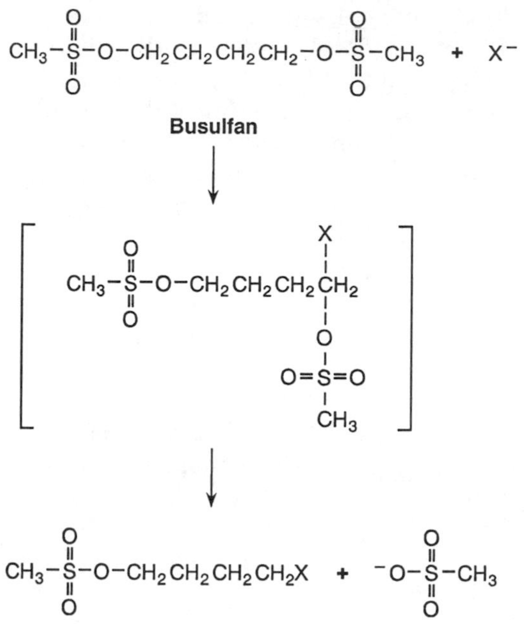

Busulfan

BCNU

$$H_2O + N_2 + \oplus CH_2CH_2Cl$$

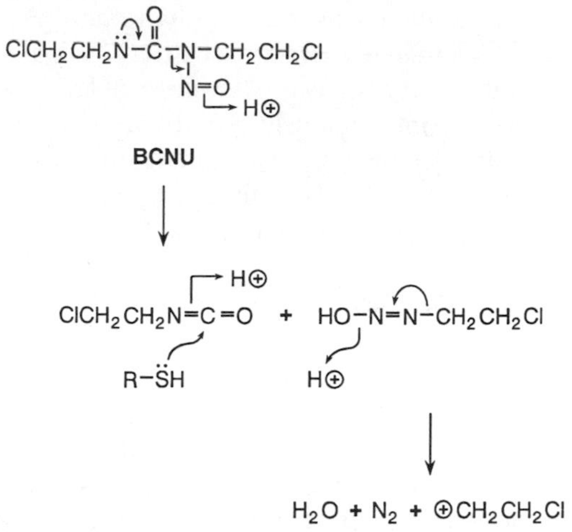

Figure 3.8 Mechanism of BCNU hydrolysis and sulfhydryl compound reaction with chlorethylisocyanate.

Figure 3.7 Mechanism of alkylation of busulfan. X represents a generic tissue nucleophile available for alkylation.

Table 3.5. Typical Pharmacokinetic Parameters Following High-Dose BCNU Administration

Measurement	Mean	Range	Std. Dev.
AUC, μg-min/ml	1620	119–10300	2072
Cmax, μg/ml	12.3	0.87–84.9	16.2
$t_{1/2}$elim, minutes	27.8	6.47–124	17.8
Cl(TB), ml/min/m²	973	58.5–503	914

solubility, 75% or more of the drug is protein bound in plasma (43).

In vivo BCNU hydrolyzes to produce chlorethylisocyanate and a chlorethyl carbonium ion or equivalent. Both have cytotoxic potential, but the ionized species is considered to be the major antitumor effector. The isocyanate carbamoylates electron-rich amino and sulfhydryl groups or can be neutralized by glutathione (Fig. 3.8). The drug has produced hepatic, pulmonary, CNS, and cardiac injuries in high-dose administration (44).

Table 3.5 shows pharmacokinetic parameters for 65 patients receiving 600 mg/m² as a 2-hour intravenous infusion. The interpatient variability of the AUC is similar to that reported for other agents used in high-dose therapy. Phase I high-dose therapy studies demonstrate that BCNU is a potent cause of VOD, and studies are underway to evaluate the association between VOD and variability in the BCNU AUC in patients undergoing high-dose therapy.

BCNU is commonly given as a 2-hour infusion in doses of 400–800 mg/m². The standard formulation produces hypotension at this dose rate of delivery. Reducing the ethanol content of the formulation may reduce this unwanted adverse effect but has not been validated by published stability data (45).

Cisplatin

Cisplatin's (cDDP's) alkylating agent properties make it attractive for use in high-dose therapy, but the ability to escalate doses is limited by its renal toxicity. The drug is activated by hydrolysis to produce a *cis*-diammine dihydroxy species capable of tissue alkylation. The hydrolysis rate is determined in part by the chloride concentration of the solubilizing media. The drug must be formulated in chloride-containing solution, and hydrolysis proceeds primarily intracellularly because of the low chloride concentration there. Some extracellular hydrolysis always occurs, however. Renal or neurologic toxicity can be exacerbated by either slow urinary flow (increased concentration × exposure time of renal tubules to extracellular hydrolyzed drug) or low urinary chloride concentration (46) (thus increasing the chloride off-rate and formation of the dihydroxy species within the tubular lumen).

cDDP is extensively protein bound, and, like all drugs, it is primarily the free-drug fraction that produces important pharmacodynamic effects (47). The $t_{1/2}$elim of the free drug is approximately 30 minutes (48), with the primary routes of elimination being renal secretion, filtration, and tissue alkylation. In high-dose therapy the drug is usually administered as 2- to 4-day continuous infusion, with total doses between 120 and 200 mg/m². At these doses, it is important to maintain urine flow above 200 mL/hr continuously during the infusion with chloride-rich intravenous fluid to avoid renal tubular toxicity.

Carboplatin

Carboplatin (CBDCA) offers an attractive alternative to cDDP for high-dose regimens because of its substantial antitumor activity overlap with cDDP. Additionally, myelosuppression is the dose-limiting toxicity at conventional doses, seemingly ideal for marrow transplant supported regimens. The chloride ligands of cDDP are replaced by a cyclobutane dicarboxylato ring structure, which renders the compound both chemically and conformationally more stable with respect to hydrolysis (displacement) of the ring structure by water (Fig. 3.9). The drug is much less protein bound than cDDP and has a plasma $t_{1/2}$elim of 2.5–4 hours (49). The drug is primarily eliminated through the kidney by filtration, with no evidence for secretion. The creatinine clearance is highly pre-

Carboplatin

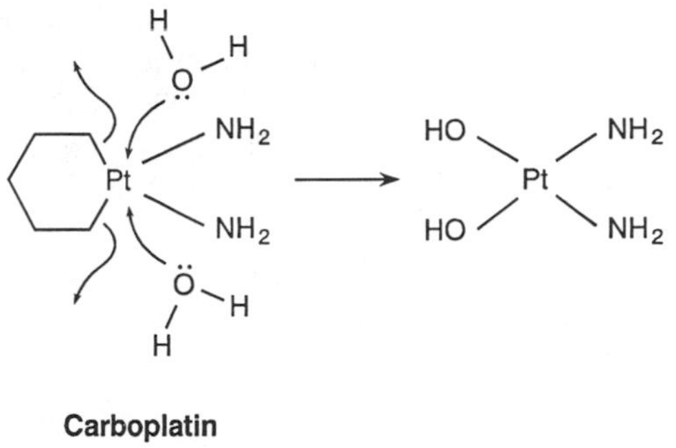

Figure 3.9 Mechanism of carboplatin hydrolysis.

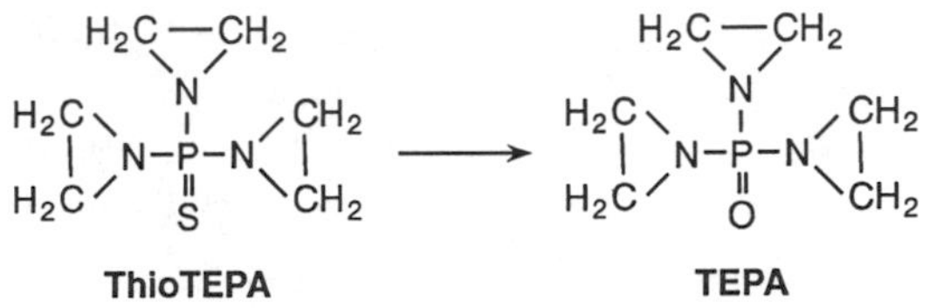

ThioTEPA   **TEPA**

Figure 3.10 Structures of thiotepa and TEPA.

dictive of drug elimination and can be used to predict the degree of thrombocytopenia produced by a given dose of this agent (50).

Difficulties have arisen when attempts have been made to add CBDCA to multiple alkylating agent regimens (51), particularly with respect to high rates of VOD in regimens already containing other agents known to cause this toxicity. It is unknown whether this is a pharmacokinetic or a pharmacodynamic effect, but care should be used when intensive CBDCA doses are added to regimens known to produce even low rates of VOD.

Thiotepa

Thiotepa (TT) was one of the earliest alkylating agents developed, producing its effects through both its alkylating properties and those of TEPA, its oxy metabolite (Fig. 3.10). While TEPA is less tumor toxic, extensive TT to TEPA conversion results in a TT/TEPA AUC ratio of 1.4 (52), indicating that TEPA may need to be accounted for in pharmacodynamic analyses. The $t_{1/2}$elim's for TT and TEPA are 1.5 hours and 10 hours, respectively. The TEPA kinetics, however, are difficult to interpret because TEPA is extensively protein bound (53) and unstable, so that unbound TEPA is usually not measured. TT freely penetrates the cerebrospinal fluid, important for both therapeutic and toxicologic considerations. Drug elimination occurs by metabolism and target tissue alkylation.

Because the conventional dose-limiting toxicity is marrow toxicity, impressive dose escalations of 10- to 50-fold over conventional doses can be achieved (54) with high-dose therapy. Gastrointestinal and CNS toxicities are then dose limiting, and the risk of VOD may be increased when this drug is used with other agents that produce hepatic toxicity. The combination of cyclophosphamide and TT is now commonly employed in the intensive treatment of solid tumors, particularly breast cancer.

Etoposide

Etoposide is the major nonalkylating agent in current use for high-dose therapy. Reasons for this use include striking activity of this drug when used in combination with platinum compounds (55) and the high degree of single-agent activity it produces with treatment of myeloid leukemia, lymphomas, and testicular cancer (56).

The $t_{1/2}$elim for etoposide is 7 hours, based upon measurement of total plasma drug concentration (57). Etoposide is extensively protein bound (>90%), however, and pharmacokinetic evaluation of the free fraction is incomplete and may be at wide variance with total drug pharmacokinetic (58). The drug is eliminated primarily by renal excretion of intact drug (30%–50%) or incompletely characterized drug metabolites (20%–30%). Unlike most alkylating agents, etoposide exhibits a marked schedule dependency in patients. A 24-hour infusion is markedly inferior to five consecutive daily infusions comprising the same total dose (59). This finding would be consistent with a short $t_{1/2}$elim for free (non-protein-bound) etoposide.

Escalation of drug dose is usually limited by mucosal toxicity and the need for prolonged infusion, because the lipid vehicle used in formulation of etoposide can cause hypotension if administered rapidly. The usual range of doses for high-dose therapy is 800–2000 mg/m^2 given in divided doses over 3–5 days.

Mitoxantrone

Mitoxantrone (DHAD) is an anthraquinone compound that is being intensively explored for use in high-dose regimens because of its predominant marrow toxicity, ability to be escalated to three to five times above conventional dose before mucosal injury becomes dose limiting, and limited cardiotoxicity compared to the structurally related anthracyclines daunorubicin and doxorubicin. While it clearly exhibits steep dose responsiveness for hematopoietic and lymphoid tumors, attempts to deliver increased doses of the single drug to patients with breast cancer produced disappointing antitumor effects and important cardiotoxicity in one trial (60).

The $t_{1/2}$elim has been reported to vary widely but seems likely to be in the range of 8 hours (61, 62). Virtually no data are available about the extent of plasma protein binding or pharmacokinetic behavior of the free fraction of the drug. One study suggests improved drug uptake by leukemia cells when DHAD is given by prolonged infusion rather than by bolus dosing (62), consistent with a short plasma half-life for the free drug fraction. The drug is eliminated from the plasma as a result of extensive tissue binding and hepatic metabolism/biliary excretion. Renal elimination of the drug is unimportant.

In high-dose therapy DHAD has been given in doses as high as 60(63) to 75(64) mg/m^2, usually in a multiple-day divided dose schedule, with mucosal and enteral injuries limiting further escalation.

Cytosine Arabinoside

Cytosine arabinoside (Ara-C) has been frequently employed in high-dose regimens, particularly for treatment of leukemias (65) and lymphomas (66). High-dose Ara-C (HI-DAC) is often limited in older patients by CNS, mucosal, or gastrointestinal toxicity in combination regimens. The $t_{1/2}$elim of Ara-C is approximately 3 hours. The major route of elimination is by catabolism to Ara-U by deoxycytidine deaminase, accomplished by many cells including hepatocytes. It is clear that prolonged exposure to the drug produces superior antitumor effects to single large boluses (67), and some of the earliest pharmacodynamic studies for any antineoplastic agent showed a correlation between Ara-C $t_{1/2}$elim and likelihood of remission induction in acute leukemia (68, 69).

In high-dose therapy Ara-C is frequently given in a dose of 750–3000 mg/m^2 every 12 hours for a total of 4–10 doses.

SUMMARY AND CONCLUSIONS

In the design of high-dose chemotherapy regimens, all available data must be evaluated to ensure maximization of the therapeutic index of the regimen. While testing of anticancer drugs in preclinical systems (in particular murine tumor models) often fails to predict activity of the drug for a specific tumor (70), pharmacokinetic parameters from such studies are often much more helpful in defining the optimal dose and dose rate of infusion of the agent. This is in part because, even if pharmacokinetic differences from mouse to man exist, the AUC for a given drug is often predictive of toxic effects irrespective of species. Additionally, the pattern of "AUC delivery," that is, a prolonged low dose-rate rate infusion versus a bolus high dose-rate administration of equal AUC, may produce toxic and therapeutic differences that trans-late across species (71). Thus preclinical pharmacokinetic data should be carefully scrutinized prior to high-dose therapy design.

During the execution of high-dose therapy trials, "sporadic" life-threatening or fatal toxicities often occur (72). While differences in the susceptibility of individual patients' organ systems to toxicity may well exist, an equally tenable hypothesis is that differences in drug disposition and exposure may be responsible. As noted above, this latter hypothesis has often proven true for antibiotics, neurotropic agents, cardiotonic drugs, and others. Because of the severity of toxicities produced with high-dose anticancer therapy and the paucity of systematic data on interpatient pharmacokinetic variability, as noted above, studies in this area are long overdue. The promise of therapeutic drug monitoring to guide drug administration makes these studies even more imperative.

In reporting the results of standard-dose treatment trials, many observers have noted the importance of describing the actual delivered dose, as opposed to the protocol-specified dose (73). Because of the potential morbidity of high-dose therapy, strict adherence to protocol-described doses seems more common than in standard dose trials. In the future, description of the actual pharmacokinetic parameters for each drug given in this setting may add greater power to our ability to analyze these trials, evaluate individual patient toxicities, and make more rational our interpretation of dose-limiting toxicities in Phase I high-dose trials. These observations in turn should provide additional impetus to delivery of more uniform high-dose anticancer therapy to patients.

REFERENCES

1. Gibaldi M, Perrier D, eds. Pharmacokinetics. New York: Marcel Dekker, 1982.
2. Evans WE, Schentag JJ, Jusko WJ, eds. Applied pharmacokinetics. Principles of therapeutic drug monitoring. Spokane, WA: Applied Therapeutics, 1986.
3. Pippenger CE, Penry JK, Kutt H. Antiepileptic drugs:

quantitative analysis and interpretation. New York: Raven Press, 1978.

4. Dhalgren JG, Anderson ET, Hewitt WL. Gentamycin blood levels: a guide to nephrotoxicity. Antimicrob Agents Chemother 1975;8:58–62.

5. Sirotnak FM. Obligate genetic expression in tumor cells of a fetal membrane property mediating "folate" transport: biological significance and implications for improving therapy of human cancer. Cancer Res 1985;45:3992–4000.

6. Baggott JE, Vaughn WH, Hudson BB. Inhibition of 5-aminoimidazole-4-carboxamide ribotide transformylase, adenosine deaminase and 5'-adenylate deaminase by polyglutamates of methotrexate and oxidized folates and by 5-aminoimidazole-4-carboxamide riboside and ribotide. Biochem J 1986;236:192–300.

7. Kamen BA, Nylen PA, Camitta BM, et al. Methotrexate accumulation in cells as a possible mechanism of chronic toxicity to the drug. Brit J Haematol 1981;49:355.

8. Refsum H, Wesenberg F, Ueland PM. Plasma homocysteine in children with acute lymphoblastic leukemia: changes during a chemotherapeutic regimen including methotrexate. Cancer Res 1991;51:828–835.

9. Fabre G, Matherly LH, Favre R, et al. In vitro formation of polyglutamyl derivatives of methotrexate and 7-hydroxymethotrexate in human lymphoblastic leukemia cells. Cancer Res 1983;43:4648–4652.

10. Bertino JR. Clinical use of methotrexate—with emphasis on the use of high doses. Cancer Treat Rep 1981;65:131–135.

11. Mallet A. A maximum likelihood estimation method for random coefficient regression models. Biometrica 1986;73:645–656.

12. Miller JA. Chromatography: concepts and contrasts. New York: John Wiley & Sons, 1988.

13. Grob R. Modern practice of gas chromatography. New York: John Wiley & Sons, 1985.

14. Snyder LR, Kirkland JJ. Introduction to modern liquid chromatography. 2nd ed. New York: Wiley-Interscience, 1979.

15. Chamberlain J, ed. Analysis of drugs in biological fluids. Cleveland: CRC Press, 1985.

16. Yost RW, Ettre LS, Conlon RD, Practical liquid chromatography: an introduction. Norwalk, CT: Perkin-Elmer Corp., 1980.

17. Schabel F, Trader M, Laster W, et al. Patterns of resistance and therapeutic synergy among alkylating agents. Antibiot Chemother 1978;23:200–215.

18. Schabel F. New experimental drug combinations with potential clinical utility. Biochem Pharmacol 1974; 23:163–176.

19. Schabel FM, Griswold DP, Corbett TH, et al. Testing therapeutic hypotheses in mice and men: observation of therapeutic activity against advanced solid tumors in mice treated with anticancer drugs that have demonstrated potential clinical utility for treatment of advanced solid tumors in man. In: DeVita VT, Bush H, eds. Methods in cancer research. Orlando, FL: Academic Press, 1979;3–51.

20. Foley GE, Friedman OM, Drolet BP. Studies on the mechanism of action of cytoxan—evidence of activation in vivo and in vitro. Cancer Res 1961;21:57–63.

21. Smith RD, Kehrer JP. Cooxidation of cyclophosphamide as an alternate pathway for its bioactivation and lung toxicity. Cancer Res 1991;51:542–548.

22. Sladek NE, Doeden D, Powers JF, et al. Plasma concentrations of 4-hydroxycyclophosphamide and phosphoramide mustard in patients repeatedly given high doses of cyclophosphamide in preparation for bone marrow transplantation. Cancer Treat Rep 1984;68:1247–1254.

23. Colvin M, Brundrett RB, Kan MNN, et al. Alkylating properties of phosphoramide mustard. Cancer Res 1976;36:1121–1126.

24. Cox PJ. Cyclophosphamide cystitis—identification of acrolein as the causative agent. Biochem Pharmacol 1979;28:2045–2049.

25. Friedman HS, Colvin OM, Aisaka K, et al. Glutathione protects against the cardiotoxicity of cyclophosphamide in the mouse. Cancer Res 1990;50:2455–2462.

26. Rollins BJ. Hepatic veno-occlusive disease. Am J Med 1986;81:297–306.

27. Cooper JAD Jr, White DA, Matthay RA. Drug-induced pulmonary disease. Am Rev Respir Dis 1986;133:321–340.

28. Colvin M. personal communication.

29. Sladek NE, Powers JF, Grage GM. Half-life of oxazaphosphorines in biological fluids. Drug Metab Dispos 1984;12:553–559.

30. Goldberg MA, Antin JH, Guinan EC, et al. Cyclophosphamide cardiotoxicity; analysis of dosing as a risk factor. Blood 1986;68:1114–1118.

31. Evans BD, Smith IE, Clutterbuck RD, Millar JL. Prevention of acute deaths after very high dose cyclophosphamide by divided dose schedule. Br J Cancer 1984;49:43–47.

32. Sladek NE, Preist J, Doeden D, Mirocha CJ, Pathre S, Krivit W. Plasma half-life and urinary excretion of cyclophosphamide in children. Cancer Treat Rep 1980;64:1061–1066.

33. Elias AD, Eder JP, Shea S, et al. High-dose ifosfamide with mesna uroprotection: a phase I study. J Clin Oncol 1990;8:170–178.

34. Alberts DS, Chen HSG, Benz D, et al. Effect of renal dysfunction in dogs on the disposition and marrow toxicity of melphalan. Br J Cancer 1981;43:330–334.

35. Cornwell GG, Pajak TF, McIntyre OR, et al. Influence of renal failure on myelosuppressive effects of melphalan: cancer and leukemia group B experience. Cancer Treat Rep 1982;66:475–481.

36. Tranchand B, Ploin Y-D, Minuit M-P, et al. High-dose melphalan dosage adjustment: possibility of using a

test dose. Cancer Chemother Pharmacol 1989;23:95–100.

37. Choi KE, Ratain ME, Williams SF, et al. Plasma pharmacokinetics of high-dose oral melphalan in patients treated with trialkylator chemotherapy and autologous bone marrow reinfusion. Cancer Res 1989; 49:1318–1321.

38. Bishop JB, Wasson JS. Toxicologic review of busulfan. Mutat Res 1986;168:15.

39. Groshow LB, Jones RJ, Brundrett RB, et al. Pharmacokinetics of busulfan: correlation with veno-occlusive disease in patients undergoing bone marrow transplantation. Cancer Chemother Pharmacol 1989; 25:55–61.

40. Vassal G, Deroussent A, Hartmann O, et al. Dose-dependent neurotoxicity of high-dose busulfan in children: a clinical and pharmacological study. Cancer Res 1990;50:6203–6207.

41. Grochow LB, Krivit W, Whitley CB, et al. Busulfan disposition in children. Blood 1990;75:1723–1727.

42. Beschorner WE, Pino J, Boitnott JK, et al. Pathology of the liver with bone marrow transplantation. Effects of busulfan, carmustine, acute graft-versus-host disease, and cytomegalovirus infection. Am J Pathol 1980;99:369.

43. Jones RB, Matthes S. Unpublished observations.

44. Phillips GL, Fay JW, Herzig GP, et al. Intensive 1,3 bis(2-chloroethyl)-1-nitrosourea (BCNU), NSC-436650 and cryopreserved autologous bone marrow transplantation for refractory cancer: a phase I–II study. Cancer 1980;52:1792–1802.

45. Herzig G. Personal communication, 1991.

46. Ozols RF, Corden BJ, Jacob J, et al. High-dose cisplatin in hypertonic saline. Ann Intern Med 1984; 100:19–24.

47. Patton TF, Himmelstein KJ, Belt R, et al. Plasma levels and urinary excretion of filterable cisplatinum species following bolus injection and IV infusion of cis-dichlorodiammineplatinum (II) in man. Cancer Treat Rep 1982;66:509–516.

48. Reece PA, Stafford I, Russell J, et al. Nonlinear renal clearance of ultrafilterable platinum in patients treated with cis-diamminedichloroplatinum (II). Cancer Chemother Pharmacol 1985;15:295–299.

49. Curt GA, et al. A Phase I and pharmacokinetic study of diamminecyclobutane-dicarboxylatoplatinum (NSC 241240). Cancer Res 1983;43:4470–4473.

50. Belani CP, Egorin MJ, Abrams JS, et al. A novel pharmacologically-based approach to dose optimization of carboplatin when used in combination with etoposide. J Clin Oncol 1989;7:1896–1902.

51. Jones RB, Shpall EJ, Ross M, et al. High-dose carboplatin, cyclophosphamide, and BCNU with autologous bone marrow support: excessive hepatic toxicity. Cancer Chemother Pharmacol 1990;26:155–256.

52. Hagen B, Neverdal G, Walstad RA, et al. Long-term pharmacokinetics of thio-TEPA, TEPA, and total alkylating activity following i.v. bolus administration of thio-TEPA in ovarian cancer patients. Cancer Chemother Pharmacol 1990;25:257–262.

53. McDermott BJ, Double JA, Bibby MC. Gas chromatographic analysis of triethylenethiophosphoramide and triethylenephosphoramide in biological specimens. J Chromatogr 1985;338:335–345.

54. Herzig G, ed. High-dose thiotepa and autologous bone marrow transplantation. Advances in Cancer Chemotherapy. New York: John Wiley & Sons, 1987.

55. Schabel FM, Trader MW, Laster WR, et al. Cis-dichlorodiammineplatinum (II): combination chemotherapy and cross-resistance studies with tumors in mice. Cancer Treat Rep 1979;63:1459–1473.

56. Fleming RA, Miller AA, Stewart CF. Etoposide, an update. Clin Pharm 1989;8:274–293.

57. Slevin ML: The clinical pharmacology of etoposide. Cancer 1991;67:319–329.

58. Stewart CF, Fleming RA, Arbuck SG, et al: Prospective evaluation of a model for predicting etoposide plasma protein binding in cancer patients. Cancer Res 1990;50:6854–6856.

59. Slevin ML, Clark PI, Osborne RJ, et al. A randomized trial to evaluate the effect of schedule on the activity of etoposide in small cell lung cancer. Abstract. Proc Am Soc Clin Oncol 1986;5:175.

60. Shpall EJ, Jones RB, Holland JF, et al. Intensive single-agent mitoxantrone for metastatic breast cancer. J Natl Cancer Inst 1988;80:204–208.

61. Hulhoven R, Dumont E, Harvengt C. Plasma kinetics of mitoxantrone in leukemic patients. Med Oncol Tumor Pharmacother 1984;1:201–204.

62. Greidanus J, de Vries EGE, Mulder NH, et al. A phase I pharmacokinetic study of 21-day continuous infusion mitoxantrone. J Clin Oncol 1989;7:790–797.

63. Ellis E, Moormeier J, Kaminer L, et al. Phase I–II study of high-dose cyclophosphamide, thiotepa, and mitoxantrone with autologous bone marrow reinfusion (ABMR) in patients with refractory malignancies [Abstract]. Proc Am Soc Clin Res 1990;9:17.

64. Mulder, PO, Sleijfer DT, Willemse PHB, et al. High-dose cyclophosphamide or melphalan with escalating doses of mitoxantrone and autologous bone marrow transplantation for refractory solid tumors. Cancer Res 1989;49:4654–4658.

65. Rudnick S, Cadman EC, Capizzi R, et al. High-dose cytosine arabinoside (HDARAC) in refractory leukemia. Cancer 1979;44:1189–1193.

66. Kantarjian H, Barlogie B, Plunkett W, et al. High-dose cytosine arabinoside in non-Hodgkin's lymphoma. J Clin Oncol 1983;1:689–694.

67. Frei E III, Bickers JN, Hewlett, et al. Dose schedule and antitumor studies of arabinosyl cytosine (NSC 63878). Cancer Res 1967;29:1325–1332.

68. van Prooijen HC. Clinical pharmacology of cytosine arabinoside in acute myeloid leukemia. In: Pinedo HM, ed. Clinical pharmacology of antineoplastic drugs. Amsterdam: Biomedical Press, 1978:177–191.

69. Baguley BC, Faulkenhaug EM. Plasma half-life of cytosine arabinoside in patients with leukemia—the effect of uridine. Eur J Cancer 1975;11:43–49.

70. Schabel FM, Griswold DP, Corbett TH, et al. Testing therapeutic hypotheses in mice and man: observations on the therapeutic activity against solid tumors of mice treated with anticancer drugs that have demonstrated or potential clinical utility for treatment of advanced solid tumors of man. Methods Cancer Res 1979;17:3–51.

71. Collins JM, Zaharko DS, Dedrick RL, et al. Potential roles for preclinical pharmacology in phase I clinical trials. Cancer Treat Rep 1986;70:73–80.

72. Peters WP, Eder JP, Henner WD, et al. Novel toxicities associated with high-dose combination alkylating agents and autologous bone marrow support. In: Dicke KA, Spitzer G, Zander AR, eds. Autologous bone marrow transplantation. Proceedings of the First International Symposium. Houston: University of Texas MD Anderson Hospital and Tumor Institute, 1985.

73. Coppin CML. The description of chemotherapy delivery: options and pitfalls. Semin Oncol 1987; 14(suppl 4):34–42.

74. Egorin MJ, VanEcho DA, Whitacre MY, et al. Human pharmacokinetics, excretion, and metabolism of the anthracycline antibiotic menogaril (7-OMEN, NSC 269148) and their correlation with clinical toxicities. Cancer Res 1986;46:1513–1520.

75. Hillcoat BL, McCulloch PB, Figueredo AT, et al. Clinical response and plasma levels of 5-fluorouracil in patients with colonic cancer treated by drug infusion. Br J Cancer 1978;38:719–724.

76. Campbell AB, Kalman SM, Jacobs C. Plasma platinum levels: relation to cisplatin dose and nephrotoxicity. Cancer Treat Rep 1983;67:169–172.

77. Egorin MJ, VanEcho DA, Olman EA, et al. Prospective validation of a pharmacologically based dosing scheme for the cisplatin analog, carboplatin. Cancer Res 1985;45:6502–6506.

78. Legha SS, Benjamin RS, MacKay B, et al. Reduction of doxorubicin cardiotoxicity by prolonged continuous intravenous infusion. Ann Intern Med 1982; 96:133–139.

79. Desai ZR, Van den Berg HW, Bridges JM, et al. Can severe vincristine neurotoxicity be prevented? Cancer Chemother Pharmacol 1982;8:211–214.

80. Priesler HV, Gessner T, Azarnia N, et al. Relationship between plasma adriamycin levels and the outcome of remission induction therapy for acute nonlymphatic leukemia. Cancer Chemother Pharmacol 1984;12:125–130.

81. Evans WE, Crom WR, Stewart CF, et al. Evidence that methotrexate systemic clearance influences the probability of relapse in children with standard-risk acute lymphocytic leukemia. Lancet 1984;1:359–362.

4

STRATEGIES FOR THE USE OF TOTAL BODY IRRADIATION AS SYSTEMIC THERAPY IN LEUKEMIA AND LYMPHOMA

Joachim Yahalom and Zvi Y. Fuks

While concepts of dose intensity are relevant to the effects of radiation on malignant tumors, the use of high-dose radiotherapy has been limited to local or loco-regional fields to reduce the risks of irreversible damage to critical organs. When total body fields have been employed in the management of malignant systemic disorders, their dose levels have been restricted by the tolerance of several critical normal tissues, thus limiting the application of this therapeutic modality to a small number of tumor types that exhibit extremely high sensitivities to radiation exposure. The most sensitive normal tissues to the effects of systemic radiotherapy are the hematopoietic and immune systems, followed by the lung and liver. While pulmonary and hepatic ratiation damage are irreversible in their chronic phase, leading to organ dysfunction or death, radiation-induced damage to hematopoietic and immune functions may be reversible even after supralethal doses of whole body exposure if appropriate marrow replacement is provided. There is thus a narrow dose window in which the hematopoietic and immune functions are severely impaired, but which is still below the threshold of pulmonary and hepatic toxicities. This dose range has been utilized in the past 2 decades for the management of leukemia and

lymphoma with total body irradiation (TBI), followed by rescue with allogeneic or autologous bone marrow transplantation (BMT). In the present review we discuss the basic radiobiologic principles that serve as guidelines in the design of TBI schemes, its role in the permanent engraftment of transplanted hematopoietic and immune progenitor cells, and its effects on normal tissue elements and on the neoplastic cells of leukemia and lymphoma.

HISTORICAL ASPECTS

The use of TBI for conditioning of patients prior to BMT has been a by-product of research on radiation sickness carried out during the late 1940s, motivated by efforts to understand the hematopoietic syndrome that occurred in nuclear exposure victims in Hiroshima and Nagasaki. Whereas the sensitivity of several large and small animals to the effects of TBI was found to vary, with LD_{50} ranging from 3–4 Gy in large animals to 6–7 Gy in rodents (1), the clinical syndrome leading to death in all experimental models was a result of an acute failure of the hematopoietic and immune systems developing over the first 30 days after exposure (1). In 1949 Jacobsen (2) discovered that mice exposed to lethal doses of TBI were rescued if the spleen was shielded during radiation exposure. While it was initially postulated that humoral factors were responsible for this phenomenon, 2 years later Lorenz (3) showed that living cells were required, and that in fact bone marrow or splenic hematopoietic cells were necessary to produce this protection. By 1956 it was demonstrated that transplanted hematopoietic cells proliferate and repopulate the depleted recipient's bone marrow cavities after TBI (4, 5), thereby replacing the immunohematopoietic system of the host and creating stable chimerism. These discoveries soon led to the first clinical applications of BMT in patients exposed accidentally to TBI (6) and in terminal leukemia patients conditioned with therapeutic doses of TBI (7). BMT after conditioning with supralethal doses of TBI and cytotoxic agents has since become a powerful clinical tool in the management of leukemia, lymphoma, aplastic anemia, and several hereditary disorders. It is estimated that nearly 20,000 patients have received allogeneic BMT since 1970 (8), most receiving some form of TBI as part of their pretransplant conditioning regimen. This experience has provided valuable information on the therapeutic and toxic effects of different dose and fractionation schemes of TBI and yielded several approaches to optimizing the therapeutic effects of TBI in the management of leukemia and lymphoma with supralethal therapies and bone marrow rescue.

THE DOSE-LIMITING TOXICITIES OF TOTAL BODY IRRADIATION

The critical dose-limiting toxicity of TBI in nontransplanted patients is bone marrow failure. The LD_{50} of whole body irradiation in the human is 300–400 cGy (9), with a peak incidence of death from hematopoietic failure occurring approximately 30 days after exposure. Since successful engraftment of hematopoietic progenitor cells after BMT overcomes this toxicity, an increase in the TBI doses to supralethal levels is feasible. Based

on observations of the experimental TBI syndrome in rodents (1, 9), the next expected dose-limiting toxicity has been the radiation-induced gastrointestinal syndrome, but routine supportive treatments with intravenous fluids, electrolytes, and antibiotics have protected patients from gastrointestinal death. Hence in practical terms, the normal organs that have limited the application of high doses of TBI have been the lungs (due to interstitial pneumonitis) and the liver (due to venoocclusive disease) (10). Although the progression and severity of the clinical syndromes that relate to these toxicities are multifactorial in nature, with several variables such as chemotherapy, infection, and graft-versus-host disease (GVHD) contributing to the development of potentially lethal pulmonary and hepatic complications after TBI, these toxicities have nonetheless limited the doses feasible with TBI to a maximum of 1000 cGy in a single fraction or 1500 cGy in dose-fractionated schemes.

While the therapeutic ratio of TBI in BMT is small, it is still sufficient to permit successful marrow engraftment. On the other hand, the tumoricidal effects of the doses feasible are unfortunately limited, and attempts to increase the dose levels of TBI to enhance its antitumor effects have resulted in unacceptable risks of pulmonary complications. A recent prospectively randomized study from Seattle (11) showed that increasing the TBI dose from 1200 cGy (200 cGy in six fractions) to 1575 cGy (225 cGy in seven fractions) in chronic myelogenous leukemia (CML) patients in first remission resulted in a decreased in leukemia relapse at 3 years from 35% to 12% ($P = .06$), but the transplant-related mortality increased from 12% to 32% ($P = .04$), leading to an overall survival for the two groups that was nearly identical. Reviews of pulmonary toxicity data in patients receiving TBI indicate that at the clinically useful dose range, a 5% increase of the lung dose could result in a 20%–50% increase in the incidence of interstitial pneumonitis (12, 13). Because of these limitations,

TBI has been used mostly in the management of malignancies that exhibit a high sensitivity to irradiation, such as leukemia, lymphoma, and Ewing's sarcoma, while its use in BMT programs for more radioresistant tumors has been limited. The relatively high toxicity of TBI emphasizes the need to optimize its dose and fractionation schemes and to base it not only on established clinical needs but also on relevant radiobiologic guidelines in an attempt to maximize the differential effects of radiation on target cells versus normal tissues.

THE CLINICAL GOALS OF TOTAL BODY IRRADIATION IN LEUKEMIA AND LYMPHOMA

TBI fulfills three functions in allogeneic BMT. It provides a powerful means of immune suppression to prevent the rejection of donor hematopoietic stem cells, it creates space within the recipient marrow to allow donor-cell engraftment, and in radiosensitive malignancies it serves as a cytotoxic agent to eradicate tumor cells. Although a few leukemia patients have been conditioned for BMT, with TBI alone (14), most recipients have received, in addition to BMT, pre- and post-transplant antileukemic and immunosuppressive drugs, such as cyclophosphamide and cyclosporine.

Whereas TBI has been used in the conditioning of the majority of patients who received allogeneic marrow transplants, its application is not essential for successful engraftment in all cases. In previously nontransfused patients with aplastic anemia, long-term engraftment is possible in a high proportion of treated patients without the use of radiation (15, 16), and conditioning with busulfan and cyclophosphamide without radiation can also produce stable chimerism in acute leukemia (17). However, most therapists have used TBI in allogeneic BMT to enhance the immunosuppressive conditioning and maximize the probability of engraftment. The most convincing evidence for the role of

TBI in improving the likelihood of engraftment is derived from experience with previously transfused aplastic anemia patients. When conditioned with high-dose cyclophosphamide alone, approximately 40% of the patients fail to engraft or have early rejections of the marrow transplant (18). However, the addition of TBI reduces the risk of graft rejection to less than 5% (18, 19). The dose of TBI administered for successful engraftment has ranged from as low as 300 cGy in aplastic anemia (18), and 500 cGy in a single fraction for leukemia (20), to 1575 cGy in a fractionated regimen for leukemia (11). Most patients with leukemia have, however, been treated with the higher doses to increase the benefits from the antileukemic effects of TBI. In addition to TBI, other techniques of high-dose and large-field radiotherapy have been used for conditioning of patients before BMT, such as total lymphoid irradiation (TLI) (21) and thoracoabdominal irradiation (22).

In advanced-stage lymphoma, there are several indications for the use of supralethal therapies with allogeneic or autologous bone marrow transplant rescue. However, most of the current transplants are carried out with autologous marrow grafts, harvested and cryopreserved when the patient achieves a complete remission from induction chemotherapy. With this approach, the issue of the effect of TBI on engraftment becomes irrelevant, and its main expected contribution is through the tumoricidal effects of radiation on lymphoma cells. The desire to use the tumoricidal effects of TBI in malignant lymphoma relates to the extraordinary sensitivity of several types of normal lymphocytes and lymphoma cells to the lethal effect of ionizing irradiation. It has been shown that human lymphocytes undergo interphase death within a few hours after radiation exposure (23), and that radiation damage is detected in vitro even after doses as low as 2–5 cGy (24). This sensitivity is shared by B and T lymphocytes of lymphoid tissues and the peripheral blood, as well as by neoplastic lymphocytes of the malignant lymphomas (25). Complete clinical remissions have indeed been observed in advanced stage nodular lymphoma with cumulative TBI doses as low as 100–150 cGy (26).

RADIOBIOLOGIC CONSIDERATIONS IN THE CLINICAL APPLICATION OF TOTAL BODY IRRADIATION

The current theories on the nature of the lethal effects of radiation in eukaryotic cells identify several types of damage to the structure and function of genomic DNA as the lethal lesions that lead to the loss of the clonogenic capacity and to cell death (27). Not all radiation lesions to DNA are, however, necessarily lethal. Some types of lesions are potentially repairable, but their ultimate fate depends upon competing processes of repair and lethal fixation (28). Thus the proportional loss of the clonogenic capacity and cell death at a given radiation dose depends on the number of primary nonrepairable lesions and on potentially repairable lesions that undergo lethal fixation. The net effect of increasing doses of radiation on the viability of mammalian cells is classically described by dose-survival curves (Fig. 4.1), which typically consist of an initial curvilinear component at the low dose range (the threshold shoulder) and an exponential component at the higher dose range (29). Several biophysical models simulate cell survival data, and parameters derived from the mathematical functions that describe these models are used to define the radiation sensitivity of mammalian cells and their potential for repair of radiation damage. Parameters that describe the slope of the exponential linear component of the dose-survival curve (Do) are commonly used to define the inherent radiosensitivity of a given cell, while parameters that describe the curvilinear threshold shoulder (Dq) reflect its capacity to repair radiation lesions and to restore clonogenicity. Target cells for TBI (i.e., immunocompetent cells,

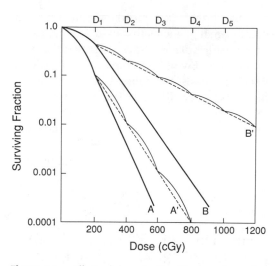

Figure 4.1. Effect of dose fractionation on the radiation survival of cells with minimal ability (A) or marked ability (B) to accumulate and repair sublethal damage. Fractionation multiplies the initial "shoulder" of the curve, resulting in a significantly shallower slope (B'-broken line) for normal tissues (e.g., lung, liver). The target cells for TBI (immunocompetent cells, leukemia, lymphoma) have a limited capacity of repair, and their survival curve is modified by dose fractionation (A'-broken line.)

leukemia and lymphoma cells) typically show little or no shoulder in their dose-survival curves and have low Do values (30) (Fig. 4.1), while cells involved in the production of the toxic effects of TBI typically have larger shoulder regions and higher Do values.

Another relevant radiobiologic factor that modulates the lethal effects of radiation in mammalian cells is the dose rate effect (31). When a given dose of radiation is delivered in a protracted fashion, at a low rate per time unit, it permits repair of potentially repairable lesions during the prolonged radiation exposure (32). Obviously, only cells capable of repair would express the dose rate effect. The effect of decreasing dose rates on the shape of the dose-survival curves in repair competent cells is a gradual disappearance of the shoulder region and an increase in the Do, both representing expressions of the radiation protective effect of a low dose rate, resulting from effective repair of potentially lethal damage. In TBI-treated patients, decreasing the dose rate results in reduction of radiation toxicity, while the radiation effect on tumor and immunocompetent target cells, which are usually deficient in repair capacity, is not affected. Dose rate effects on pulmonary toxicity have indeed been described in patients receiving single-dose TBI, but only when the dose rate was less than 5 cGy/min. Van Dyk reported that when single doses were given at high dose rates (50–400 cGy/min), the observed risk of radiation pneumonitis was 50% at a dose of 930 cGy and 95% at 1060 cGy (13). However, when a single fraction of 920–1000 cGy was administered with a dose rate of 4–6 cGy/min, the incidence of idiopathic interstitial pneumonitis was only 13% (13, 33). Similarly, Barrett et al. (32) described a 10% incidence of interstitial pneumonitis among 107 acutely ill acute myelogenous leukemia (AML) patients receiving single doses of 900–1100 cGy TBI at a dose rate of 2.5 cGy/min. Their observed incidence of interstitial pneumonitis was not significantly different from the incidence reported in severe aplastic anemia patients receiving marrow allografts after preparation with high-dose cyclophosphamide without TBI (34) but was significantly lower than the 28%–70% incidence of pneumonitis observed by other groups who pretreated leukemia patients with 1000 cGy at dose rates exceeding 5 cGy/min (references in Table 4.1). Bortin (35) showed that the rate of interstitial pneumonitis in patients with acute leukemia receiving 1000 cGy TBI at a dose rate of 2.3–5.7 cGy/min was 6%, compared to 30% in patients treated with dose rates of 6–30 cGy/min. However, the dose rate effect was limited to patients who received methotrexate for the management of GVHD, while those treated with cyclosporine for GVHD did not show a similar relationship between radiation dose rate and interstitial pneumonitis. In terms of clinical applicability, the delivery of a single treatment session of 1000 cGy at a dose rate of 2.5 cGy/min requires 400 minutes of net treatment time, which imposes significant inconviences to patients and to the treating staff and is regarded by most therapists as impractical.

An alternative method for improving the therapeutic ratio of TBI is by the use of fractionated radiation schemes (36–39). As mentioned previously, the survival curves of repair-competent cells exposed to single radiation doses are characterized by the presence of a curvilinear shoulder at the low dose region. When a course of radiation is divided into equal, small fractions separated in time by several hours, the cells surviving one dose of radiation respond to the subsequent dose as if they had never previously been irradiated (Fig. 4.1). This phenomenon is related to repair of sublethal radiation lesions, which occurs during the interval between fractions (40, 41), leading to a complete recovery of the sublethally injured cell. If the interval between fractions is sufficiently prolonged to permit a complete recovery (approximately 6 hours for most eukaryotic cells), the effective slope of the dose-survival curve of fractionated irradiation becomes progressively shallower as the dose per fraction decreases (Fig. 4.1). In other words, the total dose required to obtain a given biologic effect increases as the fraction size decreases, and for a total dose given by fractionated irradiation the ultimate effect will be smaller than that for the same total dose delivered in a single fraction. Because of normal tissue and tumor sensitivity considerations, the dose per fraction used most commonly in clinical radiotherapy is 180–200 cGy, and fraction sizes of less than 120 cGy are regarded as insufficient for providing a reasonable antitumor effect (42). Obviously, cells that are not capable of repair of sublethal damage (such as leukemia, lymphoma, and immune-competent cells) will not express the protective effect of fractionated irradiation. Therefore, in the case of TBI for leukemia, fractionated irradiation would result in decreased toxicities without impairing the therapeutic benefits of the total dose, while with hyperfractionated irradiation (fraction sizes less than 180 cGy repeated two to three times daily) the protective effect would be even further enhanced (43). Fractionated irradiation carried to maximal feasible doses of approximately 1500 cGy has indeed become a common practice in the application of TBI for BMT in leukemia and lymphoma.

THE EFFECT OF TOTAL BODY IRRADIATION DOSE FRACTIONATION ON NORMAL TISSUE TOLERANCE

There is experimental evidence that fractionating the treatment course increases the tolerance of the lungs to irradiation. Wara et al. (44) showed that the normal mouse lung can tolerate a 3.5 times higher whole lung dose if it is administered in 20 daily fractions as compared to a single dose, and that the dose ratio increase is mostly dependent on the number of fractions and to a lesser extent on the overall treatment time. Tarbell et al. (45) determined the $LD_{50/180}$ for upper-half body irradiation in mice, which measures lethality from radiation pneumonitis. When treatment was delivered in a single dose at a rate of 80 cGy/min, the $LD_{50/180}$ was 1299 cGy. Decreasing the rate of the single-dose treatment to 5 cGy resulted in protection from lung damage, expressed as an increase of the $LD_{50/180}$ to 2247 cGy (dose-modifying ratio of 1.72). However, the level of protection was even higher when the treatment was fractionated, regardless of the dose rate. When delivered by daily fractions of 200 cGy/fraction, the $LD_{50/180}$ was 3266 cGy (dose-modifying ratio of 2.51) and with hyperfractionation (120 cGy/fraction; three treatments per day), it was 2817 cGy (dose-modifying ratio of 2.16).

While these experiments provide strong evidence for the effect of fractionation on lung toxicity, the clinical data are less conclusive, with some series even failing to show a significant fractionation effect. Unfortunately, most of the data in the literature are derived from retrospective nonrandomized studies. Con-

sidering the multifactorial nature of interstitial pneumonitis in BMT, with patient selection criteria, donor-matching parameters, donor marrow treatment, pre- and posttransplant chemotherapy, TBI technique, dose rate and dose distribution inhomogeneities, and the presence of a variety of posttransplant infections, each representing an independent variable affecting the pulmonary toxicity outcome (34), a comparison of nonrandomized data even within a single database should be regarded with caution. The only prospectively randomized study that compared single-fraction TBI (1000 cGy delivered at a dose rate of 6 cGy/min) with fractionated TBI (six daily fractions of 200 cGy delivered at a dose rate of 6 cGy/min) was reported by the Seattle group (46). Fifty-three patients with AML in first remission received a non-T-depleted marrow transplant from HLA-identical siblings after conditioning with high-dose cyclophosphamide and either single-dose TBI (STBI) or fractionated TBI (FTBI), and all had sustained engraftment. Three of the 27 (11%) STBI patients developed idiopathic pneumonitis as compared to 1 of 26 (4%) of FTBI patients (statistically insignificant difference). Fourteen (52%) of the STBI patients developed venoocclusive disease of the liver, compared to 5 (19%) of the FTBI patients ($P = .02$). Leukemia relapses occurred within the 10 years after treatment in 6 of 27 (22%) of the STBI and 3 of 26 (11%) FTBI patients ($p = .09$). The authors concluded that 1200 cGy in six fractions is no less effective and perhaps more effective than 1000 cGy in a single fraction with regard to leukemic cell kill, but that FTBI is less toxic, particularly to the liver.

While most retrospective nonrandomized studies have indicated a decrease in the rate of interstitial pneumonitis in patients receiving FTBI, compared to STBI, two studies have failed to show a difference. In a large study from the International Bone Marrow Transplantation Registry, Weiner (47) reported that interstitial pneumonitis was in fact somewhat increased in patients receiving lung doses of 1200 cGy in five to six fractions (25 of 70; 36%) compared to STBI of 1000 cGy in a single fraction (29 of 121; 24%). A study from the University of Minnesota (48) showed that pulmonary toxicity in patients with acute nonlymphoblastic leukemia in first remission receiving non-T-cell-depleted BMT occurred in 19% of patients receiving STBI (750 cGy at a dose rate of 26 cGy/min) compared to 10% in patients treated with FTBI (1320 cGy delivered in fractions of 165 cGy twice daily at a dose rate of 10 cGy/min). The difference was not statistically different ($P = .37$). Several single- and multiinstitutional studies showed, however, a significant decrease in the incidence of pneumonitis with fractionated TBI (Table 4.1). A recent French cooperative study (56) of 180 patients with CML showed a 37.5% 5-year actuarial incidence of interstitial pneumonitis after 1000 cGy STBI, compared to 17.7% in patients receiving a median total dose of 1150 cGy FTBI. The Johns Hopkins hospital study (51) reported a 70% interstitial pneumonitis rate after STBI compared to 37% in patients treated with FTBI ($p = .05$). A retrospective analysis of 614 patients from Seattle (49) demonstrated pneumonitis among 44% of STBI patients compared to 29% after FTBI ($p < .001$). In a study of 208 patients from Japan, Inoue (54) demonstrated that the probability of developing interstitial pneumonitis at 3 years was 65% after STBI, and 42% after FTBI ($p = .0004$).

At Memorial Sloan-Kettering Cancer Center (MSKCC) (50) the risk of interstitial pneumonitis decreased after the introduction of hyperfractionated TBI (1320 cGy in fractions of 120 cGy three times daily) to 18% from 50% previously observed in patients receiving 1000 cGy in a single fraction. Furthermore, the mortality from interstitial pneumonitis was 26% with STBI and only 4% after hyperfractionated TBI. Based on these observations, fractionation of the TBI dose has become the common practice in treatments that include radiotherapy in the conditioning program before BMT, but the most optimal schedule has yet to be established.

The multifactorial risk of developing venoocclusive disease (VOD) of the liver is also reduced by fractionated TBI (Table 4.2). In the Seattle randomized trial (46), 52% of patients developed VOD after STBI, compared to 19% after FTBI ($P = .02$). The Villejuif group (57) reported 5 of 39 (13%) developed VOD after 1000 cGy STBI, and 0 of 31 developed it after a hyperfractionated TBI regimen (1320 cGy in 11 fractions three times daily) ($P = .07$). These data demonstrate the sparing effect of fractionated TBI on the development of hepatic VOD. Fractionation also leads to significant reductions in the risk of radiation-induced cataracts. Deeg (58) reported a 6-year cataract incidence of 75% with STBI compared to only 15% with FTBI. Data from Seattle also suggest better sparing of prepubertal ovaries with fractionated TBI and lesser impairment of total body growth in boys (59–61).

Table 4.1.   The Effect of TBI Fractionation on the Incidence of Interstitial Pneumonitis[a]

Author	IP Incidence with STBI	IP Incidence with FTBI or HFTBI	Significance
Meyers (49)	44%	29%	$P < .001$
Shank (50)	50%	18%	
Pino y Torres (51)	70%	37%	$P = .05$
Vitale (52)	58%	5%	$P = .002$
Blume (53)	28%	10%	
Inoue (54)	65%	42%	$P = .0004$
Valls (55)	35%	25%	
Socie (56)	37.5%	17.5%	$P = .02$

[a]Abbreviations: IP, interstitial pneumonitis; FTBI, fractionated total body irradiation; HFTBI, hyperfractionated total body irradiation; STBI, single dose total body irradiation.

Table 4.2.   The Effect of TBI Fractionation on the Incidence of Venoocclusive Disease of the Liver

Author	VOD Incidence with STBI	VOD Incidence with FTBI or HFTBI	Significance
Deeg (46)	14/27 (52%)	5/26 (19%)	$P = 0.02$
Cosset (57)	5/39 (13%)	0/31 (0%)	$P = 0.07$

[a]Abbreviations: VOD, venoocclusive disease; FTBI, fractionated total body irradiation; HFTBI, hyperfractionated total body irradiation; STBI, single dose total body irradiation.

THE TUMORICIDAL EFFECTS OF TOTAL BODY IRRADIATION IN LEUKEMIA

Since practically all patients conditioned for allogeneic BMT receive high doses of chemotherapy, it is nearly impossible to evaluate the true antitumor effects of TBI when used in BMT. In fact, in leukemia patients receiving allogeneic transplants without T cell separation, questions have been raised on whether increasing the TBI dose beyond the levels required to facilitate engraftment indeed decreases the eventual rates of leukemic relapses (8). There is, nonetheless, one randomized study from Seattle (11) that demonstrates decreased leukemic relapses with increase of the TBI dose. Patients with AML in first remission were randomly allocated to receive in addition to high-dose cyclophosphamide either 1200 cGy TBI in six fractions or 1575 cGy in seven fractions and were reported to have a decrease in the 3-year actuarial relapse rate from 35% to 12%, respectively ($p = .04$). Another randomized study from Seattle (46) compared the effects of 1200 cGy in six fractions with 1000 cGy in a single fraction and showed that the rate of leukemia relapse within 10 years was reduced from 6 of 27 (22%) for the patients receiving 1000 cGy to 3 of 26 (11%) for those receiving 1200 cGy. The difference, however, was not statistically significant ($p = .09$). In ALL, the use of high TBI doses (1320 cGy) delivered by hyperfractionated irradiation in combination with high-dose cyclophosphamide was shown to reduce the relapse rates in children in second remission (13% at 5 years) or third remission (25% at 5 years) when compared to historical data published in the literature for patients receiving 10 Gy (in a single fraction) (62). Although the doses used in these studies were within a relatively narrow range, these data seem to indicate a dose-response relationship of TBI and eventual relapse. On the other hand, other studies did not confirm the tumoricidal advantage of increasing the TBI dose. Cosset (63) reviewed data from several studies and demonstrated nearly identical relapse rates in patients receiving 1000 cGy in a single dose and in patients receiving 1200–1320 cGy in fractionated TBI schemes. A recent French cooperative study (56) of 180 patients with CML showed a 16% 5-year actuarial incidence of relapse after a single dose of 1000 cGy, compared to 29% in patients receiving a median dose of 1155 cGy (range, 1000–1320 cGy) by fractionated schemes of TBI. These conflicting data leave open the question of the effect of TBI dose escalation on relapse in recipients of non-T-cell-depleted allografts, in particular when fractionation schemes are used.

While radiation may in fact destroy leukemic cells, it is clear that from the existing data that the dose ranges currently in use in clinical BMT have only limited tumoricidal effects, and that in many instances leukemic cells of recipient origin most likely survive the effects of TBI. This hypothesis is supported by studies in which transplants were performed using either marrows from identical twins or cryopreserved autologous marrows collected from patients in complete remission after chemotherapy. While the overall relapse rate after non-T-cell-separated allogeneic BMT in AML patients in first remission is approximately 20% (64, 65), relapse rates in transplants across identical twin combinations conditioned with methods similar to those in allogeneic combinations have been reported to be within the 50%–60% range (66). Similarly, in autotransplanted patients the relapse rate was also reported to be approximately 60% (67). While the high rate of relapse in autologous transplant patients raises the question whether reinfusion of leukemic cells is responsible for the relapses observed, the similar high rates in identical twin combinations suggest that clinically applicable doses of TBI fail to eradicate residual leukemic cells in many patients. The differences in relapse rates between the conventional allogeneic and the syngeneic twin combinations suggest that allogeneic transplants may be associated with a substantial immune-mediated graft-versus-leukemia (GvL) effect. Whereas the GvL effect is a desirable phenomenon, it indicates the failure of TBI at clinically feasible dose levels to eradicate the last leukemic cells. On the other hand, the cytoreductive effect provided by TBI seems to contribute to the overall curative outcome, as demonstrated by the TBI dose effect, in addition to its immunosuppressive effect that facilitates engraftment of the allogeneic marrow cells.

There is one situation in which TBI is important for more than eradication of leukemia cells; that is its use to improve engraftment. There is a current need to explore the feasibility of TBI dose escalation to improve engraftment. The use of T cell depletion of donors' marrow to decrease the incidence and severity of GVHD (68, 69) is associated with a higher incidence of graft rejection and increased rates of leukemia relapses than previously observed with similar pretransplant conditioning procedures and non-T-cell-separated allografts (8, 12, 43, 63, 69). This phenomenon has been attributed to the loss of the GvL effect with regard to the increased relapse rate (70, 71) and to the loss of the "graft versus immunocompetent cell effect" of the removed T cells (63). There are several studies indicating that increasing the total FTBI dose as well as using STBI may be useful in overcoming the problems of increased rejection and relapse (63, 72, 73). Champlin (72) reported an actuarial relapse rate of 82% in patients receiving T-cell-depleted marrows after 1125 cGy of fractionated TBI (225 cGy twice daily for five times), which decreased to 15% by adding one TBI fraction and one TLI fraction. Patterson (73) reported 7% T-cell-depleted graft rejection in leukemia patients treated with 750 cGy STBI compared to 60% graft rejection with FTBI (1000–2000 cGy). Guyotat et al. (74) reported 0 of 9 graft failures after STBI (1000 cGy) and 7 of 15 (47%) after 1200 cGy FTBI ($P < .05$). Other groups have also demonstrated a decrease in graft failures by esca-

lating the total dose of FTBI (75–77). Slavin (21, 78) approached the issue of dose escalation by adding low-dose (600 cGy) fractionated TLI to 1200 cGy TBI delivered in six fractions and reported no graft rejections. These data demonstrate that the use of STBI or a relatively minor increase in the dose of FTBI is effective in decreasing relapse and graft rejection in T-cell-depleted allotransplants. The optimal dose and schedule of TBI have yet to be determined; preferably this will be done through randomized studies.

Vriesendorp (79, 80) has recently suggested that the immunosuppressive effects of TBI and its potentially lethal gastrointestinal and pulmonary toxicities are the dominant determinants of the therapeutic ratio of TBI. He used a biophysical model to predict the number of surviving target cells in critical organs with various TBI dose and fractionation schemes and demonstrated correlations between the prediction by the model and the outcome reported for the various TBI schedules. Based on this analysis, Vriesendorp recommended the use of a high fraction size (>200 cGy) in a short overall treatment time (<4 days) at the highest possible dose rate. Whether such an approach will improve the outcome with the current T-cell-depleted transplantation techniques remains to be seen.

THE TUMORICIDAL EFFECTS OF TOTAL BODY IRRADIATION IN LYMPHOMA

Although multiagent chemotherapy has been the mainstay of the management of advanced stage non-Hodgkin's lymphoma in the past 2 decades, there have been several attempts to use TBI as primary systemic therapy for low-grade lymphoma (81–84). This approach is based on the established high sensitivity of lymphoma cells to the lethal effect of ionizing irradiation (previously discussed). Based on this outstanding sensitivity phenomenon, Johnson (81) has suggested treating lymphosarcoma patients with low-dose fractionated TBI, employing fractions of 10 cGy to a total dose of 100–150 cGy, and demonstrated complete remissions in a group of previously untreated patients. This approach was subsequently adopted by the Joint Center for Radiotherapy in Boston, where Carabell et al. (82) employed TBI fractions of 15 cGy twice a week until a cumulative total dose of 150 cGy had been reached. Although most patients in this program eventually relapsed, it has become apparent that even very low doses of radiation, when administered to the entire body, can induce long remissions in advanced symptomatic lymphoma patients. Although several recent studies have confirmed these finding (83, 84), the approach has been pretty much abandoned because of the high relapse rate and the alternative availability of effective chemotherapy regimens.

Because of the high sensitivity of lymphoma cells to radiation exposure, TBI has also been used in some series to enhance the tumoricidal effects of high-dose chemotherapy prior to autologous or allogeneic BMT in advanced poor-prognosis lymphoma (85–92). Unlike the case of leukemia, the immune-mediated graft-versus-tumor effect does not seem to confer a major therapeutic effect in the management of lymphoma with allogeneic BMT. In a report by Appelbaum on the first 100 lymphoma patients transplanted in Seattle after high-dose cyclophosphamide and TBI (88), there was no difference in the outcome of treatment whether the marrow grafts were autologous or allogeneic. Because autologous stem cells from bone marrow or peripheral blood of lymphoma patients in complete remission after induction chemotherapy are more readily available than HLA-matched allogeneic stem cells from siblings, and in view of the absence of GVHD after autologous transplants and the improved techniques for autologous marrow purging and cryopreservation, most bone marrow transplantations in lymphoma have recently used autologous marrow cells (92). In this approach the immunosuppressive effects of TBI are neither required nor desirable. Hence the role of TBI in nonallogeneic BMT programs is limited to

its systemic cytotoxic potential. Since there have not been prospectively randomized studies testing the role of TBI in lymphoma treated with supralethal therapies and BMT, the true contribution of TBI in such programs is unknown. In a recent retrospective review (93) of 201 lymphoma patients from various series treated with either high-dose chemotherapy and TBI or with high-dose chemotherapy alone followed by autologous BMT, there was no difference in the outcome whether TBI was or was not used. Phillips et al. (94) performed a similar analysis but excluded cases of Burkitt's lymphoma. They concluded that although it appeared that programs involving TBI yielded improved results, a firm conclusion was not possible because the information was derived from small numbers of patients, and because of the lack of randomized studies. Since the current data indicate that the dominant factors predicting the outcome in lymphoma patient treated with BMT are the performance status and the response to previous therapies (88, 91, 92, 95), it is apparent that issues of patient selection bias preclude drawing any valid conclusions from retrospective nonrandomized studies (96).

Although a significant proportion of lymphoma patients treated with supralethal systemic therapies and autologous BMT remain free of disease, incomplete response or relapse in previously involved lymph nodes remains a major problem (85, 87, 90, 92). The Seattle group (87) reported that 59 of 62 (95%) who relapsed after autologous BMT presented their relapses at sites involved with disease before BMT. This observation would suggest that local field radiotherapy directed at such sites may improve the outcome. Phillips et al. (85) treated selected patients with 2000 cGy local field irradiation to sites of bulky disease prior to the application of high-dose cyclophosphamide and autologous BMT and observed improved survival, although the level of improvement was not statistically significant ($P = .07$). Such an approach is, however, not without risks. At MSKCC we have also observed a higher risk of pulmonary compli-cations and particularly pulmonary hemor-rhage (91, 92) in transplanted patients who presented with bulky mediastinal and/or pulmonary disease and therefore received boost radiation to the tumor area in addition to hyperfractionated TBI and high-dose che-motherapy. An analysis of toxicities of BMT in lymphoma (97) showed that the incidence of idiopathic or cytomegalovirus interstitial pneumonitis was increased (30%) in patients who received mediastinal irradiation to a dose of 2000 cGy or more before coming to trans-plant, compared to those receiving less than 2000 cGy or no irradiation (9%) ($p = .027$).

Despite the increased risk, both TBI and localized boost radiation fields may be of value in improving the outcome in lymphoma pa-tients treated with supralethal therapy and BMT rescue, provided that radiation is carefully planned to minimize the risks of complica-tion. At MSKCC we originally used a regimen of hyperfractionated TBI (1325 cGy in 11 fractions of 125 cGy, administered three times daily) and high-dose cyclophosphomide fol-lowed by autologous BMT for patients with non-Hodgkin's lymphoma. Patients with re-sidual tumor mass after induction chemo-therapy received additional radiation to areas of bulky disease (1200–1500 cGy) prior to TBI. We observed a 79% survival with a medium follow-up of 86 months in patients trans-planted in remission after induction chemo-therapy, as compared to only 13% of patients surviving after BMT in relapse or incomplete response (90). A subsequent modification of the regimen with the addition of etoposide to high-dose cyclophosphamide and hyper-fractionated TBI yielded better results in re-lapsed patients (91, 92). At a median follow-up of 44 months, 54% of relapsed patients who were salvaged with the modified regi-men are alive and disease-free. While these data are encouraging and indicate the need to achieve a complete response prior to BMT, the role of irradiation in such efforts, al-though likely positive, still needs to be firmly established.

TECHNIQUES OF TOTAL BODY IRRADIATION

There is no standard technique for the delivery of TBI, and almost every bone mar-row transplantation center has developed its own approach to accommodate its available radiation equipment and clinical facilities to the unique requirements of TBI. It should be emphasized, however, that the choice of the TBI technique applied and its dosimetry can significantly affect the success of the BMT program and in particular the rate of com-plications. Hence detailed recording and re-porting of the specific parameters of the TBI technique should not be underestimated (12, 98, 99). The equipment used in most centers is not especially dedicated to TBI and is ba-sically designed to deliver treatment to smaller and more homogeneous volumes than those employed in TBI. Since the target volume of TBI is the entire body, fitting the whole body into the limited-size radiation field frequently represents a major issue. The need to pro-vide homogeneous dose distributions to all sites despite the irregularity in body contour and tissue heterogeneity and the need to limit the dose to several critical organs also im-poses major treatment planning and radia-tion delivery difficulties. The solutions to these problems depend in most centers on modi-fications of existing facilities and thus vary widely.

A variety of patient positioning tech-niques and beam arrangements have been used to adjust the patient's size to the avail-able radiation field (Figs. 4.2, 4.3). The tech-niques for positioning the patient should be selected not only to accommodate the avail-able equipment but also to minimize incon-venience to patients during the morbid and frequently long treatment session. When frac-tionated TBI is used, the daily positioning of the patient should be reproducible to pro-vide consistency of dose distribution within each fraction. The radiation technique may involve a single or multiple field arrange-ment or a moving field technique and is de-

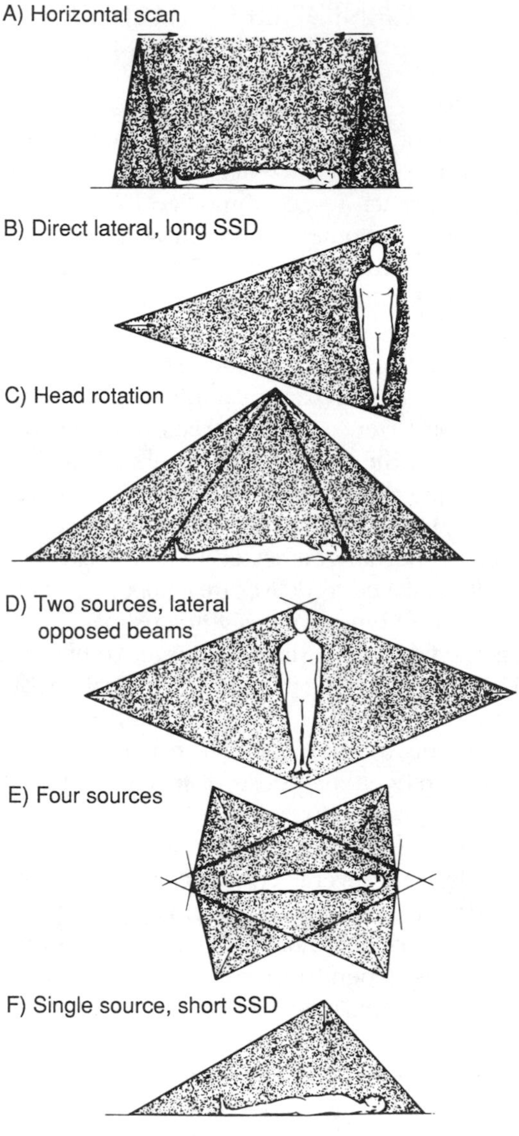

A) Horizontal scan

B) Direct lateral, long SSD

C) Head rotation

D) Two sources, lateral
   opposed beams

E) Four sources

F) Single source, short SSD

Figure 4.2. Alternative patient positioning and beam arrangements for TBI. (From Van Dyk J. Magna-field irradiation. Physical considerations. Int J Radiat Oncol Biol Phys 1983;9:1915.)

pendent on the available radiation equipment and room size. Several recent reviews have discussed aspects of the techniques in great detail (50, 98–100).

At MSKCC we have treated the patients in an upright standing position using a special stand constructed for this technique (Figs.

4.4, 4.5) (43, 101). The patient is immobilized between radiation-transparent plates that also anchor several devices that facilitate the delivery of treatment. A special radiation-transparent bicycle-like seat provides support to the patient while the patient still maintains the standing position, and special bars are available for handgrip to provide additional support. The TBI stand also provides an anchor for custom-made partial transmission lung blocks designed to decrease the total radiation dose to the lungs. A 1-cm Lexan screen is placed in front of the patient to produce electron buildup during the treatment, which is administered with 10-MeV photons to avoid underdosage to the skin. Prior to initiation of the treatment course, the patient is simulated for the design and preparation of individualized 1 half-value layer lung blocks. Anterior and posterior chest films are taken in the standing TBI position to design the shape of the blocks, and computerized tomography scan films provide tissue density information for planning of shaped electron beam boost fields for the chest wall to compensate for the underdosage of the ribs shielded by the lung blocks. The lung tissue itself receives only 60%–65% of the total dose with this technique (Fig. 4.6). The homogeneity level of the whole body field is maintained between 89% and 115% (43). Verification firms are taken during the first fractions and minor adjustments in positioning or the shape of lung blocks are made before treatment starts. At MSKCC, we also boost the testes with electrons to add 400 cGy in one fraction to the area. The testes are a sanctuary site in ALL and prior to institution of the testicular boost 4 of 28 males relapsed in the testes. No testicular relapses has been observed in over 350 male patients since the testicular boost was added to the treatment. The schedule of hyperfractionated TBI at MSKCC is illustrated in Figure 4.7 (43).

An important factor in the quality control of TBI is accurate dosimetry recording and verification (102–104). The dose should be specified at the midplane of the abdomen,

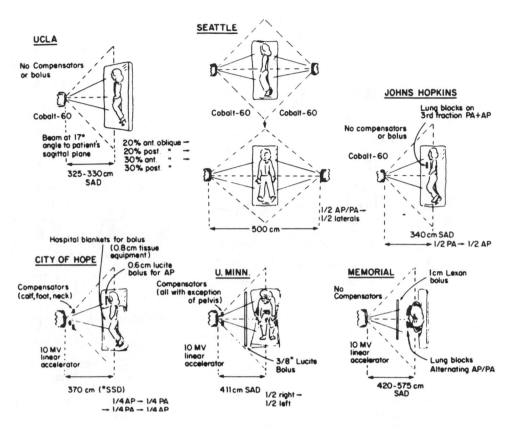

Figure 4.3.   Diagram of patient positions for TBI at various institutions. Bolus and compensators are indicated, as well as source-axis-distance (SAD) or source-skin-distance (SSD). (From Shank B. Techniques of magnafield irradiation. Int J Radiat Oncol Biol Phys 1983; 9:1926.)

and the dose to the lungs should also be calculated and reported (103). Phantom dosimetry should be performed to assess the beam quality, the dose profile, and depth dose measurements, as well as the specific transmission coefficients through the lung block under the special TBI conditions in order to ensure adherence to the quality standards of the treatments and to dose specifications. The surface dose and the exit dose should also be determined, and appropriate measures should be taken to compensate for the effects of electronic buildup when high-energy photons are used. In vivo dosimetry should also be performed to assess the absorbed dose, using appropriate detectors (103). When TBI is fractionated, in vivo dosimetry is needed at each session. At MSKCC we incorporated into

the TBI stand two cylindrical ionization chambers that provide real-time information regarding the dose during treatment (Fig. 4.5). One chamber is adjusted to measure the dose at midplane, and the other measures the exit dose. There is no ideal method for performing in vivo dosimetry, but whatever method used, it should be designed to ensure precision and reproducibility (102–104).

SIDE EFFECTS AND COMPLICATIONS OF TOTAL BODY IRRADIATION

Acute Side Effects

Standard fractionated or hyperfractionation programs are generally well tolerated

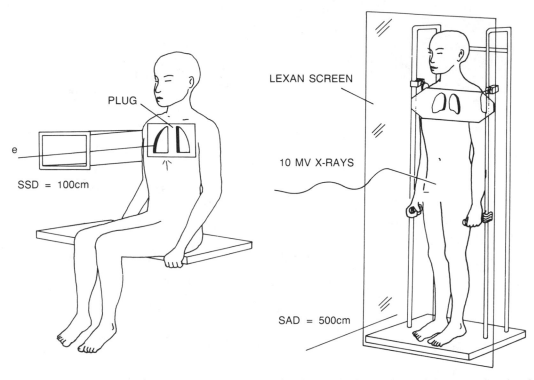

Figure 4.4. Patient position for TBI at MSKCC using a special stand for the immobilization of the patient and support of the lung shields (right). Patient position for the chest wall electron boost (left). (Reproduced with permission from Dr. G. Kutcher.)

compared to single-dose regimens (12, 43, 48). It is difficult to distinguish between the acute side effects of high-dose chemotherapy and those of TBI, particularly in regimens where intensive chemotherapy precedes TBI. Kim et al. (48) compared two regimens of TBI following high-dose cyclophosphamide. In a group of 34 patients who received single-fraction TBI without general anesthesia, radiation therapy was interrupted in 6 patients (47%) because of nausea and vomiting, despite premedication with prednisone and antiemetics. Most interruptions occurred during the second half of the treatment and lasted for an average of 45 minutes. In the hyperfractionated TBI group (165 cGy twice daily, to a total dose of 1320 cGy) only 5 of 46 patients (11%) required interruption of treatment for nausea and vomiting. Our experience at MSKCC (43) regarding acute side

effects during the 4-day hyperfractionated TBI treatment (1500 cGy in 12 three-times-daily fractions) is also excellent. Only a few patients experience nausea and vomiting, which usually occur on the 1st day approximately 2 hours after initiation of treatment. This, however, improves considerably by the 2nd day and is usually absent by the 3rd and 4th days of treatment. Diarrhea also develops during hyperfractionated TBI but subsides quickly. Patients occasionally experience salivary gland swelling, which subsides over 2–3 days. Almost all patients are fatigued by the end of the 4-day treatment course but have always been able to stand up during treatment, which lasts 10–15 minutes. Some patients may develop at the end of TBI a transient low-grade fever that is occasionally associated with chills (59). Reversible alopecia and mucositis resulting from both chemotherapy and radio-

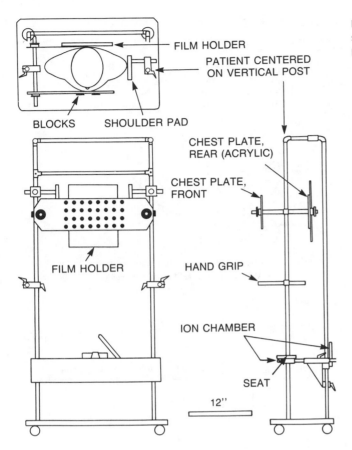

Figure 4.5. Structure of the TBI support stand used at MSKCC. (Reproduced with permission from Dr. G. Kutcher.)

FILM HOLDER
PATIENT CENTERED ON VERTICAL POST
BLOCKS   SHOULDER PAD
CHEST PLATE, REAR (ACRYLIC)
CHEST PLATE, FRONT
FILM HOLDER   HAND GRIP
ION CHAMBER
SEAT
12"

therapy are universally experienced by the 1st week after TBI. Patients may develop mild skin erythema in the first few days following irradiation. Five to 7 days after irradiation, patients may develop a reversible drop in the production of saliva and tears (105).

Pulmonary Complications

As discussed previously, pulmonary complications are a major cause of morbidity and mortality after both allogeneic and autologous BMT (47, 91, 92, 106, 107). Several factors contribute to the development of pulmonary decompensation in the transplanted patient. These factors include bacterial, fungal, and viral infections, of which cytomegalovirus pneumonia represents the most common etiology (106). GVHD increases the risk of pulmonary complications, and chemother-

apy- and/or radiation-induced pneumonitis may also contribute to risk of infection. Radiation is, however, considered to be the main cause of pneumonitis when no causative agent can be identified (idiopathic interstitial pneumonitis). As discussed previously, interstitial pneumonitis is considered to be the limiting toxicity for TBI and is used by many investigators as the main parameter for modulating the TBI dose and fractionation schemes and the design of treatment technique. The median time to diagnosis of idiopathic interstitial pneumonia after TBI is approximately 2 months, which is shorter than the usual time interval for development of radiation pneumonitis with loco-regional field radiotherapy (about 4 months). The syndrome has been diagnosed both after allogeneic and autologous BMT. In patients receiving autologous BMT for lymphoma, there is association be-

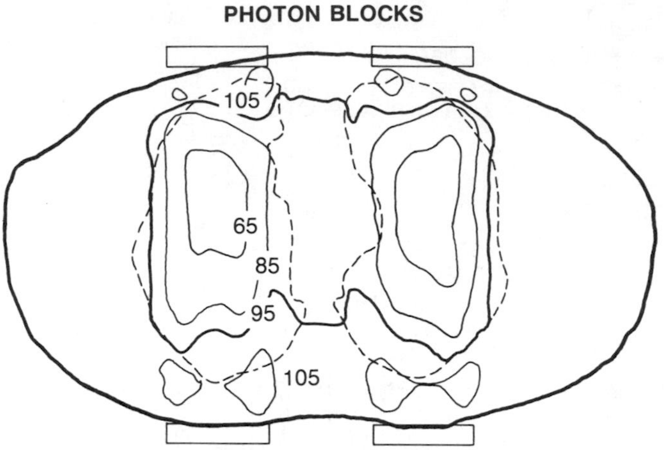

PHOTON BLOCKS

Figure 4.6. Axial dose distribution of combined photon-electron dose technique used at MSKCC to decrease the total radiation dose to the lung while delivering the full dose to the chest wall. In this case 1500 cGy with 10-MV photons were prescribed at midpelvis, and 600 cGy with 6-MeV anterior fields electrons and 11-MeV posterior field electrons were prescribed to the chest wall. (Reproduced with permission from Dr. G. Kutcher.)

SUNDAY	MONDAY	TUESDAY	WEDNESDAY	THURSDAY	FRIDAY	SATURDAY
−9	−8	−7	−6	−5	−4	−3
		TBI 125 cGy × 3	TBI 125 cGy × 3	TBI 125 cGy × 3	TBI 125 cGy × 3	Cyclophosphamide 60 mg/kg
				Chest Wall Electron Boost Ant: 300 cGy Post: 300 cGy	Chest Wall Electron Boost Ant: 300 cGy Post: 300 cGy	
		Testicular Electron Boost 400 cGy				
−2	−1	0				
Cyclophosphamide 60 mg/kg		Marrow Transplant	*Total Dose:* 1500 cGy *Dose/Fraction:* 125 cGy *Dose Rate:* 6-19 cGy/min *Interval Between Fractions:* 5h			

Figure 4.7. Schedule of the conditioning hyperfractionated TBI regimen used at MSKCC for allogeneic bone marrow transplantation. (From Shank B. Total body irradiation for bone marrow transplantation—MSKCC experience. Radiother Oncol 1990;18(suppl 1):70.)

tween pretransplant mediastinal irradiation and the development of pulmonary toxicity (97).

As discussed previously, there have been several approaches adopted to reduce the risk of radiation-induced pulmonary toxicity. In addition to decreasing the dose rate and to fractionating the treatment course, partial shielding of the lung to decrease the total lung dose has been practiced in an attempt to decrease the rate of pulmonary toxicity (43). In recent years the new approaches to decreasing the risk of GVHD with the use of T-cell-depleted marrow grafts (107), prophylactic treatment of potential pulmonary pathogens (108), and more effective management of pulmonary infections and complications have also contributed to the decrease in pulmonary toxicity after TBI.

Venoocclusive Disease of the Liver

Transient elevation of liver enzymes, such as alkaline phosphatase, serum glutamic oxaloacetic transaminase, and lactic dehydrogenase, to levels from two to four times above the normal range are observed in many patients undergoing TBI and BMT. The peak of enzyme elevation is observed at 3–5 weeks after the completion of TBI (43). These elevated enzyme levels gradually decline if no other contributing factors are present. The relative role of TBI in the etiology of this transient hepatocellular dysfunction is unknown, since other factors such as chemotherapy, antibiotics, viral infections, and total parenteral nutrition may be toxic to the liver as well.

VOD of the liver is a potentially lethal complication of BMT that may develop within a few days to a month after the procedure (109–111). While several factors contribute to the development of VOD after BMT, radiation is known to be an important contributory factor to the development of this syndrome. In a recent update of the Seattle randomized study, Deeg et al. (46) reported that 14 of 27 (52%) developed VOD after 1000 cGy single-dose TBI, compared to only 5 of 26 (19%) after 1200 cGy of fractionated TBI (P = .02). Cosset et al. (63) observed in a retrospective analysis of both allogeneic and autologous BMT that 5 of 39 (13%) patients developed VOD after 1000 cGy STBI compared to 0 of 31 patients after hyperfractionated (1320 cGy in 11 three-times-daily fractions) TBI. These data demonstrate that radiation-induced VOD can be modified by an appropriate fractionation regimen, which significantly decreases the risk of this serious complication.

Radiation-Induced Cataract Formation

The lens is one of the more sensitive organs to the effects of ionizing irradiation, developing cataracts after relatively low doses of radiation (112). However, cataracts also develop after long-term exposure to steroid therapy. Early development of cataracts has been considered an almost inevitable complication of TBI. In an analysis of the Seattle experience with single-fraction TBI, 40% of patients developed cataracts beginning 1–2 years after treatment (59). The incidence of cataracts appeared to increase with time and reached 75% at 6 years. The incidence decreased with fractionated TBI to 15% (58), which is similar to the incidence in patients who receive BMT without TBI. Nearly all patients who developed cataracts after single-exposure TBI required cataract removal, whereas after fractionated TBI only 20% have required surgery (113).

Growth Impairment in Children

Decreased growth in children receiving cyclophosphamide and single-dose TBI was documented by the Seattle group (114), while children who received transplant-preparative regimens containing cyclophosphamide without TBI show normal growth patterns (113). Several factors were found to be involved in growth retardation after BMT, including previous cranial irradiation, chronic GVHD, and TBI fractionation schemes. Subnormal levels of growth hormone (GH) have been noted in 87% of children who received both previous cranial irradiation for prophylaxis of CNS leukemia and TBI, whereas only 42% had low GH levels when only TBI was given (114). Treatment with GH resulted in some improvement in height, but less than the response usually seen in nonirradiated GH-deficient children. In the Seattle experience, boys who were treated with single-fraction TBI and evaluated 3 or more years later were found to be shorter than boys who received fractionated TBI (114). Girls showed the same trend, but the difference was not significant. A report by Barrett et al. (115) in children treated at the Royal Marsden Hospital in London showed a reduction in sitting height due to a disproportionate reduction in spinal growth, probably by an effect of TBI on the spinal epiphyses, which contribute more to growth in young children than in adolescents.

Impairment of Thyroid Function

Thyroid dysfunction has been reported in up to 43% of adult patients after TBI (116). Subclinical compensated hypothyroidism, which is manifested by elevated thyroid stimulating hormone and normal thyroxine levels, is the most common finding. Decreased thyroid function has also been observed in children treated with TBI (114). Among children who received single-dose TBI, 29%–56% had compensated hypothyroidism and 13% overt hypothyroidism. Patients who received fractionated TBI had 12%–21% compensated hypothyroidism and only had 3% overt hypothyroidism (113).

Impairment of Gonadal Function and Fertility

TBI causes primary gonadal failure in almost all patients who receive a nonfractionated treatment course (59, 113). Children frequently require the addition of sex hormone supplements to promote pubertal development. Among children who receive fractionated TBI, nearly half have normal pubertal development and normal gonadotropin levels (113). Most postpubertal women who receive TBI develop primary ovarian failure with menopausal symptoms that respond to treatment with cyclic hormones. Forty-four postpubertal women treated with allogeneic transplantation were evaluated for gynecologic abnormalities (117). Pelvic abnormalities were detected in 80% of patients and resembled atrophic changes known to

occur after ovarian failure. Atrophic abnormalities were noted in 33 of 36 recipients of TBI compared to 2 of 8 women not prepared without TBI ($P = .02$). Vasomotor symptoms were reported in 67% of TBI recipients compared to 38% of those not given TBI. These abnormalities can be corrected by early hormone replacement. Five of 139 women treated with TBI (3.6%) recovered their ovarian function between 3 and 7 years after TBI. Four of these patients conceived, but only one delivered a normal child (61). Most adult male patients treated with TBI have preservation of Leydig cell function with normal testosterone and normal serum luteinizing hormone. Sertoli cell function is usually abnormal, and spermatogenesis is absent. There is only one patient who had documented sperm production recovery (61).

Secondary Malignancies

Observations in dogs treated with 800–2100 cGy of TBI followed by autologous or allogeneic marrow grafts showed that within 10 years after TBI there was a sevenfold increase in the risk for the development of secondary malignancies (118). It was noted, however, that no lymphomas were seen and that malignancies tended to occur in the latest third of the normal dog life span. Reports by the Seattle Group (119) on 1926 patients receiving BMT for leukemia and 320 aplastic anemia patients disclosed 35 patients who developed secondary cancer between 1.5 months and 13.9 years (median, 1 year) after transplantation. Sixteen patients had non-Hodgkin's lymphoma, 6 had leukemias, and 13 had various solid tumors. The age-adjusted incidence of secondary cancer was 6.7 times higher than that of primary cancer in the general population. In a multivariate analysis, the predictors for secondary cancer were acute GVHD treated with antithymocyte globulin or anti-CD3 monoclonal antibody and TBI.

SUMMARY AND CONCLUSIONS

Although a great deal has been learned on the application of TBI as systemic therapy, in particular with regard to its effects on allogeneic bone marrow engraftment and the effects of dose fractionation in decreasing its toxicity, there are still several outstanding issues that need to be investigated. In allogeneic transplants without T cell separation, questions have been raised on whether increased doses of TBI are necessary to decrease relapse rates, particularly in view of the presumed GvL effect, which seems to contribute to the eradication of leukemia cells in transplanted patients. However, with the increasing popularity of T-cell-depleted allotransplants, which are associated with increased risks of graft rejection and relapse, there seems to be an urgent need to develop appropriate methods to increase the dose of TBI without concomitantly increasing its toxicity. In autologous BMTs, the issue of the effect of TBI on engraftment becomes irrelevant, and its main expected contribution is through its tumoricidal effects. Whereas there is little question on the efficacy of irradiation in eradicating lymphoma cells, the role of TBI and local-field boost radiotherapy in improving the current outcome of supralethal chemotherapy with autologous BMT still needs to be firmly established. It is hoped that well-designed, prospectively randomized studies will address these issues.

REFERENCES

1. Bond VP, Fliedner TM, Archambeau JO. Mammalian radiation lethality: a disturbance in cellular kinetics. New York: Academic Press, 1965.
2. Jacobsen LO, Marks EK, Gaston EO, Robson M, Zirkle RE. The role of the spleen in radiation injury. Proc Soc Exp Biol Med 1949;70:740–742.
3. Lorenz E, Uphoff DE, Reid TR, Shelton E. Modification of irradiation injury in mice and guinea pigs by bone marrow injections. J Natl Cancer Inst 1951;12:197–201.
4. Ford CE, Hamerton JL, Barnes DWH, Loutit JF. Cytological identification of radiation chimaeras. Nature 1956;177:452–454.
5. Nowell PC, Cole LJ, Habermeyer JP, Roon PL. Growth and continued function of rat marrow cells in x-radiated mice. Cancer Res 1956;16:258–261.
6. Mathe G, Jammet H, Pendic B, et al. Transfusions et greffes de moelle osseuse homologue chez des humains irradies a haute dose accidentellement. Rev Franc Etudes Clin Biol 1959;4:226–238.
7. Thomas ED, Lochte HL Jr, Lu WC, Ferrebee JW. Intravenous infusion of bone marrow in patients receiving radiation and chemotherapy. N Engl J Med 1957;257:491–496.
8. Gale RP, Butturin A, Bortin MM. What does total body irradiation do in marrow transplants for leukemia? Int J Radiat Oncol Biol Phys 1991;20:631–634.
9. Hemplemann LH, Lisco H, Hoffman JG. The acute radiation syndrome: a study of nine cases and a review of the problem. Ann Intern Med 1952,36:279–310.
10. Thomas ED. Total body irradiation regimens for marrow grafting. Int J Radiat Oncol Biol Phys 1990;19:1285–1288.
11. Clift RA, Buckner CD, Appelbaum FR, et al. Allogeneic marrow transplantation in patients with acute myeloid leukemia in first remission: a randomized trial. Blood 1990;76:1867–1871.
12. Plowman PN. A review of total body irradiation. Br J Radiol 1988;22(suppl 1):135–144.
13. Van Dyk J, Keane TJ, Kan S, Rider WD, Fryer CJ. Radiation pneumonitis following large single dose irradiation: a re-evaluation based on absolute dose to lung. Int J Radiat Oncol Biol Phys 1981;7:461–467.
14. Thomas ED, Storb R, Clift RA, et al. Medical progress. Bone marrow transplantation. N Engl J Med 1975;292:832–843, 895–902.
15. Storb R, Deeg HJ. Failure of allogencic canine marrow grafts after total body irradiation: allogeneic "resistance" vs transfusion induced sensitization. Transplantation 1986;42:571–580.
16. Champlin RE, Horowitz MM, van Bekkum DW, et al. Graft failure following bone marrow transplantation for severe aplastic anemia: risk factors and treatment results. Blood 1989;73:606–613.
17. Santos GW, Tutschka PJ, Brookmeyer R. Marrow transplantation for acute nonlymphocytic leukemia after treatment with busulfan and cyclophosphamide. N Engl J Med 1983;309:1347–1353.
18. Champlin RE, Feig SA, Gale RP. Case problem in bone marrow transplantation. I: Graft failure in aplastic anemia: its biology and treatment. Exp Hematol 1984;12:728–733.
19. Feig SA, Champlin RE, Arenson EA, et al. Improved survival following bone marrow transplantation for aplastic anemia. Br J Haematol 1983;54:509–517.
20. Messner HA, Fyles G, Meharchand J, et al. Long term survival of bone marrow transplant recipients with AML, ALL and CML after preparation with chemotherapy and total body irradiation (TBI) of 500 cGy

delivered as a single dose. J Cell Biochem 1988;(suppl 12c):92.

21. Slavin S, Or R, Weshler Z, et al. The use of total lymphoid irradiation for allogeneic bone marrow transplantation in animals and man. Surv Immunol Res 1984;4:238–252.

22. Devergie A, Gluckman E. Bone marrow transplantation in severe aplastic anemia following cytoxan and thoracoabdominal irradiation. Exp Hematol 1982;10:17.

23. Trowel OA. The sensitivity of lymphocytes to ionizing irradiation. J Pathol Bacteriol 1952;64:687–704.

24. Stefani S, Schrek R. Cytotoxic effect of 2 to 5 roentgens of human lymphocytes irradiation in vitro. Radiat Res 1964;22:126–129.

25. Cronkite EP, Chanana AD, Joel DD, Laissue J. Lymphocyte repopulation and restoration of cell mediated immunity following radiation: whole body and localized irradiation. In: Bond VP, Hellman S, Order SE, Suit HD, Withers AR, eds. Interaction of radiation and host immune defence mechanisms in malignancy. New York: Brookhaven National Laboratories, 1974:181–198.

26. Qasim MM. Blood and bone marrow response following total body irradiation in patients with lymphosarcomas. Eur J Cancer 1987;13:483–487.

27. Ward JF. DNA damage produced by ionizing radiation in mammalian cells: identities, mechanisms of formation and repairability. Prog Nucleic Acid Res 1988;3:95–125.

28. Frankenberg-Schwager M. Review of repair kinetics for DNA damage induced in eukaryotic cells in vitro by ionizing radiation. Radiother Oncol 1989; 14:307–320.

29. Alper T. Cellular radiobiology. Cambridge: Cambridge University Press, 1979.

30. Weischelbaum RR, Greenberger JS, Schmidt A, Karpas A, Moloney WC, Little JB. In vitro radiosensitivity of human leukaemia cell lines. Radiology 1981; 139:485–487.

31. Hall EJ. Radiation dose-rate: a factor of importance in radiobiology and radiotherapy. Br J Radiol 1982;45:81–97.

32. Barrett A, Depledge MH, Powles RL. Interstitial pneumonitis following bone marrow transplantation after low dose rate total body irradiation. Int J Radiat Oncol Biol Phys 1983;9:1029–1033.

33. Van Dyk J. Mah K, Cunningham JR: Iso response curves for radiation induced pulmonary damage [Abstract]. Med Phys 1986;13:615.

34. Weiner RS, Hurwitz MM, Gale PR, et al. Risk factors for interstitial pneumonia following bone marrow transplantation for severe aplastic anemia. Br J Haematol 1989;71:535–543.

35. Bortin MM, Kay HEM, Gale PR, Rimm AA. Factors associated with interstitial pneumonitis after bone marrow transplantation for acute leukemia. Lancet 1982;1:437–439.

36. Peters LJ, Withers HR, Cundiff JH, Dicke KA. Radiobiological consideration in the use of total-body irradiation for bone-marrow transplantation. Radiology 1979;131:243–247.

37. Peters LJ. The radiobiological bases of TBI. Int J Radiat Oncol Biol Phys 1980;6:785–787.

38. Evans RG. Radiobiological considerations in magnafield irradiation. Int J Radiat Oncol Biol Phys 1983;9:1907–1911.

39. O'Donoghue JA. Fractionated versus low dose-rate total body irradiation. Radiobiological considerations in the selection of regimens. Radiother Oncol 1986;7:241–247.

40. Elkind MM, Sutton HA. X-ray damage and recovery of mammalian cells in culture. Nature (Lond) 1959;184:1293–1295.

41. Elkind MM. Repair processes in the treatment and induction of cancer with radiation. Cancer 1990; 65:2165–2171.

42. Peters LJ, Ang KK. Unconventional fractionation schemes in radiotherapy. In: DeVita VT, Hellman S, Rosenberg SA, eds. Important advances in oncology. Philadelphia: JB Lippincott, 1986:269–286.

43. Shank B, O'Reilly RJ, Cunningham I, et al. Total body irradiation for bone marrow transplantation: the Memorial Sloan-Kettering Cancer Center experience. Radiother Oncol 1990;18(suppl 1):68–81.

44. Wara WM, Phillips TL, Margolis LW, et al. Radiation pneumonitis: a new approach to the derivation of time-dose factors. Cancer 1973;32:547–552.

45. Tarbell NJ, Amato DA, Down JD, Mauch P, Hellman S. Fractionation and dose rate effects in mice: a model for bone marrow transplantation in man. Int J Rad Oncol Biol Phys 1987;13:1065–1069.

46. Deeg HJ, Sullivan KM, Buckner CD, et al. Marrow transplantation for acute non lymphoblastic leukemia in first remission: toxicity and long-term follow-up of patients conditioned with single dose or fractionated total body irradiation. Bone Marrow Transplant 1986;1:151–157.

47. Weiner RS, Bortin MM, Gale RP, et al: Interstitial pneumonitis after bone marrow transplantation. Ann Intern Med 1986;104:168–175.

48. Kim TH, McGlave PB, Ramsay N, et al. Comparison of two total body irradiation regimens in allogeneic bone marrow transplantation for acute non-lymphoblastic leukemia in first remission. Int J Radiat Oncol Biol Phys 1990;19:889–897.

49. Meyers JD, Flournoy NM, Wade JD, et al. Biology of interstitial pneumonia after marrow transplantation. Recent advances in bone marrow transplantation. New York: Alan R. Liss, 1983:405–423.

50. Shank B. Techniques of magna-field irradiation. Int J Radiat Oncol Biol Phys 1983;9:1925–1931.

51. Pino y Torres JL, Bross DS, Lam WC, Wharam MD, Santos GW, Order SE. Risk factors in interstitial pneumonitis following allogeneic bone marrow

transplantation. Int J Radiat Oncol Biol Phys 1982;8:1301–1307.

52. Vitale V, Bacigalupo A, Van Lint MT, et al. Fractionated total body irradiation in marrow transplantation for leukemia. Br J Haematol 1983;55:547–554.

53. Blume KG, Forman SJ, Snyder DS, et al. Allogeneic bone marrow transplantation for acute lymphoblastic leukemia during first complete remission. Transplantation 1987;43:389–392.

54. Inoue T, Masaoka T, Shibata H. Interstitial pneumonitis following allogeneic bone marrow transplantation in the treatment of leukemia based on BMT survey in Japan. Strahlentherapie und Onkologie 1988;164:729–733.

55. Valls A, Granena A, Carreras E, Ferrer E, Algara M. Total body irradiation in bone marrow transplantation. Fractionated versus single dose. Acute toxicity and preliminary results. Bull Cancer 1989;76:797–804.

56. Socie G, Devergie A, Girinski T, et al: Influence of the fractionation of total body irradiation on complications and relapse rate for chronic myelogenous leukemia. Int J Radiat Oncol Biol Phys 1991;20:397–404.

57. Cossett JM, Baume D, Pico JL et al. Single dose versus hyperfractionated total body irradiation before allogeneic bone marrow transplantation: a non-randomized comparative study of 54 patients at the Institut Gustave-Roussy. Radiother Oncol 1989;15:151–160.

58. Deeg HJ, Fluornoy N, Sullivan KM, et al. Cataracts after total body irradiation and marrow transplantation: a sparing effect of dose fractionation. Int J Radiat Oncol Biol Phys 1984;10:957–964.

59. Deeg HJ. Acute and delayed toxities of total body irradiation. Int J Radiother Oncol Biol Phys 1983;9:1933–1939.

60. Sanders JE, Pritchard S, Mahonet P, et al. Growth and development following marrow transplantation for leukemia. Blood 1986;68:1129–1135.

61. Sanders JE. Late effects in children receiving total body irradiation for bone marrow transplantation. Radiother Oncol 1990;18:82–87.

62. Brochstein JA, Kernan NA, Groshen S, et al. Allogeneic bone marrow transplantation after hyperfractionated total body irradiation and cyclophosphamide in children with acute leukemia. N Engl J Med 1987;317:1618–1624.

63. Cosset JM, Girinsky T, Malaise E, Chaillet MP, Dutreix J. Clinical basis for TBI fractionation. Radiother Oncol 1990;18(suppl 1):60–67.

64. Clift RA, Buckner CD, Thomas ED, et al. The treatment of acute nonlymphoblastic leukemia by allogeneic marrow transplantation. Bone Marrow Transplant 1987;2:243–258.

65. Gale RP, Horowitz MM, Biggs JC, et al. For the Advisory Committee of the International Bone Marrow Transplant Registry. Transplant or chemotherapy in acute myelogenous leukemia. Lancet 1989;1:119–122.

66. Horowitz MM, Gale RP, Sondel PM. Graft-versus-leukemia reactions following bone marrow transplantation in humans. Blood 1990;75:555–562.

67. Gale, RP, Horowitz MM, Marmont A. For the International Bone Marrow Transplant Registry. Impact of T-cell depletion on transplant outcome in 3211 persons with leukemia. Exp Hematol 1989;17:484.

68. Storb R. Pathogenesis and recent therapeutic approaches to graft-versus-host disease. J Pediatr 1991;188:810–813.

69. Mitsuyasu RT, Champlin RE, Gale RP, et al. Treatment of donor bone marrow with monocloncal anti-T cell antibody and complement for the prevention of graft-versus-host disease: a prospective, randomized double-blind trial. Ann Intern Med 1986;105:20–26.

70. Champlin R, Gale RP. Bone marrow transplantation for acute leukemia: recent advances and comparison with alternative therapy. Semin Hematol 1987;24:55–67.

71. Prentice HG, Hermans J, Zwaan FR. Relapse risk in allogeneic BMT with T-cell depletion of bone marrow. Bone Marrow Transplant 1988;3:30–32.

72. Champlin R, Ho WG, Mitsuyasu RT, et al. Graft failure and leukemia relapse following T lymphocyte depleted bone marrow transplantation; effect of intensification of immunosuppressive conditioning. Transplant Proc 1987;19:2616–2619.

73. Patterson J, Prentice HG, Brenner MK, et al. Graft rejection following HLA matched T-lymphocytes depleted bone marrow transplantation. Br J Haematol 1986;63:221–230.

74. Guyotat D, Dutou L, Ehrsam A, Campos L, Archimbaum E, Fiere D. Graft rejection after T-cell depleted marrow transplantation: role of fractionated irradiation. Br J Haematol 1987;65:499–507.

75. Martin PJ, Hansen JA, Buckner CD, et al. Effects of in vitro depletion of T-cell in HLA identical allogeneic marrow grafts. Blood 1985;66:664–672.

76. Burnett AK, Hann IM, Robertson AG, et al. Prevention of graft versus host disease by ex vivo T-cell depletion: reduction in graft failure with augmented total body irradiation. Leukemia 1988;2:300–303.

77. Iriondo A, Hermosa V, Richard C, et al: Graft rejection following T lymphocyte depleted bone marrow transplantation with two different TBI regimens. Br J Haematol 1987;65:246–248.

78. Slavin S, Or R, Weshler Z, Hale G, Waldmann H. The use of total lymphoid irradiation for abrogation of host resistance to T-cell depleted marrow allografts. Bone Marrow Transplant 1986;1:98.

79. Vriesendorp HM. Radiobiological speculations on therapeutic total body irradiation. Crit Rev Hematol Oncol 1990;10:211–224.

80. Vriesendorp HM. Prediction of effects of therapeutic total body irradiation in man. Radiother Oncol 1990;18(suppl 1):37–50.

81. Johnson RE. Total body irradiation (TBI) as primary therapy for advanced lymphosarcoma. Cancer 1975;35:242–246.

82. Carabell SC, Chaffy JT, Rosenthal DS, Moloney WC, Hellman S. Results of total body irradiation in the treatment of advanced non-Hodgkin's lymphomas. Cancer 1979;43:994–1000.

83. Mendenhall NP, Marcus RB, Thar TL, Million RR. Management of advanced non-Hodgkin's lymphoma: result of prospective trial of total body irradiation [Abstract]. Am J Clin Oncol 1985;8:16.

84. Lybeert MLM, Meerwaldt JH, Deneve W. Long term results of low dose total body irradiation for advanced non-Hodgkin lymphoma. Int J Radiat Oncol Biol Phys 1987;13:1167–1172.

85. Phillips GL, Fay JW, Herzig RH, et al. The treatment of progressive non-Hodgkin's lymphoma with intensive chemoradiotherapy and autologous marrow transplantation. Blood 1990;75:831–838.

86. Armitage JO, Gingrich RD, Klassen LW, Bierman PJ, Kumar PP. Trial of high-dose cytarabine, cyclophosphamide, total-body irradiation, and autologous marrow transplantation for refractory lymphoma. Cancer Treat Rep 1986;70:871–875.

87. Peterson FB, Appelbaum FR, Hill R. Autologous marrow transplantation for malignant lymphoma: a report of 101 cases from Seattle. J Clin Oncol 1990;8:638–647.

88. Appelbaum, FR, Sullivan KM, Buckner CD. Treatment of malignant lymphoma in 100 patients with chemotherapy, total body irradiation and marrow transplantation. J Clin Oncol 1987;5:1340–1347.

89. Philip R, Armitage JO, Spitzer G, et al. High-dose therapy and autologous bone marrow transplantation after failure of conventional chemotherapy in adults with intermediate grade or high-grade non-Hodgkin's lymphoma. N Engl J Med 1987;316:1493–1498.

90. Gulati SC, Shank B, Black P, et al. Autologous bone marrow transplantation for patients with poor prognosis lymphoma. J Clin Oncol 1988;1303–1313.

91. Gulati SC, Yahalom J, Whitmarsh K, Clarkson BD, Gee T. Factors affecting the outcome of autologous bone marrow transplantation. Ann Oncol 1991; 2(suppl 1):51–55.

92. Gulati SC, Yahalom J, Portlock C. Autologous bone marrow transplantation. Curr Probl Cancer 1991; 15:1–57.

93. Singer CRS, Goldstone AH. Clinical studies of ABMT in non-Hodgkin's lymphoma. In: Goldstone AH, ed. Clinics in haematology. London: WB Saunders, 1986:105–150.

94. Phillips GL, Wolff SN, Herzig RH, et al. The role of total body irradiation in the treatment of lymphoma. In: Dicke KA, Spitzer G, Zander AR, eds. Autologous bone marrow transplantation: proceedings of the First International Symposium. Houston: University of Texas MD Anderson Hospital and Tumor Institute, 1985:117–123.

95. Cheson BD, Lacerma L, Leyland-Jones B, Sarosy G, Wittes RT. Autologous bone marrow transplantation. Ann Intern Med 1989;110:51–65.

96. Armitage JO. Bone marrow transplantation in the treatment of patients with lymphoma. Blood 1989;7:1749–1758.

97. Bearman SI, Appelbaum FR, Back A, et al. Regimen-related toxicity and early posttransplant survival in patients undergoing marrow transplantation for lymphoma. J Clin Oncol 1989;7:1288–1294.

98. Leer JWH, Broerse JJ, DeVroome H, Chin A, Noordijk EM, Dutreix A. Techniques applied for total body irradiation. Radiother Oncol 1990;18(suppl 1):10–15.

99. Quast V. Total body irradiation—review of treatment techniques in Europe. Radiat Oncol 1987;9:91–106.

100. Kim TH, Khan FM, Galvin JM. A report of the work party: comparison of total body irradiation techniques for bone marrow transplantation. Int J Radiat Oncol Biol Phys 1980;6:779–784.

101. Kutcher GJ, Bonfiglio P, Shank B, Masterson ME. Combined photon and electron technique for total body irradiation. Exhibit, International Meeting on Physical Biological & Clinical Aspects of Total Body Irradiation, The Hague, Netherlands, 1988:7–9.

102. Van Dyk J, Calvin JM, Glasgow GP, Podgorsak EB. The physical aspects of total and half body irradiation. Report of task group 29. AAPM report no. 17. New York: American Institute of Physics, 1986.

103. Briot E, Dutreix A, Bridier A. Dosimetry for total body irradiation. Radiother Oncol 1990;18(suppl 1):16–29.

104. Van Dyk J. Dosimetry for total body irradiation. Radiother Oncol 1987;9:107–118.

105. Schubert MM, Sullivan KM, Izutsu KT, Truelove EL. Oral complications of bone marrow transplantation. In: Peterson DE, Sonis ST, eds. Oral complications of cancer chemotherapy. The Hague: Martinus Nijhoff, 1983:93–112.

106. Krowda MJ, Rosenow EC, Hoagland HC. Pulmonary complications in bone marrow transplantation. Chest 1986;87:237–246.

107. Storb R. Pathogenesis and recent therapeutic approaches to graft-versus-host disease. J Pediatr 1991;118:510–513.

108. Winston DJ, Ho WG, Champlin RE. Cytomegalovirus infections after allogeneic bone marrow transplantation. Rev Infect Dis 1990;12(suppl 7):P776–792.

109. Shulman HM, McDonald GB, Matthews D, et al. An analysis of hepatic veno-occlusive disease and centrilobular hepatic degeneration following bone

marrow transplantation. Gastroenterology 1980;79:
1178–1191.

110. Woods WG, Dehner LP, Nesbit ME, et al. Fatal veno-
occlusive disease of the liver following high dose
chemotherapy, irradiation and bone marrow transplantation. Am J Med 1980;68:285–290.

111. McDonald GB, Sharma P, Matthews D, et al. Venocclusive disease of the liver after bone marrow
transplantation: diagnosis, incidence, and predisposing factors. Hepatology 1984;4:116–122.

112. Britten MJA, Halnen KE, Meredith WJ. Radiation cataract. New evidence on radiation dosage to the lens.
Br J Radiol 1966;39:612–617.

113. Sanders JE. Late effects in children receiving total
body irradiation for bone marrow transplantation.
Radiother Oncol 1990;18(suppl 1):82–87.

114. Sanders JE, Pritchard S, Mahonet P, et al. Growth

and development following marrow transplantation
for leukemia. Blood 1986;68:1129–1135.

115. Barrett A, Nicholls J, Gibson B. Late effects of total
body irradiation. Radiother Oncol 1987;9:131–135.

116. Sklar CA, Kim TH, Ramsay NKC. Thyroid dysfunction among long-term survivors of bone marrow
transplantation. Am J Med 1982;73:688–693.

117. Schubert MA, Sullivan KM, Schubert MM, et al.
Gynecological abnormalities following allogeneic
bone marrow transplantation. Bone Marrow Transplant 1990;5:425–430.

118. Deeg HJ, Storb R, Prentice R, et al. Increased cancer
risk in canine radiation chimeras. Blood 1980;55:233–
239.

119. Witherspoon RP, Fisher LD, Schoch G, et al. Secondary cancers after bone marrow transplantation
for leukemia or aplastic anemia. N Engl J Med
1989;321:784–789.

5

RADIOIMMUNOGLOBULIN THERAPY

Huib M. Vriesendorp, Syed M. Quadri, and Jerry R. Williams

GENERAL PERSPECTIVE

Radiation to the whole body—"systemic radiation"—is an attractive proposition for cancer treatment, as most human cancers are radiation responsive. However, patients can only tolerate limited amounts of uniform radiation to the whole body, i.e., ≤3.5 Gy by acutely delivered external beam without bone marrow rescue and ≤15 Gy by external beam with bone marrow rescue (1, 2). Such doses can only inactivate modest numbers of tumor cells, and higher doses cause mortality due to normal tissue damage. Radioimmunoglobulin therapy (RIT) could improve on this situation by concentrating the deposition and absorption of intravenously administered radiation to specific volumes within the body. The specificity of the immunoglobulin determines its distribution within the body, while the radioisotope connected to the immunoglobulin delivers localized radiation. RIT would thereby allow for higher tumor doses, increasing the curative potential and therapeutic ratio of systemic radiation by decreasing normal tissue irradiation.

RIT is a new extension of an older form of systemic radiation, intravenous radioactive iodine treatment for patients with metastatic thyroid cancer (3, 4). Iodine-131 treatment has an excellent therapeutic ratio due to the avid and selective uptake of iodine by thyroid tissue. The design, testing, and administration of effective RIT require interactions between many different scientific disciplines: radiochemistry, immunology, molecular biology, nuclear medicine, radiobiology, and radiation oncology. While the administration of therapeutic radioactive iodine is much less complicated and has proven almost immediately successful, RIT, considered feasible and promising since the late 1950s, is in a developmental stage.

Emerging clinical RIT results are promising, indicating that it *can* offer systemic radiation with considerable tumoricidal potential with less toxicity than large-field external beam radiation. Ten Gy and good palliation can be delivered to Hodgkin's disease without bone marrow transplantation, 30 Gy with bone marrow transplantation. Although this represents a two- to fourfold dose increase compared to external beam total body irradiation, further improvements are needed to make RIT a curative option (5). Radioimmunoglobulins can also be administered for diagnostic purposes: radioimmunoglobulin scintigraphy (RIS). RIS will not be dealt with in great detail here, except to delineate it from RIT. RIS is becoming a useful clinical tool. Diagnostic procedures are best performed with low-activity gamma-emitting isotopes in the 100–300 KeV energy range and short dwell times and physical half-lives. RIS requires rapid turnover diagnostic studies with good resolution on scans. Therapeutic (RIT) procedures, on the other hand, require localized deposition and radiation absorption, within the tumor, utilizing high-activity, beta emissions of sufficient energies, and long dwell times. Decreased deposition and short dwell times are sought in normal tissues. Ideally, RIT procedures are preceded by RIS to test tumor-targeting capability and normal tissue uptake in a given patient and to determine if the risks of a high-activity RIT procedure can be justified. Obviously, the requirements for successful RIS reagents are less stringent and easier to fulfill than for RIT reagents. However, several cogent arguments favor an expeditious continuation of the development of RIT: First, the risks of RIT (high-activity injection) can be limited to patients whose tumors are susceptible to tumor targeting as demonstrated by prior RIS. Other systemic cancer treatment such as chemotherapy is more toxic than RIT but cannot be evaluated prospectively for the efficacy of drug delivery to the tumor. Consequently, clinical application of chemotherapeutic agents is performed without this information, subjecting patients to considerable risks for normal tissue toxicity. Second, RIT does have significant tumoricidal potential. Radiobiology studies have *not* confirmed the early suspicion that the low dose rate radiation delivered by RIT can only inactivate insignificant amounts of tumor cells. In contrast, radiation doses delivered by RIT are now expected to be only slightly less effective than high dose rate radiation in daily fractions (6, 7). Third, other attractive properties of RIT are its sparing of normal tissues and its potential for inclusion in multimodality cancer treatment. The possible future role of RIT is illustrated by a comparison of drawbacks and advantages of several cancer treatment modalities in Table 5.1.

The most important remaining limitation to RIT is the relatively low uptake of radiolabeled antibody by human cancers, i.e., up to 0.01% of the injected activity per gram tumor (8). For delivery of *curative* tumoricidal radiation, an approximately fivefold selective increase of antibody uptake in the tumor needs to be obtained over currently

achievable uptake (5, 9). Animal studies with modified radiolabeled antibodies appear to indicate that such increases in radiolabeled antibody tumor uptake might be possible in humans (9–13). Dose escalation of RIT will only be rewarding if the current beneficial therapeutic ratio after low-activity RIT can be maintained by a high, selective tumor uptake of radiolabeled immunoglobulins.

VARIABLES AND ENDPOINTS

The development of RIT is incomplete. The current state of the art can be described most economically by discussing variables and endpoints one by one. Table 5.2 lists RIT variables and endpoints that will be reviewed in this chapter in separate sections. This information is followed by sections on models for RIT analysis, on current results of RIT in human patients, and a summary and conclusions section. The complexity of RIT, emphasized by the multitude of entries in Table 5.2, also accounts for the relatively slow progress made in this field.

ANTIGENIC TARGETS FOR RADIOIMMUNOGLOBULIN THERAPY

Selectivity

The antigen for targeting of RIT radiation doses should provide maximum discrimination between tumor and normal tissues. This can be achieved by the selection of antigens for RIT that only occur in tumors and not in normal tissues. The idiotypic membrane receptor of B cell lymphomas is the only known example of a tumor-*specific* antigen (14). Other antigens utilized in RIT protocols have been tumor "associated" rather than tumor specific. Tumor-associated antigens will occur in some normal tissues but are present in higher concentrations in and around tumor cells. Frequently, tumor-associated antigens are "developmental" antigens. They are associated with most cells of

Table 5.1. Advantages and Disadvantages of Radioimmunoglobulin Therapy

Competing Modality	Advantages RIT	Disadvantages RIT	Possible Solutions
Radioimmunoglobulin scintigraphy (RIS)	Therapeutic instead of diagnostic Less exposure to public and personnel	Harder to identify successful reagent Greater risks for patients	Preclinical animal work Cautious innovative clinical trials
External beam radiation therapy	Systemic Better therapeutic ratio	Low dose rate Antiantibody formation	Radiobiologic research, combined modality research Modified, less immunogenic immunoglobulins
Chemotherapy	More selective Better therapeutic ratio Prevention of ineffective administration possible Incorporation in multimodality regimen promising	Quality control more difficult Still in early developmental phase Not curative yet Antiantibody formation	Definition of safer, more reproducible, less immunogenic reagents Higher tumor dose
Immunotherapy	Pharmacokinetics analysis in vivo possible Greater tumoricidal potential	Health physics	Education of patient and personnel Appropriate monitoring and documentation of radiation exposures

Table 5.2. Variables and Endpoints in Radioimmunoglobulin Therapy

Variables	Endpoints
Antigen	Pharmacokinetics
Antibody	Radiobiology
Isotope	Tumor control
Chemical linkage	Therapeutic ratio
Route of antibody administration	
Dosimetry	
Dose escalation	
Fractionation	
Combined modality	

a given organ system in a fetus but occur only rarely in and around progenitor cells in the same organ in normal adults (e.g., α-fetoprotein [AFP, 15] and carcinoembryonic antigen [CEA, 16]). As part of the malignant process, such antigens may be overexpressed in malignant cell populations that could be considered "pathologically frozen" in an early, fetal stage and thereby provide a reasonably se-

lective target for RIT. Histocompatibility antigens and blood group antigens present a major portion of the outside cellular surface, and if cells or cell membranes are used to produce monoclonal antibodies, most often cell clones will be induced producing antibodies against histocompatibility antigens or blood groups. Such reagents are not desirable as RIT agents owing to the high density on many normal cells of the involved antigens and a corresponding lack of specificity for tumor cells.

The hematopoietic system and the lymphatic system are hierarchial systems consisting of "monocellular" suspensions in vivo. Individual cells can be teased out of their loose anatomic structures by only mild mechanical disruption, or they can be collected as ready-made monocellular suspensions directly in anticoagulated bone marrow or blood samples. The same holds for leukemias and lymphomas. Owing to the simple isolation methods for such cells, many antibodies have been raised against malignant or benign cells of blood, bone marrow, or lymphatic organs. Such antibodies are not necessarily optimal RIT reagents, because bone marrow provides the dose-limiting normal tissue to RIT (see "Dose Activity Escalation" section). Radiolabeled antibodies against antigens occurring in normal bone marrow have a priori a lower therapeutic ratio because they bring radiation directly to the dose-limiting normal tissue. Antibodies that do not target bone marrow are expected to have a better therapeutic ratio since bone marrow will receive less radiation. Antigens, present in solid tumors, have been utilized also to raise polyclonal or monoclonal antibodies. Such reagents have been reviewed recently, while new reagents continue to accumulate (17, 18). Both RIS and RIT have been applied in the diagnosis or treatment of patients with solid tumors. The endothelial barrier between circulatory system and tumor cells plays an important part of the selectivity of RIT reagents. Large molecules like IgG (150,000 MW) leave the circulatory system only with some help. When tumors reach a critical size (100–200 μm) the inefficiency of diffusion starts to limit tumor growth. Tumor cells close to blood vessels limit the utilization of nutrients and oxygen by more distal cells. Tumors overcome this limitation by secreting humoral factors that induce "tumor neovasculature" (19). Tumor neovasculature differs from normal blood vessels in many respects. For example, the endothelial barrier in tumor vessels is less complete, i.e., more leaky, facilitating diffusion of IgG molecules into the tumor interstitium. In situations where tumor-associated antigens are shared with important normal organs, the tumor/normal tissue targeting ratio of RIT reagents can still be high owing to the relative inaccessibility of antigens in normal tissues behind intact endothelial barriers (20, 21). A drawback of this selectivity mechanism for RIT is that tumors lacking neovasculature (for size or other reasons) are less susceptible to RIT.

Localization of Antigens

Tumor-associated antigens can be located within tumor cells, on tumor cell membranes, within tumor interstitium, or in the circulation. A schematic presentation of the influence of antigen location on RIT is given in Figure 5.1. Although tumors in general, including leukemias, are not limited to the circulatory system, tumor-associated antigens can be secreted in the circulatory system and quantified (e.g., AFP, CEA, and ferritin [15, 16, 22]). Combination of antigen and radiolabeled antibody in the circulation could conceivably prevent both targeting of the tumor localized outside of the circulatory system and cause immune complex disease. Antigen concentration differs between extravascular tumors and the circulatory system, being highly concentrated in the tumor. As the amount of antibody injected is considerably higher than the amount of antigen in the circulation, this in general prevents circulating antigen from interfering with tumor targeting since sufficient free antibody remains. For the same reason, immune complex disease is not observed, as the small molecular weight precipitates that are formed in antibody excess do not cause immune complex disease (23). Only in patients treated with cold antiidiotype antibodies has circulating antigen ("idiotype antibody") been shown to prevent the therapeutic antibody from reaching the malignant cells (14). In contrast, an experimental protocol in animals has been reported in which the reverse happened—i.e., circulating antigen improved tumor targeting (24). Endothelial localization of antigen would occur in malignancies originating from vascular cells. Endothelial antigens in tumor neovasculature would also be of interest as targets for cytotoxic treatment since tumor necrosis and possibly tumor sterilization might be induced by destruction of the tumor vasculature (25). Antibodies against normal endothelial cells have been demonstrated in patients with some forms of autoimmunity such as Kawasaki's syndrome (26). Serious

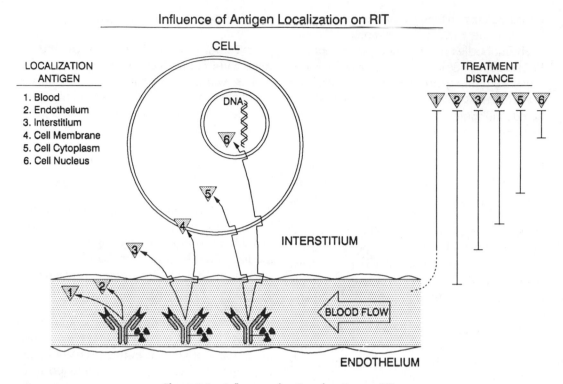

Figure 5.1.   Influence of antigen location on RIT.

antibody-induced vasculitis appears to respond to administration of cold "normal" immunoglobulins (27). It has not been determined whether the endothelium of tumor blood vessels has specific antigens that do not occur on normal endothelium. An obvious advantage of an endothelial antigen is its easy accessibility to intravenously administered antibodies. If an antigen is localized in the interstitium, such as ferritin in hepatocellular carcinoma, Kaposi's sarcoma, or Hodgkin's disease, an extra barrier is present between the intravascular antibody and the antigen. It will be more difficult and more time consuming for the antibody to reach the antigen. Important variables in this process are the size of antibody, the size of "holes" in the tumor neovasculature, and the pressure gradient between the blood vessel and interstitium (28). The best situation for RIT would be an interstitial antigen-antibody complex that would not change position. The combined molec-

ular weight of the antigen-plus-antibody lattice usually limits major movement of the complex; such complexes can be assumed to remain in the tumor. The antigen-antibody interaction, however, is dynamic, and some of the antibody will be released and diffuse back into the circulation. Interstitial antigens will not "modulate." The term "modulation" has been used to describe the behavior of some *cell-bound antigens* after antibody-antigen interaction. Antibody-antigen complexes can aggregate in one area of the cell membrane ("cap") and are subsequently internalized, leaving the cell membrane antigen-free until new antigen is synthesized. Modulation will only occur with antigens in high density on the cell membrane and with some, but not all, antibodies against the antigen (29). Modulation might increase the effectivity of RIT by bringing the isotope closer to the target (DNA in nucleus), or it might decrease the effectivity of RIT as cells temporarily devoid of the antigen cannot be targeted for a while. Antigens localized in the cytoplasm or cell nucleus require internalization and translocation for targeting and consequently develop antigen-antibody complexes at a later time after intravenous RIT administration. The number of antigenic sites required for effective targeting (in or around a cell) is estimated to be approximately 10^5–10^6 (30). It might be lower for immunoglobulins with isotopes attached that produce high-linear-energy transfer (LET) radiation (see next section).

Radionuclide to Target Cell Distance

Figure 5.1 illustrates the influence of "treatment distance," which for RIT is the distance between the target (nuclear DNA) and the isotope in the antigen-antibody complex. This relation determines the nature of the optimal isotope. The closer the proximity of the antigen to the DNA target, the shorter the required range for radioisotope emission and the greater the chance for selectivity, i.e., less radiation to normal tissues. The half-life has to be longer for isotopes with shorter ranges, as it will take a longer time (more hurdles in Fig. 5.1) to reach an antigen that is closer to the nuclear DNA. Antibodies labeled with short-range isotopes (Auger electrons) should interact with each malignant clonogenic cell. Untargeted cells outside the range of the isotope will not recieve radiation. However, when a cell is targeted by Auger electrons or alpha-emitting isotope, less isotope per cell is needed for cell kill than when a cell is targeted by a low LET (low-energy transfer) isotope (such as a beta emitter, 31). Isotopes with high-LET emissions kill cells more effectively and might successfully target and treat tumors with low numbers of tumor-associated antigens. However, within a tumor volume the density of antibody deposition can be lower for antibodies carrying long-range isotopes. Such isotopes do not have to target every cell, as they can "cross-fire," i.e., irradiate untargeted cells that are in the range of the isotope used.

ANTIBODIES

Species

Human antibodies are the best-studied antibodies but are rarely used as RIT reagents. Information obtained on human antibodies can be utilized for discussion (Fig. 5.2, Table 5.3), as many similarities and relatively few differences have been found between immunoglobulins of different mammalian species (32), with the exception of serum half-lives (33). Normal immunoglobulins of smaller species have shorter half-lives. The half-life of a transfused immunoglobulin will reflect the half-life of the species of origin, not the half-life of the corresponding normal immunoglobulin in the recipient (34; Vriesendorp, unpublished observation). In Figure 5.2, the well-known four-aminopeptide-chain model of the immunoglobulin molecule is shown: two light chains, two heavy chains, intrachain and interchain disulfide bridges, attachment for sugars, splicing site for papain—leading to three separate fragments, two of which bind antigen (F(ab), *F*ragment with *a*ntigen *b*inding)—and splicing site for pepsin leading to two fragments, one (F(ab)$_2$ binding-specific antigen, one nonspecific crystallizable fragment [F(c)] that provides effector functions for the immunoglobulin (complement binding, structure for attachment to other cells) and determines serum half-life. Molecule size is an important variable and inversely correlates with tissue penetration. Approximate molecular weights are given in Table 5.3. The generalization is that the molecule used as a RIT reagent has to be small enough and has to survive long enough in the circulation to reach the target antigen. Intuitively, one would expect that a high affinity of the immunoglobulin for the tumor-associated antigen would be advantageous. However, high-affinity antibodies might be stopped by the first tumor cells they en-

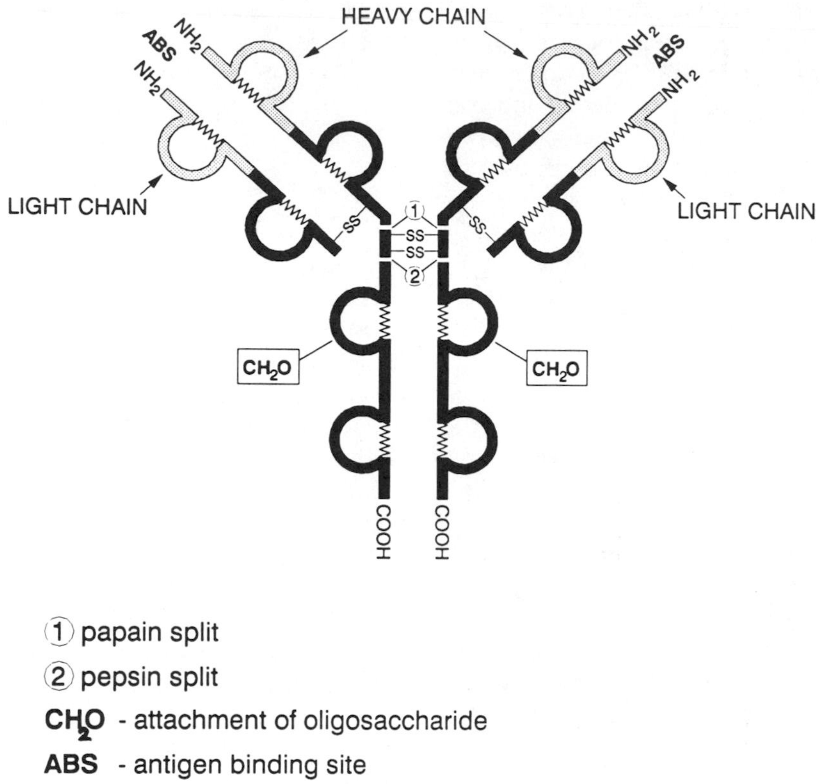

① papain split

② pepsin split

CH$_2$O - attachment of oligosaccharide

ABS - antigen binding site

Figure 5.2.   Four-peptide-chain structure of immunoglobulin.

counter and not reach less accessible parts of the tumor. Repeated RIT administrations or higher milligram amounts of administered immunoglobulin might be needed to obtain more complete tumor targeting (34). The ultimate proof of the potential of a given radioimmunoconjugate is obtained empirically in human cancer patients by pharmacokinetic and tumor-targeting studies with low-activity immunoglobulin. Animal studies can be of some help in selecting the most promising reagents for human study (35; see section on models for RIT study).

Clonality

A *mono*clonal RIT reagent will contain antibodies that are all reactive with *one* antigen only. Polyclonal antibodies will contain a mixture of antibodies against the antigens utilized for immunization and in addition contain antibodies against other antigens that the antibody-producing animal met prior to the start of the deliberate immunization schedule. The latter are estimated to amount to approximately 80% of the antibodies, while the remainder (only 20%) of the polyclonal mixture is against the specific antigen(s) used for immunization. This difference is borne out by studies in nude mice with a subcutaneously growing human malignancy. Monoclonal antibody reactive with the tumor will bring approximately five times more isotope to the tumor than a similarly labeled polyclonal antibody with reactivity against the tumor (9). There would be no reason to consider polyclonal antibodies for RIT if monoclonal antibodies were not susceptible

Table 5.3. Approximate Molecular Weights of Immunoglobulin Classes and Immunoglobulin Fragments[a]

Immunoglobulin Class or Fragment	Molecular Weight
IgM	900,000[b]
IgA	160,000[c]
	400,000[d]
IgE	190,000
IgD	180,000
IgG	150,000
F(ab)$_2$	100,000
H	50,000–70,000
F(c)	50,000
F(ab)	45,000
L	23,000

[a]Adapted from Eisen HN. Immunology, an introduction to molecular and cellular principles of the immune response. 2nd ed. Hagerstown: Harper & Row, 1980; Goodman JW. Immunoglobulin structure and function. In: Sites DP, Terr AI, eds. Basic and clinical immunology. 7th ed. Norwalk, CT: Appleton & Lange, 1991.
[b]A pentamer.
[c]Monomer; can also occur as dimer.
[d]Secretory IgA.

to very significant limitations in human patients. The linkage between monoclonal antibodies and radioisotope is frequently unstable in vivo—in particular radioactive iodine—and chelated monoclonal antibodies tend to accumulate in the normal human liver. Both complications can make the reagent lose most if not all of its potential for RIT. Research into these problems is ongoing, but until convincing reproducible solutions are obtained, polyclonal antibody will remain the reluctant standard for human RIT. (See sections on pharmacokinetics of modified and unmodified antibodies and chemical linkage.) Polyclonal antibodies could be relieved of some of their nonspecific companion antibodies by affinity purification. If successful, the purified product should demonstrate superior tumor targeting. A small trial with polyclonal antiferritin was unsuccessful in that the affinity-purified product had a very short half-life in vivo (Klein, personal communication). Gentler elution methods deserve to be tested and might yield specific, affinity-purified polyclonal antibodies with longer in vivo half-lives and better targeting, bringing higher radiation doses to the tumor.

Antiantibody Formation

Like all foreign proteins, RIT reagents will induce antibody formation in the recipient. Antiantibody formation can be detected in serum approximately 8–10 days after administration of the antigen. The interaction of antibody and antiantibody can cause allergic reactions locally, such as an Arthus reaction, or systemically, such as anaphylactic shock or serum sickness. It will interfere with targeting (the antibody will not reach the appropriate tumor antigen), and the antiantibody can remove the radiolabel from the antibody, with the toxicity risks of free radiolabel (36). A review of the determinants of antiantibody production can be of help in identifying solutions to this "show stopping" complication. The degree of foreignness of the immunoglobulin is, in all probability, important. The closer the species is to human, the lower the chance for antiantibody formation to its immunoglobulins in human patients (37). Immunoglobulins of nonhuman primates, chimeric immunoglobulins (human F(c) murine F(ab)$_2$), humanized immunoglobulin (only hypervariable region of murine origin, rest human IgG), or human monoclonal antibodies should be less immunogenic in human patients (37–39). Of the listed types, human monoclonal antibodies are the least available. They are hard to obtain, frequently high molecular weight (IgM), and of low titer. Humanized antibodies are less immunogenic than unmodified monoclonal antibodies, but patients that produced antibodies against humanized antibodies have been described (40). Antigen-antibody complexes are considered more immunogenic than antigen alone. The specificity of the antibody and the availability of its antigen-antibody complexes to the recipient's immune system are additional determinants of immunogenicity that are hard to circumvent in the RIT setting, as changes in these variables will interfere with the aims of RIT. The specificity of the antiantibody can be directed against the F(ab) parts of the immunizing antibody (antiidiotype antibody) or against its F(c) part (41, 42). Antiantibody formation is rare in patients with depressed humoral immunity, such as in patients with chronic lymphocytic lymphoma, B cell lymphoma, or Hodgkin's disease (43, 44). Patients with a T cell lymphoma or a solid tumor are frequently capable of making antiantibodies (43, 45). Possible solutions to the antiantibody problem are listed in Table 5.4. If RIT can be made so effective that a single cycle would suffice for tumor control, the antiantibody problem would become irrelevant. Obviously, this stage has not been reached and might not be a realistic goal for the future. In Johns Hopkins' RIT program for hepatocellular carcinoma, antiantibody formation problems are resolved by changing the antibody source. Rabbit, pig, baboon, or horse immunoglobulins are alternated, allowing for 10 or more RIT cycles in several patients (46). The proper antibody source is selected for each course by checking the patient for antiantibodies prior to injection. This solution cannot be applied to monoclonal RIT as the antibody specificity is usually only available in one species, in one immunoglobuin subtype. Smaller fragments of antibodies might be less immunogenic than the intact immunoglobulin, although antibodies against polypeptides as small as 5000 *MW* have been reported. Nonspecific immunosuppression can be given concurrent with RIT in an effort to prevent antibody formation. The unattractive aspects of this approach are the low efficacy and high toxicity of currently available immunosuppressive drugs. Tolerance induction or "specific" immunosuppression (i.e., suppressing the immune response of the recipient only to the injected immunoglobulin antigens) is much more attractive but difficult to achieve in the absence of previously proven, reproducible schedules of tolerance induction in human patients (47).

Pharmacokinetics of Modified and Unmodified Antibodies

Most RIT reagents take a long time to reach tumor antigens and persist for similarly long periods in circulation and normal tissues. Normal tissues will be exposed to radiation by RIT reagents in transit to the tumor or persisting in normal tissue compartments. A patient with a 100-g tumor and a tumor uptake of 0.01% of the injected activity per gram will get 99% of the administered activity in the wrong place, i.e., normal tissues. Normal tissue damage by RIT can be decreased by increasing the amount and speed of tumor targeting, removing radiolabeled antibodies from normal tissue compartments after tumor targeting has occurred, or dissociating the delivery of isotope to the tumor from the delivery of antibody to the tumor. Circulating radiolabeled antibodies can be chased out by the administration of a second antibody with specificity for the first antibody or by an extracorporeal circuit including an antibody-absorbing column (48–50). Unfortunately, the second antibody approach also decreases tumor uptake. Small immunoglobulin fragments including the antibody-binding fragment will diffuse faster and reach the antigen quicker. Small immunoglobulin fragments will wash out from normal tissues quicker than intact immunoglobulins. The quick targeting and decreased background of radiolabeled immune fragments have been utilized advantageously in tumor-imaging studies. Unfortunately, the dwell time of the small immunoglobulin fragments tested so far is also short in tumors. This prevents sufficient radiation dose deposition in the tumor

Table 5.4. Circumvention of Antiantibody Formation in Radioimmunoglobulin Therapy

1. Single cycle RIT
2. Rotation of species producing RIT reagent
3. Antibody modifications
    fragments
    humanized
4. Concurrent immunosuppression
    nonspecific
    specific

prior to elimination of the radioactive immune fragments by the kidney and increases the possibilities of radiation nephritis. The linkage of isotopes to small immunoglobulin fragments is more difficult and more prone to interfere with specificity. Another cause for short tumor dwell times of immune fragments might be the impossibility of antigen-antibody lattice formation with molecules carrying only one F(ab) part per molecule, causing a lower "avidity" of the molecule for the antigens in situ. Further studies with differently modified small immunoglobulin fragments are indicated.

Chimeric (mouse-man) monoclonal antibodies were shown to have a longer blood half-life in human patients than unmodified monoclonal antibodies, although not as long as regular human immunoglobulin (51). In general, the blood half-life of an artificially constructed antibody will be correlated to the half-life of the normal immunoglobulin in the original species that donated the F(c) fragment to the antibody. Bifunctional antibodies are another promising new twist in RIT. Two different monoclonal antibodies are synthesized; one with tumor-binding specificity and one specific for a low molecular weight hapten. Several methods have been developed to combine the two specificities into one molecule. For example, each antibody is sliced in half and one half of each antibody is allowed to reconstitute with a half of the other antibody, leading to a new composite antibody with a split (bifunctional) F(ab)$_2$ part. Such an antibody is injected cold (i.e., unlabeled) and allowed to equilibrate with the tumor. An antibody-antigen lattice can be formed by an IgM bifunctional antibody (not explored yet) but not by an IgG bifunctional antibody. IgG bifunctionals might have shorter tumor dwell times due to their lower avidity for the tumor-associated antigens. After the blood content of the antibody has significantly decreased, the second antigen (hapten) is radioactively labeled and administered. The hot hapten should target the tumor quickly due to its small size. The untargeted

remainder of the radioactive hapten will be removed by the kidney, again due to the small size of the hapten. This approach appears to hold great promise in preliminary animal and human experiments (10, 52).

RADIOISOTOPES

Isotopes for Radioimmunoglobulin Scintigraphy

The selection of the radioisotope for immunoglobulin labeling depends on the purpose of immunoglobulin administration. For diagnosis (RIS), isotope emissions need to be able to reach the diagnostic camera and provide spatial resolution. Photon emissions over 100 KeV have a range in tissue that is sufficient to reach the camera. Photon emissions over 250 KeV will decrease spatial resolution because the amount of material needed to collimate emissions cannot be accommodated in the arrays of pinhole cameras. The half-life of the isotope for RIS should be sufficiently long to permit the radioimmunoconjugate to reach the tumor before it decays and to let nonspecific radioactivity wash out of normal tissue background. On the other hand, a RIS reagent should have a short half-life isotope to limit radiation exposure of normal tissues. The upper part of Table 5.5 lists the most commonly utilized isotopes for RIS. The half-life of technetium (Tc) (0.25 days) is too short for labeling of intact immunoglobulin (MW 150,000) for RIS procedures. Most of the activity will decay prior to arrival of the immunoglobulin in the tumor (approximately 24 hours, or four half-lives). Iodine-123 has a similar problem and is not as readily available as technetium-99m. Both can be utilized for labeling of smaller immunoglobulin fragments. Indium-111 is the preferred isotope for labeling high-molecular-weight whole immunoglobulin molecules. Gallium-67 will have less spacial resolution than indium-111 and is utilized unconjugated, taking advantage of its preferential uptake in some malignancies.

Table 5.5. Isotopes for Radioimmunoglobulin Therapy and Radioimmunoglobulin Scintigraphy

Isotope	T$^1/_2$ (days)	Beta max (MeV)[a]	Gamma (MeV)
RIS			
Gallium-67	3.3	—[a]	0.093–0.388
Technetium-99m	0.25	—[a]	0.140
Indium-111	2.8	—[a]	0.173–0.247
Iodine-123	0.54	—[a]	0.159
RIS + RIT			
Copper-67	2.4	0.57	0.184
Silver-111	7.5	1.05	0.247–0.342
Iodine-131	8.0	0.61	0.080–0.723
Lutetium-177	6.7	0.50	0.113–0.208
Rhenium-186	3.8	1.07	0.137
Rhenium-188	0.7	2.12	0.155
Gold-198	2.7	0.96	0.412–0.626
RIT			
Phosphorus-32	14.3	1.71	—[b]
Nickel-66	2.9	0.20	—[b]
Strontium-89	51.6	1.46	—[b]
Yttrium-90	2.7	2.27	—[b]
Tin-121	1.1	0.38	—[b]

[a]Auger electrons ignored.
[b]Low-energy Brehmsstrahlung will occur with in vivo administration.

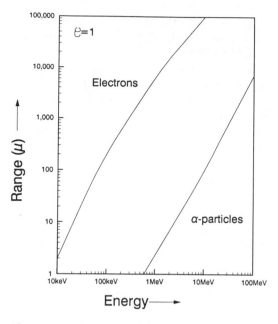

Figure 5.3. Penetration of electrons and alpha particles in tissue. (Adapted from Spiers FW Radioisotopes in the human body: physical and biological aspects. New York: Academic Press, 1968.)

Isotopes for Radioimmunoglobulin Therapy

RIT isotope performance requirements are different: localized deposition of radiation dose. A wide selection of isotopes with varying energy deposition ranges is available. Localized radiation can be obtained from soft gamma irradiation, as produced by cascades of Auger electrons, for example, or charged particle irradiation (electrons or alpha particles). Auger electrons will deposit high LET irradiation over less than one cell diameter (10 μ). Iodine-125 provides an example of such energy deposition (gamma emission of 0.035 MeV, Auger electrons and a 60-day half-life) and has been utilized alone or connected to an antibody in in vitro and in vivo experiments. The range of electron and alpha particle penetration is dependent on the energy of the particles (Fig. 5.3). The goal of RIT is to create an effective half-life in the tumor that is longer than the effective half-life

in normal tissues. Alpha emitters of lower energy (<5 MeV) have half-lives of years, too long for RIT. Alpha emitters of higher energy (>6.2 MeV) have very short half lives (seconds), too short for RIT. Intermediate-energy alpha emitters have a tissue penetration of approximately 30 μ (3–4 cell diameters), are accompanied by low abundance but high-energy gamma rays (bismuth-212, radon-222, radium-223, radium-224, astatine-211) and have half-lives between 1 hour and 12 days. The penetrating gamma rays create radiation safety problems in the radiochemistry laboratory and in vivo. Fermium-255 is an exception, with a half-life of 16 hours, 7.1 MeV alpha emission, and only low-energy gamma emissions. It is a daughter of Einsteinium-255 and not easily available. Alpha emitters have not found clinical application yet (31). The high-LET radiation of alpha emitters and the effectivity of tumor cell kill by only a few alpha particles per cell make them an attractive subject for further investigation. Owing to a much smaller size and smaller charge, electrons penetrate much more easily in tissue than alpha particles (Fig. 5.3). In early human RIT trials, isotopes with isolated beta emissions and isotopes with beta emissions admixed with gamma emissions were used most frequently (cf. lower two parts of Table 5.5). Their half-lives appear to be appropriate for clinical use. Problems with the chemical linkage of the isotope to the immunoglobulin (see next section) and the range of the isotope emissions provide the current limitations to their use. The range of the isotope emissions should fit the tumor; too long a range will deposit unnecessary irradiation in surrounding tissues, too short a range will cause dose inhomogeneities (cold spots) in the tumor (Fig. 5.4). The maximum tissue penetration of the most energetic beta particle listed in Table 5.5, yttrium-90, is approximately 11 mm. The lowest energy beta emission (nickel-66) has a tissue penetration of at most 11 μ (approx. one cell diameter). The therapeutic ra-

tio of RIT will decrease if isotopes are used with emission ranges longer than necessary for the tumors present in the patient. The radiation dose absorbed in the tumor will decrease while normal tissue toxicity will increase. In the current state of RIT the more energetic beta emitters appear to be the most useful isotopes as they can deliver the highest dose rates and higher and more homogeneous doses in larger tumors. Patients who qualify for RIT protocols will have tumors that are "scannable," i.e., larger than 1 cm. Smaller tumors frequently escape detection by RIS (30). In patients with small tumors (≤ 0.5 cm), tumor targeting cannot be verified easily, tumor dosimetry becomes problematic, and a rational, scientific development of RIT becomes more difficult. The treatment of smaller tumors with antibodies labeled with shorter range isotopes might become more acceptable when successful RIT principles have been better defined and optimized in patients with larger tumors. However, if tumor neovascu-

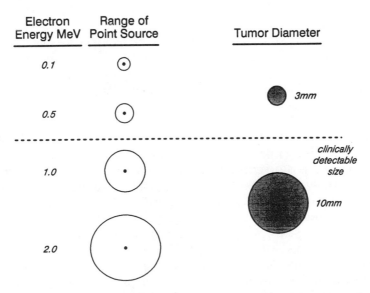

**Optimal Range of
Beta Particle for RIT**

Figure 5.4. Influence of tumor size and isotope range on isotope selection for RIT. Electron range and tumor size are depicted on the same scale. Energy spectrum of beta emitters ignored to facilitate comparisons.

lature is essential for effective RIT, patients with small tumors without neovasculature might never become candidates for RIT protocols.

Combination of Radioimmunoglobulin Scintigraphy and Radioimmunoglobulin Therapy

Optimal RIT requires a preceding RIS procedure to define tumor targeting and dosimetry. Isotopes with double emissions have been applied to this problem, one emission being a scannable gamma (RIS) and the other emission being a beta for treatment (RIT) (see Table 5.5). Patients treated with such isotopes receive a low amount of radioactivity, first to document tumor targeting and to obtain tumor dosimetry for the scheduled second, higher activity injection. A reagent that does not behave properly in vivo, demonstrating chemical instability or poor tumor targeting, will obviate the injection of unrewarding and potentially dangerous higher activities. If the reagent *does* produce desirable results, the second high-activity administration can be given within 3–4 days of the first injection (18). A combined RIS/RIT reagent has the drawback of making the patient a radiation hazard, especially in protocols using high activities. This will require inpatient management and elaborate health physics precautions.

Rhenium isotopes appear to be promising for this purpose as it has high-energy beta emissions and lower-energy gamma emissions than iodine-131, the RIS/RIT isotope most commonly used in the past. The half-life of rhenium-188 is too short for intravenous RIT with whole IgG molecules. Iodine-131 has a weak beta emission, with a tissue penetration of approximately 1 mm, and high-energy gamma emissions, which are hazardous for personnel and provide poor resolution in gamma camera views. In addition, iodine isotopes can cause dangerous radioactive vapors in the radiopharmacy and patient room. Radioactive metals will not do

so. Lutetium-177 has an even weaker beta emission but more effective and less dangerous gamma emissions than iodine-131 (53). An alternative solution to the required combination of RIS and RIT is to use the same reagent labeled with a gamma emitter first and with a beta emitter later. The first administration is at low activity for RIS. In the second administration high activity is used for RIT. Temporal separations between administrations greater than 1 week, however, may allow antiantibody formation, which could interfere with the efficacy of the second administration. The most commonly used combination of isotopes so far is indium-111 (for RIS) and yttrium-90 (for RIT) (54). Variance in biodistribution, however, may result from labeling the same antibody with different isotopes. Obviously, the double injection can be of value only if the first (RIS) injection is predictive for the second (RIT) injection. This needs to be verified and secured prior to routine clinical application.

CHEMICAL LINKAGE

Chemistry for Radioimmunoglobulin Scintigraphy Reagents

The chemistry employed for the attachment of radionuclides to immunoglobulins determines the stability of the product and can affect its biodistribution and immunospecificity. Radioisotopes can be labeled to immunoglobulins by various methods, for diagnostic or therapeutic purposes. Methods will be discussed for each isotope in the order in which they are listed in Table 5.5. Gallium-67 does not need an immunoglobulin delivery system. Gallium citrate will target malignancies such as lymphomas, melanoma, sarcoma, hepatoma, and lung cancer (55). It is a proven diagnostic tool and helpful in differentiating a recurrent residual tumor from scars resulting from prior successful chemotherapy or radiation therapy, in particular if a (SPECT) scanner is available.

Tc-99m is an ideal diagnostic radioisotope. The chemistry required for Tc-99m labeling of immunoglobulin was found to be difficult but appears to have been resolved (56). Two approaches are available for Tc-99m antibody labeling: direct labeling and labeling by conjugation. In the direct approach, disulfide bridges between the peptide chains of the immunoglobulin are reduced, and reduced Tc-99m is chelated to the endogenous sulfhydryl groups. Advantages of direct labeling are experimental simplicity and the availability of a commercial "cold kit." Both facilitate extensive use of Tc-99m-labeled immune fragments in busy nuclear medicine departments. There are, however, several disadvantages to direct labeling: instability of Tc-99m complexes and decreased affinity of the immune fragment. A second, more complicated approach to Tc-99m labeling is designed to overcome the disadvantages of direct-labeled products by the introduction of a bifunctional chelating agent between Tc-99m and the peptide chain of the immunoglobulin (56). The following agents have been employed: metallothionein (57), diamino-dithiolate (58), diamide dimercaptide (56), and DTPA (59). Conjugation methods have provided more stable and more reproducible Tc-99m immunoglobulin labeling.

Indium-111 has been attached to immunoglobulins through EDTA (56) and DTPA (60). These bifunctional chelating agents most commonly utilize the free amino group in lysine residues in the peptide chains of the immunoglobulin. More modifications have been explored for indium (56). They are diagrammed in Fig. 5.5. Two important additional considerations in the evaluation of indium chelation methods are

1. Correlation of in vivo pharmacokinetics with a similarly labeled yttrium-90 product
2. Uptake of the chelated immunoglobulin by normal liver

RIS results obtained with an indium-labeled product that does *not* correlate with the yttrium-labeled product prevent a properly controlled subsequent RIT phase. A possible source for differences in the in vitro and in vivo stability of indium- and yttrium-labeled immunoglobulins is their separate requirements for stable chelation. Yttrium appears to need eight coordination ligands, whereas indium can be complexed in a stable chelation by six or seven ligands (61). Several conjugates in Figure 5.5 have sacrificed a carboxyl group of the DTPA molecule to a peptide bond with the primary amino group of lysine (number 1: simple bifunctional chelate with cyclic dianhydride DTPA, five site-specific tripeptide DTPA linkages). Such conjugates have seven coordination points, making them stable for indium but less stable for yttrium. The problem can be solved by using a thiourea linkage (chelate number 2 in Fig. 5.5) or an aminobenzyl DTPA instead of an aminoethyleneanilide DTPA (chelates numbers 3 and 4). Linker molecules inserted between antibody and DTPA change the pharmacokinetics of the antibody (chelates numbered 3 and 4 [62]). Normal liver uptake of chelated immunoglobulins is influenced by the F(c) portion of the immunoglobulin as well as by chelation chemistry (11). The chelate-linker approach, as seen in numbers 3 and 4 of Figure 5.5, decreased liver uptake of an antibody by a factor of two in comparison to the same antibody chelated with chelate number 2. Chelated antibodies are found in parenchymal liver cells, not in Kupffer cells or in the so-called reticuloendothelial system (63). Excessive normal liver uptake will interfere with tumor targeting and cause radiation hepatitis (36). Further research is needed to prevent liver uptake of chelated antibodies. Small rodents have lower normal liver uptake than human patients, but dogs appear to experience the same problem as found in man and are the better experimental model for this problem (36). The recently developed polycyclic chelates (e.g., chelate 6 in Fig. 5.5) are immunogenic in man (64).

Iodine has the longest history as an isotope for protein labeling owing to its avail-

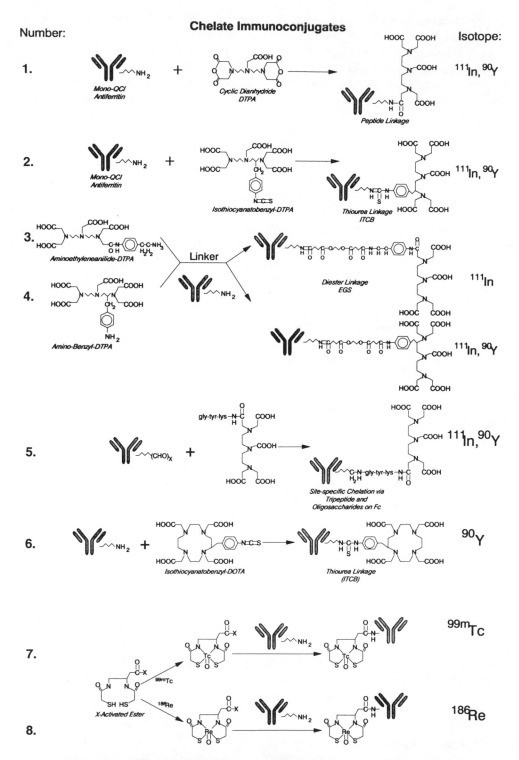

Figure 5.5.   Different chelates for immunoglobulin labeling. For references see text.

ability and the relative ease of attaching it to protein. Figure 5.6 shows diagrams for direct and indirect immunoglobulin labeling methods for iodine. The direct methods put the radioactive oxidized positive iodine in the ortho position of the tyrosine phenolic group. The drawback of this configuration is the susceptibility to "dehalogenation." It is probably an enzymatic process and due to the similarity of the iodinated tyrosine group to normal thyroid hormones (65). Indirect methods of iodine labeling probably do not have this drawback in animals but remain to be tested in human patients (66–68).

Chemistry for Radioimmunoglobulin Therapy Reagents

Some of the other isotopes listed in Table 5.5 have been administered to patients in a small molecular form not attached to an antibody or antibody fragment, i.e., iodine-131, rhenium-186, gold-198 (colloid), phosphorus-32 (phosphate or celloid), strontium-89, or yttrium-90 (colloid). The same targeting and dosimetry problems pertain to these applications as to RIT (see "Dosimetry" section). Colloids have been administered compartmentally, in the sometimes mistaken belief that this chemical configuration will remain localized (69, 70). Colloid gold-198 and phosphorus-32 have been used in the peritoneal and pleural cavity (70). Yttrium colloid has been injected in rheumatic joints (71). Ionic phosphorus-32, usually in orthophosphate form, has been given intravenously to patients with polycythemia vera. The phosphate concentrates in bone marrow and trabecular and cortical bone. Phosphorus-32 controls the disease effectively but induces

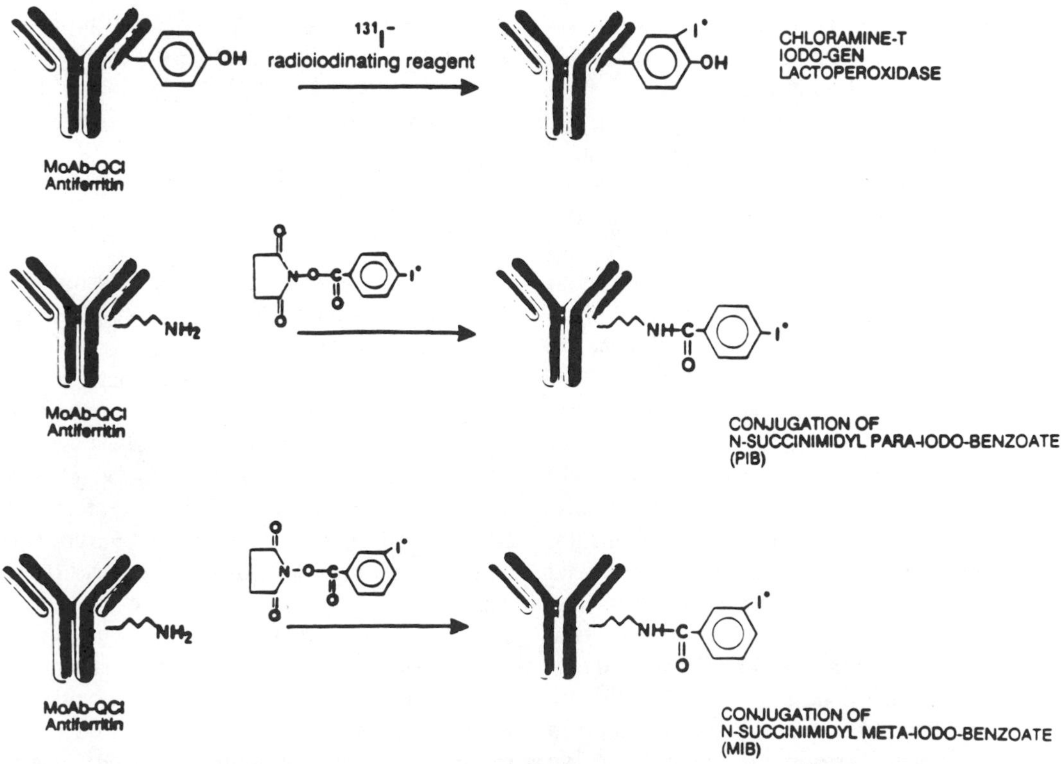

Figure 5.6.   Iodine labeling of immunoglobulins. For references see text.

leukemia after long-term use in approximately 15% of the patients (72). Rhenium and strontium isotopes show preferential bone uptake and are being evaluated for the treatment of bony metastases (73, 74). Indium-111, iodine-131, lutetium-177, rhenium-186, and yttrium-90 have been attached to high-molecular-weight antibodies for in vivo use. Indium- and iodine-labeling chemistry was summarized in prior paragraphs. Requirements for successful rhenium labeling run parallel to those for Tc and involve a bifunctional chelating agent (diamide dithiolate, 75). The chemistry for yttrium labeling is similar to the chemistry required for indium labeling, with the important provision that the immunoconjugate should have the same in vivo distribution, irrespective of the isotope used for labeling. In vivo instability dechelation could be toxic and will be dangerous if the free metal is a bone seeker, such as yttrium (76).

Chelation is also the best choice for labeling with the other metallic isotopes in Table 5.5 (lutetium, copper, silver, gold, nickel, tin) using any of the indicated methods. Clinical applications for these until now little-utilized isotopes could become interesting, if short-range beta emissions (i.e., smaller tumors) become a more important issue in RIT. The chemical linkage between isotope and antibody or other antibody modifications can change the pharmacokinetics of the administered product and the organ deposition of the radioisotope. Iodine-labeled products have a tendency to dehalogenate. This will cause deposition of radioactive iodine in the thyroid, stomach, and bladder. Most centers will try to prevent the development of hypothyroidism resulting from thyroid uptake of the radioisotope by the oral administration of cold iodine (2% Lugol solution, 20 droplets per day). European centers also recommend oral potassium perchlorate (300 mg twice daily) to prevent iodine uptake by stomach cells. The latter medication is not utilized as much in the United States, presumably due to its known side effects (aplastic anemia, hemolytic anemia, nephrotic syndrome) (77). As noted previously, indium-labeled compounds (and yttrium-labeled immunoconjugates [76]) have a tendency to disappear in the normal liver. Immunoglobulins with SH groups (e.g., F(ab) fragments) tend to be deposited in the kidney and be eliminated in urine.

ADMINISTRATION OF RADIOIMMUNOGLOBULIN THERAPY

Quality Control

Prior to in vivo administration of an RIT reagent, appropriate quality control needs to be performed and documented. New safety principles continue to emerge for RIT, delaying definitive formulation of quality control procedures (78–80). Toxicity data in several experimental animal species should be obtained. Immunologic potency, microbiologic safety, and the absence of pyrogens in the product should be documented. Impurities (chemical or radioisotope—e.g., unbound isotope) should be explored, defined, and, where necessary, removed.

Systemic Radioimmunoglobulin Therapy

The route of administration is intravenous for most RIT applications as systemic radiotherapy is usually the aim of this approach. All RIT administrations have to be performed in a setting where the appropriate radiation protection precautions can be maintained and the patient can be closely monitored for at least 2 hours after the administration. Rapid infusions (<5 minutes) of large amounts of murine proteins (10 or more mg) can lead to adverse acute reactions, pain, nausea and vomiting, chills, hypotension, and shortness of breath. Side effects are most pronounced after the administration of antibodies with unsuspected cross-reactivity with normal granulocytes (81). Large amounts of polyclonal antibodies have been administered by intravenous push without adverse side effects in many patients (5, 42, 44).

Compartmental Radioimmunoglobulin Therapy

RIT can be limited to a single compartment in the body by using administration routes other than intravenous. This has been attempted for the peritoneal cavity for ovarian and colon cancer (82, 83), for the pleural space filled with a malignant effusion (84), for the leptomeningeal space for leptomeningeal carcinomatosis (85), for liver metastases by hepatic artery infusion (86), by direct injection into malignant skin lesions (87), or by intralymphatic injection of RIT (88). A potential advantage of compartmental RIT is reduced systemic toxicity. After some intraperitoneal administrations, free isotope and/or complete radioimmunoglobulin reached the systemic circulation. When the former occurred, it was due to an yttrium chelation that was unstable in vivo. Free yttrium will be deposited in bone and deposit high radiation doses in bone marrow (89). Obviously, such administrations cannot be recommended, nor the prevention of bone uptake of yttrium by the intravenous administration of a chelating agent such as ethylenediaminetetraacetic acid (EDTA) (90). The latter will enhance kidney elimination of the chelated isotope. However, the correct solution to the problem of unstable immunoconjugate and free isotope is not to use that particular immunoconjugate and to develop an improved chelation method or immunoconjugate that provides a *stable* in vivo product.

One report indicates that radioimmunoglobulin reaches the systemic circulation after intraperitoneal administration but can be removed selectively from the systemic circulation by using neuraminidase-treated radioimmunoglobulin. Removal of sialic acid from the oligosaccharides on the F(c) part of the immunoglobulin will expose galactose. Parenchymal liver cells have a galactose re-

ceptor and remove the radioimmunoglobulin rapidly from the circulation (91). A reversal of the approach could perhaps prevent the hepatic uptake of systemically administered chelated radiolabeled immunoglobulin. Selected oligosaccharides might saturate liver receptors and thereby improve tumor targeting of subsequently injected RIS or RIT reagents (92). Intralymphatic radioactivity administration has been studied extensively in Italian patients with Hodgkin's disease (93). Radioactivity linked to antibodies has been administered intralymphatically in experimental animals (88). A "watershed" mechanism of antibody deposition has been described, in that draining lymph nodes filter out and retain antibody in order: first-echelon nodes first until they are saturated, then second echelon nodes, etc. In most cancers involvement of second-echelon nodes coincides with or is preceded by hematologic metastatic spread. Curative RIT by lymphatic administration would then be limited to cancer stages, in which a primary tumor with only first-echelon lymph node involvement is present. Usually surgery and/or external beam irradiation can provide acceptable curative treatment for such patients, negating the need for intralymphatic RIT. The intralymphatic administration of radiolabeled antibodies remains promising for diagnostic purposes.

DOSIMETRY

Dose Measurements

Progress in the application and development of RIT depends on the proper definition of doses received by important volumes within the body after the injection of radioactivity. Important volumes are tumor and dose-limiting normal tissues. The principles of RIT dosimetry are relatively simple and can be described as a logical sequence of four steps. The first step is the definition of a volume (tumor, organ, or part thereof). The second step is the determination of radioactivity in the volume as a function of time, i.e., sequential activity determination. Steps 1 and 2 permit the calculation of an area under the activity time curve for the volume (the integral of the activity time curve). This is step 3 and determines the "cumulative" activity in the volume. The fourth step is to translate activity into dose. Here one can use the so-called S values from the MIRD (*Medical Internal Radiation Dose*) schema (94). The simplified formula is Dt = A cum × St, in which Dt = the mean dose in the target volume, A cum = the cumulative activity in the target volume, and St = the value that contains all the physical parameters to translate activity in the target volume into dose. The total dose received by the target volume is higher than the calculated dose from the formula just given. Additional doses will be received from other volumes (called source volumes/organs in MIRD). The same formula (D = A × S) can be used for those dose contributions. "A cum" now indicates the cumulative activity in the source organ, and S the S(t ← s) value for the specific combination of source and target organ examined. The total dose received equals the sum of all the different D = A × S calculations. For the localized forms of radiation used in RIT, most of the radiation will come from the target organ itself, while blood is the main source organ delivering extra radiation.

The real problems of RIT dosimetry become apparent if one examines the implementation of the outlined steps 1–4 in more detail.

STEP 1: VOLUME DEFINITION

For the MIRD schema standard normal organ volumes were determined for "model" adults and children. MIRD was developed for diagnostic radioactive reagents. *Only* estimates of radiation doses to normal organs were considered, and "standardized" organs were found to suffice. The higher degree of dose precision desirable for RIT indicates the need for individual, more precise organ volumes in each patients. Computer programs

have been developed that can extract organ or tumor volumes from computerized tomography scan, magnetic resonance imaging scan, and SPECT scan data (95, 96). One of the most important normal tissues for RIT is red bone marrow (the hematopoietic system). Unfortunately, this is not a very "scannable" organ, and volume determinations remain difficult. In addition (see below), tissue inhomogeneities and small volumes complicate bone marrow dosimetry. Blood volume and flow in normal organs and tumors is another problem area in volume determinations.

STEP 2: ACTIVITY DETERMINATION

Accurately weighed biopsy samples can be counted directly in a counter calibrated for the isotope used. Repeated biopsies are required for time activity curves and quickly become an unacceptable burden to a patient. In addition, results of later biopsies might no longer reflect real activity changes due to perturbations induced by the preceding biopsies. The temporary insertion of "mini" thermoluminesence dosimeters (TLDs) circumvents part of the repeated biopsy drawbacks, as a cumulative dose is measured. Quality control in the manufacturing and reading of the TLDs is of vital importance (97). Both sampling by biopsy and TLD are subject to statistical sampling errors. One can also attempt to estimate the activity in a certain volume by external scanning. This requires isotopes emitting gamma irradiation of the appropriate energy (100–200 KeV) and corrections for attenuation. Regular gamma camera, planar front, and back views can be utilized for average organ/volume activities. SPECT scans can determine activities in different regions of the same volume (e.g., a tumor with necrotic as well as better-perfused regions). Dosimetry by external scanning (including SPECT scans) is difficult for volumes that are hard to delineate, such as tumors close to normal tissues containing high amounts of activity such as the large blood vessels in the mediastinum, the heart, or the liver. The problems of extrapolating gamma signals from a radioimmunoconjugate to a dose to be delivered by beta emissions of a similarly chelated antibody that is injected later are discussed in "Radioisotopes," above. All the activity measurements mentioned provide *macro* dosimetry. Dose inhomogeneities will exist over small volumes in critical organs that can be of great biologic importance. For example, endosteal localization of hematopoietic stem cells and hepatic vein endothelium are two radiation-sensitive volumes (or almost surfaces with a complicated geometry) that cannot be evaluated with macro dosimetry (98, 99). Microdosimetry methods, such as autoradiography, still need to be developed for such problems.

STEP 3: DETERMINATION OF CUMULATIVE ACTIVITY

This is completely dependent on the accuracy of the biologic measurements performed under step 2. Integration of the time activity function (consisting of an uptake phase and a monophasic, biphasic, or more complicated elimination phase) will provide the cumulative activity.

STEP 4: S VALUE APPLICATION

S values were determined in phantoms of "model" human beings containing artificially inoculated, homogeneously radioactive organ models. This might not be precise enough for nonmodel RIT patients with inhomogeneous activity distribution in nonstandard organs and tumors. S values for tumor of any size are not available in the MIRD schema and will have to be determined empirically.

Alternative approaches to MIRD calculations have been developed and strive for greater precision (100, 101). The simplest dosimetric assumption is that all the energy released within the target organ will be deposited in that organ. This is probably correct for most beta emitters for most organs.

For bone marrow, enmeshed in an irregular lattice of bone trabeculae of small dimension and surrounded by a thick shell of cortical bone, beta irradiation cannot be classified as nonpenetrating (i.e., all energy deposited in bone marrow). New methods based on the work of Spiers (102, 103) have taken tissue and dose inhomogeneities in bone marrow into account and have probably improved bone marrow dosimetry (103, 104). The current estimates for the precision of RIT dosimetry are the estimated dose plus or minus 50%. Most of the inaccuracy stems from the A (biologic) part of the formula $D = A \times S$ and not from the S (physical) part of the formula (105).

Radiobiologic Comparison

When "physical" dosimetry has been completed satisfactorily, radiobiologic comparisons can be initiated. Comparisons between effects of radiation doses delivered by different methods (e.g., external beam high dose rate and RIT) will allow for the determination of the relative effectiveness of each radiation modality in inducing biologic effects. This information is essential for the extrapolation of the better-known effects of fractionated external beam irradiation to RIT and also essential to the design of new RIT protocols with a better therapeutic ratio. For bone marrow and liver damage in dogs, the relative biologic effectiveness of fractionated, low LET, external beam radiation, and single-injection RIT is approximately equal (36). For tumors, no precise information is available yet. The suspicion is that RIT produces antitumor effects with a slightly lower effectiveness than low LET external beam irradiation (7). Antitumor effects of RIT are probably less susceptible to fractionation than external beam irradiation (18) and section fractionation of RIT. In vitro studies have identified several mechanisms by which RIT can kill cells (Table 5.6). The additional modes of tumor cell killing shown by RIT in comparison to classical high dose rate, low LET irradiation might

Table 5.6. Mechanisms of Cell Killing by Radioimmunoglobulin Therapy

1. Alpha component radiation survival curve
2. G-2 block sensitization by low dose rate
3. Protracted exposure sensitization by very low dose rate
4. Accelerated dose delivery

explain a relatively high biologic effectiveness of RIT. The first mechanism of RIT cell killing is the one defined previously for external beam radiation and described in classical radiation survival curve experiments. The surviving fraction (SF) after radiation is dependent on dose (D) and follows SF = $e^{-(\alpha D + \beta D^2)}$. For low dose rate radiation like RIT the beta component in the formula approaches zero. Cell killing is determined by the alpha component. One would expect RIT to be less effective than external beam irradiation at a high dose rate, due to the absence of a beta component. However, for most tumor cells with an alpha/beta ratio near 10 Gy, RIT is expected to be no more than 20% less effective than 2-Gy fractionated external beam therapy.

A second mechanism (Table 5.6) is associated with the so-called reverse dose rate effect, when a decrease in dose rate will actually increase the number of tumor cells killed. This mechanism can only occur if radiation is protracted over periods of time that are long in comparison to the cell cycle time of the irradiated cells. Therefore, the effect will not be seen after external beam irradiation but is observed regularly after RIT and applies especialy to radioresistant cells such as glioblastoma multiforme cells (106). In some low dose rate ranges cells will not be killed directly by irradiation, but their proliferation will be affected. They progress in the cell cycle until they accumulate in G-2 (so-called G-2 block). G-2, a more radiosensitive part of the cell cycle, can increase the cell killing efficiency of low dose rate radiation up to a factor of eight over an asynchronous cell population (12). High dose rate radiation will reach a given dose earlier than low dose rate radiation and be completed before surviving cells have reached the radiosensitive G-2 phase. The dose rate ranges that induce G-2 block are different for different normal tissues and different tumors, and potential therapeutic advantages cannot be extrapolated yet to clinically encountered situations.

The final and third mechanism of cell killing by RIT (Table 5.6) has only been discovered recently and labeled protracted exposure sensitization (PES). Very low dose rates ($\pm$1–9 cGy/hr) do not kill cells, do not inhibit cell proliferation, and do not induce changes in cell cycle distribution. However, after 1–3 days of very low radiation dose rates, subsequent exposure to high-dose "flash" radiation or high-dose chemotherapy will cause substantialy more cell kill in comparison to control cells that were *not* pretreated with very low dose radiation. PES is the subject of further investigation using normal as well as malignant cells (107).

Another killing mechanism of RIT is by accelerated dose delivery (number 4 in Table 5.6). It appears possible to deposit 30 Gy in Hodgkin's tumors by yttrium-90-labeled antiferritin (5). With a tumor half-life of the radioactivity of approximately 3 days, this will deliver 15 Gy to the tumor in 3 days, instead of 6 Gy by a 2 Gy/day fractionated external beam schedule. The relative contribution of each mechanism listed in Table 5.6 to tumor cell kill and normal tissue damage by RIT remains to be defined. Additional variables of importance for tumor cell kill by RIT are tumor histology and tumor size. Theoretically, it might be possible to improve on the therapeutic ratio of RIT by exploiting the uncovered radiobiologic principles in favor of more tumoricidal effects and less normal tissue damage. Predictive models have been developed to guide such efforts and await preclinical and clinical verification (108, 109).

DOSE (ACTIVITY) ESCALATION

Human Experience

The unusual character of RIT has been a source of confusion for dose escalation studies. In contrast to other potential therapeutic anticancer agents, initial RIT dose escalation studies were performed in human patients, not in experimental animals. The rationale for this daring approach was the assumption that antibody specificity would be important for therapeutic and toxic effects. Therefore, the unique, specific effects of antibody against human antigens could only be evaluated in humans. Additional semantic confusion is caused by the word "dose." For chemotherapeutic agents, "dose" describes the units or milligrams of the agent that are administered. For radiation and a radioisotope, "dose" is defined as the energy deposited in a volume of interest. In this respect, one needs to change the expression utilized by medical oncologists—of dose or dose escalation—to administered (radio) activity or activity escalation for RIT reagents. Dosimetric studies will be needed to determine the dose escalations that can be accomplished by RIT activity escalation.

Three human studies have been performed with activity escalation, one in hepatocellular carcinoma with iodine-131, one in B cell lymphoma with iodine-131, and one in Hodgkin's disease with yttrium-90 (5, 110, 111). None of the studies demonstrates a clearcut positive correlation between administered activity and tumor response. In contrast, a positive correlation was found between administered activity and normal tissue toxicity: All three studies show that higher activities lead to more bone marrow toxicity. The difference between tumor and normal tissue results is due to the unpredictability of tumor targeting and the fact that activity escalation will not always lead to tumor dose escalation. Another problem is that the doses that can be delivered to tumors with the current RIT technology are probably at the very beginning of the upslope of the dose-effect curve. In this region, the curve is relatively flat, and *many* patients per dose level will be needed to demonstrate significant differences in tumor response. The initial human activity escalation studies consist of small numbers of patients. In the hepatoma study, activity escalation was considered to cause "tumor saturation" by larger amounts of administered antibody. Fractionated RIT (day 0, day 5) was thought to have a better therapeutic ratio than single-fraction RIT because the tumor would receive a higher total amount of radioactivity by two split injections. In Hodgkin's patients, 20 mCi of yttrium-labeled antiferritin caused the same amount of bone marrow aplasia with or without the infusion of autologous bone marrow cells 18–20 days after the yttrium administration. After 30 and 40 mCi of yttrium, a bone marrow transplant appeared to shorten bone marrow aplasia (Fig. 5.7). Bone marrow transplants were also performed in patients with B cell lymphomas who did not show signs of bone marrow regeneration 1 month or later after isotope injection (111). Bone marrow transplantation appears to allow for activity escalation in man. The next ("second-level") activity-limiting normal tissue has not been defined yet in man, and the potential advantages of activity escalation for tumoricidal effects remain to be demonstrated.

Experimental Animal Experience

In contrast to prior beliefs, RIT activity escalation studies can be useful in animals, in particular for normal tissue toxicity. For that purpose antibody preparations have to be modified to obtain the same in vivo distribution as in human patients, for example, by making a similar reagent comparing rabbit antidog ferritin in dogs to rabbit antihuman ferritin in man or by taking advantage of cross-reactivity between species, in which the same reagent can be used in both species. Antibodies against human antigens can cross-react with similar antigens of many different species but will most commonly do so with antigens of subhuman primates (112, 113). In addition, larger animals than mice and rats need to be used for experimentation as the only way in which the dose distributions encountered in human patients can be approx-

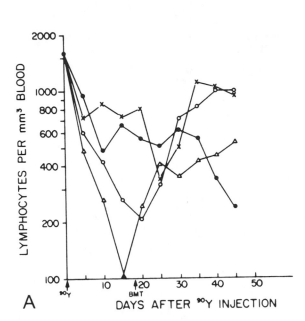

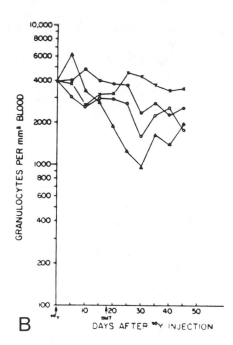

Figure 5.7. Lymphocyte (**A**) and granulocyte (**B**) levels in the peripheral blood of Hodgkin's patients after RIT with yttrium-labeled polyclonal antiferritin. O = 20 mCi, BMT = bone marrow transplantation. (O) 20 mCi; BMT −; (●) 20 mCi; BMT +; (X) 30 mCi; BMT +; (△) 40 mCi; BMT +

imated. Biodistribution of reagents and dose distribution within organs need to be observed and compared in different species to select the animal model most relevant to the human patient. In experimental animals activity escalation studies have been pushed to higher activities per kilogram than in man, and second-level activity limiting tissues have been defined. In mice, rats, and dogs, bone marrow remains the first-level activity-limiting tissue. The RIT effects observed in the peripheral blood of experimental animals are similar to the ones observed in human patients. Within 24 hours after injection, lymphocytes decrease. This appears to be due to blood rdioactivity and direct irradiation of peripheral blood lymphocytes. This almost immediate mode of death of lymphocytes has been labeled interphase death or apoptosis (114). If the amount of radioactivity is expressed per kilogram body weight, similar activities will lead to similar degrees of lymphopenia in different species (36). Several days

after the start of RIT and the start of lymphopenia, platelet and granulocyte levels decrease. The delay is caused by a different mode of cell death (radiation damage expressed in mitosis) and by the so-called bone marrow transit time (115, 116). RIT damages hematopoietic stem cells in red marrow, while the more differentiated blood cells in blood and bone marrow are radiation resistant. The damage to stem cells in the bone marrow will show up in the peripheral blood (granulopenia, thrombopenia) after the marrow transit time (the time it takes a stem cell to produce granulocytes or platelets) and the survival time of granulocytes and platelets in the peripheral blood have elapsed. Similar levels of granulopenia will be found in different species if the administered activity per kilogram is corrected for the hematopoietic stem cell concentration in the bone marrow for each species (36).

In rats activity escalation beyond the activity leading to lethal bone marrow damage with yttrium-labeled rabbit antirat ferritin leads to lethal gastrointestinal toxicity. In a dose-survival study of total body irradiation with cobalt-60, a considerable gap is found between the dose killing 50% of the rats from a bone marrow syndrome (5.5 Gy) and the dose killing 50% of the rats from a gastrointestinal syndrome (12 Gy). The bone marrow and gastrointestinal syndrome are much closer together in the RIT activity-survival study in rats (34, 107). One possible explanation for this observation is that the energy released by yttrium-90 in the bone marrow is not all absorbed in the bone marrow. The range of the yttrium beta emission and the small volumes in the rat bone marrow might lead to the absorption of radiation outside the bone marrow parenchyma. This would increase the activity needed to cause 50% mortality for the bone marrow syndrome and bring it closer to the activity required to induce a gastrointestinal syndrome. Other explanations such as the induction by RIT of radiation resistance in hematopoietic stem cells are the subject of further investigation and outside the scope of this review.

In dogs, activity escalations were performed with bone marrow transplantation, and other second-rank activity-limiting tissues could be identified. As to be expected, the second-rank activity-limiting tissues are dependent on the pharmacokinetics of the injected activity. Early studies with DTPA-chelated yttrium-90 demonstrated rapid kidney/urine elimination of the radioactivity and radiation damage to the kidney. After administration of activities higher than the one leading to kidney failure, gastrointestinal damage and early death were observed (117, 118; Table 5.7). More recent activity escalation studies with yttrium-90-labeled rabbit antidog ferritin and bone marrow transplantation identified the liver as the second-rank dose-limiting tissue under these circumstances. Approximately 15% of the injected activity ended up in the liver, depositing approximately 50 Gy there after 4 mCi/kg. This led to clinicaly detectable ascites and ele-

Table 5.7. Second-Rank Activity Limiting Normal Tissues in Dogs

1. Yttrium-90 DTPA (+ intravenously recycled urine for first 4 hours after initial administration)

Lethality	mCi yttrium/kg
Bone marrow	4
Kidney	5.5 (+ bone marrow transplantation)
Gastrointestinal	7

2. Yttrium-90 antiferritin (intravenous)

Lethality	mCi yttrium/kg
Bone marrow	2.5
Liver	4 (+ bone marrow transplantation)

vated alkaline phosphatase and liver enzyme levels in serum, but no icterus, increase in serum bilirubin, or decrease in serum protein concentrations. Animals died 150–200 days after injection of the radioimmunoglobulin. Classical veno-occlusive disease of the liver (VOD) was seen histologically in the liver at autopsy (36). The activities administered per kg body weight in the dog studies are approximately 10-fold higher than the maximum activities given to human patients. Thus it is not surprising that second-rank activity-limiting normal tissues have not been encountered yet in man. The therapeutic ratio of activity-escalated RIT might be so poor in human patients that only lower activities will be applied routinely, and second-rank dose-limiting tissues would never become an issue.

Bone Marrow Toxicity

Three manipulative procedures have been used to mitigate bone marrow toxicity after RIT. Bone marrow transplantation, the administration of hematopoietic hormones (colony-stimulating factors [CSF] and interleukins), and fractionation. Results obtained in dogs treated with RIT with or without granulocyte-CSF(G-CSF) are given in Figure 5.8. G-CSF clearly decreases the period of granulopenia. Thrombopenia and lymphopenia were of similar length in G-CSF treated

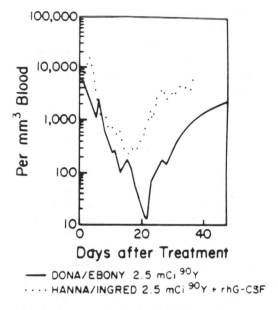

Figure 5.8. Granulocyte levels of dogs after intravenous yttrium labeled rabbit antidog ferritin. Daily 10 µg/kg human recombinant G-CSF given subcutaneously.

and control animals. Of special interest are the early granulocytosis (day 1–4) after RIT in G-CSF treated animals and the similar timing and severity of the initial granulopenia in the two groups of dogs in Figure 5.8. This appears to indicate that RIT causes the same amount of hematopoietic stem cell damage in the two groups and corroborates that RIT bone marrow damage is indeed at the hematopoietic stem cell level. G-CSF, in contrast, appears not to influence stem cells but rather early progenitor cells committed to the granulocyte lineage. In studies of Rhesus monkeys after different doses of external beam total body irradiation (TBI), CSFs were only effective in accelerating hematopoietic recovery after low or intermediate doses of TBI (119). Similarly, one would anticipate that hematopoietic hormones could only be of help after intermediate-activity RIT. After high-activity RIT only bone marrow transplantation would be of help. The timing of the bone marrow transplant is a special problem after RIT. After high-dose external beam irradiation to the whole body, bone marrow cells

are transplanted within 24 hours of the completion of the irradiation. Early bone marrow transplants after RIT will be ineffective as the transfused hematopoietic stem cells will receive too much radiation. Dog studies appear to indicate that bone marrow transplantation should be delayed until the dose rate in the bone marrow is below 1 cGy/hr (36, 120). The LD_{50} for the bone marrow syndrome of continuously irradiated beagles was not influenced by dose rate until it fell to approximately 0.6 cGy/hr. At lower dose rates animals were able to repopulate their bone marrow during irradiation (Fig. 5.9). Such animals did succumb at a later date to radiation-induced myeloproliferative disorders (120). The dose rate in the bone marrow is dependent on bone marrow targeting (i.e., initial activity in bone marrow), isotope used,

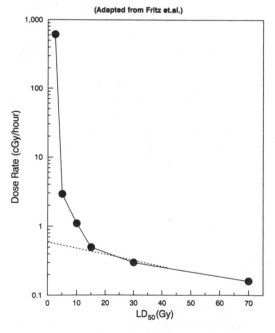

Figure 5.9. LD_{50} of beagle dogs after continuous total body irradiation at different dose rates. (Adapted from Fritz TE, Norris WP, Tolle VP, et al. Relationship of dose rate and total dose to responses of continuously irradiated beagles. In: Late biological effects of ionizing radiation. Vol. 2. IAEA-SM-2241/206. Vienna: International Atomic Energy Agency, 1978:71–83.)

activity injected, and the effective half-life of the radiolabeled immunoglobulin in bone marrow. Intense bone marrow targeting, high injected activities, high S values, and long effective half-lives all prevent early administration of bone marrow cells. In mice bone marrow transplants were ineffective 4 days after the administration of a lethal activity of gold-198 (121). In a more recent mouse study yttrium-90-labeled antibodies and a huge bone marrow cell dose were used. Bone marrow transplantation was effective around day 5 after isotope administration and became less effective from day 10 onward (122). These data are hard to extrapolate to species where such an overdose in bone marrow cells cannot be obtained, e.g., man. In dogs bone marrow transplants were effective 10 days after a supralethal activity of yttrium-90-labeled antiferritin (36). In man the shortest interval between yttrium-90 and bone marrow transplantation has been 12 days (K.A. Dicke, personal communication, 30 mCi total activity with good hematopoietic reconstitution). At some point after RIT bone marrow transplantation will become superfluous. Bone marrow transplantation can be too late to reverse complications of long-standing bone marrow aplasia, or the patient will have regenerated its own hematopoietic system. Transplanted bone marrow cells are just as sensitive as in situ bone marrow cells (123). The choice to use bone marrow transplantation after RIT is also influenced by the possibility of inducing leukemia by RIT (124). The transplantation of cryopreserved, unirradiated bone marrow cells might prevent the induction of leukemia.

Another problem of high activity RIT followed by bone marrow transplantation might be the radiation dose received by the blood-bone marrow barrier. Specific lectins on the endothelial barrier between blood and bone marrow parenchyma are expected to interact with galactosyl moieties of hematopoietic stem cell membranes to negotiate the "homing" of intravenous hematopoietic stem cells into the bone marrow (125). In Table 5.8, data are given that indicate that in dogs 5.5 mCi/kg of yttrium-90 polyclonal rabbit antiferritin will damage the blood-bone marrow barrier. Only after this high administered activity will initial bone marrow activity become higher than blood activity. Rabbit antidog ferritin is not actively deposited in dog marrow. At lower injected activities, the higher hydrostatic pressure in extravascular bone marrow spaces will decrease the diffusion of antiferritin from the low-pressure bone marrow blood vessels (126). After the highest injected activity, the pressure in the extravascular bone marrow space will decrease due to blood-bone marrow barrier damage, and the antiferritin will diffuse into the marrow more easily. Such damage might also interfere with homing by changing the lectin configuration on the endothelial barrier that is required for interaction with galactose on hematopoietic stem cells. So far only *autologous* bone marrow cells have been used for transplantation. If *allogeneic* bone marrow cells were to be required for rescue after high-activity RIT, the immunosuppressive effects of the RIT reagent used would have to be defined to determine whether they would allow for a successful allogeneic transplant and, if so, at what cell dose. Allogeneic bone marrow transplantation would not be effective after RIT administrations with little or no immunosuppressive effects, because the transplanted bone marrow cells would be rejected. With moderately immunosuppressive RIT reagents, the residual rejection potential of the host might be overcome by a high dose of bone marrow cells (127).

Table 5.8. Bone Marrow and Peripheral Blood Radioactivity after IV Yttrium-90–Labeled Antiferritin in Dogs

Injected (μCi/gm)	Initial Blood Activity (μCi/ml)	Initial Bone Marrow Activity per μCi Injected
1.0	0.96	0.59
2.5	1.07	0.97
4.0	1.01	0.92
5.5	1.07	1.22

Other organ systems—not discussed in this section—might become important in RIT toxicology if new reagents are identified with high targeting in organs, such as lung, pancreas, adrenals, etc.

FRACTIONATION OF RADIO-IMMUNOGLOBULIN THERAPY

Normal Tissues

In this review the concept of fractionation is applied to radioimmunoconjugate applications within one cycle. Repeated RIT cycles will not be considered as fractionation. The time interval available for fractionation of RIT in one cycle is limited for several reasons:

1. The host immune response can produce antidonor immunoglobulin antibodies within 8–10 days after injection of the antigen. Fractionation of RIT beyond 8 days after the first injection runs the risks of treatment being adversely affected by antiantibodies.
2. Bone marrow aplasia will be induced by the first RIT injection. Bone marrow regeneration will be delayed by subsequent RIT injections. A long interval between the first and last injection will correlate with long bone marrow depression and the toxicities thereof.
3. Bone marrow transplantation can only be helpful if the bone marrow insult is given over a short period of time and relieved as early as possible by bone marrow transplantation.

In beagle dogs, yttrium-90-labeled B72.3 injections have been compared in three groups of animals—single shot and two equally divided activity administrations on days 0 and 4 or days 0 and 8. Bone marrow toxicity was decreased by at least 15%–20% in the fractionated schedule. This is a surprising result as one would anticipate bone marrow toxicity to be dependent on total dose only and not on dose rate or fractionation (116, 120). Possible explanations for the sparing effect of RIT on bone marrow toxicity are repopulation of stem cells between fractions and/or the induction of radiation resistance by the first RIT fraction in stem cells that survive this fraction. These mechanisms are being explored in further ongoing experiments. Liver toxicity was expected and indeed found to be decreased by fractionation by about 75% (Fig. 5.10; 128). In mouse studies two or three fractionated, weekly RIT injections cause less bone marrow damage than the same total activity given in a single shot (53, 129).

Tumor Cells

Normal cells can be protected by RIT fractionation. The therapeutic ratio of RIT would be improved by fractionation if the cumulative activity in the tumor would remain the same or increase by fractionation, compared to single-shot administration, and cause similar or more extensive tumor eradication. This information is not available yet. In patients with hepatocellular carcinoma, two injections separated by 5 days seem to lead to higher total cumulative tumor activities than a single injection giving the same total radioactivity in one shot. The proposed hypothesis that temporary tumor saturation by antibody occurred after the first injection is interesting and deserves further scrutiny (110). In nude mice with s/c human colon cancer cells fractionated RIT (once a week for three times) has about the same tumoricidal effect as the same activity given as a single shot. Thus the therapeutic ratio of the fractionated RIT procedure is higher due to significantly decreased bone marrow toxicity (53, 129). Fractionation effects are expected to be different for different tumors and different normal tissues. Optimal fractionation schedules of RIT might have to be developed for each tumor type/reagent and tumor stage.

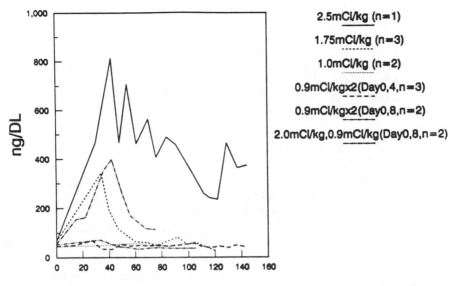

Figure 5.10. Alkaline phosphatase levels in dogs after intravenous yttrium-90-labeled B72.3.

COMBINED MODALITIES AND RADIOIMMUNOGLOBULIN THERAPY

Surgery

The resectability of primary tumor or tumor metastases is determined by preoperative diagnostic studies. During surgery tumor often looks and feels different from surrounding tissues. Subsequent resection is guided initially by the eye, hand, and mind of the surgeon. The completeness of the resection can be checked in the operating room by a provisional microscopic and histologic evaluation of resection margins. If tumor deposits can be targeted with radiolabeled immunoglobulin prior to surgery, the surgeon could use a dosimeter with a small aperture during surgery to identify suspicious areas or margins and adjust the resection margins more effectively during surgery. The feasibility of this approach has been confirmed and reported (130, 131). Studies are ongoing to define the potential role of radiolabeled antibodies in cancer surgery.

External Beam Radiation

Prior external beam irradiation at a modest dose can increase the uptake of subsequently injected radiolabeled antibodies. Presumably, this is based on endothelial changes induced by the external beam irradiation (132, 133). The dose required and the duration of the induced changes have only been defined provisionally (133, 134). The reverse—RIT preceding external beam irradiation—might also offer improvements in tumor control. As previously discussed, tumor cells can become more sensitive to radiation after protracted irradiation due either to accumulation of cells in the G-2 phase of the cell cycle or PES. Thus, especially for radioresistant cells (that do show G-2 block), RIT might enhance the response to subsequent external beam irradiation. Just the addition of RIT to external beam irradiation ("RIT boost") might be helpful in increasing local control. RIT and localized external beam irradiation do not have overlapping dose-limiting toxicity, and the therapeutic ratio of the combination should be excellent.

Chemotherapy

PES may also enhance the effects of systemic chemotherapy. Combination of two systemic modalities—RIT and chemotherapy—is worth considering, if they have different modes of action, different normal tissue side effects, and complementary effectiveness in tumor control. The mode of action of radiation differs from the various mechanisms by which chemotherapeutic agents kill tumor cells. Most chemotherapeutic agents will have bone marrow toxicity as the dose-limiting side effect (as with RIT). However, RIT might be more effective for controlling larger (>1 cm) tumor masses and have less of an effect on smaller tumor masses that have insufficient tumor neovasculature or insufficient antigen to attract the radiolabeled antibody. Chemotherapy is well known to be more effective against small tumor masses than large tumor masses (e.g., adjuvant chemotherapy). This therefore offers potential complementary action of the two modalities, RIT improving control of large tumor masses, chemotherapy sterilizing small tumor clumps. In hepatocellular carcinoma, a solid tumor, combinations of RIT and chemotherapy have been tested in large numbers of human patients (135). Unfortunately, the sensitivity of this tumor to chemotherapy and RIT is so low, that even the combined modality approach is of limited effectiveness. For the same reason, no conclusions are possible on whether the combination is more effective than either modality alone. Poor prognosis, refractory Hodgkin's disease offers a more analytical situation. Preliminary information comes from an ongoing trial at the University of Nebraska—20 to 30 mCi of polyclonal yttrium-labeled antiferritin, followed by cyclophosphamide (high dose), carmustine (BCNU), and, etoposide (VP-16) (CBV) and autologous bone marrow transplantation (K.A. Dicke, personal communication). Early results indicate that the toxicity of the combined program is similar to the toxicity of the CBV program alone. Early survival and tumor control are improved slightly in the combined program.

Hyperthermia

Hyperthermia is most effective in larger tumors, where poorly perfused tumor areas will maintain higher temperatures than well-perfused normal tissue or tumor that lose more heat from convection. In contrast, RIT will be more effective in well-perfused tumors. Again, a combination of the complementary effects of the two modalities might provide the best end result, i.e., more effective tumor control. In addition, hyperthermia might improve the uptake of radiolabeled antibody by improving perfusion. Hyperthermia will, however, not discriminate in that respect between normal tissues and tumor, possibly increasing normal tissue damage via RIT. In vitro studies indicate a much stronger interaction between low dose rate, protracted radiation, and hyperthermia than between acutely delivered radiation and hyperthermia (136, 137). Enhanced cell kill by low dose rate irradiation is also observed after hyperthermia protocols using temperatures between $37°$ and $40°$ C that are not tumoricidal on their own (138). If these observations can be confirmed in animal studies, further opportunities for clinical applications of the combination of RIT and hyperthermia would arise. Various centers have begun analysis of combined RIT and hyperthermia in experimental animal models (139, 140).

Interleukins

Many different (over nine at last count) interleukins have been identified. They are part of a larger group of diverse substances, identified by the general term "biologic response modifiers" (141). The initial identification of effects of interleukins has been within the immunohematopoietic system. However, cells from many other systems, such as endothelial cells and fibroblasts, are influenced by interleukins. Many permutations are possible between interleukins and RIT, and most remain to be investigated. It has been shown that some interleukins will increase expression of some cell membrane antigens (142). This might improve targeting of RIT reagents specific for such antigens. Studies in cancer patients indicate that endothelial damage ("vascular leak" syndrome) can be induced by interleukin-2 (IL-2) (143). This might facilitate access of the antibody to interstitial antigens. In experimental animals, tumor uptake of a RIT reagent was increased by a factor of four if both IL-2 and the radioisotope were conjugated to the same immunoglobulin (13).

MODELS FOR RADIOIMMUNOGLOBULIN THERAPY ANALYSIS

The development of RIT reagents for clinical application is a multistep process. The purpose is to identify unpromising reagents early and to limit the more time-consuming and expensive preclinical testing to the better reagents. *In vitro* RIT reagents have to pass basic safety and quality control criteria (immunologic specificity, chemical parity, microbiologic safety, and serum stability studies) (see also section "Administration of RIT reagents"). Additional in vitro tests include the confirmation of reagent tumor binding by evaluation of antibody on histologic slides of patients with the relevant tumor and verification of the absence of reagent binding to normal human tissues. Radiobiologic studies can be performed in cell cultures admixed with radiolabeled immunoglobulin or exposed to external beam radiation with dose rate patterns that mimic radiolabeled antibodies. Dillehay and Williams at Johns Hopkins have successfully designed and operated such an external beam irradiator (106).

In vivo testing of RIT reagents becomes rapidly more expensive than bench testing of cells and slides due to animal costs and higher costs of the isotopes with increased activities. Three areas of interest are pharmacokinetics, normal tissue toxicity, and tumor targeting. Small experimental animals can be used to obtain time-activity curves for all major organs by killing three or four animals at predetermined time points after RIT administration (e.g., 1, 12, 24, 48, and 96 hours after injection). The hepatoma models in rats have been very helpful in delineation of some of the specificity questions in RIT and the role played by tumor neovasculature (20, 21, 134). In larger animals, fewer animals are used and longitudinal studies (repeated biopsies in single animals) are performed. Minor modifications of a standard RIT product are best tested in small animals first. Only the more promising modifications will be further analyzed in large animal experimental models. Some characteristics are only available in larger animals (e.g., liver uptake of chelated monoclonal antibodies [36]) or cross-reactivity of antihuman lymphocyte antibodies with Rhesus monkey or chimpanzee lymphocyte antigens (112, 113).

Normal tissue toxicity is best analyzed in models that correlate well with the experience in human patients. Three aspects—(*a*) deposition of antibody, (*b*) geometry of organ and dose distribution, and (*c*) nature of normal organ responses—are of importance in preclinical toxicology. Deposition of antibody and the geometry of organ and dose distribution in human patients are most easily reproduced in *larger* experimental animals (dog, pig, monkey). The hematopoietic system and the liver of the dog appear to respond to RIT in a manner that resembles the known or anticipated response in man (36). The dog offers the additional advantage of allowing for similar individual intensive clinical care as is available to human patients. Intensive care and longitudinal studies become an important issue in activity escalation studies.

Tumor targeting can be studied in transplantable or spontaneously occurring tumors in animals. The closest approximation to the human cancer patient is the nude mouse with subcutaneously implanted human cancer cells grown out to a palpable and scannable tumor nodule. This model will overestimate the specificity of the RIT reagent and will not always predict for effective targeting in human patients (36). In addition to targeting tests, however, therapeutic trials can be performed in this model, and mechanisms that could improve human RIT can be identified. The human cancer patient with previously defined tumor masses (anatomic location and volume) is the ultimate targeting test for RIT reagents. New RIT treatment protocols are best performed in cancer patients with refractory disease for which no other curative treatment is available and in whom RIT has a chance to work (i.e., give a measurable response and increase in survival time) as a single agent. Currently, studies in patients with refractory Hodgkin's disease appear to offer such an opportunity. Patients with refractory lymphomas, in general, and, in the near future perhaps, patients with metastatic breast cancer provide additional possibilities for study. Tumor response, normal tissue toxicity, and the therapeutic ratio can be determined in RIT-sensitive patients. In RIT-resistant patients, tumor responses will be rare and minor, not providing enough information for the determination of a therapeutic ratio and the improvement of RIT. At some stage in the development of a RIT reagent, decisions have to be made on modifications of the immunoglobulin structure (e.g., fragment, chimeric antibody, humanization). In the absence of a clear-cut advantage of any of these modifications and in view of the great time and expense involved with the introduction of these modifications, it appears to be wise to wait with such investments until results obtained with complete antibodies indicate that antibody changes are required to solve one or all of the encountered problems.

RADIOIMMUNOGLOBULIN THERAPY RESULTS IN MAN

Solid Tumors

Cold monoclonal antibodies have been utilized in solid tumors. Results were re-viewed recently for melanoma and gastrointestinal malignancies (44). In a single melanoma study, 6 of 21 tumor responses were seen, while essentially no responses were seen in 45 additional patients. The most successful study utilized an IgG_3 antibody, which can be a mediating antibody for cellular cytotoxicity with human effector cells (144). The other reagents used did not have that capability. Essentially no tumoricidal effects were noted after the administration of cold antibodies to patients with gastrointestinal malignancies (145). Iodine-131 labeled F(ab) fragments with antimelanoma specificity showed reasonable targeting, but only one response was seen in 16 patients treated (146). In patients with other solid tumors, iodine-131 was again the most commonly used isotope (Table 5.9). In general, liver metastases of colon cancer are not readily imaged or treated with radioactively labeled CEA (154). Therefore, the quoted RIT study from Switzerland is remarkably successful. In 2 of 4 patients with liver metastases from colon cancer that receive intraarterial RIT and beta blockade (propranolol), a significant objective response is seen. The role of the latter drug is not clear. In recurrent ovarian cancer, bulky intraperitoneal tumors appear to be RIT resistant.

The yttrium immunoconjugate used in patients with prior ovarian cancer and a high chance for a recurrence is difficult to evaluate for antitumor effects, as the patients had no evidence of disease at the start of the RIT study. The radioimmunoconjugate in this study appears to be unstable in vivo and causes serious bone marrow toxicity. The RIT studies in liver and bile duct cancer patients (Table 5.9) are part of multimodality regimens; the contribution of RIT to response rates is unclear and might have been overestimated in the past. The brain tumor study with iodine-125 is of special interest, as it is one of the few clinical RIT studies using an isotope with a very limited range of energy deposition. Theoretically, the halogenated antibody used in this study will be internalized through the epidermal growth factor (EGF) receptor on

Table 5.9. Radioimmunoglobulin Therapy Results in Solid Tumors in Man

Tumor Type	Isotope & Antibody	Response Rate	Comments	Reference
Melanoma	I-131 Fab, p97	1/16	Good targeting but minimal responses	146
Colon	I-131 B7-25/35	2/4	Liver metastases, intraarterial RIT,	147
	I-125 CO171A	1/53	β blockade	148
Ovary	I-131 3 monoclonals	9/24	Intraperitoneal RIT, better	82, 149
	Y-90 HMFG1	12/13 NED	responses in small-volume disease	
			Adjuvant i.p. RIT, unstable chelation, bone marrow toxicity	90
Liver	I-131 polyclonal antiferritin	52/108	Multimodality treatment: external beam 7 × 3 = 21 Gy and Adriamycin and 5-fluorouracil, plus RIT	135
Bile duct	I-131 polyclonal anti-CEA	10/37	Multimodality treatment: external beam 7 × 3 = 21 Gy and Adriamycin and 5-fluorouracil plus RIT	150
Brain astrocytoma	I-125 antiepidermal growth factor receptor-425	3/15	Failure after prior cranial x-ray treatment	151
leptomeningeal carcinomatosis	I-131 5 monoclonals	6/9	12+ months response durations, selection of 1 RIT reagent for each tumor type, 20–60 mCi	85
Neuroblastoma	I-131 UJ13A	1/4	Difficult tumor volume determination	152, 153

the cell membrane. The response rates noted in the initial study in poor-prognosis, recurrent patients are encouraging. A phase 2 study is ongoing with this reagent. The RIT responses in patients with leptomeningeal carcinomatosis are long and exceed expectations based on historical controls treated with more conventional modalities for this grim oncologic condition. RIT in neuroblastoma patients has been replaced by iodine-131 meta iodobenzyl guanidine (MIBG) trials, in the hope that pharmacologic targeting is going to be as successful for this disease as iodine-131 treatment for thyroid cancer (155).

Leukemia and Lymphoma

Cold antibodies have been utilized in limited numbers of patients (44). The best response rates are seen in T cell lymphoma (approximately 25%). Response durations are short (3 to 4 months). Neither B cell lym-

phomas nor chronic lymphocytic leukemia (CLL) have responded to cold monoclonal antibodies so far, with the exception of some patients treated with antiidiotypic antibodies (14). Radiolabeled antibodies have been utilized in patients with relapsed acute myeloid leukemia in a phase 1 study of iodine-131-labeled M195. No responses were seen in 10 patients (156). In Table 5.10 RIT response rates are listed for refractory lymphoma patients. Hodgkin's disease and B cell lymphomas are probably more responsive than T cell lymphoma. The high response rates and the high activities administered indicate that in these diseases, RIT is highly active as a *single* agent and considered of interest for activity escalation studies. Optimalization of RIT reagents for tumoricidal effects and normal tissue toxicity is best performed in cautious further studies in patients with B cell lymphoma or Hodgkin's disease. The results obtained with intravenously administered MB-1 antibodies

Table 5.10. Radioimmunoglobulin Therapy Results in Lymphoma Patients

Tumor Type	Isotope & Antibody	Response Rate	Comments	Reference
B cell lymphoma				
1	I-131 LYM 1	10/18	60 mCi every 2–6 weeks until 300 mCi total; 2 complete remissions	157
2	I-131 MB1 or 1F5	5/5	5 additional patients failed to target 250–600 mCi × 1 with bone marrow transplantation	111
3	I-131 LL2	2/7	20–60 mCi	158
4	Y-90 anti Id	2/4	10–20 mCi	159
T-cell cutaneous lymphoma	I-131 T101	2/5	100–150 mCi, antigen modulation and dehalogenation	160
Hodgkin's disease				
1	I-131 polyclonal antiferritin	15/37	30 + 20 mCi; long bone marrow aplasia	161
2	Y-90 polyclonal antiferritin	22/36	20–50 mCi, bone marrow transplantation helpful more complete remissions (10) than with I-131 (1); five additional patients did not target	5

indicate that high amounts of protein (antibodies) saturate extravascular tumors better than low amounts (10 mg/kg versus 0.2 mg/kg). The antiferritin results indicate the role bone marrow transplantation can play in further RIT development (Fig. 5.7). B cell lymphoma and Hodgkin's disease patients offer the additional advantage of rarely making antibodies against the donor immunoglobulin. Obviously, many questions remain, and lymphoma patients provide exciting opportunities for further study.

The therapeutic ratio of RIT in man has been very satisfactory. Patients treated with RIT will indicate repeatedly and spontaneously that RIT compares very favorably to their previous cancer treatments, which usually include all other modalities (surgery, external beam irradiation, and multiagent chemotherapy). This is such a rewarding aspect of RIT for patients as well as their physicians that it is of utmost importance to preserve or even further improve upon the therapeutic ratio of RIT in future studies in man.

SUMMARY AND CONCLUSIONS

RIT appears to have become a viable new addition to existing cancer treatment modalities. Cold unlabeled antibodies appear to be insufficient for reproducible, clinically significant, tumoricidal effects. The addition of a radioisotope to the antibody or fragment appears to improve the analytical as well as the tumoricidal possibilities of the reagents. The slow development of RIT is due to the need for many interdisciplinary interactions that require a fairly large critical mass in terms of appropriate personnel and resources. The nuclear medicine physicians and radiation oncologists involved in this new field have to adjust to caring for patients undergoing intensive systemic cancer therapy. Some of the encountered problems have a semantic base (activity versus dose) or are based on different traditions in different disciplines. The recommended prescription method for intravenous RIT activity is per body weight, not per square meter of body surface area and not in total activity. The limited effectiveness of current RIT makes it necessary to report response rates and response durations. With improved RIT, radiation oncologists can return to the more familiar endpoints of survival and local control. The most important contribution of RIT in multimodality regimens might be improved control of bulky disease. Adjuvant applications of RIT are hard to justify under the present (imperfect) state of the art. Adjuvant studies of RIT are moreover hard to analyze or optimize, as tumor targeting and tumor dosimetry studies are usually not possible.

The limitations of RIT and, therefore, the directions for research efforts in improving RIT are clear: (a) increase deposition of radioactivity in the tumor, (b) decrease radiation exposure of normal tissues, and (c) decrease antiantibody formation. Isotope uptake in human tumors can be improved by removing the current limitations on the use of monoclonal antibodies for therapeutic applications in man. Promising leads for improvement are changes in the immunoglobulin molecule itself (such as bifunctional antibodies, changes in the F(c) part of the immunoglobulin), or changes in the chemical linkage between isotope and immunoglobulin. Normal tissue toxicity can be alleviated by bone marrow transplants, hematopoietic growth factors, protection of second-rank activity-limiting organs (liver, kidney), and fractionation of RIT. The ideal solution for the prevention of antiantibody formation would be the induction of specific immunologic tolerance for the RIT reagent. This will be accomplished more easily for small antigenic differences (humanized antibodies) than for large antigenic differences between antibody donor and host. The section on models for RIT study describes the usual chain of events in the development of a RIT reagent—laboratory bench, histologic slides of human cancers, nude mice and rats, radiotoxicity in dogs, clinical trials in B cell lymphoma or Hodgkin's disease. RIT is a refreshing exception to the philosophy developed for dose escalation of other cancer modalities. War metaphors ("blast," "superaggressive treatment," "heroic," etc.) are used to describe and justify treatments that can cure patients from previously considered lethal disorders. These same treatments, however, due to indiscriminate dose escalation, lead to high morbidity and mortality figures (>10%) from normal tissue damage. Normal tissue damage induced by anticancer agents is measured more easily and earlier in the course of treatment than anticancer effects. A potentially dangerous sequel to this state of affairs is that some physicians will see the normal tissue toxicity as a laudable aim of the treatment ("no pain, no gain"), rather than a potentially avoidable complication. RIT might become an important tool in decreasing normal tissue toxicity, while increasing tumor control. If so, it would make an enormous contribution in breaking the vicious and unproductive cycle of ever-increasing doses of cancer therapy with ever-decreasing yields for patients (little gain in tumor control and survival, steep increases in normal tissue complications).

A promising new modality has a certain ill-defined grace period, in which the scientific community is eager and optimistic regarding new applications. The scientific framework for an expeditious development of RIT appears to be in place and should guarantee the survival of RIT after the expiration of its grace period. The attraction and challenge of RIT are that further improvements are attainable by the implementation of previously proven scientific principles. Activity (dose) escalation of RIT might lead to better tumor control without extra morbidity and mortality. This sets RIT apart from other currently available cancer treatment modalities and underlines the urgent need for further studies. RIT research is an excellent investment, as it promises to deliver outpatient systemic cancer treatment with a better therapeutic ratio than previously used cancer chemotherapeutic agents. The resources required for expeditious development of RIT, however, are considerable and diverse. For the immediate future, RIT studies will probably remain limited to academic oncology centers that are willing and able to master these resource and team problems effectively.

REFERENCES

1. Vriesendorp HM, van Bekkum DW. Susceptibility to total body irradiation. In: Broerse JJ, MacVittie TJ, eds. Response to total body irradiation in different species. Boston: Martinus Nijhoff, 1984:43–53.
2. Vriesendorp HM. Prediction of effects of therapeutic total body irradiation. Radiat Oncol 1990;18(suppl 1):37–50.
3. Beierwalter WH. Therapy of thyroid carcinoma with 131-I. In: Spencer PP, Seevers RH Jr, Friedman AM, eds. Radionuclides in therapy. Boca Raton, FL: CRC Press, 1987:19–46.
4. Rawson RW, Rall JE, Peacock W. Limitations and indications in treatment of cancer of thyroid with radioactive iodine. J Clin Endocrinol 1954;11:1128–1136.
5. Vriesendorp HM, Herpst JM, Germack MA, et al. Phase I–II studies of yttrium labeled antiferritin treatment for endstage Hodgkin's disease, including RTOG 87-01. J Clin Oncol 1991;9:918–920.
6. Wessels, WB. Current status of animal radioimmunotherapy. Cancer Res 1990;50:970–973.
7. Fowler JF. Radiobiological aspects of low dose rates in immunotherapy. Int J Radiat Oncol Biol Phys 1990;18:1261–1269.
8. Vaughan ATM, Bradwell AR, Dykes PW, Anderson P. Illusions of tumor killing using radiolabeled antibodies. Lancet 1986;1:1492–1493.
9. Klein JL, Nguyen TH, Laroque P, et al. Yttrium-90 and iodine-131 radioimmunoglobulin therapy of an experimental hepatoma. Cancer Res 1989;49:63–83.
10. Stickney DR, Slater JB, Kirk GA, Ahlein C, Chang GH, Fricke JM. Bifunctional antibody. ZCE/CHH Indium-111 BLEDTA-IV clinical imaging in colorectal cancer. Antibiot Immunoconjug Radiopharmacol 1989;2:1–14.
11. Quadri SM, Vriesendorp HM, Leichner PK, Williams JR. Linker modulated biodistribution of In-111 and Y-90 labeled MOAB antiferritin immunoconjugates in nude mice and dogs. In: Dicke KA, Armitage JO, Dicke-Evinger MJ, eds. Autologous bone marrow transplantation. Proceedings of the Fifth International Symposium. Omaha, NB: University of Nebraska Medical Center, 1991:711–722.
12. Dillehay LE, Williams JR. In: Radiobiology of dose rate patterns achievable in radioimmunoglobulin therapy. In: Vaeth JM, Meyer JL, eds. The present and future role of monoclonal antibodies in the management of cancer—frontiers of radiation therapy and oncology. Vol. 24. Basel: Karger, 1990:96–103.
13. LeBerthou B, Khawli LA, Alauddin M, et al. Enhanced tumor uptake of macromolecules induced by a novel vasoactive interleukin 2 immunoconjugate. Cancer Res 1991;51:2694–2698.
14. Meeker TC, Lowder JN, Maloney DG, et al. A clinical trial of anti-idiotype therapy for B cell malignancy. Blood 1985;65:1349–1363.
15. Abelev GI. Alpha-fetoprotein in oncogenesis and its association with malignant tumors. Adv Cancer Res 1971;14:295–350.
16. Gold P, Freedman SO. Specific carcinoembryonic antigen of the human digestive system. J Exp Med 1965;122:467.
17. Boyer CM, Lidoe Y, Lottick SC, Bast RC Jr. Antigenic cell surface markers in human solid tumors. Antibiot Immunoconjug Radiopharmacol 1988;1:105–162.
18. Schlom J. Monoclonal antibodies. They are more and less than you think. In: Broder S, ed. Molecular foundations of oncology. Baltimore: Williams & Wilkins, 1991:95–134.
19. Folkman J. Tumor angiogenesis. Adv Cancer Res 1985;43:175–203.
20. Rostock RA, Klein JL, Leichner PK, Kopher KA, Order SE. Selective tumor localization in experimental hepatoma by radiolabeled antiferritin antibody. Int J Radiat Oncol Biol Phys 1983;9:1345–1350.
21. Rostock RA, Klein JL, Leichner PK, Order SE. Distribution of physiologic factors that affect 131-iodine antiferritin tumor localization in experimental hepatoma. Int J Radiat Oncol Biol Phys 1984;10:1135–1141.
22. Mori W, Asakawa H, Tagudi T. Antiplacental ferritin antiserum for cancer diagnosis. Ann NY Acad Sci 1975;259:446–449.
23. Piessens WF, David J. Immune complex disease. In: Rubenstein E, Federman DD, eds. Scientific American medicine. New York, 1990:23–35.
24. Rhodes BA, Burke DJ, Breslow K, Reed K, Austin R, Barchiel SW. Effect of circulating antigen on antibody localization in vivo. In: Burchiel SW, Rhodes BA, eds. Radioimaging and radioimmunotherapy. New York: Elsevier, 1983:25–40.
25. Denekamp J. Induced vascular collapse in tumors: a way of increasing the therapeutic gain in cancer therapy. BIR report 19. The scientific basis of modern radiotherapy. London: British Institute of Radiology, 1989:63–70.
26. Leung DY, Geha RS, Newburger JW. Two monokines, interleukin 1 and tumor necrosis factor, render cultured vascular endothelial cells susceptible to lysis by antibodies circulating during Kawasaki syndrome. J Exp Med 1986;164:1958–1972.
27. Newburger JW, Takahashi M, Burns JC. The treatment of Kawasaki syndrome with intravenous gamma globulin. N Engl J Med 1986;315:341–346.

28. Jain RK. Tumor physiology and antibody delivery. Front Radiat Ther Oncol 1990;29:37–46.

29. Boyse EA, Stockert E, Old LJ. Modification of the antigenic structure of the cell membrane by thymus—leukemia (TL) antibody. Proc Natl Acad Sci USA 1967;58:954–959.

30. Larson SM. Cancer imaging with monoclonal antibodies. In: Devita VT Jr, Hellman S, Rosenberg SA, eds. Important advances in oncology. Philadelphia; JB Lippincott, 1986:233–249.

31. Wilbur OS. Potential use of alpha emitting radionuclides in the treatment of cancer. Antibiot Immunoconjug Radiopharmacol 1991;4:85–97.

32. Porter P. Structural and functional characteristics of immunoglobulins of the common domestic species. In: Bradley CA, Cornelius CE, eds. Advances in veterinary science and comparative medicine. Vol. 23. New York: Academic Press, 1979:1–21.

33. Waldmann TA, Strober W. Metabolism of immunoglobulin. Prog Allergy 1969;13:1–110.

34. Klein JL, Ling MN, Leichner PK, et al. A model system that predicts effective half life for radiolabeled antibody therapy. Int J Radiat Oncol Biol Phys 1985;11:1489–1494.

35. Thomas DT, Chappell MJ, Dykes PW, et al. Effect of dose, molecular size, affinity, and protein binding on tumor uptake of antibody or ligand: a biomathematical model. Cancer Res 1989;49:3290–3296.

36. Vriesendorp HM, Quadri SM, Stinson RL, et al. Selection of reagents for human radioimmunotherapy. Int J Radiat Oncol Biol Phys 1991;22:37–46.

37. Klein JL, Leichner PK, Callahan KM, Kopher KA, Order SE. Effects of antiantibodies on radiolabeled antibody therapy. Antibiot Immunoconjug Radiopharmacol 1988;1:55–64.

38. Morrison SL, Johnson MJ, Harrenberg CA. Chimeric human antibody molecules: mouse antigen binding domains with human constant region domains. Proc Natl Acad Sci USA 1984;81:6851–6855.

39. Neuberger MS, Williams GJ, Fox RO. Recombinant antibodies possessing novel effector functions. Nature 1984;312:604–608.

40. Olsson L, Kaplan HS. Human-human hybridomas producing monoclonal antibodies of predefined antigenic specificity. Proc Natl Acad Sci USA 1980; 77:5429–5431.

41. Saleh MN, Wheeler RN, Khazaeli MB, et al. A phase I trial of chimeric anti GD2 monoclonal antibody C14.18 in patients with metastatic melanoma [Abstract]. Antibiot Immunoconjug Radiopharmacol 1991;4:207.

42. Shawler DL, Bartholomew RM, Smith LM. Human immune response to multiple injections of murine monoclonal IgG. J Immunol 1985;135:1530–1535.

43. Chatenoud L, Jonker M, Villermain F. The human antibody response to the OKT3 monoclonal antibody is oligoclonal. Science 1986;232:1406–1408.

44. Lowder JN. The current status of monoclonal antibodies in the diagnosis and therapy of cancer. Curr Probl Cancer 1986;10:488–551.

45. Foon KA, Schroff RW, Burn PA. Effects of monoclonal antibody therapy in patients with chronic lymphocytic leukemia. Blood 1984;64:1085–1093.

46. Order SE, Leibel SA. Radiolabeled antibodies in the treatment of primary liver cancer. Appl Radiol 1984;13:67–73.

47. Tomasi TB, Spellman C, Anderson WD. Clinically applicable procedures for producing tolerance to foreign proteins. In: Burchiel SW, Rhodes BA, eds. Radioimmunoimaging and radioimmunotherapy. New York: Elsevier, 1983:63–70.

48. Begent RHJ, Keep PA, Green AJ, et al. Liposomally entrapped second antibody improves tumor or imaging with radiolabeled (first) antitumor antibody. Lancet 1982;2:739–742.

49. Sharkey RM, Primus FJ, Goldenberg DM. Second antibody clearance of radiolabeled antibody in cancer immunodetection. Proc Natl Acad Sci USA 1984;81:2843–2846.

50. Lear JL, Kaslival RK, Feyerabend AJ, et al. Improved tumor imaging with radiolabeled monoclonal antibodies by plasma clearance of unbound antibody with anti-antibody column. Radiology 1991;179:509–512.

51. LoBuglio AF, Wheeler RH, Trang J, et al. Mouse/human chimeric monoclonal antibody in man: kinetics and immune response. Proc Natl Acad Sci USA 1989;86:4220–4224.

52. Reading CL. Hybridomas and cellular immortality. In: Tom BH, Allison JP, eds. Procedures for in vitro immunization and monoclonal antibody production. New York: Plenum Press, 1983.

53. Schlom J, Siler K, Milenic DE, et al. Monoclonal antibody-based therapy of a human tumor xenograft with a 177-lutetium labeled immunoconjugate. Cancer Res 1991;51:2889–2896.

54. Order SE, Klein JL, Leichner PK, Frincke J, Lollo C, Carlo DJ. 90-yttrium antiferritin—a new therapeutic antibody. J Radiat Oncol Biol Phys 1985;12:277–281.

55. Kaplan WD. The current status of tumor imaging. In: Zalutsky MR, ed. Antibodies in radiodiagnosis and therapy. Boca Raton, FL: CRC Press, 1988:1–12.

56. Eckelman WC, Paik CH. Labeling antibodies with metals using bifunctional chelates. In: Zalutsky MR, ed. Antibodies in radiodiagnosis and therapy. Boca Raton, FL: CRC Press, 1988:104–128.

57. Burchiel SN, Hadjian RA, Hladik, et al. Pharmacokinetic evaluation of Tc 99m methalothionein conjugated mouse monoclonal antibody B72.3 in rhesus monkeys. J Nucl Med 1989;30:1351–1357.

58. Fritzberg AR, Abrams PG, Beaumier IL, et al. Specific and stable labeling of antibodies with technetium 99m with a diamide dithiolate chelating agent. Proc Natl Acad Sci USA 1988;85:4025–4029.

59. Childs RL, Hnatowich DJ. Optimum conditions for labeling of DTPA coupled antibodies with Tc 99m. J Nucl Med 1985;26:293–299.

60. Paik CH, Hong JJ, Ebbert MA, Heald SC, Reba RC, Eckelman WC. Relative reactivity of DTPA, immunoreactive antibody—DTPA conjugates and non-immunoreactive antibody-DTPA conjugate towards [111]In. J Nucl Med 1985;26:485–492.

61. Meche HR, Riesen A, Ritter W. Molecular structure of indium DTPA. J Nucl Med 1989;30:1235–1239.

62. Paik CH, Quadri SM, Reba RC. Interposition of different chemical linkages between antibody and 111-In-DTPA to accelerate clearance from non-target organs and blood. Nucl Med Biol 1989;16:475–481.

63. Sands H, Jones PL. Methods for the study of the metabolism of radiolabeled monoclonal antibodies by liver and tumor. J Nucl Med 1987;28:390–398.

64. Kosmas C, Snook D, Verhoeyen M, et al. Immunogenicity of a macrocyclic chelating agent (DPTA) in patients receiving radiolabeled monoclonal antibodies (mAbs) for imaging and therapy. Abstract. Antibiot Immunoconjug Radiopharmacol 1991;4:212.

65. Eary JF, Krolm KA, Kishore R, Nelp WB. Radiochemistry of halogenated antibodies. In: Zalutsky MR, ed. Antibodies in radiodiagnosis and therapy. Boca Raton, FL: CRC Press, 1988:84–102.

66. Zalutsky MR, Noska MA, Colapinto EV, Garg PK, Bigner DD. Enhanced tumor localization and in vitro stability of monoclonal antibody radioiodinated using N-succinimidyl 3-(tri-n-butylstannyl)-benzoate. Cancer Res 1989;49:5543–5549.

67. Wilbur DS, Hadley SW, Hylardes MD, et al. Development of a stable radioionated reagent to monoclonal antibodies for radiotherapy of cancer. J Nucl Med 1989;30:216–226.

68. Quadri SM, Zhang YZ, Williams JR. Improvements in radioiodination of monoclonal antibodies for diagnosis and treatment of cancer. Antibiot Immunoconjug Radiopharmacol, 1991;4:283–296.

69. Seevers RH Jr. Introduction to radiocolloids. In: Spencer RP, Seevers RH Jr, Friedman AM, eds. Radionuclides in therapy. Boca Raton, FL: CRC Press, 1987:66–71.

70. Rosenshein NB, Leichner PK, Vogelsang BS. Radiocolloids in the treatment of ovarian cancer. Obstet Gynecol Survey 1979;34:708–720.

71. Bridgman JF, Bruckner F, Bleehen NM, Radioactive yttrium in the treatment of rheumatoid knee effusions. Preliminary evaluation. Ann Rheum Dis 1971;30:180–182.

72. Chaudhuri TK. 32-P therapy in polycythemia vera. In: Spencer RP, Seevers RH Jr, Friedman AM, eds. Radionuclides in therapy. Boca Raton, FL: CRC Press, 1987:103–110.

73. Maxon HR, Schroder LT, Thomas SR, et al. Re-186 (Sn) HEDP for treatment of painful osseous metastases: initial clinical experience in 20 patients with hormone-resistant prostate cancer Radiology 1990; 176:155–159.

74. Robinson RG, Blake GM, Presdon DF, et al. Strontium-89: treatment results and kinetics in patients with painful metastatic prostate and breast cancer in bone. Radiographics 1989;9:271–281.

75. Quadri SM, Wessels BW. Radiolabeled biomolecules with [186]Re: potential for radioimmunotherapy. Nucl Med Biol 1986;13:447–551.

76. Kozak RW, Raubitschek A, Mirzadeh S, et al. Nature of the bifunctional chelating agent used for radioimmunotherapy with yttrium-90 monoclonal antibodies: critical factors in determining in vivo survival and organ toxicity. Cancer Res 1989;49:2639–2644.

77. Haynes RC Jr, Murad F. Thyroid and anti-thyroid drugs. In: Goodman AG, Gilman LS, eds. The pharmacological basis of therapeutics. 6th ed. New York: Macmillan, 1980:1397–1419.

78. Kristensen K. Quality assurance for monoclonal antibodies and conjugates for clinical trials. 1991, in press.

79. Department of Health and Human Services. Points to consider in the manufacture and testing of monoclonal antibody products for human use. 1987.

80. Barber DE, Baum JW, Meinhold CB, eds. Radiation safety issues related to radiolabeled antibodies. NUREG/CR 4444. Washington, DC: Nuclear Regulatory Commission, 1991.

81. Hayes DF, Freedman EL, Kufe DW. Radioimmunoscintigraphy of human carcinoma: characterization of monoclonal antibodies. In: Zalutsky MR, ed. Antibodies in radiodiagnosis and therapy. Boca Raton, FL: CRC Press, 1988:57–82.

82. Stewart JSW, Hird V, Snook D, et al. Intraperitoneal radioimmunotherapy for ovarian cancer. Pharmacokinetics, toxicity and efficacy of 131I labeled monoclonal antibodies. Int J Radiat Biol Phys 1989;16:405–416.

83. Colcher D, Esteban J, Carrasquillo JA, et al. Complementation of intracavitary and intravenous administration of a monoclonal antibody (B72.3) in patients with carcinoma. Cancer Res 1987;47:4218–4224.

84. Courtenay-Luck N, Epenetos AA, Halnan KE, et al. Antibody-guided irradiation of malignant lesions. Three cases illustrating a new method of treatment. Lancet 1984;1:1441–1443.

85. Lashford LS, Davies AG, Richardson RB, et al. A pilot study of 131-I monoclonal antibodies in the therapy of leptomeningeal tumors. Cancer 1988;61:857–868.

86. Delaloye B, Bischof-Delaloye A, Pettavel J, et al. Intra-arterial administration of 131-I anti Cea Mab as a therapeutic approach to liver metastases. Nucl Med 1987;26:52–61.

87. Irie RF, Morton DL. Regression of cutaneous metastatic melanoma by intralesion injection with hu-

man monoclonal antibody to ganglioside GD2. Proc Natl Acad Sci USA 1986;83:8694–9698.

88. Weinstein JN. Immunolymphoscintigraphy and other nonintravenous applications of monoclonal antibodies. In: Zalutsky MR, ed. Antibodies in radiodiagnosis and therapy. Boca Raton, FL: CRC Press, 1988.

89. McLean FC, Budy AM. Radiation, isotopes and bone. New York: Academic Press, 1984.

90. Hird V, Stewart JSW, Snook D, et al. Intraperitoneally administered 90Y labeled monoclonal antibodies as a third line of treatment in ovarian cancer. A phase 1–2 trials: Problems encountered and possible solutions. Br J Cancer 1990(suppl 10):48–51.

91. Mattes MJ. Biodistribution of antibodies after intraperitoneal or intravenous injection and effect of carbohydrate modifications. JNCI 1987;79:855–862.

92. Mattes MJ, Sharkey RM, Goldenberg DM, Ong GL. Manipulation of blood clearance of antibodies by galactose conjugation [Abstract]. Antibiot Immunoconjug Radiopharmacol 1991;4:42.

93. Chiappa S, Musumeci R, Uslenghi C. Endolymphatic radiotherapy in malignant lymphomas. Recent results in cancer research. Vol. 37. New York; Springer, 1971.

94. Snyder WS, Ford MR, Watson GB. "S" absorbed dose per unit cumulated activity for selected radionuclides and organs. MIRD pamphlet no. 11. New York: The Society of Nuclear Medicine, 1975.

95. Moss AA, Christopher EC, Antonio CB. Determination of liver, kidney and spleen volumes by computed tomography: an experimental study in dogs. J Comput Assist Tomogr 1981;5:12–14.

96. Leichner PK, Vriesendorp HM, Hawkins WG, et al. Quantitative SPECT for Indium-111 labeled antibodies in the livers of beagle dogs. J Nucl Med 1991;32:1442–1444.

97. Wessels BW, Griffith MM. Miniature thermoluminescent dosimeter absorbed dose measurements in tissue phantom models. J Nucl Med 1986;27:1308–1314.

98. Lord BI, Hendry JH. The distribution of haemopoietic colony–forming units in the mouse femur and its modification by x-rays. Br J Radiol 1972;45:110–115.

99. Fajardo LF, Colby TV. Pathogenesis of veno-occlusive liver disease after radiation. Arch Pathol Lab Med 1980;104:584–588.

100. Leichner PK, Hawkins WG, Yang NC. A generalized empirical point-source function for beta-particle dosimetry. Antibiot Immunoconjug Radiopharmacol 1989;2:125–143.

101. Prestwick WV, Nunes J, Kwok CS. Beta dose point kernels for radionuclides of potential use in radioimmunotherapy. J Nucl Med 1989;30:1036–1046.

102. Spiers FW. Radioisotopes in the human body: physical and biological aspects. New York: Academic Press, 1968.

103. Whitwall JR, Spiers FW. Calculated beta ray dose factors for trabecular bone. Phys Med Biol 1976;21:16–38.

104. Eckerman KF. Aspects of the dosimetry of radionuclides within the skeleton with particular emphasis on the active marrow. In: Proceedings of the Fourth International Radiopharmaceutical Dosimetry Symposium. Oak Ridge, TN: Oak Ridge Associated Universities, 1986:514–534.

105. Siegel JA, Wessels NW, Watson EE, et al. Bone marrow dosimetry and toxicity for radioimmunotherapy. Antibiot Immunoconjug Radiopharmacol 1990;3:213–233.

106. Marin LA, Smith CE, Langston MJ, Quashie DV, Dillehay LE. Response of glioblastoma cell lines to low dose rate irradiation. Int J Radiat Oncol Biol Phys 1991;21:397–402.

107. Williams JR, Dillehay LE. Sensitization processes in human tumor cells during protracted irradiation. Possible exploitation in the clinic. Inst J Radiat Biol Phys 1991, in press.

108. Dillehay LE. A model of cell killing by low dose rate radiation including repair of sublethal damage G2 block and cell division. Radiat Res 1990;124:201–207.

109. Scott BR, Dillehay LE. A model of hematopoietic death in man from irradiation of bone marrow using radioimmunotherapy. Br J Radiat 1990;63:862–870.

110. Leichner PK, Klein JL, Siegelman SS, Ettinger DS, Order SE. Dosimetry of 131-I labeled antiferritin in hepatoma: specific activities in tumor and liver. Cancer Treat Rep 1983;67:657–658.

111. Press DW, Eary JF, Badger CC, et al. High-dose radioimmunotherapy of B cell lymphoma. Front Radiat Ther Oncol 1990;24:204–213.

112. Jonker M, van Vreeswijk W. The major histocompatibility complex of rhesus monkeys and chimpanzees. In: Zalesky MB, Abeyounis CJ, Kano K, eds. Immunobiology of the major histocompatibility complex. Basel: Karger, 1981:224–233.

113. Jonker M, Nooij FJ, den Butler G, van Lambalgen R, Fuccello AJ. Side effects and immunogenicity of murine lymphocyte-specific monoclonal antibodies in subhuman primates. Transplantation 1988;45:677–682.

114. Stefani S, Chandra S, Tomaki H. Ultrastructural events in the cytoplasmic death of lethally-irradiated human lymphocytes. Int J Radiat Biol 1977;31:215–225.

115. Bond VP, Fliedner TM, Archambeau JO. Mammalian radiation lethality. A disturbance in cellular kinetics. New York: Academic Press, 1955.

116. Vriesendorp HM. Radiation injury to hemopoietic cells: target cells, species differences and dose distribution. Antibiot Immunoconjug Radiopharmacol 1990;3:293–302.

117. Winchell HS, Pollycove M, Loughman WD, Law-

rence JII. Autologous bone marrow transplantation studies in dogs irradiated by Y-90 DTPA urine-recycling technique. Blood 1964;24:44–52.

118. Winchell HS, Pollycove M, Andersen AC, Lawrence JH. Relatively selective beta irradiation of lymphatic structures in the dog using Y-90 DTPA. Blood 1964;24:325–336.

119. Wielenga JJ. Hemopoietic stem cells in Rhesus monkeys. Surface antigens, radiosensitivity and responses to GM-CSF [Thesis]. The Netherlands; Erasmus University Rotterdam, 1990.

120. Fritz TE, Norris WP, Tolle VP, et al. Relationship of dose rate and total dose to responses of continuously irradiated beagles. In: Late biological effects of ionizing radiation. Vol. 2. IAEA-SM-2241/206. Vienna: International Atomic Energy Agency, 1978:71–83.

121. Mathe G, Hartmann L, Loverdo A, Bernard J. Essai de protection par l'injection de cellules medulaires isologues ou homologues contre la mortalité produite par l'or radioactif. Rev Franc Etudes Clin Biol 1958;3:1086–1087.

122. Morton BA, Beatty BG, Mison AP, Wanek PM, Beatty JD. Role of bone marrow transplantation in 90-Y antibody therapy of colon cancer xenografts in nude mice. Cancer Res 1990;50(suppl 3):1008–1010.

123. Vriesendorp HM, Williams JR. Radiation sensitivity of transplanted bone marrow cells. Transplantation 1988, 46:784.

124. Vriesendorp HM. Influence of radiation dose and radiation field size on the induction or treatment of leukemkia. Semin Hematol 1991;28(suppl 4):25–31.

125. Tavassoli M, Hardy CL. Molecular basis of homing of intravenously transplanted stem cells to the marrow. Blood 1990;76:1059–1070.

126. Michelsen K. Pressure relationships in the bone marrow vascular bed. Acta Physiol Scand 1967;71:16–24.

127. Vriesendorp HM. Engraftment of hemopoietic cells. In: van Bekkum DW, Lowenberg B, eds. Bone marrow transplantation. Biological mechanisms and clinical practice. New York: Marcel Dekker, 1985:73–146.

128. Vriesendorp HM, Shao Y, Stinson RL, et al. Fractionated intravenous administration of site specific yttrium-90 labeled B72.3 antibody in beagle dogs. Submitted for publication.

129. Schlom J, Molinolo A, Simpson JF, et al. Advantage of dose fractionation in monoclonal antibody targeted radioimmunotherapy. J Natl Cancer Inst 1990;82:763–771.

130. Martin EW, Mjozisik CM, Hinkle GH, et al. Radioimmunoguided surgery: a new approach to the intraoperative detection of tumor using monoclonal antibody B72.3. Am J Surg 1988;156:386–392.

131. Jager W, Feistel H, Paterok, EM, et al. Resection

guided by antibodies (REGAJ): a diagnostic procedure during second-look operation in ovarian cancer patients. Br J Cancer 1990;62(suppl 10):18–20.

132. Reinhold HS, Buisman GH. Repair of radiation damage to capillary endothelium. Br J Radiol 1975;48:727–731.

133. Krishnan L, Krishnan EC, Jewell WR. Immediate effect of irradiation on microvasculature. Int J Radiat Oncol Biol Phys 1988;15:147–150.

134. Msirikale JS, Klein JL, Schroeder J, Order SE. Radiation enhancement of radiolabeled antibody deposition in tumors. Int J Radiat Oncol Biol Phys 1987;13:1839–1844.

135. Order SE, Stillwagon GB, Klein JL, et al. 131-I antiferritin: a new treatment modality in hepatoma. An RTOG study. J Clin Oncol 1985;3:1573–1582.

136. Harisiadis L, Sung D, Kessaris N, Hall EJ. Hyperthermia and low dose rate irradiation. Radiology 1978;129:195–198.

137. Armour EP, Wang Z, Corry PM, Martinez A. Sensitization of rat ql gliosarcoma cells to low dose rate irradiation by long duration 41° C hyperthermia. Cancer Res 1991;51:3088–3095.

138. Spiro IJ, McPherson S, Cook JA, Ling CC, deGraff W, Mitchell JB. Sensitization of low dose rate irradiation by non-lethal hyperthermia. Radiat Research 1991;127:111–114.

139. Stickney DR, Gridley DS, Kirk GA, Slater JS. Enhancement of monoclonal antibody binding to melanoma with single dose radiation or hyperthermia. NCI monographs 3. Bethesda, MD: National Cancer Institute, 1987:47–52.

140. Mittal BB, Zimmer AM, Sathiaseelan B, et al. Effect of hyperthermia and 131-I antiCEA monoclonal antibody on human tumor xenografts in nude mice [Abstract]. Antibiol Immunoconjug Radiopharmacol 1991;4:217.

141. Paul WE. T cell derived interleukins. In: Broder J. Molecular foundations of oncology. Baltimore: Williams & Wilkins, 1991:135–152.

142. Greiner JW, Horan-Hand P, Noguchi P, Fisher P, Pestha S, Schlom J. Enhanced expression of surface tumor-associated antigens on human breast and colon tumor cells after recombinant human leukocyte alpha interferon treatment. Cancer Res 1989;44:3208–3214.

143. Rosenberg SA. Adoptive immunotherapy of cancer using lymphokine activated killer cells and recombinant interleukin 2. In: DeVita VT Jr, Hellman S, Rosenberg SA, eds. Important advances in oncology. Philadelphia: JB Lippincott, 1986:55–92.

144. Hougton AN, Mintzer D, Cordon-Cardo C, et al. Mouse monoclonal IgG3 antibody detecting GD3 ganglioside: a phase I trial in patients with malignant melanoma. Proc Natl Acad Sci USA 1985;82:1242–1246.

145. Sears HF, Herlyn D, Steplewski Z, et al. Phase II

clinical trial of a murine monoclonal antibody cytotoxic for gastrointestinal adenocarcinoma. Cancer Res 1985;45:5910–5913.

146. Larson SM. Lymphoma, melanoma, colon cancer: diagnosis and treatment with radiolabeled monoclonal antibodies. Radiology 1987;165:297–304.

147. Bischof-Delaloye A, Delaloye B. Rdioimmunotherapy of liver metastases from colorectal cancer. In: Seminar on radiolabeled antibodies in clinical oncology. Milan: European School of Oncology, 1990.

148. Markoe AM, Brady LW, Woo D, et al. Treatment of gastrointestinal cancer using monoclonal antibodies. Front Radiat Ther Oncol 1990;24:214–224.

149. Epenetos AA, Munro AJ, Stewart S, et al. Antibody guided irradiation of advanced ovarian cancer with intraperitoneally administered radiolabeled monoclonal antibodies. J Clin Oncol 1987;5:1890–1899.

150. Stillwagon GB, Order SE, Klein JL, et al. Multimodality treatment of primary nonresectable intrahepatic cholangiocarcinoma with 131I anti-CEA. A RTOG study. Int J Radiat Oncol Biol Phys 1987; 13:687–695.

151. Brady LW, Markoe AM, Woo DW, et al. Iodine 125 labeled anti-epidermal growth factor receptor-425 in the treatment of glioblastoma multiforme: a pilot study. Front Radiat Ther Oncol 1990;24:151–160.

152. Lashford L, Jones D, Pritchard J, Gordon I, Breatnack F, Kemshead JT. Therapeutic application of radiolabeled monoclonal antibody UJ13A in children with disseminated neuroblastoma. In: Order SE, ed. International Symposium on Labeled and Unlabeled Antibody in Cancer Diagnosis and Therapy. NCI Monographs no. 3. Bethesda, MD: National Cancer Institute, 1983:53–58.

153. Kemshead JT, Coakham HB, Lashford LS. Clinical experience of iodine-131 monoclonal antibodies in treating neural tumors. Front Radiat Ther Oncol 1990;24:166–181.

154. Carrasguillo JA. Radioimmunoscintigraphy with polyclonal or monoclonal antibodies. In: Zalutsky MR, ed. Antibodies in radiodiagnosis and therapy. Boca Raton, FL: CRC Press, 1988:169–198.

155. Beierwalter WH, Sisson JC, Shapiro B. Radionuclide therapy of adrenocortical and medullary tumors. In: Spencer RP, Seevers RH Jr, Friedman AM, eds. Radionuclides in therapy. Boca Raton, FL: CRC Press, 1987:47–64.

156. Scheinberg DA, Lovett D, Divgi CR, et al. A phase I trial of monoclonal antibody M195 in acute myelogenous leukemia: specific bone marrow targeting and internalization of radionuclide. J Clin Oncol 1991;9:478–490.

157. DeNardo GL, DeNardo SJ, O'Grady LF, Mills SL, Lewis JP, Macey DJ. Radiation treatment of B cell malignancies with immunoconjugate. Front Radiat Ther Oncol 1990;24:194–201.

158. Goldenberg DM, Horowitz JA, Sharkey RM, et al. Targeting, dosimetry and radioimmunotherapy of B cell lymphomas with iodine-131 labeled LL2 monoclonal antibody. J Clin Oncol 1991;9:548–564.

159. Parker BA, Halpern SE, Miller RA, Hupt H, Frincke J, Royston I. Radioimmunotherapy of lymphoma with auto-idiotype [Abstract]. Antibiot Immunoconjug Radiopharmacol 1991;4:203.

160. Rosen ST, Zimmer AM, Goldman-Leikink, et al. Radioimmunodetection and radioimmunotherapy of cutaneous T cell lymphomas using a 131-I labeled monoclonal antibody: An Illinois Cancer Council study. J Clin Oncol 1987;5:562–573.

161. Lenhardt R, Order SE, Spernberg J, et al. Isotopic immunoglobulin. A new systemic therapy for advanced Hodgkin's disease. J Clin Oncol 1985;3:1296–1300.

6

What Is The Best Strategy for Bone Marrow Transplants in Cancer?

Robert Peter Gale and Anna Butturini

Bone marrow transplants are increasingly used to treat cancer (1, 2). In 1991 about 12,000 transplants were performed worldwide, including equal numbers of allo- and autotransplants. Most transplants are for leukemia, lymphoma, and breast cancer. Other cancers treated by this approach include neuroblastoma, brain tumors, melanoma, Wilm tumor, Ewing sarcoma, and testicular and ovarian cancer.

Results of transplants are improving (reviewed in 3). There are several reasons for this. One is improved supportive care, including better antibiotics and transfusion techniques and, more recently, use of molecularly cloned hematopoietic growth factors like granulocyte or granulocyte-macrophage colony-stimulating factors, which accelerate bone marrow recovery and may decrease drug- and radiation-related toxicity (reviewed in 4). Another technique to accelerate hematopoietic recovery after autotransplants involves adding blood-derived stem cells to the bone marrow graft (reviewed in 5). Better techniques to identify histocompatible donors and prevent graft-versus-host disease (GVHD) (reviewed in 6) and cytomegalovirus (CMV) related interstitial pneumonia (reviewed in 7) are also important in allografts. In contrast, changes in pretransplant combinations of drugs or radiation have had little impact on disease-free survival (reviewed in 8).

Although these advances are noteworthy, considerable data suggest selection biases to a considerable extent explain improving results of transplants (reviewed in 9). Considerations involve subject selection, disease-related prognostic factors, and time-to-treatment bias (reviewed in 8). For example, transplants are now performed in persons with increasingly favorable prognostic factors for outcome with conventional therapy. Also, transplants are now often performed when the cancer is still responding to conventional therapy. Sometimes the transplant is delayed until completion of induction and/or more courses of postremission chemotherapy. Another type of delay occurs in studies involving two or more autotransplants. This study design means persons with rapidly progressing cancer do not complete the trial. These subjects are selectively censored unless there is analysis by treatment intent.

Selection biases affect transplant outcome in important but opposing directions. One is to improve the apparent results of transplants by excluding subjects least likely to benefit. However, unless these persons can be accurately identified, some subjects who might benefit will be excluded from transplantation. Also, since favorable prognostic factors for transplants are similar or identical to those predicting outcome of conventional therapy (reviewed in 10–12), using these factors to select transplant recipients means an increasing proportion of subjects are cured before the transplant. This decreases the possibility of determining whether transplants are superior to conventional therapy. Here, we consider several issues related to subject selection and transplant timing. Our object is to develop a reasonable strategy for using transplants in persons with cancer.

Issues worth considering are illustrated by the following model. Assume that 100 subjects with cancer are treated with conventional therapy, achieve remission, and are referred to a transplant center. Assume that at diagnosis 20 subjects have favorable, 40 intermediate, and 40 adverse prognostic factors. Also assume that 20 subjects were cured by the initial treatment. Although these 20 are most likely to be those subjects with favorable prognostic factors, assume their identity is unknown to the transplant center. Finally, assume that the increased intensity of therapy used with transplants cures 20% of the 80 (16 subjects) previously uncured subjects in the intermediate and adverse prognostic factor groups. These 16 cures are assumed to occur in specific subjects rather than randomly in the cohort of uncured subjects; i.e. the same 16 would be cured if the study were repeated.

Several possible treatment strategies are available to the transplant center. One is to transplant all 100 subjects. Were this done, the final outcome would be 36 cures—a cure rate of 36%. The increment in cures above conventional therapy is 16 subjects. Next, consider a strategy whereby only the 60 subjects with favorable or intermediate prognostic factors receive transplants. Assume that this includes all 20 subjects previously cured by conventional therapy and 8 of 16 subjects potentially curable by a transplant. Here, the final outcome would be 28 cures—a cure rate of 56%. This is considerably higher than the first strategy. However, the increment in cures above conventional therapy is only 8 compared to 16 when all 100 subjects were transplanted. Thus although the cure rate increases substantially, the number of subjects who benefit is less.

Using a third strategy, the transplant center selects only the 20 subjects with favorable prognostic factors to receive a transplant. The consequence would be to transplant only subjects already cured by conventional therapy. This strategy would appear to result in 100% cures, but this rate would be no greater than were the transplants not done. In fact, survival may be decreased because some persons cured by conventional therapy might die of transplant-related complications. These strategies are illustrated in Table 6.1.

The conclusion of these considerations is that increasing subject selection for transplants results in higher cure rates, but fewer lives are saved. Also, increased subject selection makes it more difficult to determine whether transplants are superior to conventional therapy. These considerations obviously apply only to settings where at least some persons are cured with conventional treatments. In other settings, like chronic myelogenous leukemia or recurrent breast cancer, which are incurable, subject selection can improve results but cannot artificially make them appear superior to conventional therapy, provided there are sufficient subjects and follow-up.

The same outcome, increased cure rates but fewer cures, occurs as the interval from remission to transplant increases (increasing

Table 6.1.   Results of Different Strategies for Transplants[a]

	Cures[b]				
Prognosis[a]	N	C	T	DFS	Total Cures
All subjects	100	20	16	36%	36
Worst subjects	60	20	8	47%	28
Best subjects	20	20	0	100%	20

[a]Prognosis of cohort based on response to chemotherapy.
[b]Definition of terms: *Cures:* those achieved with conventional therapy (C) versus those achieved with a subsequent transplant (T). *DFS:* apparent disease-free survival. *Total Cures:* sum of conventional therapy and transplants.

time-to-treatment bias). The longer the interval between diagnosis or treatment and the transplant, the greater the likelihood that subjects already cured by conventional therapy will receive transplants and the less the likelihood that subjects who might benefit from a transplant will receive it.

The strategies we discuss assume that it is not presently possible to precisely identify subjects already cured by conventional therapy or those who will benefit from a transplant. Considerable data support these notions. For example, most data suggest that variables predicting success of conventional therapy and transplants are similar. In the time-to-treatment bias model, we assumed a random loss of persons who might potentially benefit from a transplant. This is a conservative estimate since attrition of subjects in this cohort might be more or less rapid than from the cohort of subjects who would not benefit from a transplant.

What then is the best use of transplants in cancer? Increasing subject selection and time-to-treatment biases increase cure rates but decrease total cures. This is countered by the desire to avoid transplanting persons unlikely to benefit. A compromise between these extremes seems reasonable until more precise identification of the cured, the potentially curable, and the incurable is possible.

Acknowledgments

Supported in part by a grant from the center for Advanced Studies in Leukemia. RPG is the Wald Foundation Scholar in Biomedical Communications.

REFERENCES

1. Gale RP, Champlin RE, eds. New strategies in bone marrow transplantation. New York: Wiley-Liss, 1990.
2. Bortin MM, Rim A. Increasing utilization of bone marrow transplantation II. Results of 1985–1987 survey. Transplantation 1989;48:453–458.
3. Champlin RE, Bortin MM, Horowitz MM. Trends in bone marrow transplantation for leukemia [Abstract]. Exp Hematol 1991;19:569.
4. Aurer I, Ribas A, Gale RP. What is the role of recombinant colony stimulating factors in bone marrow transplantation. Bone Marrow Transplant 1990;6:79–87.
5. Henon PR, Butturini A, Gale RP. Blood derived hematopoietic cell transplants: blood to blood. Lancet 1991;337:961–963.
6. Speck B, Ringden O, Horowitz MM. Comparison of methotrexate (MTX), cyclosporine (CSA) and combined MTX and CSA to prevent graft-versus-host disease (GVHD) [Abstract]. Exp Hematol 1991;19:582.
7. Winston D, Gale RP. Prevention and treatment of cytomegalovirus infection and disease after bone marrow transplantation in the 1990's. Bone Marrow Transplant 1991;8:7–11.
8. Aurer I, Gale RP. Review: Are new conditioning regimens in AML better? Bone Marrow Transplant 1991; 7:255–261.
9. Gale RP, Horowitz MM. How best to analyze new strategies in bone marrow transplantation. Bone Marrow Transplant 1991;6:425–430.
10. Gale RP, Horowitz MM, Biggs JC, et al., for the Advisory Committee of the International Bone Marrow Transplant Registry. Transplant or chemotherapy in acute myelogenous leukemia. Lancet 1989;1:119–122.
11. Barrett AJ, Horowitz MM, Gale RP, et al. Marrow transplantation for acute lymphoblastic leukemia: factors affecting relapse and survival. Blood 1989; 74:862–871.
12. Surbone A, Armitage J, Gale RP. Autotransplants in lymphoma: better therapy or healthier patients. Ann Intern Med 1991;114:1059–1060.

7

ANALYSIS OF ECONOMIC ISSUES

Thomas J. Smith, Christopher E. Desch, and Bruce F Hillner

Cancer care is expensive (1). The estimated U.S. direct costs of cancer in 1990 were $35.3 billion; morbidity costs (days lost from work) added $11.9 billion, and mortality costs (lost income due to premature death) added $56.8 billion, for a total "economic burden" of cancer of $103 billion. Cancer care is becoming more expensive each year. From 1985 to 1990 direct costs of care rose 62%, and total costs of the economic burden rose 45%. Physicians can no longer ignore the costs of cancer therapy or concerns about its effectiveness (2, 3).

High-dose chemotherapy (HDC) with autologous bone marrow transplantation (BMT) has been at the forefront of the controversy about medical costs, as an example of a life-saving but expensive new technology (4). BMT has been used in only a small percentage of total cancer cases. However, its contribution to direct cancer costs is relatively high, and the pool of potential recipients is expanding. The interest in high-dose chemotherapy and BMT was spurred by initial success in leukemia and lymphoma and has spread to breast, testicular, and other solid tumors (reviewed in 5). BMT centers grew from a handful in 1970 to 170 in 1985, and the number of BMTs increased 24-fold between 1980 and 1985 alone (6). More than 40,000 individuals in the United States alone are candidates for HDC and autologous BMT, with estimated direct medical costs of $4.8 billion (1988 dollars) if all patients received transplantation (7).

The economic issues in HDC are paramount in planning for increased utilization. Some states and insurers already limit its use, claiming that such therapy is "experimental." However, economic factors are a major determinant in this decision, because payors are concerned that HDC will overutilize the available capital (4). Regardless, as the procedure becomes safer and more effective, more HDC will be demanded and done. As physicians and health policy makers, we must measure the cost-effectiveness of this procedure compared to conventional, less costly therapy. Is it worth the added dollars and toxicity to gain a better likelihood of response or long-term disease-free survival? To understand the financial impact of HDC for selected conditions, it is essential to analyze the following determinants: (*a*) costs, (*b*) benefits, (*c*) cost-effectiveness, (*d*) cost reduction methods, (*e*) and health care decision making, comparing alternatives in care based on cost-effectiveness. The purpose of this chapter is to examine the costs of HDC for selected conditions, relate them to established medical practices, and demonstrate the usefulness of decision analysis in determining optimal therapy. Definitions of terms commonly used in economic and decision analysis may be found in Table 7.1.

COSTS OF THERAPY

The cost of therapy is generally divided into direct and indirect costs (Table 7.2). Di-

Table 7.1. Glossary of Terms Used in Economic and Decision Analysis[a]

Costs	Resources needed to provide a service
Cost analysis	Calculating the costs incurred by a disease or medical services used to treat it
Cost-effectiveness analysis	Net cost of providing a service compared to a measure of outcomes, usually expressed as $/life-year gained
Cost-benefit analysis	Cost of providing a service and the benefit obtained, both expressed in the same unit, usually $
Quality-adjusted life year	Duration of survival modified by utility values for the value of that time, e.g., life with chemotherapy or recurrent disease may be counted as 0.7, when 0 = dead and 1 = well.

[a]Adapted for reviews by Drummond M, Stoddart G, Labelle R, et al. Health economics: an introduction for clinicians. Ann Intern Med 1987; 107:88–92; Eisenberg JA. Clinical economics. A guide to the economic analysis of clinical practice. JAMA 1989;262:2879–2886.

Table 7.2. Costs of Therapy

Direct Costs
  Hospital charges (room and board)
    Routine care
    Intensive care
    Special nursing requirements
  Pharmacy
    Antibiotics
    Hyperalimentation
    Chemotherapy
    Hematopoietins
    Antiemetics
  Physician fees
  Radiographic studies
  Operating room fees
    Anesthesia
    Sterile supplies
  Blood bank
    Random donor products
    Pheresis products
Indirect Costs
  Morbidity costs
    Income lost due to illness
    Transportation
    Lodging
    Housekeeping
    Child care
    Special diets
    Special rehabilitation needs
  Mortality Costs
    Income lost due to death

rect costs refer to medical care given during the episode of illness and include physician fees, hospital charges, medications, etc. Direct medical costs may amount to only 10% of all transplantation-related expenses (7). Indirect costs include morbidity costs (income lost from days of work missed due to illness) and mortality costs (income lost from premature death). Morbidity costs due to illness but not attributed to the health care sector, such as transportation, lodging, and special meals, may consume 30%–40% of family income and may be as high as 60% of the direct costs (7, 8). In this chapter, we will concentrate on direct medical costs.

A full accounting of the direct cost of therapy is often not available from analysis of the medical or hospital record, for the following reasons: (*a*) inadequate hospital accounting systems, (*b*) incomplete accounting of pre- and posttransplant periods, and (*c*) neglect of costs for outpatient, palliative, and supportive care. For these reasons, it has been difficult to calculate the total financial impact of HDC on society and the individual, including attention to *quality* of life, including employment, and the incremental or marginal costs of HDC.

Cost is preferred over charges to evaluate therapy or to compare alternative therapies (9). Hospital accounting systems are often inadequate to evaluate the *costs* of individual medical care. The available data are usually in *charges* (what the insurer is billed), not costs (including supplies, labor, capital equipment necessary to provide a service), but the charges can be converted to costs by standard accounting methods. Hospitals report a ratio of costs to charges (RCC) to Medicare that gives the best estimate of the cost associated with service provision. The RCC may vary from profitable (RCC < 1, or costs less than charges) to unprofitable (RCC > 1, or costs greater than charges). Table 7.3 presents some of the RCCs employed at our academic tertiary-care hospital for the range of services used by HDC patients and the impact of the RCC on hospital revenues. The accuracy of the cost data, and hence the RCC, for many institutions is unknown but represents the best available data in the absence of a true cost-accounting system. Hospital charges will vary greatly from region to region, and hospital charges for the same services vary depending on reimbursement structure. The RCCs will reflect these local factors (e.g., wages) and are influenced by the hospital used, not the resources consumed (10). RCC analysis is important in HDC planning for two reasons: (a) It is used by hospital financial planners to predict if HDC will be profitable, and whether it will be offered as part of the "product mix" of the hospital, and (b) it allows identification of high-utilization services that can be targets for cost reduction.

Costs can be measured by direct tallying of all the services used by HDC patients, but this has not been done yet for HDC patients. An alternative accounting method estimates the consumption of resources and costs in a multivariate prediction model in

Table 7.3. Cost Centers, Ratio of Cost to Charges, and Impact on Hospital Revenue[a]

Cost Center[b]	Ratio of Cost: Charge[c]	Financial Impact[d]
Pharmacy	0.50	Profitable
Room and board, ICU	1.29	Unprofitable
Room and board, non-ICU	1.29	Unprofitable
Diagnostic x-ray	0.46	Profitable
Blood bank	0.66	Profitable
OR/Sterile supplies	0.51	Profitable
Anesthesia	1.03	Unprofitable
Bone Marrow lab	0.66	Profitable

[a]Abbreviations: ICU, intensive care unit; OR, operating room
[b]"Cost center" is an accounting term for a service or group of services; it excludes professional fees.
[c]Derived from Medicare data.
[d]Financial impact on the hospital.

which charges are tallied for room and board, x-ray procedures, labs, and the operating room. This has been used to accurately estimate charges in leukemia patients (10) and general medical patients (11). This model has been successfully used to compare resource utilization but has several shortcomings: (a) It neglects physician fees, typically 27%–79% of total charges at our hospital and other institutions for HDC patients (12); (b) it neglects outpatient costs, 40% of the total (12), which are hard to capture because they are provided at separate locations; and (c) it neglects true costs. As hospitals and insurers work together to reduce costs by providing services in the least costly space or reimbursing per diem, estimates based on charges may not reflect the resources actually needed to provide HDC services.

The full cost of therapy will include all diagnosis, treatment, and follow-up costs. For HDC patients, this should include *all* costs, from diagnosis to cure or death. Hospital-based BMT and HDC typically represent only 60% of the total cost of an illness (12). The usual data presented are on the acute care costs for 1 (13) or 5 years (10). Such studies often appear to show extremely high costs for HDC: year-1 costs for BMT leukemia patients were 27 times greater than those for standard maintenance therapy. However, if the non-transplanted patients relapsed and required induction chemotherapy or BMT, costs were only 1.7 times greater (7, 13). Relapse and supportive terminal care is expensive, and costs continue to accumulate as long as the patient lives. Leukemia BMT/HDC patients live longer than standard chemotherapy patients, and the longer follow-up time is needed to "dilute" (amortize) the higher early costs.

The cost of therapy must also include expensive supportive and terminal care. Mean medical expenditures for the last year of life in cancer patients have been reported as $21,219 (1980 dollars) (14) and for the last 6 months of life as $16,280 (15). These costs are remarkably uniform across cancer diagnosis and are decreased very little by hospice or home care (14). Unfortunately, terminal care costs for cancer patients are high, with little opportunity for reduction except by withholding services. Again, HDC patients may balance high initial costs by using less terminal care, or by delaying it.

The quality of life gained also influences cost-effectiveness of therapy. The available data suggest that patients will favor the strategy that produces the most gain of life, even if some short-term toxicity is necessary to achieve it (16, 17). Early studies that addressed the issue of quality-adjusted life years used *decreased* quality of life for BMT/HDC survivors. A quality-adjusted year of life is a numerical description that combines expected survival and quality of life; it is based on the value people place on life in a given state of health. As a result of this decreased quality of life, cost per quality-adjusted life year increased when survival quality was added; for example, cost per added year of life for leukemia patients increased from $5,000–$29,000 to $8,000–$47,000 (1980 dollars) per year of life gained when adjustments were made for decreased quality of life from treatment (18). Recent studies show normal quality of life post-HDC: Of 135 autologous and allogeneic adult (mean age 27) BMT patients at Johns Hopkins, 93% reported they could do normal activities, 65% were employed, and one-third of those not working were attending school (19). Autologous HDC patients would be expected to have even *better* outcomes in the absence of graft-versus-host disease, which was a significant predictor for loss of employment. In our experience, the majority of HDC survivors return to work or school and have only a temporary decrease in quality of life from HDC. We expect that routine quality of life assessments of HDC being taken for clinical trials patients will show improved scores compared to standard chemotherapy if HDC becomes more effective and less toxic. For example, patients receiving continuous or intermittent chemotherapy for breast cancer rated their quality of life higher if their disease was kept in remission,

even despite the toxic effects of chemotherapy (20).

The cost of HDC may decrease as more is performed. The marginal cost (cost of treating an additional patient) may decrease as more patients are treated at each institution; for example, once dedicated space and staff time are available, the cost of treating each additional patient should be lower. An incremental cost analysis will show the charges and costs incurred for the operation of the program and may be performed using available charges and RCCs (Table 7.4). Full cost accounting may not translate into a cost savings for the patient or insurer, however, under current reimbursement programs. Hospitals maximize revenue by maximizing reimbursable services, and HDC with BMT can be profitable, especially in the use of inpatient ancillary services with favorable RCCs (Table 7.3), similar to routine chemotherapy (21). Most tertiary care centers desire the capability to perform HDC because of its fa-

Table 7.4. Cost of High-Dose Chemotherapy for Solid Tumor Patients (Average Charges and Average Cost)[a,b]

Description	Ave. Chg. Per Pt.	RCC[b]	Average Cost
R&B $450 rate	11,790	1.29	15,299
R&B $491 rate	7,660	1.29	9,894
R&B $1150 rate	460	1.29	594
Total R&B	**19,910**		**25,717**
Pharmacy	26,469	0.51	13,641
Pharm. Takehome	55	0.51	28
Diagnostic x-ray	654	0.46	301
Laboratory	11,638	0.40	4,729
Blood/platelets	2,555	0.66	1,694
Blood Stor./proc.	4,713	0.66	3,125
Sterile supply	4,538	0.51	2,331
OR supplies	5	0.51	3
PT	19	0.78	15
OR services	231	0.51	119
Anesthesia	134	1.03	138
Pulm. function	98	0.14	14
Bone marrow lab	2,857	0.66	1,894
Total ancillaries	**$53,967**		**$28,033**
Total	**$72,877**		**$53,750** 73%

[a]From Medical College of Virginia Hospital, 1990.
[b]Abbreviations: R + B, room and board, RCC, ratio of costs to charges; PT, physical therapy, OR, operating room.

vorable reimbursement profile (12), in addition to its high visibility and potential to bolster referral networks (7). Integrated health care systems that provide comprehensive outpatient and inpatient services are attempting to minimize the financial impact of HDC by transferring patients to specially designated "centers of excellence" with a flat per-patient or per-diem reimbursement that may help to control costs (22).

COST-EFFECTIVENESS OF THERAPY

One measure of a new technology is its cost-effectiveness compared to the standard treatment. These principles are most important in modeling cost-effectiveness of therapies:

1. Costs, not charges, matter.
2. Adverse events are important both *if* and *when* they happen. A distant event will cost less than a similar resource-consuming event now, due to discounting. Discounting reflects interest on dollars that would not be available if they were spent now. Discounting can also be applied to the value of the years gained; for many patients a current year is worth more than a future year.
3. The ideal model includes sensitivity analyses. What if, for example, therapy was twice as effective? One-half the cost? Mortality one-half of reported?
4. The ideal model establishes "thresholds," or points where a clinical choice is possible. For example, if the disease free survival (DFS) from HDC rises to 40% at 3 years, it will become the preferred choice.

We will define some commonly used terms in decision analysis and cost-effectiveness research, review the available literature, and discuss the cost-effectiveness of HDC compared to standard chemotherapy using relevant estimates of efficacy and cost. Much of this work is preliminary and has only been published in abstract form.

Decision analysis is a technique that allows the comparison of therapies for effectiveness and cost-effectiveness (23). It evaluates alternative therapies by estimating the probability of all relevant events or outcomes in the future. A decision tree is constructed to represent the typical events that happen to an oncology patient: diagnosis, therapy, follow-up, recurrence, cure, death. Costs for each event and modifiers to reflect quality of life assessments or value are added at each step. An alternative to the basic decision tree is a Markov process that is used to simulate the process over time. Cohorts of patients move from one health state to another at a set time interval, usually 1 year, based on probabilities. This may be particularly important in HDC, where therapy may produce long-term remissions compared to standard chemotherapy. A relapse 10 years after therapy would be expected to cost less than a relapse in 1 year, and the initial higher cost would be offset by the years gained.

The benchmark in cost-effectiveness research is the dollars per life-year saved ($/LY), or amount that it takes to gain an additional year of life using the new therapy. For example, if it costs $30,000 to use the new treatment with an average gain of 0.25 year, the $/LY is $120,000. The quality of that life-year saved can be estimated by using a modifier when counting years saved of a cohort of patients. For example, life with either breast cancer recurrence or major side effects of chemotherapy could be counted as 0.7 life-years rather than 1.0. There is no consensus on the best way to make quality of life adjustments (24–26). Quality of life is clearly a subjective choice, and cancer patients may feel that their life is worth all the value of a non-cancer patient's. In a randomized controlled study comparing continuous versus intermittent therapy, prolongation of life despite the side effects of chemotherapy was valued more than life with recurrence (20). Little is known about quality of life assessments in HDC patients, but patients and their physicians were close in estimates of performance status (19), suggesting that reproducible assessments of quality of life and functional status can be made. If quality adjustments are made to reflect the quality of life in a health state, the benchmark becomes quality-adjusted life-years (QALYs).

Standard cancer chemotherapy appears to be as cost-effective as other accepted medical interventions (Table 7.5). Medical interventions are usually compared to dialysis as a benchmark for acceptable cost-effectiveness; dialysis costs approximately $25,000 to gain a year of life. Chemotherapy for patients with non-small-cell lung cancer costs less than best supportive care, with the costs of drugs outweighed by savings from less frequent hospitalization. The toxicity was outweighed by the added gain in life (27). Chemotherapy plus radiation cost $28/day of additional median survival, or $10,220/year, compared to radiation alone for non-small-cell lung cancer (28). Others have questioned the magnitude of the benefits in this study, noting that only 1 of 7 patients actually benefited despite all being exposed to toxicity, and the death

rate was still 75% at 3 years (29). Alternating multiagent chemotherapy was more cost-effective than standard chemotherapy for small cell lung cancer, with an incremental cost of $3370 per life-year gained (30). The actual benefit, 6 weeks longer survival at an additional cost of $450, seems trivial since nearly all patients were dead at 18 months and treatment toxicities were similar (3).

We and others have examined the efficacy and cost-effectiveness of standard yet expensive adjuvant treatment. Adjuvant therapy of node-negative, estrogen receptor–negative breast cancer patients with chemotherapy adds an average benefit of 7–11 months, with an incremental cost of $15,400–$18,800 per quality-adjusted life-year gained (31). Tamoxifen for node-positive, estrogen receptor–positive postmenopausal women costs about $6000 per additional life-year gained; chemotherapy with doxorubicin and cyclophosphamide plus tamoxifen costs $54,000 per additional life-year gained (32). Brown has shown that adjuvant therapy with levamisole and fluorouracil in colon cancer gains 2.37 years per patient with an incremental cost of $2014 per life-year gained but

Table 7.5. Cost-Effectiveness of High-Dose Chemotherapy Compared to Other Medical Interventions[a]

Medical Intervention	Cost per Year of Life Saved ($)	Reference
Liver transplantation	43,900–250,000	48,51
HDC for limited metastatic breast cancer, cost = $100,000	85,800	39
Treatment of hypertension with captopril	72,100	48
SC for ANLL, no discounting, 5-year analysis	64,000	12
HDC/BMT for ANLL, no discounting, 5-year analysis	62,500	12
HDC for limited metastatic breast cancer, cost = $53,000	51,600	Unpublished data
Coronary artery bypass, one-vessel disease	44,500	49,51
Heart transplantation	27,200	50
HDC for recurrent Hodgkin's disease	21,500	37,38
Adjuvant chemotherapy for node-negative breast cancer	15,400–18,800	39
Treatment of moderate hypertension with propranolol	10,000	48
HDC/BMT for ANLL, 5% discounting, lifetime analysis	10,000	12
Adjuvant tamoxifen, node-positive breast cancer	6,000	32
Coronary artery bypass, left-main disease	5,600	49,51
Alternating chemotherapy for small-cell lung cancer	3,370	27
Adjuvant chemotherapy for colon cancer	2,010	33

[a]Abbreviations: SC, salvage chemotherapy; ANLL, acute nonlymphocytic leukemia.

cautions that clinical trial data are not applicable to larger populations, who may have different benefits, costs, and toxicities (33). These studies illustrate several important points for decision making about oncology care:

1. Although a treatment may be cost-effective, it may not make people live significantly longer.
2. Standard cancer care is expensive and relatively ineffective, but within the range of accepted medical interventions.
3. True gains in cost-effectiveness will be made only with vastly increased efficacy, better long-term survival, or markedly reduced costs.

COST-EFFECTIVENESS OF HIGH-DOSE CHEMOTHERAPY

There are remarkably few data on the cost-effectiveness of HDC, although the costs and efficacy have been intensely scrutinized (4). Welch and Larson studied the cost-effectiveness of allogeneic BMT/HDC for 17 patients with acute nonlymphocytic leukemia compared to 19 chemotherapy controls (10). They estimated patient charges by tallying hospital days, intensive care unit (ICU) hospital days, a per diem lab and x-ray charge, operating room (OR) procedures, and a constant. This charge estimate treats all patients as if they were in the same hospital:

Hospital charge (1983 dollars)
= ($244)(hospital days) + ($871)(ICU)
+ ($37)lab + ($345)x-ray + ($3283)(OR)
+ ($178.99)(a constant)

Total charges over 5 years (excluding physician fees) were estimated at $193,000 per patient for allogeneic transplantation and $136,000 per patient for standard chemotherapy. The costs per life-year gained were similar at $62,500 for transplantation and $64,000 for chemotherapy. The cost differences were all incurred in the first 6 months

of therapy and were largely attributable to the use of the ICU; 57% of the BMT/HDC patient days were spent in the ICU ($885/day) compared to 5% for standard chemotherapy patients. Despite the higher cost, the cost-effectiveness of BMT/HDC became more evident the longer the cohort was studied due to increased survival. As long as BMT/HDC achieved a survival advantage of 40% or more, the incremental cost-effectiveness was comparable or better than standard chemotherapy. For a typical 30-year-old patient with an otherwise normal life expectancy, and using a discount rate of 5%, the cost of saving an additional year of life by the use of HDC/BMT was $10,000, comparable to that of treating moderate hypertension in men with propranolol (Table 7.5).

The data of Welch and Larson may also be used to estimate the cost-effectiveness of HDC for solid tumors. This analysis is especially interesting because HDC for leukemia resembles HDC for solid tumors: It is expensive ($103,000 in year 1, 1989 dollars) and relatively ineffective (5 year disease-free survival of only 20% ± 13%) (34, 35). The costs are within the range of HDC for solid tumors, typically estimated at $120,000 (7). The efficacy of HDC in breast cancer is similar; typical estimates for the 5-year DFS for limited metastatic breast cancer are 5% for standard chemotherapy and 17%–40% for HDC at 3 years (36). Welch and Larson compared standard chemotherapy to HDC/BMT to *no* therapy, with all untreated patients dying immediately at no cost. In a 30-year-old patient with a lifetime expectancy of 47 years and a discount rate of 5%, standard chemotherapy for leukemia cost $22,900 to save an additional year of life compared to no therapy. High-dose chemotherapy with BMT, with better survival over a lifetime, cost only $16,600 per life-year saved despite higher initial costs. Although this charge-based model probably underestimates total cost per year of life gained by ignoring physician fees, the cost-effectiveness of HDC compared to less costly (but less effective) therapy is in line with other expensive (short-term), modestly effective (long-term) medical interventions. If all the supportive care costs for no-therapy patients were counted, estimated as at least $21,000, the advantage of HDC would be even more striking. Similarly, if HDC cost only $40,000 (12) or $53,000 (Table 7.4, Medical College of Virginia, 1990 estimated costs), rather than $100,000, it is possible that the cost per year of life gained with HDC would be decreased to an acceptable range.

We have used decision analysis to calculate the effectiveness and cost-effectiveness of HDC for relapsed Hodgkin's disease by comparing five strategies (Table 7.6) in common use (37). HDC to "sensitive responders" at first relapse gives the best overall survival compared to standard chemotherapy or HDC in second or later relapse. The incremental cost to save a life-year using HDC is $21,500, within the range of acceptable medical interventions (38).

We have examined the costs and cost-effectiveness of metastatic breast cancer treatment by HDC (39). Our decision analysis model allows the study of cohorts of women at varying risk of recurrence, efficacy of therapy, and cost. For our baseline analysis of HDC we used a 30% DFS at 2 years and 20% at 5 years. Our costs were estimated at $100,000, including physician fees and supportive care costs. We compared HDC to standard chemotherapy with a 5-year DFS rate of 5% and cost of $6,000. We used a Markov process to

follow cohorts of women from age 40 to death and a discount rate of 5%. HDC saves an additional year of life at a cost of $85,000, near the range of some medically accepted procedures (Table 7.5). If we use a cost of $53,000, our current best estimate, then HDC gains an additional year of life at a cost of $51,600, closer to the range of accepted medical procedures.

COST-BENEFIT ANALYSIS OF HIGH-DOSE CHEMOTHERAPY

Cost-benefit analysis attempts to analyze the entire economic and functional impact of therapy by measuring both costs and benefits in the same units. It typically includes earnings lost or gained and estimates of all nonmedical morbidity costs (Table 7.2). Only one cost-benefit analysis has been done of high-dose chemotherapy. Elfenbein et al. studied the impact of HDC with autologous bone marrow rescue of adjuvant treatment of poor-risk stage II breast cancer (40). They used estimates of 0.60 for probability of prolonged survival after HDC, and 0.05 for standard chemotherapy (probability of life at 5 years of 60% and 5%, respectively) with a death rate of 0.05 from HDC. HDC cost $0.34 per dollar of lifetime earning, and standard chemotherapy cost $0.46. HDC was the optimal choice as long as the probability of prolonged survival was 0.47 or greater, and probability of dying during HDC less than 0.17. They predicted HDC to be a more fruitful economic investment than standard chemotherapy but cautioned that more follow-up was needed to determine the natural history of stage II breast cancer patients after HDC. The analysis is only as strong as its assumptions, however; if HDC produces a DFS probability of less than .47, or most patients cannot return to work, or there is unexpected long-term morbidity from HDC, then standard chemotherapy may produce more benefit for the cost.

Table 7.6. Efficacy and Cost-Effectiveness of High-Dose Chemotherapy in Relapsed Hodgkin's Disease[a]

Strategy	Years Gained	Cost/Life-Year	Rank of Strategy
Immediate HDC after first relapse	9.2		3
HDC in remission after SC	8.6		4
HDC after relapse from SC	11.0	$21,500	1
HDC after any SC	9.4		2
SC alone	8.2		5

[a]SC, salvage chemotherapy.

REDUCTION OF COSTS ASSOCIATED WITH HIGH-DOSE CHEMOTHERAPY

We believe that the cost of HDC can be substantially reduced by careful attention to the most costly items listed in Table 7.4. The total cost of HDC, currently $40,200 (12) to $120,000 (7), may potentially be reduced to as little as $20–$25,000 (41). If current HDC DFS figures remain constant, with 20%–25% long-term survivors, then lower-cost HDC may be a better investment in lives gained and cost per life year. The following are recommendations for future research, as well as current application:

1. Move services to the outpatient area.
2. Use novel strategies to reduce pharmacy costs.
3. Reduce hospitalization and illness days with peripherally harvested stem cell autografts and hematopoietic colony-stimulating factors.
4. Treat only good-risk patients off-protocol.
5. Establish an HDC reimbursement system that rewards hospitals and physicians for reducing costs without sacrificing quality.

Many hospital-based services can be moved to the outpatient setting. Bone marrow harvesting can be performed safely and possibly less expensively if done in the outpatient setting with vigorous intravenous fluid support and careful aftercare; of 38 consecutive patients so treated, only 3 required hospitalization (42). Other transplant centers are giving HDC in the outpatient clinic with hospitalization only for refractory side effects such as nausea, or when febrile neutropenia is first noted (41). This has the potential to reduce as many as 5–7 pre-autologous-marrow-reinfusion hospital days although total resource consumption of pharmacy services, intravenous medications, etc., may not change appreciably.

Pharmacy costs are about 25% of our current HDC costs (Table 7.4). The use of oral rather than intravenous drugs when possible would save approximately 50% of the individual drug cost by reducing the administration cost. Enteral feeding rather than total parenteral nutrition (TPN) appears to be safe and effective, with costs only 44% of those for TPN; the average saving per patient would be $1400, with no increased morbidity or mortality (43).

Peripherally harvested stem cell autografts and hematopoietic colony stimulating factors (CSFs) appear to hasten recovery from neutropenia and would be expected to reduce total hospitalization charges by an amount proportionate to the days saved. Hospitalization room and board charges represent nearly 50% of the total patient costs (Table 7.4). Hospital days were reduced from 38 to 24 in one study, resulting in a potentially significant cost savings in room and ancillary costs (44). We have seen a substantial decrease in the use of TPN, antibiotics, and blood product support in our patients receiving peripherally harvested stem cell autografts, with a total cost of about $53,000 (excluding physician fees). In addition, the chance of dying or prolonged hospitalization from delayed engraftment appears to be reduced. Patients who die often have the highest hospitalization costs because of intensive care use, estimated at $2,500–$3,000 per day at our institution.

The use of CSFs will have a major impact on cost and toxicity of HDC, as it does for routine chemotherapy. Patients given granulocyte-CSF (G-CSF) for outpatient moderate dose chemotherapy had a 50% reduction in hospitalizations for febrile neutropenia, at a savings of $1584 (Medicare) to $2029 (private insurance) per patient; the typical cost for a several-day hospitalization for neutropenia was $5–$7,000 (45). Treatment with G-CSF reduced the number of febrile neutropenic hospital days from 35 to 1 in a study of 27 bladder cancer patients (46). Other investigators have noted similar decreases in HDC patients. For example, G-CSF reduced the number of neutropenic days requiring parenteral antibiotics from 18 to 11 (39% reduction) and parenteral nutrition days from 16 to 10 (38% reduction) (47), and should give a 35%–40% reduction in both hospital board and ancillary service costs.

The medical outcome of HDC patients can be predicted by their disease and performance status. HDC given to patients with a high likelihood of tumor response and survival will be more efficacious and cost-effective. Weider et al. found no survivors of HDC among their nine-poor-risk patients, with a median survival of only 0.6 months. These patients had a median number of 30 hospital days at a mean hospital charge of $56,500. By contrast, good-risk patients spent 34 days in the hospital at a mean charge of $44,600, with a median survival of greater than 7.5 months (12).

At least one insurer has attempted to maintain high quality and control costs by transferring patients to centers that do a large number of transplants, including HDC. Prudential has established minimum selection criteria for staff training, volume of procedures, and outcomes. Participating hospitals agree to be reimbursed at a predetermined fee, regardless of resource consumption. Although the volume of transplants has been low for most centers and restricted to heart, lung, and kidney operations, the program saved close to $2 million in its first year while maintaining quality (22). The effect of travel and isolation from support systems must be factored into the quality of life assessments, however.

The success of cost reduction in HDC depends on recognition of the competing factors of service and reimbursement. Physicians, patients, and hospitals all prefer to provide the safest, most effective service at the lowest cost that will support the HDC program and the hospital. Reimbursement systems currently do not adequately compensate the cost of room and board, and some hospitals must maximize reimbursement by emphasizing ancillary service provision. HDC

can be profitable to a hospital, but only in the use of ancillary services with favorable RCCs (Table 7.3). If the profitable service area charges are reduced to costs, the hospital will be unable to recoup losses from unprofitable services and will have less incentive to offer HDC.

HEALTH CARE POLICY ALTERNATIVES BASED ON COST-EFFECTIVENESS

Costs are a major concern of cancer patients, physicians, and insurers, regardless of efficacy (2–4). Allowing ability to pay to become the singular determinant in the treatment decision is not consonant with goals to reduce overall cancer mortality. Decisions about care are already being made on the basis of cost and potential reimbursement, and financial resources are often a reason to exclude patients from HDC. Sixty-one percent of leukemia patients eligible for human leukocyte antigen typing for bone marrow transplant in leukemia were excluded due to financial constraint, and of those typed 14% did not receive transplant for the same reason (7). How can we apply the rationality of clinical trial data and decision analysis to health care policy decisions about HDC?

The technology assessment of HDC in breast cancer has been clouded by the absence of long-term data on outcomes, the difficulty in choosing appropriate historical controls, and reimbursement issues. The longest follow-up is only 2–5 years, and trials of HDC in the adjuvant setting have only recently begun. While early results show a high DFS at 2 years, this may not translate into an overall survival benefit at 5 and 10 years. Historical control groups may not have the same survival curve of the candidates for HDC, given the broad range of biologic behaviors of cancer, especially breast cancer. The rancor of debate over experimental or standard chemotherapy has made accrual to clinical trials progressively more difficult (52). Just being part of a clinical trial may exclude reimbursement unless the patient is part of a clinical trial sponsored by the insurance industry. It is unlikely that sufficient patients will be entered on HDC clinical trials to answer the relevant questions in the next 5 years, since nationally only 1%–3% of eligible patients are accrued (52).

Decision analysis can be used to compare the efficacy and cost-effectiveness of HDC to standard chemotherapy, so these treatments can be compared to other medical interventions. We have used decision analysis in the following ways to answer relevant questions when the clinical trial data are uncertain (31, 37–39, 53):

1. Estimate efficacy and cost effectiveness when the clinical trial is not available, to establish thresholds for decisions. What if 60% DFS at 2 years is maintained at 5 years? What if 60% DFS at 2 years is 20% at 5 years? What if the death rate from toxicity is 0%? 5%? 10%? What if costs can be reduced from $120,000 to $40,000?
2. What is the optimal strategy for maximizing life-years at minimum cost? Should all eligible patients receive HDC, or those at highest risk of relapse, or just those who have "sensitive relapse"?
3. What is the cost per life-year gained of alternative strategies, e.g., two differing adjuvant therapies with differing costs and toxicities?
4. How can quality of life values be factored into the analysis, especially when two strategies have very different risks and benefits?

We have begun to analyze the costs of standard chemotherapy and HDC for patients at the Medical College of Virginia-Massey Cancer Center and have developed a model that incorporates differing assumptions about benefit, quality of life, and alternative therapies.

Patient care decisions about utilizing technology are optimally made in a rational fashion and include data on patient prefer-ence, efficacy, and cost. Decisions to limit therapy to those most likely to benefit and exclude patients with a poor prognosis are difficult to make even without financial constraints. Participants in these issues of resource allocation must include patients, physicians, and third-party payors. One final caution, however, is that the cost-effectiveness of HDC may not compare favorably to strategies to prevent cancer, reduce infant mortality, or reduce the burden of cardiovascular disease (54). Accordingly, it will be important to employ cost reduction methods where possible, develop more effective treatment, and determine the populations that are most likely to benefit.

SUMMARY AND CONCLUSIONS

HDC with autologous bone marrow support is a life-saving but expensive technology for patients with solid tumors. The direct costs of the total illness and care may vary widely, but in-hospital costs are predictable based on service consumption and range from $40,000–$120,000. The major costs are inpatient room and board, pharmacy, laboratory, blood banking, and physician fees. The long-term efficacy of most HDC is unknown, so it is not yet possible to calculate cost-effectiveness to compare with standard accepted medical technologies. Using best estimates of cost and efficacy, HDC for leukemia, lymphoma, breast cancer, and other solid tumors appears to be near or within the range of accepted medical procedures. Cost reduction may be possible with the following strategies: increased use of outpatient services, enteral nutrition, peripherally harvested stem cell autografts, hematopoietins, treatment of only good-risk patients, and designated high-volume HDC centers.

The rational allocation of resources for HDC is difficult in the absence of mature data on effectiveness and benefits. More and better data are needed from clinical trials, including disease-free and overall survival, quality of life measurements, and costs of therapy. Decision analysis can be used to define optimal clinical strategies based on efficacy and cost-effectiveness before the clinical trial data are known.

Acknowledgments
    The authors wish to thank Alan Lieber and Debra Buonaiuto for sharing cost and charge analysis data; Melanie Hillner, Roxanne Cherry, and Joann Bodurtha for constructive reading of manuscripts; and Christine Coggins for expert secretarial assistance.

REFERENCES

1. Brown ML. The national economic burden of cancer. J Natl Cancer Inst 1990;82:1811–1814.
2. McVie JC. Counting costs of care [Editorial]. J Clin Oncol 1988;6:1529–1531.
3. Markman M. An argument in support of cost-effectiveness analysis in oncology [Editorial]. J Clin Oncol 1988;6:937–939.
4. Newcomer LE. Defining experimental therapy—a third party payer's dilemma. N Engl J Med 1990;323:1702–1704.
5. Frei E III, Antman K, Teicher B, Eder P, Schnipper L. Bone marrow allotransplantation for solid tumor—prospects. J Clin Oncol 1989;7:515–526.
6. Vaughn WP, Purtillo RB, Butler D, et al. Ethical and financial issues in autologous marrow transplantation: a symposium sponsored by the University of Nebraska Medical Center. Ann Intern Med 1986; 105:134–145.
7. Durbin M. Bone marrow transplantation: economic, ethical, and social issues. Pediatrics 1988;82:774–783.
8. Bloom BS, Knorr RS, Evans AG. The epidemiology of disease expenses. The costs of caring for children with cancer. JAMA 1985;253:2392–2397.
9. Finkler SA. The distinction between cost and charges. Ann Intern Med 1982;96:102–109.
10. Welch HG, Larson EB. Cost-effectiveness of bone marrow transplantation in acute nonlymphocytic leukemia. N Engl J Med 1989;321:807–812.
11. Kukull WA, Koepsell TD, Conrad DA, Immanuel V, Prodzinski J, Franz C. Rapid estimation of hospitalization charges from a brief medical record review. Med Care 1986;24:961–966.
12. Weider PL, Walthew J, Goodwin T, Reinder A, Finstuen K. Marrow transplantation (MTX) at Virginia Mason (VM) Medical Center (tertiary care, non-university setting): cost and outcome analysis [Abstract]. Blood 1990;76(suppl):571a.
13. Armitage JO, Klassen LW, Burns WP, et al. A comparison of bone marrow transplantation with maintenance chemotherapy for patients with acute nonlymphocytic leukemia in first complete remission. Am J Clin Oncol 1984;7:273–278.
14. Gibbs JO, Narkiewicz, Moore JM. Managing the cost of terminal care in the nonelderly population. In: Scheffler RM, Andrews NC, eds. Cancer care and cost: DRGs and beyond. Ann Arbor, MI: Health Administration Press, 1989.
15. Baker MS, Kessler LG, Smucker RC. Site-specific treatment costs for cancer: an analysis of the Medicare Continuous History Sample File. In: Scheffler RM, Andrews NC, eds. Cancer care and cost: DRGs and beyond. Ann Arbor, MI: Health Administration Press, 1989.
16. O'Connor AM, Boyd NF, Warde P, Stolbach L, Till JE. Eliciting preferences for alternative drug therapies in oncology: influence of treatment outcome description, elicitation technique and treatment experience on preferences. J Chron Dis 1987;40:811–818.
17. Simes RJ, Cocker K, Glasziou P, Coates AS, Tattersall MHN. Costs and benefits of adjuvant (Adj) chemotherapy for breast cancer: an assessment of patient preferences [Abstract]. Proc Am Soc Clin Oncol 1989;8:52a.
18. Schweitzer SO, Scalzi CC. The cost-effectiveness of bone marrow transplant therapy and its policy implications. Washington, DC: Office of Technology Assessment, 1981.
19. Wingard JR, Curbow B, Baker F, Piantadus S. Health functional status, and employment of adult survivors of bone marrow transplantation. Ann Intern Med 1991;114:112–118.
20. Coates A, Gebski V, Bishop JF, et al. Improving the quality of life during chemotherapy for advanced breast cancer. A comparison of intermittent and continuous treatment strategies. N Engl J Med 1987; 317:1490–1495.
21. Desch CE, Smith TJ, Breindel CL, Beauregard DR. A rural cancer outreach program (RCOP): economic analysis from the rural hospital perspective [Abstract]. Proc Assoc Comm Cancer Centers 1991;4:11a.
22. Koska MT. Institutes of Quality experience uneven volume. Hospitals 1990;64(February 5):44,46–48.
23. Pauker SG, Kassirer JP. Decision analysis. N Engl J Med 1987;316:250–258.
24. Skeel RT. Quality of life assessments in cancer clinical trials—it's time to catch up. J Natl Cancer Inst 1989;81:472–473.
25. Moinpour CMcM, Feigl P, Metch B, Hayden KA, Meyskens FL, Crowley J. Quality of life end points in cancer clinical trials: review and recommendations. J Natl Cancer Inst 1989;81:484–491.
26. Goldhirsch A, Gelber RD, Simes RJ, Glasziou P, Coates AS, for the Ludwig Breast Cancer Study Group. Costs and benefits of adjuvant therapy in breast cancer: a quality-adjusted survival analysis. J Clin Oncol 1989;7:36–44.
27. Jaakimainen L, Goodwin PJ, Pater J, Warde P, Murray N, Rapp E. Counting the costs of chemotherapy in a National Cancer Institute of Canada randomized trial in nonsmall-cell lung cancer. J Clin Oncol 1990; 8:1301–1309.

28. Dillman RO, Seagren SL, Propert KJ, et al. A random-ized trial of induction chemotherapy plus high-dose radiation versus radiation alone in Stage III non-small cell lung cancer. N Engl J Med 1990;323:940–945.
29. Tannock IF, Boyer MB. When is a cancer treatment worthwhile? N Engl J Med 1990;323:989–990.
30. Goodwin PJ, Field R, Evans WK, et al. Cost-effective-ness of cancer chemotherapy: an economic evalua-tion of a randomized trial in small cell lung cancer. J Clin Oncol 1988;6:1537–1347.
31. Hillner BE, Smith TJ. Efficacy and cost-effectiveness of adjuvant chemotherapy in women with node-neg-ative breast cancer. A decision analysis model. N Engl J Med 1991;324:160–168.
32. Hillner BE, Smith TJ. Estimating the efficacy and cost-effectiveness of tamoxifen (TAM) versus TAM plus adjuvant chemotherapy in post-menopausal node-positive breast cancer: a decision analysis model. [Abstract] International Conference on Long-Term Antihormonal Therapy for Breast Cancer. 1991, sub-mitted.
33. Brown M. Economic considerations in adjuvant ther-apy of colon cancer. In: Proceedings of the NIH Con-sensus Conference on Adjuvant Therapy for Patients with Colon and Rectum Cancer. Bethesda, MD: NIH, 1990:73–76.
34. Applebaum FR, Dahlberg S, Thomas ED, et al. Bone marrow transplantation or chemotherapy after re-mission induction for adults with acute nonlym-phoblastic leukemia. Ann Inter Med 1984;101:581–588.
35. Chemotherapy v marrow transplantation for adults with acute nonlymphocytic leukemia: a five year fol-low-up. Blood 1988;72:179–184.
36. Antman K. High-dose studies with bone marrow sup-port in breast cancer. In: Gale RP, Champlin R (eds). Bone marrow transplantation: current controversies. New York: Alan R Liss, 1990.
37. Desch CE, Latta MR, Smith T, Hillner BE. The timing of autologous bone marrow transplantation (A-BMT) in Hodgkins disease following a chemotherapy re-lapse [Abstract]. Proc Am Soc Clin Oncol 1990;9:1055a.
38. Desch CE, Latta MR, Smith T, Hillner BE. The optimal timing of autologous bone marrow transplantation in Hodgkins disease following a chemotherapy re-lapse. J Clin Oncol, in press.
39. Hillner BE, Smith TJ, Desch CE. Estimating the cost-effectiveness of autologous bone marrow transplan-tation for metastatic breast cancer [Abstract]. Proc Am Soc Clin Oncol 1991;10:46a.
40. Elfenbein G, Fields K, Saleh R, Kalman L, Lyman G, Balducci L. High dose chemotherapy with autolo-gous bone marrow reserve (HDCBMR) as adjuvant

treatment of poor risk stage II breast cancer: a de-cision analysis [Abstract]. Blood 1990;76(suppl):536a.
41. Bitran JD. High dose chemotherapy with autologous hematopoietic stem cell support in the treatment of women with breast cancer: novel therapeutic ap-proach or passing fad? Oncol J Club 1990;2:15–16.
42. Brandwein JM, Callum J, Rubinger M, Scott JG, Keat-ing A. An evaluation of outpatient bone marrow har-vesting. J Clin Oncol 1989;7:648–650.
43. Szeluga DJ, Stuart RK, Brookmeyer R, Utermohlen V, Santos GW. Nutritional support of bone marrow transplant patients: a prospective, randomized clin-ical trial comparing total parental nutrition to an en-teral feeding program. Cancer Res 1987;47:3309–3316.
44. Elias A, Ayash L, Anderson K, et al. Hematologic sup-port during high-dose intensification for breast can-cer: recruitment of peripheral blood progenitor cells (PBPC) by GM-CSF and chemotherapy [Abstract]. Blood 1990;76(suppl):536a.
45. Glaspy JA, Bluker GC, Crawford J, Stoller RG, Strauss MJ. Decreased costs in cancer chemotherapy patients using recombinant granulocyte colony-stimulating factor [Abstract]. Clin Res 1990;39:7a.
46. Gabrilove JL, Jakubowski A, Sher H, et al. Effect of granulocyte colony stimulating factor on neutro-penia and associated morbidity due to chemother-apy for transitional cell carcinoma of the uroepi-thelium. N Engl J Med 1988;318:1414–1422.
47. Sheridan WP, Wolf M, Lusk J, et al. Granulocyte col-ony-stimulating factor and neutrophil recovery after high-dose chemotherapy and autologous bone mar-row transplantation. Lancet 1989;2:891–894.
48. Edelson JT, Weinstein MC, Tosteson ANA, Williams L, Lee TH, Goldman L. Long-term cost-effectiveness of various initial therapies for mild to moderate hy-pertension. JAMA 1990;263:407–413.
49. Russell B. Some of the tough decisions required by a national health plan. Science 1989;246:892–896.
50. Evans RW. Cost-effectiveness analysis of transplanta-tion. Surg Clin North Am 1986;66:603–616.
51. Weinstein MC, Stason WB. Cost-effectiveness of cor-onary artery bypass surgery. Circulation 1982;66(suppl 3):56-III-66.
52. American Medical Association Council on Scientific Affairs. Viability of cancer clinical research: patient accrual, coverage, and reimbursement. J Natl Cancer Inst 1991;83:254–259.
53. Hillner BE, Smith TJ. Modeling the benefits, risks, and cost-effectiveness of chemotherapy in node-neg-ative breast cancer when the data are incomplete. J Natl Cancer Inst, in press.
54. Detsky AS. Are clinical trials cost-effective. JAMA 1989;262:1795–1800.

Section II

Reestablishing Hematopoiesis after Dose-Intensive Therapy

8

THE HEMATOPOIETIC MICROENVIRONMENT

Stephen G. Emerson

The maturation of blood cells from their developmental predecessors within the bone marrow, or hematopoiesis, occurs within tightly regulated geometric niches. These niches provide elements of cell-cell contact, cell-matrix interactions, and delivery of hematopoietic growth factors essential for the processes of hematopoietic differentiation and self-renewal. In this chapter the structural and functional elements of the hematopoietic microenvironment will be described, with a particular emphasis on the impact of high-dose chemotherapy on the integrity of this critical anatomic and physiologic interface.

THE DYNAMICS OF HEMATOPOIESIS

If one takes into account the known circulating half-lives of the myeloid blood elements and the average density of these circulating cells, simple calculations show that the bone marrow produces as many myeloid cells as are circulating every other day. This figure is obviously a composite of erythropoiesis, where the red cell mass lasts approximately 4 months, thrombopoiesis, where platelets last for a week or less, and neutropoiesis, in which the granulocyte pool must be replenished every 8 hours. Looked at either from the composite perspective or from that of each lineage, hematopoiesis is an extraordinarily productive process.

These numbers, however, only begin to tell the story, as they refer only to blood cell production in the basal state. Under conditions of stress, production rates for each of the myeloid lineages can be greatly accelerated. Erythropoiesis can be increased 20- to 30-fold, for periods of decades, as seen in most patients with sickle cell anemia. Granulopoiesis can be increased at least 20-fold, and thrombopoiesis at least 3-fold. Seen from this perspective, the bone marrow has the capacity to produce as many cells as it contains in a few hours time (1).

In addition to this great productivity, hematopoiesis has the critical feature of stability. That is, despite extraordinary demands for cell production, the process never runs down. Over the past 3 decades experiments in a variety of in vivo and in vitro systems have sought to address how this can occur, with the development of the concept of the pluripotent hematopoietic stem cell. Under this scenario, rare (probably one cell per 10^6 or 10^7) stem cells exist that divide to generate one daughter cell that is programmed to differentiate and one daughter cell that becomes another stem cell. This process, which has been termed quantal mitosis, is responsible for maintaining a relatively constant pool of stem cells, permitting the continual resupply of mature bone marrow and blood cells (2).

This dynamic yet stable process occurs within the tightly packed geometric milieu of the bone marrow cavity. Within the marrow the precursor cells are packed at a density of $3-9 \times 10^8$ cells per milliliter. The bone marrow must therefore solve a major engineering problem, that is, how to supply all the nutrients and remove all the metabolic by-products produced by so many rapidly dividing cells within a confined space. This is a major problem, one not routinely solved by any neoplastic cells. In fact, when most neoplastic tumor cells reach masses or cell division rates approaching one-tenth that of bone marrow, necrotic cores develop, due either to oxygen starvation, metabolite toxicity, or both.

The functional anatomy of bone marrow solves this problem by relying on a massive flux of red cells and plasma through the bone marrow space. The best estimates from mammal studies indicate that approximately 5% of the cardiac output circulates directly to bone, and of this the majority goes to the bone marrow. Using order of magnitude estimates of 1.5 liters of bone marrow and 4.5 liters/minute for cardiac output, this means that each volume of packed bone marrow cavity is perfused with an equal volume of blood and plasma every 6 minutes. This rapid flux of oxygen-carrying capacity, plasma nutrients, and pH buffering capacity is what is responsible for the stability and viability of bone marrow cells in vivo. As described below, this rapid flux also appears to be responsible for the direct stimulation of hematopoiesis through the alembic of the nonhematopoietic, mesenchymal stromal cells lining the bone marrow cavity.

THE CELLULAR COMPONENTS OF THE BONE MARROW MICROENVIRONMENT

In addition to the hematopoietic stem cells and the progenitor and precursor cells that they produce, the bone marrow contains an additional compartment of cells that do not derive directly from the stem cells. These cells include mobile monocytes, T lymphocytes, and NK cells which course in and out of the marrow, and fixed mesenchymal cells, which are collectively termed stromal cells. The hematopoietic microenvironment, or stroma, has long been known to be a major architectural feature of bone marrow, including a complex meshwork of cells and extracellular matrix. Although the precise roles of these cells and matrix components was not early realized (3), it was immediately clear from in vitro experiments that without such a stroma hematopoiesis would rapidly die out in culture. If no attempt was made to remove these stromal elements, hematopoiesis was maintained for periods of weeks to months (4).

The stromal cells and matrix proteins appear to provide two sorts of requisites for hematopoiesis: (*a*) secreted hematopoietic growth factors (HGFs), or colony-stimulating factors (CSFs), and (*b*) an adhesive microenvironment that maintains both high local growth factor concentrations and cell-cell contact. At this time over 15 such glycoproteins have been cloned and isolated, and pharmacologic experiments in vitro and in vivo demonstrate that each has its own distinct spectrum of activities. Broadly speaking, these activities fall into several classes: (*a*) direct permissive effects on committed progenitors (e.g., erythropoietin [Epo], granulocyte colony-stimulating factor [α_1G-CSF], macrophage colony-stimulating factor [M-CSF], interleukin-5 [IL-5], IL-6) (5–8), (*b*) direct permissive effects on multilineage progenitor cells (e.g., granulocyte-macrophage colony-stimulating factor [GM-CSF], IL-3) (9), (*c*) permissive or inductive effects on primitive prepogenitors (perhaps, e.g., IL-3, IL-6, IL-7, LIF, c-kit ligand) (10–12) (*d*) direct suppressive effects on multilineage and committed progenitors (e.g., tumor necrosis factor-α[TNFα], interferon-γ [INFγ]), (13), and (*e*) indirect stimulation of CSF production via the activation of other accessory cells, [e.g., IL-1 and TNFα inducing GM-CSF and G-CSF production by fibroblasts, IFNγ inducing G-CSF production by monocytes] (14–17). Individual hormones may have activities in more than one of these classes, and distinct hormones may display overlapping activities.

While hematopoietic growth factors are necessary for hematopoietic differentiation, they are not sufficient. When immature marrow cells are placed in liquid suspension cultures with even large concentrations of CSFs, only three to four cell divisions occur; direct cell-cell (homotypic) contact is required for normal differentiation. Such contact is artificially provided in vitro in the viscous medium of short-term methylcellulose cultures. In vivo, proper cell-cell contact is thought to be achieved by virtue of adhesive proteins on differentiating marrow cells. These receptors enable cells to interact with each other as well as with external cells and matrix proteins. Key candidate receptors include the fibronectin receptor, which is present on erythroblasts and at least some erythroid progenitors but is lost as reticulocytes mature to mature red cells (18, 19). Myeloid precursors, on the other hand, may possess receptors for a novel protein unique to hematopoietic organs, termed hemonectin (20, 21). Other matrix components such as collagen and laminin may also be critical, either for the survival of the stromal cells or for the survival and differentiation of stem cells per se.

High local concentrations of both required matrix proteins and CSFs may be achieved in vivo through maintenance of a highly packed, three-dimensional geometry. For example, traditional liquid marrow cultures, relying on two-dimensional stromal supports, generate much lower effective concentrations of stromal cells, matrix proteins, and locally complexed HGFs. Naughton and Naughton have suggested that simply recreating a local three-dimensional architecture using nylon fiber meshes may enhance the ability of stromal fibroblasts to support hematopoiesis in liquid culture (22, 23). Moreover, the source of stromal cells influences the lineages of differentiation of transplanted stem cells. In mice and humans, erythroid differentiation predominates in the spleen and myeloid growth in the bone marrow (24). In addition, single murine CFU-S, which develop on the border of marrow spicules ar-

tificially implanted under the splenic capsule, show erythroid growth on the splenic side of the spleen/marrow interface but myeloid growth on the myeloid side of the boundary (25). Thus the specific cell source and configuration of the extracellular microenvironment may provide key regulatory and inductive roles in hematopoiesis.

Production of hematopoietic growth factors can be induced by the in vitro activation of hematopoietic accessory cells. To date, the major stimuli for CSF secretion by stromal accessory cells that have been identified have been products of infection or inflammation. In particular, IL-1(α or β) or TNFα will induce GM-CSF and G-CSF production by fibroblasts and endothelial cells (14, 15). While analogous results have been found for circulating cells (IFNγ and IL-3 induce G-CSF production by monocytes [16], and antigenic [α-CD3] stimulation of T cells induces the production of GM-CSF, IL-3, TNFα, LT, and IFNγ [17]), the apparent inflammatory requirement for stromal CSF secretion is a paradox. Since hematopoiesis occurs in the absence of inflammation, there must be some in vivo signal for CSF production that accounts for basal hematopoiesis. Unraveling the function of the bone marrow microenvironment thus requires considering the function of each of the cellular elements involved, both in response to activation signals and in the unactivated, basal state.

The circulating component of the bone marrow microenvironment is provided by T cells and monocytes. CSF production by *T cells* is closely linked to cellular activation. Adult T cells fail to transcribe or secrete CSFs unless activated via the antigen (CD3) receptor (17). Moreover, these T cells appear to need to be already primed in order to be able to respond to antigenic stimulation by CSF secretion. Neonatal T cells fail to transcribe or secrete detectable CSFs in response to normal antigenic mimetics, unless they have been preactivated with IL-2 (26). Naive T cells are paralyzed and only are drawn into the cytokine network once activated.

Monocytes similarly secrete cytokines only in response to activation signals. The most dramatic of these are provided by other cytokines, and by bacterial toxins themselves. As mentioned above, IFNγ or IL-3 induces G-CSF production, while LPS induces M-CSF production (16). Monocyte attachment and spreading itself is also a signal for CSF secretion, albeit at lower levels than that induced by high-affinity receptor agonists.

The largest representation within the fixed bone marrow microenvironment is that of *fibroblasts*. It has been appreciated for over 6 years now that fibroblasts can be induced to secrete CSFs by products of stimulated monocytes. Initially these observations were made using qualitative bioassays; more recently, precise molecular measurements have demonstrated that the major induced CSFs are GM-CSF and G-CSF. Together with constant quantities of kit-ligand/stem cell factor (SCF) produced constitutively by these cells, this induction appears to be largely responsible for the rise in neutrophil counts observed in inflammation (14, 15). Similar inductions of GM-CSF and G-CSF have been observed in cultured *endothelial cells,* suggesting that these cells play an analogous role to fibroblasts in the amplification of hematopoiesis during inflammation.

Until recently, however, it was not clear how or even if stromal fibroblasts contributed to the support of basal hematopoiesis, in the absence of inflammation. Experiments in many culture systems had failed to demonstrate cytokine gene expression or protein production unless the cells were stimulated with IL-1 or TNFα. Recent studies, however, have now detected cytokines secreted by basal fibroblasts when the cells are cultured under conditions simulating their physiologic environment in vivo and when sensitive detection assays are utilized. Based on the observation that the bone marrow cavity experiences such as high plasma flux, we carefully examined the behavior of bone marrow fibroblasts under conditions of rapid medium exchange. We immediately observed that this resulted in a several-fold increase in the metabolism of these cells, as measured by glucose uptake and lactate production. This implied that human bone marrow cultures not performed at the appropriate medium/serum exchange rates would perforce be suboptimal, and perhaps even doomed to failure, so that their normal CSF secretory behavior could never be determined. The converse conclusion would then also obtain, that study of human bone marrow cultures under properly optimized perfusion conditions would allow the accurate analysis and manipulation of human bone marrow stem cells and stromal cells in vitro.

We next asked whether the secretion of GM-CSF by human bone marrow stromal cells might be detected in bone marrow stromal cells cultured under rapid medium exchange conditions. Utilizing an ELISA assay with a detection limit of 0.01 ng/ml, we were unable to detect GM-CSF secreted under any of the four cultures maintained at a stable rate. However, in cultures in which the rate of medium exchange was increased from 3.5 to 7 exchanges per week, GM-CSF secretion was detectable for 2 weeks, reflecting GM-CSF secretion rates of 0.013–0.22 ng/ml/day (Fig. 8.1). Moreover, GM-CSF secretion was particularly upregulated immediately following increased serum delivery. Thus GM-CSF secretion appeared to be transiently induced by the increase in medium and serum exchange (27).

The results obtained from these measurements lead directly to several conclusions. First, metabolic, growth, and hematopoietic growth factor production rates of adherent bone marrow stromal cells are sensitive to the medium exchange protocols employed in the cultures. This result is important, because (*a*) protocols employed among different bone marrow culture laboratories vary significantly, (*b*) all exchange schedules are far from the rate of plasma exposure to bone marrow cells in vivo, and (*c*) all are submaximally supportive of stromal cell metabolism. It is interesting that some investi-

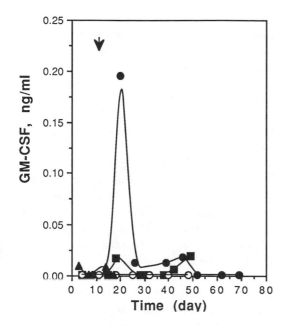

Figure 8.1. GM-CSF production as a function of the medium exchange schedule. There was transient but significant factor production in the cultures shifted from 3.5/week to 7/week. GM-CSF was undetectable in supernatants from cultures maintained with any of the other medium exchange schedules. (Reprinted from the *Journal of Cellular Physiology* 147:344–353 [1991], with permission of Wiley-Liss, Inc.)

gators have examined the effects of medium exchange rates on marrow culture function, but the most rapid exchange rates examined were equivalent to one full exchange per week. Thus according to our results the stimulatory effects of more rapid perfusion would not have been expected to be observed.

Second, upshifting of the medium exchange rates resulted in the detection of GM-CSF secretion into the culture supernatants by otherwise quiescent stromal cells. These cells had been exposed to no known inflammatory mediators. Thus the previous failure to detect CSF secretion by unstimulated stromal cell components may well have been caused, in part, by the culture conditions imposed on those experiments. The finding that GM-CSF secretion was only transiently triggered by the shift in medium exchange rate is significant but not fully explained by the

current data. The stimulation by the altered exchange schedule was accompanied by GM-CSF secretion during the time over which the cell's behavior was changing, but later ceased.

Subsequent studies, both at the protein and the RNA level, have confirmed that GM-CSF is indeed induced by serum and by serum components. IL-6 homeostasis is similar, except that there is a detectable basal secretion at nanomolar levels. No gene expression or protein secretion is detected for either IL-3 or G-CSF, however, in normal cultured bone marrow fibroblasts. These signals, if present in basal bone marrow, appear to be supplied by other cells. Although we do not yet have data at the level of secreted protein, reverse transcriptase polymerase chain reaction analyses indicate that the level of kit-ligand/SCF gene expression is also extremely responsive to serum flux.

Indeed, Singer and colleagues have recently described a subpopulation of bone marrow stromal cells that secrete extremely high quantities of CSFs (28). These cells, which are stimulated to proliferate by IL-1, TNFα, and IL-6 and appear to comprise 0.01%–1% of all adherent bone marrow cells, are termed clonally-derived stromal cells, or *CDSC.* These cells, in contrast to the background majority of bone marrow stromal fibroblasts, secrete G-CSF preferentially over GM-CSF. Low-level G-CSF secretion is detectable in the absence of stimulation either by serum or inflammatory mediators. Given the high level of CSFs produced by these cells in response to IL-1 and TNFα, it will be interesting to see what functions previously ascribed to bone marrow fibroblasts are in fact caused by this CDSC subpopulation.

In summary, the bone marrow microenvironment is comprised of several cell populations, some fixed and some transitory residents. T cells, monocytes, fibroblasts, endothelial cells, and specialized CDSC stromal cells all contribute to the maintenance of hematopoiesis both in the basal state and in response to the stresses of inflammation. These functions of the cells comprising the bone marrow microenvironment are summarized in Figure 8.2.

THE RESPONSE OF THE MICROENVIRONMENT TO HIGH-DOSE CHEMOTHERAPY

Surprisingly little is known about the precise cellular and molecular impact of high-dose chemotherapy on the bone marrow microenvironment. Classical studies using bioassays demonstrated hematopoietic-stimulating activity in the serum of patients several days following intravenous chemotherapy. More recent ELISA studies have shown that G-CSF is detectable in serum following intensive combination chemotherapy. Studies such as these clearly document that the bone marrow microenvironment, as an organ, is capable of responding to cytopenic stress by upregulating the production of critical cytokines, which then stimulate hematopoietic recovery. The cellular and molecular mechanisms by which this occurs are truly unknown at the present time. Of particular interest, the levels of cytokines produced in response to such stresses are not optimal. Supplying higher, pharmacologic doses of neutrogenic cytokines clearly accelerates the patient's recovery from the nadir.

While the increased production of CSFs acutely following chemotherapy is clear, the long-term consequences of such cytotoxic chemotherapy are less well understood. While many chemotherapeutic drugs are relatively cell-cycle specific and so might be expected to spare fixed mesenchymal stromal cells, others are not. In addition, it is entirely possible that the most important components of the microenvironment are actually proliferating, undergoing a degree of turnover similar to that of the myeloid marrow elements

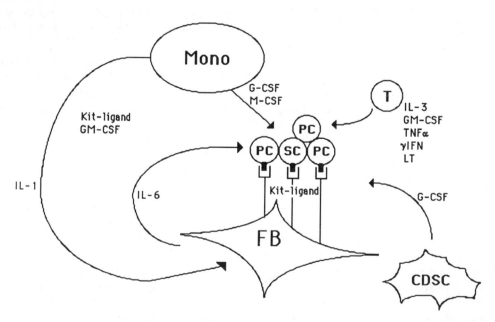

Figure 8.2. Functional anatomy of the bone marrow microenvironment. Hematopoietic stem and progenitor cells exist in a high-density microenvironment in close proximity to accessory cells that supply self-renewal and differentiation signals, in the form of soluble and membrane-bound hematopoietic growth factors. These are provided both by fixed mesenchymal fibroblasts, endothelial cells, and CDSC cells, which constitutively supply low levels of GM-CSF, G-CSF, IL-6 and kit-ligand, and by localized but mobile monocytes and T cells, which upon activation secrete many cytokines. SC, stem cell; PC, progenitor cell; FB, fibroblast.

themselves. Suspicious evidence for long-term stromal damage derives from clinical experiences in which patients who have received substantial chemotherapeutic doses fail to ever recover normal blood counts, even over years, yet never develop signs of progressive myelodysplasia. Although alternative explanations for such cases exist, they are not persuasive. For example, invoking stem cell damage for such long-term cytopenias is less likely than stromal damage. Even in allogeneic bone marrow transplantation, where few stem cells are transplanted and patients routinely have progenitor cell pools reduced 3- to 100-fold below normal levels, normal blood counts are usually reached and maintained. Since so few normal stem cells are needed for grossly normal blood counts, failure to maintain such counts rather suggests a defect in supporting proliferation from any stem cells present, i.e., a microenvironmental defect.

Nonetheless, arguments such as this are clearly only speculative. At this time, we simply do not yet have enough information on the effects of high-dose chemotherapy on the function of bone marrow microenvironmental elements. However, as described above, we now are compiling sufficient information concerning the phylogeny and function of the critical cells in the bone marrow microenvironment that these questions can be addressed, both through in vitro model systems and by evaluating cells from patients undergoing chemotherapeutic regimens. Such studies will undoubtedly be extremely important in the design of future high-dose chemotherapeutic programs for such indications as multiple autologous bone marrow transplanation.

REFERENCES

1. Emerson SG, Palsson BO, Clarke MF. The construction of high efficiency human bone marrow tissue ex vivo. J Cell Biochem 1991;45:268–272.
2. Holzer H, Biehl J, Antin P, et al. Quantal and proliferative cell cycles: how lineages generate cell diversity and maintain fidelity. Prog Clin Biol Res 1983;134:213–227.
3. Bentley SA. Bone marrow connective tissue and the haemopoietic microenvironment. Br J Haematol 1982;50(1):1–6.
4. Dexter TM, Allen TD, Lajtha LG. Conditions controlling the proliferation of haemopoietic stem cells in vitro. J Cell Physiol 1977;91:335–344.
5. Souza LM, Boone TC, Gabrilove G, et al. Recombinant human granulocyte colony-stimulating factor: effects on normal and leukemic myeloid cells. Science 1986;232:61–64.
6. Sanderson CF, O'Garra A, Warren DJ, et al. Eosinophil differentiation factor also has B-cell growth factor activity: proposed name interleukin 4. Proc Natl Acad Sci USA 1986;83:437–441.
7. Hirano T, Yasukawa K, Harada, et al. Complementary DNA for a novel human interleukin (BSF-2) that induces B lymphocytes to produce immunoglobulin. Nature 1986;324:73–76.
8. Emerson SG, Yang YC, Clark SC, et al. Human recombinant granulocyte-macrophage colony stimulating factor and interleukin 3 have overlapping but distinct hematopoietic activities. J Clin Invest 1988;82:1282–1287.
9. Leary AG, Ikebuchi K, Hirai Y, et al. Synergism between interleukin-6 and interleukin-3 in supporting proliferation of human hematopoietic stem cells: comparison with interleukin-1 alpha. Blood 1988; 71:1759–1763.
10. Namen AE, Lupton S, Hjerrild K, et al. Stimulation of B-cell progenitors by cloned murine interleukin-7. Nature 1988;333:571–573.
11. Leary AG, Wong GG, Clark SC, et al. Leukemia inhibitory factor differentiation—inhibiting activity/ human interleukin for DA cells augments proliferation of human hematopoietic stem cells. Blood 1990;75:1960–1964.
12. Zsebo KM, Williams DA, Geissler EN, et al. Stem cell factor is encoded at the Sl locus of the mouse and is the ligand for the c-kit tyrosine kinase receptor. Cell 1990;63:213–224.
13. Broxmeyer H, Lu L, Platzer E, et al. Comparative analysis of the influences of human gamma, alpha and beta interferons on human multipotential (CFU-GEMM), erythroid (BFU-E) and granulocyte-macrophage (CFU-GM) progenitor cells. J Immunol 1983;131:1300–1306.
14. Broudy VC, Kaushansky K, Harlan JM, et al. Interleukin 1 stimulates human endothelial cells to produce granulocyte-macrophage colony-stimulating factor and granulocyte colony-stimulating factor. J Immunol 1987;139:464–468.
15. Sieff CA, Tsai S, Faller DV. Interleukin 1 induces cultured human endothelial cell production of granulocyte-macrophage colony-stimulating factor. J Clin Invest 1987;79:48–51.
16. Vellenga AR, Ernst T, Ostapovicz D, et al. Independent regulation of M-CSF and G-CSF gene expression in human monocytes. Blood 1988;71:1529–1532.

17. Guba SC, Stella G, Turka LA, et al. Regulation of T cell interleukin 3 gene expression via the CD3 and CD28 pathways. J Clin Invest 1989;84:1701–1706.

18. Patel VP, Ciechanover A, Platt O, et al. Mammalian reticulocytes lose adhesion to fibronectin during maturation to erythrocytes. Proc Natl Acad Sci USA 1985;82:440–444.

19. Coulombel L, Vuillet MH, Leroy C, et al. Lineage- and stage-specific adhesion of human hematopoietic progenitor cells to extracellular matrices from marrow fibroblasts. Blood 1988;71:329–334.

20. Campbell AD, Wicha MS, Long M. Extracellular matrix promotes the growth and differentiation of murine hematopoietic cells in vitro. J Clin Invest 1985;75:2085–2090.

21. Campbell AD, Long M, Wicha MS. Haemonectin, a bone marrow adhesion protein specific for cells of granulocyte lineage. Nature 1987;329:744–746.

22. Naughton BA, Naughton GK. Establishment of long term bone marrow culture after cryopreservation in the rat [Abstract]. Blood 1986;68(suppl):474a.

23. Naughton BA, Preti RA, Naughton GK. Hematopoiesis on nylon mesh templates. I: Long-term culture of rat bone marrow cells. J Med 1987;18(3–4):219–50.

24. Bagby GC, Shaw G, Brown MA, et al. IL-1 induces GM-CSF mRNA accumulation in human stromal cells (HSC) by inducing ribonuclease inhibitory activity [Abstract]. Blood 1988;72(suppl):347a.

25. Santoli S, Yang YC, Clark SC, et al. Synergistic and antagonistic effects of recombinant human interleukin (IL) 3, IL-1 alpha, granulocyte and macrophage colony-stimulating factors (G-CSF and M-CSF) on the growth of GM-CSF-dependent leukemic cell lines. J Immunol 1987;139:3348–3354.

26. Ehlers S, Smith KA. Differentiation of T cell lymphokine gene expression: the in vitro acquisition of T cell memory. J Exp Med 1991;173:25–36.

27. Caldwell J, Locey B, Palsson BO, et al. The influence of culture perfusion conditions on normal human bone marrow stromal cell metabolism. J Cell Physiol 1991;147:344–353.

28. Singer JW. Recombinant human interleukin-6 (rhIL-6) stimulates anchorage-independent growth of marrow stromal cell (MSC) colonies which can be expanded as adherent MSC lines that constitutively produce high levels of colony-stimulating activity (CSA) [Abstract]. Blood 1989;74(7)(suppl 1):33a.

9

RECONSTITUTION OF HEMATOPOIESIS FOLLOWING ALLOGENEIC BONE MARROW TRANSPLANTATION

Nelson J. Chao and Karl G. Blume

Allogeneic bone marrow transplantation (BMT) has evolved over the past 2 decades to become an effective curative treatment modality for a variety of disorders. These include malignant diseases, dyserythropoiesis, bone marrow aplasia, immunodeficiency states, and glycolipid storage diseases (1–5). The successes of BMT have paralleled the elucidation of the major histocompatibility complex (MHC) and the development of transfusional support methods and intensive patient support measures with parenteral nutrition and broad-spectrum antimicrobial drugs.

Much of today's success in the area of BMT began 4 decades ago with a description of experimental radiation chimeras. In Greek mythology, Chimera was the offspring of Echidna and Typhon. She had the head of a lion, the body of a goat, and a snake for a tail (6). In medical terms, "chimera" is used to designate an organism whose body contains cell populations derived from genetically different individuals. The history of radiation chimera began in 1951 when Jacobson and Lorenz independently demonstrated that use of syngeneic, allogeneic, and even xenogeneic bone marrow cells could protect lethally irradiated animals (7–10). Studies of radiation-induced bone marrow chimeras have provided a vast amount of information concerning hematopoietic stem cell growth, differentiation, and function and have opened new pathways to the investigation of numerous questions in the field of hematology, oncology, and transplantation immunology.

STEM CELLS

The radiation experiments documented the existence of a hematopoietic stem cell. It was a remarkable finding that an entire organ system destroyed by radiation could be replaced by infusion of a small number of normal cells. The search for the hematopoietic stem cell began with the ability to culture progenitor cells in semisolid media (11–13). The description of various lineages of cells found in the blood and the ability to tag each of these cells specifically with a unique marker was of critical importance. Thus lymphocytes (T and B cells), monocytes and macrophages, and myeloid cells could be separated and therefore differentiated. Investigators documented that mononuclear cell fractions could give rise to colonies of mononuclear cells in vitro or to other hematopoietic cells. Thus under defined conditions, mononuclear cells gave rise to other mononuclear cells, granulocytes, and erythroid cells (14–15). Again,

151

standard in vitro assays do not allow continued propagation of these cells, and eventually, in approximately 2–4 weeks, most of these cells die. By changing some of the culture conditions, these cells can be maintained for months, but all eventually die. The final test for stem cell rests in in vivo reconstitution experiments where these cells can permanently rescue a lethally irradiated animal.

Recently the hematopoietic stem cell of the mouse has been demonstrated by depleting whole bone marrow of lineage-specific cells followed by positive selection with a new monoclonal antibody termed stem cell antigen-1 (SCA-1) (16). In this system, a single cell can give rise to multilineage colonies in the spleen and thymus. Moreover, only 25 cells can rescue 50% of lethally radiated mice. Efforts are ongoing to find the same cell in humans. Unfortunately, we are still lacking the human equivalent to the SCA-1 marker of the mouse. Isolation of stem cells in humans could help solve many problems of bone marrow transplantation, such as graft-versus-host disease, tumor contamination (when using autologous bone marrow), gene therapy, etc. Current experimental data indicate that only 1 in 2000 nucleated marrow cells is a stem cell.

GROWTH FACTORS

It became clear early on that blood cell formation, differentiation, and egress is a tightly regulated process and one of the most complex examples of multilineage differentiation. A stem cell residing in the bone marrow gives rise to red cells, granulocytes, macrophages, monocytes, basophils, eosinophils, lymphocytes, and platelets. Most of these differentiated cells are short-lived and need to be constantly replaced. Moreover, some of these cells can respond dramatically and rapidly to clinical conditions. A normal granulocyte count of 2000/ml can rise to 50,000/μl in 1 day for patients with a serious infection.

The in vitro semisolid media cell culture systems for the clonal growth of specific hematopoietic progenitors allowed the selective establishment of unique lineages. Cell division and differentiation was fully dependent on a continuous supply of specific growth factors that regulated hematopoiesis. Because these were first identified with these culture assays, they have been termed colony-stimulating factors, or CSFs (17–19). These different CSFs were defined through the analysis of cell types evolving under the influence of such factors. Many such factors have now been described. The best-characterized ones have been tested in clinical trials, and two of these have been licensed by the Food and Drug Administration. These two factors have a narrow spectrum of activity or lineage specificity, namely, stimulation only of the granulocytes (G-CSF) or granulocytes and macrophages (GM-CSF). In contrast, colonies grown in interleukin-3 (IL-3, or multi-CSF) give rise to several cell lines (20). Other growth factors, such as erythropoietin, IL-1, IL-2, and IL-4, also have specific roles and may act synergistically with other factors. Recently a multipotent growth factor, termed stem cell factor (SCF) or kit ligand, has been reported by several groups (21–23). This search began with a steel (SI) and white spotting (W) mutation found in mice. Mutation of either gene when homozygous caused embryonic death. However, compound heterozygotes carrying certain alleles of either gene are viable. These mutations are semidominant and result in similar phenotypes, particularly in the defects of hematopoiesis. Transplantation or coculture experiments between the W and SI mutations demonstrate that the defect of W mice is on a hematopoietic stem cell, whereas the SI defect is in the marrow stromal cell environment. Therefore, the SI defect is responsible for the lack of pluripotent growth factor (SCF), while the W locus codes for its receptor (c-kit tyrosine kinase receptor). SCF alone does little but in combination with GM-CSF or G-CSF results in dramatic stimulation of colony formation (23). We are only beginning to dissect the complexities of these interactions.

PREPARATORY REGIMENS FOR BONE MARROW TRANSPLANTATION

The purpose of the preparatory regimens varies according to the disease for which allogeneic BMT is being employed. For hematologic malignancies, such regimens are intended to achieve at least three purposes. The first goal in therapy of malignant diseases is to eradicate the tumor cells. The efficacy of the conditioning regimen depends on the sensitivity of the tumor cells to the agents used. The second purpose of a preparatory regimen is to decrease or remove the host resistance to transplantation—i.e., to immunosuppress the host. Host cells (T cells and natural killer [NK] cells) are present and are capable of rejecting the graft. The allogeneic graft is clearly foreign to the host, and the host defense mechanisms are set up specifically to recognize allogeneic differences and remove foreign cells. This host resistance to the donor graft can be observed by the increase in the number of cells required for a successful transplantation. Four-fold more cells are required for an allogeneic MHC identical graft as compared to autologous or syngeneic transplantation to be successful, even following high-dose total body irradiation (22, 24). When MHC-mismatched grafts are used, the number of bone marrow cells required increases 10-fold compared to the MHC-matched setting. Experiments in dogs using single agents for conditioning prior to BMT suggest that irradiation is the most effective preparatory component in MHC identical pairs. The third purpose of the conditioning regimen is to create "space," since the new donor marrow must replace the host hematopoietic system. Unless there is an area for these new cells to settle in, the new bone marrow may not grow. Figure 9.1 shows a schema for agents used in preparatory regimens.

TECHNIQUE FOR BONE MARROW GRAFTING

Bone marrow for transplantation is usually obtained by multiple marrow aspirations

PREPARATION FOR BMT

HIGH DOSE	HIGH DOSE
CHEMOTHERAPY	RADIOTHERAPY

DRUGS: CYCLOPHOSPHAMIDE
              BUSULFAN
              VP-16
              CYTOSINE-ARABINOSIDE

RADIATION: FRACTIONATED TOTAL BODY
                    IRRADIATION

Figure 9.1.   Schema of agents used in preparatory regimens.

from a healthy donor. The usual site for aspiration is the posterior iliac crest, although on rare occasions the anterior iliac crest or the sternum is also used. The bone marrow harvest is done in the operating room under general or spinal anesthesia. Each aspirate (2–5 ml) is mixed with heparin and tissue culture media (25). A total of $1-3 \times 10^8$ nucleated cells per kg recipient weight is obtained, usually in a volume of 500–1000 ml (in adult patients). The aspirate is then passed through a series of metal screens to remove larger particles (clots and bone spicules). The bone marrow is then infused intravenously into the recipient if the donor and recipients are ABO compatible. If there is a major ABO incompatibility, the marrow graft needs to be red-cell depleted by sedimentation methods (26).

HOMING

Stem cells enter the recipient's circulation and replace the recipient's endogenous cells. These donor cells then repopulate all the recipient's hematopoietic cells. Besides the normal peripheral blood cells, Langerhans cells of the skin, Kupffer cells of the liver, microglial cells of the brain, alveolar macrophages of the lung, and osteoclasts become of donor origin (27, 28). The presence of homing receptors allows intravenously infused stem cells to engraft successfully rather than requiring surgical intervention as in other organ transplantation (29). This homing process is a recognition mechanism mediated by membrane proteins, so that circulating progenitor cells bind selectively to the marrow stroma. Once settled on the marrow stromal support, these progenitor cells can divide and proliferate. As these cells divide and mature, homing receptors are diluted and lost. Mature cells do not possess homing receptors and can be released into the circulation. Studies of the homing receptors have evolved from work done in lymphocyte traffic and the development of appropriate probes that permit the dissection of this complex phenomenon. Early data from lectin mitogens suggest that the interactions of membrane lectins and membrane glycoproteins may be involved in cellular recognition and homing (30, 31). Synthetic neoglycoproteins designed by covalently linking p-amino phenyl derivatives of various active monosaccharides in pyranose form to bovine serum albumin were tested in mice subjected to lethal doses of total body irradiation (32). The presence of galactosyl and mannosyl derivatives causes a decline in CFU-S, and CFU-GM. Moreover, reconstitution of hematopoiesis in vivo was prevented in mice, suggesting a specific interaction between the synthetic probes and the ability to repopulate the bone marrow (33). Homing of these stem cells is likely to be a complex mechanism with various interactions, involving not only the specific cells but perhaps also extracellular matrix proteins. Furthermore, each receptor ligand interaction(s) may be synergistic or antagonistic in a tightly regulated system.

The bone marrow can be divided into two compartments, vascular and extravascular (34–38). In mammalian systems, hematopoiesis occurs almost exclusively in the extravascular compartment. This extravascular space does not necessarily have to be the bone marrow itself. For example, in patients with extensive myelofibrosis or malignant myelosclerosis, the infused bone marrow may give rise to normal peripheral blood counts by extramedullary hematopoiesis in splenic tissue. Only gradually, as the marrow fibrosis lessens, does hematopoiesis return to the bone marrow. Exchange between the vascular and extravascular spaces occurs at the level of the sinusoids. The sinusoids form the blood-bone marrow barrier and contain a layer of endothelium that controls the exchange between the two spaces. Thus as cells exit the bone marrow, they migrate through the body of the endothelial cells. Homing also occurs through the sinusoids. Contrary to binding of the stem cell to stromal support cells, these stem cells must first bind to endothelial cells. This is followed by internalization and subsequent externalization to the abluminal side into the stromal support system. Little is known about the binding of these stem cells to the sinusoidal endothelium.

HEMATOPOIETIC RECOVERY FOLLOWING BONE MARROW TRANSPLANTATION

By the time of donor bone marrow infusion, the patient is usually, or soon will be, severely pancytopenic in the peripheral blood and bone marrow. On day 7, random clusters of three to six nucleated cells can be found widely scattered throughout the marrow space (39). By 10–14 days, discrete colonies of hematopoietic cells are found in the bone marrow. The majority are of one cell lineage, but occasionally mixed colonies are found. This homogenous population in each cluster or colony suggests that the cells arose from a single precursor, rather than being an aggregate of circulating cells. However, cellularity early on is extremely variable, ranging from 0%–90% in one study (40). Bone marrow stroma exhibits many abnormalities, such as fibrosis, periodic-acid-Schiff-positive fat cells, interstitial edema, sinus ectasia, and granulomas. Localization of the marrow cells is also variable, being in subcortical or central areas and within intrabecular areas. In contrast, normal erythroid hematopoiesis is localized mainly centrally, and myeloid hematopoiesis is found mostly near the endosteum (41). Gradually the cellularity increases, and usually by 1 year's time, the bone marrow has returned to normal. Figure 9.2 demonstrates an example of bone marrow cellularity on days +15, +30, +100, and at 1 year after BMT.

Engraftment is generally accepted as equal or greater than 500 granulocytes/μl in the peripheral blood and varies widely from patient to patient (Fig. 9.3). It ranges from 8–30 days and depends on the underlying disease, the preparative regimen, the type of BMT (allogeneic versus autologous), and use of peripheral blood stem cells, as well as on the drugs used to prevent the development of acute graft-versus-host disease (GVHD). For example, our studies comparing cyclosporine and prednisone versus cyclosporine, prednisone, and methotrexate shows a statistically significant difference in the time to engraftment. Patients receiving methotrexate have a longer period of marrow aplasia—on the average 5 more days before engraftment is achieved (14 versus 19 days after BMT).

Red cells and platelets are transfused to maintain a clinically acceptable level, but their production also depends on the same parameters as granulocyte recovery. Red cell (reticulocyte count > 1.5%) and platelet (>25,000/μl) engraftment usually follows engraftment of granulocytes. While the median time to recovery of platelets is only slightly longer when compared to granulocytes in uncomplicated BMT patients, the range is much broader and can extend to over 100 days (Fig. 9.4). Patients with chronic GVHD may remain thrombocytopenic. Red cell recovery is fre-

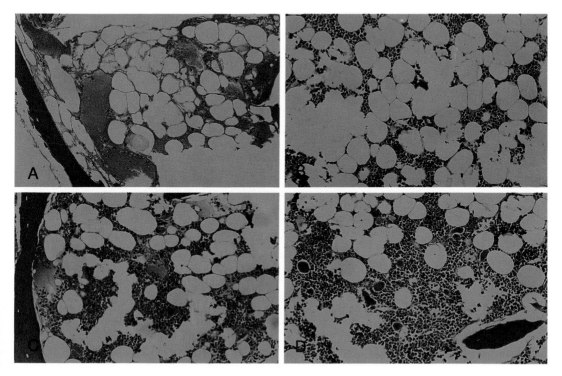

Figure 9.2.   Bone marrow biopsies done on day (**A**) +15, (**B**) +30, (**C**) +100, and (**D**) +365 following BMT. Note the increase in cellularity over time.

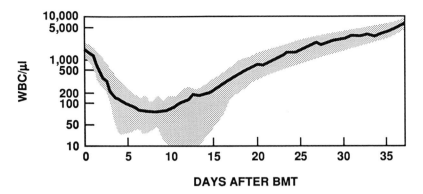

Figure 9.3. Granulocyte recovery following BMT in 10 patients transplanted for acute leukemia is shown in the solid line. Shaded area represents the observed range.

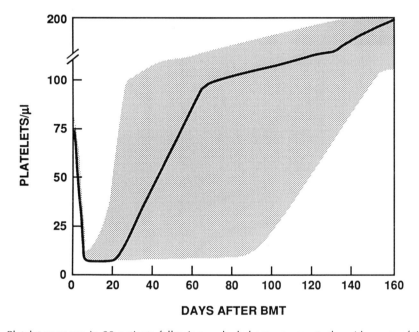

Figure 9.4. Platelet recovery in 20 patients following BMT for acute leukemia is shown in the solid line. The shaded area represents the wide range of time to platelet recovery.

quently masked by transfusion of heterologous packed red blood cells. Measurement of reticulocyte counts in a group of patients receiving allogeneic BMT for acute leukemia demonstrates that reticulocytes peak at approximately 40 days following BMT (Fig. 9.5).

There is no correlation between the number of transplanted cells or hematopoietic precursors (CFUc, CFUe, BFUe) and the recovery of nucleated cells, although some correlation exists between the number of transplanted cells and reticulocyte recovery (41, 42). There is evidence that the early findings (during the first 4 weeks) in the bone marrow are due to the outgrowth of the first wave of committed precursors, with the pro-

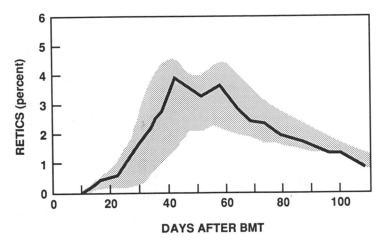

DAYS AFTER BMT

Figure 9.5. Reticulocyte counts following BMT in 10 patients transplanted for acute leukemia are shown in   the solid line. The shaded area represents the normal range.

liferation and differentiation of the pluripotent cells occurring later. Although peripheral blood granulocyte counts recover with a median of 8–30 days, bone marrow cellularity and the numbers of committed precursors can remain abnormally low for up to 3 years following BMT. This decreased bone marrow cellularity with normal peripheral blood counts may reflect hematopoiesis at extramedullary sites.

Establishment of the donor origin of the graft can be performed by the analysis of chromosomal markers, blood cell isozyme, red cell antigens, or immunoglobulin isotypes, or by restriction fragment length polymorphisms using synthetic probes to variable nuclear tandem repeat segments of DNA. Mixed hematopoietic chimerism, where both recipient and donor cells exist side by side in a stable fashion, also occurs. There is some evidence that these patients with stable mixed chimerism may have a more favorable outcome (43). Observations in experimental animals indicate that establishing mixed chimerism results in stable engraftment without evidence of GVHD (44).

With the advent of cloned growth factors, hematologic recovery after BMT is accelerated (45). As experience with these growth factors becomes available, caution must be exercised to exclude the possibility of such factors' stimulating growth of residual malignant clones (46, 47). Use of GM-CSF in allogeneic BMT has not resulted in an increased relapse rate nor in an increase of GVHD (46).

GRAFT FAILURE

Occasionally the emerging hematopoiesis is not of donor origin but of recipient origin, and the donor graft does not take. Failure to engraft or to sustain a marrow graft occurs in 1%–35% of BMT patients (48, 49). This failure rate is dependent upon the underlying disorder, the conditioning regimen employed, prior therapy, and the type of marrow graft (T cell depleted versus unmanipulated). This is most frequently observed in BMT for previously transfused patients with aplastic anemia who receive cyclosphosphamide alone as their conditioning regimen. The most frequent explanation for graft failure is residual immunocompetent host cells rejecting the allograft. Other mechanisms include relapse of the original disease and/or possibly destruction of the stromal support system. Pancytopenia during BMT may also be secondary to viral infections, especially with cytomegalovirus.

IMMUNE RECONSTITUTION

Frequent infectious complications are another risk factor in BMT. These occur, in part, due to delays in "reeducation" and recovery of normal immune function. A similar delay in normal function has been observed for granulocytes and may cause or contribute to the infectious complications (50). Abnormal granulocyte chemotaxis, phagocytic-bactericidal activity, and superoxide production have been described, particularly in patients with GVHD (Fig. 9.6). It remains unclear if such abnormalities are due to intrinsic defects from impaired cellular maturation post-BMT or due to a decrease in specific cytokine production.

As immature T cells exit from the marrow, they must be "educated" in the new thymus. Lack of functional thymic tissue is one possible explanation why GVHD occurs more frequently in the older patient population. By T cell subset analysis, most recipients of allogeneic marrow grafts require 3–4 months to achieve normal T and B cell numbers in the peripheral blood and up to a year until the ratio of CD4/CD8 cells has returned to

normal. Serum complement level reaches normal levels within 3 months following BMT. Serum IgG and IgM levels return to normal by 3–4 months, but IgA may remain low for up to 1 year in an uncomplicated BMT patient (50–54). In spite of normal levels of circulating antibody, a specific antibody reaction to a particular antigen may remain abnormally low for an extended period of time, sometimes years.

Recovery of cellular immunity takes considerably longer, as measured by delayed-type hypersensitivity, and may remain abnormal for up to 2 years (55). Responses to recall antigen may take up to 4 years before they normalize (56). The lack of response seems to be more than lack of T cell help. Co-culture experiments suggest a specific suppressor activity that can be removed by 1200 cGy. Interestingly, the pace of recovery of allogeneic and syngeneic BMT recipients is remarkably similar. Therefore, there may be other growth and/or differentiation factors that are not yet recognized. In spite of profound defects in immunity, most patients survive during this period. This is likely due to use of potent antimicrobial agents and protection derived from residual mature host and donor cells (56). The critical period of lack of defenses is the time of cross-over from

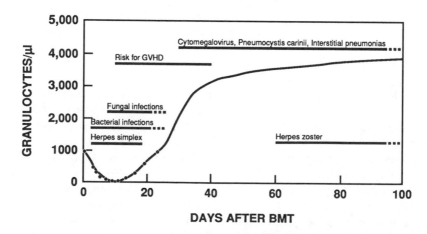

Figure 9.6.   Schematic representation of granulocyte recovery and time of increased risk of infectious complications following BMT.

residual host/donor cells to new chimeric stem cell progeny. Attempts to accelerate the immune recovery with thymus transplants or thymus extract have not yielded positive results. New factors, such as GM-CSF, IL-2, etc., are being tested in clinical trials. There is some suggestion that defective leukocyte function may be corrected with exogenous administration of GM-CSF. Future studies will concentrate on boosting or immunizing donor cells prior to grafting, with the expectation that this will afford an additional protective factor until donor stem cells have matured.

SUMMARY AND CONCLUSIONS

Recovery of normal bone marrow function is dependent on a complex interaction between the donor graft and the immunosuppressed host. The presence of homing receptors in committed hematopoietic precursors and pluripotent stem cells allows for reconstitution to occur via the blood stream. Once in the marrow environment stromal support matrix, committed precursors and stem cells are under the influence of specific growth factors in a tightly regulated process. Growth and differentiation of these transplanted cells and their egress into the blood stream results over time in a normal recovery of the peripheral blood. However, complete immunologic recovery in terms of immunoglobulin production, T and B lymphocytes, and granulocyte function may take up to 4 years to normalize. Yet in spite of apparent significant biologic obstacles, new donor-derived marrow cells seem to function sufficiently well in man to allow for excellent clinical results in many life-threatening diseases for which BMT is utilized.

REFERENCES

1. Chao NJ, Blume KG. Bone marrow transplantation. Part I: Allogeneic. West J Med 1989;151:638–643.
2. Armitage JO. Bone marrow transplantation in the treatment of patients with lymphoma. Blood 1989;73(7):1749–1758.
3. Santos GW. Marrow transplantation in acute nonlymphocytic leukemia. Blood 1989;74(3):901–908.
4. Gribben JG, Linch DL, Singer CRJ, McMillan AK, Jarrett M, Goldstone AH. Successful treatment of refractory Hodgkin's disease by high-dose combination chemotherapy and autologous bone marrow transplantation. Blood 1989;73(1):340–344.
5. Champlin R, Gale RP. Acute lymphoblastic leukemia: recent advances in etiology and therapy. Blood 1989;73(8):2051–2066.
6. Owsalt SG. Concise encyclopedia of Greek and Roman mythology. Chicago: Follet Publishing Co., 1969.
7. Lorenz E, Congdon CC. Modification of lethal irradiation injury in mice by injection of homologous and heterologous bone marrow. J Natl Cancer Inst 1954;14:955–965.
8. Lorenz E, Congdon CC, Uphoff DE. Modification of acute irradiation injury in mice and guinea pigs by bone marrow injections. Radiology 1952;58:863–877.
9. Jacobson LO, Marks EK, Robson MJ, et al. Effect of spleen protection on mortality following X-irradiation. J Lab Clin Med 1949;34:1538.
10. Jacobson LO, Simmons EL, Marks EK, Eldredge JH. Recovery from radiation injury. Science 1951;113:510.
11. Till JE, McCulloch EA. A direct measurement of the radiation sensitivity of normal mouse bone marrow cells. Radiat Res 1961;14:213.
12. Curry JL, Trentin JJ. Hematopoietic spleen colony studies. I: Growth and differentiation. Dev Biol 1967;15:395.
13. Metcalf D, Moore MAS. Haemopoietic cells. Amsterdam: North-Holland, 1971:70.
14. Trentin JJ, Curry JL, Wolf NS, Cheng V. Factors controlling stem cell differentiation and proliferation: the hematopoietic inductive micro-environment (HIM), In: The proliferation and spread of neoplastic cells, the 21st annual symposium on fundamental cancer research of the University of Texas M.D. Anderson Hospital. Baltimore: Williams & Wilkins, 1968:713–727.
15. Wolf, NS, Trentin JJ. Hemopoietic colony studies. V: Effect of hemopoietic organ stroma on differentiation of pluripotent stem cells. J Exp Med 1968;127:205.
16. Spangrude GJ, Heimfeld S, Weissman IL. Purification and characterization of mouse hematopoietic stem cells. Science 1988;241:58–62.
17. Clark SC, Kamen R. The human hematopoietic colony-stimulating factors. Science 1987;236:1229–1237.
18. Whetton AD, Dexter TM. Myeloid haemopoietic growth factors. Biochim Biophys Acta 1989;989:111–132.
19. Appelbaum FR. The clinical use of hematopoietic growth factors. Semin Hematol 1989;26(3):7–14.
20. Ganser A, Lindemann A, Seipelt G. et al. Effects of recombinant human interleukin-3 in patients with normal hematopoiesis and in patients with bone marrow failure. Blood 1990;76(4):666–676.
21. Zsebo KM, Geissler EN, Martin FH, et al. Stem cell factor is encoded at the Sl locus of the mouse and

is the ligand for the c-kit tyrosine kinase receptor. Cell 1990;63:213–224.

22. Huang E, Nocka K, Beier DR, et al. The hematopoietic growth factor KL is encoded by the Sl locus and is the ligand of the c-kit receptor, the gene product of the W locus. Cell 1990;63:225–233.

23. Martin F, Suggs S, Langley K, et al. Primary structure and functional expression of rat and human stem cell factor DNAs. Cell 1990;63:203–209.

24. Vriesendorp HM, van Bekkum DW. Role of total body irradiation in conditioning for bone marrow transplantation. Hematol Blood Transfusion 1981;25:349.

25. Thomas ED, Storb R. Technique for human marrow grafting. Blood 1970;36:507–515.

26. Bensinger WI, Buchner CD, Clift RA, Williams BM, Banaji M, Thomas ED. Comparison of techniques for dealing with major ABO-incompatible marrow transplants. Transplant Proc 1987;19:4605–4608.

27. Thomas ED, Ramberg RE, Sale GE, et al. Direct evidence for a bone marrow origin of the alveolar macrophage in man. Science 1976;192:1016–1018.

28. Gale RP, Sparkes RS, Golde DW. Bone marrow origin of hepatic macrophages (Kuppfer cells) in humans. Science 1978;201:937–938.

29. Tavassoli M, Hardy CL. Molecular basis of homing of intravenously transplanted stem cells to the marrow. Blood 1990;76(6):1059–1070.

30. Samlowski W, Daynes RA. Bone marrow engraftment efficiency is enhanced by competitive inhibition of the hepatic asialo-glycoprotein receptor. Proc Natl Acad Sci 1985;82:2508.

31. Reisner Y, Itzicovitch L, Meshorer A, Sharon N. Hemopoietic stem cell transplantation using mouse bone marrow and spleen cells fractionated by lectins. Proc Natl Acad Sci 1978;75:2933.

32. Kataoka M, Tavassoli M. Synthetic neoglycoproteins: a class of reagents for detection of sugar-recognizing substances. J Histochem Cytochem 1984;32:1091.

33. Aizawa S, Tavassoli. Molecular basis of the recognition of intravenously transplanted hemopoietic cells by bone marrow. Proc Natl Acad Sci USA 1988;85:3180.

34. DeBruyn PPH, Michelson S, Thomas TB. The migration of blood cells of the bone marrow through the sinusoidal wall. J Morphol 1971;133:417.

35. DeBruyn PPH, Becker RP, Michelson S. The transmural migration of blood cells in acute myelogenous leukemia. Am J Anat 1977;149:247.

36. Giordano GF, Lichtman MA. Marrow cell egress. The central interaction of barrier pore size and cell maturation. J Clin Invest 1973;52:1154.

37. Campbell FR. Ultrastructural studies of transmural migration of blood cells in the bone marrow of rats, mice and guinea pigs. Am J Anat 1982;135:521.

38. Weiss L. Transmural cellular passage in vascular sinuses of rat bone marrow. Blood 1970;36:189.

39. Cline MJ, Gale RP, Golde DW. Discrete clusters of

hematopoietic cells in the marrow cavity of man after bone marrow transplantation. Blood 1977;50(4):709–712.

40. van den Berg H, Kluin PM, Vossen JM. Early recognition of haematopoiesis after allogeneic bone marrow transplantation: a prospective histopathological study of bone marrow biopsy specimens. J Clin Pathol 1990;43:365–369.

41. Vellenga E, Sizoo W, Hagenbeek A, Lowenberg B. Different repopulation kinetics of erythroid (BFU-E), myeloid (CFU-GM) and T lymphocyte (TL-CFU) progenitor cells after autologous and allogeneic bone marrow transplantation. Br J Haematol 1987;65:137–142.

42. Arnold R, Schmeiser T, Heit W, et al. Hemopoietic reconstitution after bone marrow transplantation. Exp Hematol 1986;14:271–277.

43. Petz LD, Yam P, Wallace RB, et al. Mixed hematopoietic chimerism following bone marrow transplantation for hematologic malignancies. Blood 1987;70(5):1331–1337.

44. Ilstad ST, Wren SM, Bluestone JA, Barbieri SA, Sachs DH. Characterization of mixed allogeneic chimeras. Immunocompetence, in vitro reactivity, and genetic specificity of tolerance. J Exp Med 1985;162:231–244.

45. Advani R, Chao NJ, Horning SJ, et al. Granulocyte-macrophage colony-stimulating factor (GM-CSF) as an adjunct to autologous hemopoietic stem cell transplantation for lymphoma. Ann Intern Med, 1992, in press.

46. Ohno R, Masao Tomonaga M, Kobayashi T, et al. Effect of granulocyte colony-stimulating factor after intensive induction therapy in relapsed or refractory acute leukemia. N Engl J Med 1990;323(13):871–877.

47. Powles R, Smith C, Milan S, et al. Human recombinant GM-CSF in allogeneic bone-marrow transplantation for leukaemia: double-blind, placebo-controlled trial. Lancet 1990;336:1417–1420.

48. Storb R, Prentice RL, Thomas ED. Marrow transplantation for treatment of aplastic anemia: an analysis of factors associated with graft rejection. N Engl J Med 1977;296:61.

49. Thomas ED, Storb R, Clift RA, et al. Bone marrow transplantation. N Engl J Med 1985;292:832–843, 895–902.

50. Zimmerli W, Zarth A, Gratwohl A, Speck B. Neutrophil function and pyogenic infections in bone marrow transplant recipients. Blood 1991;77(2):393–399.

51. Small TN, Keever CA, Weiner-Fedus S, Heller G, O'Reilly RJ, Flomenberg N. B-cell differentiation following autologous, conventional, or T-cell depleted bone marrow transplantation: a recapitulation of normal B-cell ontogeny. Blood 1990;76(8):1647–1656.

52. Halterman RH, Graw RG Jr, Fuccillo DA, Leventhal

BG. Immunocompetence following allogeneic bone marrow transplantation in man. Transplantation 1972;14:689.

53. Elfenbein GJ, Anderson PN, Humphrey RL, et al. Immune system reconstitution following allogeneic bone-marrow transplantation in man: a multiparameter analysis. Transplant Proc 1976;8:641.

54. Noel DR, Witherspoon RP, Storb R, et al. Does graft-versus-host disease influence the tempo of immunologic recovery after allogeneic human marrow transplantation: an observation on 56 long-term survivors. Blood 1978;51:1087.

55. Witherspoon RP, Matthews D, Storb R, et al. Recovery of in vivo cellular immunity after human marrow grafting. Transplantation 1984;37:145.

56. Witherspoon RP, Lum LG, Storb R. Immunologic reconstitution after human marrow grafting. Semin Hematol 1984;21:2–10.

10

AUTOLOGOUS BONE MARROW TRANSPLANTATION

Armand Keating

Intensive therapy followed by autologous bone marrow transplantation (ABMT) is an increasingly administered form of salvage or consolidation treatment for selected patients with hematologic and other malignancies. Autotransplants have increased worldwide from 265 in 1981 at a few centers to approximately 4000 performed by 154 teams in 1989 (1–3). Indications for the procedure are also expanding, and recent investigations have focused on solid tumors, especially breast cancer (4).

The purpose of this chapter is to help evaluate the progress made in this rapidly emerging field. The rationale for ABMT will be examined, technical aspects of the procedure will be reviewed, and several of the critical issues confronting investigators performing transplants will be raised. Results of ABMT for different diseases will be briefly reviewed, and future prospects for this treatment will be explored.

THEORETICAL BASIS FOR AUTOLOGOUS BONE MARROW TRANSPLANTATION

The rationale for intensive therapy and ABMT rests with the notion that for some malignancies a steep dose-response relationship exists between the dose of treatment administered and the fraction of tumor cells killed.

For a given malignancy the slope of such curves is likely to differ with different treatment regimens. In addition to demonstrating a correlation between treatment dose and tumor kill, suitable intensive therapy should have bone marrow suppression as its dose-limiting toxicity. The strategy lies in the expectation that escalating the dose from conventional levels to those likely to require bone marrow support may result in sufficient tumor kill (at the steep portion of the dose-response curve) to be curative. Hematopoietic recovery is ensured by infusing into the patient bone marrow, or, less commonly, peripheral blood nucleated cells previously harvested and, as a rule, cryopreserved. As shown later (Table 10.1), the increase in dose leading to the probable requirement for marrow support before reaching severe extramedullary toxicity is not as high as might be anticipated. Nonetheless, since a portion of the dose-response relationship is frequently linear-log, a relatively small increase in dose may result in a large increase in tumor kill (5). Most dose-response curves have been established for single agents such as cyclophosphamide (6), melphalan (5), and total body irradiation (TBI) (7).

Figure 10.1 shows a steep response between melphalan dose and reduction in clonogenic lymphoma cells as demonstrated by von Hoff et al. (5) using an in vitro tumor

Table 10.1.   Dose Escalation of Single Agents[a]

Agent	Usual Conventional Dose	Maximum Dose without ABMT	Maximum Dose with ABMT	Limiting Extramedullary Toxicity
Cyclophosphamide mg/kg	50	200	200	Cardiac
Carmustine mg/m²	200	600	1200	Pulmonary, hepatic
Melphalan mg/m²	40	120	200	Gastrointestinal, hepatic
Etoposide mg/m²	360	1200	2400 or 60 mg/kg	Gastrointestinal
Ifosfamide mg/m²	5000	8000	18,000	Renal, bladder
Thiotepa mg/m²	50	180	1135	CNS, gastrointestinal
Carboplatin mg/m²	400	1600	2000	Hepatic, renal
Total body irradiation cGy		350	1400	Pulmonary, hepatic

[a]Based on data presented in Gulati et al., 1991 (24), and Chao and Blume, 1990 (23).

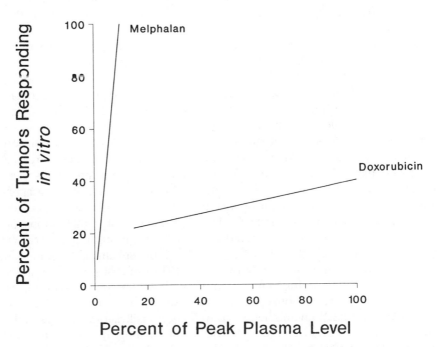

Figure 10.1. Dose-response relationship for lymphoma cells treated with melphalan and doxorubicin. (Adapted from von Hoff DD, Clark GM, Weiss GR, et al. Use of *in vitro* dose response effects to select antineoplastics for high-dose or regional administration regimens. J Clin Oncol 1986;4:1827–1834.)

colony assay. In contrast, increasing the dose of doxorubicin results in a meager increase in cytoreduction.

HISTORICAL PERSPECTIVE

Although first reports of ABMT were published over 30 years ago, in contrast to allogeneic bone marrow transplantation (allo-BMT), widespread adoption of this technique was slow until the mid to late 1980s (3). However, in providing a rationale for ABMT, early investigators anticipated some of the major problems associated with allogeneic transplantation, such as graft-versus-host disease (8). Unfortunately, the first patients selected for ABMT were particularly challenging and included individuals with teratocarcinoma, metastatic renal cell carcinoma (8), and acute lymphoblastic leukemia (ALL) in relapse (9). Nonetheless, it is of interest to note that in 1958 a child with ALL in first relapse was successfully treated with TBI (midplane dose 470 cGy at 9 cGy/min) and ABMT. Remission marrow cryopreserved in glycerol at $-70°$ C for 5 months was used as the autograft. Approximately 5×10^8 nucleated cells per kilogram were infused, and an absolute neutrophil count (ANC) of 1×10^9/liter was recorded by day 16 after transplant (9).

Unfortunately, studies conducted soon after these reports failed to show any benefit from the infusion of marrow autografts, possibly for technical reasons, and may have contributed to a hiatus in activity (10). Several studies in the 1970s failed to conclusively show a reduction in the duration of neutropenia in patients receiving marrow autografts (5, 11). In some cases this was related to rapid endogenous recovery (6). Although not a prospective randomized trial, the study by Appelbaum et al. (12) demonstrated more rapid neutrophil recovery in lymphoma patients receiving ABMT after BACT chemotherapy compared to a similar group given the same chemotherapy without marrow infusion (median 21 days versus 25 days, respectively, to ANC 0.5×10^9/liter, $P < 0.005$).

During this period, numerous single-arm phase I and phase II studies of intensive therapy regimens and ABMT were reported (reviewed in 4, 13–16). In the current decade, prospective randomized trials determining the role of ABMT in acute leukemia, lymphoma, and breast cancer should be completed.

INTENSIVE THERAPY REGIMENS

Intensive therapy regimens for ABMT appear to have developed as a result of several different approaches:

1. dose escalation of single agents in standard phase I studies
2. phase II studies employing agents previously tested in phase I trials
3. using combinations of non-cross-resistant alkylating agents
4. the application of conditioning regimens for allo-BMT
5. employing agents that lack overlapping extramedullary side effects in otherwise empirical combinations.

Alkylating agents are the mainstay of intensive therapy regimens for several reasons. Alkylators show a steep dose-response curve for hematologic and some other malignancies (see Fig. 10.1). Also, for most, the dose-limiting toxicity is marrow suppression. Based on the studies by Schabel and others (17), the notion of non-cross-resistance between different alkylating agents (i.e., a neoplasm resistant to one alkylating agent is not resistant to others) is well accepted and has led to the use of combinations of these drugs, such as carmustine and melphalan (18) and cyclophosphamide, cisplatin, and carmustine (19) in intensive therapy protocols.

Earlier phase I dose escalation studies examined a variety of single agents (including nonalkylators) such as cyclophosphamide (5), melphalan (20), carmustine (21), etoposide (22), and others. Many of these studies were not designed to demonstrate a critical requirement for marrow support. Nonetheless, accumulated evidence indicates that for most agents the myeloablative dose is rarely more than threefold the maximum tolerated dose (MTD) without hematopoietic rescue. Table 10.1, constructed from data presented in two excellent reviews of ABMT (23, 24), compares conventional and high doses of single agents with levels requiring marrow rescue. Of the single chemotherapy agents investigated, thiotepa appears to demonstrate the highest dose escalation—fivefold over the MTD without marrow support. Surprisingly, agents such as melphalan can be escalated by less than twofold before extramedullary toxicity supervenes. However, as previously mentioned, it should be appreciated that for agent-disease combinations giving steep dose-response curves, a relatively small dose escalation can translate into an additional log in tumor cell kill.

The MTD for a single agent listed in Table 10.1 may exceed the MTD for the same drug when used in combination with other agents. For example, in the phase I dose escalation study for the STAMP-5 protocol, the MTD for thiotepa was 500 mg/m^2 and 800 mg/m^2 for carboplatin (25).

Other combinations have been devised using agents with different (nonoverlapping) extramedullary toxicities so that the MTD for the single agent may be used in the combination. For example, etoposide can be given at 60 mg/kg when combined with TBI 1000 cGy (26) or with melphalan 140 mg/m^2 and TBI 500 cGy (27).

Several relatively common intensive therapy protocols have evolved for particular indications and are listed in Table 10.2.

TECHNICAL ASPECTS OF AUTOLOGOUS BONE MARROW TRANSPLANTATION

Bone Marrow Harvesting

Bone marrow is almost invariably harvested from both posterior iliac crests using multiple needle aspirations. For infants, an orthopaedic procedure involving curettage of cleaved iliac crests has been successfully developed (33). The standard aspiration procedure is usually conducted under general anesthesia but can also be successfully performed with an epidural anesthetic. In a minority of patients (approximately 10%) who require additional cells to obtain an adequate autograft, some teams perform aspirations from the anterior iliac crests. Alternatively, the patient can undergo repeat harvesting from the posterior iliacs 8–10 weeks later.

The mode of practice for harvesting autografts is based on procedures developed for marrow donors providing allografts. Marrow donors are frequently hospitalized 2–3 days for the procedure. This may be unnecessary, since Brandwein et al. (34) have shown that marrow autografts can be safely and effectively obtained in a surgical day unit on an outpatient basis.

The quantity of marrow required for successful ABMT has not been definitively established. Most teams aim to harvest 2.5 × 10^8 nucleated cells/per kilogram. Attempts to correlate autograft-related variables with the rate of engraftment have been largely unsuccessful. Poor correlation between nucleated cell count in the autograft and marrow recovery posttransplant may be due to the possibility that a minimum threshold cell dose is exceeded in the autografts of most patients (35). Some studies (36, 37) indicate that CFU-GM levels correlate with reconstitution, but because 12–14 days are required to complete the assay, the results can only be employed retrospectively.

Most practitioners advocate harvesting small volumes (1–2 ml) of marrow from as many different puncture sites as possible, since larger volumes become contaminated with peripheral blood. Batinic et al. (38) showed that the nucleated cell concentration was 3-fold lower and CFU-GM levels 10-fold lower in the final autograft as compared to the first 1.0-ml sample from normal marrow donors. It remains unclear whether small-volume aspirations (as compared to the more practical

Table 10.2.   Common Intensive Therapy Regimens

Regimen	Agents	Disease	Reference
CBV	Cyclophosphamide Carmustine Etoposide	HD	28
Cyclophosphamide TBI		Lymphoma AML	29
BEAC	Carmustine Etoposide Cytarabine Cyclophosphamide	NHL	30
BEAM	Carmustine Etoposide Cytarabine Melphalan	HD NHL	31
Busulphan Cyclophosphamide		AML	32
BACT	Carmustine Cytarabine Cyclophosphamide Thioguanine	Lymphoma Leukemia	12
Cyclophosphamide Thiotepa Carboplatin		Breast cancer	25

3- to 5-ml aliquots) lead merely to a reduced volume for further processing or actually provide a better autograft because of a higher concentration of vital cells.

Autograft Cryopreservation

After harvesting, most teams cryopreserve the autograft. A few centers, lacking cryopreservation facilities, store the marrow at 4° C, usually for no more than 54 hours (39). Consequently, centers that do not cryopreserve autografts are restricted to intensive therapy regimens comprising agents that are rapidly cleared from the body, such as melphalan (or TBI), but not etoposide.

Prior to freezing, the marrow cells are further processed to enrich for the nucleated cell fraction either by obtaining a buffy-coat preparation using automated cell separator instrumentation (e.g., IBM 2991) (40) or by density-gradient centrifugation (with Ficoll or Percoll).

Most institutions freeze the nucleated cells by controlled-rate freezing in the presence of a cryoprotectant. The mechanism of action of cryoprotectants is not fully known but is in part due to retardation of ice crystal formation as a result of binding of water molecules by the agent (41). It is unclear whether entry of the agent into cells is required. The most commonly used cryoprotectant is dimethylsulfoxide (DMSO), but glycerol and hydroxyethyl starch have also been employed (42). The use of cryoprotective agents enables the autograft to be frozen at a slow rate in order to avoid intracellular damage. However, other groups have shown adequate viability when cells are cryopreserved rapidly without controlled rate freezing (43). The duration of the transition phase—the point at which the latent heat of fusion is released when liquid water is transformed to ice—is a major variable of cell viability, and reducing this interval is particularly important, either by manual operation or when constructing controlled-rate freezing programs. Most groups freeze autografts at 1° C per minute in 10% DMSO and cryopreserve the cells in the liquid phase of liquid nitrogen at $-196°$ C. Although long-term storage may be superior at this temperature, adequate cryopreservation has been demonstrated at -120 to $-140°$ C (44). At our center, of the most recent 100 autografts cryopreserved that were subsequently infused, 90% were used after less than 6 months in storage. In such a setting, freezers operating at $-135°$ C may provide a less costly alternative to the use of liquid nitrogen.

There is general agreement that the cryopreserved marrow should be thawed rapidly (in a water bath at $40°$ C) at the bedside and infused immediately into the patient (42).

CRITICAL ISSUES IN AUTOLOGOUS BONE MARROW TRANSPLANTATION

The rapid deployment of hematopoietic growth factors for clinical use, improvements in hematopoietic progenitor cell collection, and increasing acceptance of ABMT by the medical and lay communities suggest that more transplants will be conducted, with less morbidity. With this background of optimism, it is particularly important to appreciate that studies must be completed, or are required to demonstrate, a definitive role of ABMT in the treatment of any disease. In this context, several important issues confronting investigators in the field can be identified and are discussed below.

Timing of Autologous Bone Marrow Transplantation

Timing of ABMT is an important determinant of outcome after transplant. Contributory factors are complex and include the following.

TIME-TO-TREATMENT BIAS

Entry of patients into ABMT protocols (or indeed into any other single-arm treatment trial) may be subject to inadvertently unspecified exclusion criteria. A frequently discussed example is acute myeloid leukemia in first remission (AML in CR1) (45). Here, ABMT performed increasingly later after remission-induction selects for a group enriched with individuals already cured by conventional chemotherapy. A corollary is that patients relapsing early after achieving remission do not proceed to transplant in CR1 and thus unfavorably influence the conventional therapy arm that is usually compared with the ABMT group (time censoring).

In order to appropriately compare results of ABMT studies in acute leukemia, the interval from remission-induction to transplant should be known; most protocols stipulate that the interval not exceed 6 months.

TREATMENT DURING LESS- OR MORE-ADVANCED DISEASE

Results are best when ABMT is performed early in the disease course (14). However, the efficacy of primary therapy and the ability to accurately determine unfavorable prognostic features at diagnosis that predict for relapse after transplant are confounding factors when analyzing outcome. Nonetheless, suggestive evidence is available. For example, Gulati et al. (46) transplanted a high-risk group with intermediate grade non-Hodgkin's lymphoma (NHL), identified at diagnosis by the presence of a lactate dehydrogenase (LDH) level >500 u/ml or a mass $>8 \times 8$ cm. ABMT was administered after induction therapy and the outcome compared with results of a cohort that underwent transplant after relapse following conventional dose induction therapy. Results favor early ABMT when historical data are taken into account, showing a 20% long-term disease-free survival after conventional induction therapy for the poor-prognosis group. Similarly, studies of ABMT in AML can be identified that suggest a benefit to early transplant (47–49). However, analysis of single-arm studies to determine whether ABMT should be performed in CR1 or in second remission (CR2) may be problematic, as the following exercise looking at best- and worst-case scenarios demonstrates. ABMT for AML in CR1 results in 45%–50% long-term disease-free survival (DFS) according to several studies (15). Relapse rates after conventional remission-induction chemotherapy range from 60% (49) to 80% (50, 51), and reinduction of AML in first relapse varies considerably, from 22% to 88% (52), but in one study was approximately 60% in the age group eligible for ABMT (52). Since long-term DFS of patients undergoing ABMT in CR2 varies from 14% (53) to 36% (54), then studies can be selected that show a major benefit for ABMT in CR1 (ABMT in CR1 giving 50% DFS versus 23% overall DFS from CR1 already cured + reinduction therapy + ABMT in CR2) or that indicate an advantage to transplanting patients in CR2 (DFS 45% in CR1 versus 53% overall DFS in CR2, if cures by conventional remission-induction therapy are included).

Thus the important issue of timing of transplantation—early versus late—can only be addressed in controlled prospective trials. Other factors are also likely to have an impact on outcome, such as performance status, which is an independent prognostic variable in patients undergoing ABMT for Hodgkin's disease (HD) (55).

Disease Status at Treatment

In addition to timing of ABMT, two other related issues are important in determining outcome after transplant: chemotherapy-sensitive disease and tumor bulk at transplant.

THE ISSUE OF CHEMOTHERAPY-SENSITIVE DISEASE

Earlier studies of ABMT in NHL indicate that outcome posttransplant is highly dependent upon the sensitivity of relapsed disease to conventional doses of salvage chemotherapy (30). Apart from patients with an excellent partial response to frontline therapy (56), the best results are obtained in patients with

intermediate- or high-grade NHL who achieved CR with an anthracycline-containing regimen and whose relapsed disease responded to salvage chemotherapy. This observation has since been confirmed in follow-up studies (57, 58). Results are likely to be due to the combined effects of salvage and high-dose therapy before transplant. For relapsed NHL, DHAP (59) is well documented as salvage chemotherapy and is administered to determine sensitivity of the relapsed disease to chemotherapy as well as to reduce tumor burden prior to intensive therapy and ABMT (30). At many centers, patients with NHL resistant to salvage chemotherapy are ineligible for ABMT. Consequently, a desirable property of a salvage regimen would be to identify prospectively as many patients with relapsed disease as possible, who will become long-term disease-free survivors after ABMT. To address this issue, studies must be undertaken with different salvage regimens while retaining the same intensive therapy protocol. The strategy is to incorporate into the new salvage chemotherapy-sensitive group as many patients as possible from cases resistant to the previous salvage regimen that are destined to remain disease-free after transplant.

As a first step toward achieving this goal, Stewart et al. (60) challenged lymphoma (HD and NHL) patients unresponsive to DHAP or other frontline salvage chemotherapy with the mini-BEAM protocol. Twelve of 22 patients underwent transplant (allo-BMT as well as ABMT), and 5 remain disease-free. In a study of relapsed HD, Jagannath et al. (55) showed that responsiveness to the last salvage regimen was a factor in determining prognosis after ABMT. However, strategies to improve salvage regimens are unlikely to increase DFS by more than 15%. To improve outcome further, other approaches that decrease relapse after ABMT, especially at sites of prior bulky disease, are necessary.

TUMOR BURDEN AT AUTOLOGOUS BONE MARROW TRANSPLANTATION

Further investigation is required to determine the effect of tumor burden at the time of intensive therapy and transplant on DFS. Patients with measurable residual HD before intensive therapy who achieve CR posttransplant have improved DFS (55). Whether or not results are further improved posttransplant for patients achieving CR with additional aggressive salvage therapy prior to intensive treatment is not entirely clear. However, Crump et al. (61) indicate that for patients with relapsed HD, attaining CR with salvage before intensive therapy and ABMT confers a favorable outcome. An alternative explanation is that aggressive salvage therapy merely identifies a group with biologically favorable disease that responds to intensive therapy.

Purging the Autograft

Considerable effort and resources are devoted to devise and improve methods that selectively eliminate neoplastic cells from marrow autografts. Despite animal transplant models showing the value of marrow purging (62), prospective studies demonstrating the clinical utility of purging in ABMT are lacking. Moreover, for lymphoma and the solid tumors, relapse patterns after ABMT suggest a failure to eradicate disease in the patient rather than from the autograft. Also, relapse rates for AML in CR1 are similar for syngeneic transplants and autotransplants using unpurged grafts (45, 63). However, if new intensive therapy regimens can be found that improve outcome posttransplant, then relapse rates may be further decreased by eliminating residual clonogenic neoplastic cells in the autograft.

A multitude of different approaches have been taken to eliminate residual malignant cells from marrow (64). The most common clinically feasible methods are listed in Table 10.3. It is unclear which method is superior for the elimination of a particular tumor type. With some exceptions (72), few in vitro studies have attempted to compare the efficacy of different purging modalities while demon-

Table 10.3. Practical Methods of Marrow Purging in Autologous Bone Marrow Transplantation

	Reference
A. Pharmacologic	
4-Hydroperoxycyclophosphamide (4-HC)	65
Mafosfamide	48
B. Immunologic	
Monoclonal antibodies and complement	66
Immunotoxins	67
Monoclonal antibodies and magnetic microspheres	68
C. Biophysical	
Photoactive agents	69
D. Culture	
Long-term bone marrow culture	70
E. Positive selection for normal early progenitors	
Enrichment for CD34+ cells	71

strating multipotent hematopoietic progenitor cell viability.

Many single-arm trials of different purging modalities have been conducted in a wide variety of diseases, usually with a small number of subjects. Interpretation of such studies is problematic because of the common problems of time censoring (73), patient selection bias (74), and reduced statistical significance as a result of small numbers (75).

The most extensive experience in clinical marrow purging is with acute leukemia. Two studies claim a clinical benefit to marrow purging, both for AML and both retrospective. In one, Gorin et al. (76) performed a retrospective analysis of ABMT for AML in CR1 with purged or unpurged autografts and identified a subgroup with a favorable outcome. Patients who received intensive therapy with a TBI-containing regimen and ABMT with purged marrow within 6 months of achieving CR1 had a probability of relapse of 20%. In contrast, for a similar group receiving unpurged autografts, the probability of relapse was 61%.

In another study, Rowley et al. (77) conducted a retrospective analysis of patients with AML at high risk of relapse and showed that lower levels of CFU-GM correlated with a more favorable outcome (CFU-GM <1% of original value, n = 22, DFS = 36%; CFU-GM >1%, n = 23, DFS = 12%).

These data need to be reconciled with results of syngeneic transplants for AML in CR1. In a preliminary analysis of 44 twin transplants, almost all of whom received a TBI-containing regimen, the probability of relapse was 51% (78). The usual caveats regarding comparisons of single-arm trials apply. However, one conclusion is that the decreased relapse rate after purged ABMT may not be due to elimination of residual leukemia from the autograft but results from the induction of a graft-versus-leukemia-like effect as a consequence of employing purged marrow (73, 79).

Whatever the explanation, sufficient data are available to warrant the initiation of a prospective randomized trial. Such an endeavor would be feasible if conducted by a large cooperative group as a multicenter study.

Improving Hematopoietic Recovery after Autologous Bone Marrow Transplantation

Since much of the morbidity and most of the mortality associated with ABMT is related to neutropenia and thrombocytopenia, attempts to hasten marrow recovery after transplant may result in clinical benefit. The use of recombinant hematopoietic growth factors to address this issue has been tackled with alacrity by many investigators. Studies have employed GM-CSF, G-CSF, and M-CSF after ABMT, mostly for lymphoma or solid tumors (80). Phase I/II studies are underway with IL-3 and trials with IL-6 are likely in the near future.

None of the studies showed a reduction in the period of agranulocytosis after transplant. This can be explained by the absence of committed growth-factor-responsive progenitors in the marrow after therapy and before similar cells in the infused autograft have differentiated in response to the factor. Most

phase II trials showed accelerated granulopoiesis after neutrophils appeared but did not demonstrate an effect on platelet recovery. Results were confirmed in several prospective randomized trials of GM-CSF (81–84). Granulocyte recovery to an ANC of $>0.5 \times 10^9$/liter was accelerated by 7–13 days compared to the control group. In the study by Nemunaitis et al. (81), patients receiving GM-CSF reached an ANC of 0.5×10^9/liter 7 days earlier, had fewer infections, required 3 fewer days of antibiotics, and were hospitalized 6 fewer days than patients given placebo. There were no toxic effects specifically ascribed to GM-CSF at a dose of 250 $\mu g/m^2$/day administered as a 2-hour infusion.

A 1-year follow-up was conducted of patients with lymphoid malignancies who received GM-CSF after ABMT (85). Accepting the potential limitations of a small study (n = 27), there was no evidence of stem cell depletion or overt late graft failure, and the relapse rate was similar to results in historical controls.

Several phase II studies but not randomized trials of G-CSF after ABMT have been completed (86, 87). Granulocyte but not platelet recovery is accelerated compared to historical controls, and the treatment had little toxicity (mostly myalgia and bone pain). M-CSF (nonrecombinant) also hastens neutrophil recovery, but probably to a lesser extent than do either G- or GM-CSF (88).

Results suggest that growth factors administered singly after transplant are unlikely to reduce the period of agranulocytosis. Combinations, either together or sequential, of early- and later-acting factors may reduce the interval and should be tested.

Another approach is to provide autografts with increased concentrations of early and very late hematopoietic progenitors. This may be accomplished, in part, with peripheral blood stem cell transplants (89, 90). Increased levels of late progenitors such as CFU-GM can be documented during the recovery phase after chemotherapy (91) or after administration of GM-CSF (92).

Chemotherapy (93) or GM-CSF-mobilized (94) peripheral blood stem cells in conjunction with marrow autografts may lead to even more rapid and sustained engraftment. If such approaches are further combined with in vivo administration of growth factors as well as with in vitro priming of the autograft, the agranulocytopenic interval after ABMT may be abrogated, and the notion of outpatient-based transplants becomes feasible.

Improving Results of Autologous Bone Marrow Transplantation with Immunomodulators

Allo-BMT is associated with lower relapse rates than are autologous or syngeneic transplants for similar cases (95, 96). This effect is also observed in patients with AML who lack clinical manifestations of graft-versus-host disease (GVHD) (97) but appears to be abolished in chronic myeloid leukemia (CML) patients receiving T-cell-depleted allotransplants (97). Such clinical evidence of a graft-versus-leukemia (GVL) effect is supported by animal studies (98) and suggests a basis for separating GVHD from the GVL effect (99).

In order to overcome the lack of a GVL effect in ABMT, several avenues have been explored. In one, Jones and the Baltimore group have used cyclosporine to induce skin manifestations indistinguishable from GVHD in patients with lymphoma undergoing ABMT (100). Acute GVHD of the skin was demonstrated in a minority of patients with AML in CR2 (101). Rat (102) and mouse (103) models for syngeneic GVHD have been developed and require thymic damage in addition to cyclosporine. The phenomenon is attributed to CD8+ T cells reacting to autologous or syngeneic class II MHC molecules (104). Expression of these forbidden autoreactive T cells may be permitted by the suppressive effects of cyclosporine and thymic dysfunction. A GVL effect was demonstrated in a rat tumor model involving neoplastic cells expressing class II determinants (105). Studies are in progress to determine if a clinical GVL effect accompanies autologous GVHD.

Another approach is the administration of IL-2 after ABMT (106, 107). IL-2 induces tumor regression in animal models and in some patients with advanced malignancies (108, 109). The interleukin promotes T cell reconstitution after transplant and is known to activate NK cells and support proliferation of LAK cells (110). Phase I studies indicate that toxicity is acceptable; effects on the graft were transient (107). In addition to effects on T cells, IL-2 may exhibit secondary antitumor effects by inducing the release of γ-interferon and TNF-α (111).

The carboxamide-quinoline, Linomide, enhances NK cell number and activity (112–114), appears to be well tolerated, and is currently in trials to determine its effect on relapse after ABMT for AML.

A desirable goal in all these approaches is to induce a GVL effect in ABMT without the attendant morbidity and mortality associated with allogeneic transplantation.

RESULTS OF AUTOLOGOUS BONE MARROW TRANSPLANTATION

Acute Myeloid Leukemia

Intensive therapy and ABMT are attractive treatment options for AML in CR1 since leukemic cells show a steep dose-response relationship with alkylating agents and TBI, the disease is at an early stage, tumor burden is minimal, and the method largely overcomes the restrictions of allogeneic marrow transplantation. Despite such advantages, ABMT for AML is central to the controversial issues involving this treatment modality.

The two most important controversies concern the superiority of ABMT over optimal conventional therapy and whether or not autograft purging results in decreased relapse after transplant. The issue of marrow purging and the need for prospective trials were discussed earlier. It is likely not possible to determine the former from results of published single-arm trials of conventional therapy or ABMT, since most accrue relatively small numbers of patients, involve heterogeneous groups, and exhibit survival rates with wide confidence limits (75).

Reports of long-term DFS after ABMT for AML in CR1 range from 35% to 61%, with a median follow-up of at least 24 months and a median interval from CR to ABMT of between 3.8 and 6 months (76, 116–119). Either purged or unpurged autografts were used, and most centers used cyclophosphamide-TBI combinations or busulphan and cyclophosphamide.

Reiffers et al. (51) addressed the issue of the role of ABMT in this disease in a prospective controlled trial. Eighty-five patients under age 50 received standard remission induction therapy, and after one consolidation course, 58 were assigned to allo-BMT with cyclophosphamide and fractionated TBI, if a suitable sibling donor was available, or were randomized to ABMT consisting of a double autotransplant with single-agent high-dose melphalan and unpurged marrow, or to four monthly cycles of a complex chemotherapy regimen including etoposide, high-dose cytosine arabinoside, and amsacrine. The actuarial relapse rates were significantly different ($p < .0002$): 18% for allotransplants, 50% for autotransplants, and 83% for patients receiving the chemotherapy regimen. The same group has provided preliminary data to address the question of the role of intensive therapy in AML (120). In a prospective trial, individuals in CR1 after a single mild consolidation course were allocated to allogeneic transplantation only or to intensive consolidation chemotherapy (121) and then randomization to ABMT with a busulphan-melphalan regimen or to maintenance chemotherapy. Patients receiving the most intensive treatment—consolidation chemotherapy then intensive therapy with ABMT—had a higher risk of relapse than patients undergoing only allogeneic transplantation. These studies need to be confirmed by others but suggest that ABMT is superior to conventional therapy and also that further treatment

intensification cannot produce the reduced relapse rates that result from the immune-mediated mechanisms of allo-BMT.

Results of ABMT for advanced leukemia are highly variable and in general less satisfactory than for AML in CR1. However, the treatment remains an important option since few long-term survivors have been reported after conventional-dose chemotherapy (52). Intensive therapy regimens similar to those for AML in CR1 were employed, and purged as well as unpurged marrows were administered. DFS ranges from 14% to 28% for studies with a median follow-up of more than 24 months (53, 65, 66, 122).

The Yeager study (65) employed busulphan/cyclophosphamide intensive therapy and autografts purged with 4-hydroperoxycyclophosphamide (4-HC) for patients with AML in CR2 and CR3. The study was recently updated (54); of 88 patients entered, 35 remain in unmaintained remission at a median of 26 months after ABMT. Actuarial DFS for CR2 is 36% and for CR3 23%.

At present it is unknown whether these relatively high survival rates for advanced AML are due to the intensive regimen, to 4-HC purging, or to both. If recent excellent results (122) using unpurged marrow can be maintained with longer follow-up, then the role of marrow purging becomes less clear and may only become apparent when intensive regimens improve.

Acute Lymphoblastic Leukemia

Results of ABMT for ALL are difficult to compare to results for similar groups receiving conventional therapy alone (123–126). Interpretation is confounded by inclusion of pediatric with adult cases and by the bias of time censoring. Since a recent study showed no advantage to allo-BMT over conventional chemotherapy for ALL in CR1 (127), it is unlikely that similar patients would benefit from ABMT. For high-risk ALL patients (including CR2 and CR3 cases), Kersey et al. (126) indicated an estimated relapse rate of 37% in recipients of allotransplants with GVHD, 75% for patients receiving allografts without GVHD, and 79% in patients receiving autografts. However, results of conventional-dose salvage chemotherapy in a similar group, especially in individuals with a brief CR1, are dismal (126). These data indicate that a minority of patients with high-risk ALL will become long-term disease-free survivors after ABMT. Once again, it is unclear whether or not purging the autografts with a cocktail of monoclonal antibodies recognizing lymphoid determinants contributed to relapse rates that were comparable to those after allo-BMT in patients without GVHD. These data also suggest that improvements after ABMT are more likely to come from introducing immunotherapy, as discussed previously, than from improving intensive therapy regimens.

Non-Hodgkin's Lymphoma

The role of ABMT in the treatment of NHL can be examined according to the stage of disease. For intermediate- and high-grade NHL the categories are as follows:

1. *High-risk NHL in CR1:* There is a lack of consensus on prognostic factors identifying patients at high risk of relapse, as distinct from factors identifying the risk of not achieving remission (58). Once these factors are established, patients should be recruited into prospective trials.
2. *Primary refractory NHL:* The Philip study (30) showed that all patients in this group relapsed after ABMT. The data strongly suggest that at present, there is no role for ABMT in these patients.
3. *NHL in resistant relapse:* Patients who achieved CR with frontline therapy but are unresponsive to salvage chemotherapy have 10%–14% long-term DFS (30). This group should be the subject of investigation using new approaches, including more aggressive salvage regimens that demonstrate a reduction in tumor bulk.
4. *NHL in sensitive relapse:* Patients who

achieve CR with frontline therapy and are responsive to salvage chemotherapy have up to 45% long-term DFS (30, 57, 58). Similar results may be achieved with aggressive salvage chemotherapy in the absence of ABMT. A prospective randomized study to address this question is underway (128, 129). At present ABMT appears appropriate therapy for this group.
5. *NHL with partial response to frontline therapy:* Philip et al. (56) showed excellent survival in patients with partial remission after frontline therapy for NHL. Since results with conventional therapy for this group are poor (130), ABMT is indicated. Salvage therapy prior to intensive therapy and ABMT may further improve outcome, but this has not been established.

Autograft purging is unlikely to have a major influence on outcome posttransplant for intermediate-grade lymphoma since 80%–90% of relapses occur at sites of previous, especially bulky, disease (58).

The role of ABMT in low-grade lymphoma is of considerable interest since patients are not cured after conventional treatment. Morbidity and mortality are low (131), and transplants have been performed in CR1 or in first relapse. Prospective trials with a long follow-up will be required to definitively address the role of ABMT for low-grade disease.

Hodgkin's Disease

ABMT is increasingly employed in the treatment of patients with relapsed or refractory HD, the continuing controversy regarding the nature of optimal therapy notwithstanding. Since the disease-free interval after conventional salvage may extend to years, and because ABMT in HD is associated with moderately high treatment-related mortality—from 4% (132) to 23% (133)—timing of transplantation is an important issue. At present, indications at many centers include partial response after optimal frontline chemotherapy, relapse after MOPP/ABVD-containing regimens, and relapse after salvage chemotherapy following failure of local radiotherapy.

Three regimens are widely used: (*a*) CBV (cyclophosphamide, carmustine [BCNU], and etoposide [VP-16]) (28), (*b*) BEAM (BCNU, etoposide, cytosine arabinoside [ara-C], melphalan) (134), and (*c*) cyclophosphamide and TBI (29). Dose escalation of agents in CBV results in improved CR rate after transplant (135) but is also associated with increased treatment-related mortality (132, 136). TBI is usually avoided in intensive therapy regimens in patients previously treated with mantle irradiation because of a high incidence of fatal interstitial pneumonitis (133, 29).

DFS in relatively heterogeneous groups ranges from 22% to 57% with a follow-up of at least 24 months (24). Recent reports of long-term follow-up indicate that 10% of patients may relapse late (2–3 years) after transplant (137). Adverse risk factors for survival after ABMT with CBV include poor performance status at transplant and failure of more than two prior chemotherapy treatments (55).

An interesting study from the Vancouver group (138) identifies patients with a low probability of remaining disease-free after ABMT. Individuals with one or more of the following risk factors had only a 19% chance of remaining disease-free: stage IV disease at diagnosis, B symptoms at relapse, and a time from primary treatment to relapse of less than 1 year.

Prospective randomized trials of ABMT in relapsed or refractory HD would be very helpful to determine optimal therapy for this condition but will be hampered by poor accrual because of good results reported in single-arm studies and by the changing nature of alternative salvage therapy that will be increasingly used in conjunction with hematopoietic growth factors.

Chronic Myeloid Leukemia

Over 200 autotransplants have been performed in CML (139). Results are best in chronic phase. Two studies are of particular interest. In one, Goldman's group (140) demonstrated Ph-negative hematopoiesis for more than 1 year in 3 of 18 patients who underwent intensive therapy with busulphan/melphalan and autologous peripheral blood stem cells. In the other, Barnett and colleagues (70) have employed the long-term bone marrow culture system as a means of purging Ph(+) clonogenic cells from the autograft. Of 8 evaluable patients, 6 have 0%–6% Ph(+) marrow 2–27 months after transplant. In view of the high relapse rate after syngeneic transplants for CML, longer follow-up in a large number of patients will be required to determine the curative potential of this innovative approach.

Solid Tumors

Based on results with hematologic malignancies, it is reasonable to investigate the possibility that intensive therapy and ABMT may produce remissions, or even cures, in patients with advanced solid tumors, provided the latter respond to conventional doses of chemotherapy and exhibit a steep dose-response curve with some agents. Examples of malignancies suitable for investigation include breast cancer, testicular cancer, neuroblastoma, selected sarcomas such as Ewing sarcoma, and small cell lung cancer.

A pilot study in small cell lung cancer appeared to be unrewarding (141). Preliminary reports of refractory germ cell tumors with etoposide and carboplatin indicate that further studies are warranted (142). Over 600 children with advanced neuroblastoma have been treated with intensive therapy and ABMT (143), and initial promising studies (144) led to a European randomized trial that suggests a benefit to the transplant arm (145).

Further randomized trials are in progress (143), but long-term follow-up will be necessary because relapses up to 10 years after therapy have been documented (146). Marrow purging for neuroblastoma is sophisticated but remains of unproven value (68).

Interest in ABMT for breast cancer has been particularly high recently. The disease is common, dose intensity at conventional levels appears to increase remission rates (147), and survival of premenopausal patients receiving adjuvant chemotherapy is increased compared to control groups (148). Several single agents in high dose followed by ABMT have been tested in advanced breast cancer and include melphalan (149, 150) etoposide (23), hydroxyurea (151), and thiotepa (152) and have resulted in complete responses in a few. Results of multiagent therapy have been more rewarding, particularly combinations of different alkylating agents. Antman and colleagues have studied combinations of cyclophosphamide, carmustine, and cisplatin in phase I studies (19). More recently, the same group has conducted phase II studies (STAMP-25) of four cycles of doxorubicin, 5-fluorouracil, and methotrexate induction followed by intensive therapy with cyclophosphamide, thiotepa, and carboplatin and hematopoietic cell rescue (25). High response rates were reported (15 of 16 patients), and mortality was low (4%). Peters and colleagues treated 22 patients with previously untreated metastatic disease with high-dose cyclophosphamide, cisplatin, and melphalan or carmustine and ABMT. Treatment-related mortality was 22%, but 14% are disease-free a minimum of 4 years posttransplant (153, 154).

The same group has investigated the role of intensive therapy and ABMT as consolidation of adjuvant therapy for high-risk primary breast cancer (stage II or III with 10 or more involved axillary nodes). Using the cyclophosphamide, carmustine, and cisplatin protocol, 7% died of treatment-related causes but 72% of patients remained free of disease a median 14 months after transplant (154).

These studies indicate that intensive therapy and ABMT produces DFS in many patients and prolonged survival in a minority with high-risk breast cancer. Studies are suf-ficiently mature to warrant phase III trials. At present, multicenter cooperative groups have organized prospective randomized trials of ABMT in high-risk primary breast cancer as well as in metastatic disease.

FUTURE PROSPECTS

This is a particularly vital time for investigators in ABMT. Numerous avenues hold promise. After many years of single-arm studies, prospective randomized trials are now in progress to determine the role of ABMT in AML, NHL, neuroblastoma, and breast cancer, among others. The application of fundamental observations regarding hematopoietic progenitor cell and growth factor interactions may enable clinical investigators to devise protocols for manipulating autografts and treating patients that will further reduce the period of neutropenia and thrombocytopenia or abrogate it entirely. Immunotherapy after ABMT is in its infancy but should be pursued vigorously because the goal of reducing relapse rates to levels observed with allo-BMT is worthwhile and feasible, especially if the low morbidity and mortality of autotransplants is retained.

Acknowledgments

The author wishes to thank Rose Ierullo for ably typing the manuscript. The work was supported by the Medical Research Council of Canada and the National Cancer Institute of Canada (NCIC). Dr. Keating is a Senior Research Scientist of the NCIC.

REFERENCES

1. Report of an international cooperative study: bone marrow autotransplantation in man. Lancet 1986; 2:960–962.
2. Gorin NC, Gale RP, Armitage JO, for the Advisory Committee of the International Transplant Registry (ABMTR). Autologous bone marrow transplants: different indications in Europe and North America. Lancet 1989;2:312–318.
3. Gorin NC. Autologous bone marrow transplantation in hematological malignancies. Am J Clin Oncol (CCT) 1991;14(suppl 1):S5–S14.
4. Frei E, Antman K, Teicher B, et al. Bone marrow autotransplantation for solid tumors—prospects. J Clin Oncol 1989;7:515–526.

5. von Hoff DD, Clark GM, Weiss GR, et al. Use of *in vitro* dose response effects to select antineoplastics for high-dose or regional administration regimens. J Clin Oncol 1986;4:1827–1834.
6. Buckner CD, Rudolph RH, Fefer A, et al. High dose cyclophosphamide therapy for malignant disease. Cancer 1972;29:357–365.
7. Hewitt HB, Wilson CW. A survival curve for mammalian leukemia cells irradiated *in vivo* (implications for the treatment of mouse leukemia by whole body irradiation). Br J Cancer 1959;13:69–75.
8. Kurnick NB, Montano A, Gerdes KC, et al. Preliminary observations on the treatment of postirradiation hematopoietic depression in man by the infusion of stored autogenous bone marrow. Ann Intern Med 1958;49(5):973–986.
9. McGovern JJ, Russell PS, Atkins L, Webster EW. Treatment of terminal leukemic relapse by total-body irradiation and intravenous infusion of stored autologous bone marrow obtained during remission. N Engl J Med 1959;260:675–683.
10. Kurnick NB. Autologous and isologous bone marrow storage and infusion in the treatment of myelosuppression. Transfusion 1962;2:178–187.
11. Tobias JS, Weiner RS, Griffiths CT, et al. Cryopreserved autologous marrow infusion following high-dose cancer chemotherapy. Eur J Cancer 1977;13:269–277.
12. Appelbaum FR, Herzig GP, Ziegler JL, et al. Successful engraftment of cryopreserved autologous bone marrow in patients with malignant lymphoma. Blood 1978;52:85–95.
13. Cheson BD, Lacerna L, Leyland-Jones B, et al. Autologous bone marrow transplantation. Ann Intern Med 1989;110:51–65.
14. Armitage JO, Gale RP. Bone marrow autotransplantation. Am J Med 1989;86:203–206.
15. Burnet AK. Autologous bone marrow transplantation in acute leukemia. Leuk Res 1988;12:531–536.
16. Canellos GP, Nadler L, Takvorian T. Autologous bone marrow transplantation in the treatment of malignant lymphoma and Hodgkin's disease. Semin Hematol 1988;25(suppl 2):58–65.
17. Schabel FM, Trader MW, Laster WR, et al. Patterns of resistance and therapeutic synergism among alkylating agents. Antibiot Chemother 1978;23:200–215.
18. Herzig RH, Phillips GL, Lazarus HM, et al. Intensive chemotherapy and autologous bone marrow transplantation for the treatment of refractory malignancies. In: Dicke KA, Spitzer G, Zander AR, eds. Autologous bone marrow transplantation. Houston: University of Texas M.D. Anderson Hospital and Tumor Institute, 1985;197–202.
19. Antman K, Eder J, Elias A, et al. High-dose combination alkylating agent preparative regimen with autologous bone marrow support: the Dana-Farber Cancer Institute/Beth Israel Hospital experience. Cancer Treat Rep 1987;71:119–125.
20. McElwain TJ, Hedley DW, Burton G, et al. Marrow autotransplantation accelerates haematological recovery in patients with malignant melanoma treated with high-dose melphalan. Br J Cancer 1979;40:72–80.
21. Phillips GL, Fay JW, Herzig GP, et al. Intensive 1,3-bis(2-chloroethyl)-1-nitrosourea (BCNU), NSC #4366650 and cryopreserved autologous marrow transplantation for refractory cancer. A phase I–II study. Cancer 1983;52:1792–1802.
22. Wolff SN, Fer MF, McKay CM, et al. High-dose VP-16-213 and autologous bone marrow transplantation for refractory malignancies: a phase I study. J Clin Oncol 1983;1:701–705.
23. Chao NJ, Blume KG. Bone marrow transplantation, part II—autologous. West J Med 1990;152:46–51.
24. Gulati S, Yahalow J, Portlock C. Autologous bone marrow transplantation. Curr Prob Cancer 1991;15:5–56.
25. Antman K, Eder JP, Elias A, et al. Dose intensive regimens in breast cancer: the Dana Farber Cancer Institute and Beth Israel experience. In: Dicke KA, Armitage JO, Dicke-Evinger MJ, eds. Autologous bone marrow transplantation: proceedings of the Fifth International Symposium. Omaha, NE: University of Nebraska Medical Center, 1990;305–311.
26. Blume KG, Forman SJ, O'Donnell MR, et al. Total body irradiation and high dose etoposide: a new preparatory regimen for bone marrow transplantation in patients with advanced hematologic malignancies. Blood 1987;69(4):1015–1020.
27. Keating A, Brandwein J. Autologous marrow transplantation for non-Hodgkin's lymphoma: high-dose etoposide and melphalan with or without TBI. In: Dicke KA, Armitage JO, Dicke-Evinger MJ, eds. Autologous bone marrow transplantation: proceedings of the Fifth International Symposium. Omaha, NE: University of Nebraska Medical Center, 1990;427–431.
28. Jagannath S, Dicke KA, Armitage JO, et al. High-dose cyclophosphamide, carmustine and etoposide and autologous bone marrow transplantation for relapsed Hodgkin's disease. Ann Intern Med 1986;104:163–168.
29. Appelbaum FR, Sullivan KM, Buckner CD, et al. Treatment of malignant lymphoma in 100 patients with chemotherapy, total body irradiation and marrow transplantation. J Clin Oncol 1987;5:1340–1347.
30. Philip T, Armitage J, Spitzer G, et al. High dose therapy and autologous bone marrow transplantation in 100 adults with intermediate and high grade non-Hodgkin's lymphoma. N Engl J Med 1987; 316:1493–1498.
31. Biron P, Goldstone A, Colombat P, et al. A new cytoreductive conditioning regimen before ABMT for lymphomas: the BEAM protocol—a phase II study. In: Dicke KA, Spitzer G, Zander AR, eds. Autologous

bone marrow transplantation: proceedings of the Second International Symposium. Houston: University of Texas MD Anderson Hospital and Tumor Institute, 1987.

32. Santos GW, Tutschka PJ, Brookmeyer R, et al. Marrow transplantation for acute nonlymphocytic leukemia after treatment with busulfan and cyclophosphamide. N Engl J Med 1983;309:1347–1353.

33. Kapelushnik J, Kirby M, Saunders EF, et al. Incidence of graft-versus-host disease in allogeneic bone marrow transplant patients using surgical procurement of bone marrow as compared to aspiration. UCLA Symposia on Molecular and Cellular Biology. J Cell Biochem 1990;(suppl 14A):296.

34. Brandwein JM, Callum J, Rubinger M, et al. An evaluation of outpatient bone marrow harvesting. J Clin Oncol 1989;7:648–650.

35. Brandwein JM, Callum J, Sutcliffe SB, et al. Analysis of factors affecting hematopoietic recovery after autologous bone marrow transplantation for lymphoma. Bone Marrow Transplant 1990;6:291–294.

36. Spitzer G, Verma DS, Fisher R, et al. The myeloid progenitor cell—its value in predicting hematopoietic recovery after autologous bone marrow transplantation. Blood 1980;55:317–323.

37. Douay L, Gorin N-C, Mary J-Y, et al. Recovery of CFU-GM from cyropreserved marrow in vivo evaluation after autologous bone marrow transplantation are predictive of engraftment. Exp Hematol 1986;14:358–365.

38. Batinic D, Marusic M, Pavletic Z, et al. Relationship between differing volumes of bone marrow aspirates and their cellular composition. Bone Marrow Transplant 1990;6:103–107.

39. Takahashi M, Singer JW. Effects of marrow storage at 4 degrees C on the subsequent generation of long-term marrow cultures. Exp Hematol 1985;13(7):691–695.

40. Gilmore M, Prentice H, Blacklock H, et al. A technique for rapid isolation of bone marrow mononuclear cells using Ficoll-metrizoate and the IBM 2991 blood cell processor. Br J Haematol 1982; 50:619.

41. Rowe AW. Biochemical aspects of cryoprotective agents in freezing and thawing. Cryobiology 1966;3:12–18.

42. Gorin NC. Collection, manipulation and freezing of haemopoietic stem cells. Clin Haematol 1986; 15(1):19–48.

43. Stiff PJ, DeRisi MF, Langleben A, et al. Autologous bone marrow transplantation using unfractionated cells without rate-controlled freezing in hydroxyethyl starch and dimethyl sulfoxide. Ann NY Acad Sci 1983;411:378–380.

44. Gulati S, Shank B, Yahalom J, et al. Autologous BMT for patients with poor-prognosis lymphoma and Hodgkin's disease. In: Dicke KA, Spitzer G, Jagan-

nath S, eds. Autologous bone marrow transplantation: Proceedings of the Fourth International Symposium. Houston: MD Anderson Hospital Publishers, 1988;231–239.

45. Gale RP, Butturini A. Autotransplants in leukemia. Lancet 1989;2:315–317.

46. Gulati SC, Shank B, Black P, et al. Autologous bone marrow transplantation for patients with poor-prognosis lymphoma. J Clin Oncol 1988;6(8):1303–1313.

47. Dicke KA, McCredie KB, Spitzer G, et al. Autologous bone marrow transplantation in patients with adult acute leukemia in relapse. Transplantation 1978;26:169–173.

48. Gorin NC, Douay L, Laporte JP, et al. Autologous bone marrow transplantation using marrow incubated with asta Z 7557 in adult acute leukemia. Blood 1986;67:1367–1376.

49. Gale RP, Butturini A, Horowitz MM. Does more intensive therapy increase cures in acute leukemia? Semin Hematol 1991;28(3)(suppl 4):93–94.

50. The Toronto Leukemia Study Group. Results of chemotherapy for unselected patients with acute myeloblastic leukemia: effect of exclusions on interpretation of results. Lancet 1986;1:786–788.

51. Reiffers J, Gaspard MH, Maraninchi D, et al. Comparison of allogeneic or autologous bone marrow transplantation and chemotherapy in patients with acute myeloid leukaemia in first remission: a prospective controlled trial. Br J Haematol 1989;72:57–63.

52. Angelov L, Brandwein JM, Baker MA, et al. Results of therapy for acute myeloid leukemia in first relapse. Leukemia Lymphoma 1991;6:15–24.

53. Spinolo JA, Dicke KA, Horwitz LJ, et al. High-dose chemotherapy and unpurged autologous bone marrow transplantation for acute leukemia in second or subsequent remission. Cancer 1990;66:619–626.

54. Yeager AM, Rowley SD, Jones RJ, et al. Autologous transplantation with chemopurged bone marrow in patients with acute myelocytic leukemia in second and third remission. In: Dicke KA, Armitage JO, Dicke-Evinger MJ, eds. Autologous bone marrow transplantation: Proceedings of the Fifth International Symposium. Omaha, NE: University of Nebraska Medical Center, 1990;91–98.

55. Jagannath S, Armitage JO, Dicke KA, et al. Prognostic factors for response and survival after high-dose cyclophosphamide, carmustine, and etoposide with autologous bone marrow transplantation for relapsed Hodgkin's disease. J Clin Oncol 1989; 7(2):179–185.

56. Philip T, Hartmann O, Biron P, et al. High-dose therapy and autologous bone marrow transplantation in partial remission after first-line induction therapy for diffuse non-Hodgkin's lymphoma. J Clin Oncol 1988;6(7):1118–1124.

57. Brandwein JM, Sutcliffe SB, Scott JG, et al. Clinical outcome of patients with relapsed/refractory non-Hodgkin's lymphoma referred for autologous bone marrow transplantation. Leukemia Lymphoma 1991; 4:231–238.

58. McMillan AK, Goldstone AH. Autologous bone marrow transplantation for non-Hodgkin's lymphoma. Eur J Haematol 1991;46:129–135.

59. Velasquez WS, Cabanillas F, Salvador P, et al. Effective salvage therapy for lymphoma with cisplatin in combination with high-dose Ara-C and dexamethasone (DHAP). Blood 1988;71(1):117–122.

60. Stewart AK, Brandwein JM, Sutcliffe SB, et al. Mini-BEAM as salvage chemotherapy for refractory Hodgkin's disease and non-Hodgkin's lymphoma. Leukemia Lymphoma 1991;5:111–115.

61. Crump M, Brandwein J, Sutcliffe S, et al. Autologous bone marrow transplants (ABMT) for relapsed Hodgkin's disease (HD): CR at transplant in the most important prognostic factor [Abstract]. Blood 1991;78(10, suppl 1):96.

62. Sharkis SJ, Santos GW, Colvin M. Elimination of acute myelogenous leukemic cells from marrow and tumor suspensions in the rat with 4-hydroperoxycyclophosphamide. Blood 1980;55:521–523.

63. Fefer A. Current status of syngeneic marrow transplantation and its relevance to autografting. Clin Haematol 1986;15:49–65.

64. Gross S. Perspectives in marrow purging. In: Gross S, Gee A, Worthington-White D, eds. Progress in clinical and biological research: bone marrow purging and processing, vol. 333. New York: Alan R. Liss, 1990;xxix–xxxiv.

65. Yeager AM, Kaizer H, Santos GW, et al. Autologous bone marrow transplantation in patients with acute nonlymphocytic leukemia, using in vivo marrow treatment with 4-hydroperoxycyclophosphamide. N Engl J Med 1986;315:141–147.

66. Ball ED, Mills LE, Cornwell GG, et al. Autologous bone marrow transplanation for acute myeloid leukemia using monoclonal antibody-purged bone marrow. Blood 1990;75:119–1206.

67. Roy DC, Griffin JD, Belvin M, et al. Anti-My9-blocked-ricin: an immunotoxin for selective targeting of acute myeloid leukemia cells. Blood 1991;77:2404–2412.

68. Treleaven JG, Gibson FM, Ugelstad J, et al. Removal of neuroblastoma cells from bone marrow with monoclonal antibodies conjugated to magnetic microspheres. Lancet 1984;1:70–73.

69. Sieber F. Merocyanine 540 as a marrow purging agent: interactions of merocyanine 540 with normal and neoplastic cells. In: Dicke KA, Spitzer G, Jagannath S, Evinger-Hodges MJ, eds. Autologous bone marrow transplantation: proceedings of the Fourth International Symposium. Houston: University of Texas MD Anderson Cancer Center, 1989;763–767.

70. Barnett MJ, Eaves CJ, Phillips GL, et al. Successful autografting in chronic myeloid leukemia after maintenance of marrow in culture. Bone Marrow Transplant 1989;4:345–351.

71. Berenson RJ, Bensinger WI, Hill RS, et al. Engraftment after infusion of CD34+ marrow cells in patients with breast cancer or neuroblastoma. Blood 1991;77:1717–1722.

72. Jones RJ, Miller CB, Zehnbauer BA, et al. In vitro evaluation of combination drug purging for autologous bone marrow transplantation. Bone Marrow Transplant 1990;5:301–307.

73. Gale RP, Armitage JO, Butturini A. Is there a role for autotransplants in acute leukemia? Bone Marrow Transplant 1989;4:217–219.

74. Keating A, Baker MA. Effect of exclusion criteria on interpretation of clinical outcome in AML. In: Gale RP, ed. UCLA symposia on molecular and cellular biology: acute myelogenous leukemia, new series. Vol. 134. New York: Wiley-Liss, 1990;235–237.

75. Keating A, Gale RP. Evaluating therapy for AML. In: Gale RP, ed. UCLA symposia on molecular and cellular biology: acute myelogenous leukemia, new series. Vol. 134. New York: Wiley-Liss, 1990;163–164.

76. Gorin NC, Aegerter P, Auvert B, et al. Autologous bone marrow transplantation for acute myelocytic leukemia in first remission: a European survey of the role of marrow purging. Blood 1990;75(8):1606–1614.

77. Rowley SD, Jones RJ, Piantadosi S, et al. Efficacy of ex vivo purging for autologous bone marrow transplantation in the treatment of acute nonlymphoblastic leukemia. Blood 1989;74(1):501–506.

78. Keating A. Is marrow purging necessary or clinically useful? Bone Marrow Transplant 1991;7(suppl 1):61–65.

79. Mangoni L, Carlo-Stella C, Carella AM, et al. Autologous bone marrow transplantation (ABMT) in ANLL in first remission: chemical and immunological properties of mafosfamide for minimal residual disease control. Blood 1990;76(suppl 1):2194A.

80. Aurer I, Ribas A, Gale RP. What is the role of recombinant colony stimulating factors in bone marrow transplantation? Bone Marrow Transplant 1990;6:79–87.

81. Nemunaitis J, Rabinowe SN, Singer JW, et al. Recombinant granulocyte-macrophage colony-stimulating factor after autologous bone marrow transplantation for lymphoid cancer. N Engl J Med 1991;324(25):1773–1778.

82. Gorin NC, Coiffier B, Pico J. Granulocyte-macrophage colony-stimulating factor (GM-CSF) shortens aplasia duration after autologous bone marrow transplantation (ABMT) in non-Hodgkin's lymphoma. A randomized placebo-controlled double-blind study. Blood 1990;76(suppl 1):542A.

83. Link H, Boogaerts M, Carella A, et al. Recombinant human granulocyte-macrophage colony stimulating

factor (RH-GM-CSF) after autologous bone marrow transplantation for acute lymphoblastic leukemia and non-Hodgkin's lymphoma: a randomized double blind multicenter trial in Europe. Blood 1990; 76(suppl 1):152A.

84. Advani R, Greenberg P, Gulati S, et al. Randomized placebo controlled trial of granulocyte-macrophage colony stimulating factor in patients undergoing autologous bone marrow transplantation (BMT). Blood 1990;76(suppl 1):525A.

85. Nemunaitis J, Singer JW, Buckner CD, et al. Long-term follow-up of patients who received recombinant human granulocyte-macrophage colony stimulating factor after autologous bone marrow transplantation for lymphoid malignancy. Bone Marrow Transplant 1991;7:49–52.

86. Sheridan WP, Wolf M, Lusk J, et al. Granulocyte colony-stimulating factor and neutrophil recovery after high-dose chemotherapy and autologous bone marrow transplantation. Lancet 1989;2:891–894.

87. Taylor KM, Jagannath S, Spitzer G, et al. Recombinant human granulocyte colony-stimulating factor hastens granulocyte recovery after high-dose chemotherapy and autologous bone marrow transplantation in Hodgkin's disease. J Clin Oncol 1989; 7:1791–1799.

88. Masaoka T, Motoyoshi K, Takaku F, et al. Administration of human urinary colony stimulating factor after bone marrow transplantation. Bone Marrow Transplant 1988;3:121–127.

89. Juttner CA, To LB, Ho JQK, et al. Early lymphohemopoietic recovery after autografting using peripheral blood stem cells in acute non-lymphoblastic leukemia. Transplant Proc 1988;20:40–43.

90. Kessinger A, Armitage JO. The evolving role of autologous peripheral stem cell transplantation following high-dose therapy for malignancies. Blood 1991;77:211–213.

91. To LB, Shepperd KM, Haylock DN, et al. Single high doses of cyclophosphamide enable the collection of high numbers of hemopoietic stem cells from the peripheral blood. Exp Hematol 1990;18:442–447.

92. Gianni AM, Siena S, Bregni M, et al. Granulocyte-macrophage colony-stimulating factor to harvest circulating haemopoietic stem cells for autotransplantation. Lancet 1989;2:580–585.

93. Gianni AM, Bregni M, Siena S, et al. Rapid and complete hemopoietic reconstitution following combined transplantation of autologous blood and bone marrow cells. A changing role for high dose chemoradiotherapy? Hematological Oncology 1989;7: 139–148.

94. Gianni AM, Brengni M, Siena S, et al. Very rapid and complete hematopoietic reconstitution following combined transplantation of autologous bone marrow and GM-CSF-exposed stem cells. Bone Marrow Transplant 1989;4(suppl 2):78.

95. Butturini A, Bortin MM, Gale RP. Graft-versus-leukemia following bone marrow transplantation. Bone Marrow Transplant 1987;2:233–242.

96. Gale RP, Champlin RE. How does bone marrow transplantation cure leukaemia? Lancet 1984;2:28–30.

97. Horowitz MM, Gale RP, Sondel PM, et al. Graft-versus-leukemia reactions after bone marrow transplantation. Blood 1990;75:555–562.

98. Barnes DWH, Loutit JF. Treatment of murine leukaemia with x-rays and homologous bone marrow: II. Br J Haematol 1957;3:241–252.

99. Slavin S, Ackerstein A, Naparstek E, et al. The graft-versus-leukemia (GVL) phenomenon: Is GVL separable from GVHD? Bone Marrow Transplant 1990;6:155–161.

100. Jones RJ, Vogelsang GB, Hess A, et al. Induction of graft-versus-host disease after autologous bone marrow transplantation. Lancet 1989;1:754–757.

101. Talbot DC, Powles RL, Sloane JP, et al. Cyclosporine-induced graft-versus host disease following autologous bone marrow transplantation in acute myeloid leukemia. Bone Marrow Transplant 1990; 6:17–20.

102. Glazier A, Tutschka PJ, Farmer ER, et al. Graft-versus-host disease in cyclosporin A-treated rats after syngeneic and autologous bone marrow reconstitution. J Exp Med 1983;158:1–8.

103. Cheney RT, Sprent J. Capacity of cyclosporine to induce auto-graft-versus-host disease and impair intrathymic T cell differentiation. Transplant Proc 1985;17:528.

104. Hess AD, Horwitz L, Beschorner WE, et al. Development of graft vs host disease like syndrome in cyclosporine-treated rats after syngeneic bone marrow transplantation. J Exp Med 1985;161:718–730.

105. Geller RB, Esa AH, Beschorner WE, et al. Successful in vitro graft-versus-tumor effect against an Ia-bearing tumor using cyclosporine-induced syngeneic graft-versus-host disease in the rat. Blood 1989; 74:1165–1171.

106. Heslop HE, Gottlieb DJ, Reittie JE, et al. Spontaneous and interleukin 2 induced secretion of tumour necrosis factor and gamma interferon following autologous marrow transplantation or chemotherapy. Br J Haematol 1989;72(2):122–126.

107. Blaise D, Olive D, Stoppa AM, et al. Hematologic and immunologic effects of the systemic administration of recombinant interleukin-2 after autologous bone marrow transplantation. Blood 1990;76:1092–1097.

108. Rosenberg S, Mule J, Spiess P, et al. Regression of established pulmonary metastases and subcutaneous tumor mediated by the systemic administration of high dose recombinant interleukin-2. J Exp Med 1985;161:1169.

109. Rosenberg S, Lotze M, Muul L, et al. A progress re-

port on the treatment of 157 patients with advanced cancer using lymphokine activated killer cells and interleukin 2 or high-dose interleukin 2 alone. N Engl J Med 1987;316:889–897.

110. Ettinghausen S, Moore J, White D, et al. Hematologic effects of immunotherapy with lymphokine-activated killer cells and recombinant IL2 in cancer patients. Blood 1987;6:1654.

111. Heslop HE, Gottlieb DJ, Alessandra CM, et al. In vivo induction of gamma interferon and tumor necrosis factor by interleukin-2 infusion following intensive chemotherapy or autologous marrow transplantation. Blood 1989;74:1374–1380.

112. Kalland T. Effects of the immunomodulator LS2616 on growth and metastasis of the murine B16-F10 melanoma. Cancer Res 1986;46:3018–3022.

113. Larsson E-L, Joki A, Stalhandske T. Mechanism of action of the immunomodulator LS2616 on T-cell responses. Int J Immunopharmacol 1987;9(4):425–431.

114. Bengtsson M, Simonsson B, Carlsson K, et al. Immunostimulation post autologous bone marrow transplantation with the novel drug linomide: augmentation of T- and NK-cell functions. In: Dicke KA, Armitage JO, Dicke-Evinger MJ, eds. Autologous bone marrow transplantation: proceedings of the Fifth International Symposium. Omaha, NE: University of Nebraska Medical Center, 1990;771–782.

115. Lowenberg B, Verdonck LJ, Dekker AW, et al. Autologous bone marrow transplantation in first remission: results of a Dutch prospective study. J Clin Oncol 1990;8:287–294.

116. McMillan AK, Goldstone AH, Linch DC, et al. High-dose chemotherapy and autologous bone marrow transplantation in acute myeloid leukemia. Blood 1990;76:480–488.

117. Carella AM, Gaozza E, Santini G, et al. Autologous unpurged bone marrow transplantation for acute non-lymphoblastic leukemia in first complete remission. Bone Marrow Transplant 1988;3:537–541.

118. Spinolo JA, Dicke KA, Horwitz LJ, et al. Double intensification with amsacrine/high-dose ara-C and high-dose chemotherapy with autologous bone marrow transplantation produces durable remission in acute myelogenous leukemia. Bone Marrow Transplant 1990;5:111–118.

119. Korbling M, Hundstein W, Fliedner TM, et al. Disease-free survival after autologous bone marrow transplantation in patients with acute myelogenous leukemia. Blood 1989;74:1507–1516.

120. Reiffers J, Maraninchi D, Rigal-Hoguet F, et al. Does more intensive treatment cure more patients with acute myeloid leukemia? In: Gale RP, ed. Keystone symposia workshop: curing leukemia. Semin Hematol 1991;28(3)(suppl 4):90–92.

121. Champlin R, Gajewski J, Nimer S, et al. Post remission chemotherapy for adults with acute myelogenous leukemia: improved survival with high-dose cyarabine and daunorubicin consolidation treatment. J Clin Oncol 1990;8:1199–1206.

122. Meloni G, De Fabritiis P, Petti MC, et al. BAVC regimen and autologous bone marrow transplantation in patients with acute myelogenous leukemia in second remission. Blood 1990;75:2282–2285.

123. Blaise D, Gaspard MH, Stoppa AM, et al. Allogeneic or autologous bone marrow transplantation for acute lymphoblastic leukemia in first relapse. Bone Marrow Transplant 1990;5:7–12.

124. Simonsson B, Burnett AK, Prentice HG, et al. Autologous bone marrow transplantation with monoclonal antibody purged marrow for high risk acute lymphoblastic leukemia. Leukemia 1989;3:631–636.

125. Sallan SE, Niemeyer CM, Billett AL, et al. Autologous bone marrow transplantation for acute lymphoblastic leukemia. J Clin Oncol 1989;7:1594–1601.

126. Kersey JH, Weisdorf D, Nesbit ME, et al. Comparison of autologous and allogeneic bone marrow transplantation for treatment of high-risk refractory acute lymphoblastic leukemia. N Engl J Med 1987;317(8):461–467.

127. Horowitz MM, Messerer D, Hoelzer D, et al. Chemotherapy compared with bone marrow transplantation for adults with acute lymphoblastic leukemia in first remission. Ann Intern Med 1991;115:13–18.

128. Philip T, Chauvin F, Armitage J, et al. Parma international protocol: pilot study of DHAP followed by involved-field radiotherapy and BEAC with autologous bone marrow transplantation. Blood 1991; 77:1587–1592.

129. Philip T, Armitage J, Spitzer G, et al. An international randomized study of relapsed diffuse intermediate and high grade lymphoma in adults. In: Dicke KA, Spitzer G, Zander AR, eds. Autologous bone marrow transplantation: proceedings of the Third International Symposium. Houston: University of Texas MD Anderson Hospital and Tumor Institute 1987;313.

130. Philip T, Biron P. Role of high-dose chemotherapy and autologous bone marrow transplantation in the treatment of lymphoma. Eur J Cancer 1991; 27(3):320–322.

131. Friedman AS, Takvorian T, Anderson KA, et al. Autologous bone marrow transplantation in B cell non-Hodgkin's lymphoma: very low treatment-related mortality in 100 patients in sensitive relapse. J Clin Oncol 1990;8:784–791.

132. Carella AM, Congin AM, Gaozza E, et al. High-dose chemotherapy with autologous bone marrow transplantation in 50 advanced resistant Hodgkin's disease patients. An Italian group report. J Clin Oncol 1988;6:1411–1416.

133. Phillips GL, Wolff SN, Herzig RH, et al. Treatment of progressive Hodgkin's disease with intensive chemoradiotherapy and autologous bone marrow transplantation. Blood 1989;73:2086–2092.

134. Gribben JG, Linch DC, Singer CRJ, et al. Successful treatment of refractory Hodgkin's disease by high dose combination chemotherapy and autologous bone marrow transplantation. Blood 1989;73:340–344.

135. Phillips GL, Barnett M, Buskard N, et al. Augmented cyclophosphamide (C), BCNU (B) and etoposide (V) = CBV and autologous bone marrow transplantation for progressive Hodgkin's disease. Blood 1986;68:277.

136. Carella AM, Carlier P, Mandelli F, et al. High dose chemotherapy and autologous bone marrow transplantation for Hodgkin's disease in Italy. Bone Marrow Transplant 1990;5(suppl 2):195.

137. Bierman P, Jagannath S, Armitage J, et al. High dose cyclophosphamide, carmustin, and etoposide in Hodgkin disease: follow-up of 128 patients. In: Dicke KA, Armitage JO, Dicke-Evinger MJ, eds. Autologous bone marrow transplantation: proceedings of the Fifth International Symposium. Omaha, Neb: University of Nebraska Medical Center, 1990;519–527.

138. Lohri A, Barnett M, Fairey RN, et al. Outcome of treatment of first relapse of Hodgkin's disease after primary chemotherapy: identification of risk factors from the British Columbia experience 1970 to 1988. Blood 1991;77:2292–2298.

139. Butturini A, Keating A, Goldman J, et al. Autotransplants in chronic myelogenous leukaemia: strategies and results. Lancet 1990;335(1):1255–1258.

140. Brito-Babapule F, Apperley F, Rassool F, et al. Complete remission after autografting for chronic myeloid leukemia. Leuk Res 1987;11:1115–1117.

141. Ihde DC, Deisseroth AB, Lichter AS, et al. Late intensive combined modality therapy followed by autologous bone marrow infusion in extensive-stage small-cell lung cancer. J Clin Oncol 1986;4:1443–1454.

142. Nichols CR, Tricot G, Williams SD, et al. Dose intensive chemotherapy in refractory germ cell cancer—a phase I/II trial of high dose carboplatin and etoposide with autologous bone marrow transplantation. J Clin Oncol 1989;7:932–939.

143. Graham-Pole J. Outcome for children with neuroblastoma receiving marrow-ablative treatments supported by autologous marrow infusions. In: Dicke KA, Armitage JO, Dicke-Evinger MJ, eds. Autologous bone marrow transplantation: proceedings of the Fifth International Symposium. Omaha, NE: University of Nebraska Medical Center, 1990;587–597.

144. Hartmann O, Benhamon E, Beanjean F, et al. Repeated high-dose chemotherapy followed by purged autologous bone marrow transplantation as consolidation therapy in metastatic neuroblastoma. J Clin Oncol 1987;5:1205–1211.

145. Pritchard J, Germond S, Jones D, et al. Is high-dose melphalan of value in treatment of advanced neuroblastoma? Preliminary results of a randomized trial by the European Neuroblastoma Study Group. Proc Am Soc Clin Oncol 1986;5:205.

146. Philip T, Bernard JM, Zucker R, et al. High-dose chemoradiotherapy with bone marrow transplantation as consolidation in neuroblastoma: an unselected group of stage IV patients over 1 year of age. J Clin Oncol 1987;5:266–271.

147. Hryniuk W, Levine MN. Analysis of dose intensity for adjuvant chemotherapy trials in stage II breast cancer. J Clin Oncol 1986;4:1162–1170.

148. Fisher B, Fisher ER, Redmond C. Ten year results from NSABP clinical trial evaluating the use of phenylalanine mustard in the management of primary breast cancer. J Clin Oncol 1986;4:929–941.

149. Lazarus H, Herzig R, Graham-Pole J, et al. Intensive melphalan chemotherapy and cryopreserved autologous bone marrow transplantation for the treatment of refractory cancer. J Clin Oncol 1983;2:359–367.

150. Corringham R, Gilmore M, Prentice H, et al. High-dose melphalan with autologous bone marrow transplant: treatment of poor prognosis tumors. Cancer 1983;52:1783–1787.

151. Ariel I. Treatment of disseminated cancer by intravenous hydroxyurea and autogenous bone marrow transplants: experience with 35 patients. J Surg Oncol 1975;7:331–335.

152. Brown R, Herzig R, Fay J, et al. A phase I–II study of high-dose N,N', N''-triethylenethiophosphoramide (thiotepa) and autologous marrow transplantation (AMT) for refractory malignancies. Proc Am Soc Clin Oncol 1986;4:127.

153. Peters WP, Shpall EJ, Jones RB, et al. High dose combination alkylating agents with bone marrow support as initial treatment for metastatic breast cancer. J Clin Oncol 1988;6:1368–1376.

154. Peters WP, Ross M, Vredenburgh JJ. High dose combination alkylating agents with autologous bone marrow transplantation for primary and metastatic breast cancer. In: Dicke KA, Armitage JO, Dicke-Evinger MJ, eds. Autologous bone marrow transplantation: proceedings of the Fifth International Symposium. Omaha, NE: University of Nebraska Medical Center, 1990;313–321.

11

REESTABLISHING HEMATOPOIESIS AFTER DOSE-INTENSIVE THERAPY WITH PERIPHERAL STEM CELLS

Anne Kessinger

The discovery that hematopoietic progenitor cells routinely travel with the mononuclear cell fraction of peripheral blood leukocytes in laboratory animals (1) and humans (2) led investigators to explore the possibility that these cells, when transplanted, might function like bone marrow cells to reverse bone marrow aplasia. After animal studies demonstrated that transplanted peripheral stem cells reliably restored radiation-ablated marrow function (3–5), clinical studies began. A series of patients in the aggressive phase of chronic myelogenous leukemia (CML) were treated with high-dose therapy and autologous peripheral stem cell transplantation (6). The circulating stem cells had been collected and cryopreserved earlier, when the disease was in the chronic phase. Transplantation of the leukemic autologous stem cells resulted in restoration of the chronic phase of the disease for nearly all of the patients, thereby demonstrating that leukemic peripheral stem cells could reestablish myelopoiesis.

Reports of two unsuccessful attempts to restore marrow function with transplanted syngeneic peripheral stem cells at the turn of the 1980s (7, 8) caused some concern about the ability of transplanted nonleukemic human peripheral stem cells to restore bone marrow function. However, in the mid-1980s, successful autologous peripheral stem cell autografts for patients with diseases other than CML were reported by investigators from a number of centers (9–14). Since that time, autologous peripheral stem transplants have been performed with increasing frequency.

APHERESIS FOR PERIPHERAL STEM CELL COLLECTION

Hematopoietic progenitors constitute a larger percentage of the marrow mononuclear cell population than of the peripheral blood mononuclear cell pool (6). Approximately 750–1000 cm^3 of harvested marrow contains sufficient numbers of stem cells to perform a successful autologous bone marrow transplant in an adult (15), while peripheral stem cells collected for the same purpose are typically extracted from 40 or more liters of blood (16). Apheresis is used to procure stem cells from a blood volume of this magnitude. Compared with a standard marrow collection procedure performed in an operating suite while the donor receives general anesthesia, apheresis is an outpatient procedure that requires no anesthesia. Peripheral stem cell apheresis also avoids the discomfort associated with aspirating marrow numerous times from the pelvic bones. On the other hand, peripheral stem cell collections are much more time consuming than marrow collections, requiring several days to complete.

The vascular access needed for efficient apheresis often is a problem for patients who have been extensively treated with chemotherapy prior to initiating a peripheral stem cell collection. To circumvent this predicament, central venous catheters can be used, placed either in the subclavian vein (17) or the inferior vena cava (18).

Any commercially available apheresis device can be used to collect peripheral stem cells, using machine settings designed to collect lymphocytes or low-density mononuclear cells. Depending upon the protocol selected, each apheresis procedure requires approximately 2.5–4 hours to complete, and the collections can be repeated on a daily basis until a sufficient number of cells have been harvested.

PROCESSING AND CRYOPRESERVATION

Stem cell apheresis products taken directly from the blood cell separator have been cryopreserved and successfully transplanted (16). Most investigators, however, have employed purification techniques to remove cellular contamination prior to cryopreservation because larger volumes of stem cell products are associated with an increased likelihood of side effects at the time of reinfusion (19). The particular method employed depends upon the characteristics of stem cell product collected (e.g., the granulocyte, platelet, and/or red cell content), but care must be taken to ensure the purification method does not decrease the effectiveness of the graft (20). Centrifugation or "soft spin" to remove platelets (17), elutriation to concentrate low-density cells (20), density gradients to remove red cells (21), and repeat apheresis of the product to remove red cells and granulocytes (19) are all methods that

have been used to purify peripheral stem cell apheresis products.

One of two basic cryopreservation techniques, or minor modifications thereof, can be used to prepare the stem cells for long-term storage. Both of these methods were modeled after methods that are used to cryopreserve marrow. The method most commonly used employs the addition of the cryoprotectant dimethyl sulfoxide (DMSO) to the product at a concentration of 10% by volume. The cellular concentration of the stem cell product is adjusted to approximately 1–2 $\times$ 10^8 cells/cm^3 with autologous serum, and the mixture is cooled in a controlled rate freezer and then stored in a liquid nitrogen freezer (16). The second method uses hydroxyethyl starch and DMSO as cryoprotectants, and the final concentration of DMSO is 5% by volume. The cell concentration of the mixture is adjusted as described above, and the cells are placed directly into a $-80°$ C freezer for cooling and storage without controlled rate freezing (22). No study has been performed to determine if one cryopreservation technique is superior to the other, but the method utilizing 5% DMSO has been suggested only for short-term storage (4 months or less) of stem cells (22).

PERIPHERAL STEM CELL MOBILIZATION

Mobilized stem cells can accelerate the rate of marrow function recovery following peripheral stem cell transplantation. Mobilized stem cells are peripheral stem cells whose circulating numbers have been deliberately increased during their collection. When transplants are done with mobilized peripheral stem cells, marrow function recovery occurs about a week sooner than when nonmobilized peripheral stem cells or autologous bone marrow is transplanted (23) (Table 11.1). Clinically useful mobilization of hematopoietic stem cells from extravascular sites into the circulation occurs when myelopoiesis is stimulated in response to administration of

Table 11.1. Time to Recovery of $0.5 \times 10^9/l$ Granulocytes in Circulating Blood Following Transplantation of Mobilized and Nonmobilized Peripheral Stem Cells

	No. Patients	Median Day
Mobilized		
Juttner et al. (21)	8	11
Gianni et al. (24)	2	12
Korbling et al. (25)	12	20.5
Reiffers et al. (26)	44	17
Nonmobilized		
Kessinger et al. (20)	33	25
Lasky et al. (27)	7	24
Williams et al. (28)	16	16

myelotoxic chemotherapy (29) or by specific cytokines (30) or both (24, 31).

Unfortunately, the universal employment of mobilized cells is not yet possible because mobilization methods do not always produce clinically important increases in circulating stem cells. Patients who are not likely to demonstrate a response to chemotherapy-induced mobilization attempts are those with a history of receiving extensive prior chemotherapy and patients who have histopathologic evidence of malignant cells in bone marrow; some patients with no apparent risk factors fail to increase circulating stem cell numbers following mobilization attempts (23, 32, 33). Whether these risk factors will also be valid for attempted mobilization with cytokines is uncertain since very few patients with bone marrow metastases or a history of prior extensive therapy have been studied thus far.

Currently, mobilized peripheral stem cell harvesting is a somewhat unpredictable process. Once chemotherapy-induced mobilization has been attempted, recognition of the success of the effort occurs 2 weeks after the fact, since culture assays for stem cell quantification require 14 days to complete. Estimating the best time to begin collections after attempted chemotherapy-induced mobilization is difficult. Criteria such as the initial recovery of platelet numbers and the return of

a specific number of neutrophils or specific percentage of monocytes in the neutrophil fraction have been used but are not precise in defining the optimum time of mobilization, which generally extends over only 3–4 days. Reports of a quantitative assay for stem cell content that requires just a few hours are encouraging and may reliably indicate the best time to collect the mobilized cells (34). Cytokine-induced mobilization may produce an increased number of peripheral stem cells for a more predictable and prolonged time period.

Another difficulty with mobilized stem cell harvesting is determining the point when sufficient cells for transplantation have been collected. Traditionally, the definition of an adequate graft has centered around the number of colony-forming units, granulocyte-macrophage (CFU-GM) present, as determined by culture assays. Unfortunately, these assays are not standardized; therefore the optimum number of CFU-GM in a transplant product is necessarily different at each transplant center. If flow cytometric methods are able to measure stem cell content in a clinically useful way and can be standardized (34), the definition of an adequate mobilized peripheral stem cell product for transplantation will become obvious.

STEM CELL INFUSION

One or 2 hours before the peripheral stem cell transplant, patients receive intravenous hydration to optimize renal function. At the time of transplantation, the cryopreserved cells are removed from the freezer and thawed in a 37° C water bath in the processing laboratory or at the patient's bedside. At some transplant centers, the cells are diluted in autologous plasma immediately after thawing (10) or washed with a mixture of saline, albumin, and acid citrate dextrose (12) and then infused. Most transplants are done with cells that have been thawed at the bedside and immediately infused. Some investigators have transfused the product through a filter

(10), but more often, filters are not used. No studies have been done to determine if the different thawing and infusion methods have an impact on clinical outcome. Since peripheral stem cells are collected with multiple apheresis procedures, the cells are stored in several bags. Most centers infuse all the cells in less than 4 hours.

Infusion of thawed cryopreserved stem cells, whether collected from the marrow (35) or peripheral blood (19), can be associated with toxicity. Toxicities have been reported more frequently with peripheral stem cell infusion than with marrow infusion (19). This may be because the volume of the peripheral stem cell graft is generally larger than the autologous bone marrow graft. These adverse events, which include hemoglobinuria, nausea, fever, chills, vomiting, and increased blood pressure, are short-lived and resolve without therapeutic intervention. Prior to the use of purification techniques that removed contaminating red cells from the product, side effects of important clinical consequence such as renal failure were seen (19). These toxicities have been ameliorated and even eliminated with the use of purification methods. Administration of diphenhydramine hydrochloride and meperidine hydrochloride just prior to the beginning of stem cell infusion may lessen the severity of the reactions such as fever and chilling.

ADVANTAGES OF PERIPHERAL STEM CELL TRANSPLANTATION

Although only two indications for peripheral stem cell autografting have emerged thus far, this technique may eventually prove to have a number of advantages over autologous marrow transplantation. One indication for use of peripheral stem cells pertains to patients who are candidates for high-dose therapy but have neither a suitable allogeneic marrow donor nor an autologous marrow suitable for transplantation. In this instance, an autologous marrow unsuitable for transplantation contains malignant cells or is sufficiently hypocellular to prevent an adequate marrow harvest. The most common causes of hypocellularity are prior chemotherapy and prior pelvic irradiation. Thus autologous circulating mononuclear cells serve as an alternative source of hematopoietic progenitors for transplantation. Oncologists also have used peripheral stem cells rather than autologous marrow for transplantation if restoration of marrow function is judged likely to be accelerated. As described above, accelerated recovery can be anticipated only if the transplant is done with mobilized stem cells.

Other potential advantages that await the demonstration of clinical relevance include the probability that contaminating tumor cells are less likely to be collected from autologous peripheral blood than from marrow. Two separate laboratories have reported that peripheral stem cell collections from patients with metastatic marrow disease and no recognizable tumor cells on routine microscopic examination of their peripheral blood films rarely contained tumor cells that could be detected with long-term culture, immunochemical, flow cytometric, molecular probing, and karyotyping techniques (36, 37). The clinical significance, if any, of reinfusing tumor cells that are not detectable with routine histopathologic microscopic examination is unknown. However, autologous peripheral stem cell transplants have been used as an alternative to purged autologous bone marrow transplants for patients with proven or suspected marrow metastases (38, 39).

Because a peripheral stem cell transplant contains a larger number of immunocompetent lymphocytes than a marrow harvest (the apheresis protocols used to collect peripheral stem cells are nearly identical to those used to collect lymphocytes for lymphokine-activated killer [LAK] cell production), the assumption has been made that infusion of peripheral stem cells will hasten immune recovery in the autologous setting (40). No studies are yet available to establish this potential advantage as fact, however.

Thus far, peripheral stem cells have been

transplanted strictly for their restorative powers, but suggestions that these cells may have therapeutic value as well are beginning to appear (41). No randomized prospective trials have been done comparing the tumor response and long-term event-free survival among patients with similar diseases treated with similar high dose therapy who receive either autologous peripheral stem cell transplants or autologous bone marrow transplants.

ENGRAFTMENT AND HEMATOLOGIC RECONSTITUTION

In general, if successful mobilization techniques are used during stem cell collection, recovery of circulating granulocytes following peripheral stem cell transplantation is more rapid than with transplantation of autologous bone marrow or nonmobilized peripheral stem cells (Table 11.1). Platelet and red cell recovery also have been accelerated for some patients, but delayed platelet recovery has been reported for others. Whether megakaryocyte precursors mobilized to circulate are proportionally fewer in number than other lineage-specific progenitors is unknown.

When nonmobilized peripheral stem cells are used, the speed of engraftment is generally comparable to what would be expected following an autologous bone marrow transplant, provided at least 6.5×10^8 mononuclear cells per kilogram collected with a minimum of six apheresis procedures are transfused and the patient has not received total body irradiation (16). When total body irradiation is added to high-dose chemotherapy, recovery of circulating blood cells following nonmobilized peripheral stem cell transplantation is predictably prolonged for patients with histopathologic evidence of lymphomatous marrow involvement (36). Our experience has shown that more than 98% of patients, including those with delayed engraftment, eventually recover marrow function following nonmobilized autologous peripheral stem cell transplantation.

GROWTH FACTORS IN PERIPHERAL STEM CELL TRANSPLANTATION

There are several points in the course of a peripheral stem cell transplant when growth factors might be inserted in an attempt to shorten the period of aplasia following high-dose therapy. As described earlier, growth factors have been used singly and in combination with chemotherapy to produce peripheral stem cell mobilization. Erythropoietin (42), interleukin-3 (43), granulocyte-macrophage colony-stimulating factor (44), and granulocyte colony-stimulating factor (45) have all been shown to increase the number of circulating human hematopoietic progenitors. Ten heavily pretreated patients who received granulocyte-macrophage colony stimulating factor (GM-CSF) as the only method of mobilization during stem cell collection have been transplanted (25, 30). Although mobilization did occur as measured by progenitor culture assays, return of marrow function was no faster than would have been expected with transplantation of nonmobilized stem cells. One patient who experienced rapid progression of tumor growth in the marrow and elsewhere following high-dose therapy failed to engraft. The other nine patients had a sustained recovery of marrow function, suggesting that either pluripotent stem cells capable of indefinite self-renewal were collected and transplanted or recovery of endogenous marrow occurred. Two previously untreated patients who were transplanted with stem cells that had been mobilized with GM-CSF and chemotherapy had rapid, sustained recovery of marrow function. (24)

Peripheral stem cells mobilized with chemotherapy and/or growth factors have been collected from patients who were not heavily pretreated and transplanted along with autologous bone marrow following high-dose therapy (46, 47). This technique was designed to ensure that stem cells capable of continuous self-renewal supplied from the bone marrow would be combined with a large number of committed stem cells from the peripheral blood that possessed the potential to produce rapid recovery of myelopoiesis for transplantation. Initial reports suggest that this transplantation technique, when combined with GM-CSF administration after transplantation, can reduce the time required to recover circulating white blood cells by 3 days when compared with the white cell recovery of patients who received the same high-dose therapy and autologous bone marrow transplantation. In contrast, the addition of non-mobilized peripheral stem cells from heavily pretreated patients to autologous bone marrow at the time of transplant does not result in a more rapid return of marrow function (48).

Use of growth factors in nonmobilized peripheral stem cell transplants at the time of reinfusion to hasten engraftment has not been reported. GM-CSF has been used successfully in patients who received nonmobilized peripheral stem cell transplants and experienced delayed engraftment, even though the patients were heavily pretreated (49).

CLINICAL RESULTS

Patients with a number of different malignancies have been treated with high-dose therapy and autologous peripheral stem cell transplantation. The most commonly reported diseases include chronic myelogenous leukemia, acute lymphocytic leukemia, acute myelogenous leukemia, multiple myeloma, non-Hodgkin's lymphoma, and Hodgkin's disease. Fewer patients with breast cancer, ovarian cancer, sarcoma, and cervical carcinoma have also received peripheral stem cell transplants. Some patients have been followed for a sufficient period of time to permit comments about the possibility of long-term event-free survival.

Chronic Myelogenous Leukemia

The first series of successful human peripheral stem cell transplants was done for patients with this disease beginning in 1977 (50). The number of circulating progenitor cells in patients with this disease is much larger than normal, a situation presumably analogous to the expansion of circulating stem cell numbers following administration of growth factors or myelotoxic chemotherapy. The patients had their peripheral stem cells collected and cryopreserved while the disease was in chronic phase. When the disease became aggressive, high-dose therapy was administered, followed by infusion of the autologous cells. Forty-seven of 50 patients experienced restoration of bone marrow function with reapperance of the chronic phase of the disease. Unfortunately, for most patients, the second chronic phase persisted for only a short time (median, 13 weeks), thereby limiting the value of the procedure (6). A smaller series of patients from a different center described seven patients in CML blast crisis who received peripheral stem cell autografts. Marrow function returned for five patients, and their median time of remission before disease acceleration returned was 11 months (51). Recently, high-dose therapy and autologous peripheral stem cell transplantation was used for CML patients before transformation to an accelerated phase occurred (52). These studies are quite preliminary, but a small number of patients became Ph-negative and remained so during a 3-year follow-up period. Confirmation of these findings is necessary before conclusions can be drawn regarding the utility of this approach.

Acute Leukemia

In 1984, To et al. (53) suggested that peripheral stem cells mobilized with induction chemotherapy in newly diagnosed acute myelogenous leukemia might be relatively free of leukemic contamination for responding patients. They reasoned that since leukemic cells are more susceptible to cytotoxic killing, the initial cells that repopulate peripheral blood following induction or consolidation chemotherapy are more likely to be normal. If later in the disease course the patient became a candidate for high-dose therapy, transplantation of these mobilized peripheral stem cells might function as well as purged autologous marrow. In 1989 Reiffers et al. reviewed the tumor responses of 55 patients who had received high-dose therapy and autologous peripheral stem cell transplantation for acute leukemia (54). Twenty-one patients with acute myelogenous leukemia (AML) in first remission, 16 patients with acute lymphocytic leukemia in first remission (12 adults and 4 children), and 18 patients with acute leukemias in second remission underwent transplantation. Six patients had early toxic deaths. Nine first-remission AML patients were in continuous complete remission 3–41 months (median, 13 months) after transplant, while 11 patients relapsed 3 to 13 months after transplant. Four patients with first-remission ALL remained in continuous complete remission 13–26 months after transplant, and 9 patients relapsed 2–15 months after transplant. For the patients transplanted in second remission, 12 relapsed at a median time of 4 months after transplant, and 4 continued in complete remission 6 to 33 months after transplant. The authors concluded that these results were roughly equivalent to results obtained with high-dose therapy and autologous marrow transplantation for acute leukemias, and that superiority of autologous peripheral stem cell transplantation had yet to be demonstrated.

Multiple Myeloma

The use of peripheral stem cell transplantation in the management of multiple myeloma is being reported with increasing frequency. About 400 patients with this disease, considered incurable until now, have received high-dose therapy and hematopoietic stem cell transplantation in hopes of eradicating the malignancy (55). No consensus has been reached regarding the preferred source of autologous stem cells (marrow or peripheral blood) in this setting. However, patients with extensive marrow involvement or those who had received prior pelvic irradiation would be obvious candidates for peripheral stem cell support if they were also candidates for high-dose therapy and autologous stem cell transplantation. Suitable candidates for high-dose therapy have been suggested to be those who have received a minimal amount of prior therapy, have malignancies that are responsive to chemotherapy, have in AgG myeloma isotype, and are 65 years of age or less (55). Patients who are less than 50 years and have a suitable allogeneic donor may be considered for an allogeneic bone marrow transplant.

Barlogie and Gahrton (55) have compiled a series of 69 multiple myeloma patients treated at three different centers (56–58) with high-dose therapy and autologous peripheral stem cell transplantation. Consequently, this composite series represents a heterogeneous group of patients who were at different points in their disease courses when treated with different high-dose regimens. Summarizing the results of this diverse population reveals that 3 patients experienced an early death due to engraftment failure, 18 had a complete remission (i.e., disappearance of monoclonal gammopathy), and 48 had a partial response. With a median follow-up of 12–18 months after transplantation, 45 of 58 patients remained in partial or complete remission. The ultimate outcome for these patients awaits longer follow-up, but the results thus far suggest that high-dose therapy and peripheral stem cell transplantation can at least improve the disease course for some patients.

Non-Hodgkin's Lymphoma

The treatment of refractory non-Hodgkin's lymphomas with high-dose therapy and autologous peripheral stem cell transplantation has been reported by a number of investigators (9, 28, 39, 59–61). Most of the patients received peripheral stem cell transplants because the autologous marrow was hypocellular or was known to contain lymphomatous cells (9, 28, 39). Mobilized peripheral stem cells were used for some of the transplants in hopes of achieving a rapid engraftment and decreasing the likelihood of inadvertent transplantation of tumor cells (59–61). The largest series of patients has been reported from the University of Nebraska Medical Center (39) and recently has been updated.

Twenty-nine patients (16 male and 13 female) with relapsed or refractory nontransformed low-grade lymphomas and a bone marrow abnormality (lymphomatous marrow involvement during the disease course or hypocellularity due to prior pelvic irradiation) had peripheral stem cell transplantation following high-dose therapy. High-dose cyclophosphamide (60 mg/kg × two doses) and total body irradiation (12 Gy in six fractionated doses) were used for 24 patients who had not received prior irradiation. Five patients received only high-dose chemotherapy (carmustine, cyclophosphamide, etoposide, and cytarabine). The median age was 43 years (range, 26–63 years). Three patients had a toxic death 35, 69, and 102 days after transplantation. Seventeen patients achieved a complete remission, 4 a partial remission, 3 patients failed to respond, and 3 more had not yet been restaged. Two patients who had an early death were not evaluated for response. The actuarial event-free survival (EFS, survival without tumor progression) for all 29 patients was 41% at 41 months (Fig. 11.1). Their actuarial survival at 41 months was 51% (Fig. 11.2). The follow-up of this series of patients with indolent lymphomas is not long enough to be certain that cures can result from high-dose therapy and autologous peripheral stem cell transplantation, but long-term survival free of disease progression has been observed for some patients.

Forty-one patients (25 male and 16 fe-

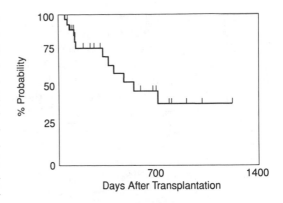

Figure 11.1. Actuarial event-free survival for 29 patients with low-grade non-Hodgkin's lymphoma.

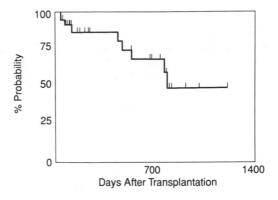

Figure 11.2. Actuarial survival for 29 patients with low-grade non-Hodgkin's lymphoma.

male) have been treated for refractory intermediate- and high-grade lymphomas with high-dose therapy and autologous peripheral stem cell transplantation. The median age of the patients was 42 years, with a range of 17–59 years. The high-dose therapy they received varied according to the histologic subtype of lymphoma being treated. All patients had marrow hypocellularity in traditional harvest sites or evidence of tumor cells in the bone marrow during the course of their disease. At 57 months, the actuarial EFS for all 41 patients was 28% (Fig. 11.3), and the actuarial survival was 39% (Fig. 11.4). Some of these patients may have achieved cure of their disease.

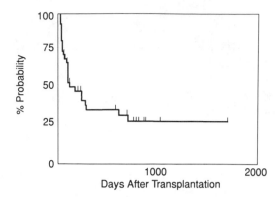

Figure 11.3. Actuarial event-free survival for 41 patients with intermediate- and high-grade non-Hodgkin's lymphoma.

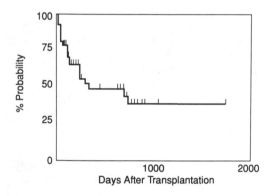

Figure 11.4. Actuarial survival for 41 patients with intermediate and high-grade non-Hodgkin's lymphoma.

Hodgkin's Disease

Hodgkin's disease is the most commonly reported tumor treated with high-dose therapy and autologous peripheral stem cell transplantation. At least 83 Hodgkin's disease patients managed with this strategy are documented in the literature (25, 27, 28, 61–63). Interestingly, the majority of these patients received cyclophosphamide, carmustine, and etoposide (CBV) in approximately the same doses. Descriptions of clinical outcome are available for 82 patients (Table 11.2). Nearly all of these 82 reported patients had a marrow abnormality, either hypocellularity or metastatic disease, which precluded the use

Table 11.2. High-Dose Therapy and Peripheral Stem Cell Transplantation for Hodgkin's Disease

Reference	No. Patients	% Patients with EFS	No. Patients with EFS	Months EFS (Range)
Lasky et al. (27)	7	29	2	?
Zander et al. (62)	4	25	1	7
Williams et al. (28)	3	67	2	9 (6–13)
Korbling et al. (25)	12	60	8	12 (6–34)
Kessinger et al. (41)	56	50	28	13 (3–39)

of autologous bone marrow transplantation. Fourteen patients received stem cells that had been mobilized prior to collection. Four reports described series of fewer than 10 patients followed no longer than 13 months (27, 28, 61, 63). Two larger reported series with maximum patient follow-up beyond 3 years include 68 patients.

Korbling et al. (25) described 12 patients with refractory Hodgkin's disease and no evidence of bone marrow metastases who had received prior pelvic irradiation that precluded autologous bone marrow collection. Peripheral stem cell mobilization was attempted using either chemotherapy (8 patients) or GM-CSF (4 patients). One patient had an early toxic death, and 7 were in an unmaintained complete remission at the time of the report. These patients in complete remission had been followed for a median of 318 days (range, 187–1033 days). Although the follow-up is short, these results are comparable and perhaps superior to the outcome of relapsed Hodgkin's disease patients treated with CBV and autologous bone marrow transplantation at other institutions (63).

The largest reported series of refractory Hodgkin's disease patients treated with CBV and peripheral stem cell transplantation includes 56 patients who were followed for a median of 13 months after transplant (41). All patients had a marrow abnormality that prevented autologous bone marrow transplant.

No attempt to mobilize stem cells prior to collection was made. Twenty-six of the patients had bone marrow involvement at the time of stem cell harvesting, and the other 30 patients had some other marrow abnormality (hypocellularity or prior history of bone marrow metastases). The actuarial EFS for all 56 patients was 37% at 3 years. The 3-year projected survival of the 30 patients without marrow metastases at the time of transplant was 47% compared to a projected survival of 27% for those patients with marrow involvement. Those patients without bone marrow involvement, a group somewhat analogous to the series reported by Korbling (25) described above, experienced an outcome better than might have been expected if they had received autologous bone marrow transplants (63). Although a randomized prospective trial will be required to answer the question, the results from these two trials suggest that a peripheral stem cell transplant might be therapeutic as well as restorative.

ALLOGENEIC PERIPHERAL STEM CELL TRANSPLANTATION

Does the pluripotent peripheral stem cell circulate in humans, and are pluripotent stem cells responsible for the durability of autologous peripheral stem cell transplants? The answers to these questions are not available since no method to identify the human pluripotent stem cell exists. Allogeneic peripheral stem cell transplants in animals where donor hematopoietic cells can be distinguished from recipient cells suggest that the pluripotent stem cell does circulate and can be used for successful allogeneic transplants (64). Sustained hematopoietic recovery has been observed after autologous peripheral stem cell transplantation for patients who had received total body irradiation, but this observation does not prove that pluripotent stem cells were transplanted. In those instances, eventual resurgence of autochthonous marrow stem cells may have been responsible for the sustained recovery, rather than transplan-

tation of stem cells capable of perpetual self-renewal. Since no method exists to determine whether the hematopoiesis observed years after transplantation was a result of autologous circulating stem cells or bone marrow stem cells, the source of the cells responsible for sustained engraftment remains unknown. To determine whether peripheral stem cell transplants can restore sustained marrow function, transplantation of either autologous peripheral stem cells that have been marked to distinguish them from marrow stem cells or an allogeneic peripheral stem cell graft where donor cells can be distinguished from recipient cells is required.

One human allogeneic peripheral stem cell transplant has been reported (65). For this transplant, the number of T lymphocytes in the allograft was reduced to approximately the number that would be present in a routine allogeneic bone marrow transplant to avoid excessive graft-versus-host disease. The myelopoiesis established after the transplant was a pure donor cell population, but the patient died of an infection a month after transplantation, so that sustained hematopoiesis could not be evaluated.

The advantages of allogeneic peripheral stem cell transplantation versus allogeneic bone marrow transplantation include avoidance of general anesthesia and the discomfort that accompanies a bone marrow collection procedure for normal donors. Allogeneic peripheral stem cell donation might be more attractive than bone marrow donation to some potential unrelated donors.

CONCLUSIONS

The peripheral blood can serve as an alternate source of hematopoietic progenitors for autologous transplantation. Peripheral stem cell transplantation can be used for patients who are candidates for high-dose therapy but not for allogeneic transplant and who have bone marrow abnormalities that preclude autologous bone marrow transplantation. If techniques are used to mobilize the stem cells into the circulation prior to their collection, peripheral stem cell transplantation results in earlier recovery of hematopoietic function than would be expected with autologous bone marrow transplantation.

Methods to improve the transplantation process are needed. Reducing the number of apheresis procedures required to collect a sufficient number of cells, decreasing the period of aplasia following transplantation, and improving the mobilization procedures to make them universally applicable and reproducible are all issues currently being investigated. Whether peripheral stem cell transplantation will eliminate the need for bone marrow purging or have a therapeutic component is an issue that awaits resolution.

REFERENCES

1. Goodman JW, Hodgson GS. Evidence for stem cells in the peripheral blood of mice. Blood 1962;19:702–714.
2. Barr RD, Whang-Peng J, Perry S. Hemopoietic stem cells in human peripheral blood. Science 1975;190:284–285.
3. Nothdurft W, Bruch C, Fliedner TM, et al. Studies on the regeneration of the CFUc population in blood and bone marrow of lethally irradiated dogs after autologous transfusion of cryopreserved mononuclear blood cells. Scand J Haematol 1977;17:470–481.
4. Sarpel SC, Zander AR, Harvath L et al. The collection, preservation and function of peripheral blood hematopoietic cells in dogs. Exp Hematol 1979;7:113–120.
5. Storb R, Graham TC, Epstein RB et al. Demonstration of hemopoietic stem cells in the peripheral blood of baboons by cross circulation. Blood 1977;50:537–542.
6. McCarthy DM, Goldman JM. Transfusion of circulating stem cells. CRC Crit Rev Clin Lab Sci 1984;20:1–24.
7. Hershko C, Gale RP, Ho WG, et al. Cure of aplastic anemia in paroxysmal nocturnal hemoglobinuria by marrow transfusion from identical twin; failure of peripheral-leukocyte transfusion to correct marrow aplasia. Lancet 1979;1:945–947.
8. Abrams RA, Glaubiger D, Appelbaum FR, et al. Result of attempted hematopoietic reconstitution using isologous peripheral blood mononuclear cells: a case report. Blood 1980;56:516–520.
9. Korbling M, Dorken B, Ho AD, et al. Autologous transplantation of blood-derived hemopoietic stem cells after myeloablative therapy in a patient with Burkitt's lymphoma. Blood 1986;67:529–532.
10. Reiffers J, Bernard P, David B, et al. Successful autologous transplantation with peripheral blood hemopoietic cells in a patient with acute leukemia. Exp Hematol 1986;14:312–315.
11. Castaigne S, Calvo F, Douay L, et al. Successful haematopoietic reconstitution using autologous peripheral blood mononucleated cells in a patient with acute promyelocytic leukaemia [Letter]. Br J Haematol 1986;62:209–211.
12. Tilly H, Bastit D, Lucet JC, et al. Haemopoietic reconstitution after autologous peripheral blood stem cell transplantation in acute leukaemia [Letter]. Lancet 1986;2:154–155.
13. Bell AJ, Figes A, Oscier DG, et al. Peripheral blood stem cell autografting [Letter]. Lancet 1986;1:1027.
14. Kessinger A, Armitage JO, Landmark JD, et al. Reconstitution of human hematopoietic function with autologous cryopreserved circulating stem cells. Exp Hematol 1986;14:192–196.
15. Kessinger A, Armitage JO. Harvesting marrow for autologous transplantation from patients with malignancies. Bone Marrow Transplant 1987;2:15–18.
16. Kessinger A, Armitage JO, Landmark JD, et al. Autologous peripheral hematopoietic stem cell transplantation restores hematopoietic function following marrow ablative therapy. Blood 1988;71:723–727.
17. Lasky LC, Hurd DD, Smith JA, et al. Clinical collection and use of peripheral blood stem cells in pediatric patients. Transplantation 1989;47:613–616.
18. Haire WD, Lieberman RP, Lund GB, et al. Translumbar inferior vena cava catheters: safety and efficacy in peripheral blood stem cell transplantation. Transfusion 1990;30:511–515.
19. Kessinger A, Schmit-Pokorny K, Smith D, et al. Cryopreservation and infusion of autologous peripheral blood stem cells. Bone Marrow Tranplant 1990;5(suppl 1):25–220.
20. Kessinger A, Armitage JO, Smith DM, et al. High-dose therapy and autologous peripheral blood stem cell transplantation for patients with lymphoma. Blood 1989;74:1260–1265.
21. Juttner CA, To LB, Ho JQK, et al. Early lympho-hemopoietic recovery after autografting using peripheral blood stem cells in acute non-lymphoblastic leukemia. Transplant Proc 1988;20:40–43.
22. Stiff PJ, Koester AR, Weidner MK, et al. Autologous bone marrow transplantation using unfractionated cells cryopreserved in dimethylsulfoxide and hydroxyethyl starch without controlled-rate freezing. Blood 1987;70:974–978.
23. Kessinger A, Armitage JO. The evolving role of autologous peripheral stem cell transplantation following high-dose therapy for malignancies [Editorial]. Blood 1991;211–213.
24. Gianni AM, Tarella C, Siena S, et al. Durable and complete hematopoietic reconstitution after autografting of rhGM-CSF exposed peripheral blood pro-

genitor cells. Bone Marrow Transplantation 1990; 6:143–145.

25. Korbling M, Holle R, Haas R, et al. Autologous blood stem-cell transplantation in patients with advanced Hodgkin's disease and prior radiation to the pelvic site. J Clin Oncol 1990;8:978–985.

26. Reiffers J, Castaigne S, Tilly H, et al. Hematopoietic reconstitution after autologous blood stem cell transplantation: a report of 46 cases. Plasma Ther Transfus Technol 1987;8:360–362.

27. Lasky LC, Hurd DD, Smith JA, et al. Peripheral blood stem cell collection and use in Hodgkin's disease. Comparison with marrow in autologous transplantation. Transfusion 1989;29:323–327.

28. Williams SF, Bitran JD, Richards JM, et al. Peripheral blood-derived stem cell collections for use in autologous transplantation after high dose chemotherapy: an alternative approach. Bone Marrow Transplant 1990;5:129–133.

29. To LB, Shepperd KM, Haylock DN, et al. Single high doses of cyclophosphamide enable the collection of high numbers of hemopoietic stem cells from the peripheral blood. Exp Hematol 1990;18:442–447.

30. Haas R, Ho AD, Bredthaues U, et al. Successful autologous transplantation of blood stem cells mobilized with recombinant human granulocyte-macrophage colony-stimulating factor. Exp Hematol 1990;18:94–98.

31. Tarella C, Ferrero D, Bregni M, et al. Peripheral blood expansion of early progenitor cells after high-dose cyclophosphamide and reGM-CSF. Eur J Cancer 1991;27:22–27.

32. Korbling M, Martin H. Transplantation of hemapheresis-derived hemopoietic stem cells: a new concept in the treatment of patients with malignant lymphohemopoietic disorders. Plasma Ther Transfus Technol 1988;9:119–132.

33. Cantin G, Marchand-Laroche D, Leblond PF. Blood-derived stem cell collection in acute nonlymphoblastic leukemia: predictive factors for a good yield. Exp Hematol 1989;17:991–996.

34. Siena S, Bregni M, Brando B, et al. Flow cytometry for clinical estimation of circulating hematopoietic progenitors for autologous transplantation in cancer patients. Blood 1991;77:400–409.

35. Davis JM, Rowley SD, Braine HG, et al. Clinical toxicity of cryopreserved bone marrow graft infusion. Blood 1990;75:781–786.

36. Sharp JG, Kessinger A, Pirruccello SJ, et al. Frequency of detection of suspected lymphoma cells in peripheral blood stem cell collections. In: Dicke KA, Armitage JO, eds. Autologous bone marrow transplantation. Proceedings of the Fifth International Symposium. Omaha, NE: University of Nebraska Medical Center, 1991:801–810.

37. Langlands K, Craig JIO, Parker AC, et al. Molecular determination of minimal residual disease in pe-

ripheral blood stem cell harvests. Bone Marrow Transplant 1990;5(suppl 1):64.

38. Kessinger A, Vose JM, Bierman PJ, et al. High dose therapy and autologous peripheral stem cell transplantation for patients with relapsed lymphomas and bone marrow metastases. In: Dicke KA, Armitage JO, eds. Autologous bone marrow transplantation. Proceedings of the Fifth International Symposium. Omaha, NE: University of Nebraska Medical Center, 1991:837–840.

39. Kessinger A, Nademanee A, Forman SJ, et al. Autologous bone marrow transplantation for Hodgkin's and non-Hodgkin's lymphoma. Hematol Oncol Clin North Am 1990;4:577–587.

40. Zander AR, Cockerill. Autologous transplantation with circulating hemopoietic stem cells. J Clin Apheresis 1987;3:191–201.

41. Kessinger A, Bierman PJ, Vose JM, et al. High-dose cyclophosphamide, carmustine, and etoposide followed by autologous peripheral stem cell transplantation for patients with relapsed Hodgkin's disease. Blood 1991;77:2322–2325.

42. Ganser A, Bergmann M, Volkers B, et al. In vivo effects of recombinant human erythropoietin on circulating human hemopoietic progenitor cells. Exp Hematol 1989;17:433–435.

43. Alter R, Welniak AL, Jackson JD, et al. In-vitro clonogenic monitoring of peripheral blood stem cell collections following interleukin-3 administration [Abstract]. Blood 1990;76(suppl 1):129a.

44. Socinski MA, Cannistra SA, Elias A, et al. Granulocyte-macrophage colony stimulating factor expands the circulating haemopoietic progenitor cell compartment in man. Lancet 1988;1:1194–1198.

45. Duhrsen U, Villeval JL, Boyd J, et al. Effects of recombinant human granulocyte colony-stimulating factor on hematopoietic progenitor cells in cancer patients. Blood 1988;72:2074.

46. Gianni AM, Siena S, Bregni M, et al. Granulocyte-macrophage colony-stimulating factor to harvest circulating haemopoietic stem cells for autotransplantation. Lancet 1989;2:580–585.

47. Peters WP, Kurtzberg J, Kirkpatrick G, et al. GM-CSF primed peripheral blood progenitor cells coupled with autologous bone marrow transplantation will eliminate leukopenia following high dose chemotherapy [Abstract]. Blood 1989;74(suppl 1):50a.

48. Lobo F, Kessinger A, Landmark JD, et al. Does the addition of peripheral blood stem cells shorten the period of aplasia in patients receiving myeloablative therapy and autologous bone marrow transplantation? [Abstract]. Proc Am Assoc Cancer Res 1989;30:234.

49. Vose JM, Bierman PJ, Kessinger A, et al. The use of recombinant human granulocyte-macrophage colony stimulating factor for the treatment of delayed engraftment following high dose therapy and autologous hematopoietic stem cell transplantation for

lymphoid malignancies. Bone Marrow Transplant 1991;7:139–143.

50. Goldman JM, Catovsky D, Hows J, et al. Cryopreserved peripheral blood cells functioning as autografts in patients with chronic granulocytic leukaemia in transformation. Br Med J 1979;1:1310–1313.

51. Karp DD, Parker LM, Binder N, et al. Treatment of blastic transformation of chronic granulocytic leukemia using high-dose BCNU chemotherapy and cryopreserved autologous peripheral blood stem cells. Am J Hematol 1985;18:243–249.

52. Goldman JM, Autografting for CML: is there a role? In: Champlin RE, Gale RP, eds. New strategies in bone marrow transplantation. New York: Wiley-Liss, 1991:155–162.

53. To LB, Haylock DN, Kimber RJ, et al. High levels of circulating haemopoietic stem cells in very early remission from acute non-lymphoblastic leukaemia and their collection and cryopreservation. Br J Hematol 1984;58:399–410.

54. Reiffers J, Leverger G, Castaigne S, et al. Tumor response after autologous blood stem cell transplantation in leukemic patients. In: Dicke KA, Spitzer G, Jagannath S, Evinger-Hodges MJ, eds. Autologous bone marrow transplantation, proceedings of the Fourth International Symposium. Houston: University of Texas MD Anderson Cancer Center, 1989:719–722.

55. Barlogie B, Gahrton G. Bone marrow transplantation in multiple myeloma. Bone Marrow Transplant 1991;7:71–79.

56. Fermand JP, Levy Y, Gerota J, et al. Treatment of aggressive multiple myeloma by high-dose chemotherapy and total body irradiation followed by blood stem cells autologous graft. Blood 1989;73:20–23.

57. Reiffers J, Marit G, Boiron JM. Peripheral blood stem-cell transplantation in intensive treatment of multiple myeloma [Letter]. Lancet 1989;2:1336.

58. Ventura GJ, Barlogie B, Hester JP, et al. High dose cyclophosphamide, BCNU and VP-16 with autologous blood stem cell support for refractory multiple myeloma. Bone Marrow Transplant 1990;5:265–268.

59. Takaue Y, Watanabe T, Hoshi Y, et al. Effectiveness of high-dose MCNU therapy and hematopoietic stem cell autografts treatment of childhood acute leukemia/lymphoma with high risk features. Cancer 1991;67:1830–1837.

60. Bell AJ, Figes A, Oscier DG, et al. Peripheral blood stem cell autografts in the treatment of lymphoid malignancies: initial experience in three patients. Br J Haematol 1987;66:63–68.

61. Reiffers J, Leverger G, Marit G, et al. Haematopoietic reconstitution after autologous blood stem cell transplantation. In: Gale RP, Champlin RE, eds. Bone marrow transplantation: current controversies. New York: Alan R. Liss, 1989:313–320.

62. Zander AR, Lyding J, Cockerill KJ, et al. Autologous blood stem cell transplantation. In: Dicke KA, Spitzer G, Jagannath S, Evinger-Hodges MJ, eds. Autologous bone marrow transplantation, proceedings of the Fourth International Symposium. Houston: University of Texas MD Anderson Cancer Center, 1989:713–717.

63. Jagannath S, Armitage JO, Dicke KA, et al. Timing of high dose CBV and autologous bone marrow transplantation in the management of relapsed or refractory Hodgkin's disease. In: Dicke KA, Spitzer G, Jagannath S, Evinger-Hodges MJ, eds. Autologous bone marrow transplantation, proceedings of the Fourth International Symposium. Houston: University of Texas MD Anderson Cancer Center, 1989:275–283.

64. Korbling M, Fliedner TM, Calvo W, et al. Albumin density gradient purification of canine hemopoietic blood stem cells (HBSC): long-term allogeneic engraftment without GVH-reaction. Exp Hematol 1979;7:277–288.

65. Kessinger A, Smith DM, Strandjord SE, et al. Allogeneic transplantation of blood-derived, T cell-depleted hemopoietic stem cells after myeloablative treatment in a patient with acute lymphoblastic leukemia. Bone Marrow Transplant 1989;4:643–646.

12

HIGH-DOSE CANCER THERAPY WITHOUT STEM CELL SUPPORT—HUMAN SOLID TUMORS

Robert B. Livingston

BACKGROUND AND RATIONALE

It is important first to define what is implied by the term "high-dose therapy." For the purpose of this discussion, the implication is that hospitalization for supportive care is required. Thus by definition, most "dose-intensive" programs, intended as they are for outpatient administration at frequent intervals, are not high-dose." In a volume that is largely devoted to the use of high-dose therapy in the context of autologous stem cell support, usually derived from marrow that was previously harvested and stored, one must ask first why there should be an interest in approaches that exclude marrow infusion as a supportive technique. The most important reason is to avoid the inadvertent administration of viable tumor cells that may contaminate the bone marrow collection.

Tumor cells may be found in marrow specimens that appear histologically negative. Using monoclonal antibody techniques, Stahel et al. found marrow involvement in 69% of samples from patients with small cell lung cancer, while standard histochemical stains detected it in only 16%; this included 8 of 16 patients with limited disease by the usual staging criteria (1). Similarly, Cheung et al. reported that marrow involvement in neu-roblastoma could be detected in 74% of patients with stage III and IV disease, while the sensitivity of conventional stains was 27% (2), and that as few as 0.01% tumor cells could be detected by the antibody technique. Detection of "micrometastases" in the marrow of patients with primary breast cancer was reported by Redding et al. in 1983 (3) using antibody technology, and subsequent reports by Cote et al. (4) and Ellis et al. (5) have confirmed that monoclonal antibodies to membrane and cytoskeletal antigens can detect fewer than one cancer cell in 10^4 hematopoietic cells. Porro et al. have used a less sensitive monoclonal antibody to a membrane antigen that is not universally expressed in breast cancer (6). The reported frequency of marrow positivity in patients with primary breast cancer at the time of operation varies from 16%–35% (see Table 12.1).

Are the tumor cells detected by such techniques really "micrometastases" to bone marrow, with prognostic significance? The available evidence suggests that they are. In a followup of Redding's initial report, Coombes et al. reported that the group with detected micrometastases was relapsing at a faster rate (7), and Mansi et al. from the same group (8) reported relapse in 32 of 81 breast cancer patients with positive marrows,

Table 12.1.   Primary Breast Cancer—Frequency of Marrow Positivity for Tumor by Immunocytochemical Methods[a]

Series	Reference	Number of Patients	Number Positive	% Positive	Type of Antibody
Mansi	8	307	81	26	Polyclonal EMA
Cote	4	51	18	35	Monoclonal-membrane + cytokeratin
Ellis	5	6	2	33	Monoclonal-cytokeratin
Porro	6	159	25	16	Monoclonal-membrane antigen

[a]Abbreviations: EMA, epithelial membrane antigen.

versus 45 of 226 who were antibody negative (30% versus 10%). Salvadori et al., using the antibody described by Porro, have detected relapse in the same proportion of "positive" and "negative" patients (9), but their initial frequency of positives remains only about half of that reported by investigators who used anticytokeratin antibodies. Moss et al. recently reported that antibody-detected micrometastases are a powerful, independent predictor of relapse in children with neuroblastoma (10).

When tumor cells grow in a culture established from marrow harvest, one might expect an even stronger correlation with subsequent relapse. Vaughan et al. from the University of Nebraska established Dexter-type, long-term cell cultures using the materials scraped from the marrow collection screens in primary breast cancer patients undergoing elective marrow storage because of other identified poor prognostic factors (11). Overall, 16 of 28 (57%) of histologically negative marrows contained malignant cells that could be detected in culture, using cytologic evaluations of cytospin preps. Relapse had occurred in 8 of 16 with positive cultures and 0 of 12 with negative cultures ($p < .05$), in a preliminary analysis.

The most persuasive evidence that marrow contamination produces marrow relapse would come from a study in which patients received the same intensive chemotherapy, but half the patients were randomized to receive autologous marrow support and the other half not. If the relapse rate were substantially higher in the former group, such a

conclusion would prove inescapable. Such a study has been done. The preliminary analysis, reported by Huan et al. (12), indicates that 14 of 18 stage IV breast cancer patients transplanted in complete response (CR) had relapsed, versus 7 of 17 who received the same chemotherapy without a transplant. It is too early to draw a definitive conclusion from this analysis, but the results are suggestive.

One approach to the problem of marrow contamination is to attempt "purging" of the tumor cells ex vivo. Antibody with complement, lectin separation, immunomagnetic separation, and cytotoxic drug treatment have been described. The general problem to date with methods that employ antibody with complement is variable degrees of tumor-cell depletion and low potency (13). Shpall et al. recently reported the use of 4-hydroperoxycyclophosphamide (4-HC) to treat the collected marrow in a phase I trial among patients with stage IV breast cancer, who underwent subsequent high-dose chemotherapy and infusion of the "purged" marrow (14). Compared to unpurged historical controls who received the same high-dose regimen, levels up to 60 µg/ml did not delay engraftment significantly. However, 80 µg/ml did result in such a delay, and further escalation of 4-HC was not attempted. The 60 µg/ml level of 4-HC produced a 2.0 log reduction in breast cancer cells in clonogenic assay by the same investigators, while 40 µg/ml produced only 1.0 log. Immunomagnetic purging coupled to 4-HC, studied by the same group of investigators, produced a higher level of cytoreduction, but affected CFU-C GM recovery in vitro (15). Monoclonal antibodies conjugated to *Pseudomonas* exotoxin A (16) or ricin immunotoxin (17) are newly described, promising approaches to purging. Whether they will be superior to the complement-antibody methods remains to be seen. As yet, it is fair to say that no method of marrow treatment to eliminate contamination has established clinical efficacy. Inadequate tumor cell kill and/or damage to normal hematopoietic precursors remain potential problems with each.

Two final reasons to avoid regimens that ablate all of the host's endogenous hematopoietic stem cells bear mention. The first is preservation of marrow reserve, should the patient require subsequent chemotherapy at the time of relapse. The second is that, should a patient have long-term survival after the use of high-dose chemotherapy, prior exposure to certain stem cell toxins may be associated with a higher risk of second malignancy (18–20).

CYTOTOXIC AGENTS—EXTRAMEDULLARY TOXICITY IS DOSE LIMITING

The first group of compounds that fit this description are DNA cross-linkers: cyclophosphamide, cisplatin, and streptozocin. Cyclophosphamide at high dose is limited by acute hemorrhagic carditis, rather than myelosuppression (21). Its inability to completely eradicate hematopoietic progenitors at tolerated doses in vivo is probably related to the production by stem cells of aldehyde dehydrogenase, an enzyme that inactivates 4-HC; production of this enzyme is lost in the more committed progenitors (22). Cisplatin at standard doses (up to 100 mg/m^2) is only slightly myelosuppressive and is limited by acute toxicities of renal damage, nausea, and vomiting. When these are overcome by techniques of forced intravenous hydration and intensive parenteral antiemetics, its dose-limiting toxicity shifts to either myelosuppression and neuropathy (23) or neuropathy and ototox-

icity (24), depending on whether the drug is delivered by a daily × 5 schedule or a day 1, 8, schedule on a monthly basis. In either case, the maximum tolerated dose for a single course is 200 mg/m^2. Both cyclophosphamide and cisplatin lend themselves well to high-dose protocols without marrow support, combined with each other or with other drugs (Table 12.2). Streptozocin, on the other hand, appears synergistic with other nitrosoureas in the production of hepatic toxicity (25) and myelosuppression (26).

A second class to consider are topoisomerase-II inhibitors. Etoposide (VP-16) is clearly limited by oropharyngeal mucositis at doses that permit complete bone marrow recovery. If the dose is divided over three fractions, 2.7 gm/m^2 is dose limiting (27); if in six fractions over 3 consecutive days, 3.5 gm/m^2 (28). Hepatotoxicity is not a feature of high-dose etoposide therapy, and neurotoxicity is also absent (28, 29), with the probable exception of glioma patients who sustain a peculiar syndrome of CNS deterioration, responsive to dexamethasone (30). Doxorubicin (Adriamycin) has hematologic dose-limiting toxicity that can be partially overcome by the use of granulocyte colony-stimulating factor (G-CSF), only to be replaced by dose-limiting epithelial toxicity involving the oral and vaginal mucosa, palms, and soles (31). Even without growth factor support, doxorubicin is sometimes acutely dose limited by mucosal or cardiac toxicity (32), making it a suboptimal candidate for inclusion in high-dose combination regimens.

Vincristine is nonmyelosuppressive, but its limited spectrum, schedule dependence, and the appearance of dose-limiting peripheral neuropathy with repeated dosing have made it unattractive for incorporation with high-dose combinations. Glucocorticoids share the problem of a narrow spectrum of sensitive malignancies and include among their protean complications a propensity to promote infectious complications. Thus most investigations of high-dose therapy without marrow support have focused on cyclophos-

Table 12.2.   Toxicity Characteristics—Drugs Used in High-Dose Therapy

Drug	Necessity for Myeloid Stem Cell Support	Extramedullary Organ Toxicity	
		Dose Limiting	Other Major
Thiotepa	+	CNS	Mucositis, skin
Cyclophosphamide	−	Cardiac	
Ifosfamide	−	Renal	
Melphalan	+	Mucositis	Diarrhea, renal
BCNU	+	Lung, liver	CNS
Carboplatin	+	Renal, liver	Ototoxicity
Mitomycin C	?	Kidney, liver	Cardiac, gastrointestinal
Busulfan	+	Mucositis	Pulmonary, anorexia, rash, "autoimmune"
Etoposide	−	Mucositis	Cardiac?
Mitoxantrone	+	Mucositis	Cardiac
Cisplatin	−	Neuropathy	Renal, ototoxicity

phamide, cisplatin, etoposide, or a combination of these agents.

DRUG-ORIENTED INVESTIGATIONS

High-dose cyclophosphamide (CTX) was investigated in a series of drug-oriented studies, beginning with the work of Finklestein et al. (33) who reported the administration of oral cyclophosphamide (10 mg/kg daily) to 31 children with a variety of solid tumors, 21 as initial therapy and 10 as salvage therapy for progressive disease. Leukopenia was dose limiting after approximately 120 mg/kg of cyclophosphamide per cycle. The overall response rate in the 26 evaluable patients who received cyclophosphamide as initial therapy was 80%. Two patients with sarcoma who failed previous lower daily doses of cyclophosphamide achieved significant tumor responses.

Buckner et al. reported a series of 25 patients with various refractory solid tumor malignancies who were treated with single or multiple courses of high-dose cyclophosphamide (60–120 mg/kg), with two treatment-related deaths (34). Eight patients, including 3 with ovarian carcinoma, responded for a median of 2 months (range, 1 to 12+ months), for an overall response rate of 32%.

Mullins and Colvin treated 11 patients with refractory solid tumors with 60 mg/kg of cyclophosphamide for 18 courses and 16 patients with 100 mg/kg of cyclophosphamide for 26 courses (35). There were 2 patients with a partial response (PR) (18%) in the first group and two PRs (13%) in the second. In a second series of 10 evaluable patients treated with 120 mg/kg of cyclophosphamide over 2 days, 2 patients achieved a PR for a response rate of 20% (36). The toxicity of the therapy was tolerable, with one treatment-related death in the 37 patients in the two series.

Collins et al. gave high-dose cyclophosphamide to 22 patients with refractory solid tumors or lymphoma, at 120 mg/kg over 2 days (37). Nineteen patients had received prior cyclophosphamide; among those with lymphoid malignancies and prior cyclophosphamide, 22% achieved a CR and 78% responded, but the median response duration was only 2 months.

Postmus et al. examined etoposide in a phase I study of 22 patients (28) and observed PR in 9 of 17 evaluable for response, including 1 of 4 breast, 3 of 7 small cell lung carcinoma, and 5 of 5 germ cell tumors. He and his group combined cyclophosphamide and etoposide, in doses of 7 gm/m^2 over 3 days for cyclophosphamide and 0.9–2.5 gm/

m^2 over 3 days (in six doses) for etoposide, in a trial that included autologous marrow infusion (38). Mucositis became evident at 1.5 gm/m^2 total etoposide dose (250 mg/m^2/ fraction) and was dose limiting at 2.5 gm/m^2. Eight of 11 patients with refractory small cell, ovarian cancer, or germ cell tumors had responses. Notably, two "older patients" in their fifties succumbed to a syndrome of "erythematous dermatitis, fever, and fluid retention, finally leading to multiple organ failure," at total etoposide doses of 1.5 gm/m^2 and 2.5 gm/m^2, respectively.

The three-drug combination of cyclophosphamide, etoposide, and cisplatin (CEP) was examined in a phase I study of repeated cycles, administered without bone marrow transplantation, by Neidhart et al. (39). Forty-two patients with advanced cancer were studied; slightly more than half received a second cycle, and 8 received three or more cycles of therapy. Doses and schedule for the maximum tolerated dose are shown in Table 12.3. Hematologic toxicity was not dose dependent. The dose-limiting toxicities were cardiac and/or pulmonary side effects, which proved fatal in 5 of 9 patients treated at the highest dose level. The overall response rate was 61%, including 9 of 11 lymphomas, 5 of 11 "lung cancer," and 1 of 3 breast cancers. The author pointed out that "the ability to repeat dose-intensive cycles of treatment may be critical to obtain durable responses. . . . The total dose delivered in the present study is two- to fourfold that given in most bone marrow transplant regimens."

DISEASE-ORIENTED INVESTIGATIONS

Ovary

Because of dramatic tumor responses in three patients with ovarian carcinoma from their initial study (34), Buckner et al. subsequently treated nine patients with ovarian carcinoma with multiple courses of high-dose cyclophosphamide (120 mg/kg), delivering a median number of six cycles (40). The overall response rate was 89%, with a 67% CR rate, without any toxic deaths. Median duration of response was 10 months (range, 2 to 40+ months). A later series comparing high-dose cyclophosphamide to standard oral melphalan (L-PAM) as initial therapy in ovarian cancer did not result in a significantly higher response rate or prolonged survival (41). A third series (42) exploring the use of high-dose cyclophosphamide as a single agent in refractory ovarian carcinoma only produced a PR in one of eight patients.

It should be noted that both of these last two series used lower doses of cyclophosphamide, total doses of 80 mg/kg and 70 mg/kg, respectively. Osborne et al. gave the highest dose of cyclophosphamide as a single agent, 7 gm/m^2 with mesna, for two cycles to 20 patients with previously untreated ovarian cancer (43). This was followed by five courses of standard-dose cisplatin at 100 mg/m^2. Eleven of 20 demonstrated an initial response to cyclophosphamide, with three pathologic CRs (15%). The

Table 12.3. CEP Programs (Cyclophosphamide, Etoposide, Cisplatin) in High-Dose Consolidation[a]

| Series | Ref. | Tumor Type(s) | No. Pts. | Dose and Schedule | | |
				C (gm/m^2)	E (mg/m^2)	P (mg/m^2)
Neidhart	39	Various	42	[b]2.5 × 2, d 1 + 2	[b]500 × 3, d 1 − 3	[b]50 × 3, d 1 − 3
Johnson	52	SCLC	20	1.85 × 2, d 1 + 2	400 × 3, d 1 − 3	40 × 3, d 1 − 3
Dunphy	83	Breast	58	[b]1.75 × 3, d 1 − 3	[b]200 × 6, d 1 − 3	[b]60 × 3, d 1 − 3
Collins	45	Breast, ovary	34	2.2 × 2, d 5 + 6	125 × 6, d 1 − 3	60 × 2, d 1 + 6

[a]Abbreviations: C, cyclophosphamide; E, etoposide; P, cisplatin.
[b]Maximum tolerated dose (MTD).

overall response rate to the sequential regimen was 14 of 20 (70%), with five pathologic CRs (25%), a result judged to be "no more effective than conventional treatment in advanced ovarian cancer." High-dose cyclophosphamide was associated with "cumulative, fatal" hematologic toxicity in two patients.

It is now recognized that etoposide is an active agent in alkylator-refractory patients with ovarian cancer (44). Given the present reliance on platinum-based regimens to induce remission, coupled with the suggestive evidence for a dose-response to cyclophosphamide, Collins et al. have initiated a trial of high-dose CE±P (cyclophosphamide + etoposide ± cisplatin) in patients with refractory ovarian cancer, using the same dose and schedule described elsewhere in this chapter under breast cancer (45).

Small Cell Lung Carcinoma

Three approaches to high-dose therapy have been taken: as induction, as intensification, or as salvage. Induction attempts will be reviewed first.

Souhami and associates treated 16 patients with small cell lung cancer (SCLC) with high-dose cyclophosphamide (160–200 mg/kg) with autologous marrow infusion and reported an overall response rate of 81% with a 44% CR rate (46). However, after consolidation with thoracic irradiation (4000 rad), the median survival time was 69 weeks, similar to results obtained with standard combination chemotherapy. In a second series of 18 patients, two courses of cyclophosphamide (200 mg/kg) with marrow infusion did not improve the response rate, decrease the incidence of local recurrence, or prolong the median duration of response as compared to a single cycle, and there were three septic deaths in this group (47). As calculated by computerized tomographic scans, the reduction in tumor volume was considerably less after the second course of high-dose cyclophosphamide compared to the first course.

A pilot study of single-agent etoposide

was carried out at Vanderbilt University in 16 patients with extensive disease, using a dose of 400 mg/m^2 day for 3 consecutive days: A 60% overall response rate was achieved, with a 30% CR and a median survival of 7.5 months (48, 49). Subsequently, however, Luikart et al. for the Cancer and Leukemia Group B reported on results of the same dose and schedule in 21 previously untreated patients with extensive disease (50). Only five PR were achieved (24%), and there was a treatment-related death rate of 28% due to myelosuppression and pneumonia. The discrepancy between these reports is not readily explained.

Johnson et al. from Vanderbilt (51) next constructed a two-drug regimen of high-dose cyclophosphamide (50 mg/kg/day × 2) plus high-dose etoposide (400 mg/m^2/day × 3). This "CE" was given once, followed by four cycles of standard CAV (cyclophosphamide, Adriamycin, and vincristine). After induction therapy 16 of 17 had responded, including five CR (29%). The median survival was 10 months, with two survivors beyond 2 years. Treatment-related mortality was seen in 6%. Building on this program, Johnson et al. (52) proceeded to CEP, in which cisplatin at 120 mg/m^2 was added to the CE regimen, with the other two drugs in the same dose and schedule as before (see Table 12.3). Twenty patients with extensive SCLC were treated, and 17 received two induction cycles of CEP, given at approximately 4-week intervals. Subsequently, four cycles of outpatient CAV were administered. The CR rate to initial CEP was 65%, with CR ultimately achieved in 83% of patients who went on to the CAV program. The average hospital stay was 23 days for each cycle, and delays were not required for the second course. However, only half the patients were able to complete all four subsequent cycles of CAV chemotherapy, and the others required dosage modification secondary to persistent leukopenia and/or prolonged thrombocytopenia. This observation suggests that the "nonablative" high-dose CEP combination is nonetheless associated with stem cell impairment. Two patients (10%) had early deaths related to neutropenic infection and subsequent adult respiratory disease syndrome (ARDS). Nonhematopoietic toxicity was mild to moderate mucositis, seen in 57% of courses. The median survival on this trial was 11 months, with 3 survivors beyond 18 months (15%).

Souhami et al. (53) reported on a small study in which carboplatin at 400–600 mg/m² was combined with etoposide (120 mg/m²/day × 4) and either high-dose cyclophosphamide (40 mg/kg/day × 4) or melphalan (140 mg/m²), followed by autologous marrow (such a program would probably be possible with cyclophosphamide, but not with melphalan, in the absence of stem cell infusion). Nine of nine responded, but there were no CRs to a single cycle; all had limited disease.

These conclusions appear tentatively justified regarding the use of high-dose induction programs in SCLC: (*a*) Overall and complete response rates are higher than expected with "standard" doses of the agents, used alone or in combination; (*b*) high-dose CEP is the most active regimen yet reported in terms of CR for patients with extensive disease (see Table 12.4); (*c*) median survival is not strikingly superior, nor are long-term survival results very encouraging, compared to other programs of induction therapy that do not require hospitalization.

A second approach in this disease has been late intensification with high-dose che-motherapy when the disease has been cytoreduced by induction, following a rationale similar to that for marrow-ablative therapy applied to leukemia in remission. Smith et al. (54) administered four cycles of standard chemotherapy, followed by high-dose cyclophosphamide at 7 gm/m² over 12 hours by infusion, combined with mesna. A total of 27 patients were treated, the first 17 receiving autologous bone marrow infusion and the last 10 none: There was no difference in the time to marrow recovery. Transient cardiac arrhythmias were observed in four patients (15%), but no other cardiotoxicity from this dose (equivalent to 260 mg/kg), which suggests that peak blood level must be important in producing hemorrhagic carditis, and that the prolonged infusion prevented this. Unfortunately, no durable responses were seen; however, local failure was a major problem, and chest irradiation was not used.

Additional studies of a single cycle of high-dose cyclophosphamide as late intensification have now been reported by Souhami et al. (53), using 50 mg/kg/day × 4 with autologous marrow after two cycles of standard induction chemotherapy (doxorubicin, vincristine, and etoposide); by Banham et al., using 160–240 mg/kg plus autologous marrow after induction (55); and by Goodman et al. for the Southwest Oncology Group, using 50 mg/kg/day × 3 (no marrow infusion) after a prolonged period of induction chemoradiotherapy and consolidation chemotherapy at standard dose (56). The results are sum-

Table 12.4. Complete Response (CR) and Survival in Extensive Small Cell Lung Cancer—"Standard" Versus High-Dose Therapy for Induction[a]

Series	Reference	Type Treatment	Number Patients	Regimen	CR %	MST (Mo.)	2-Year Survival
Evans	87	"Standard"	145	CAV/PE	39	10	<10
Ettinger	88	"Standard"	283	CAV/HEM	23	10.5	10
Jackson	89	"Standard"	70	CAVE	29	10	16
Johnson	51	High-dose	17	CE→CAV	29	10	12
Johnson	52	High-dose	20	CEP→CAV	65[b]	11	15

[a]Abbreviations: MST, median survival time; PE, *cis*-platinum, etoposide; HEM, hexamethylmelamine, etoposide, methotrexate; CAVE, cyclophosphamide, Adriamycin, vincristine, etoposide.
[b]To initial CEP × 2.

marized in Table 12.5. Essentially, none of these programs exploring a single cycle of high-dose cyclophosphamide produced results suggesting an improvement in overall therapeutic outcome compared to standard therapy. Only the study by Goodman et al. employed local chest irradiation. That trial was also confined to patients with limited disease and, like Souhami's, avoided prior exposure to alkylator therapy in the induction phase.

High-dose cyclophosphamide plus etoposide has been employed as late intensification in two trials for SCLC. Sculier et al. (57) conducted a pilot study in 15 patients, 11 with limited disease. After three courses of standard induction therapy that involved lower doses of cyclophosphamide and etoposide, patients received cyclophosphamide at 50 mg/kg every 12 hours for four doses, combined with etoposide at doses of 250 to 875 mg/m^2, also every 12 hours for four doses. Bone marrow infusion was employed for the higher doses of etoposide. Five of 10 PR patients were converted to CR, but median response duration was only 8 months and median survival, 11 months. Cardiac toxicity was observed in seven instances, with one death from "irreversible cardiac failure" at the highest etoposide dose: The high incidence of cardiac complications may be related to coadministration of cyclophosphamide and an etoposide dose equal to or exceeding 500 mg/m^2 (58). Cunningham et al. studied 22 patients, 16 with limited disease (59). After three cycles of cyclophosphamide-containing standard induction chemotherapy, patients received 45 mg/kg every 5 hours for four doses of cyclophosphamide (total dose, 180 mg/kg). Etoposide was given in five divided doses, the last four as a 4-hour infusion after each infusion of cyclophosphamide, to a total dose of 1000 mg/m^2. Radiotherapy to the primary tumor site was variably employed after high-dose consolidation in the limited stage patients. Two of 11 PR converted to CR, and there were no treatment-related deaths. However, the median survival was only 11 months (12 for limited, 10 for extensive), and 19 of 22 had relapsed.

Taken at face value, the CE high-dose consolidation programs appear disappointing. However, it bears mention that the trial by Sculier et al. involved a phase I design, was associated with cardiac toxicity, had associated infusion of autologous (potentially contaminated) marrow, and did not include any form of local treatment. The study by Cunningham involved exposure to etoposide only over a 24-hour period. It is now clear that etoposide is a schedule-dependent drug in SCLC, with superior efficacy for a total dose of 500 mg/m^2 administered over five consecutive daily fractions, as opposed to a single infusion of the same dose over 24 hours (60). The optimal schedule of administration for this agent in the setting of high-dose chemotherapy is not clear, but it seems likely that longer duration may be more important than higher dose. Indeed, in patients with chemorefractory SCLC treated on a randomized basis with etoposide at 300, 600, or 900 mg/m^2 over 3 days by Wolff et al. (61), there was

Table 12.5. High-Dose Cyclophosphamide as Consolidation for Small Cell Lung Carcinoma[a]

Series	Ref.	No. Pts.	Stage: Lim/Ext	PR → CR Proportion	MST (Mo.) Lim/Ext	Mortality %
Smith	54	27	16/11	4/10	—	4
Banham	55	23	—	16/20[b]	12.5/8	5
Souhami	53	15	14/1	4/8	10/0	13
Goodman	56	58	58/0	5/27	11/0	19
Total		**123**			**10–12.5[c]**	

[a]Abbreviations: Lim, limited stage; Ext, extensive stage.
[b]"Further tumor regression."
[c]Limited.

no evidence of a dose-response effect, except for hematologic toxicity: Only four responses were seen in a study of 77 patients with 26, 27, and 26 entered at each respective dose level.

Japanese investigators recently reported on high-dose etoposide combined with cisplatin to treat relapsed SCLC (62). Each of 20 patients received etoposide at 500 mg/m^2/day, as an intravenous infusion over 24 hours, for 3 consecutive days, coupled with cisplatin at 80 mg/m^2 on day 1. No bone marrow was infused, although 5 patients received G-CSF. An encouraging response rate of 50% (9 of 18 evaluable) was observed, with one CR. This result is particularly impressive since 12 patients had previously received etoposide in conventional doses, of whom five had PR. Median response duration was 8 weeks and median survival 20 weeks. Reported response rates for "standard" doses of cisplatin and etoposide in the salvage setting range from 12% to 55% (63–65). However, the 55% response rate was for a patient population without prior exposure to either agent.

In summary, high-dose consolidation without marrow support produced disappointing results for cyclophosphamide as a single agent in SCLC. High-dose consolidation with CE was interpreted as unpromising, but results may have been compromised by the schedule of etoposide and the lack of local therapy. CEP has not been investigated in the setting of consolidation. These results may all be viewed in the context of the trial reported by Humblet et al. (66), a randomized study in which CE was combined with BCNU (1,3-*bis*-(2-chloroethyl)-1-nitrosourea) as remission intensification and a "standard" dose of this consolidation regimen was compared to one involving autologous marrow support. Doses for the latter were 6 gm/m^2 for cyclophosphamide (over 4 days), 300 mg/m^2 for BCNU, and 500 mg/m^2 for etoposide (125 mg/m^2/day × 4). In the high-dose intensified group, the CR rate increased from 39% to 79%, and relapse-free survival was statistically superior postrandomization for this group (28

versus 10 weeks, $p = .003$). However, most patients relapsed at the primary site (no local therapy was given), and 4 of 23 among the intensified patients had deaths while aplastic (17%). The median survival of 16 limited disease patients who received high-dose, late intensification was 19 months, a result comparable to the best reported with standard, concurrent combined modality therapy (67).

Breast Cancer

As in SCLC, high-dose therapy has been used in both the induction and intensification modes for the treatment of stage IV breast cancer. Such studies have been generally aimed at patients with estrogen- and progesterone-receptor (ER and PR) negative disease, or whose disease was ER/PR-positive but no longer responded to hormone manipulation (hormone refractory), who have an especially poor prognosis. This is also true for ER/PR-positive patients with liver or lymphangitic lung involvement. Although their chance of responding to initial chemotherapy is greater than 50%, the median survival is between 12 and 18 months, and disease-free survival beyond 2 years is rare (<5%) with standard therapy, utilizing outpatient drug regimens.

Both retrospective analysis (68) and a prospective, randomized trial (69) indicate the importance of dose intensity (mg/m^2/wk) in the initial chemotherapy of metastatic breast cancer, and active investigation of this concept is ongoing in a number of treatment centers with programs that are suitable for outpatient use. However, an attempt to deliver a "high-dose" regimen of FAC (5-fluorouracil, Adriamycin, cyclophosphamide) as induction therapy in a manner sufficiently intensive to require hospitalization for supportive care proved no more efficacious than "standard" FAC in a randomized trial, but with significantly more frequent and severe complications (70). Jones et al., in a study of single-agent Adriamycin which pushed that agent to the limits of toxicity, demonstrated a high overall and complete response rate, but the median time to progression and survival were similar to other experience (71). Peters et al. employed a single course of induction therapy with doses of cyclophosphamide, cisplatin, and BCNU (CPB) so intensive that autologous bone marrow infusion was required to prevent lethal myelosuppression; in a selected group of premenopausal, ER-negative patients, 54% achieved CR, and 3 of 22 (14%) remain on a plateau of disease-free survival (72; unpublished data presented at National Cancer Institute strategy meeting, Rockville, MD, October 1990). The treatment-related death rate, however, exceeded 20%, and the median time to progression was only 5 months.

A more promising approach appears to be the use of very high doses of drugs in "consolidation" after a remission has been induced with outpatient chemotherapy. (See Tables 12.6 and 12.7). Single alkylating agents have been attempted (cyclophosphamide after 5-fluorouracil [5-FU], vincristine, and Adriamycin [73]; melphalan plus autologous bone marrow transplantation [ABMT] after varied induction [74]), with disappointing results. However, the combination of cyclophosphamide and a single dose of total body irradiation and ABMT resulted in 1 of 7 long-term CRs (now in excess of 5 years) (75, 76). With a two-drug combination of cyclophosphamide and thiotepa plus ABMT after LOMAC (leucovorin, Oncovin [vincristine], methotrexate, Adriamycin, cyclophosphamide) in-

duction, Williams et al. reported an apparent "plateau" of 14% remaining disease-free beyond 2 years (77, 78). The Johns Hopkins groups has also used cyclophosphamide and thiotepa with ABMT as consolidation, after a 16-week program of dose-intensive induction, with a similar early plateau of 17% (79). Jones et al. have used their combination of CPB in more than 40 patients with poor prognosis (but excluding those with pelvic bone metastases) who had received induction with AFM (Adriamycin, 5-FU, and methotrexate) for two to four cycles; the median time to progression is 19 months, with a plateau of 20% to 25% disease-free beyond 2 years (80; RB Jones, EJ Shpall, M Ross, et al., personal communication, 1990). Antman et al. also utilized four cycles of AFM induction in a prospectively studied poor-risk patient population, but consolidation was with the 4-day "STAMP V" program of cyclophosphamide, thiotepa, and carboplatin plus ABMT; among 29 patients entered, seven (24%) remain disease-free, but with follow-up in most still between 2 and 4 years (81). The fatal toxicity of these transplant programs is variable: 4% to 18% for cyclophosphamide plus thiotepa (77, 79); 18% for CPB in Jones's experience (80), and 3% for STAMP V, as reported by Antman (81). All are associated with the potential for long-term disease-free survival in a small proportion of patients. This potential was not realized when such programs were attempted in the "salvage" setting, after disease progression on standard chemotherapy, although objective

Table 12.6. High-Dose Consolidation (HDC) for Stage IV Breast Cancer in Remission—Programs Involving Autologous Bone Marrow Transplant[a]

Series	Ref.	Year	No. Pts.	HDC Regimen and Frequency	Deaths from HDC	Median Time to Failure (Mo.)	Long-Term DFS
Livingston	75	1987	7	CTX + TBI × 1	0	7	1/7 (5+ yr)
Vincent	74	1988	15	L-PAM × 1	3(20%)	7	1/15 (18+ mo)
Williams	77	1989	22	CTX + TT × 1 after LOMAC	4(14%)	6	4/22 (14%) at 13 +−22+ mo.
Peters	72	1990	39	CTX + DDP + BCNU × 1 after AFM	"13%"	—	9/39 (22%) at 24+ mo.

[a]Abbreviations: DFS, disease-free survival; TBI, total body irradiation; TT, thiotepa; DDP, cisplatin.

Table 12.7. High-Dose Consolidation for Stage IV Breast Cancer in Remission—Programs Not Requiring ABMT[a]

Series	Ref.	Date	No. Pts.	HDC Regimen and Frequency	Deaths from HDC	Median Time to Failure (Mo.)	MST (Mo.)	Long-Term DFS
Ellis	73	1989	26	CTX × 1	0	5	15	None
Dunphy	83	1990	58	CEP × 2	5 (9%)	13	25	25%[b]
Collins	45	1990	15	CEP × 2	1 (7%)	TE	TE	TE

[a]Abbreviations: TE, too early.
[b]At 24 months.

remissions of short duration were often obtained (82). Therefore, it appears that the use of such an approach is most likely to succeed when the patient's cancer is in remission (PR or CR) already; however, to date, the achievement of intitial CR has not been a prerequisite to long-term survival (W Peters, K Antman, personal communication).

Is it essential to perform ABMT (or provide an alternative source of "harvested" stem cells) to deliver high-dose consolidation that is effective? This question was addressed at the M.D. Anderson Hospital by Dunphy, Spitzer, et al., using two cycles of the three-drug combination of CEP after FAC-type induction in 58 poor-prognosis patients. Three dose levels of CEP were used, with incremental increase in each drug from level 1 to level 3. Marrow was harvested in all patients, but they were randomized to receive or not to receive ABMT immediately after completion of CEP. In patients randomized to the no-marrow arm, "salvage" ABMT was given if the patient had not recovered to 500 neutrophils/mm^3 by day 28 or 50,000 platelets/mm^3 by day 35 after day 1 of each chemotherapy cycle (about 3 and 4 weeks, respectively, from the completion of chemotherapy). Using these criteria, 6 of 26 (23%) of the "no marrow" group required ABMT. Although blood count recovery was significantly faster in the group randomized to ABMT initially, no difference was observed in treatment-related morbidity or mortality. Overall, the long-term disease-free survival from high-dose CEP × 2 is approximately 25% (83, 84). Interestingly, preliminary analysis of relapse indicates a higher rate of failure among those CR patients who received initial ABMT than among those who did not (77% versus 41%), suggesting the possibility that tumor cells with metastatic potential may have been infused in some patients (12). Observations by Vaughan et al. of the Nebraska group that cancer cells from some patients with primary breast cancer can be grown in vitro from washing of the wire mesh used to sieve the marrow at the time of elective harvest, and that such patients are more likely to relapse early (11), would support this possibility.

Collins et al. at the University of Washington have now employed high-dose CEP at the same dose intensity as the M.D. Anderson "level 1" in 34 patients; 19 with persistent or relapsed ovarian cancer after initial, platinum-based chemotherapy; and 15 with ER-negative or hormone-refractory stage IV breast cancer, in remission after Adriamycin-based induction treatment (45). Bone marrow was not harvested or infused. As shown in Table 12.8, there is no evidence of cumulative myelosuppression, and both the duration of grade 4 count depression and the incidence of sepsis compare favorably to the M.D. Anderson experience. No patient has had delayed marrow recovery to the degree specified as an indication for "salvage" ABMT (q.v.). The four deaths (12%) were all related to the period of profound, universal neutropenia within 2 weeks after completion of drug treatment, which is observed with or without ABMT. The mortality rate in breast cancer is 7%, comparable to the 9% observed at M.D. Anderson. It is too early to comment on treatment efficacy of this program, but "level 1" CEP was associated with long-term disease-free sur-

Table 12.8.   Hematologic Toxicity of CEP × 2: A Comparison of Three Programs[a]

Series	Ref.	Number Patients		Days <500 ANC Median (range)		Days to ≥20,000 Platelets: Median (range)		Sepsis (%)	
		Cycle 1	Cycle 2	Cycle 1	Cycle 2	Cycle 1	Cycle 2	Cycle 1	Cycle 2
MDAH[b]	83	58	48	23(15–34)	23(17–56)	18(13–28)	24(14–65)	35	44
UWMC[c]	45	27	13	16(6–23)	15(11–19)	21(14–32)	19(15–28)	26	23
Vanderbilt	52	20	17	10[d]	10[d]	15	15	24[e]	

[a]Abbreviations: ANC, Absolute neutrophil count.
[b]Levels 1, 2, 3.
[c]Level 1.
[d]WBC < 1000/mm³.
[e]Combined.

vival in 6 of 15 patients reported by Dunphy. Collins has not observed any cardiac or non-infectious pulmonary toxicity of the type reported by Neidhart and believes the explanation may be related to the difference in peak levels of etoposide, associated with glutathione depletion (58).

Although CEP for two cycles can be safely given at level 1 without the need for ABMT, the use of granulocyte-macrophage colony-stimulating factor (GM-CSF) may improve its therapeutic index. Neidhart recently reported the use of GM-CSF at 500–750 $\mu g/m^2$, divided into two doses subcutaneously each day, after a CEP regimen of slightly greater intensity than level 1. The duration of profound neutropenia was shortened, and the incidence of febrile neutropenia requiring antibiotics was reduced to about 50% (virtually 100% of patients required them previously) (85). Although concern has been expressed in the past about the possibility that tumor cells may have functional receptors for GM-CSF, a recent study indicates that at least for human solid tumors in cell culture, no such effect could be demonstrated (86).

In summary, there is suggestive evidence from multiple phase II trials that high-dose, multiple-drug chemotherapy consolidation, performed in poor-prognosis breast cancer patients in remission, can improve the disease-free survival at 2 years from the 5% expected on standard therapy (75) to the range of 20%. However, under the best of circumstances, 5% to 10% of patients may be ex-

pected to die sooner than they otherwise would have, related to the acute myelosuppressive toxicity of these programs. Furthermore, patient selection may be argued to have favorably influenced the results; the effect of high-dose consolidation on an "unselected" denominator of such patients is unknown. It is likewise unclear whether programs that employ agents like thiotepa, carboplatin, and BCNU, which are "obligate stem cell toxins" in high doses and therefore mandate a source of exogenous stem cell support to allow for bone marrow recovery, are superior to regimens like CEP, which do not require such support, even when given twice. It does appear that GM-CSF may speed recovery from neutropenia in either setting. Based on these considerations, an intergroup trial has been initiated to test "standard" chemotherapy as it is currently practiced in the community versus either of two approaches with high dose consolidation: CEP × 2 (no ABMT) or STAMP V + ABMT.

SUMMARY AND CONCLUSIONS

High-dose therapy without stem cell support is feasible, provided that the agents chosen are appropriate. Cyclophosphamide, etoposide, and cisplatin are the best-studied representatives of such agents, and the combination of all three (CEP, CVP) is currently the most promising "non-ablative" regimen. For SCLC, it can produce CR in greater than 50% of patients as an induction program.

However, most of these remissions are not durable, and the role of high-dose therapy in that disease remains undefined. In breast cancer, stage IV with poor prognosis (hormone receptor negative or hormone refractory), CEP as late intensification for patients in remission has been reported to yield long-term disease-free survival in 25% with mortality of 9% related to the treatment, a result that is comparable to those reported for "obligate stem cell" programs. Theoretical advantages of programs that can be administered without stem cell support include a lower risk of contamination by infused, potentially clonogenic tumor cells; greater tolerance for subsequently administered radiation or chemotherapy; and a lesser chance of long-term hematopoietic damage, of the type that may eventuate in chronic dysplasia or leukemia. Since "nonablative" programs are still substantially myelotoxic, supportive care including the use of hematopoietic growth factors is an appropriate avenue of clinical research for them, as well as for those that rely on stem cell support. Future considerations include (a) prospective, randomized comparison to "standard" (non-high-dose) therapy and to "obligate stem cell" combinations (e.g., in consolidation therapy for breast cancer), and (b) investigation of these programs in a "non-cross-resistant" sequence with treatments that involve the infusion of host-derived hematopoietic stem cells.

REFERENCES

1. Stahel RA, Mabry M, Skarin AT, et al. Detection of bone marrow metastasis in small-cell lung cancer by monoclonal antibody. J Clin Oncol 1985;3:455–461.
2. Cheung N-KV, Von Hoff DD, Strandjord SE, et al. Detection of neuroblastoma cells in bone marrow using G_{D2} specific monoclonal antibodies. J Clin Oncol 1986;4:363–369.
3. Redding WH, Coombes RC, Monaghan P, et al. Detection of micrometastases in patients with primary breast cancer. Lancet 1983;2:1271–1274.
4. Cote RJ, Rosen PP, Hakes TB, et al. Monoclonal antibodies detect occult breast carcinoma metastases in the bone marrow of patients with early stage disease. Am J Surg Pathol 1988;12:333–340.
5. Ellis G, Ferguson M, Yamanaka E, et al. Monoclonal antibodies for detection of occult carcinoma cells in bone marrow of breast cancer patients. Cancer 1989;63:2509–2514.
6. Porro G, Menard S, Tagliabue E, et al. Monoclonal antibody detection of carcinoma cells in bone marrow biopsy specimens from breast cancer patients. Cancer 1988;61:2407–2411.
7. Coombes RC, Berger U, Mansi J, et al. Prognostic significance of micrometastases in bone marrow in patients with primary breast cancer. NCI Monogr 1986;1:51–53.
8. Mansi JL, Powles TJ, Coombes RC. The detection and evaluation of bone marrow micrometastases in primary breast cancer. In: Paterson AHG, Leis AW, eds. Fundamental problems in breast cancer. Boston: Martinus Nijhoff, 1987;299–301.
9. Salvadori B, Squicciarini P, Rovini D, et al. Use of monoclonal antibody MBr1 to detect micrometastases in bone marrow specimens of breast cancer patients. Eur J Cancer 1990;26:865–867.
10. Moss TJ, Reynolds CP, Sather HN, et al. Prognostic value of immunocytologic detection of bone marrow metastases in neuroblastoma. N Engl J Med 1991;324:219–216.
11. Vaughn WP, Mann SL, Garvey J, et al. Breast cancer detected in cell culture of histologically negative bone marrow predicts systemic relapse in patients with stage I, II, III and locally recurrent disease [Abstract]. Proc Am Soc Clin Oncol 1990;9:9.
12. Huan S, Dunphy F, Yau J, et al. Comparison of relapse patterns following high dose chemotherapy with or without autologous bone marrow infusion in breast cancer patients [Abstract]. Proc. Am Assoc Cancer Res 1990;31:185.
13. Gee AP, Boyle MD. Purging tumor cells from bone marrow by use of antibody and complement: a critical appraisal. J Natl Cancer Inst 1988;80:154–159.
14. Shpall EJ, Jones RB, Bast RC, et al. 4-Hydroperoxy-cyclophosphamide purging of breast cancer from the mononuclear cell fraction of bone marrow in patients receiving high-dose chemotherapy and autologous marrow support: a phase I trial. J Clin Oncol 1991;9:85–93.
15. Anderson IC, Shpall EJ, Leslie DS, et al. Elimination of malignant clonogenic breast cancer cells from human bone marrow. Cancer Res 1989;49:4659–4664.
16. Bjorn MJ, Manger R, Sivam G, et al. Selective elimination of breast cancer cells from human bone marrow using an antibody-Pseudomonas exotoxin A conjugate. Cancer Res 1990;50:5992–5996.
17. Tondini C, Pap SA, Hayes DF, et al. Evaluation of monoclonal antibody DF3 conjugated with ricin as a specific immunotoxin for in vitro purging of bone marrow. Cancer Res 1990;50:1170–1175.
18. Witherspoon RP, Fisher LD, Schoch G, et al. Secondary cancers after bone marrow transplantation for leukemia or aplastic anemia. N Engl J Med 1989;321:784–789.

19. Greene MH, Harris EL Gershenson DM, et al. Melphalan may be a more potent leukemogen than cyclophosphamide. Ann Intern Med 1986;105:360–367.
20. Boice JD, Greene MH, Killen JY, et al. Leukemia and preleukemia after adjuvant treatment of gastrointestinal cancer with semustine (methyl-CCNU). N Engl J Med 1983;309:1079–1084.
21. Appelbaum FR, Strauchen JA, Graw RG, et al. Acute lethal carditis caused by high-dose combination chemotherapy: a unique clinical and pathological entity. Lancet 1976;1:58–62.
22. Sahovic EA, Colvin M, Hilton J, et al. Role for aldehyde dehydrogenase in survival of progenitors for murine blast cell colonies after treatment with 4-hydroperoxycyclophosphamide in vitro. Cancer Res 1988;48:1223–1226.
23. Gandara DR, Perez EA, Phillips WA, et al. Evaluation of cisplatin dose intensity: current status and future prospects. Anticancer Res 1989;9:1121–1128.
24. Mortimer JE, Schulman S, MacDonald JS, et al. High-dose cisplatin in disseminated melanoma: a comparison of two schedules. Cancer Chemother Pharmacol 1990;25:373–376.
25. Lokich JJ, Drum DE, Kaplan W. Hepatic toxicity of nitrosourea analogues. Clin Pharmacol Ther 1974; 16:363–367.
26. Micetich KC, Erickson LC, Fisher RI. A phase I trial of streptozotocin followed by BCNU [Abstract]. Proc Am Assoc Cancer Res 1989;30:275.
27. Wolff SN, Fer MF, McKay C, et al. High dose VP 16-213 and autologous bone marrow transplantation for refractory malignancies—a phase I study. J Clin Oncol 1983;1:701–705.
28. Postmus PE, Mulder NH, Sleijfer DT, et al. High-dose etoposide for refractory malingnancies: a phase I study. Cancer Treat Rep 1984;68:1471–1474.
29. Littlewood TJ, Bentley DP, McQueen INF. High dose etoposide does not cause peripheral neuropathy. Cancer Chemother Pharmacol 1987;19:180–181.
30. Leff RS,Thompson JM, Daly MB, et al. Acute neurologic dysfunction after high-dose etoposide therapy for malignant glioma. Cancer 1988;62:32–35.
31. Bronchud MH, Howell A, Crowther D, et al. The use of granulocyte-stimulating factor to increase the intensity of treatment with doxorubicin in patients with advanced breast and ovarian cancer. Br J Cancer 1989;60:121–125.
32. Jones RB, Holland JF, Bhardwaj S, et al. A phase I–II study of intensive-dose adriamycin for advanced breast cancer. J Clin Oncol 1987;5:172–177.
33. Finklestein JZ, Hittle RE, Hammond GD. Evaluation of a high dose cyclophosphamide regimen in childhood tumors. Cancer 1969;23:1239–1242.
34. Buckner CD, Rudolph RH, Fefer A, et al. High-dose cyclophosphamide therapy for malignant disease. Cancer 1972;29:357–365.
35. Mullins GM, Colvin M. Intensive cyclophosphamide (NSC-26271) therapy for solid tumors. Cancer Chemother Rep 1975;59:411–419.
36. Mullins GM, Anderson PN, Santos GW. High dose cyclophosphamide therapy in solid tumors. Cancer 1975;59:411–419.
37. Collins C, Mortimer J, Livingston RB. High-dose cyclophosphamide in the treatment of refractory lymphomas and solid tumor malignancies. Cancer 1989;63:228–232.
38. Postmus PE, De Vries EGE, De Vries-Hospers HG, et al. Cyclophosphamide and VP-16-213 with autologous bone marrow transplantation. A dose escalation study. Eur J Cancer Clin Oncol 1984;20:777–782.
39. Neidhart JA, Kohler W, Stidley C, et al. Phase I study of repeated cycles of high-dose cyclophosphamide, etoposide, and cisplatin administered without bone marrow transplantation. J Clin Oncol 1990;8:1728–1738.
40. Buckner CD, Briggs R, Clift RA, et al. Intermittent high-dose cyclophosphamide (NSC-26371) treatment of stage III ovarian carcinoma. Cancer Chemother Rep 1974;58:697–703.
41. Young RC, Canellos GP, Chabner BA, et al. Chemotherapy of advanced ovarian carcinoma: a prospective randomized comparison of phenylalanine mustard and high dose cyclophosphamide. Gynecol Oncol 1974;2:489–497.
42. Piver MS, Barlow JJ, Chung WS. High-dose cyclophosphamide (NSC-26271) for recurrent or progressive ovarian adenocarcinoma. Cancer Chemother Rep 1975;59:1157–1158.
43. Osborne R, Evans B, Gallagher C, et al. High-dose cyclophosphamide followed by cisplatinum in the treatment of ovarian cancer. Cancer Chemother Pharmacol 1987;20:48–52.
44. Kuhnle H, Meerpohl HG, Lenaz L, et al. Etoposide in cisplatin-refractory ovarian cancer [Abstract]. Proc Am Soc Clin Oncol 1988;7:137.
45. Collins C, Cain J, Livingston R. High dose cyclophosphamide, VP-16 and cisplatin (CEP) does not require bone marrow infusion. Proc Am Soc Clin Oncol 1991; in press.
46. Souhami RL, Harper PG, Linch DC, et al. High dose cyclophosphamide with autologous bone marrow transplantation as initial treatment of small cell carcinoma of the bronchus. Cancer Chemother Pharmacol 1982;8:31–35.
47. Souhami RL, Finn G, Gregory WM, et al. High-dose cyclophosphamide in small-cell carcinoma of the lung. J Clin Oncol 1985;3:958–963.
48. Wolff SN. High-dose etoposide as a single-agent chemotherapy for small cell carcinoma of the lung. Cancer Treat Rep 1983;67:957–958.
49. Greco A. Personal communication.
50. Luikart SD, Propert KJ, Modeas CR, et al. High-dose etoposide therapy for extensive small cell lung cancer: a Cancer and Leukemia Group B study. Cancer Treat Rep 1987;71:533–534.

51. Johnson DH, Wolff SN, Hainsworth JD, et al. Extensive-stage small-cell bronchogenic carcinoma: intensive induction chemotherapy with high-dose cyclophosphamide plus high-dose etoposide. J Clin Oncol 1985;3:170–175.
52. Johnson DH, DeLeo MJ, Hande KR, et al. High-dose induction chemotherapy with cyclophosphamide, etoposide, and cisplatin for extensive-stage small-cell lung cancer. J Clin Oncol 1987;5:703–709.
53. Souhami RL, Hajichristou HT, Miles DW, et al. Intensive chemotherapy with autologous bone marrow transplantation for small-cell lung cancer. Cancer Chemother Pharmacol 1989;24:321–325.
54. Smith IE, Evans BD, Harland SJ, et al. High-dose cyclophosphamide with autologous bone marrow rescue after conventional chemotherapy in treatment of small cell lung carcinoma. Cancer Chemother Pharmacol 1985;14:120–124.
55. Banham S, Cunningham D, Hutcheon A, et al. High dose chemotherapy as late dose-intensification in small cell lung cancer [Abstract]. In: Proceedings of the Fourth World Conference on Lung Cancer, Northbrook, IL: American College of Chest Physicians, 1985:124.
56. Goodman GE,Crowley JC, Livingston RB, et al. Treatment of limited small cell lung cancer with concurrent VP-16/cisplatin radiotherapy followed by intensification with high-dose cyclophosphamide. A Southwest Oncology Group study. J Clin Oncol 1991;9:453–457.
57. Sculier JP, Klastersky J, Stryckmans P, et al. Late intensification in small-cell lung cancer: a phase I study of high doses of cyclophosphamide and etoposide with autologous bone marrow transplantation. J Clin Oncol 1985;3:184–191.
58. Livingston R, Collins C. Cardiopulmonary toxicity from high dose cyclophosphamide etoposide and cisplatin is related to dose of etoposide. Proc Am Soc Clin Oncol 1991;10:104.
59. Cunningham D, Banham SW, Hutcheon AH, et al. High-dose cyclophosphamide and VP-16 as late dosage intensification therapy for small cell carcinoma of the lung. Cancer Chemother Pharmacol 1985;15:303–306.
60. Slevin ML, Clark PI, Joel SP, et al. A randomized trial to evaluate the effect of schedule on the activity of etoposide in small-cell lung cancer. J Clin Oncol 1989;7:1333–1340.
61. Wolff SN, Birch R, Pudipeddi S, et al. Randomized dose-response evaluation of etoposide in small cell carcinoma of the lung: a Southeastern Cancer Study Group trial. Cancer Treat Rep 1986;70:583–587.
62. Masuda N, Fukuoka M, Matsui K, et al. Evaluation of high-dose etoposide combined with cisplatin for treating relapsed small cell lung cancer. Cancer 1990;65:2635–2640.
63. Batist G, Carney DN, Cowan KH, et al. Etoposide (VP-
16) and cisplatin in previously treated small-cell lung cancer: clinical trial and in vitro correlates. J Clin Oncol 1986;4:982–986.
64. Lopez JA, Mann J, Grapski RT, et al. Etoposide and cisplatin salvage chemotherapy for small cell lung cancer. Cancer Treat Rep 1985;69:369–371.
65. Evans WK, Osoba D, Feld R, et al. Etoposide (VP-16) and cisplatin: an effective treatment for relapse in small-cell lung cancer. J Clin Oncol 1985;3:65–71.
66. Humblet Y, Symann M, Bosly A, et al. Late intensification chemotherapy with autologous bone marrow transplantation in selected small-cell carcinoma of the lung: a randomized study. J Clin Oncol 1987;5:1864–1873.
67. McCracken JD, Janaki LM, Crowley JJ, et al. Concurrent chemotherapy/radiotherapy for limited small cell lung carcinoma: a Southwest Oncology Group study. J Clin Oncol 1990;8:892–898.
68. Hryniuk W, Bush H. The importance of dose intensity in chemotherapy of metastatic breast cancer. J Clin Oncol 1984;2:1281–1288.
69. Tannock I, Boyd N, DeBoer G. A randomized trial of two dose levels of cyclophosphamide, methotrexate and fluorouracil chemotherapy for patients with metastatic breast cancer. J Clin Oncol 1988;6:1377–1387.
70. Hortobagyi GN, Bodey GP, Buzdar AU, et al. Evaluation of high-dose versus standard FAC chemotherapy for advanced breast cancer in protected environment units: a prospective randomized study. J Clin Oncol 1987;5:354–364.
71. Jones RB, Holland JF, Bhardwaj S, et al. A phase I-II study of intensive-dose Adriamycin for advanced breast cancer. J Clin Oncol 1987;5:172–177.
72. Peters WP, Shpall EJ, Jones RB, et al. High-dose combination alkylating agents with bone marrow support as initial treatment for metastatic breast cancer. J Clin Oncol 1988;6:1368–1376.
73. Ellis GK, Green S, Schulman S, et al. Combination chemotherapy and high-dose cyclophosphamide intensification for poor prognosis breast cancer. A Southwest Oncology Group study. Cancer 1989;64:2409–2415.
74. Vincent MD, Powles TJ, Coombes RC, et al. Late intensification with high-dose melphalan and autologous bone marrow support in breast cancer patients responding to conventional chemotherapy. Cancer Chemother Pharmacol 1988;21:255–260.
75. Livingston RB, Schulman S, Griffin BR, et al. Combination chemotherapy and systemic irradiation consolidation for poor prognosis breast cancer. Cancer 1987;59:1249–1254.
76. Livingston R. Unpublished data. November 1990.
77. Williams SF, Mick R, Desser R, et al. High-dose consolidation therapy with autologous stem cell rescue in stage IV breast cancer. J Clin Oncol 1989;7:1824–1830.

78. Bitran J. Data presented at NCI strategy meeting, Rockville, MD, October 1990.
79. Data presented at NCI strategy meeting, San Antonio, TX, November 1990.
80. Jones RB, Shpall EJ, Ross M, et al. AFM induction chemotherapy, followed by intensive alkylating agent consolidation with autologous bone marrow support (ABMS) for advanced breast cancer. Current results. Proc Am Soc Clin Oncol 1990;9:9.
81. Antman K. Data presented at NCI strategy meeting, Rockville, MD, October 1990.
82. Antman K, Gale RP. Advanced breast cancer: high-dose chemotherapy and bone marrow autotransplants. Ann Intern Med 1988;108:570–574.
83. Dunphy FR, Spitzer G, Buzdar AU, et al. Treatment of estrogen receptor-negative or hormonally refractory breast cancer with double high-dose chemotherapy intensification and bone marrow support. J Clin Oncol 1990;8:1207–1216.
84. Spitzer G. Data presented at NCI strategy meeting, Rockville, MD, October 1990.
85. Neidhart J. Data presented at San Antonio Breast Conference, Growth Factor Symposium, November 1990.
86. Foulke RS, Marshall MH, Trotta PP, et al. In vitro assessment of the effects of granulocyte-macrophage colony-stimulating factor on primary human tumors and derived lines. Cancer Res 1990;50:6264–6267.
87. Evans WK, Feld R, Murray N, et al. Superiority of alternating non-cross-resistant chemotherapy in extensive small cell lung cancer. A multicenter, randomized clinical trial by the National Cancer Institute of Canada. Ann Intern Med 1987;107:451–458.
88. Ettinger DS, Finkelstein DM, Abeloff MD, et al. A randomized comparison of standard chemotherapy versus alternating chemotherapy and maintenance versus no maintenance therapy for extensive-stage small-cell lung cancer: a phase III study of the Eastern Cooperative Oncology Group. J Clin Oncol 1990;8:230–240.
89. Jackson DV, Case LD, Zekan PJ, et al. Improvement of long-term survival in extensive small-cell lung cancer. J Clin Oncol 1988;6:1161–1169.

13

IMMUNOLOGIC RECONSTITUTION AFTER HIGH-DOSE CHEMORADIOTHERAPY AND ALLOGENEIC OR AUTOLOGOUS BONE MARROW OR PERIPHERAL BLOOD HEMATOPOIETIC STEM CELL TRANSPLANTATION

Robert P. Witherspoon

All patients receiving marrow-ablative chemotherapy or chemoradiotherapy followed by marrow support experience substantial risk of infection, anemia, or hemorrhage until engraftment and myeloid, erythroid, and platelet precursors evolve into mature blood cells to restore normal protective mechanisms. Myeloid engraftment takes place in 2–3 weeks. Lymphoid repopulation occurs more slowly. Even after lymphocytes have returned to normal levels, their function is impaired. As a result, recovery of humoral and cellular immunity may take 1 year or longer depending on whether the patient received an autologous or allogeneic graft and whether the recipient developed chronic graft-versus-host disease (GVHD). Presently, randomized studies show a clear benefit of addition of myeloid growth factors to treatment in the 1st 3 weeks after autologous transplantation to hasten the time to durable engraftment of myeloid cells. Factors that could speed recovery of lymphocytes are now in early stages of evaluation, and, if effective,

could lead to enhancement of humoral and cellular immunity to pathogens. The purpose of this review is to highlight the events of immunologic reconstitution in autologous and allogeneic marrow transplant recipients and underscore differences in recovery that have clinical implications.

THE CLINICAL PROBLEM

Bacterial, viral, and fungal infection in the 1st 3 months after allogeneic or autologous marrow transplantation is a major cause of morbidity and mortality (1–3). Bacterial infection results in mortality in as many as 10% of patients early after grafting (4). Interstitial pneumonitis from cytomegalovirus (CMV) infection, once a cause of death in nearly 30% of transplant recipients, can now be substantially prevented by administration of blood products from CMV-seronegative donors if the recipient is fortunate enough to not have been previously exposed to the virus and has a marrow donor who is seronegative (5). For patients who are CMV seropositive, the risk of CMV pneumonitis is still 20% in spite of the use of prophylactic administration of acyclovir (6). A current study in Seattle of ganciclovir administration to prevent CMV pneumonia in CMV-seropositive patients when they begin excreting CMV after transplant shows encouraging results and has the potential to reduce the incidence of CMV pneumonia to 12% (JM Goodrich, unpublished observations). Treatment of CMV interstitial pneumonia with ganciclovir and CMV immune globulin has reduced the mortality of this infection from 90% to 50% (7, 8). However, CMV pneumonia not responsive to therapy and fungal infection from *Aspergillus* species organisms continue to be a threat to transplant recipients early after grafting.

When patients become long-term survivors beyond 3 months from transplant, two-thirds of them are healthy and have few infections. However, one-third develop chronic GVHD, and these patients have a higher incidence of infection, mainly from bacterial organisms (9–11). Chronic GVHD is the main predictor of infection among recipients of HLA matched or mismatched family member marrow. For example, the Kaplan-Meier probability of developing the first pulmonary infection by 4 years after transplant is 0.50 among recipients of HLA-identical marrow with chronic GVHD. Recipients of marrow from HLA-nonidentical family members with chronic GVHD have a 0.51 probability of developing the first pulmonary infection. Patients without chronic GVHD with HLA-identical family member donors have a probability of developing a pulmonary infection of 0.21, whereas the probability for pulmonary infection among recipients with HLA-nonidentical family member donors is 0.18. These differences are not significant (Fig. 13.1). Recipients of unrelated donor marrow, however, have a high incidence of infection that is unaffected by chronic GVHD. The cumulative incidence of bacteremia or septicemia in recipients of unrelated phenotypically HLA-

identical marrow is 30%, a figure that is higher than the 12% in recipients of the HLA-identical sibling marrow ($p = .001$) (Fig. 13.2). These infections contribute heavily to the nonrelapse mortality in long-term survivors of marrow transplantation who have chronic GVHD and of those who receive grafts from unrelated donors (Fig. 13.3). Recipients of autologous marrow are equally troubled with infections in the 1st 3–4 months after transplant. The relapse rate after autologous transplantation is high, owing perhaps to the lack of chronic GVHD and associated graft-versus-malignancy effect. The high relapse rate after autologous transplantation is the target of immune therapies to reduce relapse and improve long-term survival.

CELLULAR REPOPULATION AFTER TRANSPLANTATION

Mature B lymphocytes bearing surface immunoglobulin achieve normal levels in peripheral blood by 3 months after grafting (12). Earlier precursors to mature B cells appear prior to this time. For example, CD19 B cells and B cells coexpressing CD19 and CD20 as well as CD19 and CD5 have been identified within the 1st 3 months (13, 14). The CD19–CD5 immature B cells may not be able to secrete immunoglobulin in normal quantitative or qualitative terms, as evidenced by poor correlation between numbers of CD5 B cells and serum immunoglobulin levels. During acute GVHD, CD5 B cells are reduced in the peripheral blood, although their role in the etiology of the GVH reaction is not known (14). With greater elapsed time after transplant, the immature B cells diminish and are replaced by B cells with normal adult surface phenotype. Ig subclass deficiencies for IgG2 and IgG4 are common in patients within the 1st 3–4 months of transplantation, when infection with bacterial organisms bearing polysaccharide antigens is common (15, 16). During the first several months after transplantation, disordered Ig synthesis is also manifested by transient appearance of mono-

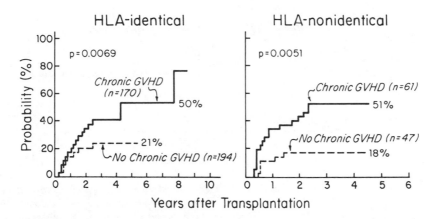

Figure 13.1. Probability of developing pulmonary infection among patients who survived more than 3 months after transplantation who were discharged from the transplant center. The left panel shows data for HLA-identical recipients, 170 of whom had chronic GVHD and 194 of whom did not have chronic GVHD. The right panel shows data from HLA-nonidentical recipients, 61 of whom had chronic GVHD and 47 of whom did not have chronic GVHD. (From Sullivan KM, Agura E, Anasetti C, et al. Chronic graft-versus-host disease and other late complications of bone marrow transplantation. Semin Hematol 1991;28:250–259.)

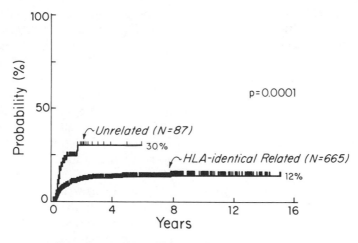

Figure 13.2. Cumulative incidence of bacteremia-septicemia among patients who survived more than 3 months after transplantation who were discharged from the transplant center. Data are shown from 87 recipients of HLA phentoypically identical unrelated marrow and from 665 recipients of HLA-identical related marrow.

clonal and oligoclonal gammopathy, which subsides with time. Syngeneic marrow graft recipients also develop these transient abnormalities, suggesting that the appearance of monoclonal Ig is associated with development of the immune system in a new host rather than an effect of major or minor histocompatibility differences between host and donor (17, 18).

T lymphocytes recover to normal levels, but subtypes of T cells, helper-inducer cells, and suppressor-cytotoxic cells are imbalanced initially with excessive numbers of suppressor T lymphocytes (19, 20). These suppressor T cells are capable of blocking in vitro Ig production following stimulation by pokeweed mitogen. The lower number of helper lymphocytes is associated with dimin-

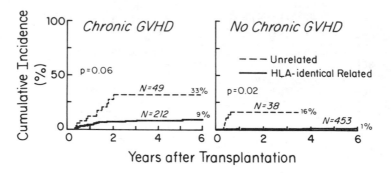

Figure 13.3.   Nonrelapse mortality in patients who survived 3 months and were discharged from the transplant center. The left panel shows data from patients with chronic GVHD, 49 of whom received HLA phenotypically identical unrelated marrow and 212 of whom received HLA-identical related marrow. The right panel shows data from patients without chronic GVHD, 38 of whom received HLA phenotypically identical unrelated marrow and 453 of whom received HLA-identical related marrow.

ished in vitro Ig production following pokeweed mitogen stimulation of peripheral blood B and T cells (20–23).

Natural killer (NK) cells and cells capable of mediating antibody-dependent and lectin-dependent cytotoxicity are normal by 30 days after transplantation (24, 25). Large granular lymphocytes appear to recover initially in elevated numbers and are responsible for lymphokine production in recipients who receive T-lymphocyte-depleted grafts (26, 27). Monocytes recover as early as 41 days after transplant and demonstrate normal in vitro accessory function for pokeweed-mitogen-induced Ig production, antigen presentation, and interleukin-1 (IL-1) production (28–30).

T cell repopulation of soybean lectin T-lymphocyte-depleted marrow graft recipients is similar to repopulation in conventional grafts and is complete by 5–6 months. No differences were detected in ratios of CD4 and CD8 T cells between the groups. In vitro responses of T cells to mitogens were similar in conventional and T-depleted grafts with follow-up beyond 1 year. Thus although mature T cells were removed from the infused marrow, the subsequent repopulation and function of T cells clinically was not impaired long term. The incidence of posttransplant infectious episodes in recipients of T-cell-de-

pleted and conventional marrow grafts with respect to culture-positive septicemia, localized infections, pneumonia from fungal or viral organisms, herpes zoster infection, or *Candida* mucositis was not statistically significant, supporting the similarity in the tempo of immune reconstitution between the groups (31). In vitro studies, however, point out some T cell dysfunctions in lymphocytes of T-depleted marrow grafts. T cell activation, intracellular calcium flux, and proliferation following CD6 depletion of marrow grafts were abnormal for 6 months after transplant (32). More sensitive methods of evaluating T cell repopulation reveal lower numbers of T cells by limiting dilution techniques, but the tritiated thymidine uptake and IL-2 production in response to phytohemagglutinin (PHA) stimulation and cytotoxic function of the T cells were the same as that of an equal number of normal T cells (33). Therefore, while sensitive methods of testing repopulation and function of T cells disclose some differences in quantitative transfer of T cell clones and their in vitro function from those of conventional grafts, these differences are apparently less important clinically for protection from infection.

Recipients of autologous grafts experience cellular repopulation remarkably similar to the repopulation seen in allogeneic marrow graft recipients (34). Functional studies of B lymphocyte proliferation and Ig secretion in vitro show no differences in the patterns of response to antigen and growth factors among autologous marrow or peripheral blood stem cell transplant recipients and allogeneic marrow graft recipients (35–38).

Autologous recipients of depleted marrow for lymphoma experience some differences in immune recovery from the immune recovery seen in allogeneic recipients. Patients transplanted for non-Hodgkin lymphoma with autologous B-lymphocyte-depleted marrow had normal engraftment of myeloid cells, but return to normal serum Ig levels and recovery of B cell proliferation in vitro to stimulation with anti-µ were impaired for more than a year. In vitro proliferation of T lymphocytes to mitogens and growth-factor-conditioned media was lower compared to that of lymphocytes from normal controls for more than a year. These in vitro and in vivo deficiencies were not associated with adverse clinical toxicities or infection (39). However, the same group has reported a high rate of posttransplant infection in 14 patients treated by T-cell-depleted autologous marrow transplantation for T cell non-Hodgkin lymphoma or T cell leukemia. Thirty-six percent of the patients developed bacteremia in the early posttransplant period. Additional infections were herpes zoster, hepatitis, and *Pneumocystis carinii.* Two of the patients developed Epstein-Barr virus-associated lymphoproliferative syndromes (40). While the pattern of T cell repopulation of lymphocyte subsets in the peripheral blood was similar to the patterns seen with B-cell-depleted marrow, the infectious complications were clearly different from those of patients given B-lymphocyte-depleted marrows for non-Hodgkin lymphoma. There were no apparent differences in the techniques of depletion other than the cell type targeted for elimination. The difference in immune deficiency reflected in the higher incidence of infection was probably related to immune suppression of T cell functions, although specific T cell functions were not formally tested in vitro or in vivo.

REGAINING FUNCTIONAL COMPETENCE IN VIVO AND IN VITRO

Serum Ig levels are low initially after transplant. By 1 year serum IgG and IgM have achieved normal levels. IgA is low often for 2 years even among autologous, syngeneic, or allogeneic recipients without GVHD, and rises to normal thereafter (41). Patients with chronic GVHD often have normal levels of serum IgG and normal Ig subclass levels by 1 year. Yet chronic GVHD patients experience higher incidence of infection. Therefore, the quality of the antibody produced may be abnormal and result from disturbed expression of the immunoglobulin gene repertoire, leading to ineffective regulation of Ig idiotype synthesis. Lack of T cell regulation of Ig synthesis has been shown by the synthesis of monoclonal Ig following grafting. These abnormalities subside in those patients who do not develop chronic GVHD.

Lower than normal serum antibody response to specific antigens bacteriophage ΦX174, keyhole limpet hemocyanin (KLH), and pneumococcal and meningococcal antigens has been shown for patients early after grafting and for long-term patients with chronic GVHD (42–44). Delayed-type hypersensitivity to the recall antigens *Candida,* mumps, *Trichophyton,* and the neoantigen dinitrochlorobenzene (DNCB) measured by skin testing, which provides an indication of in vivo cellular immunity, demonstrates that early patients and patients with chronic GVHD have diminished reactivity (45). These data indicate that recipients of allogeneic marrow grafts have combined humoral and cellular immune deficiencies most common in the early posttransplant period and in the long-term survivors with chronic GVHD. The deficiencies in humoral immunity involve both T-dependent and T-independent systems. Polysaccharide antigens are thought to be processed by T-independent mechanisms of the immune response, suggesting that the poor response to polysaccharide antigens in transplant recipients is the result of B lymphocyte deficiencies. Protein antigen, on the other hand, utilizes T-dependent mechanisms for antigen presentation and switching from IgM to IgG in the secondary response to antigen. Chronic GVHD patients demonstrate poor serum antibody responses to immunization with the T-dependent antigens bacteriophage ΦX174 and KLH as well. T cells from these patients also secrete low amounts of IL-2 in vitro after stimulation with PHA (46–49). Lymphocytes in vitro show failure of B cell function, failure of helper T cell function, or excessive T cell suppression in assays of pokeweed mitogen (PWM)-induced Ig production. Lymphocytes from patients with chronic GVHD may have any or a combination of these deficiencies, whereas healthy long-term survivors have fewer deficiencies (50).

Deficient in vivo cellular immunity may be responsible for the late infection from viral organisms, principally varicella infection. Any marrow transplant patient regardless of GVHD is at risk for disseminated or localized varicella infection for 2 or more years after transplant (51).

In summary, the principal predictors of immunologic recovery are time elapsed from transplant and the presence of chronic GVHD. Syngeneic and autologous recipients have clinical courses and immunologic recovery similar to that seen in allogeneic transplant recipients without GVHD. Treatment of autologous marrow may impair some immune function long-term principally due to type of antibody treatment and whether the antibody damages early precursors. Further studies are needed to understand the effect of autologous marrow treatment on immune recovery and the clinical implications with regard to protection from infection.

TRANSFER OF IMMUNITY FROM DONOR TO RECIPIENT

Following transplantation, the immunoglobulin synthesized becomes donor in type

(52). It is not surprising that recipients of marrow from donors sensitized to specific antigens would develop immunity to the specific antigen. The first example in humans was reported in the syngeneic setting and showed transfer of immunity to KLH from a sensitized twin to the previously nonimmunized recipient (53). Transfer of immune reactivity from the donor to the marrow graft recipient has been shown in most of 60 patients for tetanus, diphtheria, and measles antigens in the absence of postgrafting immunization within the 1st 3 months after grafting, as well as 1 year and later after transplantation (54, 55). These studies have been confirmed and extended in a report of 235 patients less than 100 days from grafting and 149 patients more than 6 months from transplant (56). In vitro cultures of recipient T lymphocytes (donor derived) showed transfer of antigen-specific helper activity when they were cultured with normal tetanus-immune B cells (57). Recipient (donor derived) B cells cultured with Epstein-Barr virus produced anti-tetanus toxoid antibody in culture supernatants (58). These data show that donor immunity was adoptively transferred from HLA-identical donors to recipients via the marrow inoculum and persisted in the recipients for years in the absence of recent immunization of donor or recipient before or after grafting (59). Transfer of immunity to tetanus and diphtheria antigens also occurs in spite of HLA nonidentity between donor and recipient or removal of mature T cells from the donor graft (60). Chronic GVHD appeared to lower the percentage of patients who had normal antibody production to tetanus, diphtheria or measles, compared to patients without chronic GVHD (54, 60). Transfer of cellular immunity to varicella from seropositive donors to transplant recipients was not effective unless the recipient experienced a pretransplant varicella-zoster infection (61). These findings indicate that memory cells in the marrow are transferred and are capable of either long life or self-replication in response to antigen stimulation (62). Additional evidence for this view is shown by the reduction of donor-derived isohemagglutinin in recipients of lymphocyte-depleted marrow early after grafting, followed by recovery of donor isohemagglutinin 6 months after transplant when mature lymphocytes reappear (63).

Allergin-specific IgE-mediated hypersensitivity is adoptively transferred by bone marrow transplantation from donor to recipient by B cells with allergin-specific memory (64). These data suggest that allergic diseases may be acquired by recipients of bone marrow from atopic donors. Such transfer could be of particular clinical importance in the posttransplantation identification of recipients who acquire asthma or drug allergy. Transfer of other immunologic conditions from donors to recipients has been responsible for the development of some unusual complications in transplant recipients, including myasthenia gravis (65) and autoimmune thyroiditis (66, 67). In each of these cases, clinical or subclinical disease was found in the donor after the recipient became symptomatic or showed abnormal thyroid function.

We have demonstrated transfer of immunity to the neoantigen KLH from immunized donors to allogeneic sibling recipients. One patient received marrow from an HLA-identical sibling who had been immunized to KLH 2 weeks before transplant. Serum was collected from the patient 9 months after transplant and assayed for the presence of KLH IgM and IgG. The serum KLH IgG titer from the patient was elevated 3 $\log_2$ dilutions above the pretransplant baseline for the patient. This titer was also 3 $\log_2$ dilutions higher than the maximum titer from 36 recipients of marrow from donors who had not been immunized with KLH. Three other patients received marrow from donors immunized with KLH 4 weeks before transplant. One recipient received the first injection of KLH 1 year after transplant, and the serum anti-KLH antibody response was IgG in type with no change in KLH IgM antibody production, indicating transfer of immunity. The other two patients did not demonstrate transfer of immunity. In contrast, nine individuals who received mar-

row from donors not immunized with KLH were given the initial injection of KLH after transplant, and their serum antibody response consisted of anti-KLH IgM but very little KLH IgG. These data indicate that immunity to neoantigens can be transferred with marrow from sensitized donors. In the cases where transfer did not occur, the likely explanation is that transfer is accomplished most effectively when both donor and recipient have been sensitized to KLH (68). In this way antigen present in the recipient is available to stimulate and expand sensitized clones transferred with the immunized marrow inoculum. Similar results have been shown for other antigens tetanus, diphtheria, *Pseudomonas aeruginosa,* and cytomegalovirus (69–72).

These findings have implications for immunization of transplant recipients. It is clear that immunity can be transferred from donors to recipients, and that immunity to tetanus, diphtheria, and measles serum antibody levels in the normal range can be detected for several years after transplant, even when the donor or the recipient was not boosted before or after transplantation. However, levels of serum antibody to these antigens decrease with time, suggesting that periodic boosting may be needed. One recent study of 48 marrow transplant recipients showed that among patients who were seropositive to tetanus before transplant, 51% lost their seropositivity 1 year after transplant. After one injection of tetanus toxoid, 7 of 14 boosted individuals were seropositive 1 year after the boost, whereas when given two or three tetanus toxoid boosters, the response rate increased to 90% and 100%, respectively, and the recipients remained seropositive for 2 more years after vaccination (73). Of course, the incidence of infection with tetanus in marrow transplant recipients must be very low, and no cases have been reported. It is possible that boosting is not necessary to convey protection from tetanus infection and that transferred immunity is sufficient. The situation for measles vaccination may be different. One study reported vaccination of marrow transplant recipients with measles vaccine more than 2 years from grafting. The patients did not have chronic GVHD and were not on immunosuppressive treatment. The response rate to the vaccine in 20 transplant recipients was lower than the response rate in normal controls (77% versus 90%). There was no vaccine-associated morbidity (74). This number of patients is clearly too small to draw conclusions about the wider application of live attenuated vaccines in marrow transplant recipients. The safety and efficacy of the vaccines in patients less than 2 years from grafting or patients with chronic GVHD are unknown. At the time of writing, this author is aware of only one case of measles in a marrow transplant patient who received marrow from a non-immunized HLA-identical sibling donor (10). Later, when the recipient had chronic GVHD, the donor developed measles and subsequently infected the recipient who died of disseminated measles pneumonia. In recent years there has been concern in the United States that the early vaccines against measles were not as effective as current vaccines (75). Measles infection may therefore become a problem in the communities where transplant recipients live, leading to risk of infection.

Immunization with pneumococcal vaccine results in a serum antibody response in patients without chronic GVHD but is usually not effective in producing a serum antibody response in patients with chronic GVHD (42). Polysaccharide vaccines conjugated to protein carriers such as the *Haemophilus influenza* b-diphtheria vaccine may have advantages in transplant recipients in whom T cell function is normal (76, 77). For those with abnormal T cell function and diminished IL-2 production, administration of the vaccine with IL-2 may be an effective strategy similar to that demonstrated for hepatitis B vaccine in chronic renal failure patients (78). Results of studies using different strategies to overcome poor responses of chronic GVHD patients to bacterial polysaccharide antigens will greatly aid in setting clear recommendations

for the use of vaccines to prevent bacterial infection in marrow transplant recipients.

At present, exposure to tetanus infection within the 1st year after transplant should be treated with injection of tetanus immune globulin. Beyond that time, patients without chronic GVHD may receive tetanus toxoid booster injection. More than one injection is likely to increase serum antibody level and the response rate. Exposure to measles should be treated with Ig injection. The inactivated polio vaccine is recommended if there is an outbreak in the patient's community or area of travel. The use of live vaccines routinely is not recommended.

PERSISTENCE OF HOST IMMUNITY

In allogeneic marrow transplant recipients, the persistence of host immunity can be demonstrated. Recipients of ABO-incompatible marrow have a gradual decline in serum isohemagglutinins by about 6 weeks after transplant (42). Occasionally, the original host isohemagglutinin persists longer. Detection of original host isohemagglutinin 5 months, 11 months, and longer than 3 years has been reported (79, 80). These times are much longer than what can be expected due to diffusion of antibody from tissue spaces into the serum and suggest that production of antibody by host cells is the likely explanation. In these rare cases, erythropoiesis of the donor-derived red cells is suppressed, delaying the recovery of a normal hematocrit. In the reported cases, eventual decline of the isohemagglutinin occurred. After decline in isohemagglutinin titer, reticulocytosis of the donor red cells ensued, restoring the hematocrit to normal.

Whether host immunity can play an effective role in protecting allogeneic transplant recipients from infection is not clear. Generally, the host cells cease function, and immune reactions against pathogens are donor derived. Host immunity itself probably plays no protective role against infection in marrow recipients beyond 1–2 months after transplantation. The role of host effects is probably the expression of specific antigen on the surface of host cells, which stimulates incoming donor cells to expand their clones to specific antigens (68).

Whether immunization of autologous marrow transplant recipients before marrow harvest will aid in protection from infection after transplantation has not been tested. The intensity of the conventional chemotherapy or radiotherapy delivered to treat the primary disease is an important factor. If immunity to pathogens were well established in the host before a marrow harvest, memory cells would be harvested and reinfused with the marrow. This marrow and immune system may or may not function well depending upon the underlying disease or treatment the patient received before immunization and storage of the autologous marrow.

CAN IMMUNE RECOVERY BE HASTENED AFTER MARROW TRANSPLANTATION?

The two most important factors in the tempo of immune reconstitution are time after transplant and the presence of chronic GVHD. The origin of the marrow is apparently less important because recovery in syngeneic recipients is similar to that of allogeneic recipients without GVHD. Why does it take so long for immune recovery to occur? In normal children, the thymus plays an important role in the developing immune system. In marrow transplantation, unless the recipient is very young, the thymus has involuted, leaving no place for intrathymic instruction of developing T cells. One hypothesis for the disordered balance of T cell subset repopulation, immune deficiency, and chronic GVHD is the lack of a functioning thymus in older transplant patients. In support of this hypothesis is the lower incidence of chronic GVHD among children as compared to adults receiving HLA-identical sibling grafts for leukemia or aplastic anemia, and the lower lev-

els of thymic factor in the serum of patients who have chronic GVHD (81, 82). The conditioning regimen may further destroy thymic remnants (83), and once chronic GVHD ensues, additional thymic destruction occurs (84). Trials in human marrow transplant recipients to correct thymic deficiency with the use of thymic implants or thymic factors have been ineffective to normalize immune responses or to prevent or ameliorate chronic GVHD (85–88). Perhaps a combination of thymic factors is needed rather than a single factor, or thymic implants are required that are phenotypically identical for HLA with the donor. This goal is not possible in human beings unless thymic tissue banks could be established. The role of the thymus would be expected to be more crucial in recipients of HLA-nonidentical sibling marrow. The patterns of infection in patients without chronic GVHD suggest minor differences in rates of infection with respect to receiving HLA-identical and HLA-nonidentical marrow (Fig. 13.1). These clinical events suggest sufficient cooperation occurs between antigen-presenting cells, T cells, and B cells in recipients of HLA-nonidentical marrow that immune reactivity against pathogens is possible and effective. Therefore, T cell programming appears to take place either in a nonthymic pathway or in some residual thymic remnants not totally destroyed by the conditioning therapy or GVHD.

Another hypothesis regarding immune recovery after grafting is that GVHD affects immune recovery completely independent of the thymus. This hypothesis is supported by the normal recovery of patients without GVHD who have HLA-identical or nonidentical donors contrasted to the delayed immune recovery associated with chronic GVHD. In this case, a rationale to prevent delayed immune recovery could be based on prevention of GVHD. At present prevention of acute GVHD in recipients of conventional grafts is accomplished through treatment with a combination of the agents methotrexate and cyclosporine or the use of intravenous immunoglobulin infusions during the 1st 3 months after transplant (89, 90). Passive transfer of antibodies in the infused globulin has also resulted in reduced incidence of bacterial infection in the early posttransplant period. Continuation of Ig infusions beyond the 1st 3 months to reduce infection is under investigation.

The role of growth factor administration for recovery of hematopoietic cells is now emerging. T lymphocytes and other accessory marrow cells produce granulocyte-macrophage colony-stimulating factor (GM-CSF) in normal individuals. However, in marrow transplant recipients studied up to 18 months after receiving untreated or treated marrows, T cells express little or no mRNA for GM-CSF after PHA stimulation in vitro, and GM-CSF secretion is reduced or absent (91). As shown in a placebo-controlled randomized trial, GM-CSF administration to recipients of autologous grafts hastens the time to peripheral blood neutrophil count of 500×10^{-6}/ml by 7 days, shortens the period of hospitalization by 6 days, reduces episodes of infection from opportunistic bacterial organisms, and shortens the duration of antibiotic administration by 3 days. While there was no difference in survival between the treated and placebo groups, morbidity was reduced by GM-CSF (92). Trials in allogeneic recipients are ongoing to determine if a similar effect can be obtained without exacerbation of acute GVHD (93).

Deficiencies of growth factors important for lymphocyte recovery have been documented. In particular, IL-2 is diminished in the supernatants of T cells taken from recipients of conventional untreated marrow in the early posttransplant period and from long-term survivors with chronic GVHD, but not from patients without chronic GVHD (30, 46–48, 94). IL-2 provides signals for cooperation between antigen-presenting cells and effector cells to produce normal cellular and humoral immunologic defense against pathogens as well as responses to alloantigens. IL-2 added to culture restores normal alloreac-

tivity in cell-mediated lympholysis of effector cells from acute GVHD patients (47). Peripheral blood mononuclear cells from recipients of allogeneic marrow that has been depleted of T cells have normal to elevated levels of in vitro PHAC- or OKT3-induced IL-2 secretion produced by the large number of large granular lymphocytes with NK activity that repopulate the blood of these patients in the 1st 2 months post grafting (27). IL-2 administration may benefit cooperation between T and B cells for antibody production to bacterial pathogens in patients with deficient IL-2 production. Of course, administration of IL-2 to recipients of allogeneic marrow may stimulate the appearance of GVHD.

A group of patients who might benefit from IL-2 administration are the recipients of autologous marrow grafts. Here the aim is to augment antitumor effects mediated by lymphokine-activated killer (LAK) cells, as has been described in patients with advanced cancer (95). In spite of posttransplant immunosuppressive treatment, peripheral blood mononuclear cells taken from autologous marrow graft recipients can be induced in vitro by IL-2 to generate cytolytic activity against Daudi cell line, Raji cell line, and fresh ovarian carcinoma cells (96). NK activity of mononuclear cells taken from recipients of HLA-identical marrow for treatment of chronic myelogenous leukemia (CML) against K562 CML targets was augmented by in vitro culture with IL-2 (97). When infused in vivo to autologous marrow recipients treated for hematologic malignancy 14–91 (median 30) days after grafting, IL-2 resulted in elevation of lymphocyte counts and NK and LAK lymphocyte subsets expressing CD16 and CD56, elevated activity against Daudi and K562 cell lines, and leukemia blast cell colonies. The administration of IL-2 resulted in moderate toxicities. The toxicities were fever ($>39°$ C), diarrhea, skin rash, nausea, hypotension, and thrombocytopenia. These toxicities ended when IL-2 infusions were stopped (98). These studies by several groups indicate that IL-2 can be administered safely to patients within the

1st 2–3 months after grafting and that cyto-lytic function against tumor cell lines and fresh leukemic cells is augmented in vitro (99, 100). Further studies will be needed to establish the most effective dose and schedule of administration of IL-2 or IL-2 and LAK cells and to assess the efficacy of this therapy to reduce posttransplant relapse of hematologic malignancy.

IL-4, also known as B cell stimulatory factor 1, is one of the lymphokines important for maturation of B cells to proliferate and secrete Ig in response to antigens (101). Pro-duction of factors important for B lympho-cyte development may, like IL-2 and GM-CSF, be deficient. Factors important for B cell growth and maturation to Ig-producing cells include IL-7, IL-1, IL-3, IL-4, IL-5, IL-6, and IL-11 (102–104). We have preliminary evidence of deficiency of IL-4 production by periph-eral blood mononuclear cells taken from pa-tients early after grafting and from long-term patients with chronic GVHD, but not from patients without chronic GVHD (unpub-lished observations). B lymphocytes from chronic GVHD patients, however, were re-sponsive when IL-4 was added to culture (105). These in vitro data suggest that B cells of chronic GVHD patients have appropriate re-ceptors for interaction with IL-4 and that ex-ogenous IL-4 replaces the deficiency of IL-4 production and permits B lymphocyte growth and development to begin. A knowledge of deficiencies of production of other interleu-kins and deficiencies of response to interleu-kins would greatly aid in development of clinical trials aimed at restoration of immune competence of B cells in marrow transplant recipients. Restoration of humoral immunity in marrow transplant recipients with chronic GVHD will reduce the incidence of bacterial infection after transplant, thereby reducing mortality and improving the quality of life.

CONCLUSIONS

Marrow transplantation was initially re-stricted to patients with syngeneic donors and allogeneic HLA-identical siblings for treat-ment of hematologic malignancies or aplastic anemia. Autologous marrow transplantation is now emerging as treatment of these ma-lignancies after the patient has been induced into first remission. Extension of the suit-ability of donors to partially matched family member donors and unrelated donors in-creases the potential for application of this therapy to more patients and to nonmalig-nant diseases such as thalassemia, congenital immune deficiencies, and inborn errors of metabolism. To be safe, the immune system must be competent to protect the marrow re-cipient from pathogens. At present, this result is achieved with sufficient time after trans-plant in patients with syngeneic grafts and al-logeneic recipients who do not develop chronic GVHD. Graft manipulation and pre-transplant treatment in recipients of autolo-gous marrow conspire to delay normal re-covery in this growing population of marrow graft recipients. The role of HLA matching in determining the risk of developing infection, especially in recipients of unrelated marrow, is poorly understood and should be studied. Strategies to accelerate the immune reactivity to pathogens by vaccine design, delineation of specific deficiencies of production, and re-sponse to growth factors will lead to clinical trials to augment immune recovery and pro-tect patients from serious and fatal posttrans-plant infections.

Acknowledgments
    Supported in part by grants CA 18221 and CA 18029 of the National Cancer Institute and grant HL 36444 of the National Heart, Lung and Blood Institute, awarded by the National Institutes of Health, D.H.H.S. The author wishes to acknowledge the skilled word processing of Bonnie Larson in preparation of the manuscript.

REFERENCES

1. Winston DJ, Gale RP, Meyer DV, et al. Infectious complications of human bone marrow transplan-tation. Medicine 1979;58:1–31.
2. Petersen FB, Buckner CD, Clift RA, et al. Infectious complications in patients undergoing marrow transplantation: a prospective randomized study of

the additional effect of decontamination and laminar air flow isolation among patients receiving prophylactic systemic antibiotics. Scand J Infect Dis 1987;19:559–567.

3. Wingard JR, Chen DY-H, Burns WH, et al. Cytomegalovirus infection after autologous bone marrow transplantation with comparison to infection after allogeneic bone marrow transplantation. Blood 1988;71:1432–1437.

4. Paulin T, Ringden O, Nilsson B, et al. Variables predicting bacterial and fungal infections after allogeneic marrow engraftment. Transplantation 1987; 43:393–398.

5. Bowden RA, Sayers M, Flournoy N, et al. Cytomegalovirus immune globulin and seronegative blood products to prevent primary cytomegalovirus infection after marrow transplantation. N Engl J Med 1986;314:1006–1010.

6. Meyers JD, Reed EC, Shepp DH, et al. Acyclovir for prevention of cytomegalovirus infection and disease after allogeneic marrow transplantation. N Engl J Med 1988;318:70–75.

7. Reed EC, Bowden RA, Dandliker PS, et al. Treatment of cytomegalovirus pneumonia with ganciclovir and intravenous cytomegalovirus immunoglobulin in patients with bone marrow transplants. Ann Intern Med 1988;109:783–788.

8. Emanuel D, Cunningham I, Jules-Elysee K, et al. Cytomegalovirus pneumonia after bone marrow transplantation successfully treated with the combination of ganciclovir and high-dose intravenous immune globulin. Ann Intern Med 1988;109:777–782.

9. Sullivan KM, Agura E, Anasetti C, et al. Chronic graft-versus-host disease and other late complications of bone marrow transplantation. Semin Hematol 1991; 28:250–259.

10. Sullivan KM, Shulman HM, Storb R, et al. Chronic graft-versus-host disease in 52 patients: Adverse natural course and successful treatment with combination immunosuppression. Blood 1981;57:267–276.

11. Sullivan KM, Witherspoon RP, Storb R, et al. Prednisone and azathioprine compared with prednisone and placebo for treatment of chronic graft-v-host disease: prognostic influence of prolonged thrombocytopenia after allogeneic marrow transplantation. Blood 1988;72:546–554.

12. Noel DR, Witherspoon RP, Storb R, et al. Does graft-versus-host disease influence the tempo of immunologic recovery after allogeneic human marrow transplantation? An observation on 56 long-term survivors. Blood 1978;51:1087–1105.

13. Ault KA, Antin JH, Ginsburg D, et al. Phenotype of recovering lymphoid cell populations after marrow transplantation. J Exp Med 1985;161:1483–1502.

14. Antin JH, Ault KA, Rappeport JM, et al. B lymphocyte reconstitution after human bone marrow transplan-

tation. Leu-1 antigen defines a distinct population of B lymphocytes. J Clin Invest 1987;80:325–332.

15. Aucouturier P, Barra A, Intrator L, et al. Long lasting IgG subclass and antibacterial polysaccharide antibody deficiency after allogeneic bone marrow transplantation. Blood 1987;70:779–785.

16. Sheridan JF, Tutschka PJ, Sedmak DD, et al. Immunoglobulin G subclass deficiency and pneumococcal infection after allogeneic bone marrow transplantation. Blood 1990;75:1583–1586.

17. Mitus AJ, Stein R, Rappeport JM, et al. Monoclonal and oligoclonal gammapathy after bone marrow transplantation. Blood 1989;74:2764–2768.

18. Fischer AM, Simon F, Le Deist F, et al. Prospective study of the occurrence of monoclonal gammapathies following bone marrow transplantation in young children. Transplantation 1990;49:731–735.

19. Atkinson K, Hansen JA, Storb R, et al. T-cell subpopulations identified by monoclonal antibodies after human marrow transplantation. I: Helper-inducer and cytotoxic-suppressor subsets. Blood 1982;59:1292–1298.

20. Witherspoon RP, Goehle S, Kretschmer M, et al. Regulation of immunoglobulin production after human marrow grafting: the role of helper and suppressor T cells in acute graft-versus-host disease. Transplantation 1986;41:328–335.

21. Witherspoon RP, Lum LG, Storb R, et al. In vitro regulation of immunoglobulin synthesis after human marrow transplantation. II: Deficient T and non-T lymphocyte function within 3–4 months of allogeneic, syngeneic, or autologous marrow grafting for hematologic malignancy. Blood 1982;59:844–850.

22. Korsmeyer SJ, Elfenbein GJ, Goldman CK, et al. B cell, helper T cell, and suppressor T cell abnormalities contribute to disordered immunoglobulin synthesis in patients following bone marrow transplantation. Transplantation 1982;33:184–190.

23. Pahwa SG, Pahwa RN, Friedrich W, et al. Abnormal humoral immune responses in peripheral blood lymphocyte cultures of bone marrow transplant recipients. Proc Natl Acad Sci USA 1982;79:2663–2667.

24. Livnat S, Seigneuret M, Storb R, et al. Analysis of cytotoxic effector cell function in patients with leukemia or aplastic anemia before and after marrow transplantation. J Immunol 1980;124:481–490.

25. Lopez C, Kirkpatrick D, Livnat S, et al. Natural killer cells in bone marrow transplantation (Letter). Lancet 1980;2:1025.

26. Brenner MK, Reittie JE, Grob J-P, et al. The contribution of large granular lymphocytes to B cell activation and differentiation after T-cell-depleted allogeneic bone marrow transplantation. Transplantation 1986;42:257–261.

27. Welte K, Keever CA, Levick J, et al. Interleukin-2 production and response to interleukin-2 by peripheral blood mononuclear cells from patients af-

ter bone marrow transplantation. II: Patients receiving soybean lectin-separated and T cell-depleted bone marrow. Blood 1987;70:1595–1603.

28. Tsoi M-S, Dobbs S, Brkic S, et al. Cellular interactions in marrow-grafted patients. II: Normal monocyte antigen-presenting and defective T-cell-proliferative functions early after grafting and during chronic graft-versus-host disease. Transplantation 1984;37:556–561.

29. Shiobara S, Witherspoon RP, Lum LG, et al. Immunoglobulin synthesis after HLA-identical marrow grafting. V: The role of peripheral blood monocytes in the regulation of in vitro immunoglobulin secretion stimulated by PW mitogen. J Immunol 1984;132:2850–2856.

30. Brkic S, Tsoi M-S, Mori T, et al. Cellular interactions in marrow-grafted patients. III: Normal interleukin 1 and defective interleukin 2 production in short-term patients and in those with chronic graft-versus-host disease. Transplantation 1985;39:30–35.

31. Keever CA, Small TN, Flomenberg N, et al. Immune reconstitution following bone marrow transplantation: comparison of recipients of T-cell depleted marrow with recipients of conventional marrow grafts. Blood 1989;73:1340–1350.

32. Soiffer RJ, Bosserman L, Murray C, et al. Reconstitution of T-cell function after CD6-depleted allogeneic bone marrow transplantation. Blood 1990;75:2076–2084.

33. Rozans MK, Smith BR, Burakoff SJ, et al. Long-lasting deficit of functional T cell precursors in human bone marrow transplant recipients revealed by limiting dilution methods. J Immunol 1986;136:4040–4048.

34. Singer CRJ, Tansey PJ, Burnett AK. T lymphocyte reconstitution following autologous bone marrow transplantation. Clin Exp Immunol 1983;51:455–460.

35. Small TN, Keever CA, Weiner-Fedus S, et al. B cell differentiation following autologous, conventional, or T-cell depleted bone marrow transplantation: a recapitulation of normal B cell ontogeny. Blood 1990;76:1647–1656.

36. Kiesel S, Pezzutto A, Moldenhauer G, et al. B-cell proliferative and differentiative responses after autologous peripheral blood stem cell or bone marrow transplantation. Blood 1988;72:672–678.

37. Matsue K, Lum LG, Witherspoon RP, et al. Proliferative and differentiative responses of B cells from human marrow graft recipients to T cell-derived factors. Blood 1987;69:308–315.

38. Kagan JM, Champlin RE, Saxon A. B-cell dysfunction following human bone marrow transplantation: functional-phenotypic dissociation in the early posttransplant period. Blood 1989;74:777–785.

39. Anderson KC, Ritz J, Takvorian T, et al. Hematologic engraftment and immune reconstitution posttransplant with anti-B1 purged autologous bone marrow. Blood 1987;69:597–604.

40. Anderson KC, Soiffer R, DeLage R, et al. T-cell-depleted autologous bone marrow transplantation therapy: analysis of immune deficiency and late complications. Blood 1990;76:235–244.

41. Witherspoon RP, Kopecky K, Storb RF, et al. Immunological recovery in 48 patients following syngeneic marrow transplantation for hematological malignancy. Transplantation 1982;33:143–149.

42. Witherspoon RP, Storb R, Ochs HD, et al. Recovery of antibody production in human allogeneic marrow graft recipients: influence of time posttransplantation, the presence or absence of chronic graft-versus-host disease, and antithymocyte globulin treatment. Blood 1981;58:360–368.

43. Witherspoon RP, Deeg HJ, Lum LG, et al. Immunologic recovery in human marrow graft recipients given cyclosporine or methotrexate for the prevention of graft versus-host disease. Transplantation 1984;37:456–461.

44. Quinti I, Velardi A, Le Moli S, et al. Antibacterial polysaccharide antibody deficiency after allogeneic bone marrow transplantation. J Clin Immunol 1990;10:160–166.

45. Witherspoon RP, Matthews D, Storb R, et al. Recovery of in vivo cellular immunity after human marrow grafting: influence of time postgrafting and acute graft-versus-host disease. Transplantation 1984;37:145–150.

46. Welte K, Ciobanu N, Moore MAS, et al. Defective interleukin 2 production in patients after bone marrow transplantation and in vitro restoration of defective T lymphocyte proliferation by highly purified interleukin 2. Blood 1984;64:380–385.

47. Mori T, Tsoi M-S, Gillis S, et al. Cellular interactions in marrow-grafted patients. I: Impairment of cell-mediated lympholysis associated with graft-vs-host disease and the effect of interleukin 2. J Immunol 1983;130:712–716.

48. Tsoi M-S, Mori T, Brkic S, et al. Ineffective cellular interaction and interleukin 2 deficiency causing T cell defects in human allogeneic marrow recipients early after grafting and in those with chronic graft-versus-host disease. Transplant Proc 1984;16:1470–1472.

49. Warren HS, Atkinson K, Pembrey RG, et al. Human bone marrow allograft recipients: production of, and responsiveness to, interleukin 2. J Immunol 1983;131:1771–1775.

50. Lum LG, Seigneuret MC, Storb RF, et al. In vitro regulation of immunoglobulin synthesis after marrow transplantation. I: T-cell and B-cell deficiencies in patients with and without chronic graft-versus-host disease. Blood 1981;58:431–439.

51. Atkinson K, Meyers JD, Storb R, et al. Varicella-zoster virus infection after marrow transplantation for aplastic anemia or leukemia. Transplantation 1980;29:47–50.

52. Witherspoon RP, Schanfield MS, Storb R, et al. Immunoglobulin production of donor origin after marrow transplantation for acute leukemia or aplastic anemia. Transplantation 1978;26:407–408.
53. Starling KA, Falletta JM, Fernbach DJ. Immunologic chimerism as evidence of bone marrow graft acceptance in an identical twin with acute lymphocytic leukemia. Exp Hematol 1975;3:244–248.
54. Lum LG, Munn NA, Schanfield MS, et al. The detection of specific antibody formation to recall antigens after human bone marrow transplantation. Blood 1986;67:582–587.
55. Lum LG, Seigneuret MC, Storb R. The transfer of antigen-specific humoral immunity from marrow donors to marrow recipients. J Clin Immunol 1986;6:389–396.
56. Lum LG, Seigneuret MC, Shiobara S, et al. Adoptively transferred immunity persists in human marrow graft recipients. In: Truitt RL, Gale RP, Bortin MM, eds. Cellular immunotherapy of cancer. New York: Alan R. Liss, 1987:449–460.
57. Shiobara S, Lum LG, Witherspoon RP, et al. Antigen specific antibody responses of lymphocytes to tetanus toxoid after human marrow transplantation. Transplantation 1986;41:587–592.
58. Jin N-R, Lum LG. IgG anti-tetanus toxoid antibody production induced by Epstein-Barr virus from B cells of human marrow transplant recipients. Cell Immunol 1986;101:266–273.
59. Lum LG. A review: the kinetics of immune reconstitution after human marrow transplantation. Blood 1987;69:369–380.
60. Lum LG, Noges JE, Beatty P, et al. Transfer of specific immunity in marrow recipients given HLA-mismatched, T cell-depleted, or HLA-identical marrow grafts. Bone Marrow Transplant 1988;3:399–406.
61. Kato S, Yabe H, Yabe M, et al. Studies on transfer of varicella-zoster-virus specific T-cell immunity from bone marrow donor to recipient. Blood 1990;75:806–809.
62. Cooley MA, Atkinson K, Adamthwaite D. In vitro function of CD4+ cells of naive and memory phenotype in bone marrow transplant recipients. Transplant Proc 1991;23:165–166.
63. Bär BMAM, Santos GW, Donnenberg AD. Reconstitution of antibody response after allogeneic bone marrow transplantation: effect of lymphocyte depletion by counterflow centrifugal elutriation on the expression of hemagglutinins. Blood 1990;76:1410–1418.
64. Agosti JM, Sprenger JD, Lum LG, et al. Transfer of allergen-specific IgE-mediated hypersensitivity with allogeneic bone marrow transplantation. N Engl J Med 1988;319:1623–1628.
65. Bolger GB, Sullivan KM, Spencer AM, et al. Myasthenia gravis after allogeneic bone marrow transplantation: relationship to chronic graft-versus-host disease. Neurology 1986;36:1087–1091.
66. Aldouri M, Ruggier R, Epstein O, et al. Adoptive transfer of hyperthyroidism and autoimmune thyroiditis following allogeneic bone marrow transplantation for chronic myeloid leukaemia. Br J Haematol 1990;74:118–120.
67. Wyatt DT, Lum LG, Casper J, et al. Autoimmune thyroiditis after bone marrow transplantation. Bone Marrow Transplant 1990;5:357–361.
68. Wimperis JZ, Gottlieb D, Duncombe AS, et al. Requirements for the adoptive transfer of antibody responses to. J Immunol 1990;144:541–547.
69. Saxon A, Mitsuyasu R, Stevens R, et al. Designed transfer of specific immune responses with bone marrow transplantation. J Clin Invest 1986;78:959–967.
70. Wimperis JZ, Brenner MK, Prentice HG, et al. Transfer of a functioning humoral immune system in transplantation of T-lymphocyte-depleted bone marrow. Lancet 1986;1:339–343.
71. Wimperis JZ, Brenner MK, Prentice HG, et al. B cell development and regulation after T cell-depleted marrow transplantation. J Immunol 1987;138:2445–2450.
72. Gottlieb DJ, Cryz SJ, Jr., Furer E, et al. Immunity against *Pseudomonas aeruginosa* adoptively transferred to bone marrow transplant recipients. Blood 1990;76:2470–2475.
73. Ljungman P, Wiklund-Hammarsten M, Duraj V, et al. Response to tetanus toxoid immunization after allogeneic bone marrow transplantation. J Infect Dis 1990;162:496–500.
74. Ljungman P, Fridell E, Lönnqvist B, et al. Efficacy and safety of vaccination of marrow transplant recipients with a live attenuated measles, mumps, and rubella vaccine. J Infect Dis 1989;159:610–615.
75. Markowitz LE, Preblud SR, Orenstein WA, et al. Patterns of transmission in measles outbreaks in the United States, 1985–1986. N Engl J Med 1989;320:75–81.
76. Insel RA, Anderson PW. Response to oligosaccharide-protein conjugate vaccine against *Hemophilus influenzae* b in two patients with IgG$_2$ deficiency unresponsive to capsular polysaccharide vaccine. N Engl J Med 1986;315:499–503.
77. Eskola J, Peltola H, Takala AK, et al. Efficacy of *Haemophilus influenzae* type b polysaccharide-diphtheria toxoid conjugate vaccine in infancy. N Engl J Med 1987;317:717–722.
78. Meuer SC, Dumann H, Zum Buschenfelde K-HM, et al. Low-dose interleukin-2 induces systemic immune responses against HBsAg in immunodeficient non-responders to hepatitis B vaccination. Lancet 1989;1:15–18.
79. Barge AJ, Johnson G, Witherspoon R, et al. Antibody-mediated marrow failure after allogenic bone marrow transplantation. Blood 1989;74:1477–1480.
80. Volin L, Ruutu T. Pure red-cell aplasia of long du-

ration after major ABO-incompatible bone marrow transplantation. Acta Haematol 1990;84:195–197.

81. Storb R, Prentice RL, Sullivan KM, et al. Predictive factors in chronic graft-versus-host disease in patients with aplastic anemia treated by marrow transplantation from HLA-identical siblings. Ann Intern Med 1983;98:461–466.

82. Atkinson K, Incefy GS, Storb R, et al. Low serum thymic hormone levels in patients with chronic graft-versus-host disease. Blood 1982;59:1073–1077.

83. Shulman HM, Sullivan KM, Weiden PL, et al. Chronic graft-versus-host syndrome in man. A long-term clinicopathologic study of 20 Seattle patients. Am J Med 1980;69:204–217.

84. Seddik M, Seemayer TA, Lapp WS. T cell functional defect associated with thymic epithelial cell injury induced by a graft-versus-host reaction. Transplantation 1980;29:61–66.

85. Atkinson K, Storb R, Ochs HD, et al. Thymus transplantation after allogeneic bone marrow graft to prevent chronic graft-versus-host disease in humans. Transplantation 1982;33:168–173.

86. Witherspoon RP, Hersman J, Storb R, et al. Thymosin fraction 5 does not accelerate reconstitution of immunologic reactivity after human marrow grafting. Br J Haematol 1983;55:595–608.

87. Witherspoon RP, Navari R, Storb R, et al. Treatment of marrow graft recipients with thymopentin. Bone Marrow Transplant 1987;1:365–371.

88. Witherspoon RP, Sullivan KM, Lum LG, et al. Use of thymic grafts or thymic factors to augment immunologic recovery after bone marrow transplantation: brief report with 2 to 12 years' follow-up. Bone Marrow Transplant 1988;3:425–435.

89. Storb R, Deeg HJ, Whitehead J, et al. Methotrexate and cyclosporine compared with cyclosporine alone for prophylaxis of acute graft versus host disease after marrow transplantation for leukemia. N Engl J Med 1986;314:729–735.

90. Sullivan KM, Kopecky KJ, Jocom J, et al. Immunomodulatory and antimicrobial efficacy of intravenous immunoglobulin in bone marrow transplantation. N Engl J Med 1990;323:705–712.

91. Thomas S, Clark SC, Rappeport JM, et al. Deficient T cell granulocyte-macrophage colony stimulating factor production in allogeneic bone marrow transplant recipients. Transplantation 1990;49:703–708.

92. Nemunaitis J, Rabinowe SN, Singer JW, et al. Recombinant granulocyte-macrophage colony-stimulating factor after autologous bone marrow transplantation for lymphoid cancer. N Engl J Med 1991;324:1773–1778.

93. Nemunaitis J, Buckner CD, Appelbaum FR, et al. Phase I/II trial of recombinant human granulocyte-macrophage colony-stimulating factor following allogeneic bone marrow transplantation. Blood 1991; 77:2065–2071.

94. Azogui O, Gluckman E, Fradelizi D. Inhibition of IL 2 production after human allogeneic bone marrow transplantation. J Immunol 1983;131:1205–1208.

95. Rosenberg SA, Lotze MT, Muul LM, et al. A progress report on the treatment of 157 patients with advanced cancer using lymphokine-activated killer cells and interleukin-2 or high-dose interleukin-2 alone. N Engl J Med 1987;316:889–897.

96. Higuchi CM, Thompson JA, Cox T, et al. Lymphokine-activated killer function following autologous bone marrow transplantation for refractory hematological malignancies. Cancer Res 1989;49:5509–5513.

97. Hauch M, Gazzola MV, Small T, et al. Anti-leukemia potential of interleukin-2 activated natural killer cells after bone marrow transplantation for chronic myelogenous leukemia. Blood 1990;75:2250–2262.

98. Higuchi CM, Thompson JA, Petersen FB, et al. Toxicity and immunomodulatory effects of interleukin-2 after autologous bone marrow transplantation for hematologic malignancies. Blood 1991;77:2561–2568.

99. Gottlieb DJ, Prentice HG, Heslop HE, et al. Effects of recombinant interleukin-2 administration on cytotoxic function following high-dose chemo-radiotherapy for hematological malignancy. Blood 1989;74:2335–2342.

100. Blaise D, Olive D, Stoppa AM, et al. Hematologic and immunologic effects of the systemic administration of recombinant interleukin-2 after autologous bone marrow transplantation. Blood 1990; 76:1092–1097.

101. Paul WE. Interleukin-4: a prototypic immunoregulatory lymphokine. Blood 1991;77:1859–1870.

102. Uckun FM. Regulation of human B-cell ontogeny. Blood 1990;76:1908–1923.

103. Paul SR, Bennett F, Calvetti JA, et al. Molecular cloning of a cDNA encoding interleukin 11, a stromal cell-derived lymphopoietic and hematopoietic cytokine. Proc Natl Acad Sci USA 1990;87:7512–7516.

104. Barut B, Morimoto C, Paul S, et al. Interleukin 11 augments immunoglobulin secretion through selective stimulation of the T cell helper inducer (CD4 + CD45RA−) subset [Abstract]. Blood 1990;76:201a.

105. Witherspoon RP, McGregor BA, Mori M, et al. B-lymphocytes of marrow graft recipients with chronic graft-versus-host disease respond to in vitro proliferative signals [Abstract]. Exp Hematol 1990;18:686.

14

MARROW CONTAMINATION: DETECTION AND SIGNIFICANCE

J. Graham Sharp and David A. Crouse

In the adult, hematopoietically active bone marrow is distributed throughout the axial skeleton; in children and some pathologic conditions, it is found at additional sites. Consequently, lymphohematopoietic tissue, including the marrow, is a model systemic tissue and as such can serve as the surrogate for detection of metastatic disease. Although not all metastases involve the marrow, the situation of tumor cells in the marrow provides a suitable contrast to strictly localized disease. In the latter, the challenge of high-dose therapy is to eliminate tumor locally while permitting survival of adequate numbers of normal marrow clonogenic cells. When tumor is metastatic to marrow, elimination must be accomplished in a situation where the tumor cells and marrow cells reside in the same microenvironment.

Primary myeloid diseases, such as leukemia, present a unique challenge because the malignant cells closely resemble normal populations. They often share the same phenotype and growth factor receptor expression, although sometimes they can be distinguished genotypically. This emphasizes the application of molecular techniques to detect the genetic deviations from normal that may be present in leukemic populations. Unfortunately, identifying increasingly small genetic deviations raises questions about the ultimate clinical relevance of the small numbers of cells with such abnormalities. Not surprisingly, therefore, marrow contamination with tumor has an impact on outcome that establishes the importance of detecting marrow contamination in candidates for high-dose therapy.

An alternative strategy that permits a further escalation of therapy is the use of autologous bone marrow transplantation (ABMT) (1, 2) or peripheral stem cell transplantation (PSCT) (3). Removal, freezing, and storing of hematopoietic products prior to therapy permits escalation of marrow-toxic drugs to levels at which toxicity to other systems (usually mucosal epithelium) becomes the most frequent life-threatening complication. The marrow aplasia induced by high-dose therapy is corrected by reinfusion of the stored hematopoietic cells. In this approach to high-dose therapy, philosophical, ethical, and practical considerations dictate that every effort be made to ensure that the reinfused product (marrow or blood mononuclear cells) is free of tumor cells. Consequently, detection of metastatic contamination (occult tumor) in such harvests is of some significance. We should perhaps note at this point that although contamination of such products even with minimal tumor cells is associated with a poorer clinical outcome, residual tumor at sites of bulk disease, relatively, is of much greater clinical importance.

BIOLOGIC CONSIDERATIONS

Elimination of tumor cells either locally or metastatic to marrow without induction of fatal aplasia requires that the product of the number of clonogenic tumor cells and their surviving fraction at the selected doses of chemotherapy be lower than the similar product for marrow clonogenic cells. A number of factors influence this calculation. The cell kinetic characteristics of drug killing are important (4). Most, but not all, are cycle-specific agents. In the hematopoietic system, this results in elimination of many of the more differentiated progenitor populations, which are comprised of more actively cycling cells (5). These are also the cells that respond to the well-defined colony-stimulating factors/interleukins. In contrast, the more primitive marrow stem cells, which are largely non-cycling cells (at least when in contact with microenvironmental stromal cells) are less sensitive to high-dose therapy and usually survive to repopulate the hematopoietic system (6, 7). This is particularly true of the most primitive hematopoietic stem cell population. Such cells probably require a different class of cytokines for activation prior to responding to the better-characterized lineage specific growth and differentiation factors. However, these cells take a significant time to differentiate to functional cells, and, since they do not respond initially to most individual colony-stimulating factors/interleukins, the consequent period of aplasia cannot be significantly shortened by these factors combined with "purified/enriched" stem cells. The characteristics of dependence upon some form of stromal cell contact, short-range interactions, or paracrine/juxtacrine factors exhibited by more primitive hematopoietic stem cells (6) is apparently shared by some types of tumor cells, particularly lung tumors and breast cancer cells (8, 9). The exact nature of these interactions is currently uncertain. Although such cellular intercourse is not well understood, the similarities in kinetics and microenvironmental dependence for both primitive hematopoietic cells and at least some tumor cells complicates the therapeutic elimination of the latter cells without irreparable damage to the former. At the same time, it provides an opportunity to detect tumor cells contaminating marrow by employing culture systems that have been developed to maintain primitive hematopoietic cells. The similarities in kinetic characteristics of primitive hematopoietic cells and most tumor cells mean that the number of clonogenic tumor cells is a significant determinant in clinical outcome. The presence of bulky residual tumor at any nonmarrow site usually makes the degree of marrow contamination irrelevant. However, in circumstances in which the bulk of tumor can be eliminated, marrow contamination can become a critical determinant of outcome.

TECHNICAL CONSIDERATIONS IN THE DETECTION OF MARROW CONTAMINATION

Experience of the Pathologist

The ability to achieve a high sensitivity in the detection of minimal residual disease (MRD) against a background of bone marrow cells is heavily dependent on the experience of the pathologist examining the material. The identification of tumor cells in these circumstances can be complicated by the altered composition of the background marrow cells following prior chemotherapy of the patient. Immunocytochemical stains can pinpoint cells that possess a particular epitope, e.g., cytokeratin in breast cancer cells. However, the quality of the morphology of such preparations is often much poorer than that of Romanowsky-stained cells. Furthermore, when cells metastatic to the bone marrow are examined, often the tissue-specific features that help to confirm the nature of the particular cell type in situ are missing. Additionally, macrophages and their precursors, which are common in bone marrow, can stain nonspecifically under some circumstances, or they may contain epitope-positive phagocytosed material, which may be confusing (10). Some of these problems can be circumvented by the use of nonmammalian enzymes in the staining process. Others can only be distinguished with experience. When other special techniques are used, such as cell and tissue culture or in situ hybridization, morphologic preservation can be compromised and potentially misleading artifacts introduced. All such studies, but particularly immunocytochemical analysis, should be approached critically with a high degree of cynicism so that the danger of overinterpretation, which carries potential undue risk to the patient, can be avoided or minimized.

Sampling Problems

Several studies have indicated that the likelihood of observing metastatic tumor in bone marrow is increased by including a greater number of sites for sampling of the bone marrow (11). In the Brown Norway rat leukemia model, Martens et al. (12) demonstrated the inhomogeneous distribution of leukemia in the marrow. This is probably the case for many tumors metastatic to the marrow. Traditionally, we employ bilateral iliac crest core biopsies and aspirates. Mansi et al. (13) examined aspirates from eight different sites. We have been more successful in detecting tumor cells, particularly breast cancer cells, on the material that remains on the stainless steel screens (14) used to filter a marrow harvest than on aspirated samples. The composition of the harvests changes rapidly as the amount of blood contamination increases. The ability to detect MRD is probably quite dependent upon both the quality of the aspirate and the number of aspirates studied. Each program should develop a standard protocol for this procedure in order to maintain consistency of data collection, and the priority assigned to detection of MRD must be determined. The detection of MRD has prognostic significance, as, for example, does cytogenetic analysis. Which of these is most

important is a function of both disease and program emphasis. Cytogenetic studies may have greater prognostic value in leukemia than in breast cancer, while the culture-based observation of MRD may be more informative in breast cancer than in cytogenetic studies. In lymphoma, we have found that a significant sample (approximately 10 ml at the 200-ml total volume) of a marrow harvest is probably as useful as the screens employed to filter the harvest. These screens are, however, probably better sources of material for detecting breast cancer cells. Overall, the ability to detect tumor contamination in the marrow by any technique is improved by use of as many high-quality biopsies or aspirates as can be reasonably obtained.

Flow Cytometry

Several attempts have been made to employ flow cytometry to detect rare tumor cells. In general, the results have been disappointing (15, 16). Although flow cytometry can be employed with some success in model systems where characteristics such as size, DNA content, or surface phenotype of the tumor cells are known, the situation is much less satisfactory with studies of patient samples. If the frequency of the tumor cells is low (e.g., 1 in 10^5 bone marrow cells), the positive event rate in flow cytometry is low, and the coefficient of variation determined from the histogram of the detected cells is high. For example, it is possible to detect CD34+ stem cells in the bone marrow, where they have a frequency of 1%–4% of the nucleated cells in a normal individual. However, attempts to quantitate CD34+ cells in unmobilized blood samples where the frequency is at least 10-fold lower have been technically complex and only marginally successful (17). Enrichment steps to solve the problems associated with detecting the cells present in a very low frequency (18), unfortunately, introduce additional variables such as the efficiency of separation of the tumor cells versus the nucleated marrow cells. This in turn complicates the estimation of frequency. Possibly, and only when relatively specific markers are available (e.g., cytokeratin), flow cytometry could be employed to enrich tumor cells and, by sorting, deposit these cells on a slide for more efficient morphologic examination. This might reduce the time needed to screen such samples from a couple of hours to a few minutes. This approach has only been employed in small-scale studies to date (16, 18).

A problem that arises in all antibody-based detection systems (e.g., flow cytometry and immunocytochemistry) is that of epitope-negative tumor cells or cells with low epitope density (19). The traditional approach to this problem has been to employ additional antibodies as a "battery" or "cocktail" (16, 19). Unfortunately, the nonspecific background staining increases as more antibodies are employed, with consequent risk of increased false-positives. We suggest the critical evaluation of any antibody that is considered for inclusion in a battery or cocktail. More is not necessarily better, and at some point the risk of false-positives outweighs the proportion of tumor cells that will be missed because of low epitope density or negativity.

These concerns are especially relevant to leukemias, in which there is considerable overlap in epitope expression between normal and malignant cells. Not only does this have practical consequences in terms of making it difficult to distinguish between normal and leukemic cells, but also, if there is epitope overlap between such populations, use of some of these antibodies for purging may lead to prolonged engraftment times for transplanted patients. A final concern in the use of antibodies for tumor cell detection is the possible problem associated with antigen modulation and activation of antigen expression. In these situations, antigens may be transiently expressed or down modulated because of the status of the patient (recent prior chemotherapy) or as a result of in vitro handling of the cell product.

Molecular Approaches

Molecular techniques are increasingly attractive because of their exquisite sensitivity and precision. Southern analysis of T cell or B cell receptor-associated gene rearrangements have become routine procedures to confirm the diagnosis of lymphoma (20). The level of sensitivity for detection of clonal populations by this technique when optimally performed is probably 1% of the total population. Other genes have been studied for other malignancies, including *myc*, *sis*, and *raf* in acute myelogenous leukemia (21) and *c-erB-2* in breast cancer (22). As experience has grown, the impact of their sensitivity has also been recognized. Such techniques should be applied rigorously using appropriate controls. Contamination in polymerase chain reaction (PCR) studies can be devastating. These techniques, particularly PCR amplification of oncogene-associated sequences, detect tumor-related genotypes in cells that are strongly suspected to be nonmalignant, and these techniques may detect tumor cells in patients who are clinically well and who remain so for many years after the detection of the tumor cells. Thus, molecular techniques appear to be too sensitive a method for detecting tumor cells in some instances. The clinician has a major dilemma when tumor cells appear to be detected in the marrow of a patient who seems clinically well. Our approach has been conservative. We follow such patients very closely without intervention unless other indicators appear. An attempt to clarify the relevance of detection of cells with abnormal molecular genotypes in bone marrow is being made by combining in situ techniques for the detection of these cells with in situ analysis of RNA expression, on the assumption that cells expressing an abnormal message may be more likely to express their malignant phenotype. It is still too early to evaluate the clinical importance of the application of these techniques.

Culture Studies

A technique for detecting tumor cells in bone marrow that has had some success in the hands of a variety of investigators is to place the bone marrow into culture and allow the tumor cells to grow and amplify, permitting their detection by the other techniques described above (23). The primary rationale for this approach seems to be that it works. One might speculate that it should work because tumor cells have a greater degree of autonomy than normal cells and therefore should survive preferentially. However, the underlying biology is probably much more complicated. Although culture systems permit the outgrowth of lymphoid leukemia, lymphoma, and solid tumor cells, nearly all myeloid leukemia cells placed in such cultures show evidence of differentiation (24, 25). We believe these cultures provide an environment in which combinations of cytokines are presented to target cells, potentially at close range and in some instances while the target cell is adherent to the cell that is the source of the growth factor(s). This would explain the tumor-specific patterns of growth in these cultures. Breast cancer cells tend to grow attached to the adherent layer of the cultures. In contrast, non-Hodgkin's lymphoma (NHL) cells expand as the supernatant cells of the culture. Myeloid leukemic cells may be defective in their ability to participate in such short-range interactions, possibly because they are defective in adhesion molecule expression (26). Consequently, they behave differently from other tumor types in these culture systems.

The identification of tumor cells from cultures employs the techniques described above: immunocytochemistry for breast cancer, Southern analysis for NHL. A concern in the application of these techniques to cultured cells is the possibility of culture-induced artifacts. This could include antigen modulation, although probably the greatest documented concern is the induction of cytogenetic abnormalities (27). When cytogenetic markers for tumor identification are employed, we require three identical abnormal metaphases that were present in the fresh tumor sample. This limits the application of cytogenetics with cultured cells. The cells in the cultures, particularly those associated with the adherent layers, are relatively quiescent, and metaphases are infrequent. Culture conditions can also mask cytogenetic abnormalities (28). This limits the sensitivity of confirmation of tumor cell presence by cytogenetic techniques. The same, of course, is true for fresh samples. The requirement of three identical abnormal metaphase plates in cells present at 1 in 10^5 nucleated cells illustrates the limits of this approach.

MODEL SYSTEMS VERSUS PATIENT STUDIES

Model systems in which known numbers of tumor cells (almost always well-established cell lines) are added to normal bone marrow have been widely used to evaluate and calibrate the sensitivity of methods of tumor cell detection. An example of the use of such a model system is presented below. In this study, varying numbers of the cell line CEM T lymphoma cells were added to normal apheresis product. The mixtures were cultured for up to 4 weeks. Every week samples were drawn, blind coded, and examined for the presence of lymphoblastoid cells. Lower numbers of seeded cells required longer culture periods to assure detection. These data are shown in Figure 14.1 and can be interpreted as the proportion of CEM cells necessary for them to become evident after a given period of culture. An unknown sample evident in the same time period can now be interpreted as a level of tumor cell contamination equivalent to a percentage of CEM cells. Although we have data relating positivity for tumor cells in such cultures to clinical outcome, we have not yet evaluated whether this type of estimate of tumor burden will correlate with clinical outcome. Anecdotally, we have noted that tumor cells which quickly become apparent in cultures of histologically negative marrows are more likely to be associated with a poorer clinical course. This type of tumor is also more likely to give rise to a cell line that will grow in an immuno-

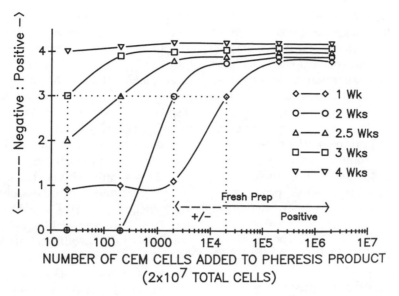

Figure 14.1 An example of a model system employed to calibrate the sensitivity of detection of T lymphoma cells using an in vitro culture technique. Cells of the CEM line were added in various proportions to a normal apheresis product, and this mixture was placed into culture. Cell preparations were made before culture and at weekly demidepopulation of the cultures. The CEM cells can be observed morphologically on cytospin preparations or detected with a similar sensitivity by Southern analysis of their clonal rearrangement. The samples were graded as 1: no evidence of CEM cells; 2: suspicious, but no clear evidence of CEM cells; 3: clear evidence of CEM cells; and 4: predominance of CEM cells. The time of appearance of detectable CEM cells in the cultures according to these criteria was noted. There is a clear inverse relationship between the number of CEM cells originally added and the time at which they become evident. This permits an estimate to be made of the sensitivity of this model system. In this case 20 CEM cells added to 2×10^7 cells of apheresis product became evident by 3 weeks (i.e., 1 CEM cell in 10^6 normal cells). In contrast when 2×10^4 CEM cells were added (i.e., 1 in 10^3), they were immediately evident in the fresh preparation.

deficient mouse (29). An association of successful heterotransplantation in the nude mouse, poor prognosis, and amplification of the *HER-2/neu* oncogene has recently been reported for breast carcinomas (30). Our observations also suggest that the ability to grow the detectable tumor cells in an immunodeficient mouse is a strong indicator of poor prognosis. We have been able to grow primary or early passage cells from NHL, melanoma, and acute myelogenous leukemia (AML) in various types of immunodeficient mouse models. Note that the optimal host (nu/nu, SCID, etc.) varies with tumor type, for reasons that are not understood. In all instances, the survival of patients from whom the transplantable neoplastic cells were de-

rived was only weeks to months, and all died in relapse.

Model systems are useful for initial establishment of a technique, for comparisons of various techniques, and for calibration of techniques in terms of defined cell lines. However, the sensitivity of assays performed using model systems represents the best that can be achieved with that particular method and likely overestimates the sensitivity of the same technique applied to patient samples. For example, in immunocytochemical studies, the staining characteristics of the added tumor cell line can be optimized, and positive- and negative-stained controls are available for comparative purposes. In patient samples, a positive preparation is often not as convincingly positive as the positive control, and the background staining is more variable. In culture studies, the tumor cell lines employed are culture adapted and most probably amplify faster than fresh primary or metastatic tumor cells. Again, this is likely to lead to an overestimate of sensitivity of the technique. However, there are many established techniques using model systems. Studies in the future should emphasize evaluation of patient samples and clinical outcome. This information may be employed prospectively to plan the optimum therapy and improve overall patient outcome.

SPECIFIC DISEASE EXAMPLES

Solid Tumors

BREAST CANCER

The primary approach for the detection of breast cancer micrometastases in bone marrow has been the use of monoclonal antibodies (MoAb) to epithelial-cell-associated antigens that have minimal cross-reactivity with cells normally present in the marrow. The detection systems have employed fluorescence microscopy, immunocytochemistry and, to a lesser extent, flow cytometry.

The pioneering studies of investigators at the Ludwig Institute in London (31, 32) showed that in a study of 110 women with primary breast cancer, tumor cells were observed in bone marrow by immunocytochemistry for epithelial membrane antigen (EMA) in 31 patients (28%) who had no other evidence of metastases. Patients for whom conventional criteria indicated a poor prognosis were more likely to have EMA-positive cells in their marrow. Subsequently, this group reported the outcome of 307 patients with primary breast cancer (33). Micrometastases were found in 81 cases (26.4%). The presence of micrometastases was related to other poor prognostic factors such as spread to lymph nodes, vascular invasion, T stage, and pathologic size. With a median follow-up of 28 months, 75 patients had relapsed, 60 at

distant sites. Of these 60, 26 had micrometastases at presentation. They concluded that the relapse-free-interval was significantly shorter for patients with micrometastases, and these patients had a shorter survival. However, the usefulness of this aproach has been disputed. Blamey et al. (34) claim that when the other prognostic variables were taken into account, the prognostic value of EMA-positive cells in marrow was eliminated.

In response to this criticism, Untch et al. (35) reported their observations employing a cocktail of MoAbs to EMA and cytokeratin. Their study involved 68 patients, and they found 25 (36.7%) with marrow micrometastases. There was a correlation with T stage but not menopausal state. They also, unlike Mansi et al. (33), found a correlation with the presence of estrogen receptors but not with spread to lymph nodes. Mansi et al. (13) then reported a further follow-up of 350 patients with a median of 35 months, including studies in which repeat multiple marrow aspirates were obtained from a subset of 82 patients. Micrometastases were found in 26% of patients at the time of the initial surgery. When multiple marrow aspirates were obtained in the subset at a median time of 18 months after surgery but prior to "overt relapse," patients with no evidence of disease had a low incidence of micrometastases (2%–3%), but in patients with local recurrence, the incidence of micrometastases was 3 of 16 (19%), with distant disease other than in bone 3 of 10 (30%) and in 19 of 19 (100%) of patients with radiologically proven bone disease. They concluded that many micrometastases are the result of shedding of cells from the primary carcinoma, and that a portion are not viable. They also noted that this technique was insufficiently sensitive to accurately monitor adjuvant therapy in breast cancer patients. Ceci et al. (36) studied bone marrow biopsies on 173 unselected breast cancer patients and concluded that positive bone x-rays and scans correlated better than marrow biopsies to metastatic disease.

Other investigators have attempted similar approaches although generally with small patient groups. Giai et al. (37) found 2 of 45 (4%) patients positive, confirming the observation of others that a single bone marrow sample is inadequate for accurate evaluation of the presence of micrometastases. A similar conclusion was reached by Mathieu et al. (38). Ellis et al. (39) studied bilateral aspirates of 25 patients and found 4 positive (16%) but with no correlation with disease stage. Ginsbourg et al. (40) combined immunofluorescence for mammary epithelial antigens with a MoAb to bromodeoxyuridine to study bone marrow samples from 200 patients with breast cancer after a period of 30 minutes of in vitro culture with bromodeoxyuridine. This technique should permit not only detection of metastatic cells but also an assessment of their DNA-synthetic phase fraction. They reported that mammary cells could be detected in the marrow of 60% of cases studied, and 50% had a high labeling index. This is the highest frequency of marrow contamination reported and raises some methodologic concerns. Clinical outcome was not reported.

One possible reason for the wide variability in outcome is that the tumor cells vary in their reactivity with the MoAbs used in the detection system (19). Additionally, the patients are not of uniform disease stage. Because most of the above studies have been performed at initial diagnosis, the data tend to be biased to early stages of disease, which makes correlation with stage difficult to detect, particularly in studies with small patient numbers. Clearly, studies of single aspirates or biopsy specimens contribute little because the sampling is inadequate. Furthermore, in the above studies, no attempt has been made, other than in limited model studies, to estimate the frequency at which tumor cells are being detected.

These issues have been addressed in some recent studies. Cote and colleagues have employed a fluorescent antibody technique to detect cytokeratin-positive cells in marrow aspirates (41). They attempted to estimate the frequency of detection of cells in the marrow

sample both by estimating the number of positive cells and by using a model system. They found that none of 44 control bone marrows showed positive cells. However, antigen-positive cells were present in the marrow of 35% (18 of 51) patients with operable breast cancer in which no abnormal cells were seen by routine bone marrow cytology. We have employed long-term culture of bone marrow samples to detect breast cancer cells in bone marrow harvests. This technique amplifies the tumor cells from the cell population scraped from the stainless steel screens used to filter the entire marrow harvest. It permits their detection in part because of the loss of the majority of differentiated cells during the culture period and, based on the observation that after culture the tumor cells appear as small clumps that are usually not observed in the initial sample, probably by growth of the cells. We estimate that this technique detects breast cancer cells in bone marrow at about 1 in 10^5 nucleated cells. Using this technique with samples from patients with stage I, II or III disease or with locally or regionally recurrent disease, we have found that 50% of the culture-positive patients have recurred with metastatic disease, compared to 8.5% of the culture negative patients ($P \leq$ .05, log rank test) (42).

Employing the same model system of MCF-7 breast cancer cells added to normal bone marrow, the immunofluorescence technique of the Sloan-Kettering group (43) and our culture method give similar sensitivities of detection of about one tumor cell in 10^6 bone marrow cells. This is probably one log greater than the sensitivity applied to patient samples. Because of the similar sensitivities of the methods, we believe we can combine the Sloan-Kettering data, which have a greater proportion of stage I and II patients, with our data, which are biased toward stage III patients. The results are shown in Table 14.1. It is also possible to compare the clinical outcome from the two studies for all patients who are lymph node positive (LN[pos]) and either bone marrow negative (BM[neg]) or positive

Table 14.1. Frequency of Suspected Tumor Cell Contamination of Histologically Normal Bone Marrow of Patients with Breast Cancer at Various Stages[a]

Frequency (Patients with Tumor Cells Detected/Total)	Clinical Stage of Disease			
	I	II	III	IV—With No Other Evidence of Marrow Involvement
Number	4/16	21/50	8/14	7/13
(%)	25%	42%	57%	54%

[a]From combined data from Cote RJ, Rosen PP, Hakes TB, et al. Monoclonal antibodies detect occult breast carcinoma metastases in the bone marrow of patients with early stage disease. Am J Surg Pathol 1988;12:333–340; and Sharp JG, Vaughan WP, Kessinger A, et al. Significance of detection of tumor cells in hematopoietic stem cell harvests of patients with breast cancer. In: Dicke KA, Armitage JO, Dicke-Evinger MJ, eds. Autologous bone marrow transplantation, V. Omaha: University of Nebraska Medical Center, 1991:385–391.

Table 14.2. Influence of Bone Marrow Positivity on Clinical Outcome for Untransplanted Lymph Node–Positive Patients with Breast Cancer[a,b]

Status	Sloan Kettering		Nebraska		Combined	
	Relapsed Total	%	Relapsed Total	%	Relapsed Total	%
LN[pos] BM[neg]	1/14	7	1/11	9	2/25	8
LN[pos] BM[pos]	6/12	50	7/15	47	13/27	48

[a]Data from Cote RJ, Rosen PP, Lesser ML, et al. Detection of occult bone marrow micrometastases (BMM) in patients with operable breast cancer predicts early recurrence. Proc US Cancer Acad Pathol 1990;23A (Sloan Kettering); and Sharp JG, Vaughan WP, Kessinger A, et al. Significance of detection of tumor cells in hematopoietic stem cell harvests of patients with breast cancer. In: Dicke K, Armitage JO, Dicke-Evinger MJ, eds. Autologous bone marrow transplantation, V. Omaha: University of Nebraska Medical Center, 1991:385–391 (Nebraska).
[b]Median follow-up at least 30 months.

(BM[pos]) and not transplanted (44). These data are presented in Table 14.2.

The data in Tables 14.1 and 14.2 show that bone marrow positivity established by sensitive techniques is a frequent occurrence in women with breast cancer. Up to one quarter of the patients with stage I disease and cytologically normal-appearing bone marrow have tumor cells in their marrow detected by these techniques. This suggests that although lymphatic spread clearly is the more common route of spread of breast cancer, at least some tumors spread directly by a hema-

togenous route. The clinical outcome for these patients is not known because this group is too small for analysis. However, the group of stage II and III patients (LN[pos]) is large enough for analysis. There is an excellent correspondence between two separate studies of these patients (Table 14.2). The BM[pos] patients in this group are about six times more likely to relapse within about 3 years than BM[neg] negative patients. Clearly, the data raise concerns over the likelihood of reinfusing tumor if high-dose therapy is combined with ABMT for these patients. Currently, there is no absolute evidence that reinfusion of such cells will lead to reestablishment of tumor or early systemic relapse in such patients. This is a risk whose frequency and significance are not yet known. There is a hint that not all breast tumor cells lead to metastatic disease (13). At the same time it is possible that reinfusion of tumor cells may, in some instances, cause the death of the patient.

In summary, immunofluorescence or immunocytochemical detection of breast cancer cells in bone marrow can be applied successfully and appears to be more sensitive than morphologic analysis, although historically this has been controversial. However, this approach *must be applied to multiple marrow aspirates* and/or biopsies to increase the likelihood of finding positive cells and accurately evaluating their frequency. This technique can also be applied to marrow harvests, but unless these harvests are cultured for a period of several weeks to amplify the tumor cells, it is necessary to examine a large number of cells (approximately 10^6) to achieve sensitivity. When a highly sensitive technique is applied to a moderate number of patient samples (30 patients plus) or a less-sensitive technique to a much larger patient sample (several hundred), a correlation is seen both between marrow positivity and stage and clinical outcome. A proportion of patients (perhaps up to 25%) classified clinically as stage I already have metastatic disease in marrow, and women whose marrow is initially negative can develop marrow metastases after local recurrence of their tumor. Women who are both LN^{pos} and BM^{pos} are six times more likely to relapse within 3 years than women who were BM^{neg}. ABMT in breast cancer carries a significant likelihood of reinfusing tumor cells, although the clinical relevance of this risk is currently unknown. *A thorough evaluation of the marrow of breast cancer patients at all stages for tumor cell contamination is justified* and will likely lead to more accurate staging and therefore the most appropriate selection of therapy and optimal clinical result.

COLON CANCER

Only limited studies have been performed to determine the frequency and importance of bone marrow contamination in colon cancer. Because of the relative refractoriness of the primary tumor to most types of high-dose therapy and probable metastatic spread in advanced cases to abdominal lymph nodes, liver, and elsewhere, there has not been a major interest in the detection of marrow contamination. However, if new and improved high-dose regimens can be devised, this will become an important task. The detection of marrow metastases in colon cancer could be of relevance in studies employing MoAbs to target radioisotopes, toxins, or drugs to the tumor. Studies by Schlimok et al. (45) employing MoAbs to cytokeratins and the 17-1A antigen and Schneider et al. (46) employing a MoAb to cytokeratin component 18 concluded that the immunocytologic approach was superior to conventional cytology. The former study indicated 8 of 39 (20.5%) colon cancer patients with no clinical evidence of metastatic disease (stage M_0) and who were cytologically BM^{neg} had immunocytochemically detectable epithelial cells that were likely tumor cells in their marrow, since such cells were not seen in 75 normal controls. In colon cancer, as in breast cancer, the frequency of marrow positivity correlated with lymph node positivity in that 2 of 22 (9.1%) of lymph-node-negative (LN^{neg}) pa-

tients had tumor cells in marrow, compared to 6 of 17 (35.3%) of LN^{pos} patients ($P \leq .05$). Also, 9 of 17 patients with cytokeratin-positive cells in their marrow also had 17-1A positive cells in their marrow. Schneider et al. (46) reported that 14 of 61 (23%) of stage M_0 patients had cytokeratin-positive cells in their marrow. The frequency of marrow contamination in LN^{neg} patients was 2 of 31 (6%) and in LN^{pos} patients 12 of 30 (40%). Both of these studies concluded that the incidence of tumor cell contamination of bone marrow was correlated with conventional risk factors such as tumor size, lymph node involvement, and the presence of distant metastases. The specific clinical outcome for BM^{pos} versus BM^{neg} patients appears not to have been reported. Although the clinical significance of these findings is unknown, these data must be considered when applying therapies that target tumor cells and are locally toxic, such as radioimmunotherapy, and might lead to enhanced localization in marrow with increased hematologic toxicity.

LUNG CANCER

Bone marrow metastases of lung cancer, like breast cancer metastases, have been detected using immunocytochemical and culture techniques. Lung tumor cells, similar to breast cancer cells as well as some other epithelial tumor cells, appear to have an affinity in culture for marrow stromal cells (8, 9). Hunter et al (47) employed discontinuous gradients to process histologically negative bone marrow from 36 patients with small cell lung cancer (SCLC) for a tumor culture assay. Tumor colony growth was observed in 8 of 36 (22%) of these patients. The clinical outcome for these patients was not reported. Hay et al. (48) in Edinburgh employed a panel of MoAbs useful for detecting SCLC that did not cross-react significantly with normal marrow elements. They reported that this approach markedly increased the detection of marrow micrometastases. There was a close correlation between immunolocytochemical positivity and the ability to grow SCLC-like cells in culture. They reported clinical outcome for a limited sample of patients with short follow-up. Of 10 patients studied, 2 were BM^{neg} and had not relapsed at 6 or 10 months. Five of the 8 BM^{pos} patients relapsed within 2–6 months. In contrast, tenVelde et al. (49) investigated whether immunohistochemical analysis of routinely processed bone marrow biopsy specimens could detect marrow metastases more effectively than conventional microscopy. They found that immunohistochemistry did not yield any additional tumor positive cases (to those detected by conventional microscopy) and further that histologic evaluation of a bone marrow biopsy specimen, even by immunohistochemistry, did not contribute information relevant for staging, therapy evaluation, or prognosis of SCLC. A subsequent report by the Edinburgh group (50) described the use of immunocytochemistry to detect SCLC-like cells in the marrow of 8 of 12 patients who were disease-free by conventional criteria. These probably include the 10 patients discussed above; however, this is not apparent from the authors' report. Six of the 12 patients ultimately relapsed. Two of the 4 patients with negative marrows also relapsed. In serum-free cultures, samples from 9 of the 12 patients grew SCLC-like colonies. The authors concluded that "bone marrow positivity using these techniques appears to predict a high risk of metastatic relapse regardless of further therapy." Based on the available data, we feel this is a strong overstatement of the case. The evidence that immunocytochemical detection of tumor cell contamination of the marrow in patients with SCLC predicts clinical outcome needs additional study. As noted for breast cancer, it is important that multiple aspirates/biopsies be studied in a sufficient number of patients with adequate follow-up.

In summary, there are indications that in SCLC immunocytochemical or culture techniques can detect tumor cells in histologically negative marrows. Although there are hints that this information might be relevant clinically, currently the data are inadequate to reach such a conclusion. Additional studies of this topic are warranted.

NEUROBLASTOMA

Because about 65% of children with neuroblastoma present with disseminated disease at diagnosis, there has long been an interest in techniques for the detection of neuroblastoma cells contaminating marrow and purging techniques to eliminate these to permit high-dose therapy with ABMT (51). Favrot et al. (52) compared histologic, cytologic, and immunologic analyses for the detection of neuroblastoma cells in bone marrow *employing multiple core biopsies and aspirates.* There was a difference in sensitivity of detection between the core biopsies (more frequently positive [63%] than the aspirates [13%]. In 24% of the cases, both were positive. In only 1 of 33 pathologic cases was marrow involvement diagnosed on a core biopsy imprint preparation. These authors concluded that the immunocytochemical method of tumor cell detection was more sensitive. Essentially similar conclusions were reached by Gussetis et al. (53). They were able to detect neuroblastoma cells in bone marrow in 11 of 16 patients by immunocytochemical techniques, whereas marrow biopsies on 6 of these patients were normal. Aspirates stained conventionally were only positive in 3 patients.

The clinical relevance of immunocytologic detection of bone marrow contamination by neuroblastoma cells has recently been reported (54). In a study of 197 patients with newly diagnosed neuroblastoma, routine marrow examination for tumor contamination was positive in 46% of patients, whereas immunocytologic studies detected tumor in 67%. Immunocytologic study detected bone marrow metastases in 34% of patients diagnosed clinically with only localized or regional disease. Patients over 1 year of age with marrow metastases did more poorly ($P = .006$) than those without marrow metastases.

Patients with stage IV disease did more poorly if there was a large number of tumor cells (greater than 0.02%) in their marrow (P = .03). The authors concluded that the immunocytochemical analysis of bone marrow was a more sensitive predictor of clinical outcome than conventional analysis.

An alternative to ABMT for rescue from the marrow aplasia and blood cytopenias following high-dose therapy is PSCT. In this regard, Moss et al. (55) examined blood samples drawn from neuroblastoma patients at the time of marrow sampling and studied these blood samples by the same immunocytologic technique. They observed tumor cells in 75% of specimens at diagnosis, 36% during therapy, and in 14% of PSCT harvests. Six of 13 patients with minimal or no marrow involvement had positive blood specimens. Consequently, in neuroblastoma, there appears to be a significant risk of tumor cell contamination in PSCT harvests, and they recommended that chemotherapy be administered before peripheral blood stem cell (PSC) collection. No data on clinical outcome of PSCT in neuroblastoma with or without tumor cell contamination were reported.

In summary, immunocytochemical detection of marrow contamination by neuroblastoma cells is more sensitive than conventional techniques. Patients with marrow contamination do significantly less well than patients without marrow contamination. Patients with stage IV disease and extensive marrow contamination (>0.02% tumor cells) do less well than patients with lesser amounts of marrow contamination. PSC collections from neuroblastoma patients have a significant likelihood of being contaminated with tumor cells, although the clinical relevance of these cells has not been determined.

Leukemias

Since both leukemia and lymphoma represent neoplastic diseases of cell types whose normal counterparts may be found in the blood or marrow, the ability to detect cancerous cells against a background of normal cells with very similar phenotypes has always been a problem. The increasing use of autologous hematopoietic transplantation has rekindled the need to identify morphologically indistinct cells that may be present at a very low frequency and, if transplanted, lead to a significant adverse outcome in the patient. Leukemias are, by concensus, most likely to be present in marrow and blood, even when the patient is in remission. This has led to the extensive use of purging of autologous transplants in leukemia and the parallel need to employ sensitive detection approaches on the hematopoietic product both before and after purging procedures. Since there is a range of leukemias that are treated by high-dose therapy and/or transplantation or cytokine treatment, this section will consider them individually.

ACUTE LYMPHOCYTIC LEUKEMIA

The detection of minimal residual disease in acute lymphocytic leukemia (ALL) has received a major share of the attention in recent years. Part of this focus is related to its relatively common nature and overall good prognosis for all but a small "high-risk" group, including many T-ALLs. To identify this group of patients, routine phenotyping employing surfacer markers and DNA flow cytometry, cytogenetics, and leukemic colony assays can now be extended with a variety of molecular approaches. Specialized flow cytometric techniques have been reported by several groups (15, 56, 57). The report that terminal deoxynucleotidyl transferase (TdT) can be quantitatively detected using two-color flow cytometric methods and standard surface markers (CD5, CD15, CD10) may allow this approach to efficiently follow or screen potential T-ALL-containing samples (15). In standardization assays with mixed normal and leukemic patient samples, the detection limit for this method was reported to be 3.5 cells/ 10,000 (15). Equivalent sensitivity recently has been reported by another group using a similar two-color flow method (58).

The ability to follow unique gene rearrangements of clonally derived neoplastic cells of the T and B lymphoid lineages has provided a new and sensitive method to evaluate MRD in leukemic patients. If the technique is applied to marrow or blood without any additional technical preparation, the detection limit has been reported to be in the range of 2%–5% (59). Modifications to this technique that include an immunoselection step prior to the Southern analysis extended the detection limit to approximately 1 in 10^3 marrow cells for T-ALL (60). The further addition of PCR to sample DNA prior to Southern analysis has, in a number of laboratories, extended the detection limit even further to 1 in 10^4 or 10^6 cells (57, 61, 62). It should be pointed out, however, that the PCR of such samples may lead to false-negative results, particularly where samples contain heterogenous (oligoclonal) heavy chain gene rearrangements in precursor-B-ALL. Since TCR and γ and δ genes also rearrange in about 60% of these samples, probes for these regions may be more reliable, even in precursor-B-ALL (63).

CHRONIC LYMPHOCYTIC LEUKEMIA

In view of the slowly progressing course of this disease, less effort has been directed at the detection and quantitation of MRD. However, considering the emerging relevance of early detection of MRD in the more aggressive leukemias, recent efforts to apply these techniques to chronic lymphocytic leukemia (CLL) have appeared. The monoclonal nature of CLL allows the examination of samples for unique gene rearrangements, chromosome abnormalities, surface phenotype, or some combination of these characteristics. The use of $SIg_{\kappa/\lambda}$ ratios alone for estimating excess clonality appeared to correlate well with duration of remission (e.g., normal ratios associated with extended remission; 64). In most of these same patients, however, the persistence of the neoplastic clone could be detected by the more sensitive DNA probing techniques. This emphasizes the difficulty in

completely eliminating the CLL clone(s) and suggests that the long-term follow-up of such patient populations may ultimately be more revealing if correlated to repeated DNA analysis.

ACUTE MYELOGENOUS LEUKEMIA

As with most hematologic malignancies, marrow smears and biopsies form the primary basis of diagnosis, classification, and monitoring of the neoplastic cells. In the case of MRD, however, these methods become less sensitive, especially when the marrow is hypoplastic. Trephine biopsy was shown to be necessary in such cases to accurately describe the nature and extent of the disease (65). In parallel to morphologic evaluation, extensive evaluation of the classification of AML using MoAbs has been reviewed recently by Foon et al. (66). The majority of the studies acknowledge that the surface molecules detected on AML cells are not unique to the leukemic clones and are shared by various normal cell types in the marrow and blood. Like other lymphohematopoietic cancers, however, when a panel of reagents is combined with morphologic evaluation, it is possible to gain insights into the phenotype(s) of the malignant cells (67–69). The heterogeneous nature of AML clones appears to correlate with the similar distribution of normal myeloid precursors. In some of these studies, the AML cells were distinguished by their unique level of expression of CD34 (My-10) and Vim-2 (69). Indeed, using a flow cytometric approach combined with sorting and subsequent mitotic analysis, the investigators were able to detect AML cells with a sensitivity of 10^{-2}–10^{-3}. As a final point, AML is one of the few lymphohematopoietic malignancies with an accepted animal parallel, the Brown Norway rat myelogenous leukemia (BNML), used in a variety of experimental models to detect MRD and assess therapeutic effectiveness (70). In the BNML system, the nonhomogeneous distribution of the disease (12) and application of flow cytometric approaches to detect

MRD (71) paralleled the findings in patients and provides a useful tool for further studies.

CHRONIC MYELOGENOUS LEUKEMIA

Chronic myelogenous leukemia (CML) is a myeloproliferative disease characterized commonly by a reciprocal translocation between chromosomes 9 and 22 (i.e., t[9; 22] that results in the presence of the Philadelphia chromosome (Ph^1). Since the chromosomal alteration is present in all hematopoietic lineages, the malignancy is considered to occur at the level of the stem cell. After variable periods of time, the disease loses its maturing phenotype and enters into an acute or blast phase that resembles acute leukemia of either lymphoid or myeloid lineages. The response of these different presentations varies widely; thus it is important to be able to accurately assess the presence and phenotype of any MRD following therapy.

Until recently, the presence of the Ph^1 clone was the primary confirmation of residual disease (72). In the past few years, however, emphasis has been placed on applying combined cytogenetic and molecular cytogenetic approaches (73). Although the appearance of the Ph^1 chromosome and *bcr/abl* rearranged transcripts can be followed by cytogenetic and Southern blot analysis, these approaches have limited sensitivity (74). The application of the PCR to amplify the specific *bcr/abl* mRNA has extended the sensitivity of detection (75). Indeed, the results of PCR analysis of both blood and marrow samples have correlated well with the clinical status of the patients. In a study of long-term (5–7 years) cytogenetic and hematologic remission patients, Morgan et al. were not able to find evidence of the *bcr/abl* leukemic transcripts and thus considered these patients "truly cured" (76). Arnold et al. (77), Martiat et al. (78), and Hughes et al. (79) have reported similar correlation between PCR analysis and clinical (relapse/remission) status of the patient. Unfortunately, the PCR technique is technically demanding and subject to significant criticism (80, 81). This has led in turn to new PCR approaches that are more rapid and reliable in the diagnosis of Ph^1-positive disease (82).

Unlike some other tumors that grow in culture, CML does not appear to have this capacity to any significant extent. Indeed, the loss of CML clones in culture has led to the use of prior short-term culture for purging neoplastic cells prior to transplant (83). The long-term effectiveness of this procedure is yet to be determined.

ACUTE NONLYMPHOCYTIC LEUKEMIA

The absence of leukemic-specific antibodies in this disease category, like many others, significantly limits the ability to detect malignant clones. Critical morphologic approaches, however, have been reported to identify patients with residual marrow leukemic cells posttherapy (84). Additionally, acute nonlymphocytic leukemia (ANLL) cells are among the few neoplastic types that may be uniquely detected by in vitro clonal assays. Findley et al. (85) have reported that the in vitro clonal growth characteristics of childhood ANLL studied in soft agar assay correlate well with the response to therapy and may identify a subset of patients with poor prognosis. However, there are no reports that propose theoretical or present actual detection limits for such cells.

HAIRY CELL LEUKEMIA

Hairy cell leukemia (HCL) is a chronic lymphoproliferative disorder of B cells characterized by an infiltration of morphologically unique cells into the marrow and spleen. The cells appear to represent preplasma cells bearing a characteristic set of surface markers (66, 86). The ability to identify HCL cells by sampling combined with MoAb reagents has prompted a number of studies related to detecting MRD in the blood and marrow of such patients.

The hypocellular marrow of patients, which is typical following therapy, prevents the characteristic morphology of HCL from being a reliable screening method for residual disease. On the other hand, in the same group of patients, marrow biopsies and aspirates have been studied extensively with a variety of different MoAbs. Most of the reagents were not described as being completely specific for HCL cells; however, unique combinations of surface marker positivity, particularly when it involved the "HCL-associated trimeric protein," were relatively specific (87–90). Among this latter group of reagents, positive reaction with the B-Ly7 MoAb was superior to all other antibodies or morphologically related techniques for identifying HCL. Identification of as little as 1%–2% B-Ly7-positive cells in the marrow was suggested to be strongly indicative of residual marrow infiltration of the HCL (normal BM approximately 0.3%+). This could be an even more selective probe when combined with HCL morphologic characteristics (90). However, the use of MoAbs directed against the HCL trimeric protein is only indicated when 100% of the HCL cells are positive at initial diagnosis (approximately 75% of the HCL cases) (89). Since it is known that the B-Ly7 MoAb retains its reactivity for HCL after interferon treatment of the patient, it can be an effective tool for monitoring disease status in these patients.

Lymphomas

NON-HODGKIN'S LYMPHOMA

Lymphoma cells also are difficult for the pathologist to detect in bone marrow because of the overlap of their morphology and surface markers with normal cells. Consequently, they are not usually detectable using conventional light microscopy with aspirates until the tumor cells are several percent of the total cells (15). There appear to be no differences in sensitivity between biopsies and aspirates from iliac crests providing bilateral biopsies were obtained, but sternal aspirates gave a greater sensitivity of detection of marrow involvement (91). Inhomogeneity of marrow involvement with disease probably complicates detection and emphasizes the need for multiple biopsies (12). Flow cytometric analysis of these populations is also complicated by heterogeneity (92) and the overlap in phenotype of the lymphoma cells and normal cells. Flow cytometry can provide a clue about the presence of a B cell tumor if there is dominance of a clone expressing a particular light chain. Generally, the sensitivity of Southern analysis for detecting a clonal T cell receptor or immunoglobulin heavy chain rearrangement is about 1%–2% when applied with DNA standards expressing a known rearrangement. These techniques applied alone are only slightly more sensitive (fivefold at best) than the pathologist can achieve by visual inspection. Consequently, a number of other approaches have been attempted to try and increase the sensitivity of detection of NHL. These have included the use of various culture techniques (23, 93) and attempts to use immune selection (18) or PCR (94) to increase the sensitivity of the molecular approaches.

Benjamin et al. (93) presented evidence based on an in vitro culture technique that at least 17% of normal-appearing bone marrow cells from patients with undifferentiated lymphomas contained occult tumor cells. Smith et al. (95) also noted, using a soft agar colony assay, that 6 of 35 histologically negative bone marrow specimens showed lymphoma growth. Lymphoma colony growth was associated statistically with both a short duration of complete remission and a short duration of survival. Philip et al. (96) and Favrot and Herve (59) have also described a liquid culture system that permits the sensitive detection of Burkitt's lymphoma cells. This technique has been used to monitor purging procedures.

We have employed a period of liquid culture in the presence of a mixed growth factor preparation to amplify lymphoid populations. Samples from these cultures were subjected to Southern analysis and/or immunophenotyping by flow cytometry. Any clonal populations that become evident are compared to and must match those of the patient's original tumor (97). Confirmation of the malignant nature of the cells was attempted by growth in an immunodeficient (nude or SCID) mouse model (29). Generally, only more aggressive lymphomas will grow readily in nude mice (98). As new techniques to immunosuppress or tolerize such mice to human cells are developed, potentially a wider group of tumors can be studied by this approach. With this method, about one-third of histologically normal appearing marrow harvests contained NHL cells. As shown in Table 14.3, the presence of such cells was associated with a higher relapse rate in recipients of high-dose therapy and ABMT. Surprisingly, the relapses in the ABMT group were largely associated with sites of prior bulky disease rather than with systemic relapses that one would have anticipated if reinfused tumor cells were the cause of relapse. This suggests that either reinfused tumor cells home to sites of prior disease or, alternatively, that marrow positivity is simply an indicator of biologically more aggressive disease. We suspect the latter hypothesis is correct. In terms of population size, the reinfused tumor cells are small in number compared to the likely number of tumor cells that survive even high-dose therapy in patients with bulky disease (97, 99).

Bregni et al. (18) employed immunoselection to enrich the proportion of malignant cells in the sample prior to application

of Southern analysis. They have reported the ability to detect marrow relapses in 4 of 7 patients with ALL 1.5 to 9 months prior to hematologic relapse. This technique does not appear to have been applied extensively in NHL. PCR has been used to detect samples containing t(14:18) NHL cells (100). This technique was used to monitor purging in a model system.

In summary, marrow contamination in NHL can be detected at a level of about 1% by Southern analysis under ideal conditions. This sensitivity can be increased by up to two logs by a period of in vitro culture prior to the application of Southern analysis. The tumor cells detected by this approach are clinically relevant since patients who are marrow positive have a poorer outcome without or with ABMT.

HODGKIN'S DISEASE

The exact nature, origins, and lineage derivation of the malignant cell of Hodgkin's disease (HD), the Reed-Sternberg (R-S) cell, are still highly controversial (101–105). In our studies of apheresis harvests from HD patients placed into long-term culture, we have noted that in about a third of cases the cultures develop a mononuclear cell population at 3–6 weeks that immunocytochemically is CD30 positive, with some cells also CD15 positive. Such cultures accumulate large uninucleate and binucleate cells with this phenotype, which morphologically resemble R-S

Table 14.3. Influence of Marrow Positivity on Clinical Outcome of Non-Hodgkin's Lymphoma Patients Undergoing High-Dose Therapy and Transplantation

Marrow Status	Intermediate & High-Grade NHL Predicted 3-Year Survival		Poor Prognosis NHL (all grades) Predicted 5-Year Survival			
	Poor Prognosis Achieving CR[a] with ABMT	All Patients[b]	Achieving CR[a] with ABMT	All Patients[b]	Achieving CR[a] with PSCT	All Patients[b]
—	77%	22%	50%	14%	N/A	N/A
+	9%	2%	27%	7%	83%	50%

[a]Analysis was restricted to patients who achieved a complete clinical remission (CR) in order to be able to detect the influence of occult tumor in the harvest on outcome.
[b]Includes patients who had treatment-related mortality or failed to achieve a CR. These data are included to provide a realistic comparison of overall outcomes.

cells. The cultures go on, long-term, to generate B cells that can be clonal, but since different clones arise in different cultures from the same patient, they are initially polyclonal in most cases. It is likely that Epstein-Barr virus (EBV) and/or human herpes virus-6 (HHV-6) is involved in the generation of these B cells (106). The relevance of these cells to HD tumors is currently uncertain; however, EBV genome is present with a high incidence in HD tissues (107, 108). Also, HHV-6 has been detected in a small proportion of Hodgkin's lymphomas (109).

In the absence of specific markers of R-S cells, it is essentially impossible to confirm the presence of HD in bone marrow other than by histologic techniques. Since it appears that R-S cells can be potent cytokine producers (110), many of the cells associated with R-S cells were originally normal cells and their progeny. In the presence of sustained proliferative stimuli as seen with the cultured cells, these can be driven to clonal expansion and, potentially, expression of generally random chromosome abnormalities. This would account for the lack of consistency in reports of gene rearrangements (111–114) and chromosome abnormalities (115). Our studies of R-S-like cells obtained in culture have not been helpful in predicting clinical outcome for HD patients since the actuarial 3-year survival for patients with or without these cells is the same. It appears that the only report currently that indicates that marrow contamination in HD as determined by conventional techniques is clinically significant is that of Kessinger et al. (116). They reported the outcome of HD patients who underwent high-dose therapy and PSCT either because of histologically evident marrow involvement, prior pelvic irradiation, or inadequate marrow harvests. The patients who underwent PSCT because of marrow involvement had a poorer outcome than patients without marrow involvement, suggesting marrow involvement was a significant detrimental prognostic indicator. Note that the overall survival of these patients was at least as good as that observed for similar patients who underwent ABMT.

In summary, since there are no specific markers that can be used to positively identify the malignant R-S cell of HD, current detection of marrow contamination is limited to conventional histologic examination. There are limited clinical data to indicate that marrow contamination is a poor prognostic sign.

CONTAMINATION OF BLOOD STEM CELL COLLECTIONS

As described elsewhere (117), PSCT is being increasingly employed as an alternative to ABMT for rescue of patients from marrow aplasia and blood cytopenias attendant to high-dose therapy (3, 118, 119). Historically, it has been known that tumor cells can be found, on occasion, in the blood of patients (120–122). Only recently have studies been initiated to examine PSC harvests for the presence of tumor cells using sensitive methods similar to those employed to study bone marrow. In breast cancer, preliminary immunocytochemical studies and culture studies (19, 123) have been attempted. These studies confirm that breast tumor cells are present in the blood of some patients. However, the overall incidence of patients with tumor cells in their blood appears to be lower than in bone marrow (19% versus 52%).

In NHL, direct comparison by Southern analysis of blood and bone marrow in a small series of 5 patients showed that although 2 of the 5 patients had clonal rearrangements detectable in their bone marrow, none were detected in their blood (124). In culture studies of apheresis harvests (PSC) of NHL patients, only 1 of 20 (5%) were positive for tumor cells. The recipient of this harvest failed to achieve a complete remission after high-dose therapy and died after 78 days. In contrast, recipients of negative PSC harvests who achieved a complete remission had an 83% actuarial survival (Table 14.3) even though they had positive marrows (106). Overall, such patients had a significantly better outcome than recipients of marrow (Table 14.3; see also 125).

In summary, although studies of tumor cell contamination of PSC harvests are in their infancy, techniques developed to study bone marrow contamination can be applied successfully. In breast cancer and NHL, preliminary data suggest that PSC harvests may be less likely to be contaminated with tumor cells than the bone marrow, and PSCT is associated with a better outcome in marrow-positive patients. It remains to be demonstrated that the use of such harvests will translate into a clinical benefit, although this appears possible.

CYTOKINES AND TUMOR CELL CONTAMINATION

Increasingly, cytokines such as erythropoietin (EPO), granulocyte colony-stimulating factor (G-CSF), and granulocyte-monocyte colony-stimulating factor (GM-CSF) are being employed to permit the escalation of chemotherapy doses without transplantation, to facilitate harvest of stem cells, and to accelerate recovery of hematopoiesis after transplantation. In general, it remains to be determined if the use of such factors will have an impact on marrow contamination. Two quite different scenarios can be envisaged. Many myeloid tumor cells have receptors for the colony-stimulating factors, as do some neuroectodermal and other tumors for GM-CSF. There is a concern that the use of these factors will stimulate tumor growth. As well as being a risk, this property might be employed positively for the patient by scheduling cycle-specific chemotherapy to kill the newly proliferating tumor cells. At the same time, factors such as GM-CSF can functionally activate macrophages and theoretically stimulate their antitumor effectiveness. There is much research to be done to assess the true risk:benefit ratio of the impact of cytokines on marrow contamination. At the present time, preliminary data are encouraging. In our studies of interleukin-3 (IL-3) in patients, largely with HD, we have seen no promotion of tumor growth in a small sample of six pa-

tients. Similarly, adverse reports of stimulation of tumor growth have been very few considering the large number of patients who have now been treated with cytokines. Nonetheless, the full spectrum of the in vivo effects of cytokines is not readily predicted on the basis of their effects in in vitro clonal assays, and there are reports of IL-3 and GM-CSF stimulation of tumor cell growth, predominantly epithelial cancers associated with the abdomen (126, 127). Caution should be the watchword in the current application of cytokines until more is known.

SUMMARY AND CONCLUSIONS

Marrow contamination may be the most important prognostic indicator of a poor outcome in breast cancer, NHL, HD, neuroblastoma, and possibly lung cancer in patients who achieve a remission with high-dose therapy. Occult marrow contamination can be detected using immunocytochemical, culture, or molecular techniques in histologically normal marrows. In poor-prognosis patients who are candidates for high-dose therapy and transplantation, the frequency of tumor-contaminated marrow is about 25%–50% for breast cancer patients, 33% for NHL patients, 46% for HD patients, 67% for neuroblastoma patients, and 50% for lung cancer patients. Molecular techniques, particularly PCR for translocated oncogene sequences, can detect minimal residual disease in many leukemia patients, including patients who appear clinically well. The absence of cells with such molecular abnormalities is a good prognostic sign, but the presence of small numbers of such cells may not be clinically important.

Despite the clinical evidence that marrow contamination is a poor prognostic indicator for patients undergoing high-dose cancer therapy, the mechanisms underlying these associations are not clear. If the straightforward concern that tumor cells capable of reestablishing disease were being reinfused in transplanted hematopoietic harvests was correct, we could predict a high incidence of early systemic relapses. For most transplanted patients, including those with documented marrow positivity, relapse in sites of preexisting disease and systemic relapse is rare. Furthermore, marrow-positive nontransplanted patients have similarly high relapse rates. Also, significant number of patients undergoing allotransplants relapse. Consequently, we postulate that marrow positivity is a surrogate indicator of biologically aggressive disease. Speculatively, stromal cells in the marrow microenvironment favor the maintenance of cells with or induce multidrug resistance. Careful attention to the negative influence of marrow contamination on outcome for patients undergoing high-dose therapy should permit the development of therapeutic protocols designed to further improve clinical outcome.

Acknowledgments

We acknowledge the American Cancer Society, the Nebraska Department of Health, and the National Institutes of Health (grants CA 46686, AI25820, and RR05908) for research support. We thank Mrs. Sally Mann and Ms. Joanne DeBoer for excellent technical assistance, Martin Bast and Jene Pierson and the Nebraska Lymphoma Project for data tracking, and Ms. Roberta Anderson for typing the manuscript. We thank our colleagues Anne Kessinger, M.D., William Haire, M.D., Elizabeth Reed, M.D., and Jule Vose, M.D. for helpful comments. This review was completed 8/28/91.

REFERENCES

1. Armitage JO. Bone marrow transplantation in the treatment of patients with lymphoma. Blood 1989;73:1749–1758.
2. Frei E III, Antman K, Teicher et al. Bone marrow autotransplantation for solid tumors—prospects. J Clin Oncol 1989;7:515–526.
3. Kessinger A, Armitage JO, Landmark JD, et al. Autologous peripheral hematopoietic stem cell transplantation restores hematopoietic function following marrow ablative therapy. Blood 1988;71:723–727.
4. Skipper HE. Criteria associated with destruction of leukemia and solid tumor cells in animals. Cancer Res 1987;27:2636–2645.
5. Spangrude GJ. Hematopoietic stem-cell differentiation. Curr Opinion Immunol 1991;3:171–178.
6. Gordon MY. Hemopoietic growth factors and receptors: bound and free. Cancer Cells 1991;3:127–133.
7. Chaudhary PM, Roninson IB. Expression and activity of P-glycoprotein, a multidrug efflux pump, in human hematopoietic cells. Cell 1991;66:85–94.
8. Zipori D, Krupsky M, Resnitzky P. Stromal cell effects on clonal growth of tumors. Cancer 1987; 60:1757–1762.
9. Strobel E-S, Stobel HG, Bross KJ, et al. Effects of human bone marrow stroma on the growth of human tumor cells. Cancer Res 1989;49:1001–1007.
10. Joshi SS, Novak DJ, Messbarger L, et al. Levels of detection of tumor cells in human bone marrow with or without prior culture. Bone Marrow Transplant 1990;6:179–183.
11. Kamby C, Guldhammer B, Vejborg I, et al. The presence of tumor cells in bone marrow at the time of first recurrence of breast cancer. Cancer 1987; 60:1306–1312.
12. Martens ACM, Schultz FW, Hagenbeek A. Nonhomogeneous distribution of leukemia in the bone marrow during minimal residual disease. Blood 1987;70:1073–1078.
13. Mansi JL, Berger U, McDonnell T, et al. The fate of bone marrow micrometastases in patients with primary breast cancer. J Clin Oncol 1989;7:445–449.
14. Sharp JG, Mann SL, Kessinger A, et al. Detection of occult breast cancer cells in cultured pretransplantation bone marrow. In: Dicke KA, Spitzer G, Jagannath S, eds. Autologous bone marrow transplantation, III. Houston: The University of Texas MD Anderson Cancer Center, 1987:497–502.
15. Gore SD, Kastan MB, Goodman SN, et al. Detection of minimal residual T cell acute lymphoblastic leukemia by flow cytometry. J Immunol Methods 1990;132:275–286.
16. Leslie DS, Johnston WW, Daly L, et al. Detection of breast carcinoma cells in human bone marrow using fluorescence-activated cell sorting and conventional cytology. Am J Clin Pathol 1990;94:8–13.
17. Serke S, Sauberlich S, Abe Y, et al. Analysis of CD34-positive hemopoietic progenitor cells from normal human adult peripheral blood: flow-cytometrical studies and in vitro colony (CFU-GM, BFU-E) assays. Ann Haematol 1991;62:45–53.
18. Bregni M, Siena S, Dalla-Favera R, et al. High sensitivity and specificity assay for detection of leukemia/lymphoma cells in human bone marrow. Ann NY Acad Sci 1987;511:473–482.
19. Taha M, Ordonez NG, Kulkarni S, et al. A monoclonal antibody cocktail for detection of micrometastatic tumor cells in the bone marrow of breast cancer patients. Bone Marrow Transplant 1989;4:297–303.
20. Naeim F, Gatti RA, Yunis JJ. Recent advances in diagnosis and classification of leukemias and lymphomas. Dis Markers 1990;8:231–264.

21. Evinger-Hodges MJ, Spinolo JA, Cox I, et al. Detection of minimal residual disease in acute myelogenous leukemia by RNA-in situ hybridization. In: Dicke K, Spitzer G, Jagannath S, Evinger-Hodges MJ, eds. Autologous bone marrow transplantation, IV. Houston: The University of Texas MD Anderson Cancer Center, 1989:179–186.

22. Ro J, El-Naggar A, Ro JY, et al. c-erB-2 amplification in node-negative human breast cancer. Cancer Res 1989;49:6941–6944.

23. Joshi SS, Kessinger A, Mann SL, et al. Detection of tumor cells in histologically normal bone marrow using culture techniques. Bone Marrow Transplant 1987;1:303–310.

24. Schiro R, Coutinho LH, Will A, et al. Growth of normal versus leukemic bone marrow cells in long term culture from acute lymphoblastic and myeloblastic leukemias. Blut 1990;61:267 270.

25. Pirruccello SJ, Lang MS, DeBoer J, et al. OMA-AML-1: a leukemic myeloid cell line with stem cell and spontaneously differentiating cell compartments. Blood 1991, submitted.

26. Gordon MY, Dowding CR, Riley GP, et al. Altered adhesive interactions with marrow stroma of haematopoietic progenitor cells in chronic myeloid leukaemia. Nature 1987;328:342–344.

27. Morten JEN, Hay JH, Steele CM, et al. Tumorigenicity of human lymphoblastoid cell lines, acquired during in vitro culture and associated with chromosome gains. Int J Cancer 1984;34:463–470.

28. Sun G, Koeffler HP, Gale RP, et al. Use of conditioned media in cell culture can mask cytogenetic abnormalities in acute leukemia. Cancer Genet Cytogenet 1990;46:107–113

29. Joshi SS, DeBoer JM, Strandjord SJ, et al. Characterization of a newly established human Burkitt's lymphoma cell line, OMA-BL-1. Int J Cancer 1991; 47:643–648.

30. Giovanella BC, Vardeman DM, Williams LJ, et al. Heterotransplantation of human breast carcinomas in nude mice. Correlation between successful heterotransplants, poor prognosis and amplification of the Her-2/neu oncogene. Int J Cancer 1991;47:66–71.

31. Neville AM. Some immunobiochemical approaches for the detection of metastases. Invasion Metastasis 1982;2:2–11.

32. Redding WH, Monaghan P, Imrie SF, et al. Detection of micrometastases in patients with primary breast cancer. Lancet, 1983;2:1271–1274.

33. Mansi JL, Berger U, Easton D, et al. Micrometastases in bone marrow in patients with primary breast cancer: evaluation as an early predictor of bone metastases. Br Med J 1987;295:1093–1096.

34. Blamey RW, Robertson JFR, Locker AP. Micrometastases in bone marrow in patients with breast cancer. Br Med J 1987;295:1487.

35. Untch M, Harbeck N, Eiermann W. Micrometastases in bone marrow in patients with breast cancer. Br Med J 1988;296:290.

36. Ceci G, Franciosi V, Nizzoli R, et al. The value of bone marrow biopsy in breast cancer at time of diagnosis: a prospective study. Cancer 1988;61:96–98.

37. Giai M, Natoli C, Sismondi P, et al. Bone marrow micrometastases detected by a monoclonalantibody in patients with breast cancer. Anticancer Res 1990;10:119–122.

38. Mathieu M-C, Friedman S, Bosq J, et al. Immunohistochemical staining of bone marrow biopsies for detection of occult metastasis in breast cancer. Breast Cancer Res Treatment 1990;15:21–26.

39. Ellis G, Ferguson M. Yamanaka E, et al. Monoclonal antibodies for detection of occult carcinoma cells in bone marrow of breast cancer patients. Cancer 1989;63:2509–2514.

40. Ginsbourg M, Musset M, Misset JL, et al. Identification of mammary metastatic cells in the bone marrow as a marker of a minimal residual disease and of their proliferative index as a factor of prognosis—an immunocytologic study with monoclonal antibodies. Suppl J Med Oncol Tumor Pharmacother 1988;1:51–54.

41. Cote RJ, Rosen PP, Hakes TB, et al. Monoclonal antibodies detect occult breast carcinoma metastases in the bone marrow of patients with early stage disease. Am J Surg Pathol 1988;12:333–340.

42. Sharp JG, Vaughan WP, Kessinger A, et al. Significance of detection of tumor cells in hematopoietic stem cell harvests of patients with breast cancer. In: Dicke K, Armitage JO, Dicke-Evinger MJ, eds. Autologous bone marrow transplantation, V. Omaha: University of Nebraska Medical Center, 1991:385–391.

43. Osborne MP, Asina S, Wong GY, et al. Immunofluorescent monoclonal antibody detection of breast cancer in bone marrow: sensitivity in a model system. Cancer Res 1989;49:2510–2513.

44. Cote RJ, Rosen PP, Lesser ML, et al. Detection of occult bone marrow micrometastases (BMM) in patients with operable breast cancer predicts early recurrence. Proc US Canad Acad Pathol 1990;23A.

45. Schlimok G, Funke I, Holzmann B, et al. Micrometastatic cancer cells in bone marrow: in vitro detection with anti-cytokeratin and in vivo labeling with anti-17-1A monoclonal antibodies. Proc Natl Acad Sci USA 1987;84:8672–8676.

46. Schneider BM, Schlimok G, Riethmuller G, et al. Knochenmarksmikrometastasen bei kolorektalen Karzinomen. Onkologie Originalie 1989; Fortschr Med 107, Jg, Nr. 2:59/23–63/31.

47. Hunter RF, Broadway P, Sun S, et al. Detection of small cell lung cancer bone marrow involvement by discontinuous gradient sedimentation. Cancer Res 1987;47:2737–2740.

48. Hay FG, Ford A, Leonard RCF. Clinical applications of immunocytochemistry in the monitoring of the bone marrow in small cell lung cancer (SCLC). Int J Cancer 1988;2(suppl):8–10.
49. tenVelde GPM, Kuypers-Engelen BTMJ, Volovics A, et al. Examination of bone marrow biopsy specimens and staging of small cell lung cancer. Eur J Cancer 1990;26:1142–1145.
50. Leonard RCF, Duncan LW, Hay FG. Immunocytochemical detection of residual marrow disease at clinical remission predicts metastatic relapse in small cell lung cancer. Cancer Res 1990;50:6545–6548.
51. Saarinen UM, Coccia PF, Gerson SL, et al. Eradication of neuroblastoma cells in vitro by monoclonal antibody and human complement: method for purging autologous bone marrow. Cancer Res 1985;45:5969–5975.
52. Favrot MC, Frappaz D, Maritaz O, et al. Histological, cytological and immunological analyses are complementary for the detection of neuroblastoma cells in bone marrow. Br J Cancer 1986;54:637–641.
53. Gussetis E, Ebener U, Wehner S, et al. Immunological detection and definition of minimal residual neuroblastoma disease in bone marrow samples obtained during or after therapy. Eur J Cancer Clin Oncol 1989;25:1745–1753.
54. Moss TJ, Reynolds CP, Sather HN, et al. Prognostic value of immunocytologic detection of bone marrow metastases in neuroblastoma. New Engl J Med 1991;324:219–226.
55. Moss TJ, Sanders DG, Lasky LC, et al. Contamination of peripheral blood stem cell harvests by circulating neuroblastoma cells. Blood 1990;76:1879–1883.
56. Tsurusawa M, Kaneko Y, Katano N, et al. Flow cytometric evidence for minimal residual disease and cytological heterogeneities in acute lymphoblastic leukemia with severe hypodiploidy. Am J Hematol 1989;32:42–49.
57. Campana D, Yokota S, Coustan-Smith E, et al. The detection of residual acute lymphoblastic leukemia cells with immunologic methods and polymerase chain reaction: a comparative study. Leukemia 1990;4:609–614.
58. Drach J, Gattringer C, Huber H. Combined flow cytometric assessment of cell surface antigens and nuclear TdT for the detection of minimal residual disease in acute leukemia. Br J Haematol 1991;77:37–42.
59. Favrot MC, Herve P. Detection of minimal malignant cell infiltration in the bone marrow of patients with solid tumours, non-Hodgkin lymphomas and leukaemias. Bone Marrow Transplant 1987;2:117–122.
60. Bregni M, Siena S, Neri A, et al. Minimal residual disease in acute lymphoblastic leukemia detected by immune selection and gene rearrangement analysis. J Clin Oncol 1989;7:338–343.
61. Yokota S, Hansen-Hagge TE, Ludwig W-D et al. Use of polymerase chain reactions to monitor minimal residual disease in acute lymphoblastic leukemia patients. Blood 1991;77:331–339.
62. Yamada M, Wasserman R, Lange B, et al. Minimal residual disease in childhood B-lineage lymphoblastic leukemia: persistence of leukemic cells during the first 18 months of treatment. New Engl J Med 1990;323:448–455.
63. Beishuizen A, Hahlen K, van Vering ER, et al. Detection of minimal residual disease in childhood leukemia with the polymerase reaction. New Engl J Med 1991;324:772–773.
64. Brugiatelli M, Callea V, Morabito F, et al. Immunologic and molecular evaluation of residual disease in B-cell chronic lymphocytic leukemia patients in clinical remission phase. Cancer 1989;63:1979–1984.
65. Islam A, Catovsky D, Goldman JM, et al. Bone marrow biopsy changes in acute myeloid leukaemia. I: Observations before chemotherapy. Histopathology 1985;9:939–957.
66. Foon KA. Laboratory and clinical applications of monoclonal antibodies for leukemias and non-Hodgkin's lymphomas. Curr Probl Cancer 1989;13:63–128.
67. Wouters R, Lowenberg B. On the maturation order of AML cells: a distinction on the basis of self-renewal properties and immunologic phenotypes. Blood 1984;63:684–689.
68. Griffin JD, Larcom P, Schlossman SF. Use of surface markers to identify a subset of acute myelomonocytic leukemia cells with progenitor cell properties. Blood 1983;62:1300–1303.
69. Delwel R, van Gurp R, Bot F, et al. Phenotyping of acute myelocytic leukemia (AML) progenitors: an approach for tracing minimal numbers of AML cells among normal bone marrow. Leukemia 1988;2:814–819.
70. Martens ACM, van Bekkum DW, Hagenbeek A. Minimal residual disease in leukemia: studies in an animal model for acute myelocytic leukemia (BNML). Int J Cell Cloning 1990;8:27–38.
71. Martens ACM, Hagenbeek A. Detection of minimal disease in acute leukemia using flow cytometry: studies in a rat model for human acute leukemia. Cytometry 1985;6:342–347.
72. Rowley J. A new consistent chromosomal abnormality in chronic myleogenous leukemia identified by quinicrine fluorescence and Giemsa staining. Nature 1973;243:290–293.
73. Rowley J. Molecular cytogenetics: Rosetta stone for understanding cancer—Twenty-ninth G.H.A. Clowes Memorial Award Lecture. Cancer Res 1990;50:3816–3825.
74. Delfau M-H, Kerckaert J-P, d'Hooghe MC, et al. Detection of minimal residual disease in chronic mye-

loid leukemia patients after bone marrow transplantation by polymerase chain reaction. Leukemia 1990;4:1–5.

75. Fey MF, Kulozik AE, Hansen-Hagge TE, et al. The polymerase chain reaction: a new tool for detection of minimal residual disease in haematological malignancies. Eur J Cancer 1991;27:89–94.

76. Morgan GJ, Janssen JWG, Guo A-P, et al. Polymerase chain reaction for detection of residual leukaemia. Lancet 1989;1:928–929.

77. Arnold R, Bartram CR, Heinze B, et al. Evaluation of remission state in chronic myeloid leukemia patients after bone marrow transplantation using cytogenetic and molecular genetic approaches. Bone Marrow Transplant 1989;4:389–392.

78. Martiat P, Maisin D, Philippe M, et al. Detection of residual BCR/ABL transcripts in chronic myeloid leukaemia patients in complete remission using the polymerase chain reaction and nested primers. Br J Haematol 1990;75:355–358.

79. Hughes TP, Morgan GJ, Martiat P, et al. Detection of residual leukemia after bone marrow transplant for chronic myeloid leukemia: role of polymerase chain reaction in predicting relapse. Blood 1991;77:874–878.

80. Wright PA, Wynford-Thomas D. The polymerase chain reaction: miracle or mirage? A critical review of its uses and limitations in diagnosis and research. J Pathol 1990;162:99–117.

81. Hughes TP, Goldman JM. Biological importance of residual leukaemic cells after BMT for CML: does the polymerase chain reaction help? Bone Marrow Transplant 1990;5:3–6.

82. Dhingra K, Talpaz M, Riggs MG, et al. Hybridization protection assay: a rapid, sensitive, and specific method for detection of Philadelphia chromosome-positive leukemias. Blood 1991;77:238–242.

83. Barnett MJ, Eaves CJ, Phillips GL et al. Successful autografting in chronic myeloid leukemia after maintenance of marrow in culture. Bone Marrow Transplant 1989;4:345–351.

84. Cassileth PA, Gerson SL, Bonner H, et al. Identification of early relapsing patients with adult acute nonlymphocytic leukemia by bone marrow biopsy after initial induction chemotherapy. J Clin Oncol 1984;2:107–111.

85. Findley HW Jr, Steuber CP, Krischer JP, et al. Pediatric oncology group study of in vitro clonal growth patterns of leukemic cells in childhood acute non-lymphocytic leukemia as a predictor of induction response. Cancer Res 1987;47:4225–4228.

86. Anderson KC, Boyd AW, Fisher DC, et al. Hairy cell leukemia: a tumor of pre-plasma cells. Blood 1985;65:620–629.

87. Schwarting R, Stein H, Wang CY. The monoclonal antibodies, anti-S0HCL1 (anti-Leu-14) and anti-S-HCL3 (anti-Leu-M5) allow the diagnosis of hairy cell leukemia. Blood 1985;65:974–983.

88. Soligo D, Lambertenghi-Deliliers G, Berti E, et al. Immunohistochemical evaluation of bone marrow involvement in hairy cell leukemia during interferon therapy. Blut 1987;55:121–126.

89. Falini B, Pileri SA, Flenghi L, et al. Selectiion of a panel of monoclonal antibodies for monitoring residual disease in peripheral blood and bone marrow of interferon-treated hairy cell leukemia patients. Br J Haematol 1990;76:460–468.

90. Thaler J, Dietze O, Faber V, et al. Monoclonal antibody B-ly7: a sensitive marker for detection of minimal residual disease in hairy cell leukemia. Leukemia 1990;4:170–176.

91. Horlyck A, Thorling K. Bone marrow examination in non-Hodgkin's lymphoma: comparison of the diagnostic value of marrow aspirations and trephine biopsy. Eur J Haematol 1991;46:54–56.

92. Winter JN, Marder RJ, Mankad B, et al. Heterogeneity among the non-Hodgkin's lymphomas: implications for autologous bone marrow transplantation with in vitro purging using monoclonal antibodies. Cancer 1988;61:1081–1090.

93. Benjamin D, Magrath IT, Douglas EC, et al. Derivation of lymphoma cell lines from microscopically normal bone marrow in patients with undifferentiated lymphomas: evidence of occult bone marrow involvement. Blood 1983;61:1017–1019.

94. McCormick F. The polymerase chain reaction and cancer diagnosis. Cancer Cells 1989;1:56–61.

95. Smith SD, Kisker S, Bush L, et al. Utilization of a human tumor cloning system to monitor for bone marrow involvement in children with non-Hodgkin's lymphoma. Cancer 1983;53:1724–1729.

96. Philip I, Philip T, Favrot MC, et al. Establishment of lymphomatous cell lines from bone marrow samples from patients with Burkitt's lymphoma. J Natl Cancer Inst 1984;73:835–840.

97. Sharp JG, Joshi SS, Armitage JO, et al. Significance of detection of occult non-Hodgkin's lymphoma in histologically uninvolved bone marrow by a culture technique. Blood 1992, in press.

98. Igarashi T, Oka K, Miyamoto T. Human non-Hodgkin's malignant lymphomas serially transplanted in nude mice conditioned with whole-body irradiation. Br J Cancer 1989;59:356–360.

99. Schultz FW, Martens ACM, Hagenbeek A. The contribution of residual leukemic cells in the graft to leukemia relapse after autologous bone marrow transplantation: mathematical considerations. Leukemia 1989;3:530–534.

100. Negrin RS, Kiem H-P, Schmidt-Wolf IGH, et al. Use of the polymerase chain reaction to monitor the effectiveness of ex vivo tumor cell purging. Blood 1991;77:654–660.

101. Diehl V, Kirchner HH, Burrichter H, et al. Characteristics of Hodgkin's disease-derived cell lines. Cancer Treat Rep 1982;66:615–632.

102. Drexler HG, Amlot PL, Minowada J. Hodgkin's disease-derived cell lines—conflicting clues for the origin of Hodgkin's disease? Leukemia 1987;1:629–637.
103. Kennedy ICS, Hart DNJ, Colls BM, et al. Nodular schlerosing, mixed cellularity and lymphocyte-depleted variants of Hodgkin's disease are probable dendritic cell malignancies. Clin Exp Immunol 1989;76:324–331.
104. Naumovski L, Smith SD. Origin of Reed-Sternberg cells in Hodgkin's disease. New Engl J Med 1989;321:543.
105. Andreesen R, Bross KJ, Brugger W, et al. Origin of Reed-Sternberg cells in Hodgkin's disease. New Engl J Med 1989;321:543–544.
106. Sharp JG, Kessinger A, Armitage JO, et al. Clinical significance of occult tumor cell contamination of hematopoietic harvests in non-Hodgkin's lymphoma and Hodgkin's disease. In: Zander A, ed. Autologous bone marrow transplantation in lymphoma, Hodgkin's disease and multiple myeloma. Berlin: Springer-Verlag, 1991, in press.
107. Herbst H, Niedobitek G, Kneba M, et al. High incidence of Epstein-Barr virus genomes in Hodgkin's disease. Am J Pathol 1990;137:13–18.
108. Masih A, Weisenburger D, Duggan M, et al. Epstein-Barr viral genome in lymph nodes from patients with Hodgkin's disease may not be specific to Reed-Sternberg cells. Am J Pathol 1991;139:37–43.
109. Torelli G, Marasca R, Luppi M, et al. Human herpesvirus-6 in human lymphomas: identification of specific sequences in Hodgkin's lymphomas by polymerase chain reaction. Blood 1991;77:2251–258.
110. Samoszuk M, Nansen L. Detection of interleukin-5 messenger RNA in Reed-Sternberg cells of Hodgkin's disease with eosinophilia. Blood 1990;75:13–16.
111. Griesser H, Feller A, Lennert K, et al. Rearrangement of the β chain of the T cell antigen receptor and immunoglobulin genes in lymphoproliferative disorders. J Clin Invest 1986;78:1179–1184.
112. Sundeen J, Lipford E, Uppenkamp M, et al. Rearranged antigen receptor genes in Hodgkin's disease. Blood 1987;70:96–103.
113. Roth MS, Schnitzer B, Bingham EL, et al. Rearrangement of immunoglobulin and T-cell receptor genes in Hodgkin's disease. Am J Pathol 1988;131:331–338.
114. Herbst H, Tippelmann G, Anagnostopoulos I, et al. Immunoglobulin and T-cell receptor gene rearrangements in Hodgkin's disease and Ki-1-positive anaplastic large cell lymphoma: dissociation between phenotype and genotype. Leukemia Res 1989;13:103–116.
115. Schouten HC, Sanger WG, Duggan M, et al. Chromosomal abnormalities in Hodgkin's disease. Blood 1989;73:2149–2154.
116. Kessinger A, Bierman PJ, Vose JM, et al. High-dose cyclophosphamide, carmustine, and etoposide followed by autologous peripheral stem cell transplantation for patients with relapsed Hodgkin's disease. Blood 1991;77:2322–2325.
117. Henon PR, Butturini A, Gale RP. Blood-derived cell transplants: blood to blood. Lancet 1991:337:961–963.
118. Bell AJ, Hamblin TJ, Oscier DG. Peripheral blood stem cell autografting. Hematol Oncol 1987;5:45–55.
119. Juttner CA, To LB, Haylock DN, et al. Autologous blood stem cell transplantation. Transplant Proc 1989;21:2929–2931.
120. Pruitt JC, Hilberg AW, Kaiser RF. Malignant cells in peripheral blood. New Engl J Med 1958;259:1161–1164.
121. Scheinin TM, Koivuniemi AP. The occurrence of cancer cells in blood. Surgery 1962;51:652–657.
122. Carey RW, Taft PD, Bennett JM, et al. Carcinocythemia (carcinoma cell leukemia): an acute leukemia-like picture due to metastatic carcinoma cells. Amer J Medicine 1976;60:273–278.
123. Sharp JG, Kessinger A, Pirruccello SJ, et al. Frequency of detection of suspected lymphoma cells in peripheral blood stem cell collections. In: Dicke K, Armitage JO, Dicke-Evinger MJ eds. Autologous bone marrow transplantation, V. Omaha: University of Nebraska Medical Center, 1991:801–810.
124. Langlands K, Craig JIO, Parker AC, et al. Molecular determination of minimal residual disease in peripheral blood stem cell harvests. Bone Marrow Transplant 1990;5(suppl 1):64–65.
125. Kessinger A, Vose JM, Bierman PJ, et al. High dose therapy and autologous peripheral stem cell transplantation for patients with bone marrow metastases and relapsed lymphomas: an alternative to bone marrow purging. Exp Hematol 1991;19:1013–1016 (1991) in press.
126. Dippold WG, Klingel R, Kerlin M, et al. Stimulation of pancreas and gastric carcinoma cell growth by interleukin 3 and granulocyte-macrophage colony-stimulating factor. Gastroenterology 1991;100:1338–1344.
127. Joraschkewitz M, Depenbrock H, Freund M, et al. Effects of cytokines on in vitro colony formation of primary human tumor specimens. Eur J Cancer 1990;26:1070–1074.

15

BONE MARROW PURGING

Elizabeth J. Shpall, Charles Johnston, and Lisa Hami

INTRODUCTION

High-dose therapy with autologous bone marrow support (ABMS) has become the treatment of choice for certain patients with acute leukemia (1), Hodgkin's disease (2), non-Hodgkin's lymphoma (NHL) (3), neuroblastoma (4), and selected breast cancer patients who have a poor prognosis with standard therapy (5). Autologous marrow may contain clonogenic tumor cells that could contribute to relapse of cancer if reinfused into the patient. To minimize this risk, marrow is usually collected from patients when they are in remission. However, recent studies with molecular (6), tissue culture (7), or immunohistochemical (8) techniques have demonstrated that occult tumor cells can often be found in the marrow of patients with a variety of malignancies when routine histologic evaluation suggests no evidence of disease. Animal studies have documented the potential to transplant a variety of malignancies when reinfused marrow contains tumor cells (9). Recently a patient with chronic myelogenous leukemia received allogeneic marrow from his brother that unknowingly contained acute leukemia (10). The patient subsequently developed the brother's acute myelogenous leukemia and died, providing clinical evidence that tumor infused in marrow can be transplanted and lead to lethal consequences in humans.

Purging the bone marrow "ex vivo" before giving it back to the patient may eradicate the residual tumor. There are several problems, however, in evaluating whether or not purging the marrow is beneficial. First, the extent of tumor cell depletion after purging is difficult to determine, given the current limitations in the technology of minimal residual disease detection. Second, there is the potential for damaging the normal marrow progenitor cells with the purging procedure, thereby putting patients at risk for infection and/or bleeding as a consequence of delayed marrow recovery. Third, the clinical outcomes of trials that include purging, compared to trials that do not, are hard to interpret. At this point the clinical end points that might justify purging, other than relapse rate, are controversial. To date no randomized trials of purging versus no purging have been performed.

In spite of these obstacles, the theoretic possibility of reinfusing clonogenic tumor and compromising otherwise curative therapy stimulates ongoing development of purging regimens. Different purging methods have been developed that have varying strengths and limitations. Many clinical studies of single modality marrow purging, summarized in Table 15.1, have been performed in an attempt to remove clonogenic tumor cells from patient bone marrow. In combined modality purging studies involving several malignancies, summarized in Table 15.2, superior tumor cell depletion is usually produced when compared to using either method alone.

Table 15.1. Bone Marrow Purging Methods[a,b]

Pharmacologic methods:	4-HC/mafosfamide
	Cisplatin
	VP-16
	Vincristine
	Methylprednisolone
	Merocyanine 540
Immunologic methods:	Monoclonal antibodies plus:
	Complement
	Magnetospheres
	Toxins
Physical methods:	Lectin agglutination
	Counterflow elutriation

[a]Reprinted with permission from Shpall E, Bast RC, Johnston CS, et al. Combined purging approaches in autologous transplantation. In: Gee A, ed. Bone marrow processing and purging: a practical guide. Copyright 1991 CRC Press, Inc., Boca Raton, FL.
[b]Abbreviations: 4-HC, 4-hydroperoxycyclophosphamide; VP-16, etoposide.

Table 15.2. Combination Purging Methods[a,b]

Investigator	Method	Disease
Shpall (132)	4-HC+IMP	Breast cancer
Morecki (127)	4-HC+IMP	Breast cancer
Uckun (59)	4-HC+IT	ALL, B cell
Uckun (85)	4-HC+IT	ALL, T cell
DeFabritiis (42)	4-HC+MoAb/C'	NHL, Burkitt's
Chao (35)	VP-16+MoAb/C'	AML
Haleem (103)	MoAb/C'+DCF-DCA	NHL, T cell
Rowley (88)	4-HC+VCR+IMP	ALL
Gulati (113)	4-HC+VP-16	AML
Horwitz (36)	4-HC+VCR	AML, ALL
Marchetti (86)	Mafos+MC-540	ALL

[a]Reprinted with permission from Shpall E, Bast RC, Johnston CS, et al. Combined purging approaches in autologous transplantation. In: Gee A, ed. Bone marrow processing and purging: a practical guide. Copyright 1991 CRC Press, Inc., Boca Raton, FL.
[b]Abbreviations: ALL, acute lymphocytic leukemia; AML, acute myelogenous leukemia; DCF-DCA, deoxycorformycin-deoxyadenosine; 4-HC, 4-hydroperoxycyclophosphamide; IMP, immunomagnetic purging; IT, immunotoxin; MC-540, merocyanine 540; MoAbs/C', monoclonal antibodies and complement; VCR, vincristine; NHL, non-Hodgkin's lymphoma.

In order to evaluate a purging regimen one must consider how effectively it eradicates tumor cells, as well as how toxic it is for the normal marrow progenitor cells.

Tumor Cell Depletion

The preclinical benefit of marrow purging has been demonstrated with tissue culture methods, or in animal models, for a number of malignancies. Tumor cell elimination is most commonly evaluated in culture with clonogenic assays. In this system an admixture of bone marrow and tumor cells from a particular cell line is purged and then incubated with supplemented media for 10–14 days, at which time tumor colony growth is evaluated. Statistical analysis of the tumor cell colonies remaining is performed and will allow one to estimate the log-depletion of the clonogenic tumor cells produced by the purging method being studied (11). A variety of techniques for the detection of minimal residual disease in marrow before and after purging are being developed and are discussed in another chapter.

Bone Marrow Recovery

Tissue culture techniques have been used by many investigators to assess bone marrow stem cell viability following ex vivo purging. Marrow samples from before and after the purge are incubated in methylcellulose- or agarose-based culture systems with a variety of growth factors such as interleukin-3 (IL-3), granulocyte-macrophage colony-stimulating factor (GM-CSF), or tumor cell line, placental, or phytohemagglutinin-lymphocyte conditioned media (PHA-LCM). After 7–14 days in culture, the colony-forming units granulocyte-macrophage (CFU-GM), and/or CFU-granulocyte-erythroid-megakaryocyte-macrophage (CFU-GEMM), as well as burst-forming unit-erythroid (BFU-E)-derived colonies, are scored for growth. CFU-GEMM, or more commonly CFU-GM, remaining after the purge have been evaluated for their ability to predict bone marrow reconstitution kinetics. Kaizer reported that CFU-GM growth in short-term tissue culture assays was not predictive of hematologic reconstitution (12). More recently, however, several investigators have shown that the CFU-GM content of an autograft does predict for the reconstitution of leukocytes both with and without purging marrow in a variety of malignancies (13–16).

Clinically, the toxic end point of most phase I purging studies is the time to acceptable marrow reconstitution, referred to as engraftment. Engraftment is commonly defined as the number of days following marrow infusion required for a patient to achieve a white blood cell count ≥ 1000 cells per microliter, or a granulocyte count of ≥ 500 cells per microliter. Platelet reconstitution is generally defined as the number of days following marrow infusion required for a patient to become platelet transfusion independent, or to achieve a platelet count $\geq 20,000$ cells per microliter without transfusional support. This chapter will review the preclinical results of the purging procedures most commonly in use, emphasizing tumor cell elimination (clonogenic assay results) and normal marrow stem cell damage (CFU-GM recovery). In addition the major clinical trials where marrow purging has been employed will be discussed, with emphasis on engraftment kinetics.

PURGING METHODS

The three most commonly employed purging techniques involve pharmacologic, immunologic, and physical methods and will be discussed in detail. Other methods, including alkyl-lysophospholipid treatment, which reportedly has selective anticancer activity (17), lymphokine-activated killer (LAK) cell purging (18), and hyperthermia (19) show promise but are in earlier stages of development than the methods discussed in this chapter.

Pharmacologic Methods

CYCLOPHOSPHAMIDE DERIVATIVES

Bruce first reported that cyclophosphamide was more toxic for neoplastic cells than for normal cells, using a murine spleen-colony assay to determine the relative sensitivities of normal hematopoietic stem cells and

clonogenic lymphoma cells to various doses of antitumor agents in vivo (20). 4-Hydroperoxycyclophosphamide (4-HC) is the synthetic analogue of 4-hydroxycyclophosphamide, the active metabolite of cyclophosphamide produced by hepatic microsomal activation (21, 22). 4-HC hydrolyzes spontaneously in vitro to produce 4-hydroxycyclophosphamide. Mafosfamide (Asta-Z 7557) is a more stable cyclophosphamide derivative that also hydrolyzes to produce 4-hydroxycyclophosphamide in vitro. Marrow purging with either 4-HC (12) or Asta-Z (23) has been shown to decrease the amount of tumor in the bone marrow of patients with acute leukemia. 4-HC has also been used to purge the bone marrow of lymphoma (24) and breast cancer (16).

4-HC and Asta-Z have several properties that make them attractive candidates for use as purging agents. They are relatively easy to formulate, stable in vitro, and only require a short treatment time. Time becomes an important consideration when using human bone marrow, which often must be harvested and frozen on the same day. In a typical procedure the marrow cells are incubated for 30 minutes in a 37° C water bath with the appropriate concentration of 4-HC or Asta-Z dissolved in tissue culture media, usually in a final concentration of 2×10^7 marrow cells per milliliter. Following the incubation, the cell suspension is rapidly cooled to 4° C, washed, and then resuspended in the media prior to cryopreservation.

In an initial phase I purging study with a buffy coat fraction of bone marrow containing red blood cells and granulocytes, Kaizer et al. determined that the maximally tolerated dose of 4-HC in patients with acute myelogenous leukemia was 100 μg/ml (12). More recently Jones et al. showed that the erythrocytes and granulocytes present in the buffy coat decrease the efficacy of 4-HC (25). Hervé et al. noted similar results with Asta-Z, where the leukemic cell and CFU-GM recovery postpurge is dependent upon the nucleated and red cell concentration of the autograft (26). The authors postulate that the cellular aldehyde dehydrogenase present in the erythrocytes and granulocytes degrades cyclophosphamide to inactive metabolites, thereby decreasing the effective concentration of the drug in the incubation mixture. Perhaps as a result, the variable erythrocyte content of the incubation mixtures has produced a wide variation in marrow progenitor cell survival and time to marrow reconstitution following 4-HC treatment of the buffy coat. In clinical studies Rowley et al. demonstrated that the higher the erythrocyte content in the 4-HC-purged autograft, the higher the probability of leukemic relapse (27). For these reasons the use of a purified mononuclear cell (MNC) marrow fraction has been of recent interest.

Ficoll-Hypaque density gradient separation of bone marrow produces an erythrocyte- and neutrophil-free product that contains the MNCs necessary for marrow reconstitution. With the Ficoll-separated marrow the variability in postpurge marrow progenitor cell viability has been shown to be less than for buffy-coat-treated cells, with no difference in the engraftment kinetics (28). Several bone marrow transplant centers are now purging the MNC fraction of marrow with 4-HC. The maximally tolerated dose of 4-HC when using an MNC fraction of marrow is reported to be 60 μg/ml for patients with acute leukemia or NHL (28), and 80 μg/ml for patients with breast cancer (16). It is important to note that with the MNC fraction, the removal of erythrocytes and granulocytes steepens the dose-response curve for 4-HC (25) and Asta-Z (29), making changes in drug concentration and/or incubation time more critical than when a buffy coat fraction is purged.

Gorin et al. addressed the issue of interpatient variability by attempting to use a uniform incubation hematocrit (5%) in the autografts they were purging. Additionally, in one series of leukemic patients they adjusted the dose of Asta-Z according to the patient's postpurge CFU-GM recovery (23). The au-

thors defined the optimal dose of Asta-Z as that which produced 5% recovery of prepurge CFU-GM in each patient's marrow. This allowed for dose escalation in some patients, but resulted in the dosing deescalation in others. The clinical results in such patients, discussed below, are quite promising. Other investigators have noted that it is difficult to achieve a uniform incubation hematocrit consistently and prefer the use of an MNC layer to avoid the issue of interpatient variability (28).

Protection of Normal Marrow Progenitors from 4-Hydroperoxycyclophosphamide

In addition to killing tumor cells, 4-HC is toxic to normal marrow progenitor cells (CFU-GM). CFU-GM recovery of $\geq$1% of unpurged control samples produces consistent engraftment in patients receiving high-dose chemotherapy with ABMS (15). The lower the CFU-GM content in the purged marrow autograft, the longer the time to marrow recovery. Low CFU-GM content in the purged marrow autograft (<1% of preincubation levels) has produced lower relapse rates and increased disease-free survival rates in acute myelogenous leukemia patients when compared to autografts that contain >1% CFU-GM (27). Nevertheless, delays in marrow engraftment increase the risk of infection and bleeding in patients receiving high-dose chemotherapy and ABMS.

Methods to reduce engraftment delays without compromising the antitumor effects of 4-HC are being investigated. Ethiofos (WR-2721) is an organic thiophosphate that has been reported to selectively protect normal bone marrow and other tissues from the cytotoxicity of alkylating agents (30). Preclinical studies demonstrated that pretreatment of the marrow with WR-2721 followed by 4-HC produced a 1–2 log higher CFU-GM recovery than 4-HC alone, without reducing the log-elimination of breast cancer cells (31). Clinical studies are underway to determine the effects of WR-2721 plus 4-HC on marrow reconstitution. Preclinical studies suggest that recombinant growth factors such as interleukin-3 may stimulate 4-HC-purged marrow and increase engraftment rates, but clinical data are too preliminary to discuss.

OTHER CHEMOTHERAPEUTIC AGENTS

Cisplatin has activity against a variety of human tumors. Since the dose-limiting renal toxicity associated with in vivo administration is not an issue when cisplatin is employed ex vivo, it has the potential to become a very useful purging agent. Preliminary preclinical data suggest that cisplatin may be a valuable drug for elimination of neuroblastoma (32) and small cell lung cancer (33) cells from bone marrow. Cisplatin in combination with 4-HC has shown impressive antitumor effects against leukemic cell lines (34). Other chemotherapeutic agents, including etoposide (VP-16) (35), vincristine (36), and methylprednisolone (37), have been used to purge the marrow of leukemia and lymphoma.

MEROCYANINE 540

Sieber et al. have extensively evaluated merocyanine 540 (MC-540), an amphipathic dye that preferentially binds to and photosensitizes malignant cells, which are then killed by white light (38). This method has little adverse effect on normal marrow progenitor cells and has been used clinically to purge marrow of leukemia and lymphoma.

Immunologic Methods: Monoclonal Antibodies

Monoclonal antibodies (MoAbs) are extremely useful marrow-purging agents because they can be targeted to the unwanted tumor cells, while theoretically sparing the normal progenitor cells. Additionally, a "cocktail" of multiple MoAbs recognizing different epitopes can be utilized to broaden the tumor cell recognition. This may improve the purging of tumor cells that have heterogeneous antigen expression (39). Once the tumor cells are identified by the MoAbs, they can be destroyed in situ with complement or toxins, or they can be physically removed with polyclonal antibodies linked to magnetic microspheres. Thus the appropriate antibodies that react with the tumor and not the normal progenitor cells theoretically represent a more selective marrow-purging procedure than pharmacologic or physical methods. The majority of MoAb-containing purging regimens employ the MNC fraction of marrow. This allows for more direct antibody-tumor cell interactions, and decreases the amount of antibody as well as the other reagents required for treatment.

MONOCLONAL ANTIBODIES PLUS COMPLEMENT

Antibody and complement have been used to purge the marrow of a variety of tumors including acute lymphocytic leukemia (ALL) (40), acute myelogenous leukemia (AML) (41), and NHL (42). IgM antibodies bind complement most effectively. Complement derived from baby rabbits is felt to be the most effective for killing antibody-sensitized human cell targets, but human serum complement has been employed as well (43). Once the MoAb binds the tumor cell, the complement cascade is activated through the MoAb's Fc receptor, with eventual lysis and tumor cell death (44).

Although initially promising, more recent studies demonstrated that subpopulations of tumor cells were resistant to complement-mediated lysis (45). Gee et al. extensively characterized the major factors responsible for the development of complement resistance. These include the elaboration of an anticomplementary factor by the normal bone marrow cells (46), the ability of tumor cells expressing low levels of target antigen to avoid destruction by complement (47), and the difficulty obtaining reproducible batches of complement that lack nonspecific toxicity to the normal marrow cells (48). Complement resistance stimulated the development of alternative MoAb-based purging methods such as immunomagnetic purging and immunotoxin therapy.

MONOCLONAL ANTIBODIES PLUS MAGNETIC MICROSPHERES: IMMUNOMAGNETIC PURGING

Unlike complement-mediated purging, immunomagnetic purging (IMP) does not require antibodies of a particular isotype, is unaffected by anticomplementary factors associated with normal bone marrow cells, and can eliminate tumor cells expressing low levels of target antigen. As with complement-mediated purging, IMP requires an effective antibody or a panel of antibodies.

Initially the marrow/tumor cell suspensions are incubated with MoAbs, most commonly of the IgG subclass. The cells are then washed to remove unbound antibody, and an aliquot of sheep or goat antimouse immunoglobulin-coated magnetic microspheres is added to the suspension. Some methods employ IgM antibodies directly attached to the magnetospheres, and then only one incubation step is required. This "direct" linkage usually yields an inferior target-cell depletion when compared to the "indirect" method (49).

The most commonly employed magnetospheres, Dynal M450, originally constructed by Ugelstadt et al., are available commercially (50). They are 4.5 μm in diameter, 20% magnetite at the core, and can be obtained with the polyclonal sheep or goat antimouse antibody covalently linked to the surface. An example using IMP to purge breast cancer cells from marrow is depicted in Figure 15.1. In practice the anti-breast-cancer MoAbs are added to the marrow/tumor cell suspension where they react with the CAMA-1 breast cancer cells. The polyclonal antibodies linked to the magnetospheres are then added, and they bind to the MoAbs. In preclinical studies the entire suspension is subjected to the magnetic field generated by a small permanent samarium-cobalt magnet. The magnetospheres are rapidly attracted to the

magnet, binding the tumor cells to the side of the tube. Nonadherent cells are poured off and assayed for residual tumor cells in a limiting dilution assay, or for bone marrow progenitor cell recovery in tissue culture assays, depending upon the experiment.

For the clinical studies a magnetic separation device that can handle the large volumes of marrow is employed. Several different devices have been developed (51–53). Some of the early devices were of the flow-through variety, as shown in Figure 15.2. Stationary magnetic separation devices, as shown in Figure 15.3, have also been developed. With the stationary configuration, the marrow is purged in a blood bag that sits on top of the magnetic array. The nonadherent cells are then pumped into a collection pack with a peristaltic pump. This system is less cumbersome and more sterile than the flow-through technique.

With the IMP method, nucleated cell recoveries in most studies are generally 55%–75% of the prepurge value, with insignificant loss of CFU-GM (54).

MONOCLONAL ANTIBODIES PLUS TOXINS: IMMUNOTOXIN PURGING

Immunotoxins (ITs) are constructed by covalent binding of an MoAb to a potent toxin. Cross-linking reagents include midobenzoyl-N-hydroxysuccinimide ester (MBS), which forms a thioether bond, and N-succinamidyl-3 (2-pyridyldithio)-propionate (SPDP), which results in a disulfide bond between the antibody and the toxin (55). Plant toxins are most commonly used, including ricin and abrin, which have two chains, as well as the ricin A chain, saporin, momordin, gelonin, and pokeweed antiviral protein (PAP), all of which have a single chain (56). Additionally, *Pseudomonas* exotoxin has been frequently employed.

The most common intracellular targets of the toxins are the cellular ribosomes, which are irreversibly inactivated, terminating subsequent protein synthesis and resulting in cell

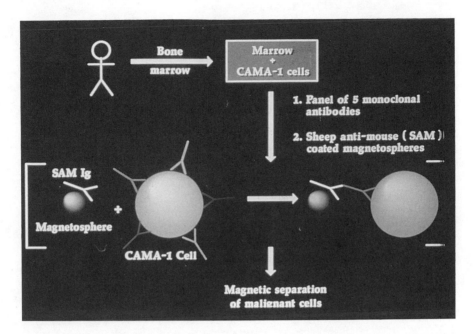

Figure 15.1. Immunomagnetic purging to remove CAMA-1 breast cancer cells from normal bone marrow.

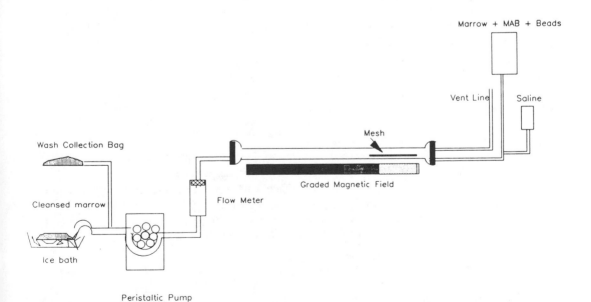

Figure 15.2. Flow-through immunomagnetic purging apparatus for clinical use with large volumes of bone marrow.

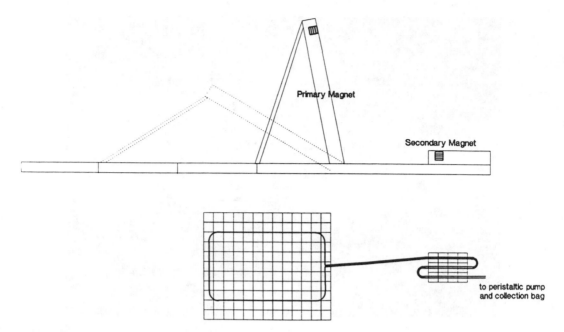

Figure 15.3. Stationary immunomagnetic purging apparatus for clinical use with large volumes of bone marrow. Top figure: Side view of apparatus. Bottom figure: Front view of apparatus with primary and secondary magnet.

death (57). With the two-chain toxins such as ricin, the A chain is the potent enzyme responsible for ribosomal inhibition, while the B chain simply facilitates the entry of the A chain into cells. Since the MoAb subserves the normal B chain function and facilitates specific tumor binding, the A chain alone is often used. Given the catalytic nature of ricin, very few molecules must be internalized to kill the cell (58).

ITs have been developed to purge bone marrow of leukemia (59), lymphoma (60), and breast cancer (61–63). They have also been used to selectively deplete the T lymphocytes responsible for graft-versus-host disease (GVHD) in allogeneic bone marrow transplantation (BMT) (64, 65). As with IMP, nucleated cell recoveries in most IT studies are 60%–75% of the prepurge value, with minimal loss of CFU-GM (62).

Although extremely effective in purging tumor cells, the preparation of appropriate reagents is very labor intensive. Each anti-

body must be individually conjugated to the toxin. This does not allow for the flexibility inherent in the IMP system, where the antibodies can easily be interchanged provided they interact with the magnetic microspheres and do not interfere with each other in the process of membrane binding.

Physical Methods

LECTIN AGGLUTINATION

Lectins are nonimmunoglobulin glycoproteins that can bind specifically to cell surface carbohydrates and stimulate agglutination of these cells. The agglutination can be reversed in the presence of an excess of the corresponding sugar. Soybean agglutinin (SBA) is the most commonly used lectin. It was used as part of the T cell depletion procedure in marrow used for allogeneic BMT, after studies had revealed that SBA is nontoxic to normal marrow progenitor cells (66). Similar techniques using lectin-based regimens have been developed to purge breast cancer and lymphoma from bone marrow, as described below.

COUNTERFLOW ELUTRIATION

Counterflow centrifugation elutriation allows separation of large numbers of cells on the basis of size and sedimentation properties (67). Cells suspended in media are pumped into a spinning chamber in a direction opposing the centrifugal field. By loading cells into a chamber at a counterflow rate, which balances the centrifugal forces, the cells remain in suspension and align themselves with respect to sedimentation properties. The MNC compartment contains the smaller cells such as T lymphocytes, which have elutriation characteristics different from those of the larger granulocytes. The majority of T cells are eluted initially. The remaining cells can then be collected separately and infused as an allogeneic T-cell-depleted marrow graft in patients with leukemia. The procedure has not been reported for purging tumor cells from marrow.

PURGING METHODS USED FOR SPECIFIC DISEASES

Acute Myelogenous Leukemia

RATIONALE

Age and donor availability restrict HLA-matched allogeneic BMT to less than 20% of adults with AML (68). This has generated considerable interest in the development of regimens with ABMS for high-risk patients with this disease. The use of ex vivo marrow purging for patients with AML was stimulated by data demonstrating higher relapse rates following unpurged ABMS when compared with allogeneic BMT (68). Although some investigators postulate that the absence of a graft-versus-leukemia (GVL) effect following regimens using ABMS may contribute to the higher recurrence rate, it is possible that some of

the relapses following ABMS are due to reinfusion of leukemia in the graft.

PRECLINICAL STUDIES

Pharmacologic

Pharmacologic treatment with 4-HC or Asta-Z is currently the most widely employed purging method for AML. Initial preclinical studies in rats revealed that incubation of mixtures of leukemic cells and normal bone marrow cells with 4-HC led to a dose-dependent antitumor effect, without damaging the repopulating ability of the marrow cells (69). Similar observations were later obtained with Asta-Z (70).

Monoclonal Antibodies Plus Complement

The development of immunologic purging methods has been limited by the possibility that MoAbs to AML cells may cross-react with normal hematopoietic progenitor cells. In addition the phenotype of leukemic stem cells may differ from that of their progeny (71). However, Ball et al. described a panel of MoAbs that recognize antigens expressed on AML blast cells, without reacting to normal marrow progenitor cells (72). The two most reactive antibodies, AML-2-23 and PM-81, were noted to bind the leukemic cells in more than 95% of the AML patients tested. In the presence of complement, these antibodies were shown to be cytotoxic to the leukemic cells bearing the appropriate surface antigen(s). DeFabritiis et al. also described a murine MoAb, S4-7, that reacted with human myelomonocytic cells but not with the less differentiated pluripotent stem cells (73). About 35% of AML patients were found to express the S4-7 antigen on more than 90% of their leukemic cells.

Combinations

Chao combined VP-16 with an MoAb against P-glycoprotein plus complement (35), Horowitz combined 4-HC plus vincristine (36), and Gulati has combined 4-HC plus VP-16 (74) to purge AML cells from human bone marrow. In all three studies the combination regimen produced superior tumor cell depletion than either method alone.

CLINICAL STUDIES

The clinical AML purging studies are summarized in Table 15.3. Gorin et al. analyzed the European Cooperative Group for Bone Marrow Transplantation (EBMT) data from 263 patients with AML autografted in first complete remission (CR) and found that the leukemia-free survival following total body irradiation (TBI) was superior for patients who received Asta-Z-purged versus unpurged marrow (63% versus 34%, respectively; $P = .002$), as shown in Figure 15.4 (75). The benefit was most pronounced in the group who received individually adjusted doses of Asta-Z (probability of relapse with dose-adjusted purge: 17%; standard-dose purge: 56%; and no purge: 59%; $P = .0002$ at 3 years). The kinetics of engraftment were slower for patients who received purged versus unpurged marrow.

Yeager et al. reported 88 patients with AML in second or third CR who received high-dose cyclophosphamide, busulfan, and ABMS, using a 4-HC-purged autograft (1). At latest follow-up, 35 patients remain in unmaintained remission at a median of 26.5 months following treatment (76). Figure 15.5 shows the actuarial disease-free survival of 36% for

patients transplanted in second CR and 23% in third CR. This actuarial disease-free survival rate is similar to that seen with syngeneic BMT and is higher than that usually reported for patients who receive high-dose therapy and unpurged ABMS in second or third CR. More recently the same investigators extended their 4-HC purging study to include 34 high-risk patients (poor-prognosis chromosomal abnormalities, FAB M4-M7, or difficulty achieving CR) with AML in first CR. Seventeen patients remain in unmaintained remission at a median of 381 days following therapy, with an actuarial disease-free survival of 46% as shown in Figure 15.6 (77).

Ball et al. purged the bone marrow of AML patients who expressed antigens reactive with the antibodies employed in the purge on ≥20% of their blast cells. Their initial report included 10 AML patients who received marrow purged with the MoAbs AML-2-23 and PM-81 plus rabbit complement (72). Eight of 10 patients engrafted successfully, while 2 patients did not have adequate platelet recovery. A more recent report includes 30 AML patients (8 from the initial report) transplanted in first (6 patients), second (18 patients), and third CR (6 patients) (78). The actuarial relapse-free survival for these patients is shown in Figure 15.7.

Acute Lymphoblastic Leukemia

RATIONALE

Unlike the encouraging results in patients with AML, purging marrow with 4-HC

Table 15.3. Acute Myelogenous Leukemia: Marrow Purging Clinical Results

Purging Method	Disease Status	Prep. Regimen	Leukocyte Recovery (Days)	2 Yr DFS (%)	Principal Investigator
Asta-Z	CR1	Cy/TBI	≥15	63	Gorin (75)
None	CR1	Cy/TBI	<15	34	
4-HC	CR2	Bu/Cy	43	36	Yeager (76)
	CR3	Bu/Cy	43	23	
4-HC	CR1	Bu/Cy	39	46	Yeager (77)
MoAbs,C'	CR1	Bu/Cy	35	67	Ball (78)
	CR2,3	Bu/Cy	35	18	

[a]All results expressed as the median.
[b]Abbreviations: Bu/Cy, busulfan and cyclophosphamide; C', complement; CR, complete remission; DFS, disease-free survival; Cy/TBI, cyclophosphamide and total body irradiation.

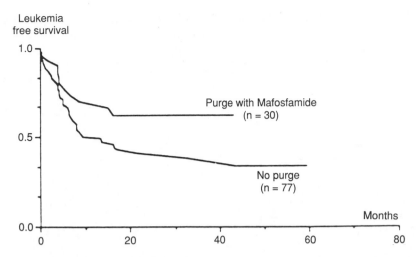

Figure 15.4. Cumulative probability of leukemia-free survival in patients with standard risk AML autografted in CR1 after TBI, according to whether the bone marrow was or was not purged ex vivo with mafosfamide ($P < .005$ in multivariate analyses). (From Gorin NC, Aegerter B, Auvert G, et al. Autologous bone marrow transplantation for acute myelogenous leukemia in first remission: a European survey of the role of marrow purging. Blood 1990;75:1606–1614.)

alone resulted in 80% relapse rates for patients in ALL in second or third CR, which is lower than the 50% relapse rate achieved with syngeneic BMT in a comparable patient population, and suggests that tumor in the marrow might have contributed to the recurrence of disease (79). Alternatives to 4-HC that have been investigated include other chemotherapeutic drugs plus 4-HC, complement-mediated purging, and IT therapy to eradicate ALL cells from bone marrow. Combined immunopharmacologic regimens have also been developed for ALL.

PRECLINICAL STUDIES

Pharmacologic

Jones et al. reported that the combination of 4-HC, vincristine, and methylprednisolone was significantly superior to 4-HC alone when used as a purging regimen for ALL cells (37).

Monoclonal Antibodies Plus Complement

CD9 is found on most ALL cells. CD19, CD24, and CD10, which is the common acute leukemia antigen (CALLA), are found on most B-ALL cells. MoAbs to CD9, CD10, CD19, and CD24 plus complement have been used by several investigators to eliminate ALL cells from marrow while sparing the normal progenitors (58). The combination of CD9 and CD10 antibodies plus complement was more effective in purging the ALL cells than either antibody individually (80). CD9, CD10, and CD24 antibodies plus complement produced superior clonogenic tumor cell depletion than any one or two of the antibodies (81).

Immunotoxins

An anti T-cell leukemia MoAb conjugated to intact ricin was used to treat the syngeneic marrow of lethally irradiated rats, which contained 3.0 logs of tumor cells (82). None of the recipients of IT-purged marrow developed ALL, while all the rats who received unpurged marrow died of leukemia. Marrow progenitor cell recovery following the IT treatment was 50% of control.

Fauser et al. purged marrow/ALL cell suspensions with a ricin A chain-conjugated anti-T-cell IT (T101) (83). They demonstrated

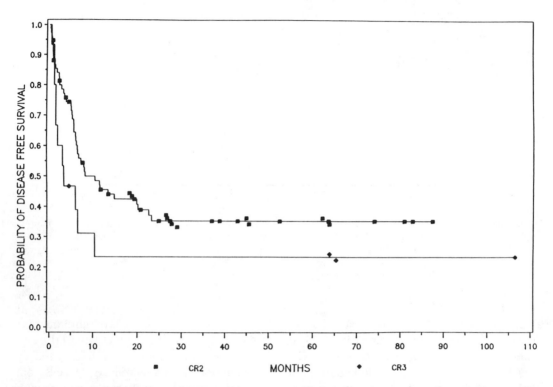

AUTOLOGOUS BMT IN PATIENTS WITH AML
23–AUG–90

Figure 15.5 Probability of disease-free survival for patients treated in CR2 (*squares*) or CR3 (*diamonds*) with high-dose cyclophosphamide, busulfan, and 4-HC-purged ABMS. (From Yeager A, Rowley S, Jones RJ, et al. Autologous transplantation with chemopurged bone marrow in patients with acute myelocytic leukemia in second or third remission. In: Dicke KA, ed. Autologous bone marrow transplantation: proceedings of the Fifth International Symposium. Omaha, NE: University of Nebraska Press, 1990:91–98.)

that marrow progenitor cell recovery following IT treatment was far greater than that achieved in the untreated suspensions. The authors suggested that the presence of ALL cells inhibits normal hematopoiesis.

Immunomagnetic Purging

Purging with the combination of CD9 and CD10 MoAbs plus magnetospheres demonstrated that more than 4.0 logs of Nalm 6 pre-B human ALL cells could be removed from marrow under optimal conditions (84).

Combinations

Using a combination of complement-mediated purging with the MoABs BA-1, BA-2, and BA-3 (to antigens CD9, CD10, and CD24, respectively) plus Asta-Z, LeBien et al. demonstrated superior ALL tumor cell depletion than that achieved with either method individually (81). In similar studies Ukun et al. demonstrated that ITs in combination with a cyclophosphamide derivative were superior to either modality alone when used to purge marrow of T (85) and B (59) cell leukemia.

The radiolabeling of IT (RIT) is currently being investigated. T101-ricin has been labeled with iodine-125, iodine-131, and yttrium-90 (55). These RITs appear to retain selective binding to T ALL cells, with 3–4 logs of tumor cell depletion noted in clonogenic assay. With the cytotoxic potential of both a

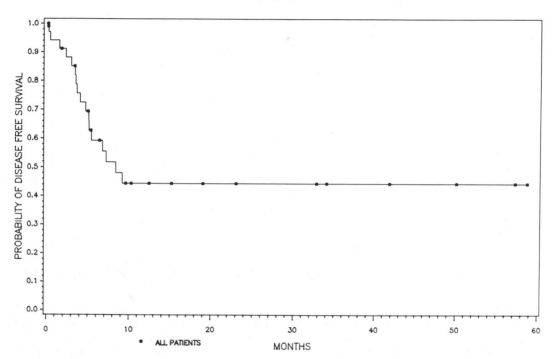

Figure 15.6.   Probability of disease-free survival for patients treated in CR1 with high-dose cyclophosphamide, busulfan, and 4-HC-purged ABMS. (From Yeager A, Rowley S, Santos G. Autologous bone marrow transplantation with acute nonlymphocytic leukemia, using ex vivo marrow treatment with 4-hydroperoxycyclophosphamide: an update. In: Powles R, Gordon-Smith EC, eds. Critical papers in bone marrow transplantation: an anthology. In press.)

radiolabeled antibody plus an IT, the RIT may be superior to IT alone for marrow purging.

The combinations of 4-HC plus cisplatin (34), vincristine (36), or MC-540 (86) were found to be more active against ALL cells than the agents individually and are being evaluated in clinical trials.

CLINICAL STUDIES

The ALL clinical purging trials are summarized in Table 15.4. The studies are characterized by generally rapid engraftment rates following high-dose therapy, but less than optimal disease-free survival in those studies with adequate follow up. Gilmore et al. used anti-CD7 and anti-CD10 and/or anti-CD19 MoAbs, respectively, with complement, to purge the marrow of high-risk T cell and B cell ALL patients in first CR (87). The other studies on Table 15.4 included ALL patients in second or subsequent CR. Rowley et al. demonstrated that the MNC fraction of marrow could be safely purged with the combination of 4-HC (60 μg/ml), vincristine (3.0 μg/ml), and methylprednisolone (5.0 mg/ml) (88). The engraftment rates were comparable to those of patients whose marrow is purged with 4-HC alone. It is of interest that the CFU-leukemia cultured from the marrow grafts of 12 of the patients was considerably more sensitive to the combination regimen than to 4-HC alone, while the sensitivity of the CFU-GM from these patients did not differ between the two regimens.

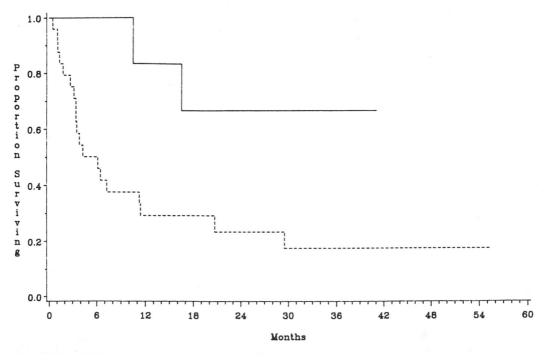

Figure 15.7. Relapse-free survival, computed as time to relapse or death in 30 AML patients in first CR (*solid line*) or second or third CR (*dashed line*) who received high-dose therapy and ABMS using marrow purged with monoclonal antibodies and complement. (From Ball ED, Mills LE, Cornwell GC III, et al. Autologous bone marrow transplantation in acute myelogenous leukemia using monoclonal antibody-purged bone marrow. Blood 1990;75:1119–1206.)

Table 15.4. Acute Lymphoblastic Leukemia: Marrow Purging Clinical Results[a,b]

Purging Method	Prep. Regimen	Leukocyte Recovery (Days)	3-Yr DFS (%)	Principal Investigator
Chemical	Cy/TBI	35	—	Rowley (88)
MoAbs,C'	Cy/TBI	24	21	Ramsey (90)
MoAbs,C'	Cy/TBI	23	32	Gilmore (87)
MoAbs,C'	Cy/TBI	59	27	Ritz (89)
MoAbs,C'	Cy/TBI	20	17	Vallera (55)

[a]All results expressed as the median.
[b]Abbreviations: C', complement; Chemical, 4-HC, vincristine, and methylprednisolone; Cy/TBI, cyclophosphamide and total body irradiation; DFS, disease-free survival.

Ritz et al. demonstrated prompt engraftment in ALL patients whose marrow was purged with the anti-CALLA MoAb J5, plus complement, with a relapse-free survival at 5 years reported to be 27% (89).

Ramsay and colleagues from the Uni-

versity of Minnesota used the cocktail of BA-1, BA-2, and BA-3 MoAbs plus complement to purge the marrow of similar patients (90). Vallera et al. from the same group purged the marrow of T cell ALL patients with a cocktail of ITs including T101-ricin, TA1-ricin, and UCHT4-ricin (55). Prompt engraftment occurred in both studies, with 21% and 17% long-term disease-free survivals reported (58). Given the relatively high relapse rates of these studies and the preclinical data suggesting that a combined-modality purging regimen is superior to individual methods, a combined approach evaluating IT plus 4-HC marrow purging is currently in progress at the University of Minnesota.

ALLOGENEIC BONE MARROW TRANSPLANTATION FOR LEUKEMIA: T CELL DEPLETION

GVHD is the major cause of morbidity and mortality in patients who receive allogeneic marrow grafts. Several marrow-purging procedures are currently employed to remove the T cells that cause GVHD from the marrow graft, prior to infusion in the patient. The most widely used method is complement-mediated purging with one, or frequently a cocktail of pan-T-cell antibodies, including CD2 plus CD3, CD2, CD5, and CD7 (91), and Campath-1 (92). IMP using an anti-T-cell antibody with magnetospheres (93) and IT treatment with ricin-conjugated antibodies such as CD3, CD5, and CD11a (64) have also been employed. Other methods of T cell depletion include soybean lectin agglutination with E-rosette depletion (94) and counterflow elutriation (95). Rapid marrow reconstitution is a consistent finding with marrow that has been T-depleted (96). Recent data, however, suggest that T cell depletion may diminish the GVL effect of allogeneic BMT, resulting in higher relapse rates than those achieved with unpurged allogeneic marrow grafts (97). Research is underway to further separate the subsets of T cells and ultimately purge those responsible for GVHD, without depleting those that may cause a GVL effect.

COMMON DISEASES

Non-Hodgkin's Lymphoma/Burkitt's Lymphoma

RATIONALE

Twenty percent to 75% of NHL patients will have histologic evidence of marrow involvement at the time of initial relapse, which is when patients are typically evaluated for marrow-supported high-dose regimens (98). Benjamin et al. showed that 17% of NHL patients with histologically normal bone marrow had occult marrow metastases that were demonstrated by tissue culture techniques (99). Using clonal immunoglobulin gene rearrangements, Hu et al. found evidence of lymphomatous involvement in the peripheral blood of 76% of their NHL patients, all of whom had histologically normal bone marrow biopsies (100). In addition, Vaughan et al. have shown that diffuse leukemic and bone marrow relapses can occur following infusion of histologically normal marrow in patients with NHL who receive high-dose chemotherapy with ABMS (7). Since it is becoming increasingly evident that bone marrow metastases are more common than histologic evaluation alone would suggest, techniques for purging NHL from marrow are being used with increasing frequency.

PRECLINICAL STUDIES

Preclinical studies have generally used Burkitt's lymphoma cell lines, which are widely available. 4-HC has produced a 4–5 log reduction in B cell NHL (101). MoAbs and complement have been used to purge bone marrow of NHL cells of both B (102) and T cell origin (103). Bast et al. reported 5 logs of NHL cell depletion following treatment with the MoAbs J2, J5, and B1 plus complement, with no significant inhibition of marrow progenitor cells (80). In their study, two MoAbs produced more tumor cell depletion than one MoAb, but the combination of three antibodies was no more effective than J2 and B1 or J2 and J5.

Bregni et al. conjugated an MoAb reactive with the immunoglobulin heavy chain (TEC IgM) to the plant toxin saporin-6 (104). Clongenic assays and [^{3}H]thmidine incorporation studies demonstrated that a 2-hour incubation with the IT killed 3 logs of the Bjab 113 Burkitt's lymphoma cells. CFU-GM recovery following the IT incubation with normal marrow was 75% of control.

Favrot et al. used the IMP technique with a panel of three MoAbs to eliminate more than 4 logs of Burkitt's lymphoma cells (105). In similar experiments Kvalheim et al. used magnetic beads coated with an IgM anti-HLA-DR antibody (AB4) to produce a 4 log depletion of Burkitt's lymphoma cells (106). The depletion was increased to 5 logs when two additional anti-B-cell antibodies were added to the regimen. The procedure required two incubations with the magnetospheres for optimal depletion. Bone marrow progenitor cell recovery in the latter study was 80%.

Other

Using SBA-coated magnetic beads, Mumcuoglu et al. demonstrated that more than 4 logs of lymphoma cells could be depleted from marrow, with no decrease in the CFU-GM (107).

Combinations

Chemotherapeutic agents have been combined with monoclonal antibodies plus complement for eradication of T lymphoma cells (103). DeFabritiis et al. combined 4-HC with an anti-B-cell monoclonal antibody plus complement for purging of Burkitt's lymphoma cells (42). In both studies the combination produced NHL depletion superior to either method alone.

CLINICAL STUDIES

The clinical NHL purging studies are summarized on Table 15.5. Immunologic methods have been used most commonly to purge the marrow of NHL patients. The B1 MoAb recognizes a pan-B-cell-restricted antigen, which is expressed on the surface of most mature normal and malignant B lymphocytes but is not present on the surface of hematopoietic stem cells (108). Takvorian et al. purged the marrow of 49 NHL patients with B1 plus complement (109). Marrow reconstitution occurred promptly in all patients. Of interest is that immunologic reconstitution took longer than hematologic engraftment. The number of circulating B cells became normal in the majority of patients by 5 months following transplant, but in a few patients it took as long as 1 year.

In an update of that study Freedman et al. reported on 100 NHL patients (which included the initial 49) (110). The patients were treated as described for the original group except that the marrows of one third of the patients were purged with more than one MoAb, including B1, B5, J5, and/or J2. Freedman reported that 35% of the patients had relapsed, the majority in sites of bulk disease. However, 14% of the relapsed patients developed metastases in both old and new sites, and 20% of them relapsed solely in new sites. Widespread leukemic relapse, particularly in new sites not previously involved, suggests that tumor may have been infused. Of interest is that none of the patients who relapsed solely in new sites had histologic evidence of tumor in the harvested marrow. Thirty-seven of the 100 patients actually had histologic evidence of NHL in the marrow at harvest (prior to purging), which has not adversely affected disease-free survival, as shown in Figure 15.8.

Philip et al. (111) and Negrin et al. (112) have developed purging regimens for NHL patients with MoAbs and complement. They report engraftment and disease-free survival rates similar to those of Freedman's group, as shown on Table 15.5.

Chemical methods have also been employed to purge NHL from bone marrow. Gulati et al. used 4-HC to purge the marrow of 14 NHL patients who had histologic evi-

Table 15.5. Non-Hodgkin's Lymphoma: Marrow Purging Clinical Results[a,b]

Purging Method	Prep. Regimen	Leukocyte Recovery (Days)	Platelet Recovery (Days)	2-Yr DFS (%)	Principal Investigator
MoAb,C'	Cy/TBI	24	28	—	Takvorian (109)
MoAbs,C'	Cy/TBI	27	29	50	Freedman (110)
MoAbs,C'	HDC	17	24	46	Philip (111)
MoAbs,C'	HDC/TBI	18	28	63	Negrin (112)
4-HC	Cy/TBI	19	34	—	Gulati (101)
4-HC	Cy/TBI or HDC	20	35	—	Rowley (114)

[a]All results expressed as the median.
[b]Abbreviations: C', complement; Cy/TBI, cyclophosphamide and total body irradiation; DFS, disease-free survival; HDC, high-dose chemo therapy.

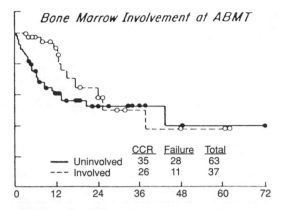

Figure 15.8. Kaplan-Meier estimate of disease-free survival probability with respect to lymphomatous bone marrow involvement (*dashed line*) or not (*solid line*), at the time of marrow harvest in NHL patients receiving high-dose therapy and ABMS using marrow purged with monoclonal antibodies and complement. (From Freedman AS, Takvorian T, Anderson K, et al. Autologous bone marrow transplantation in B-cell non-Hodgkin's lymphoma: very low treatment-related mortality in 100 patients in sensitive relapse. J Clin Oncol 1990;8:874–891.)

dence of tumor in the marrow at presentation (101). A buffy coat fraction of marrow was treated with 4-HC in concentrations of 60–120 μg/ml. In subsequent NHL patients the investigators have added VP-16 to the 4-HC regimen. Preliminarily it appears that there is no difference in time to reconstitution for marrows purged with 4-HC plus VP-16 compared to 4-HC alone, or to the unpurged marrow of NHL patients without marrow metastases (113). Rowley et al. purged the MNC fraction of NHL patients' marrows with 60 μg/ml 4-HC. The median time to leukocyte engraftment of 20 days was significantly faster than the engraftment rate of 40 days noted for patients with AML who had their MNC marrow fraction purged with 60 μg/ml 4-HC ($P < .001$) (114).

Neuroblastoma

RATIONALE

High-dose chemotherapy regimens with ABMS are used to treat poor-prognosis pa-

tients with stage IV neuroblastoma. Since 75% of stage IV neuroblastoma patients have bone marrow metastases, purging has been a major component in the design of intensive regimens for this disease.

PRECLINICAL STUDIES

The original technique for IMP was developed for patients with stage IV neuroblastoma by Treleaven et al. using a panel of seven antineuroblastoma monoclonal antibodies (115). They demonstrated that 3 logs of neuroblastoma cells could be consistently removed from bone marrow with the IMP technique. In depletion experiments with Hoechst dye-labeled neuroblastoma cells, Kemshead et al. demonstrated that no residual neuroblasts could be identified in marrow samples containing 1%–5% of the tumor cells before purging (116). Similar results have been obtained by others, using alternative combinations of anti-neuroblastoma MoAbs (51, 117).

CLINICAL STUDIES

The high-dose regimens in the majority of these studies, summarized in Table 15.6, include combination chemotherapy alone or in conjunction with TBI (118). Seeger et al. sedimented, filtered, and then purged the marrow of neuroblastoma patients with the IMP technique, using a panel of four anti-neuroblastoma MoAbs (119). All evaluable patients have engrafted successfully. Tumor could not be detected in any of the post-purge marrows, using an immunocytochemical method that detects one tumor cell per 10^5 normal cells.

Graham-Pole et al. have shown that marrow recovery in neuroblastoma patients following the IMP procedure is generally rapid and similar to that for age- and disease-matched patients who receive comparable high-dose chemotherapy with an unpurged autograft (120, 121). Although rare patients had a prolonged (8-week) engraftment period, this has been attributed to the preparative regimen or correlated significantly with

Table 15.6. Neuroblastoma: Marrow Purging Clinical Results[a,b]

Purging Method	Prep. Regimen	Leukocyte Recovery (Days)	Platelet Recovery (Days)	2-Yr DFS (%)	Principal Investigator
IMP	HDC/TBI	23	34	47	Seeger (119)
IMP	HDC/TBI	34	46	32	Graham-Pole (120)
4-HC	HDC/TBI	26	37	48	Hartmann (123)

[a]All results expressed as the median.
[b]Abbreviations: HDC/TBI, high-dose chemotherapy and total body irradiation.

the amount of chemotherapy administered prior to transplant (122).

Hartmann et al. used Asta-Z-purged marrow for neuroblastoma patients in their study (123). Their reported disease-free survival of 48% at a median of 28 months is superior to the 12% 2-year disease-free survival rate of a historically controlled group receiving standard therapy.

Breast Cancer

RATIONALE

Bone and bone marrow involvement with breast cancer is common. In women with primary breast cancer, 20% (124)–28% (125) had tumor cells detected in their bone marrow with an immunochemical method staining for specific breast cancer-associated antigens. Forty percent to 60% of patients with stage IV breast cancer have evidence of bone marrow metastases using routine histologic techniques (126). In a comparative study of radionuclide bone scans and random bone marrow biopsies, increasing sites of positivity on the bone scan correlated with increasing frequency of histologically positive bone marrows, as shown on Table 15.7.

PRECLINICAL STUDIES

Morecki et al. performed a series of preclinical purging studies using normal bone marrow mixed with a human breast cancer cell line (127). By magnetically purging the suspension with SBA-linked magnetic microspheres, in combination with 4-HC, a 4–5 log depletion of breast cancer cells was achieved, which was superior to either method alone.

Table 15.7. Bone Marrow Involvement in Newly Diagnosed Stage IV Breast Cancer[a]

No. Bone Metastases	% Pts. with + Marrows
1	44
2	48
3	73
>3	94

[a]From Kamby C. Clinical and radiologic characteristics of bone metastases in breast cancer. Cancer 1987;60:2524–2531.

Coombes et al. developed an IT (LICR-LON-Fib 75/abrin A-chain) that depleted five of seven breast cancer cell lines from marrow, with an 83% recovery of control CFU-GM (62). Yu et al. conjugated each of three anti-breast-cancer MoAbs to ricin A-chain (61). Simultaneous treatment with two ITs produced additive antitumor activity against the SKBr-3 breast cancer cell line with each of the possible combinations. Tondini et al. conjugated the anti-breast-cancer MoAb DF3 to intact ricin and demonstrated a 1.6 log reduction of MCF-7 cells with a 2.6–2.8 log reduction of both the ZR-75-1 and BT-20 cell lines (63). A 30% reduction in CFU-GM was noted when bone marrow was treated with DF3-IT.

An IMP regimen was developed using a panel of five MoAbs that reacted with breast cancer but not with human bone marrow (128). Preclinical studies demonstrated depletion of 3–4 logs of clonogenic breast cancer cells using the IMP technique. In similar experiments 2.5 logs of breast cancer cells were eliminated with 4-HC (129). Breast cancer cells were then treated sequentially with the IMP regimen followed by 4-HC; this treatment was then repeated in the reverse order (4-HC followed by IMP). As shown in Figure 15.9, 4.5 logs of clonogenic tumor cells were eliminated with the combined treatments, regardless of their sequence. The elimination was greater with the combinations than with either individual treatment (130). The CFU-GM recovery was sequence-dependent, with superior recovery noted when 4-HC was used first, followed by IMP. In comparative preclinical studies, treatment with five different ITs in combination proved less consistently effective than treatment with a 4-HC plus IMP in depleting breast cancer cells from bone marrow (131).

CLINICAL STUDIES

These data, summarized on Table 15.8, describe trials where high-dose alkylating agent chemotherapy with purged ABMS was administered to patients with stage IV breast cancer. Shpall et al. performed a phase I study to assess the impact of 4-HC, IMP, and 4-HC plus IMP on time to engraftment, using the purged MNC fraction of bone marrow for the autograft (132). Figure 15.10 shows that at the first three 4-HC dose levels of 20, 40, and 60 μg/ml, there was no statistically significant

Table 15.8. Breast Cancer: Marrow Purging Clinical Results[a,b]

Purging Method	Prep. Regimen	Leukocyte Recovery (Days)	Platelet Recovery (Days)	Principal Investigator
4-HC	HDC	28	33	Shpall (16)
IMP	HDC	21	27	Shpall (52)
4-HC	HDC	23	25	Kennedy (133)
IT	HDC	17	24	Coombes (62)

[a]All results expressed as the median.
[b]Abbreviations: IT, immunotoxin LICR-LON 75/abrin A-chain; HDC, high-dose chemotherapy.

difference in time to engraftment (19, 20, and 23 days, respectively) compared to the unpurged historical controls (17 days). At 80 μg/ml engraftment was significantly delayed (28 days) ($P = .027$), and further escalation of 4-HC was not attempted (16). The immunomagnetically purged group experienced no difference in engraftment (21 days) compared to the unpurged controls (52). Accrual to the trial continues using IMP plus 4-HC purged marrow.

Kennedy et al. purged a buffy coat fraction of bone marrow with 100 μg/ml 4-HC and noted that leukocyte and platelet recovery was prompt (133).

Coombes purged the marrow of breast cancer patients using the IT LICR-LON-Fib 75/abrin A-chain (62). The time to leukocyte and platelet recovery was comparable to that noted in a group of patients who received the same high-dose therapy with unpurged marrow support. The impact on the disease-free survival for the breast cancer purging trials will require longer follow-up.

Small Cell Lung Cancer

RATIONALE

Small cell lung cancer (SCLC) has been detected with monoclonal antibodies in the histologically normal bone marrow of 50% and 80% of patients with limited and extensive disease, respectively (134). Although the role of high-dose therapy with ABMS for SCLC remains unclear, several interesting marrow-

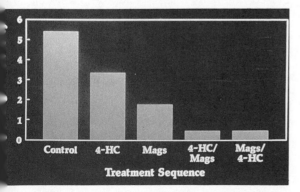

Figure 15.9. Effect of sequential treatment with 4-HC and immunomagnetic purging (Mags) on clonogenic elimination of breast cancer cells from human bone marrow. (From Anderson I, Shpall EJ, Leslie D, et al. Elimination of malignant clonogenic breast cancer cells from human bone marrow. Cancer Res 1989;49:4659–4664.)

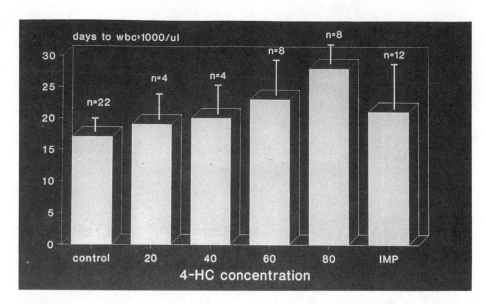

Figure 15.10. Median days to leukocyte engraftment (white blood cell count ≥1000 cells per microliter) in breast cancer patients receiving high-dose therapy and 4-HC-purged or immunomagnetically purged ABMS.

purging regimens have been evaluated in preclinical studies for this disease.

PRECLINICAL STUDIES

Using the IMP technique in conjunction with panels of MoAbs reactive with SCLC, Elias et al. (135) and Vredenburgh et al. (136) removed 2–3 logs and 4–5 logs, respectively, of SCLC cells from bone marrow. Meagher et al. reported that WR-2721 and MC-540 eliminated all detectable SCLC cells in their assay without affecting the hematopoietic progenitor cells (137). Benard et al. demonstrated effective eradication of SCLC cells using cisplatin as a purging agent (138).

CLINICAL STUDIES

No clinical studies have been performed with purged marrow in SCLC patients.

SUMMARY AND CONCLUSIONS

With current technology and available clinical studies it is not yet possible to determine whether relapse of malignancy results from endogenous tumor and/or from infusion of tumor along with the autologous marrow. Therefore, the question of whether purging is or is not clinically necessary remains unanswered. Although the majority of patients receiving intensive marrow-supported regimens relapse at sites of bulk disease, the follow-up time for most of the trials discussed in this chapter is relatively short (less than 5 years). With longer follow-up and continued improvements in the cytoreductive regimens several investigators have reported unexpected patterns of relapse that may be due to infusion of clonogenic tumor cells (101).

There are preliminary studies suggesting that marrow purging may benefit certain patients. The data of Gorin suggest that higher disease-free survival rates and lower relapse rates can be achieved in recipients of chemopurged grafts when compared to unpurged autografts for certain patients with AML in first or subsequent CR (68). The data of Yeager (76) and Ball (78) suggest that patients with AML in second or third CR can experience durable relapse-free survival with purged ABMS therapy, which is not the case for the majority of similar patients who have received unpurged marrow (139, 140).

Obviously, a randomized trial comparing purged to unpurged marrow is desirable to validate the importance of purging. Such trials have been very difficult to organize. Patient refusal, the large numbers of patients that would be required, the lack of agreement on the optimal purging regimen, and even the lack of agreement on the need to purge at all are obstacles that have thus far prevented the development of such a trial.

Marrow-supported intensive treatments are being employed with increasing frequency earlier in the course and stage of malignant disease. In this setting, marrow contamination by tumor may be less frequent, but the potential to eradicate tumor in the marrow and the patient will be increased. Therefore, the penalty for reinfusion of viable tumor with the marrow theoretically becomes more severe. Since multiple studies have demonstrated a reduction of clonogenic tumor from the marrow and a lack of associated major morbidity following this procedure (23), many investigators have concluded that the routine use of marrow purging for autotransplants is justified in patients known to be at substantial risk for marrow involvement with their disease. It is hoped that randomized trials will be performed in the future to determine whether purging bone marrow is necessary or desirable, and in what settings the benefit is maximal.

REFERENCES

1. Yeager A, Kaizer H, Santos G, et al. Autologous bone marrow transplantation in patients with acute nonlymphocytic leukemia, using ex vivo marrow treatment with 4-HC. New Engl J Med 1986;315:14–147.
2. Jagannath S, Dicke K, Armitage JO, et al. High-dose cyclophosphamide, carmustine, and etoposide and autologous bone marrow transplantation for relapsed Hodgkin's disease. Ann Intern Med 1986; 104:163–168.
3. Philip T, Armitage JO, Spitzer G, et al. High-dose therapy and autologous bone marrow transplantation after failure of conventional chemotherapy in adults with intermediate-grade or high-grade non-Hodgkin's lymphoma. New Engl J Med 1987; 316:1493–1498.
4. Seeger RC, Reynolds PC, Moss TJ, et al. Autologous bone marrow transplantation for poor-prognosis neuroblastoma. In: Dicke K, Spitzer G, Jagannath S, eds. The Third International Symposium on Autologus Bone Marrow Transplantation. Houston: University of Texas MD Anderson Hospital and Tumor Institute, 1987:375–381.
5. Antman K, Gale RP. Advanced breast cancer: high dose chemotherapy and bone marrow autotransplants. Ann Intern Med 1988;108:570–574.
6. Lee MS, Chang KS, Cabanillas F, et al. Detection of minimal residual cells carrying the t(14;1B) by DNA sequence amplification. Science 1987;237:175–178.
7. Vaughan WP, Weisenburger DD, Sanger W, et al. Early leukemic recurrence of non-Hodgkin's lymphoma after high-dose antineoplastic therapy. Bone Marrow Transplant 1987;1:373–379.
8. Redding WH, Monaghan P, Imrie SF, et al. Detection of micrometastases in patients with primary breast cancer. Lancet 1983;3:1271–1273.
9. Trigg ME, Poplack DG. Transplantation of leukemic bone marrow treated with cytotoxic antileukemic antibodies and complement. Science 1982;217:259–261.
10. Niederwieser DW, Appelbaum FR, Gastl G, et al. Inadvertent transmission of a donor's acute myeloid leukemia in bone marrow transplantation for chronic myelocytic leukemia. New Engl J Med 1990;322:1794–1795.
11. Johnson E, Brown WB. The Spearman estimator for serial dilution assays. Biometrics 1961;March:79–88.
12. Kaizer H, Stuart R, Brookmeyer R, et al. Autologous bone marrow transplantation in acute leukemia: a phase I study of in vitro treatment of marrow with 4-hydroperoxycyclophosphamide to purge tumor cells. Blood 1985;65:1504–1510.
13. Douay L, Gorin N-C, May J-Y, et al. Recovery of CFU-GM from cryopreserved marrow and in vivo evaluation after autologous bone marrow transplantation are predictive of engraftment. Exp Hematol 1986;14:358–365.
14. Spitzer G, Verma D, Fisher R, et al. The myeloid progenitor cell—its value in predicting hematopoietic recovery after autologous transplantation. Blood 1980;55:317–323.
15. Rowley S, Zuehlsdorf M, Braine H, et al. CFU-GM content of bone marrow graft correlates with time to hematologic reconstitution following autologous bone marrow transplantation with 4-HC-purged bone marrow. Blood 1987;70:271–275.
16. Shpall EJ, Jones RB, Bast RC, et al. 4-HC purging of breast cancer from the mononuclear cell fraction

of bone marrow in patients receiving high-dose chemotherapy and autologous marrow support: a phase I trial. J Clin Oncol 1991;9:85–93.

17. Vogler WR, Olson AC, Berdel WE, et al. Purging leukemia remission marrows with alkyl-lysophospholipids, pre-clinical and clinical results. In: Gross S, Gee S, Worthington-White D, eds. Bone marrow purging and processing. New York: Wiley-Liss, 1990:1–20.

18. Long GS, Cramer DV, Harnaha JC, Hiserodt JC. Lymphokine-activated killer (LAK) cell purging of leukemic bone marrow: range of activity against different hematopoietic neoplasms. Bone Marrow Transplant 1990;6:169–177.

19. Gidali J, Szamosvolgyi S, Feher I, et al. Survival and characteristics of murine leukemic and normal stem cells after hyperthermia: a murine model for human bone marrow purging. Leukemia Research 1990;14:453–457.

20. Bruce WR, Meeker BE, Valeriote FA. Comparison of the sensitivity of normal hematopoietic and transplanted lymphoma colony-forming cells to chemotherapeutic agents administered in vivo. J Natl Cancer Inst 1966;37:233–237.

21. Peter G, Wagner T, Hohorst H. Studies on 4-hydroperoxycyclophosphamide: a simple preparation method and its application for the synthesis of a new class of "activated" sulfur-containing cyclophosphamide derivatives. Cancer Treat Rep 1976; 60:429–435.

22. Takimazawa A, Matsumoto S, Iwata T, et al. Studies On cyclophosphamide metabolites and their related compounds II. Preparation of an acute species of cyclophosphamide and related compounds. J Am Chem Soc 1973;95:985–986.

23. Gorin N, Douay L, Laporte M, et al. Autologous bone marrow transplantation using marrow incubated with Asta Z 7557 in adult acute leukemia. Blood 1986; 67:1367–1376.

24. Gulati S, Fedorciw R, Gopal A, et al. Autologous stem cell transplant for poor prognosis diffuse histiocytic lymphoma. In: Dicke K, Spitzer G, Zander A, eds. Proceedings from the First International Symposium on ABMT. Houston: The University of Texas M.D. Anderson Hospital and Tumor Institute, 1985:75–81.

25. Jones RJ, Zuehlsdorf M, Rowley SD, et al. Variability in 4-HC activity during clinical purging for autologous bone marrow transplantation. Blood 1987; 70:1490–1494.

26. Herve P, Cahn JY, Plouviere E, et al. Autologous bone marrow transplantation for acute leukemia using transplant chemopurified with metabolite of oxazaphosphorines (ASTA Z 7557, INN mafosfamide): first clinical results. Invest New Drugs 1984;2:245–252.

27. Rowley S, Jones RJ, Piantadosi S, et al. Efficacy of ex vivo purging for autologous bone marrow transplantation in the treatment of acute nonlymphoblastic leukemia. Blood 1989;74:501–596.

28. Rowley S, Davis JM, Piantadosi S, Jones RJ, Yeager AM, Santos GW. Density gradient separation of autologous bone marrow grafts before ex-vivo purging with 4-hydroperoxycyclophosphamide. Bone Marrow Transplant 1990;6:321–327.

29. Douay L, Mary JY, Giarratana MC, et al. Establishment of a reliable experimental procedure for bone marrow purging with mafosfamide (Asta Z 7557). Exp Hematol 1989;17:429–432.

30. Wasserman TH, Phillips TL, Ross G, et al. Differential protection against chemotherapeutic effects on bone marrow CFUs by WR-2721. Cancer Clin Trials 1981;4:3–6.

31. Shpall EJ, Jones RB, Johnston C, et al. Purging of breast cancer cells from bone marrow using WR-2721 and 4-HC. Proc Am Assoc Cancer Res 1990; 31:337.

32. Bettan-Renaud L, de Vathaire F, Benard J, et al. Potential therapeutic role of cisplatin in autologous bone marrow transplantation: in vitro eradication of neuroblastoma cells from bone marrow. Br J Cancer 1989;60:529–532.

33. Benard J, Bettan-Renaud L, Gavoille A, et al. In vitro chemical eradication of small cell lung cancer: application in autologous bone marrow transplantation. Eur J Cancer Clin Oncol 1988;24:1561–1566.

34. Peters RH, Brandon CS, Avila LA, et al. In vitro synergism of 4-HC and cisplatin: relevance for bone marrow purging. Cancer Chemother Pharmacol 1989;23:129–134.

35. Chao N, Aihara M, Blume KG, et al. Bone marrow purging combining a monoclonal antibody against P-glycoprotein and VP-16. Exp Hematol 18:674, 1990.

36. Horwitz LJ, Auber ML, Khorana S, et al. 4-HC and vincristine as ex vivo marrow treatment for acute leukemia in second remission. In: Dicke K, Spitzer G, Jagannath S, eds. The Third International Symposium on Autologus Bone Marrow Transplantation. Houston: University of Texas M.D. Anderson Hospital and Tumor Institute, 1987:143–150.

37. Jones RJ, Miller CB, Zehnbauer BA, et al. In vitro evaluation of combination purging for autologous bone marrow transplantation. Bone Marrow Transplant 1990;5:301–307.

38. Sieber F, Spivak JL, Sutcliffe AM. Selective killing of leukemic cells by merocyanine 540-mediated photosensitization. Proc Natl Acad Sci USA 1984;81: 7584.

39. Malpas J, Kemshead J, Pritchard J, Greaves M. Variability of surface antigen expression on neuroblastoma cells as revealed by monoclonal antibodies. In: Raybard C, Clement R, Lebreuil G, Benard J, eds. Proceedings of the thirteenth meeting of the International Society of Pediatric Oncologists. Amsterdam: Excerpta Medica, 1981:90–95.

40. Bast C, Ritz J, Lipton JM, et al. Elimination of leukemic cells from human bone marrow using monoclonal antibody and complement. Cancer Res 1983;43:1389–1394.
41. Ball ED, Mills LE, Coughlin CT, et al. Autologous bone marrow transplantation in acute myelogenous leukemia: in vitro treatment with myeloid cell-specific monoclonal antibodies. Blood 1986;68:1311–1315.
42. DeFabritiis P, Bregni M, Lipton J, et al. Elimination of clonogenic Burkitt's lymphoma cells from human bone marrow using 4-HC in combination with monoclonal antibodies and complement. Blood 1985;65:1064–1079.
43. Ohanian SH, Schlager SI. Humoral immune killing of nucleated cells: mechanisms of complement-mediated attack and target cell defense. CRC Crit Rev Immunol 1981;1:165–209.
44. Green H, Goldberg B. The action of antibody and complement on mammalian cells. Ann NY Acad Sci 1960;87:352–362.
45. Winter J, Marder R, Mankad B, et al. Heterogeneity among non-Hodgkin's lymphomas: implications for autologous bone marrow transplantation with in vitro purging using monoclonal antibodies. Cancer 1988;61:1082–1090.
46. Gee A, Bruce K, Morris T, et al. Evidence for an anticomplementary factor associated with normal bone marrow cells. J Natl Cancer Inst 1985;75:441–445.
47. Gee AP, Bruce K, Van Hilten J, et al. Selective loss of expression of a tumor-associated antigen on a human leukemia cell clone induced by treatment with monoclonal antibody and complement. J Natl Cancer Inst 1987;78:29–35.
48. Gee AP, Boyle MD. Purging tumor cells from bone marrow by use of antibody and complement: a critical appraisal. J Natl Cancer Inst. 1988;80:154–159.
49. Kemshead J, Gibson F. Monoclonal antibodies and magnetic microspheres used for depletion of tumor cells from bone marrow. In: Gee A, Gross S, eds. Proceedings of the First International Workshop on Bone Marrow Purging. Orlando, FL: Scientific and Medical Macmillan Press, 1987:84–89.
50. Ugelstad J, Mfutakamba HR, Mork PC. Preparation and application of monodisperse polymer particles. J Polymer Sci 1985;72:225–240.
51. Gee AP, Lee C, Bruce K. Graham-Pole JR, et al. Immunomagnetic purging and autologous transplantation in stage D neuroblastoma. Bone Marrow Transplant 1987;2:89–93.
52. Shpall EJ, Bast RC, Joines WT, et al. Immunomagnetic purging of breast cancer from bone marrow for autologous transplantation. Bone Marrow Transplant 1991;7:145–151.
53. Ball E, Powers F, Vredenburgh J, Heath C, Converse A. Purging of small cell lung cancer cells using immunomagnetic beads and a flow-through device. Bone Marrow Transplant 1991;8:35–40.
54. Kemshead J, Elsom G, Patel K. Immunomagnetic manipulation of bone marrow. Prog Clin Biol Res 1990;333:238–251.
55. Vallera DA. Immunotoxins for ex vivo bone marrow purging in human bone marrow transplantation. In: Frankel AE, ed. Immunotoxins. Hingham, MA: Kluwer Academic Publishers, 1988:515–531.
56. Barbieri L, Stripe F. Ribosome-inactivating proteins from plants: properties and possible uses. Cancer Surv 1982;1:489–520.
57. Olnes S, Pihl A. Different biologic properties of the two constituent peptide chains of ricin, a toxic protein inhibiting protein synthesis. Biochemistry 1973;12:3121–3126.
58. Ramsay NK, Kersey JH. Bone marrow purging using monoclonal antibodies. J Clin Immunol 1988;8:81–88.
59. Uckun F, Ramakrishnan S, Houston L. Increased efficiency in selective elimination of leukemia cells by a combination of a stable derivative of cyclophosphamide and a human B-cell specific immunotoxin containing pokeweed antiviral protein. Cancer Res 1985;45:69–75.
60. Bregni M, Lappi DA, Siena S, et al. Activity of a monoclonal antibody-saporin-6 conjugate against B-lymphoma cells. J Natl Cancer Inst 1988;80:49–55.
61. Yu YH, Crews JR, Cooper S, et al. Use of immunotoxins in combination to inhibit clonogenic growth of human breast carcinoma cells. Cancer Res 1990;50:3231–3238.
62. Coombes RC, Buckman R, Forrester A, et al. In vitro and in vivo effects of a monoclonal-antibody-toxin conjugate for patients with breast cancer. Cancer Res 1986;46:4217–4220.
63. Tondini C, Pap SA, Hayes DF, et al. Evaluation of monoclonal antibody DF3 conjugated with ricin as a specific immunotoxin for in vitro purging of human bone marrow. Cancer Res 1990;50:1170–1175.
64. Filipovich AH, Vallera DA, Youle RJ, et al. Graft-vs-host disease prevention in allogeneic bone marrow transplantation. A pilot study using immunotoxins for T cell depletion in donor marrow. Transplantation 1987;44:62–69.
65. Fauser AA, Lothar K, Casellas P, et al. Reconstitution of hematopoiesis after bone marrow purging with ricin A chain immunotoxin. Transplantation 1986; 41:356–360.
66. Reisner Y, Kapoor N, Kirkpatrick D. Transplantation for severe combined immunodeficiency (SCID) with histocompatible parental marrow fractionated by soybean agglutinin and sheep red blood cells: experience in six consecutive cases. Transplant Proc 1983;15:1431–1435.
67. Noga SJ, Wagoner JE, Rowley SD, et al. Using elu-

triation to engineer bone marrow allografts. In: Gross S, Gee A, Worthington-White D, eds. Bone marrow purging and processing. New York: Wiley-Liss, 1990:344–368.

68. Singer CRJ, Linch DC, Bown SG, et al. Differential phthalocyanine photosensitization of acute myeloblastic leukemia progenitor cells: a potential purging technique for autologous bone marrow transplantation. Br J Haematol 1988;68:417–422.

69. Sharkis S, Santos G, Colvin M, et al. Elimination of acute myelogenous leukemic cells from marrow and tumor suspensions in the rat with 4-HC. Blood 1980;55:521–524.

70. Hagenbeek A, Martens ACH. Toxicity of Asta Z (INN Mafosfamide) to normal and leukemic stem cells: Implications for autologous marrow transplantation. Invest New Drugs 1984;2:237–241.

71. Lowenberg B, Bauman J. Further results in understanding the subpopulation of structure of AML: clonogenic cells and their progeny identified by differentiation markers. Blood 1985;66:1225–1232.

72. Ball ED, Fanger MW. The expression of myeloid-specific antigens on myeloid leukemia cells: correlation with leukemia subclass and implications for myeloid differentiation. Blood 1983;61:456–461.

73. DeFabritiis PD, Ferrero D, Sandrelli A, et al. Monoclonal antibody purging and autologous bone marrow transplantation in acute myelogenous leukemia in complete remission. Bone Marrow Transplant 1989;4:669–674.

74. Gulati SC, Whitmarsh K, Reich L, et al. Results of autologous bone marrow transplantation for acute leukemia. Bone Marrow Transplant 1989;4:61–64.

75. Gorin NC, Aegerter B, Auvert G, et al. Autologous bone marrow transplantation for acute myelogenous leukemia in first remission; a European survey of the role of marrow purging. Blood 1990;75:1606–1614.

76. Yeager A, Rowley S, Jones RJ, et al. Autologous transplantation with chemopurged bone marrow in patients with acute myelocytic leukemia in second or third remission. In: Dicke KA, ed. Autologous bone marrow transplantation: proceedings of the Fifth International Symposium. Omaha, NE: University of Nebraska Press, 1991:90–98.

77. Yeager A, Rowley S, Santos G. Autologous bone marrow transplantation with acute nonlymphocytic leukemia, using ex vivo marrow treatment with 4-hydroperoxycyclophosphamide: an update. In: Powles R, Gordon-Smith EC, eds. Critical papers in bone marrow transplantation: an anthology. 1991, in press.

78. Ball ED, Mills LE, Cornwell GC III, et al. Autologous bone marrow transplantation for acute myelogenous leukemia using monoclonal antibody-purged bone marrow. Blood 1990;75:1119–1206.

79. Kersey JH, Weisdor D, Nesbit ME, et al. Comparison of autologous and allogeneic bone marrow transplantation for treatment of high-risk refractory acute lymphoblastic leukemia. New Engl J Med 1987; 317:461–467.

80. Bast RC, DeFabritiis P, Lipton J, et al. Elimination of malignant clonogenic cells from human bone marrow using multiple monoclonal antibodies and complement. Cancer Res 1985;45:499–503.

81. LeBien TW, Anderson JM, Vallera DA, Uckun F. Increased efficacy of selective elimination of leukemic cells by a combination of monoclonal antibodies BA-1, BA-2, BA-3 plus complement and mafosfamide (Asta-Z-7557). Leuk Res 1985;10:139–143.

82. Thorpe PE, Matson DW, Brown AN, et al. A selective killing of malignant cells in a leukemic rat bone marrow using an antibody-ricin conjugate. Nature 1982;297:594–596.

83. Fauser AA, Lothar K, Casellas P, Laurent G, Cooper BA, Lohr GW. Reconstitution of hematopoiesis after bone marrow purging with ricin A chain immunotoxin. Transplantation 1986;41:356–360.

84. Trickett AE, Ford DJ, Lam-Po-Tang, Vowels MR. Comparison of magnetic particles for immunomagnetic bone marrow purging using an acute lymphoblastic leukemia model. Transplant Proc 1990;22:2177–2178.

85. Uckun F, Kazimiera G, Meyers D, et al. Marrow purging in autologous bone marrow transplantation for T-lineage ALL: efficacy of ex vivo treatment with immunotoxins and 4-hydroperoxycyclophosphamide against fresh leukemic marrow progenitor cells. Blood 1987;69:361–366.

86. Marchetti-Rossi M, Centis F, Talevi N, Manna A, Sparaventi G, Porcellini A. Decontaminating bone marrow with Merocyanine 540, Mafosfamide or both. In: Dicke K, Spitzer G, Jagannath S, eds. The Third International Symposium on autologous bone marrow transplantation. Houston: University of Texas M.D. Anderson Hospital and Tumor Institute, 1987: 151–157.

87. Gilmore M, Hamon H, Prentice H, et al. Failure of purged autologous bone marrow transplantation in high risk acute lymphoblastic leukemia in first complete remission. Bone Marrow Transplant 1991;8:19–26.

88. Rowley SD, Jones RJ, Miller CB, Santos GW. Acute lymphoblastic leukemia (ALL): a phase I study of autologous bone marrow transplantation with combination drug purging. Proc Am Soc Clin Oncol 1990;9:202.

89. Ritz J, Sallan SE, Bast RC, et al. Autologous bone marrow transplantation in CALLA-positive acute lymphoblastic leukemia after in vitro treatment with J5 monoclonal antibody and complement. Lancet 1982;2:60–63.

90. Ramsey N, LeBien T, Nesbit M, et al. Autologous bone marrow transplantation for patients with ALL in second or subsequent remission: results of bone marrow treated with monoclonal antibodies with BA-1, BA-2, and BA-3 plus complement. Blood 1985;66:508–513.

91. Herve P, Cahn JY, Flesch M. Successful graft-vs-host disease prevention without graft failure in 32 HLA identical allogeneic bone marrow transplants with marrow depleted of T cells by monoclonal antibodies and complement. Blood 1987;69:388–393.

92. Waldmann H, Polliak A, Hale G. Elimination of graft versus host disease by in vitro depletion of alloreactive lymphocytes with a monoclonal rat anti-human lymphocyte antibody (Campath-1). Lancet 1984;2:483–486.

93. Vardtal F, Albrechtsen D, Ringden O, et al. Immunomagnetic purging of bone marrow allografts. In: Gee A, Gross S, eds. Proceedings of the First International Workshop on Bone Marrow Purging. Orlando, FL: Scientific and Medical Macmillan Press, 1987:94–99.

94. O'Reilly RJ, Collins N, Brochstein J, et al. Transplantation of marrow depleted of T cells by soybean lectin agglutination and E rosette depletion: major histocompatability complex-related graft resistance in leukemia transplant recipients. Transplant Proc 1985;17:445–459.

95. Wagner JE, Noga SJ, Vogelsang GB, Hess AD, Santos GW, Donnenberg AD. Elutriation: model for studying the effects of lymphocyte depletion on engraftment, graft versus host disease and graft versus leukemia. Bone Marrow Transplant 1987;2(suppl 2):145.

96. Kernan MA, Collins NH, Cunningham I, Castro-Malaspina H, Flomenberg N. Prevention of GVHD in HLA-identical marrow grafts by removal of T-cells with soybean agglutinin and SRBCs. Bone Marrow Transplant 1987;2(suppl 2):13–18.

97. Butturini A, Bortin MM, Seeger RC, Gale RP. Graft-vs-leukemia following bone marrow transplantation: a model of immunotherapy in man. Prog Clin Biol Res 1987;244:371–390.

98. Foucar K, McKenna RW, Frizzera G, et al. Incidence and patterns of bone marrow involvement by lymphoma in relation to the Lukes-Collins classification. Blood 1979;54:1417–1422.

99. Benjamin D, Magrath IT, Douglass EC, Corash LM. Derivation of lymphoma cell lines from microscopically normal bone marrow in patients with undifferentiated lymphomas: evidence of occult bone marrow involvement. Blood 1983;61:1017–1019.

100. Hu E, Trela M, Thompson J. Detection of B cell lymphoma in peripheral blood by DNA hybridisation. Lancet 1985;2:1092–1095.

101. Gulati S, Shank B, Black P, et al. Optimum timing of autologous bone marrow transplantation for patients with large B-cell lymphoma. In: Dicke K, Spitzer G, Jagannath S, eds. The Third International Symposium on Autologous Bone Marrow Transplantation. Houston: University of Texas M.D. Anderson Hospital and Tumor Institute, 1987:279–293.

102. Favrot M, Philip T, Philip I, et al. Bone marrow purging procedure in Burkitt lymphoma with monoclonal antibodies and complement. Quantification by a liquid culture monitoring system. Br J Cancer 1986;64:161–166.

103. Haleem A, Kurtzberg J, Olsen G, et al. Combined chemoseparation and immunoseparation of clonogenic T lymphoma cells from human bone marrow using 2'deoxycorformycin, deoxyadenosine, 3A-1 monoclonal antibody and complement. Cancer Res 1987;47:4608–4612.

104. Bregni M, Lappi D, Siena S, et al. Activity of a monoclonal antibody-saporin-6 conjugate against B-lymphoma cells. J Natl Cancer Inst 1980;80:511–517.

105. Favrot M, Philip I, Combaret O, Philip T. Experimental evaluation of an immunomagnetic bone marrow purging procedure using the Burkitt lymphoma model. Bone Marrow Transplant 1987;2:59–66.

106. Kvalheim G, Fostad O, Pihl A, et al. Elimination of B-lymphoma cells from human bone marrow: model experiments using monodisperse magnetic particles coated with primary monoclonal antibodies. Cancer Res 1987;47:846–851.

107. Mumcuoglu M, Favrot M, Slavin S. Lectin-binding properties of Burkitt's lymphoma cell lines: application to bone marrow purging. Exp Hematol 1990;18:55–60.

108. Nadler L, Stashenko P, Ritz J, Hardy R, Pesando J, Schlossman S. A unique cell surface antigen identifying lymphoid malignancies of B cell origin. J Clin Invest 1981;67:134–140.

109. Takvorian T, Canellos GC, Ritz J, et al. Prolonged disease free survival after autologous bone marrow transplantation in patients with non-Hodgkins lymphoma with poor prognosis. New Engl J Med 1987;316:1499–1505.

110. Freedman AS, Takvorian T, Anderson K, et al. Autologous bone marrow transplantation in B-cell Non-Hodgkins lymphoma: very low treatment-related mortality in 100 patients in sensitive relapse. J Clin Oncol 1990;8:874–891.

111. Philip T, Biron P, Philip I, et al. Massive therapy and ABMT in pediatric and young adults with Burkitt's lymphoma. Eur J Cancer Clin Oncol 1986;22:1015–1021.

112. Negrin RS, Chao NJ, Horning SJ, Long GD, O'Connor PO, Blume KG. Autologous bone marrow transplantation with monoclonal antibody plus complement "purged" bone marrow for high-risk non-Hodgkin's lymphoma: low transplant related mortality. Blood 1990;76:557a.

113. Gulati S, personnal communication (data submitted for publication).
114. Rowley SD, Miller CB, Piantadosi S, Davis JM, Santos GW, Jones RJ. Phase I study of combination drug purging for autologous bone marrow transplantation. J Clin Oncol, 1991, in press.
115. Treleaven J, Ugelstad J, Philip T, et al. Removal of neuroblastoma cells from bone marrow with monoclonal antibodies conjugated to magnetic microspheres. Lancet 1984;1:70–75.
116. Kemshead J, Heath L, Gibson FM, et al. Magnetic microspheres and monoclonal antibodies for the depletion of neuroblastoma cells from bone marrow: experiences, improvements and observations. Br J Cancer 1986;54:771–778.
117. Reynolds PC, Seeger RC, Co DD, Black AT, Wells J, Ugelstad J. Model system for removing neuroblastoma cells from bone marrow using monoclonal antibodies and magnetic immunobeads. Cancer Res 1986;46:846–851.
118. Gee A, Lee C, Bruce K, et al. Immunomagnetic purging and autologous transplantation in stage D neuroblastoma. In: Gee A, Gross S, eds. Proceedings of the First International Workshop on Bone Marrow Purging. Orlando, FL: Scientific and Medical Macmillan Press, 1987:89–93.
119. Seeger RC, Villablanca JG, Matthay KK, et al. Intensive chemoradiotherapy and autologous bone marrow transplantation for poor prognosis neuroblastoma. Prog Clin Biol Res 1991;366:527–533.
120. Graham-Pole J, Casper J, Elfenbein G, et al. High-dose chemoradiotherapy supported by marrow infusions for advanced neuroblastoma: a Pediatric Oncology Group Study. J Clin Oncol 1991;9:152–158.
121. Graham-Pole J, Gee A, Gross S, et al. Bone marrow transplantation for advanced neuroblastoma: a multicenter POG pilot study. In: Evans A, D'Angio H, Seeger R, Knudsen A, eds. Advances in neuroblastoma research. New York: Liss, 1988:215–223.
122. Graham-Pole J, Gee A, Gross S, et al. What factors affect hematologic recovery after myeloablation and autologous marrow rescue in neuroblastoma patients. Proc Am Soc Clin Oncol 1988;7:267.
123. Hartmann O, Benhamou E, Beaujean F, et al. Repeated high-dose chemotherapy followed by purged autologous bone marrow transplantation as consolidation therapy in metastatic neuroblastoma. J Clin Oncol 5:1205–1211, 1987.
124. Porro G, Menard S, Tagliabue E, et al. Monoclonal antibody detection of carcinoma cells in bone marrow biopsy specimens from breast cancer patients. Cancer 1988;61:2407–2411.
125. Redding H, Monaghan P, Ormerod M, et al. Detection of micrometastases in patients with primary breast cancer. Lancet 1983;2:1271–1273.
126. Buzdar AU. Natural history of stage IV breast cancer. In: Dicke K, Spitzer G, Zander A, eds. The First International Symposium on Autologous Bone Marrow Transplantation. Houston: University of Texas M.D. Anderson Hospital and Tumor Institute, 1985:185–188.
127. Morecki S, Pavlotsky S, Margel S, Slavin S. Purging breast cancer cells in preparation for autologous bone marrow transplantation. Bone Marrow Transplant 1987;1:357–363.
128. Frankel A, Ring D, Tringale F, et al. Tissue distribution of breast cancer-associated antigens defined by monoclonal antibodies. J Biol Response Mod 1987;4:273–286.
129. Shpall E, Jones R, Bast R, et al. 4-hydroperoxycyclophosphamide (4-HC) of breast cancer from the Ficolled mononuclear cell fraction (FMNCF) of bone marrow. Proc Am Soc Clin Oncol 1989;8:12.
130. Anderson I, Shpall EJ, Leslie D, et al. Elimination of malignant clonogenic breast cancer cells from human bone marrow. Cancer Res 1989;49:4659–4664.
131. Cooper KL, Shpall EJ, Peters WP, Bast RC. Elimination of clonogenic breast cancer cells from human bone marrow: comparison of immunotoxin treatment with chemoseparation and immunoseparation using 4-hydroperoxycyclophosphamide (4-HC) and immunomagnetic separation. Proc Am Assoc Cancer Res 1989;30:237.
132. Shpall EJ, Bast RC, Joines W, et al. Immunopharmacologic bone marrow purging in metastatic breast cancer patients receiving high-dose chemotherapy with autologous bone marrow support. Proc Am Soc Clin Oncol 1990;9:9.
133. Kennedy MJ, Beveridge R, Rowley S, et al. High dose consolidation chemotherapy and rescue with purged autologous bone marrow following dose-intense induction for metastatic breast cancer. Proc Am Soc Clin Oncol 1989;8:19.
134. Stahel R, Mabry M, Skarin A, Speak J, Bernal S. Detection of bone marrow metastases in small cell lung cancer by monoclonal antibody. J Clin Oncol 1985;3:455–461.
135. Elias A, Pap S, Bernal S. Purging of small cell lung cancer-contaminated bone marrow by monoclonal antibodies and magnetic beads. In: Gross S, Gee A, Worthington-White D, eds. Bone marrow purging and processing. New York: Wiley-Liss, 1990:263–275.
136. Vredenburgh JJ, Ball ED. Elimination of small cell carcinoma of the lung from human bone marrow by monoclonal antibodies and immunomagnetic beads. Cancer Res 1990;50:7216–7220.
137. Meagher R, Rothman S, Paul S, Koberna P, Wilmer C, Baucco P. Purging of small cell lung cancer cells using ethiofos (WR-2721) and light-activated merocyanine 540 phototreatment. Cancer Res 1989;49:3637–3641.

138. Benard J, Bettan-Renaud L, Gavoille A, et al. In vitro chemical eradication of small cell lung cancer: application in autologous bone marrow transplantation. Eur J Cancer Clin Oncol 1988;24:1561–1566.

139. Dicke KA, Spitzer G. Evaluation of the use of high-dose cytoreduction with autologous marrow rescue in various malignancies. Transplantation 1986;41:4–12.

140. Goldstone A, Anderson C, Linch D, Franklin I, Boughton B, Cawley J, Richards J. Autologous bone marrow transplantation following high-dose chemotherapy for treatment of adult patients with AML. Br J Haematol 1986;64:529–532.

16

Marrow Contamination: Positive Selection

*Peter M. Lansdorp, Terry E. Thomas, Christian R. Schmitt,
and Connie J. Eaves*

High-dose chemotherapy regimens in combination with transplantation of autologous hematopoietic cells are being used increasingly for the treatment of a variety of malignancies. In cases where a tumor-free source of autologous hematopoietic cells is available and is adequate to ensure hematologic rescue, this approach is limited by only two other factors. These are (a) inability of the high-dose treatment regimen to eliminate sufficient tumor cells in vivo to achieve a lasting remission (cure) and (b) potentially unacceptable side effects on non-hematopoietic tissues. The latter can be more or less defined, but the response of a particular tumor to dose escalation is not always predictable. The extent of the therapeutic advantage provided by dose escalation in combination with autologous transplantation is therefore likely to vary from patient to patient. On the other hand, this drawback is also likely to be less significant when aggressive treatment regimens are introduced at earlier stages of disease, a therapeutic principle that is receiving increasing attention.

All strategies that depend on hematologic rescue by transplantation of autologous marrow or blood are, however, also potentially complicated by the possibility of contaminating tumor cells. Methods for obtaining autologous hematopoietic cells free of tumor cells are thus clearly desirable, and techniques to remove tumor cells from blood or marrow harvests while retaining the cells required for hematologic rescue are of considerable interest. Approaches to achieve this goal tend to emphasize either one or the other of these requirements and are, accordingly, described as positive or negative (purging) selection procedures (1). Both approaches involve the selection or targeting of cells, but in negative selection procedures the targeted (tumor) cells are killed or removed from the autograft, whereas with positive selection the targeted (hematopoietic) cells must be recovered using nontoxic physical methods.

Currently available purging techniques use a variety of pharmacologic, biophysical, and/or immunologic agents either alone or in combination with physical cell separation techniques (1, and this volume). A major drawback to this approach is the natural diversity of different tumor types as well as the extensive heterogeneity that characterizes tumor cells of the same type, or even from the same individual. Thus a procedure that efficiently removes one type of tumor cells may be of limited value for a different type of tumor, and even within a single tumor, heterogeneity in pharmacologic, immunologic, and physical parameters can be expected. In contrast, heterogeneity between normal hematopoietic cells from different individuals is likely to be small in comparison. For this reason "positive selection" is an attractive alternative to purging techniques. In principle, a single positive selection technique should be applicable to many tumors, assuming criteria can be identified to distinguish primitive normal hematopoietic cells from tumor cells. Because with positive selection techniques the selected cells are physically removed from the tumor cells, the presence of the latter within the selected population can be analyzed using a variety of sensitive diagnostic procedures (including PCR methodology, flow cytometry, in situ hybridization, and immunohistochemistry). This allows quality control each time a selection procedure is used with a sensitivity that is difficult to achieve with most purging techniques.

Given these considerations, it may come as a surprise and a disappointment that large-scale positive selection techniques appropriate for general clinical use are not yet available. A small number of centers, including our own, have initiated programs to develop this technology, but for a variety of reasons (some of which are detailed in this paper) progress in this field has been relatively slow. This reflects in part our ignorance until recently of what cells need to be selected, even in animal models. Nevertheless, recent studies with experimental animals have now established that hematologic rescue with highly purified hematopoietic cell populations is feasible (2–5), and preliminary efforts along these lines in the clinical setting of autologous transplantation are encouraging (6–8).

In this review we will summarize recent progress in the development of positive selection techniques designed for wide clinical applicability and discuss major remaining obstacles. The focus will be on techniques for the isolation of cells that express CD34. This marker is selectively expressed on primitive human hematopoietic cells and is not expressed on most nonhematopoietic cells (6, 9). Thus most positive selection strategies for primitive human hematopoietic cells have

been based on the use of monoclonal antibodies against CD34. The proportion of cells in normal marrow that express CD34 as determined by flow cytometry is of the order of only a few percent, and this value is even lower for normal peripheral blood. Thus the potential enrichment of primitive hematopoietic cells obtainable using this marker alone is at least 20-fold. This marker may be of less value in patients whose malignant stem cells also express CD34, although it may be possible to effectively utilize CD34-based separation strategies in conjunction with other markers in such situations. However, this will require more detailed information about the composition of the CD34 compartment in patients with normal, perturbed, and malignant hematopoiesis.

SOURCES OF HEMATOPOIETIC CELLS

Hematopoietic cells from a variety of sources have been used to protect against hematologic failure after extensive chemoradiotherapy, and any of these might, in principle, serve as "crude material" for the isolation of specific hematopoietic cell subpopulations. These include autologous bone marrow, autologous peripheral blood mononuclear cells obtained by leukapheresis of patients that have or have not received previous chemotherapy, growth factors (or combinations of these), and allogeneic bone marrow from related, unrelated, or organ donors, fetal liver, and cord blood. Recently, marrow cells that have been maintained in vitro for 10 to 14 days have also been used successfully as autografts (10–12), and additional in vitro manipulations to achieve stem cell expansion are under investigation in many laboratories. Obviously there are differences in the quality and quantity of hematopoietic cells that can be obtained from each of these sources. Even if all possible sources of allogeneic cells are excluded from this discussion and only autologous marrow and peripheral blood are considered, differences between the relative numbers of different types of CD34-positive cells obtainable from these latter two sources may be expected. Hematopoietic progenitors detectable by standard in vitro colony assays are present in large numbers in leukapheresis harvests obtained from patients treated with some combinations of chemotherapy and certain growth factors, and transplantation of such cell populations results in rapid hematologic recovery (13–15). However, in the absence of data on the long-term reconstitution of patients transplanted with peripheral blood cells alone, particularly in the autologous setting, some caution regarding this approach seems warranted. Data from murine experiments suggest that transplantation of more mature progenitor cells contributes to early hematologic recovery but that these cells are distinct from and can be separated from more primitive hematopoietic cells that are responsible for long-term hematopoietic reconstitution (16, 17). This functional heterogeneity of hematopoietic cells is an important consideration as both the relative and absolute numbers of these subtypes of hematopoietic cells would be expected to vary in autologous leukapheresis samples. Because all of these, as well as most lineage-restricted clonogenic progenitor cells, express CD34, analyses of the various subpopulations of CD34-positive cells that can now be distinguished using directly labeled antibodies against CD34 (18) may allow important predictive correlations to be established between CD34 phenotype and short- and long-term reconstituting potential.

An example of the types of subpopulations of CD34-positive cells that can be demonstrated in normal marrow by flow cytometry is illustrated in Figure 16.1. This particular three-color staining experiment displays CD34-positive and CD34-negative subpopulations defined by differences in their expression of CD45RA, CD33, and CD10. The results shown confirm earlier observations that CD34-positive cells can be subdivided into two populations of about equal size (18). These previous studies also showed that normal marrow cells capable of initiating sustained (≥5 weeks) clonogenic progenitor output in long-term cultures (LTC-IC) (19) are enriched in the CD34-positive, CD45RA-negative cell fraction. The results shown in Figure 16.1 would thus predict that LTC-IC would be found to express some CD33 but not CD10. Whether such cells can eventually be quantitated directly by phenotype analysis and their in vivo engraftment potential determined by correlative studies of rates of recovery of different types of primitive hematopoietic cells is an area of active investigation. Ultimately, however, genetic marking of cells in the autograft, for example using retrovirus-mediated gene transfer, should provide definitive information about the in vivo reconstituting potential of selected marrow subpopulations by allowing the progeny of cells within the autograft to be followed and characterized over time.

PHYSICAL CELL SEPARATION TECHNIQUES

Given the low frequency of CD34-positive cells in normal bone marrow and peripheral blood, the use of a preliminary step to allow their bulk enrichment is of considerable interest. Unfortunately, considerable heterogeneity among CD34-positive cells with respect to most physical characteristics has been found, and this has limited the overall enrichment that can be obtained with methods such as counterflow centrifugational elutriation or density centrifugation. However, a two- to fivefold enrichment of CD34-positive cells with a good yield (>90%) can be readily and reproducibly obtained by density centrifugation (20). Because such a separation also removes the majority of red blood cells, it constitutes a very useful first step in positive selection procedures. For large-scale separations of bone marrow (typically 1 to 2 liters of pooled cells from many individual aspirates), it is also convenient to first concentrate the nucleated cells to a 100- to 200-ml volume of buffy coat by standard centrifuga-

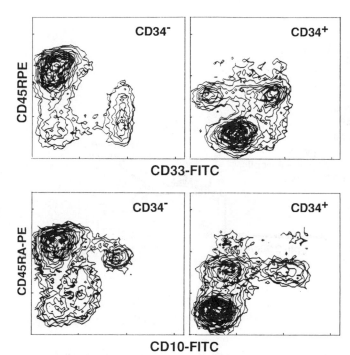

Figure 16.1. Bivariate contour histograms of nucleated bone marrow cells stained with the indicated antibody conjugates as well as cyanine-5 (Cy-5) labeled anti-CD34. Cells stained by three-color immunofluorescence were analyzed on a two-laser flow cytometer and divided into CD34-negative and CD34-positive cells based on Cy-5 fluorescence (excited with an He-Ne laser). Orange fluorescence from R-phycoerythrin (RPE) linked to anti-CD45RA of individual cells was then correlated with green fluorescence of FITC linked to either anti-CD33 or anti-CD10 antibodies to obtain the bivariate contour plots shown. Note that the overall staining patterns of CD34-negative and CD34-positive cells differ dramatically and that cells that express CD34-positive are highly heterogeneous.

tion. In our laboratory we have developed a large-scale density separation technique for such bone marrow buffy coat preparations using Percoll (21). The principle of this method is illustrated in Figure 16.2. In seven experiments, 44% (23% to 72%) of the nucleated cells were recovered from the buffy coat without significant loss of in vitro clonogenic progenitors, which were thereby enriched an initial twofold. This method, like other density separation protocols that have been described (22, 23), typically yields a concentrated suspension of light-density nucleated cells within 1 to 2 hours and thus provides a useful preenrichment step prior to the use of other immunoselection procedures.

Counterflow centrifugal elutriation allows cells to be separated primarily on the basis of size differences and, to a lesser extent, differences in density. The majority of clonogenic cells and cells classified morphologically as blasts can be recovered in fractions that are enriched for large cells and

relatively depleted of lymphocytes and erythrocytes. Such preparations have recently been used successfully in the transplant setting (24). However, it seems likely that the most primitive hematopoietic cells with long-term in vivo repopulating ability are smaller cells (16, 20) and hence may be relatively depleted in the large cell (Rotor off) fraction (16).

IMMUNOSELECTION

The introduction of monoclonal antibodies against cell surface antigens has greatly expanded possibilities for distinguishing and separating functionally distinct populations (25). Well-known examples are monoclonal antibodies directed against the CD4 and CD8 antigens that are expressed on functionally distinct subpopulations of lymphocytes and that, as a group, are characterized by expression of the CD3 antigen. Monoclonal antibodies can be produced in unlimited quantities, and this feature of monoclonal antibodies, together with their exquisite

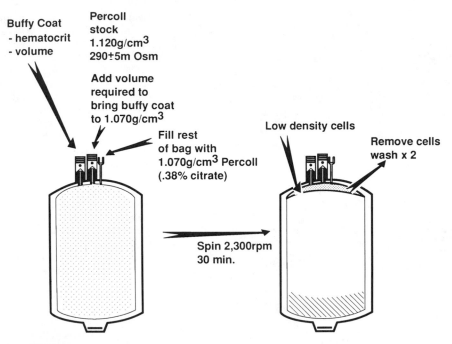

Figure 16.2. Principle of the "in bag" Percoll density separation procedure developed by the authors (21). Nucleated cells from a typical 1- to 2-liter bone marrow harvest are concentrated into a buffy coat suspension of 100 to 200 ml using a COBE cell centrifuge. The buffy coat cells are then transferred into a 600-ml transfer bag and a calculated volume of Percoll stock solution added to suspend the cells in a Percoll solution that has a final density of 1.070 g/cm³. The bag is then filled with Percoll of this density and spun. Low-density (d ≤ 1.070 g/cm³) cells are recovered from the top of the bag. Compared to methods in which cells are layered on top of a density gradient medium, this procedure has a high capacity, is rapid, and uses relatively small volumes of density gradient medium for efficient and reproducible separations.

specificity, makes them attractive tools for the development of cell separation techniques.

Recognition of the requirement for transplantation of hematopoietic stem cells to achieve long-term reconstitution of hematopoiesis in recipients of supralethal doses of chemoradiotherapy prompted research aimed at stem cell isolation more than 20 years ago (reviewed in 2). It is therefore not surprising that many investigators started to explore the possibility of using monoclonal antibodies to isolate primitive human hematopoietic cells in the early 1980s (26, 27). A significant milestone was the development of monoclonal antibodies that bind CD34 (18). These antibodies react with a heavily glycosylated transmembrane protein of 110 kD (28) that is selectively expressed on immature lympho-hematopoietic cells (reviewed in 29). Strong expression (>50,000 molecules per cell) is restricted to only a few percent of low-density marrow cells, and CD34 expression appears to decrease with maturation and/or differentiation (24, 30). Although only a small fraction of all marrow cells express levels of CD34 detectable by flow cytometry, this CD34-positive compartment is, nevertheless, itself highly heterogeneous, as discussed above (see Figure 16.1). Expression of CD34 on non-hematopoietic cells appears to be restricted to cells of the vascular endothelium and ontologically related mesenchymal cells (e.g., in fetal skin) (9). Anti-CD34 antibodies have therefore been widely used for enrichment of primitive human hematopoietic cells.

The most powerful tool for the separation of cells using monoclonal antibodies is the fluorescence-activated cell sorter (FACS). With this machine cells can be purified on the basis of multiple parameters including different levels of fluorescence intensity that can be objectively and reproducibly distinguished by the FACS. This combination of analysis and separation allows the isolation of highly purified populations of cells with defined surface and light-scattering properties. The purity of the FACS-sorted cells can also be easily measured by reanalysis of their staining properties indicated by the same fluorescent-labeled antibodies used for sorting. For these reasons the FACS is currently the preferred laboratory tool for purification of cells that express CD34 or subpopulations thereof. Limitations of the FACS for the large-scale positive selection of CD34-positive cells for therapeutic applications are the costs of the machine, practical limitations in the total number of cells that can be analyzed and sorted (approximately 2×10^7 cells per hour), as well as the technical skill required for the maintenance and operation of an FACS. For these reasons considerable effort has been put into the development of batch-wise immunoabsorption procedures that can be scaled up to handle the large numbers of cells required for clinical autologous transplantation protocols (i.e., usually >1 to 2×10^{10} nucleated bone marrow cells or peripheral blood leucocytes).

IMMUNOADSORPTION TECHNIQUES

The major challenge that any immunoadsorption technique must address is to transfer the molecular specificity of a particular monoclonal antibody to the physical separation of whole cells (that have a mass >10^9 times that of antibody molecules). This challenge is considerable because marrow cells are neither inert (or even rigid) nor homogeneous particles with constant physical properties, but highly heterogeneous entities

with complex and continuously changing surface properties.

For immunoabsorption to be possible, the desired cell-surface-specific antigen-antibody interaction has to be coupled to another defined surface (i.e., particle, bead, or dish) that can then be used to achieve a physical separation between antibody-labeled and -unlabeled cells. Immunoadsorption procedures must therefore incorporate a number of features that are not easily combined. For example, interactions of the cells and the immunoadsorption surface in the absence of antibodies must be minimal, but repulsive forces (which are advantageous) should not be stronger than the attraction provided by (multiple) antibody-antigen interactions. If antibodies are immobilized on a surface, the kinetics of the antigen-antibody interactions will be altered, and it may be difficult to obtain sufficient binding to take full advantage of the specificity provided by a particular monoclonal antibody. Shearing forces may also favor dissociation of specifically bound antibody, whereas the increased chances of multivalent interactions with immobilized antibody may favor association. Both shearing forces and multivalent interactions are likely to change the reactivity pattern observed with the original, typically bivalent, monoclonal antibody as analyzed by standard indirect immunofluorescence.

A variety of surfaces, varying in size from a panning dish to submicron magnetic particles, have been used for immunoadsorption of cells (Fig. 16.3). Whatever the surface, it must allow physical separation of the bound cells from the remaining cell suspension. This is most easily achieved with large surfaces (e.g., as in panning methods). On the other hand, nonspecific interactions with unlabeled cells also typically increase with larger surfaces. For these reasons it could be argued that the "ideal" surface for positive selection would probably be as small as is compatible with the physical properties required for separation of bound from unbound cells. In Figure 16.3 approximate volumes of different types

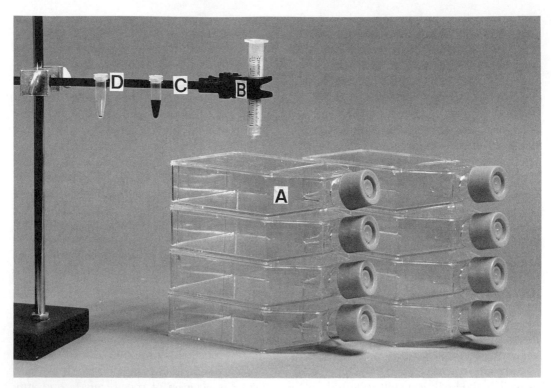

Figure 16.3.   Packed volumes of various particles currently in use for positive selection of cells that express CD34 in relation to a fixed surface area (600 cm²). Compared to eight 75 cm² culture tissue flasks used for panning (**A**), a 3-ml column of 200 μm diameter beads (**B**), 0.3 ml of 3.4-μm diameter magnetic beads (**C**) and 10 μl of 100-nm diameter iron-dextran particles (**D**) are required to yield the same total immunoadsorption surface area (600 cm², sufficient for separtion of approximately 10⁹ cells).

of packed beads currently used for cell separations in relation to a fixed (600 cm²) surface area are shown. The smallest (iron-dextran) particles clearly have the best volume-to-surface-area ratio, but separation of cells labeled with these beads requires special high-gradient magnetic filters (30, 31) and stronger magnets than those useful for separation of cells labeled with commercially available particles, paramagnetic polystyrene coated particles (32, 33). Whether the theoretical advantages of the smaller-sized iron dextran beads (rapid antigen-antibody kinetics, minimal nonspecific binding) outweigh the advantage of using larger beads that can be recovered with a simple magnet is currently under study.

Panning

The basic principles of some of the current techniques for positive selection of cells that express CD34 are illustrated in Figure 16.3. Adsorption of bone marrow cells labeled with anti-CD34 to the plastic surface of petri dishes or tissue culture flasks coated with anti-mouse immunoglobulin and recovery of the adherent cells by vigorous pipetting ("panning") is the first positive selection technique that was applied for the purification of cells that express CD34 (18). Although clearly advantageous in its simplicity and cost (expensive beads, magnets, and other equipment are not required), the separation of a typical 2×10^{10} bone marrow cell harvest would demand a very large number of flasks to provide sufficient surface area (i.e., at 2×10^6 cells per cubic centimeter, 130 flasks would be required). In addition the nonspecific binding of cells to plastic and difficulties in reproducibly removing specifically bound cells have effectively limited this approach to laboratory settings, where it probably has a place as a simple, rapid, and inexpensive, albeit rather crude, enrichment procedure.

Immunoadsorption Columns

Immunoadsorption columns for the selection of CD34-positive cells have been developed by at least two groups (7, 34). The technique developed by Berenson and his colleagues (7) has recently been tested clinically, and this method will therefore be discussed here in some detail. The method they have developed is based on high-affinity interaction between biotin-labeled antibodies on cells and avidin coupled to polyacrylamide beads. Bone marrow cells are labeled with biotinylated anti-CD34 or unlabeled anti-CD34 followed by biotinylated antiimmunoglobulin and then passed at a constant flow rate over a column containing avidin-labeled polyacrylamide beads (average diameter 200 μm). The constant flow minimizes chances for nonspecific interactions between cells and beads that are already low with polyacrylamide beads. Apparently the biotin-avidin interaction is sufficiently strong to withstand the shearing forces acting upon labeled cells during their passage through the column, resulting in an efficient depletion step. For positive selection, labeled cells can be recovered by mechanical disruption of the column and "vigorous pipetting" of the resulting polyacrylamide bead slurry. The purity of cells expressing CD34 obtained from these columns has been reported to range from 62% to 92% in five patients that were transplanted with selected cells. The total number of cells for recovered transplantation in these patients varied from 56 to 260 $\times$ 10^6 (1.2% of

the harvested nucleated bone marrow cells). Despite apparent adequate recovery of CD34-positive cells with this procedure, hematologic recovery was relatively slow (7, 8). Whether this delayed hematologic recovery was due to the infusion of reduced numbers of, or damaged, cells is not yet clear. Another possibility is that many of the primitive antibody-labeled cells were "opsonized" and captured in the reticuloendothelial system.

The purity of the cells isolated for transplant applications may be an important consideration for the success of positive selection strategies in many settings. The relationship between the purity of isolated cells and the efficiency of depletion of CD34-negative cells (including tumor cells in this theoretical example) is illustrated in Table 16.1. It can be seen that for a 2 to 4 log depletion of CD34-negative cells (including tumor cells that could present a minor fraction of these cells), the purity of the selected cells rapidly needs to exceed 70% when only a few percent of cells in the starting cell suspension express CD34.

Table 16.1.   Depletion of CD34- Cells during Positive Selection of CD34+ Cells[a]

Starting Material % of CD34+ Cells	Purified Fraction (50% Recovery of CD34+ Cells) % CD34+ Cells)	Log Depletion of CD34− Cells
0.1	50	3.3
	70	3.7
	90	4.2
	95	4.5
	99	5.3
1.0	50	2.3
	70	2.7
	90	3.2
	95	3.5
	99	4.3
5.0	50	1.6
	70	1.9
	90	2.5
	95	2.9
	99	3.6

[a]These calculations are based on theoretical purifications that assume 50% recovery of CD34+ cells.

Magnetic Beads

Positive selection of CD34-positive cells using paramagnetic (polystyrene coated) microspheres with a diameter of 3.4 μm was described by Civin et al. (33). These authors used sheep anti-mouse IgG$_1$-coated beads for removal of bone marrow cells that were reactive with My10 anti-CD34 monoclonal antibodies. After incubation, the cells were separated in a tissue culture flask, using a strong magnet to hold the magnetic beads and cells bound to such beads to the wall of the flask while unbound cells were poured off. Release of the cells from the microspheres was achieved using chymopapain (see below). Efficiency of removal and recovery was evaluated using colony assays to quantitate progenitors. These measurements indicated that a progenitor enrichment of up to a 100-fold could be achieved using this method. The possibility of scaling up this technique for clinical transplantation purposes is now being evaluated as is the possibility of directly coupling anti-CD34 antibodies to the beads.

Submicron Magnetic Particles

As argued above, the ideal particle for large-scale positive selection techniques is one that is as small as possible and yet allows bound and unbound cells to be physically separated. Molday described the use of iron-dextran particles with a mean diameter of 50–100 nm for cell separation techniques (35). With this approach, cells are indirectly labeled with such particles. Because of their small size, they provide a weak magnetic moment to the cells to which they are bound. The latter is, however, sufficient to retain cells in a high-gradient magnetic filter inside a strong magnetic field generated by an electromagnet or a strong samarian-cobalt magnet (35, 36).

We have recently started to explore this approach for the isolation of cells that express CD34, and preliminary results are encouraging. Up to 2×10^8 cells are incubated with tetrameric antibody complexes (37) in which anti-CD34 monoclonals are cross-linked to antibodies that react with the iron-dextran particles (38). The cells are then washed and loaded into a 3-ml syringe that has been loosely packed with stainless steel wire. The syringe is then placed inside a strong (e.g., 10 kG) magnetic field generated by an electromagnet. Unbound cells are washed away with several column volumes of buffer, after which bound cells are recovered by turning off the electromagnet. The result of a typical experiment using this procedure is shown in Figure 16.4. Compared to immunoadsorption of CD34-positive cells to glass beads using tetrameric antibody complexes (34, 37), the most striking observation has been that essentially *all* selected cells are recovered with this technique at ≥55 to 85% purity. Mechanisms of nonspecific cell entrapment are currently under study in an attempt to further increase purity.

Thus far we have shown that the presence of iron-dextran particles on cells that express CD34 does not alter their capacity for in vitro colony formation in semisolid medium nor their ability to initiate the long-term output of clonogenic cells on competent irradiated feeders. If it can be established that the homing and growth potential of these cells in vivo is similarly unaffected, and if the purity of the selected CD34-positive cells can be increased further, the use of submicron magnetic particles (which do not change light-scatter properties of cells as analyzed by flow cytometry) could become the method of choice for positive selection of cells that express CD34.

PROCESSING OF SELECTED CELLS

The various methods for positive selection of CD34-positive cells described above all yield cells that are more or less modified by the cell separation procedure (Fig. 16.5). However, little is known about the subsequent behavior in vivo of cells modified as required for their isolation. Studies of mice

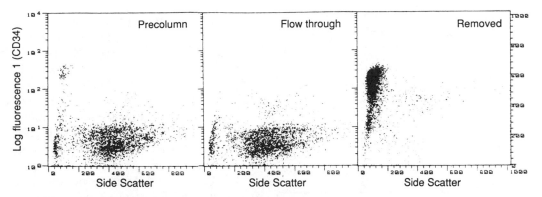

Figure 16.4. Positive selection of cells that express CD34 using iron-dextran particles (38). For this experiment low-density bone marrow cells were labeled with tetrameric antibody complexes in which mouse IgG$_1$ antiperoxidase antibodies were cross-linked to mouse IgG$_1$ anti-CD34 using F(ab')$_2$ fragments of rat monoclonal anti-mouse IgG$_1$ (37). Cells were then passed through a 3-ml syringe loosely packed with stainless steel wool in a 10-kG magnetic field generated by an electromagnet. Precolumn and flow-through cells were labeled with anti-mouse-Ig-FITC, as were the cells recovered from the column after the magnet was turned off. Dot plot profiles of green fluorescence (CD34) plotted against the side scatter of individual cells are shown. Note that cells that express CD34 were efficiently depleted in the flow-through fraction and that such cells are highly enriched in the removed cell fraction.

transplanted with purified stem cells to which tetrameric antibody complexes or magnetic beads have been attached (39, 40), or rats transplanted with chymopapain-treated bone marrow (32) indicate that even extensive cell surface modifications do not obliterate the hematopoietic repopulating ability of these cells. In theory, both the cell number used for transplantation as well as the modification of the cell surface of CD34-positive cells resulting from the isolation procedure could change homing patterns and functional properties in vivo. The effects of infusion of limited cell numbers could be minimized by mixing the selected cells with irradiated CD34-negative cells, but changes at the cell surface may be more difficult to avoid. Perhaps competition with soluble CD34, relevant peptides, or anti-CD34 anti-idiotype antibodies could be used to yield purified CD34-positive cells with no antibodies attached. As an alternative approach, the use of a highly specific glycoprotease enzyme (41) that abolishes reactivity of some anti-CD34 monoclonals by cleavage of the CD34 molecule might be considered. However, in the absence of convincing data to demonstrate significant advantages to the use of unmodified cells as compared to cells with antibodies (or even beads) still attached, perfection of techniques to yield unmodified selected cells is unlikely to receive much attention as a research priority.

CONCLUSIONS

In this chapter we have attempted to give an overview of current techniques for the selection of cells that express CD34. Some of the basic problems with various approaches have been outlined to explain the limited use of existing technology for clinical purposes and to define areas for futher study. To obtain efficient batch-wise separation of cells that express CD34, it is necessary to carefully balance specific and nonspecific interactions of cells with the immunoadsorption surface. The separation efficiency can be affected by many different factors, including antigen expression-turnover, antigen/antibody interactions, coupling of the antibody to separation particle, interaction between cell surfaces and the

Methods For Recovery Of CD34+ Cells
From Immunoadsorbents

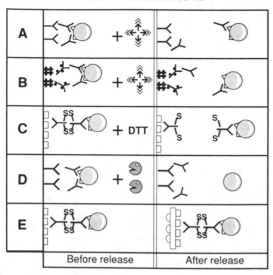

| | Before release | After release |

Figure 16.5. Positive selection alters the surface of cells that express CD34. The effects of various isolation procedures currently in use for the positive selection of CD34-positive cells are illustrated. Positive selection by means of panning (**A**) most likely results in some anti-CD34 antibodies at the surface of CD34-positive cells. Some antibody would also be expected on cells selected on columns using biotinylated antibodies (**B**) (6–8) or tetrameric antibody complexes (34). Conditions for reductive cleavage (**C**) of tetramers (34, 37) will also change some cell surface proteins on CD34-positive cells and enzymes (**D**) that cleave CD34 (32, 41) may also cleave other cell surface glycoproteins. Such modifications or the presence of iron-dextran particles at the surface of the selected cells (**E**) could change the properties of cells upon transplantation.

separation particle, strength of the forces used to separate cells labeled with particles, and flow characteristics of the separation chamber. All of the above are dynamic processes that need to be controlled simultaneously to obtain a desirable and reproducible result. At the moment no single positive selection technique allows the reproducible isolation of suspensions of CD34-positive cells at a high purity (>90% CD34-positive) without substantial losses of the cells desired (e.g., ≥30%). However, growing interest and efforts to develop this type of technology are likely to yield

solutions to the remaining obstacles in the near future. Reproducible technology for the purification of hematopoietic cells could increase the use of autologous transplantation significantly and even has the potential to become a standard clinical procedure that could be used routinely before subsequent manipulations of the cells. For these applications the time, labor, and cost of such a cell-processing step would, however, have to be carefully considered. At the same time progress in the development of more selective antitumor therapies and the use of growth factor treatment in vivo following high-dose chemotherapy may reduce or alter the type of hematologic rescue or support required. In addition, culture conditions will eventually be defined to enable the selective expansion in vitro of both short- and long-term reconstituting cells. The availability of procedures for the large scale isolation of highly purified suspensions of these cells will undoubtedly facilitate these developments as well as contribute to the realization of clinical gene therapy protocols and other novel therapeutic strategies that exploit hematopoietic stem cell transplants.

Acknowledgments

The authors wish to thank Sara Abraham, Colleen McAloney, and Cam Smith for excellent technical assistance. The manuscript was typed by Karen Windham. These studies were supported by the National Cancer Institute of Canada (NCIC) and the British Columbia Health Care and Research Foundation as well as by grant A129524 from the U.S. National Institutes of Health. Christian Schmitt was supported by the Institut National de la Sante et de la Recherche Medicale (INSERM) and the Association pour la Recherche sur le Cancer (France). Connie Eaves is a Terry Fox Cancer Research Scientist of the NCIC.

REFERENCES

1. Gross S, Gee AP, Worthington-White DA eds. Bone marrow purging and processing. New York: Wiley-Liss, 1990.
2. Visser JWM, van Bekkum DW. Purification of pluripotent hemopoietic stem cells: past and present. Exp Hematol 1990;18:248–256.
3. McCarthy KF, Hale ML, Fehnel PL. Purification and analysis of rat hemopoietic stem cells by flow cytometry. Cytometry 1987;8:296–305.

4. Berenson RJ, Andrews RG, Bensinger WI, et al. Antigen CD34+ marrow cells engraft lethally irradiated baboons. J Clin Invest 1988;81:951–955.
5. Wagemaker G, van Gills FCJM, Bart-Baumeister JAK, Wielenga JJ, Levinsky RJ. Sustained engraftment of allogeneic CD34 positive hemopoietic stem cells in Rhesus monkeys [Abstract]. Exp Hematol 1990; 18(suppl 6):704.
6. Berenson RJ, Andrews RG, Bensinger WI, et al. Selection of CD34+ marrow cells for autologous marrow transplantation. In: Dicke KA, Spitzer G, Jagannath S, Evinger-Hodges MJ, eds. Autologous bone marrow transplantation. Houston: M.D. Anderson Cancer Center, 1989:55–60.
7. Berenson RJ, Bensinger WI, Hill R, et al. Stem cell selection—clinical experience. In: Gross S, Gee AP, Worthington-White DA, eds. Bone marrow purging and processing. New York: Wiley-Liss, 1990:403–413.
8. Bensinger WI, Berenson RJ, Andrews RG, et al. Positive selection of hemopoietic progenitors from marrow and peripheral blood for transplantation. J Clin Apheresis 1990;5:74–76.
9. Fina L, Molgaard HV, Robertson D, et al. Expression of the CD34 gene in vascular endothelial cells. Blood 1990;75:2417–2426.
10. Barnett MJ, Eaves CJ, Phillips GL, et al. Successful autografting in chronic myeloid leukemia after maintenance of marrow in culture. Bone Marrow Transplant 1989;4:345–351.
11. Barnett MJ, Eaves CJ, Phillips GL, et al. Autografting with curative intent for patients with chronic myeloid leukemia. In: Dicke KA, Armitage JO, Dicke-Evinger MJ, eds. Autologous bone marrow transplantation: proceedings of the fifth annual symposium. Omaha, NE: University of Nebraska Medical Center, 1991:237–240.
12. Chang J, Morgenstern G, Coutinho L, et al. The use of bone marrow cells grown in long-term culture for autologous bone marrow transplantation in acute myeloid leukemia: an update. Bone Marrow Transplant 1989;4:5–9.
13. To LB, Haylock DN, Kimber RJ, Juttner CA. High levels of circulating haemopoietic stem cells in very early remission from acute non-lymphoblastic leukaemia and their collection and cryopreservation. Br J Haematol 1984;58:399–410.
14. Juttner CA, To LB, Haylock DN, Dyson PG. Peripheral blood stem cell selection, collection and auto-transplantation. In: Gross S, Gee AP, Worthington-White DA, eds. Bone marrow purging and processing. New York: Wiley-Liss, 1990:447–460.
15. Gianni AM, Bregni M, Stern AC, et al. Granulocyte-macrophage colony-stimulating factor to harvest circulating haemopoietic stem cells for autotransplantation. Lancet 1989;2:580–584.
16. Jones RJ, Wagner JE, Celano P, Zicha MS, Sharkis SJ. Separation of pluripotent haematopoietic stem cells from spleen colony-forming cells. Nature 1990; 347:188–189.
17. Eaves CJ, Sutherland HJ, Szilvassy SJ, et al. Phenotypic and functional characterization of primitive haematopoietic stem cells. In: Sachs L, Abraham NG, Wiedermann CJ, Levine AS, Konwalinka G, eds. Molecular biology of haematopoiesis. Andover, Hants, U.K.: Intercept Ltd., 1990:87–98.
18. Lansdorp PM, Sutherland HJ, Eaves CJ. Selective expression of CD45 isoforms on functional subpopulations of CD34+ hemopoietic cells from human bone marrow. J Exp Med 1990;172:363–366.
19. Sutherland HJ, Lansdorp PM, Henkelman DH, Eaves AC, Eaves CJ. Functional characterization of individual human hemopoietic stem cells cultured at limiting dilution on supportive marrow stromal layers. Proc Natl Acad Sci USA 1990;87:3584–3588.
20. Sutherland HJ, Eaves CJ, Eaves AC, Dragowska W, Lansdorp PM. Characterization and partial purification of human marrow cells capable of initiating long-term hemopoiesis in vitro. Blood 1989;74:1563–1570.
21. Thomas TE, Abraham SJR, Phillips GL, Lansdorp PM. A simple procedure for large scale density separation of bone marrow cells for transplantation. Transplantation, in press.
22. Rowley SD, Davis JM, Braine H, et al. Density-gradient separation for 4-hydroperoxycyclophosphamide purging of autologous bone marrow grafts. In: Gross S, Gee AP, Worthington-White DA, eds. Bone marrow purging and processing. New York: Wiley-Liss, 1990:369–378.
23. Areman EM, Sacher RA, Deig HJ. Cryopreservation and storage of human bone marrow: a survey of current practices. In: Gross S, Gee AP, Worthington-White DA, eds. Bone marrow purging and processing. New York: Wiley-Liss, 1990:523–530.
24. Noga SJ, Wagner JE, Rowley SD, et al. Using elutriation to engineer bone marrow allografts. In: Gross S, Gee AP, Worthington-White DA, eds. Bone marrow purging and processing. New York: Wiley-Liss, 1990:345–361.
25. Knapp W, Dorken B, Gilks WR, et al. Leucocyte typing IV. White cell differentiation antigens. Oxford: Oxford University Press. 1989.
26. Beverley PCL, Linch D, Delia D. Isolation of human haematopoietic progenitor cells using monoclonal antibodies. Nature 1980;287:332–333.
27. Young NS, Hwang-Chen S-P. Anti-K562 cell monoclonal antibodies recognize hemopoietic progenitors. Proc Natl Acad Sci USA 1981;78:7073–7077.
28. Civin CI, Strauss LC, Brovall C, Fackler MJ, Schwartz JF, Shaper JH. Antigenic analysis of hematopoiesis. III: A hemopoietic progenitor cells surface antigen defined by a monoclonal antibody raised against KC-1a cells. J Immunol 1984;133:157–165.
29. Civin CI, Trischmann TM, Fackler MJ, et al. Report on the CD34 cluster workshop. In: Knapp W, Dorken

B, Gilks WR, Ruber EP, Schmidt RE, Stein H, eds. Leucocyte typing IV. White cell differentiation antigens. 1989:818–825.

30. Molday RS. Cell labeling and separation using immunospecific microspheres. In: Pretlow TG II, Pretlow TP, eds. Cell separation: methods and selected applications. Vol. 3. New York: Academic Press, 1984:237–263.

31. Civin CI, Banquerigo ML, Strauss LC, Loken MR. Antigenic analysis of hematopoiesis. VI: Flow cytometric characterization of My-10-positive progenitor cells in normal human bone marrow. Exp Hematol 1987;15:10–17.

32. Miltenyi S, Muller W, Weichel W, Radbruch A. High gradient magnetic cell separation with MACS. Cytometry 1990;11:231–238.

33. Civin CI, Strauss LC, Fackler MJ, Trischmann TM, Wiley JM, Loken MR. Positive stem cell selection—basic science. In: Gross S, Gee AP, Worthington-White DA, eds. Bone marrow purging and processing. New York: Wiley-Liss, 1990:387–402.

34. Thomas TE, Sutherland HJ, Lansdorp PM. Specific binding and release of cells from beads using cleavable tetrameric antibody complexes. J Immunol Methods 1989;120:221–231.

35. Molday RS, Molday LL. Separation of cells labeled with immunospecific iron dextran microspheres using high gradient magnetic chromatography. FEBS Lett 1984;170:232–237.

36. Miltenyi S, Muller W, Weichel W, Radbruch A. High gradient magnetic cell separation with MACS. Cytometry 1990;11:231–238.

37. Lansdorp PM, Thomas TE. Purification and analysis of bispecific tetrameric antibody complexes. Mol Immunol 1990;27:659–666.

38. Thomas TE, Lansdorp PM. Unpublished observations.

39. Fraser CC, Eaves CJ, Svilvassy SJ, Humphries RK. Expansion in vitro of retrovirally marked totipotent hematopoietic stem cells. Blood 1990;76:1071–1076.

40. Spangrude GJ, Heimfeld S, Weissman IL. Purification and characterization of mouse hemopoietic stem cells. Science 1988;241:58–62.

41. Sutherland DR, Abdullah KM, Mellors A, Davidson J, Baker MA. Cleavage of the lymphohemopoietic progenitor cell antigen CD34 by a novel glycoproteinase from P. Haemolytica. Blood 1990;76(suppl 1):122a.

17

HEMATOPOIETIC GROWTH FACTORS

Rosemary Mazanet and James D. Griffin

The growth and differentiation of blood-forming cells (hematopoiesis) involves complex mechanisms that are only beginning to be understood. This system provides for the ongoing replenishment of short-lived cellular blood elements and allows for prompt and specific differentiation of target cells in response to stress states such as blood loss or infection. This process is regulated by a series of glycoprotein hormones termed hematopoietic growth factors (HGF). Some of these HGFs are also referred to as "colony-stimulating factors" (CSFs). The CSFs induce proliferation of hematopoietic progenitor cells, activate mature blood cells, enhance mature effector cell function (1, 2), and initiate the production of other hematopoietic growth factors (3–5).

CSFs are produced by a variety of cell types in response to different stimuli, and have multiple biologic activities on different target cells. This has led to the realization that intricate cytokine interactions are employed in cell growth, differentiation, and function. As a result, when HGFs are administered as pharmacologic agents, the clinical effects are the result of both the direct actions of the factor and the indirect actions due to activation of other cytokines or networks.

Over the last few years, a large number of HGF genes have been cloned, and their products have been purified, cloned, and produced in bacteria or yeast. Although all of these molecules merit discussion, we will focus our attention on the CSFs known to regulate the production of myeloid cells now in clinical trials: granulocyte colony-stimulating factor (G-CSF), monocyte colony-stimulating factor or colony-stimulating factor 1 (M-CSF or CSF-1), granulocyte-monocyte colony-stimulating factor (GM-CSF), and multilineage colony-stimulating factor (multi-CSF), also known as interleukin-3 (IL-3). The first hematopoietic growth factor to be described, erythropoietin (EPO), will also be discussed. Other HGFs, such as the c-kit ligand (MGF, stem cell growth factor, or Steel factor) and a fusion protein of GM-CSF and IL-3 (FP or PIXY) are just entering clinical trials and show great promise on the basis of in vitro testing.

In the context of dose-intensive chemotherapy and bone marrow transplantation, this chapter will provide an overview of the biologic characteristics of the HGF family, up through selected preclinical results of their administration that illustrate their mechanisms of action. The effects of these agents in stimulating solid tumor cells, abnormal marrow cells, and peripheral blood progenitor cells will also be discussed briefly, as background for the following chapters dealing separately with each CSF. The clinical use of CSFs to abrogate cytopenias, whether idiopathic or therapy related (i.e., chemotherapy for malignancies or azidothymidine [AZT] for AIDS) has been reviewed elsewhere (6, 7) and will not be presented here.

BACKGROUND

Over 3 decades ago, in vitro methods of bone marrow culture in semisolid media such as agar or methylcellulose were developed (8, 9). Marrow cells did not spontaneously proliferate in these culture systems, but colonies of single or multiple lineages resulted when media (conditioned by various sources: placenta, lectin-stimulated spleen cells, peripheral blood mononuclear cells, and tumor cell lines) was continuously supplied (10). Because these specific protein factors that induce colony growth were initially identified through these colony formation assays, they were named colony-stimulating factors (11). Considerable progress has been made in determining the cell types contained within the hematopoietic colonies and in characterizing the different CSFs in both murine and human systems. The in vitro assays continue to be refined and have identified the lineage hierarchy of normal hematopoietic progenitor cells, and the CSFs involved at each level (Fig. 17.1).

Many of these cytokines are produced by marrow stromal cells and are undoubtedly involved in hematopoietic stem cell development at specific sites within the marrow. Several CSFs also act on end stage cells, promoting their survival and stimulating functional activities. Local production of CSFs by cells in areas of inflammation is likely important for attracting and activating neutrophils, monocytes, eosinophils, and basophils. Some of the locally produced CSFs may enter the vascular system and affect neutrophil margination, adhesiveness, and release from the marrow. Potentially, they would ultimately increase marrow production of granulocytes and monocytes. From this perspective, we must consider the double role that CSFs may have in high-dose chemotherapy: The first is to stimulate early hematopoietic reconstitution; the second is to increase the functional effectiveness of neutrophils, monocytes, and macrophages.

NORMAL HEMATOPOIESIS

The development of the human hematopoietic system begins in the blood islands of the yolk sac. Later, stem cells migrate to the fetal liver and finally to the bone marrow, which becomes the major site of hematopoiesis (12). Umbilical cord blood is rich in hematopoietic progenitors (13) and can be used as a source of stem cells for transplantation.

Hematopoietic Stem Cells

The hematopoietic stem cell is defined as having the capacity for both self-renewal and differentiation along multiple lineages. In most hematopoietic lineages, differentiation is associated with a loss of the potential for self-renewal. It has been suggested that the lineage commitment decision is stochastic and thus not likely to be influenced by differentiation factors such as the CSFs (14, 15). Others argue that CSFs induce proliferation and maturation among cells that express specific receptors and thus are capable of modulating the output of end stage cells by stimulating additional divisions of maturing progenitor cells (16, 17). Little is known about the mechanism of commitment of individual stem cells toward differentiation. Evidence suggests, however, that the most primitive stem cells are, under steady-state conditions, proliferatively inactive and multipotent in their differentiation potential. They serve mainly as a reserve compartment, providing a mechanism of protection from premature marrow exhaustion.

Bone marrow stem cells vary greatly in self-renewal and proliferative capacity and can be divided into fractions with different self-renewal capacities by centrifugation, separation of adherent and nonadherent cells in culture, or cell sorting based on antigenic differences. In addition to colony-forming assays, there are several important in vivo murine assays that are used to characterize immature hematopoietic cells. The most

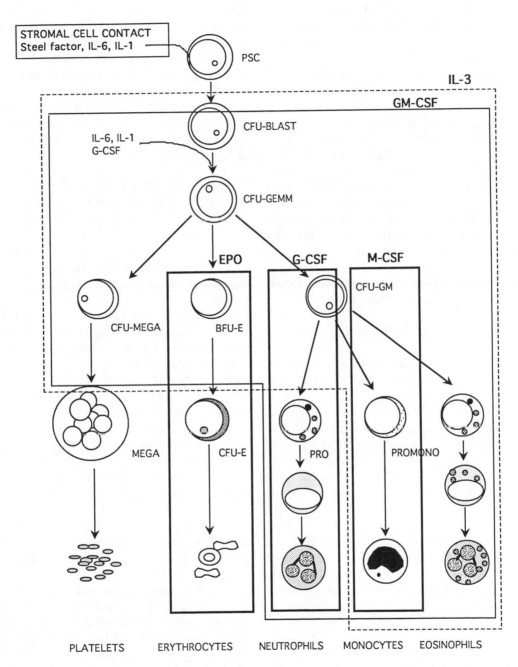

Figure 17.1. Abbreviations: PSC, primitive stem cell; CFU-GEMM, colony-forming unit, granulocyte-erythrocyte-monocyte-megakaryocyte; CFU-MEGA, colony-forming unit, megakaryocyte; BFU-E, burst-forming unit, erythrocyte; CFU-GM, colony-forming unit, granulocyte, macrophage; mega, megakaryocyte; CFU-E, colony-forming unit, erythrocyte; pro, promyelocyte; promono, promonocyte.

common in vivo technique is the spleen colony assay described initially almost 30 years ago (18). Injection of syngeneic marrow into irradiated recipient mice produces macroscopic colonies (nodules) of hematopoietic cells in the spleen in 7–14 days. These clonal colonies contain large numbers of differentiated cells but also daughter cells capable of forming a limited number of similar colonies upon retransplantation. The assay for measuring early stem cell content is based on the ability of very primitive stem cells to sustain hematopoiesis in vitro when seeded onto preformed marrow-derived stromal layers in multiple-well culture plates. Other complex assays have been used to assay even earlier stem cells. For example, stem cells capable of reconstituting long-term hematopoiesis can be assayed by serial transplantation of competitive repopulation assays (19).

Hematopoietic Progenitor Cells

There are a number of in vitro colony assays for human hematopoietic progenitor cells, which include the CFU-GM, BFU-E, CFU-GEMM, and CFU-blast assays. The cells defined by these assays have extensive proliferative capacity, and the CFU-blast and CFU-GEMM (colony-forming unit, granulocyte-erythrocyte-monocyte-megakaryocyte) are multipotent. The CFU-blast is the most primitive human stem cell detected in the cell colony assays and has some capacity for self-renewal (20), whereas the CFU-GEMM generates committed progenitor cells of various lineages and has little self-renewal capability (21). The CFU-GM assay identifies progenitors that give rise to colonies of granulocytes or monocytes. Other lineage-specific assays include the burst-forming units of erythrocytes (BFU-E) and CFU-E for the erythroid lineage and the CFU-mega for megakaryocytes. Various subpopulations of hematopoietic progenitor cells may serve different functions in reestablishing hematopoiesis after bone marrow transplant. The more committed stem cells, such as CFU-GM, CFU-E, and most CFU-

S in the mouse, appear to be important for early engraftment and hematopoietic recovery. In contrast, the primitive stem cells appear to be responsible for long-term hematopoiesis following transplantation. Thus achieving both short-term hematopoietic recovery and long-term hematopoiesis and recipient survival after bone marrow transplantation may depend on both the committed stem cell and the primitive stem cell content of the donor marrow.

MOLECULAR CHARACTERISTICS OF COLONY-STIMULATING FACTORS

Molecular cloning studies have enabled researchers to determine the genomic arrangement of the human CSF genes and to produce large quantities of purified factors in order to assess their in vitro activity. It is interesting to note that chromosome 5_q contains a family of genes involved in hematopoietic regulation (22–24). The genes for GM-CSF, IL-3, M-CSF and the M-CSF and the M-CSF receptor, IL-4, IL-5, and the receptor for platelet-derived growth factor (PDGF) all map to the long arm of chromosome 5, prompting the speculation that additional genes involved in hematopoiesis will be discovered in this region. It is noteworthy that deletions involving chromosome 5_q have been described in various hematopoietic disease states (22, 25). The gene encoding for G-CSF is on chromosome 17, near the 15:17 translocation breakpoint characteristic of acute promyelocytic leukemia (26).

The known sources and targets of specific CSFs are summarized in Table 17.1. Although many cells can produce CSFs, different CSFs are produced by different cells. In the majority of mature cell types investigated, transcription of the GM-CSF, G-CSF, and M-CSF genes is constitutive even in the absence of specific stimuli (55–58), although the transcripts are rapidly degraded in the cytoplasm and do not become useful protein unless the stabilization of mRNAs leads to induction.

Table 17.1 Characteristics of Human Hematopoietic Growth Factors[a]

Growth Factor	Protein Size (kD)	Chromosome	Cellular Source	Progenitor-Cell Targets	Mature-Cell Target
GM-CSF	14–35 127AA	5q23–31[27]	T lymphocytes, monocytes, fibroblasts endothelial cells[27–29,59,60]	CFU-blast, CFU-GEMM, CFU-GM CFU-Meg, BFU-E[27,30–37]	Granulocytes, eosinophils monocytes[34,38–40]
G-CSF	18–22 177AA	17q11.2–21[26]	Monocytes, fibroblasts, endothelial cells[28,29,41,59,60]	CFU-G[27]	Granulocytes[42]
Interleukin-3 (multi-CSF)	14–28 133AA	5q23–31[43]	T lymphocytes[44]	CFU-blast, CFU-GEMM, CFU-GM CFU-E, CFU-Meg, BFU-E[30–33,45]	Eosinophils, monocytes, basophils[46]
M-CSF (CSF-1)	Dimer 35–40 × 2 189AA	5q33.1[47]	Monocytes, fibroblasts endothelial cells[41,48]	CFU-M[49]	Monocytes[50,51]
Erythropoietin	34–39 166AA	7q11–22[52]	Renal peritubular cells[53,54]	CFU-E, BFU-E, CFU-Meg[30–32]	None

[a]Abbreviations: CFU-E =, colony-forming unit-erythroid; CFU-G, colony-forming unit-granulocyte; CFU-M =, colony-forming unit-macrophage

There is little evidence for constitutive production of CSFs except that fibroblast and endothelial cell lines spontaneously produce M-CSF (59, 60). Even less is known about the mechanisms required to shut off CSF production, although there is evidence for downregulation of transcription after induction (61).

The biologic effects of the cytokines are mediated through binding to a low number of high-affinity receptors on target cells (62–66). These cell surface receptors appear to also be widely expressed by abnormal hematopoietic cells (65, 67–69) and also by nonhematopoietic cells (70–72). The potential significance of this ligand binding will be discussed later in the text.

In vitro data predict that IL-3 might affect more cell types than either GM-CSF or G-CSF, specifically eosinophils and platelets. Although all three factors are likely to stimulate neutrophil production, only GM-CSF and G-CSF enhance their function. Additional data indicate that combining CSFs synergistically stimulates hematopoietic progenitors; for example, combining IL-3 with G, M, or GM-CSF may be more potent in stimulating granulocyte recovery than any one alone.

GRANULOCYTE-MONOCYTE COLONY-STIMULATING FACTOR

Structural Features

GM-CSF is a monomeric protein with two internal disulfide bridges that maintain the three-dimensional configuration (73). The mature protein consists of 127 amino acids with two arginine-linked glycosylation sites, resulting in a total molecular weight that can vary between 14 and 35 kD (27, 74, 75). The human GM-CSF gene maps to chromosome 5q-21-32 and is composed of four exons and three introns, spanning 2.5 kb (22, 25, 27, 36, 76). The protein sequence homology between human and murine GM-CSF is low, only 60% (27). Normally glycosylated sites on the native protein are exposed in proteins produced in yeast and *E. coli* vectors (77) and have led to the clinical development of GM-CSF antibodies.

GM-CSF exerts its effects through interaction with specific high-affinity receptors on the plasma membrane of granulocytes and macrophages (78). Receptor expression is characterized by low number (20–200 per cell) and high affinity, with mature neutrophils and eosinophils having the highest density (approximately 500–800 binding sites per cell), whereas the receptor density on monocytes is approximately 150 per cell, with leukemic cell lines having the lowest receptor density (79). There is a linear correlation between receptor saturation and effectiveness. Ligand binding results in downmodulation of the GM-CSF receptor due to internalization.

At least two different functional classes of GM-CSF receptor have been identified. The neutrophil GM-CSF receptor exclusively binds GM-CSF, while IL-3 competes for binding of GM-CSF to a second class of receptors detected on some leukemic cell lines, such as KG1 and MO-7E (63, 80). Signal transduction may involve activation of a tyrosine kinase (81–85). The receptor is believed to be composed of at least two subunits, both of which have recently been cloned (86–88).

Sources

GM-CSF is made by endothelial cells, fibroblasts, marrow stromal cells, and T lymphocytes (89–91). Activated T cells can also produce GM-CSF as well as IL-3 but produce little or no G-CSF or M-CSF (92). GM-CSF production by human monocytes is controversial; however, mature human macrophages can synthesize GM-CSF (93). In a variety of cells, the production of GM-CSF is highly regulated, primarily by mediators of inflammation. In individual cell types, the CSF genes can be independently regulated (29, 41, 55–57, 89, 94, 95).

Human GM-CSF was purified from conditioned medium from a T lymphoblast cell line (27, 38). Glycosylated GM-CSF is produced by cloning of the gene into mammalian (Chinese hamster ovary) cells (27) or yeast (74). A nonglycosylated form is produced in *E. coli* (96). Clinically significant differences in either activity or toxicity between the two products have not been demonstrated (73), but the degree of glycosylation of GM-CSF has been shown to be inversely related to the binding affinity of the molecule (97).

Hematopoietic Target Cells

GM-CSF is a consistent inducer of differentiation of normal granulocytes and monocytes in semisolid media (27, 38). This factor provides a potent in vitro stimulus for the growth of committed bone marrow progenitor cells, including CFU-GEMM, CFU-E, and CFU-GM. Its proliferative effects on the CFU-blast, the earliest bone marrow progenitor defined in vitro, are modest when compared to those of IL-3, and similarly it is less active on CFU-GEMM. In addition to effects on the myeloid lineage, GM-CSF also stimulates the growth of human BFU-E in the presence of erythropoietin when adherent and E-rosette-forming cells are removed from preparations (34, 38). It may be involved in concert with other CSFs in the regulation of megakaryopoiesis (31).

GM-CSF enhances proliferation of myeloid precursor cells from both normal bone marrow and human myeloid leukemia cell lines, HL-60 and KG-1 (34, 36), resulting in increased numbers of cells displaying monocytic and eosinophilic characteristics. GM-CSF induces the synthesis of other cytokines by myelomonocytic cells including M-CSF, tumor necrosis factor α (TNF α) IL-1, G-CSF and IL-6 (48, 98–100).

Effect on Cell Migration

GM-CSF had been previously described as a neutrophil migration-inhibition factor from T lymphoblasts (38, 39). Patients receiving continuous infusions of GM-CSF have been reported to have impaired neutrophil migration into sterile skin windows, although the clinical implications of this are unclear (101–103). Inhibition of migration of neutrophils may relate to the rapidly induced surface expression of MO1 antigen (cell surface adhesion protein CD11b) by GM-CSF (40, 104, 105). The MO1 protein functions as the receptor for the complement component C3bi; and is a member of an adhesion molecule family including LFA-1 (CD11a) and GP150,95 (CD11c), heterodimers that each share a common β chain (CD18) but differ in their α chain subunits (106). Induction of MO1 surface expression on neutrophils has been associated with neutrophil aggregation in vitro, suggesting an additional mechanism by which neutrophils are immobilized (40).

In addition, both GM-CSF and G-CSF cause a rapid transient increase in leukocyte adhesion molecule-1 (LAM-1) affinity on granulocytes that may enhance neutrophil endothelial binding. On longer exposures, however, GM-CSF induces shedding of LAM-1, which might contribute to the observed impairment of granulocyte migration into skin windows (107).

The observation of a rapid decline in circulating neutrophils after initiation of GM-CSF in clinical trials may be interpreted as a leukocyte-endothelial interaction (104). The short-term rebound of circulating granulocytes during continued administration of GM-CSF shows that other signals must be present for the effect to be maintained.

Effect on Cellular Function

GM-CSF also exerts profound effects on the function of mature myeloid cells. GM-CSF stimulates superoxide anion generation in response to the bacterial chemoattractant f-met-leu-phe (39, 108) and augments neutrophil oxidative metabolism important in neutrophil microbicidal and tumoricidal activities (38). Thus granulocytes exposed to GM-CSF appear to be more efficient in killing bacteria and to be primed for activation (109–111).

GM-CSF modulates the number and af-

finity of neutrophil N-formyl-methionyl-leucyl-phenylalamine (FMLP) receptors, which is associated with an enhanced response to the bacterially produced ligand (112). GM-CSF-induced priming of neutrophils for the bacterial chemoattractant peptide FMLP may support the arrest of neutrophils at the inflammatory sites. Moreover, rapidly induced release of membrane-associated arachidonic acid by GM-CSF may contribute to neutrophil activation in vitro (113). There is enhanced eosinophil cytotoxicity and leukotriene synthesis (114). By enhancing the function of antigen-presenting cells, GM-CSF also augments the primary antibody response (115).

Additionally, this cytokine prolongs the viability of both neutrophils and eosinophils in vitro by an average of 6–9 hours and may thereby contribute to enhanced granylocyte function (32, 116). However, neither GM-CSF nor G-CSF affects the respiratory burst in adherent monocytes (117).

It has been noted that GM-CSF enhances the killing of *Leishmania tropica* by murine peritoneal macrophages (118), activates intracellular killing of *Leishmania donovani* by human monocyte-derived macrophages (119), and enhances tumoricidal activity against cell line A375 (120). There is also a role in the activation of macrophages to inhibit *Trypanosoma cruzi* (121). A TNF-dependent mechanism is operational in vitro for the human monocyte tumoricidal activity on a murine fibrosarcoma line (122).

INTERLEUKIN-3

Structural Features

IL-3 is a 14- to 20-kD glycoprotein, with various degrees of glycosylation. Recombinant human IL-3 is expressed in *E. coli* and is nonglycosylated.

The human IL-3 gene is closely linked to the GM-CSF gene on chromosome 5q and has five exons and four introns (45). Some aspects of transcriptional regulation of the two genes are similar (75). Biologic activities of human and murine IL-3 share similar features, but there is no cross-reactivity between both species-specific proteins. The murine IL-3 receptor is 140 kD and may become tyrosine phosphorylated upon binding (123). Some data suggest that IL-3 may mediate its proliferative effects through activating protein kinase C (124). Like GM-CSF, IL-3 activates a tyrosine kinase in all responding cells (85).

Sources

The activated T lymphocyte appears to be the primary source of IL-3 (90), although murine brain cells have recently been shown to have IL-3 transcripts (125).

Hematopoietic Target Cells

IL-3 appears in vitro to have activity at an earlier stage than GM-CSF, stimulating the growth of early multipotential progenitor cells such as CFU-blast and CFU-GEMM, but also inducing the proliferation of more committed progenitor cells, including CFU-GM, CFU-EO, and CFU-mega (35). This multilineage hematopoietic growth factor requires the participation of later-acting factors for optimal stimulation of hematopoiesis. Neutrophils lack responsiveness to IL-3 (126), and possible lack of a direct action of IL-3 on mature neutrophil function needs to be kept in mind. Monocytes, eosinophils, and basophils, however, do express IL-3 receptors. The IL-3 receptor has been cloned and shares structural homology with the GM-CSF receptor. Recent data suggest that the IL-3 and GM-CSF receptors may even share a common subunit (88). All of the HGF receptors except c-fms (the M-CSF receptor) and c-kit (the Steel factor) receptor belong to a superfamily of receptors with some common structural features such as a W-S-X-W-S motif near the transmembrane domain (127, 128).

Effect on Cellular Function

IL-3 appears to exert its effect at a specific stage of the cell cycle prior to the S phase

(129). It induces morphologic changes in bone-marrow-derived and peritoneal macrophages, including increases in size, spreading vacuolation, and the number of cytoplasmic processes (130). It can also influence blood monocyte proliferation and modulate M-CSF receptors on these cells and tissue-derived macrophages (131). Several synergistic and overlapping actions of multi-CSF and GM-CSF have been described (100, 132), possibly due to ligation of both factors to similar receptor structures (133). IL-3, like GM-CSF, has been shown to stimulate monocyte cytotoxicity through a TNF-dependent mechanism (122, 134). In a murine model, IL-3 injected into the peritoneal cavity resulted in an increased number of activated macrophages and monocytes (135).

GRANULOCYTE COLONY-STIMULATING FACTOR

Structural Features

G-CSF is a 24–28 kD hydrophobic protein with internal disulfide bridges. G-CSF has only o-glycosylation (no arginine-linked carbohydrate sites) and a narrower range of molecular weights (18–22 kD) (69, 136) than other CSFs. Recombinant human G-CSF expressed in E. coli differs from native G-CSF by the addition of an N-terminal methionine and absence of glycosylation, resulting in a lower molecular weight. Alternative splicing results in two versions, the longer with less biologic activity. It is found on human chromosome 17q22 and has five exons and four introns with mRNA of 2.0 kb (26, 137). G-CSF binds to a receptor molecule of 150,000 kD present on cells of the neutrophil lineage.

Sources

G-CSF was first identified by its capacity to induce granulocyte-macrophage differentiation of a murine myelomonocytic cell line (138). Human G-CSF was originally purified from conditioned media from the 5637 bladder carcinoma cell line (139), and a longer (by three amino acids) G-CSF protein was cloned from a squamous cell carcinoma line (137) and may be less biologically active in vitro. Purified recombinant r-HuG-CSF and highly purified native human G-CSF have identical activity (28, 69, 140, 141).

G-CSF is produced by activated monocytes, macrophages, activated neutrophils, fibroblasts and endothelial cells (3, 35, 91, 142), in response to IL-1, TNF, and bacterial endotoxin.

Hematopoietic Target Cells

The major in vitro activity of G-CSF is to promote the growth of granulocyte colonies (56, 69) by affecting neutrophil progenitor proliferation (143, 144) and differentiation (69, 143). G-CSF is a CSF that has minimal direct in vivo or in vitro effects on the production of other hematopoietic cell lines (138, 141), although there may be some in vitro activity on CFU-GEMM and BFU-E (91) and even early progenitor cells (145), especially in concert with other cytokines (146). Unlike GM-CSF, which activates both mature neutrophils and eosinophils (147), G-CSF activates only neutrophils.

Effect on Cell Migration

Like GM-CSF, G-CSF causes a rapid transient increase in LAM-1 affinity on granulocytes that may enhance neutrophil endothelial binding, although the levels of LAM-1 expression on the surface of mature neutrophils is unchanged (107, 148). G-CSF does not affect surface expression of other common adhesion molecules by neutrophils and monocytes (142), although increased surface expression of the CD11b antigen on neutrophils has been reported (149). As with GM-CSF, the rapid changes in cell surface adhesion molecules may partially explain the acute and transient neutropenia following the administration of G-CSF (150). Additionally, G-CSF may act as a chemotactic signal for phagocytes, including neutrophils and monocytes.

Effect on Cellular Function

Exposure to G-CSF results in a functional activation of selected neutrophil end-cell functional activation, including enhanced phagocytic ability (151), enhancement of antibody-dependent cellular cytotoxicity (ADCC) (152), expression of FMLP receptors and FC receptors for immunoglobulin A (1, 39, 112, 119, 153, 154), and priming of the cellular metabolism associated with respiratory burst (155). After exposure to G-CSF, neutrophils increased, and there was more sustained free radical production in response to FMLP (142).

MONOCYTE COLONY-STIMULATING FACTOR

Structural Features

M-CSF is distinct from the other CSFs in terms of gene/protein structure and biologic activity. The M-CSF gene is located in a single copy on chromosome 5q33 and is associated with the gene coding for its receptor (25, 156). The M-CSF receptor, a 165-kD protein, is encoded by the c-fms protooncogene (62). The human gene has 10 exons and 9 introns (47, 156). At least three different forms of M-CSF protein have been identified with different translation sizes and have been termed M-CSF α, β, and γ. The homodimer protein is heavily glycosylated, resulting in a range of molecular weights of 36–90kD, and exists as secreted or membrane-anchored protein. Differential splicing results in two active forms of M-CSF with molecular weights of 45,000 and 85,000, both of which are heavily glycosylated.

Sources

M-CSF was initially purified from two sources, urine and a pancreatic carcinoma cell line (157–159), having two active forms of cDNA (47, 49).

M-CSF is produced by monocytes, granulocytes, fibroblasts, marrow stromal cells, and endothelial cells, (3, 90, 91, 142), and possibly B lymphocytes (160). M-CSF production can be increased by other cytokines, including γ interferon, IL-1 and TNF, or bacterial endotoxin.

Hematopoietic Target Cells

Although M-CSF supports monocyte-macrophage progenitor development in vitro in the murine system, its potentiation of macrophage colony formation from human bone marrow is relatively weak. M-CSF increases monocyte and macrophage number, increases macrophage antitumor (both antibody directed and antibody independent) and antimicrobial activity, and stimulates the secondary release of other cytokines, including G-CSF, GM-CSF, IL-1, TNF, and interferon. It may function primarily in the activation of microbicidal and tumoricidal capacity of monocytes and macrophages, rather than in the potentiation of growth.

Effects on Cellular Function

Human M-CSF acts primarily on the growth of macrophage colony formation from normal human bone marrow cells in vitro (73), where it induces the secretion of IL-1, TNF, interferon, and plasminogen activator (161–163). These actions may potentially enable M-CSF to prime monocytes and macrophages to combat infectious disease. M-CSF exhibits the capacity to prime murine peritoneal macrophages for the killing of the TU-5 sarcoma cell line in vitro (164), and induces antibody-independent monocyte tumoricidal activity against a murine fibrosarcoma cell line (122).

ERYTHROPOIETIN

Structural Features

Erythropoietin (EPO), the first human hematopoietic growth factor to be purified, is a 166-amino-acid glycoprotein with a molecular weight of 34–39 kD and a 24%–31% carbohydrate content. Although the carbohydrate moieties are not essential for in vitro activity, the nonglycosylated form is rapidly cleared by the liver and therefore ineffective in vivo (52, 165). For this reason, recombinant EPO produced in bacteria was not active in vivo. These difficulties in the production of active EPO were solved when the gene was expressed in Chinese hamster ovary (CHO) cells (166–168). Recombinant EPO from CHO cells is heavily glycosylated, like the natural hormone. The gene for EPO is located on chromosome 7q11-q22 (70, 169) and consists of four introns and five exons. EPO is both constitutively expressed and inducible in response to hypoxia and cobalt. Isolation, purification, and cloning of the human gene have permitted production of large quantities of recombinant human EPO, as well as the availability of an accurate radioimmunoassay using a polyvalent rabbit antihuman EPO antibody.

Sources

EPO was purified from a protein found in the urine of patients with aplastic anemia (169). EPO circulates in minute quantities and is measurable in plasma (170, 171). In utero, EPO is produced primarily in the liver, but during the last trimester the renal peritubular interstitial cell becomes the major source (53, 54), although the liver continues to produce a small amount of EPO even in adult life. In response to local tissue hypoxia, transcription of the gene is increased, and more interstitial cells are recruited to produce EPO in a feedback mechanism.

Hematopoietic Target Cells

EPO is a regulatory growth factor for terminal erythrocyte development and red cell production (172). Immature erythroid cells like BFU-E are also subject to control by other CSFs such as IL-3 and GM-CSF, but more committed CFU-E are acted upon primarily by EPO. CFU-E have two classes of EPO receptors, both low and high affinity. The EPO receptor has been cloned by D'Andrea and is a member of the HGF superfamily (127, 128).

EPO is essential for the development of erythroid cells (173) and can, when used in concert with multilineage cytokines, also promote the differentiation of megakaryocyte progenitors in vitro (30, 31). High-affinity binding sites are present on a human erythroleukemia cell line (67), and autocrine production of EPO has been reported to contribute to autonomous proliferation of erythroleukemia cells in humans (173).

EFFECTS OF COLONY-STIMULATING FACTORS ON NONHEMATOPOIETIC CELLS

Many nonhematopoietic cells in culture maintain CSF receptors on their surface (70, 71, 174, 175), as is evidenced by the fact that M-CSF, G-CSF, and GM-CSF were isolated from transformed human cell lines. Both G-CSF and GM-CSF can stimulate the migration and proliferation of cultured human vascular endothelial cells (72).

With regard to neoplastic cells, small cell lung cancer lines possess both G-CSF and GM–CSF receptors (71); however, the clinical significance of this is unknown. Interestingly, there is evidence that GM-CSF at high concentrations may inhibit the proliferation of these cells (176). Laboratory studies have suggested that GM-CSF may enhance monocyte antitumor cytotoxicity in some cell lines (177–179). It is interesting that some investigators have observed that G-CSF and GM-CSF stimulate the growth of some malignant cell lines (175, 180–182). Two studies, one of lymphoma cell lines and one of lymphocyte stimulation in humans receiving GM-CSF, both concluded that GM-CSF enhanced the growth of malignant and normal lymphoid cells (183, 184). A large series found that 4 fresh solid tumors and cell lines were moderately stimulated by GM-CSF, but 10 were

distinctly inhibited and 19 were not affected (185).

Case reports have documented patients with malignancy-associated leukemoid reactions and high serum growth factor levels, presumably of tumor origin (186). There are also data to suggest that the presence of a neoplasm in vivo may increase the number of circulating CFU-GM (187).

In clinical trials, GM-CSF alone (with no chemotherapy) has been administered to more than 100 patients; only one sarcoma patient had a partial response. There is no evidence that exposure to IL-3 in a screening of 25 different cell lines (tritiated thymidine proliferation assay) results in any convincing growth-promoting effects in solid tumors or lymphomas.

EFFECTS OF COLONY-STIMULATING FACTORS ON MARROW FAILURE/DISEASE STATES

Myelodysplasia

In laboratory studies of granulocytes from patients with myelodysplasia, GM-CSF stimulated proliferation. While the absolute number of blasts increased, the percentage of blasts decreased in many cases because of the increased absolute number of granulocytes (188, 189). The stimulation of clonogenic cell proliferation from myelodysplastic marrow cells was less with G-CSF than with GM-CSF; however, the induction of granulocytic differentiation was more readily seen with G-CSF (190, 191).

The use of G-CSF and GM-CSF in myelodysplasia and in leukemias requires caution prior to the availability of data from large randomized trials. Preliminary data from small randomized trials suggest that the incidence of evolution to leukemia in patients with myelodysplasia and the number of patients with regrowth of leukemia after induction treatment in relapsed patients with acute myeloid leukemia (AML) is not significantly different.

As predicted from in vitro experiments, the preliminary phase I/II data of IL-3 in patients with marrow failure states and myelodysplasia demonstrate an impact of the drug on the three major hematopoietic lineages that are suppressed by chemotherapy (192–194).

Acute Myeloid Leukemia

Cultured human leukemia cells have mixed responses to CSFs, reflecting the heterogeneous biology of AML. Although a subset of leukemic cells (AML) in vitro can produce small quantities of CSFs (G- and GM-CSF), these quantities appear insufficient to support optimal in vitro growth (195, 196). G-CSF has been known to differentiate murine leukemia cells, and an initial proliferative effect of IL-3, GM-CSF, and G-CSF on human leukemic specimens has been noted as well, although this differentiation capacity has been less striking (181, 197, 198). The clinical implications of these observations are unclear. Currently, both G- and GM-CSF are being studied after reinduction therapy in refractory AML patients, or in elderly patients with newly diagnosed AML, in an attempt to decrease the period of neutropenia. Whether the fraction of AML patients who have regrowth of leukemic cells after induction is increased by treatment with myeloid CSFs will require a randomized trial.

Taking advantage of the noted differentiative potential of G- and GM-CSF on AML cells, these CSFs are being used to synchronize leukemic cells or to enhance the activity of a phase-specific cytotoxic drug such as cytosine arabinoside against AML by increasing the proliferation of leukemic cells (199–203).

POTENTIAL CLINICAL APPLICATIONS

Initial Clinical Observations

Preclinical studies with bacterially synthesized human GM-CSF are limited by the lack of cross-species activity, and even in monkeys only short-term studies can be undertaken because antibodies develop (77). Nonhuman primate studies have demonstrated that the administration of recombinant human GM-CSF augments the number and function of circulating leukocytes in normal animals (204, 205). Preclinical in vivo studies have been carried out in mice and monkeys, where G-CSF caused a rapid increase in circulating neutrophils of up to 20-fold but had no consistent effects on lymphocytes, monocytes, platelets, or red cells (143). The direct effects of the CSFs are largely confined to cells that contain CSF receptors; however, the stimulated cells may be induced to secrete other cytokines.

Purified recombinant human GM-CSF has been available for clinical investigation for over 4 years (206). *E. coli*-derived rhGM-CSF at a dose of 5 μg/kg/d subcutaneously produces an initial neutropenia within the first 30 minutes, associated with pooling of neutrophils in the lung (207). During this time period, the expression of the CD11b adhesion protein (Mo1) by neutrophils is rapidly upregulated, although it is unclear whether this is involved in the mechanism of GM-CSF-induced neutropenia (105). The neutropenia is rapidly reversible within 1 hour, followed by a gradual daily increase in the absolute neutrophil count that initially is thought to occur through mobilization of preformed neutrophils from sequestered vascular sites, followed by production of newly formed neutrophils via GM-CSF-induced progenitor cell proliferation. Within 1 week of GM-CSF administration, circulating progenitor cell levels increase over baseline values, and bone marrow CFU-GM are mobilized into S phase as documented by thymidine suicide studies (208). These hematologic effects of GM-CSF are rapidly reversible after drug discontinuation. Significantly increased leukocytes, granulocytes, monocytes, lymphocytes, and eosinophils were observed (as well as platelets and reticulocytes in a few) in patients treated with GM-CSF. Toxicity includes bone pain as well as sporadic fever, chills, myalgias, headache, and anorexia. Accumulation of granulocytes and monocytes in lungs, liver, pericardium, pleura, and peritoneum can be seen in a dose-related fashion. The chronic overproduction of GM-CSF or IL-3 results in multisystem tissue damage (209, 210).

Unlike GM-CSF, the maximal tolerated dose (MTD) for G-CSF has not been established, despite asymptomatic high levels of neutrophilia. Pulmonary infiltration by mature neutrophils was observed, but without pulmonary dysfunction (211).

Combination Colony-Stimulating Factors

In vitro data predict that IL-3 might affect more cell types than either GM-CSF or G-CSF, specifically eosinophils and platelets. Although all three factors are likely to stimulate neutrophil production, only GM-CSF and G-CSF enhance their function. Additional data indicate that combining CSFs synergistically stimulates hematopoietic progenitors; for example, combining IL-3 with G, M, or GM-CSF may be more potent in stimulating granulocyte recovery than any one alone.

The sequential administration of IL-3 and GM-CSF suggests that the range of IL-3 activity may include an early population of hematopoietic progenitor cells that subsequently becomes responsive to GM-CSF. The nonhuman primate data for recombinant human IL-3 contrast with those of GM-CSF or G-CSF, in that the administration of IL-3 to nonhuman primates with normal hematopoiesis results in only minimal to modest increases in the circulating leukocyte count but an increase in the bone marrow cellularity and in the myeloid to erythroid ratio (132, 212–216). However, if administration of IL-3 is immediately followed by nonoverlapping administration of GM-CSF, the value of circulating leukocytes increases significantly and is higher than those observed when GM-CSF is administered alone. This effect is only noted when the IL-3 treatment is initiated 24 hours

after chemotherapy (215, 216). These in vivo data suggest that IL-3 when administered early primes a population of myeloid progenitor cells to respond to later-acting hematopoietic growth factors, such as GM-CSF or even G-CSF.

Hematopoietic Growth Factors in Autologous Bone Marrow Transplantation

There is a steep correlation between the dose of many chemotherapeutic agents (particularly alkylating agents, for which kinetic resistance does not apply) and tumor cytotoxicity in many laboratory models and in clinical studies. In tumors such as lymphomas including Hodgkin's disease, high-dose chemotherapy with autologous marrow support appears to result in prolonged disease-free survival compared to treatment with conventional chemotherapy regimens for patients failing initial therapy. The concept of removal and storage of sufficient numbers of hematopoietic stem cells to reestablish normal marrow function is well established in both animal models and in many human trials. The major morbidity of high-dose chemotherapy remains prolonged neutropenia. While anemia and thrombocytopenia can be treated by transfusion, no effective method restores granulocyte and monocyte levels. The incidence of bacterial and fungal infection correlates with both duration and severity of neutropenia. In patients provided with marrow support, the first neutrophil is detectable on day 9–11. An absolute neutrophil count (ANC) > 500 is achieved at a median of 18–26 days after transplant, with platelet transfusion independence at a median of 21–28 days and discharge at a median of 30–50 inpatient days.

The mechanism of hematopoietic engraftment is not well characterized. We do not understand how various types of progenitor cells contribute to this process and how the progenitor cells and microenvironment may have been changed by prior chemotherapy.

In particular, little is known about how to optimally use different compartments of stem cells (in the blood and the marrow), nor how to alter these compartments in clinically useful ways. Recent studies have indicated that cytokines may substantially increase the size of the blood or marrow stem cell pool. Many of these cytokines are produced by marrow stromal cells and are undoubtedly involved in hematopoietic stem cell development at specific sites within the marrow. An analysis of cytokine activity on progenitor cells in vitro may predict likely in vivo effects, thus pointing toward potential clinical use. Various techniques are now possible to determine the cytokine requirements of these primitive cells.

In primates, both G- and GM-CSF increased levels of granulocytes and monocytes and enhanced the rate of regeneration following bone marrow transplantation (BMT). Nonhuman primate studies have demonstrated that the administration of recombinant human GM-CSF may accelerate hematopoietic reconstitution in animals undergoing total body irradiation and autologous bone marrow transplantation (217, 218).

IL-3 administration increased the white blood cells primarily by increasing basophil and eosinophil counts. However, IL-3 and GM-CSF were synergistic on neutrophil, platelet, and erythroid recovery following BMT. Similar effects were observed in phase I human studies. G- and GM-CSF increased neutrophil counts, whereas GM-CSF stimulated monocytes and eosinophils as well. No effects on platelet counts were noted with G-CSF, but GM-CSF was associated with enhanced platelet recovery following BMT in primates.

Of note, endogenous human GM-CSF levels initially fall after marrow-ablative therapy and then rise between days 7 and 21 after bone marrow reinfusion (219, 220), and increased serum levels are also measured in patients with graft-versus-host disease (GVHD) (221). Monokines recover early, lymphokines late (222). T cell production of GM-CSF in response to mitogens remains blunted 18 months after allogeneic BMT, perhaps partly explaining the poor response to infection post transplant (223). Trials of hematopoietic growth factors in patients undergoing allogeneic transplantation require considerable caution since growth factors may indirectly activate T cells (through TNF and IL-1 by macrophages in the case of GM-CSF), exacerbating GVHD. Canine studies suggest that G-CSF accelerates engraftment in BMT from matched littermates, but a trend toward increased GVHD was noted. The use of immune-modulating drugs as GVHD prophylaxis further complicates this issue.

A few investigators are attempting to culture marrow incubated with cytokines for use as hematopoietic rescue after high-dose chemotherapy, in an attempt to further accelerate engraftment (224, 225).

Peripheral Blood Progenitor Cells

The reason for peripheral blood to contain circulating hematopoietic progenitor cells is incompletely understood. Less well known is how this population of cells is regulated. The circulating progenitor cell population is apparently quite immature compared to marrow cells, is in the G-0 phase of the cell cycle, and does not actively contribute to hematopoiesis. Peripheral blood progenitor cells (PBPCs) express the CD34 differentiation marker and can be quantitated by colony assay (226).

Stem cells collected from the peripheral blood of laboratory animals by cytophoresis have successfully reconstituted myelopoiesis following marrow-lethal treatment (227, 228). Weiner et al. demonstrated that PBPCs could be collected via established techniques for harvesting platelets (228), but 5–8 leukaphereses are required for adequate stem cell collection in humans (229, 230). The larger number of CFU-GM required for PBPC hematopoietic rescue compared to autologous bone marrow transplant (ABMT) may reflect a lower ratio of pluripotent to committed stem cells in peripheral blood, or to the few stromal cells transplanted with the pheresed cells. Investigators using PBPCs as the sole source for hematopoietic rescue must consider the possibility that PBPCs may contain enough mature progenitors to support patients through acute myelosuppression of multiple high-dose courses but might not be sufficient to prevent cumulative myeloablative effects.

Previous efforts to augment circulating progenitor cell numbers have had limited success. It was first observed more than 15 years ago that patients had an increased concentration of peripheral blood CFU-GM at the time of leukocyte recovery following chemotherapy, and this phenomenon has been confirmed in other patients (231–235). Nonetheless, over five leukaphereses are required for adequate stem cell collection, making PBPCs impractical as a routine source of stem cells. One interesting technique currently under investigation is to positively select CD34 cells (hematopoietic stem cells) with monoclonal antibody (236).

Effect of Colony-Stimulating Factors on Peripheral Blood Progenitor Cells

In a Dana-Farber Cancer Institute (DFCI) trial of GM-CSF in patients with sarcoma prior to the delivery of chemotherapy, nine patients were studied during 3- to 7-day continuous intravenous infusions of GM-CSF at doses of 4, 8, 16, and 64 μg/kg/day. PBPCs were quantitated during cycles 1 (with GM-CSF) and 2 (without GM-CSF) of MAID (mesna, doxorubicin, ifosfamide, and dacarbazine [DTIC]) chemotherapy in three of these patients. Immediately following chemotherapy, circulating CFU-GM were not detectable. The stem cell recovery after cycle 1 (with GM-CSF) was increased 30-fold in CFU-GM and 14-fold for BFU-E, compared to recovery after cycle 2 (without GM-CSF, $p = .001$). In addition to

Table 17.2.   The Stimulation of Progenitor Cells in Peripheral Blood by GM-CSF ± Chemotherapy

Factor	dl	Cycle 0	Cycle 1 + GM-CSF	Cycle 2 − GM-CSF
PB CFU-GM/ml	36	469	2251	74
PB BFU-E/ml	68	242	1125	80

higher numbers of peripheral blood CFU-GM, the peak level occurred earlier in the cycle with GM-CSF than in the cycle without GM-CSF (day 16, 16, 16, versus day 19, 22, 27). Marrow CFU-GM and BFU-E showed no significant change in response to chemotherapy, GM-CSF, or the combination (Table 17.2) (208).

This finding that GM-CSF will further increase the absolute number of circulating CFU-GM enhanced by chemotherapy rebound suggested that this augmentation may facilitate collection of adequate numbers of PBPCs with fewer leukaphereses. More recently, G-CSF has been reported to increase the numbers of circulating progenitor cells by up to 200-fold as well (144, 237, 238). This phenomenon was taken into clinical trials to evaluate the feasibility of PBPC autografting following high-dose chemotherapy (239–242).

While there is a theoretical concern that the administration of CSFs may deplete marrow stem cell populations, there has been no clinical evidence of stem cell exhaustion.

CONCLUSIONS

The available data suggest that growth factors will be a significant addition to the clinician's armamentarium. In addition they provide laboratory researchers with new tools for examining the process of hematopoiesis, clinically and at the molecular level. One of the limitations of dose-intensive chemotherapy is the toxicity of prolonged myelosuppression. If hematologic reconstitution could be hastened, this should substantially reduce mortality, morbidity, and the expense of high-dose therapy.

Whether the decreased incidence of febrile neutropenia or numbers of antibiotic days results from earlier granulocyte recovery or from more functionally efficient neutrophils is currently impossible to assess. Because the financial aspects of CSFs are only now emerging, it is difficult to determine at what level these drugs will be cost-effective. They may be cost-effective in the setting of intensive therapy such as BMT, where the reliable recovery of patients even a few days earlier would save several thousand dollars per patient.

REFERENCES

1. Weisbart RH, Gasson JC, Golde DW. Colony-stimulating factors and host defense. Ann Intern Med 1989;110(4):297–303.
2. Wang JM, Chen ZG, Golella S, et al. Chemotactic activity of recombinant G-CSF. Blood 1988;72:1456–1460.
3. Fibbe WE, Damme JV, Biolliau A, et al. Human fibroblasts produce granulocyte-CSF, macrophage-CSF, and granulocyte-macrophage-CSF following stimulation by interleukin-1 and poly(rI). poly(rC). Blood 1988;72:860–866.
4. Motoyoshi K, Yoshida K, Hatake K. Recombinant and native human urinary colony-stimulating factor directly augments granulocytic and granulocyte-macrophage colony-stimulating factor production of human peripheral blood monocytes. Exp Hematol 1989;17:68–71.
5. Wieser M, Bonifer R, Oster W. Interleukin-4 induces secretion of CSF for granulocytes and CSF for macrophages by peripheral blood monocytes. Blood 1989;73:1105–1108.
6. Groopman J. Status of colony-stimulating factors and AIDS. Semin Oncol 1990;17:31–41.
7. Glaspy J, Golde D. Clinical trials of myeloid growth factors. Exp Hematol 1990;18:1137–1141.
8. Pluznik D, Sachs L. The cloning of normal "mast" cells in tissue culture. J Cell Comp Physiol 1965;66:319–324.
9. Bradley T, Metcalf D. The growth of mouse bone marrow cells in vitro. Aust J Exp Biol Med Sci 1966;44:287–299.
10. Dexter T, Allen T, Lajtha L. Conditions controlling the proliferation of haemopoietic stem cells in vitro. J Cell Physiol 1977;91:335–344.
11. Metcalf D. In-vitro cloning techniques for hemopoietic cells: clinical applications. Ann Intern Med 1977;87(4):483–488.
12. Broxmeyer HE. Hematopoietic stem cells. In: Tru-

bowitz S, Davis E, ed. Human bone marrow. Boca Raton, FL: CRC Press, 1982:145–208.
13. Broxmeyer HE, Douglas GW, Hangoc G, et al. Human umbilical cord blood as a potential source of transplantable hematopoietic stem/progenitor cells. Proc Natl Acad Sci 1989;86:3828–3832.
14. Till J, McCulloch E, Siminovitch L. A stochastic model of stem cell proliferation, based on growth of spleen-colony forming cells. Proc Natl Acad Sci USA 1964;51:29–36.
15. Ogawa M, Porter P, Nakahata T. Renewal and commitment to differentiation of hemopoietic stem cells (an interpretive review). Blood 1983;61:823–829.
16. Koike K, Stanley E, Ihle J, Ogawa M. Macrophage colony formation supported by purified CSF-1 and/or interleukin-3 in serum-free culture; evidence for hierarchical difference in macrophage colony forming cells. Blood 1986;67:859–864.
17. Metcalf D, Burgess A. Clonal analysis of progenitor cell commitment to granulocyte or macrophage production. J Cell Physiol 1982;111:275–283.
18. Till J, Culloch EM. A direct measurement of the radiation sensitivity of normal mouse bone marrow. Radiat Res 1961;14:213–222.
19. Siminovitch L, McCulloch E, Till J. The distribution of colony-forming cells among spleen colonies. J Cell Comp Physiol 1963;62:327–336.
20. Leary A, Ogawa M. Blast cell colony assay for umbilical cord blood and adult bone marrow progenitors. Blood 1987;69:953–959.
21. Fauser A, Messner H. Identification of megakaryocytes, macrophages and eosinophils in colonies of human bone marrow containing neutrophilic granulocytes and erythroblasts. Blood 1979;53:1023–1027.
22. LeBeau MM, Westbrook CA, Diaz MO, et al. Evidence for the involvement of GM-CSF and FMS in the deletion (5q) in myeloid disorders. Science 1986;231:984–987.
23. LeBeau M, Pettenati M, Lemons R. Assignment of the GM-CSF, CSF-1 and FMS genes to human chromosome 5 provides evidence for linkage of a family of genes regulating hematopoiesis and for their involvement in the deletion 5q in myeloid disorders. Cold Spring Harb Symp Quant Biol 1986;51:899.
24. LeBeau M, Lemons R, Espinosa R. Interleukin-4 and interleukin-5 map to human chromosome 5 in a region encoding growth factors and receptors and are deleted in myeloid leukemias with a del (5q). Blood 1989;73:647–650.
25. Pettenati MJ, LeBeau MM, Lemons RS, et al. Assignment of CSF-1 to 5q32.1: evidence for clustering of genes regulating hematopoiesis and for their involvement in the deletion of the long arm of chromosome 5 in myeloid disorders. Proc Natl Acad Sci 1987;83:2970–2974.
26. Simmers RN, Webber LM, Shannon MF, et al. Localization of the G-CSF gene on chromosome 17

proximal to the breakpoint in the t(15;17) in acute promyelocytic leukemia. Blood 1987;70(1):330–332.

27. Wong G, Witek J, Temple P, et al. Human GM-CSF: molecular cloning of the complimentary DNA & purification of natural and recombinant proteins. Science 1985;228:810.

28. Koeffler H, Gasson J, Raynard J. Recombinant human TNF stimulates production of granulocyte colony-stimulating factor. Blood 1987;70:55–59.

29. Bagby G, Dinarello C, Wallace P, Wagner C, Hefeneider S, McCall E. Interleukin-1 stimulates granulocyte-macrophage colony-stimulating activity release by vascular endothelial cells. J Clin Invest 1986;78:1316–1323.

30. Long M, Hutchinson R, Gragowski L, Heffner C, Emerson S. Synergistic regulation of human megakaryocyte development. J Clin Invest 1988;82:1779–1786.

31. Bruno E, Miller M, Hoffman R. Interacting cytokines regulate in vitro human megakaryopoiesis. Blood 1989;73:671–677.

32. Metcalf D, Bagley CG, Johnson GR, et al. Biologic properties in vitro of recombinant human granulocyte-macrophage colony-stimulating factor. Blood 1986;67:37–45.

33. Hoang T, Haman A, Goncalves O, Wong GG, Clark SC. Interleukin-6 enhances growth factor-dependent proliferation of the blast cells of acute myeloblastic leukemia. Blood 1988;72(2):823–826.

34. Sieff C, Emerson S, Donahue R, et al. Human recombinant granulocyte-macrophage colony-stimulating factor: a multilineage hematopoietin. Science 1985;230:1171.

35. Sieff CA, Niemeyer CM, Nathan DG, et al. Stimulation of human hematopoietic colony formation by recombinant gibbon multi-colony-stimulating factor or interleukin-3. J Clin Invest 1987;80:818–823.

36. Tomonaga M, Golde GW, Gasson JC., Biosynthetic (recombinant) human granulocyte-macrophage colony-stimulating factor: effect on normal marrow and leukemia cell lines. Blood 1986;67:31–35.

37. Paquette RL, Zhou JY, Yang YC, Clark SC, Koeffler HP. Recombinant gibbon interleukin-3 acts synergistically with recombinant human G-CSF and GM-CSF in vitro. Blood 1988;71(6):1596–1600.

38. Gasson J, Weisbart R, Kaufman S, et al. Purified human granulocyte-macrophage colony-stimulating factor. Direct action on neutrophils. Science 1984; 226:1339.

39. Weisbart R, Golde D, Clark S, Wong G, Gasson J. Human granulocyte-macrophage colony-stimulating factor is a neutrophil activator. Nature 1985; 314:361–363.

40. Arnaout MA, Wang EA, Clark SC, Sieff CA. Human recombinant granulocyte-macrophage colony-stimulating factor increases cell-to-cell adhesion and surface expression of adhesion-promoting surface glycoproteins on mature granulocytes. J Clin Invest 1986;64:328–334.

41. Vellenga E, Rambaldi A, Ernst T, Ostapovicz D, Griffin J. Independent regulation of M-CSF and G-CSF gene expression in human monocytes. Blood 1988;71:1528–1532.

42. Delwel R, Dorssers L, Touw I, Wagemaker G, Lowenberg B. Human recombinant multilineage colony stimulating factor (interleukin-3): stimulator of acute myelocytic leukemia progenitor cells in vitro. Blood 1987;70(1):333–336.

43. Yang Y, Kovacic S, Kriz R. The human genes for GM-CSF and IL-3 are closely linked in tandem on chromosome 5. Blood 1987;71:958–961.

44. Otsuka T, Miyajima A, Brown N. Isolation and characterization of an expressible cDNA encoding human IL-3: induction of IL-3 mRNA in human T cell clones. J Immunol 1988;140:2288–2295.

45. Yang YC, Ciarletta AB, Temple PA, et al. Human IL-3 (multi-CSF): identification by expression cloning of a novel hematopoietic growth factor related to murine IL-3. Cell 1986;47:3–10.

46. Kelleher C, Miyauchi J, Wong G, Clark S, Minden MD, McCulloch EA. Synergism between recombinant growth factors, GM-CSF and G-CSF, acting on the blast cells of acute myeloblastic leukemia [published erratum appears in Blood 1987;70(1):339]. Blood 1987;69(5):1498–1503.

47. Ladner MB, Martin GA, Noble JA, et al. Human CSF-1: gene structure and alternative splicing of mRNA precursors. EMBO J 1987;6:2693–2698.

48. Horiguchi J, Warren K, Kufe D. Expression of the macrophage specific colony-stimulating factor in human monocytes treated with GM-CSF. Blood 1987;68:1251–1261.

49. Wong CG, Temple PA, Leary AC, et al. Human CSF-1: molecular cloning and expression of 4 kb cDNA encoding the human urinary protein. Science 1987;235:1504–1509.

50. Hoang T, Nara N, Wong G, Clark S, Minden MD, McCulloch EA. Effects of recombinant GM-CSF on the blast cells of acute myeloblastic leukemia. Blood 1986;68(1):313–316.

51. Griffin J, Young D, Herrmann F, Wiper D, Wagner K, Sabbath K. Effects of recombinant human GM-CSF on proliferation of clonogenic cells in acute myeloblastic leukemia. Blood 1986;67:1448–1453.

52. Law M, Lai G, Lin F. Chromosomal assignment of the human erythropoietin gene and its DNA polymorphism. Proc Natl Acad Sci USA 1986;83:6920–6924.

53. Koury S, Bondurant M, Koury M. Localization of erythropoietin synthesizing cells in murine kidneys by in situ hybridization. Blood 1988;71:524–527.

54. Lacombe C, DaSilva J, Bruneval P. Peritubular cells are the site of erythropoietin synthesis in the murine hypoxic kidney. J Clin Invest 1988;81:620–623.

55. Koeffler H, Gasson J, Tobler A. Transcriptional and post-transcriptional modulation of colony-stimulating factor expression by tumor necrosis factor and other agents. Mol Cell Biol 1988;8:3432–3438.

56. Thorens B, Mermod JJ, Vassally P. Phagocytosis and inflammatory stimuli induce GM-CSF mRNA in macrophages through posttranscriptional regulation. Cell 1987;48:671–679.

57. Ernst T, Ritchie A, Demetri G, Griffin J. Regulation of granulocyte- and monocyte colony-stimulating factor mRNA levels in human blood monocytes is mediated primarily at a post-transcriptional level. J Biol Chem 1989;264:5700–5703.

58. Shaw G, Kamen R. A conserved AU sequence from the 3' untranslated region of GM-CSF mRNA mediates selective mRNA degradation. Cell 1986;46:659–667.

59. Sieff CA, Schickwann T, Faller V. Interleukin-1 induces cultured human endothelial cell production of granulocyte-macrophage colony-stimulating factor. J Clin Invest 1988;79:48–51.

60. Yang Y, Tsai S, Wong G, Clark S. Interleukin-1 regulation of hematopoietic growth factor production by human stromal fibroblasts. J Cell Physiol 1988; 134:292–296.

61. Tobler A, Gasson J, Reichel H, Norman AW, Koeffler HP. Granulocyte-macrophage colony-stimulating factor. Sensitive and receptor-mediated regulation by 1,25-dihydroxyvitamin D3 in normal human peripheral blood lymphocytes. J Clin Invest 1987; 79(6):1700–1705.

62. Sherr CJ, Rettenmier CW, Sacca R, Roussel MF, Look AP, Stanley ER. The C-FMS protooncogene product is related to the receptor for the mononuclear phagocyte growth factor CSF-1. Cell 1985;41:665–676.

63. Park LS, Waldron PE, Friend D, et al. Interleukin-3, GM-CSF, and G-CSF receptor expression on cell lines and primary leukemia cells: receptor heterogeneity and relationship to growth factor responsiveness. Blood 1989;74(1):56–65.

64. Sawada K, Krantz S, Kans J. Purification of human erythroid colony-forming units and demonstration of specific binding of erythropoietin. J Clin Invest 1987;80:357–366.

65. Gasson J, Kaufman S, Weisbart R, Tomonaga M, Golde D. High affinity binding of granulocyte-macrophage colony-stimulating factor to normal and leukemic human myeloid cells. Proc Natl Acad Sci USA 1986;83:669–673.

66. DiPersio J, Billing P, Kaufman S, Eghtesady P, Williams RE, Gasson JC. Characterization of the human granulocyte-macrophage colony-stimulating factor receptor. J Biol Chem 1988;263(4):1834–1841.

67. Fraser J, Lin F-K, Berridge M. Expression and modulation of specific, high affinity binding sites for erythropoietin on the human erythroleukemic cell line K562. Blood 1988;71:204–209.

68. Rambaldi A, Wakamiya N, Vellenga E, et al. Expression of the macrophage colony-stimulating factor and c-fms genes in human acute myeloblastic leukemia cells. J Clin Invest 1988;81(4):1030–1035.

69. Souza LM, Boone TC, Gabrilove J, et al. Recombinant human granulocyte colony-stimulating factor: effects on normal and leukemic myeloid cells. Science 1986;232:61–65.

70. Rettenmier C, Sacca R, Furman W. Expression of the human c-fms proto-oncogene product (colony-stimulating factor-1 receptor) on the peripheral blood mononuclear cells and choriocarcinoma cell lines. J Clin Invest 1986;77:1740–1746.

71. Baldwin GC, Gasson JC, Kaufman SE, et al. Nonhematopoietic tumor cells express functional GM-CSF receptors. Blood 1989;73(4):1033–1037.

72. Bussolino F, Wang JM, Defelippi P, et al. Granulocyte and granulocyte-macrophage colony-stimulating factors induce human endothelial cells to migrate and proliferate. Nature 1989;337:471–473.

73. Clark SC, Kamen R. The human hematopoietic colony stimulating factors. Science 1987;236:1229–1237.

74. Cantrell MA, Anderson D, Cerretti DP, et al. Cloning, sequence and expression of the human granulocyte macrophage colony stimulating factor. Proc Natl Acad Sci 1985;82:6250–6254.

75. Miyatake S, Otzuka T, Yokota T, Lee F, Erait K. Structure of the chromosomal gene for granulocyte-macrophage colony-stimulating factor: comparison of the mouse and human genes. EMBO J 1985;4:2561–68.

76. Huebner K, Isobe M, Croce CM, Golde DW, Kaufman SE, Gasson JC. The human gene encoding GM-CSF is at 5q21-32, the chromosome region deleted in the 5q-anomaly. Science 1985;230:1282–1285.

77. Gribben JG, Devereux S, Thomas NS, et al. Development of antibodies to unprotected glycosylation sites on recombinant human GM-CSF. Lancet 1990; 335:434–437.

78. Cannistra SA, Koenigsmann M, DiCarlo J, Groshek P, Griffin JD. Differentiation-associated expression of two functionally distinct classes of granulocyte-macrophage colony-stimulating factor receptors by human myeloid cells. J Biol Chem 1990;265(21):12656–12663.

79. Griffin JD, Colony stimulating factors and their receptors: a comparison of normal and leukemic myeloid cells. Mol Biother 1989;1:9a.

80. Gesner T, Mufson R, Norton C, Turner K, Yang Y-C, Clark S. Specific binding, internalization and degradation of human recombinant interleukin-3 by cells of the acute myelogenous leukemia line KG-1. J Cell Physiol 1988;136:493–499.

81. Gomez-Cambronero J, Yamazaki M, Metwally F. Granulocyte-macrophage colony-stimulating factor and human neutrophils; role of guanine nucleotide regulatory proteins. Proc Natl Acad Sci USA 1989;86:3569–3573.

82. Morla A, Schreurs J, Miyajima A, Yang J. Hematopoietic growth factors activate the tyrosine phosphorylation of distinct sets of proteins in interleukin-3 dependent murine cell lines. Mol Cell Biol 1988;8:2214–2218.
83. Isfort R, Stevens D, May W, Ihle J. Interleukin-3 binds to a 140-kDa phospho-tyrosine-containing cell surface protein. Proc Natl Acad Sci USA 1988;85:7982–7986.
84. Ferris D, Willet-Brown J, Ortaldo J, Farrar W. Interleukin-3 stimulation of tyrosine kinase activity in FDC-P1 cells. Biochem Biophys Res Commun 1988;154:991–996.
85. Kanakura Y, Druker B, Cannistra S, Furukawa Y, Torimoto Y, Griffin J. Signal transduction of the human granulocyte-macrophage colony-stimulating factor and IL-3 receptors involves tyrosine phosphorylation of a common set of cytoplasmic proteins. Blood 1990;76:706–715.
86. Gearing D, King J, Gough N, Nicola N. Expression cloning of a receptor for human granulocyte-macrophage colony-stimulating factor. EMBO J 1989; 8:3667–3676.
87. Chiba S, Shibuya K, Piao Y-F, et al. Identification and cellular distribution of distinct proteins forming human GM-CSF receptor. Cell Regulation 1990;1:327–335.
88. Hayashida K, Kitamura T, Gorman D, Arai K-I, Yokota T, Miyajima A. Molecular cloning of a second subunit of the receptor for human granulocyte-macrophage colony-stimulating factor (GM-CSF): reconstitution of a high-affinity GM-CSF receptor. Proc Natl Acad Sci USA 1990;87:9655–9659.
89. Munker R, Gasson J, Ogawa M, Koeffler HP. Recombinant human TNF induces production of granulocyte-monocyte colony-stimulating factor. Nature 1986;323:79–82.
90. Oster W, Lindemann A, Mertelsmann R, Herrmann F. Production of macrophage-, granulocyte-, granulocyte-macrophage- and multi-colony-stimulating factor by peripheral blood cells. Eur J Immunol 1989;19:543–547.
91. Sieff CA. Hematopoietic growth factors. J Clin Invest 1987;79:1549–1557.
92. Herrmann F, Oster W, Meuer S, Lindemann A, Mertelsmann R. Interleukin-1 stimulates T lymphocytes to produce granulocyte-monocyte colony-stimulating factor. J Clin Invest 1988;81:1415–1418.
93. Scheibenbogen C, Zenke G, Faggs B, et al. Secretion of colony-stimulating factors for macrophages (M-CSF) and granulocyte-macrophages (GM-CSF) is developmentally regulated in human macrophages. Mol Biother 1989;1:52a.
94. Broudy V, Kaushansky K, Segal G, Harlan J, Adamson J. Tumor necrosis factor type alpha stimulates human endothelial cells to produce granulocyte-macrophage colony-stimulating factor. Proc Natl Acad Sci USA 1986;83:7467–7471.
95. Chan J, Slamon D, Nimer S, Golde D, Gasson J. Regulation of expression of human granulocyte-macrophage colony-stimulating factor. Proc Natl Acad Sci USA 1986;83:8669–8673.
96. Burgess A, Begley C, Johnson G. Purification and properties of bacterially synthesized human granulocyte-macrophage colony stimulating factor. Blood 1987;69:43–51.
97. Cebon J, Dempsey P, Nice E, Layton J, Burgess AW, Morstyn G. Granulocyte macrophage colony-stimulating factor for human lymphocytes: purification and characterization of differently glycosylated forms. Proc Am Soc Cancer Res 1989;30:71.
98. Cicco NA, Lindemann A, Content J, et al. Inducible production of interleukin-6 by human polymorphonuclear neutrophils: role of granulocyte-macrophage colony-stimulating factor and tumor necrosis factor-alpha. Blood 1990;15(75):2049–2052.
99. Lindemann A, Riedel D, Oster W, Ziegler-Heitbrock J, Mertelsmann R, Hermann F. GM-CSF induces cytokine secretion by polymorphonuclear neutrophils. J Clin Invest 1989;83:1308–1312.
100. Oster W, Lindemann A, Mertelsmann R, Herrmann F. Granulocyte-macrophage colony-stimulating factor (CSF) and multi-lineage CSF recruit human monocytes to express granulocyte CSF. Blood 1989;73:64–68.
101. Peters WP, Stuart A, Affronti ML, Kim CS, Coleman RE. Neutrophil migration is defective during recombinant human granulocyte-macrophage colony-stimulating factor infusion after autologous bone marrow transplantation in humans. Blood 1988; 72(4):1310–1315.
102. Linch DC, Devereux S, Addison IE. The effects of recombinant human granulocyte-macrophage colony-stimulating factor on phagocyte kinetics in man. Behring Inst Mitt 1988;83:320–332.
103. Addison IE, Johnson B, Devereux S, Goldstone AH, Linch DC. Granulocyte-macrophage colony-stimulating factor may inhibit neutrophil migration in vivo. Clin Exp Immunol 1989;76(2):149–153.
104. Herrmann F, Schulz G, Lindemann A, et al. Hematopoietic responses in patients with advanced malignancy treated with recombinant human granulocyte-macrophage colony-stimulating factor. J Clin Oncol 1989;7(2):159–167.
105. Socinski MA, Cannistra SA, Sullivan R, et al. Granulocyte-macrophage colony-stimulating factor induces the expression of the CD11b surface adhesion molecule on human granulocytes in vivo. Blood 1988;72(2):691–697.
106. Miller LJ, Schwarting R, Springer TA. Regulated expression of the Mac-1, LFA-1, T150.95-glycoprotein family during leukocyte differentiation. J Immunol 1986;137:2891–2900.
107. Demetri GD, Spertini O, Prat ES, et al. GM-CSF and G-CSF have different effects on expression of the

neutrophil adhesion receptors LAM-1 & CD11b. Blood 1990;76:178a.

108. Sullivan R, Fredette JP, Socinski M. et al. Enhancement of superoxide anion release by granulocytes harvested from patients receiving granulocyte-macrophage colony-stimulating factor. Br J Haematol 1989;71(4):475–479.

109. Baldwin GC, Gasson JC, Quan SG, et al. Granulocyte-macrophage colony-stimulating factor enhances neutrophil function in acquired immunodeficiency syndrome patients. Proc Natl Acad Sci USA 1988;85(8):2763–2766.

110. Sullivan R, Griffin JD, Wright J, et al. Effects of recombinant human granulocyte-macrophage colony-stimulating factor on intracellular pH in mature granulocytes. Blood 1988;72(5):1665–1673.

111. Mayani H, Baines P, Bowen DT, Jacobs A. In vitro growth of myeloid and erythroid progenitor cells from myelodysplastic patients in response to recombinant human granulocyte-macrophage colony-stimulating factor. Leukemia 1989;3(1):29–32.

112. Weisbart RH, Golde DW, Gasson JC. Biosynthetic human GM-CSF modulates the number and affinity of neutrophil f-Met-Leu-Phe-receptors. J Immunol 1986;137:3584–3587.

113. Sullivan R, Griffin JD, Simons ER, et al. Effects of recombinant human granulocyte and macrophage colony-stimulating factors on signal transduction pathways in human granulocytes. J Immunol 1987;139:3422–3430.

114. Silberstein DS, Owen WF, Gasson JC, et al. Enhancement of human eosinophil cytotoxicity and leukotriene synthesis by biosynthetic (recombinant) granulocyte-macrophage colony-stimulating factor. J Immunol 1986;137:3290–3294.

115. Morrissey PJ, Bressler L, Tark LS, Alpert A, Gillis S. Granulocyte-macrophage colony stimulating factor augments the primary antibody response by enhancing the function of antigen presenting cells. J Immunol 1987;139:1113–1119.

116. Lopez AF, Williamson DJ, Gamble JR, et al. Recombinant human granulocyte macrophage-colony stimulating factor stimulates in vitro mature human neutrophil and eosinophil function, surface receptor expression, and survival. J Clin Invest 1986;78:1220–1228.

117. Nathan CF. Respiratory burst in adherent human neutrophils: triggering by colony-stimulating factors CSF-GM and CSF-G. Blood 1989;73:301–306.

118. Handman E, Burgess AW. Stimulation by granulocyte-macrophage colony stimulating factor of Leishmania tropica killing by macrophages. J Immunol 1979;122:1134–1137.

119. Weiser WY, Niel AV, Clark SC, David JR. Recombinant human GM-CSF activates intracellular killing of Leishmania donovani by human monocyte-derived macrophages. J Exp Med 1987;166:1436–1446.

120. Grabstein KH, Urdal DL, Tushinski RJ. et al. Induction of macrophage tumoricidal activity by granulocyte-macrophage colony-stimulating factor. Science 1986;232:506–508.

121. Reed SG, Nathan CF, Pihl DL, et al. Recombinant granulocyte-macrophage colony stimulating factor activates macrophages to inhibit Trypanosoma cruzi and release hydrogen peroxide: comparison with interferon-gamma. J Exp Med 1987;166:1734–1746.

122. Cannistra SA, Vellenga E, Groshek P, Rambaldi A, Griffin JD. Human granulocyte-monocyte colony stimulating factor and interleukin-3 stimulate monocyte cytotoxicity through a tumor necrosis factor-dependent mechanism. Blood 1988;71:672–676.

123. Sorensen P, Mui A, Krystal G. Tyrosine phosphorylation of the 140 kD interleukin-3 receptor. Exp Hematol 1989;17:351a.

124. He Y, Hewlett E, Temels D, Quesenberry P. Inhibition of interleukin-3 and colony-stimulating factor 1-stimulated marrow cell proliferation by pertussis toxin. Blood 1988;71:1187–1195.

125. Farrar W, Vinocour M, Hill J. In situ hybridization histochemistry localization of interleukin-3 mRNA in mouse brain. Blood 1989;73:137–140.

126. Lopez AF, Dyson PG, To LB, et al. Recombinant human interleukin-3 stimulation of hematopoiesis in humans: loss of responsiveness with differentiation in the neutrophilic myeloid series. Blood 1988;72:1797–1804.

127. Bazan J. A novel family of growth factor receptor: a common binding domain in the growth hormone, prolactin, erythropoietin and IL-6 receptors, and the p75 IL-2 receptor beta chain. Biochem Biophys Res Commun 1989;164:788–795.

128. Cosman D, Lyman S, Idzerda R, et al. A new cytokine receptor superfamily. Trends Biochem Sci 1990;15:265.

129. Kelvin DJ, Chance S, Shreeve M, Axelrad AA, Connolly JA, McLeod D. Interleukin-3 and cell cycle progression. J Cell Physiol 1986;127:403–409.

130. Crapper RM, Vairo G, Hamilton JA, Clark-Lewis I, Schrader JW. Stimulation of bone marrow-derived and peritoneal macrophages by a T lymphocyte-derived hemopoietic growth factor, persisting cell-stimulating factor. Blood 1985;66:859–866.

131. Chen BDM, Clark CR. Interleukin-3 (IL-3) regulates the in vitro proliferation of both blood monocytes and peritoneal exudate macrophages: synergism between a macrophage lineage-specific colony-stimulating factor (CSF-1) and IL-3. J Immunol 1986;137:563–570.

132. Donahue RE, Seehra J, Metzger M, et al. Human IL-3 and GM-CSF act synergistically in stimulating hematopoiesis in primates. Science 1988;241:1820–1823.

133. Mofson RA, Gesner TG, Turner K, Norton C, Yang YC, Clark SC. Characterization of IL-3 receptors on

human acute myelogenous leukemia cell-line KG-1. Blood 1987;70:181a.

134. Whetton AD, Bazill GW, Dexter TM. Stimulation of hexose uptake by hemopoietic cell growth factor occurs in WEHI-3 myelomonocytic leukaemia cells. A possible mechanism for loss of growth control. J Cell Physiol 1985;123:73–78.

135. Metcalf D, Begley C, Johnson G, Nicola N, Lopez A, Williamson D. Effects of bacterially synthesized murine multi-CSF (IL-3) on hematopoiesis in normal adult mice. Blood 1987;68:46–57.

136. Nagata S, Tsuchiya M, Asany S, et al. Molecular cloning and expression of cDNA for human granulocyte colony stimulating factor. Nature 1986;319:415–418.

137. Nagata S, Tsochiya M, Asano S, et al. The chromosomal gene structure and mRNAs for human granulocyte colony-stimulating factor. EMBO J 1986;5:575–581.

138. Burgess A, Metcalf D. Characterization of a serum factor stimulating the differentiation of myelomonocytic leukemic cells. Int J Cancer 1980;26:647–654.

139. Welte K, Platzer E, Lu L. Purification and biochemical characterization of human pluripotent hematopoietic colony stimulating factor. Proc Natl Acad Sci USA 1985;82:1526–1530.

140. Zsebo KM, Yuschenkoff VN, Schiffer S, et al. Vascular endothelial cells and granulopoiesis: interleukin-1 stimulates release of G-CSF and GM-CSF. Blood 1988;71:99–103.

141. Seelentag W, Mermod J, Montesano R. Additive effects of interleukin-1 and tumor necrosis factor-alpha on the accumulation of the three granulocyte and macrophage colony-stimulating factor mRNAs in human endothelial cells. EMBO J 1987;6:2261–2265.

142. Lindemann A, Hermann F, Oster W, et al. Haematologic effects of recombinant human granulocyte colony stimulating factor in patients with malignancy. Blood 1989;74:2644–2657.

143. Welte K, Bonilla MA, Gillio AP, et al. Recombinant human granulocyte colony-stimulating factor. Effects on hematopoiesis in normal and cyclophosphamide-treated primates. J Exp Med 1987;165(4):941–948.

144. Duhrsen U, Villeval JL, Boyd J, Kannourakis G, Morstyn G, Metcalf D. Effects of recombinant human granulocyte colony-stimulating factor on hematopoietic progenitor cells in cancer patients. Blood 1988;72(6):2074–2081.

145. Ogawa M. Characterization of primitive hemopoietic progenitors in man. Exp Hematol 1989;17:1a.

146. Leary A, Wong G, Clark S. Leukemia inhibitory factor differentiation-inhibiting activity/human interleukin for DA cells augments proliferation of human hematopoietic stem cells. Blood 1990;75:1960–1964.

147. Vadas M, Varigos G, Nicola N. Eosinophil activation by colony-stimulating factor in man: metabolic effect and analysis by flow cytometry. Blood 1983;61:1232–1241.

148. Spertini O, Kansas G, Munro J, Griffin J, Tedder T. Regulation of leukocyte migration by activation of the leukocyte adhesion molecule-1 (LAM-1) selectin. Nature 1991;349:691–694.

149. Yuo A, Kitagawa S, Oshaka A. Recombinant human granulocyte colony-stimulating factor as an activator of human granulocytes; potentiation of responses triggered by receptor-mediated agonists and stimulation for C3bi receptor expression and adherence. Blood 1989;74:2144–2149.

150. Morstyn G, Campbell L, Souza LM, et al. Effect of granulocyte colony stimulating factor on neutropenia induced by cytotoxic chemotherapy. Lancet 1988;1:667–672.

151. Weisbart RH, Kacena A, Shuh A, Golde DW. GM-CSF induces human neutrophil IgA-mediated phagocytosis by an IgA Fc-receptor activation mechanism. Nature 1988;332:647–648.

152. Glaspy JA, Baldwin GC, Robertson PA, et al. Therapy for neutropenia in hairy cell leukemia with recombinant human granulocyte colony-stimulating factor. Ann Intern Med 1988;109(10):789–795.

153. Platzer E, Welte K, Gabrilove J, Harris T, Mertelsmann R, Moore M. Biological activities of a pluripotent hematopoietic colony stimulating factor on normal and leukemic cells. J Exp Med 1985;162:1788.

154. Platzer E, Oez S, Welte K, et al. Human pluripotent hematopoietic colony stimulating factor: activities on human and murine cells. Immunobiology 1986;172:185–193.

155. Kitagawa S, Yuo A, Souza L. Recombinant human granulocyte colony-stimulating factor enhances superoxide release in human granulocytes stimulated by chemotactic peptide. Biochem Biophys Res Commun 1987;144:1143.

156. Nienhuis AW, Bunn JF, Turner TH, et al. Expression of the human C-FMS protoncogene in hematopoietic cells and its deletion in the (5q-) syndrome. Cell 1985;42:421–425.

157. Das S, Stanley E, Guilbert L, Forman L. Human colony-stimulating factor (CSF-1) radioimmunoassay; resolution of three subclasses of human colony-stimulating factors. Blood 1981;58:630–641.

158. Motoyoshi K, Suda T, Kusumoto K, Takaku F, Miura Y. Granulocyte-macrophage colony stimulating and binding activities of purified human urinary colony-stimulating factor to murine and human bone marrow cells. Blood 1982;60:1378–1386.

159. Wu M, Cini J, Yunis A. Purification of a colony-stimulating factor from cultured pancreatic carcinoma cells. J Biol Chem 1979;254:6226–6228.

160. Pistoia V, Ghio R, Roncella S, Cozzolino F, Zupo S, Ferrarini M. Production of colony-stimulating activity by normal and neoplastic human B lymphocytes. Blood 1987;69:1340–1347.

161. Warren MK, Ralph P. Macrophage growth factor CSF-1 stimulates human monocyte production of interferon, tumor necrosis factor and colony stimulating activity. J Immunol 1986;137:2281–2285.

162. Fleit H, Rabinovitch M. Interferon induction in marrow-derived macrophages: regulation by L cell conditioned medium. J Cell Physiol 1981;108:347–352.

163. Lin H-S, Gordon S. Secretion of plasminogen activator by bone marrow-derived mononuclear phagocytes and its enhancement by colony stimulating factors. J Exp Med 1979;150:231–245.

164. Ralph P, Nakoinz I. Stimulation of macrophage tumoricidal activity by the growth and differentiation factor CSF-1. Cell Immunol 1987;105:270–279.

165. Zanjani E, Ascensao J. Erythropoietin. Transfusion 1989;29:46–57.

166. Browne J, Cohen A, Egrie J. Erythropoietin: gene cloning, protein structure and biological properties. Cold Spring Harb Symp Quant Biol 1986;51:693.

167. Jacobs K, Shoemaker C, Rudersdorf R. Isolation and characterization of genomic and cDNA clones of human erythropoietin. Nature 1988;313:806.

168. Lin F, Suggs S, Lin C. Cloning and expression of the human erythropoietin gene. Proc Natl Acad Sci USA 1988;82:7580.

169. Miyake T, Kung C, Goldwasser E. Purification of human erythropoietin. Biol Chem 1977;252:5558–5564.

170. Garcia J, Ebbe S, Hollander L, Cutting H, Miller M, Cronkite E. Radioimmune assay of erythropoietin: circulating levels in normal and polycythemic human beings. Lab Clin Med 1982;99:624–635.

171. Cotes P, Core C, Liu JY. Determination of serum immunoreactive erythropoietin in the investigation of erythrocytosis. N Engl J Med 1986;315:283–287.

172. Eaves C, Eaves A. Erythropoietin dose-response curves for three classes of erythroid progenitors in normal human marrow and in patients with polycythemia vera. 1978;52:1196–1210.

173. Mitjavila M-T, LeCouedic J-P, Casadevall N, et al. Autocrine stimulation by erythropoietin and autonomous growth of human erythroid leukemic cells in vitro. J Clin Invest 1991;88:789–797.

174. Uzumaki H, Okabe T, Sasaki N, et al. Identification and characterization of receptors for granulocyte colony-stimulating factor on human placenta and trophoblastic cells. Proc Natl Acad Sci USA 1989;86:9323–9326.

175. Dedhar S, Gaboury L, Galloway P, Eaves C. Human granulocyte-macrophage colony-stimulating factor is a growth factor active on a variety of cell types of nonhemopoietic origin. Proc Natl Acad Sci USA 1988;85(23):9253–9257.

176. Ruff M, Farrar W, Pert C. Interferon gamma and granulocyte-macrophage colony-stimulating factor inhibit growth and induce antigens characteristic of myeloid differentiation in small cell lung cancer cells. Proc Natl Acad Sci USA 1986;83:6613–6617.

177. Wing EJ, Magee DM, Whiteside TL, Kaplan SS, Shadduck RK. Recombinant human granulocyte/macrophage colony-stimulating factor enhances monocyte cytotoxicity and secretion of tumor necrosis factor alpha and interferon in cancer patients. Blood 1989;73(3):643–646.

178. Kleinerman ES, Knowles RD, Lachman LB, Gutterman JU. Effect of recombinant granulocyte/macrophage colony-stimulating factor on human monocyte activity in vitro and following intravenous administration. Cancer Res 1988;48(9):2604–2609.

179. Cannistra SA, Socinski MA, Groshek P, et al. In vivo administration of human granulocyte-monocyte colony stimulating factor enhances monocyte tumoricidal activity. Proc Am Soc Clin Oncol 1988;7:167(abstract 645).

180. Nachbaur D, Denz H, Zwierzina H, Schmalzl F, Huber H. Stimulation of colony formation of various human carcinoma cell lines by rhGM-CSF and rhIL-3. Cancer Lett 1990;50(3):197–201.

181. Avalos BR, Gasson JC, Hedvat C, et al. Human granulocyte colony-stimulating factor: biologic activities and receptor charcterization on hematopoietic cells and small cell lung cancer cell lines. Blood 1990;75(4):851–857.

182. Berdel WE, Danhauser-Riedi S, Steinhauser G, Winton EF. Various human hematopoietic growth factors (interleukin-3, GM-CSF, G-CSF) stimulate clonal growth of nonhematopoietic tumor cells. Blood 1989;73(1):80–83.

183. Ho AD, Haas R, Wulf G, et al. Activation of lymphocytes induced by recombinant human granulocyte-macrophage colony-stimulating factor in patients with malignant lymphoma. Blood 1990;75(1):203–212.

184. Paul CC, Baumann MA. Modulation of spontaneous outgrowth of Epstein-Barr virus immortalized B-cell clones by granulocyte-macrophage colony-stimulating factor and interleukin-3. Blood 1990;75(1):54–58.

185. Salmon SE, Liu R. Effects of granulocyte-macrophage colony-stimulating factor on in vitro growth of human solid tumors. J Clin Oncol 1989;7(9):1346–1350.

186. Enomoto T, Sugawa H, Inoue D, et al. Establishment of a human undifferentiated thyroid cancer cell line producing several growth factors and cytokines. Cancer 1990;65(9):1971–1979.

187. Crouse DA, Changnian L, Kessinger A, Ogren F, Sharp JG. Modulation of stem and progenitor cell number in the marrow, spleen and peripheral blood of tumor bearing mice. J Cell Biochem 1990;14A:326.

188. Tohyama K, Ohmori S, Michishita M, et al. Effects of recombinant G-CSF and GM-CSF on in vitro differentiation of the blast cells of RAEB and RAEB-T. Eur J Haematol 1989;42(4):348–353.

189. Carlo SC, Cazzola M, Bergamaschi G, et al. Growth of human hematopoietic colonies from patients with

myelodysplastic syndromes in response to recombinant human granulocyte-macrophage colony-stimulating factor. Leukemia 1989;3(5):363–366.

190. Nagler A, Ginzton N, Negrin R, Bang D, Donlon T, Greenberg P. Effects of recombinant human granulocyte colony stimulating factor and granulocyte-monocyte colony stimulating factor on in vitro hemopoiesis in the myelodysplastic syndromes. Leukemia 1990;4:193–202.

191. Nagler A, Binet C, Mackichan M, et al. Impact of marrow cytogenetics and morphology in in vitro hematopoiesis in the myelodysplastic syndromes: comparison between recombinant human granulocyte colony-stimulating factor (CSF) and granulocyte-monocyte CSF. Blood 1990;76:1299–1307.

192. Ogawa M. Hemopoietic stem cells: stochastic differentiation and humoral control of proliferation. Environ Health Perspect 1989;80:199–207.

193. Ganser A, Seipelt G, Lindemann A, et al. Effects of recombinant human interleukin-3 in patients with myelodysplasia. Blood 1990;76:455–462.

194. Ganser A, Lindemann A, Seipelt G, et al. Effects of recombinant interleukin-3 in patients with normal hematopoiesis and in patients with bone marrow failure. Blood 1990;76:666–676.

195. Young DC, Wagner K, Griffin JD. Constitutive expression of the granulocyte-macrophage colony-stimulating factor gene in acute myeloblastic leukemia. J Clin Invest 1987;79(1):100–106.

196. Young D, Demetri G, Ernst T, Cannistra S, Griffin J. In vitro expression of colony-stimulating factor genes by human acute myeloblastic leukemia cells. Exp Hematol 1988;16:378–382.

197. Vellenga E, Ostapovicz D, O'Rourke B, Griffin J. Effects of recombinant IL-3, GM-CSF and G-CSF on proliferation of leukemic clonogenic cells in short-term and long-term cultures. Leukemia 1987;1:584–589.

198. Vellenga E, Young D, Wagner K, Wiper D, Ostapovicz D, Griffin J. The effects of GM-CSF and G-CSF in promoting growth of clonogenic cells in acute myeloblastic leukemia. Blood 1987;69:1771–1776.

199. Estey E, Freireich E, Deisseroth A, Gutterman J. Treatment of poor prognosis AML with ara-C and GM-CSF. Proc Am Assoc Cancer Res 1989;30:282 (Abstract 1121).

200. Estey EH, Dixon D, Kantarjian HM, et al. Treatment of poor-prognosis, newly diagnosed acute myeloid leukemia with ara-C and recombinant human granulocyte-macrophage colony-stimulating factor. Blood 1990;75(9):1766–1769.

201. Estey EH, Kantarjian HM, Beran M, et al. Treatment of poor-prognosis, newly diagnosed acute myelogenous leukemia with high-dose cytosine arabinoside (Ara-C) and rHUGM-CSF. Haematol Bluttransfus 1990;33:732–736.

202. Cannistra SA, Groshek P, Griffin JD. Granulocyte-macrophage colony-stimulating factor enhances the cytotoxic effects of cytosine arabinoside in acute myeloblastic leukemia and in the myeloid blast crisis phase of chronic myeloid leukemia. Leukemia 1989;3(5):328–334.

203. Ciaiolo C, Ferrero D, Pugliese A, et al. Enhancement of methotrexate cytotoxicity by modulation of proliferative activity in normal and neoplastic T lymphocytes and in a myeloid leukemia cell line. Tumori 1988;74(5):537–542.

204. Donahue R, Wang E, Stone D, et al. Stimulating of hematopoiesis in primate by continuous infusion of recombinant human GM-CSF. Nature 1986;321:872–875.

205. Mayer P, Lam C, Obenaus H, Liehl E, Besemer J. Recombinant human GM-CSF induces leukocytosis and activates peripheral blood polymorphonuclear neutrophils in nonhuman primates. Blood 1987;70:206–213.

206. Antman KS, Griffin JD, Elias A, et al. Effect of recombinant human granulocyte-macrophage colony-stimulating factor on chemotherapy-induced myelosuppression. N Engl J Med 1988;319(10):593–598.

207. Devereux S, Linch D, Campos CC, et al. Transient leucopenia induced by GM-CSF. Lancet 1987;1:1523–1524.

208. Socinski MA, Cannistra SA, Elias A, Antman KH, Schnipper L, Griffin JD. Granulocyte-macrophage colony stimulating factor expands the circulating haemopoietic progenitor cell compartment in man. Lancet 1988;1:1194–1198.

209. Lang R, Metcalf D, Cuthbertson R, et al. Transgenic mice expressing a hemopoietic growth factor gene (GM-CSF) develop accumulations of macrophages, blindness and a fatal syndrome of tissue damage. Cell 1987;51:675–686.

210. Chang J, Metcalf D, Lang R, Gonda T, Johnson G. Non-neoplastic hemopoietic myeloproliferative syndrome induced by dysregulted multi-CSF (IL-3) expression. Blood 1989;73:1487–1497.

211. Pojda Z, Molineux G, Dexter T. Hemopoietic effects of short-term in vivo treatment of mice with various doses of rhG-CSF. Exp Hematol 1990;18:27–31.

212. Krumwieh D, Weinmann E, Seiler EH. Human recombinant derived IL-3 and GM-CSF in hematopoiesis of normal cynomolgus monkeys. Behring Inst Mitt 1988;83:250–257.

213. Mayer P, Valent P, Schmidt G, Liehl E, Bettelheim P. The in vivo effects of recombinant human interleukin-3: demonstration of basophil differentiation factor um histamine producing activity, and priming of GM-CSF-responsive progenitors in nonhuman primates. Blood 1989;74:613.

214. Geissler K, Valent P, Mayer P, et al. Recombinant human interleukin-3 expands the pool of circulating hemopoietic progenitor cells in primates—synergism with recombinant human granulocyte-mac-

rophage colony-stimulating factor. Blood 1990; 75:2305–2310.

215. Zeidler C, Krumwieh D, Seiler F, Welte K. Effects of recombinant human interleukin-3 (rh IL-3) in chemotherapy induced myelosuppression in primates. Blood 1988;72(suppl 1):140.

216. Gillio AP, Laver J, Abboud M, et al. IL-3 prevents neutropenia following 5-fluorouracil and cyclophosphamide induced myelosuppression in cynomolgus primates [Abstract 469]. Blood 1988; 72(suppl 1):117.

217. Nienhuis AW, Donahue RE, Karlsson S, et al. Recombinant human granulocyte macrophage colony-stimulating factor (GM-CSF) shortens the period of neutropenia after autologous bone marrow transplantation in a primate model. J Clin Invest 1987;80:573–577.

218. Monroy RL, Skelly RR, MacVittie TJ, et al. The effect of recombinant GM-CSF on the recovery of monkeys transplanted with autologous bone marrow. Blood 1987;70:1696–1699.

219. Yamasaki K, Solberg LAJ, Jamal N, et al. Hemopoietic colony growth-promoting activities in the plasma of bone marrow transplant recipients. J Clin Invest 1988;82(1):255–261.

220. Geissler D, Niederwieser D, Aulitzky WE, et al. Serum colony stimulating factor in patients undergoing bone marrow transplantation: enhancing effect of recombinant human GM-CSF. Behring Inst Mitt 1988;83:289–300.

221. Kanamaru A, Hara H. Hematopoietic factors in graft-versus-host reaction. Int J Cell Cloning 1987;5(6):450–462.

222. Atkinson K. Production of growth factors for the hemopoietic and immune systems after marrow transplantation. J Cell Biol 1990;14A:259.

223. Thomas S, Clark SC, Rappeport JM, Nathan DG, Emerson SG. Deficient T cell granulocyte-macrophage colony stimulating factor production in allogeneic bone marrow transplant recipients. Transplantation 1990;49(4):703–708.

224. Meagher RC, Herzig RH. Effects of recombinant human hematopoietic growth factors in vitro. In: UCLA symposia on molecular & cellular biology. Los Angeles, Wiley-Liss, 1990:330.

225. Haas R, Ogniben E, Kiesel S, et al. Enhanced myelopoiesis in long-term cultures of human bone marrow pretreated with recombinant granulocyte-macrophage colony-stimulating factor. Exp Hematol 1989;17(3):235–239.

226. Siena S, Bregni M, Brando B, et al. Flow cytometry for clinical estimation of circulating hematopoietic progenitors for autologous transplantation in cancer patients. Blood 1991;77(2):400–409.

227. Sarpel SC, Axel Z, Harvath L, et al. The collection, preservation & function of peripheral blood hematopoietic cells in dogs. Exp Hematol 1979;7:113–120.

228. Weiner R, Richman C, Yankee R. Semicontinuous flow centrifugation for the pheresis of immunocompetent cells & stem cells. Blood 1977;49:391–397.

229. Juttner CA, Haylock DN, Branford A, et al. Haemopoietic reconstitution using circulating autologous stem cells collected in very early remission from acute non-lymphoblastic leukemia. Exp Hematol 1986;14:465 (abstract 312).

230. Goldman JR, Th'ng K, Park D, Spiers A, Lowenthal R, Ruutu T. Collection, cryopreservation and subsequent viability of haemopoietic stem cells intended for treatment of chronic granulocytic leukaemia in blast-cell transformation. Br J Haematol 1978;40:185–195.

231. Richman CM, Weiner RS, Yankee RA. Increase in circulating stem cells following chemotherapy in man. Blood 1976;47:1031–1039.

232. To LB, Haylock DN, Kimber R, Juttner CA. High levels of circulating hematopoietic stem cells in very early remission from acute non-lymphocytic leukaemia & their collection & cryopreservation. Br J Haematol 1984;58:399–410.

233. Ruse-Riol F, Legros M, Bernard D, et al. Variations in committed stem cells in the peripheral blood of cancer patients treated by sequential combination chemotherapy for breast cancer. Cancer Res 1984;44:2219–2224.

234. Lohrmann HP, Schreml W, Lang M, Betzler M, Fliedner TM, Heimpel H. Changes of granulopoiesis during & after adjuvant chemotherapy of breast cancer. Br J Haematol 1978;40:369–381.

235. Abrams RA, Johnston-Early A, Kramer C, Minna JD, Cohen MH, Deisseroth AB. Amplification of circulating granulocyte-monocyte stem cell numbers following chemotherapy in patients with extensive small cell carcinoma of the lung. Cancer Res 1981;41:35–41.

236. Lebkowski JS, Schain L, Strand V, Warren D, Levinsky R, Okarma T. Positive selection of human hematopoietic stem cells using the AIS stem stem collector. J Cell Biochem 1990;14A:330.

237. Toki H, Shimokawa T, Okabe K, Ishimitsu T. Recombinant human granulocyte colony-stimulating factor (fG-CSF) amplifies the number of peripheral blood stem cell (PBSC) of lymphoma patients on chemotherapy. Proc Am Soc Clin Oncol 1990;9:188 (Abstract 728).

238. Sheridan WP, Morstyn G, Wolf M, et al. Granulocyte colony-stimulating factor and neutrophil recovery after high-dose chemotherapy and autologous bone marrow transplantation. Lancet 1989;2:891–895.

239. Gianni AM, Bregni M, Siena S, et al. Very rapid and complete hematopoietic reconstitution following combined transplantation of autologous bone marrow and GM-CSF exposed stem cells [Abstract]. Bone Marrow Transplant 1989;4S:78.

240. Gianni AM, Bregni M, Siena S, ct al. Rapid and complete hematopoietic reconstitution following combined transplantation and autologous blood and bone marrow cells. A changing role for high dose chemoradiotherapy. Hemat Oncol 1989;7:139–148.

241. Gianni AM, Siena S, Bregni M, et al. Granulocyte-macrophage colony-stimulating factor to harvest circulating haemopoietic stem cells for autotransplantation. Lancet 1989;2:580–585.

242. Bonadonna G. Karnofsky Memorial Lecture: conceptual and practical advances in the management of breast cancer. J Clin Oncol 1989;10:1380–1397.

18

GRANULOCYTE-MONOCYTE COLONY-STIMULATING FACTOR

L. Kanz, W. Brugger, K. Bross, J. Frisch, and R. H. Mertelsmann

The hematopoietic growth factors have provided exciting new possibilities for cancer treatment. Following extensive in vitro studies, it has only recently become possible to study recombinant hematopoietic growth factors in vivo. Several of these cytokines have entered clinical trials. Granulocyte colony-stimulating factor (G-CSF), granulocyte-monocyte colony-stimulating factor (GM-CSF), and erythropoietin (Epo) are currently in an advanced stage of testing and have recently been approved. Interleukin-1 (IL-1), IL-3, and macrophage colony-stimulating factor (M-CSF) have also been introduced and are studied for their clinical potential. The main questions to be asked are whether these molecules may mitigate cancer therapy-related side effects, augment nonspecific mechanisms of host resistance, and indirectly improve antitumor responses and survival by reducing toxicity and thus altering the definition of the maximum tolerated doses of conventional chemotherapeutic regimens.

GM-CSF is currently under active investigation to define its role in the following:

1. enhancing hematopoietic recovery following chemo- or radiotherapy and bone marrow transplantation
2. increasing the circulating pool of peripheral blood hematopoietic stem cells
3. stimulating hematopoiesis in patients with primary or secondary bone marrow failure syndromes
4. activating mature blood cells to possibly prevent or accelerate recovery from infections
5. treating acute leukemia, particularly in combination with cytotoxic drugs

This article will summarize the preclinical biology of GM-CSF and focus on the role of this cytokine in the acceleration of bone marrow recovery following chemo/radiotherapy and bone marrow transplantation, as well as its potential to facilitate cell harvesting for peripheral stem cell transplantation.

PRECLINICAL BIOLOGY

Molecular Biology

The gene for GM-CSF has been localized to chromosome 5q21-32 (1) near the genes for other cytokines such as IL-3, IL-4, IL-5, and IL-9. It is approximately 2.5 kbp in length and is composed of four exons and three introns (2). The 5'-flanking region plays an important role in the inducible expression of the GM-CSF gene (for review of GM-CSF gene regulation see 3, 4).

The gene encodes a protein of 144 AA, including a signal sequence of 17 residues and two sites for N-glycosylation (5–8); glycosylation is not essential for the biologic activity of the protein. Complementary DNA encoding GM-CSF has been expressed in Chinese hamster ovarian (CHO) cells, *E. coli*, and in yeast, with all forms of recombinant GM-CSF displaying the activity of the nonrecombinant native molecule.

Under steady-state conditions, GM-CSF is constitutively expressed in monocytes, endothelial cells, and fibroblasts, and following activation many more cells types, including T and B cells, mast cells, mesothelial cells, and osteoblasts, express GM-CSF messenger RNA (9–18).

GM-CSF binds with high and low affinities to its receptor (19). This receptor belongs to the cytokine receptor family (20), which includes the receptors for IL-2β, IL-3/4/5/6/7, G-CSF, and Epo. Current evidence indicates that the GM-CSF receptor is a multisubunit complex with a molecularly defined low-affinity binding subunit (21, 22) and a 120-kD protein that confers a high-affinity receptor complex when coexpressed with the low-affinity receptor (23, 24). Tyrosine phosphorylation and expression of c-fos and c-myc genes play an important role in the GM-CSF signaling pathway, though the receptor does not contain a kinase domain (25, 26).

High-affinity GM-CSF receptors are widely expressed by hematopoietic cells, with mature granulocytes expressing the highest number of receptors (19, 27); low-affinity receptors are expressed in human small cell carcinoma lines as well as other tumor cells (28–31). However, there is no in vivo evidence for accelerated growth of nonhematopoietic tumor cells when patients with solid tumors are given colony-stimulating factors (CSFs) in order to stimulate bone marrow recovery after chemo/radiotherapy.

GM-CSF and IL-3 have been shown to partially cross-compete with each other for binding to receptors on KG-1 cells, eosinophils, and some fresh leukemia cells (32–35); this might be of practical importance when IL-3 and GM-CSF are combined or used in a sequential mode in clinical trials.

Recent evidence indicates that the GM-CSF receptor may be naturally secreted and may play an important role in immune function (36).

Biologic Activities

GM-CSF stimulates granulocyte, monocyte, and eosinophil colony formation in vitro (37, 38) and—in concert with Epo—also has erythroid burst-promoting activity (39). Megakaryocytic colony formation, either alone or in concert with IL-3, has also been reported to be stimulated by GM-CSF (40–43). Its effect on nuclear polyploidization of developing megakaryocytes has not been reported. Recently megakaryocytic progenitor cells in S-phase were shown to increase upon GM-CSF therapy in patients with normal hematopoiesis; however, this was not accompanied by enhanced platelet production (44).

At least in our assay system (45, 46), GM-CSF can only induce suboptimal stimulation of colony-forming units, megakaryocyte (CFU-Meg) as analyzed by colony numbers and size of individual colonies when compared to colony-stimulating activities present in aplastic anemia plasma. These observations suggest that GM-CSF might stimulate only a subpopulation of CFU-Meg; additional factor(s) are necessary to stimulate the entire population of CFU-Meg progenitors.

In addition to the proliferation-stimulating activities on hematopoietic progenitor cells, GM-CSF induces a broad range of functional changes in mature effector cells. In monocytes/macrophages it induces the production of other cytokines (e.g., tumor necrosis factor [TNF], IL-1, IL-6, G-CSF), prostaglandins, and major histocompatibility (MHC) class II molecules; in vitro tumor cell cytotoxicity is also increased, and GM-CSF augments intracellular killing of parasites (47–54). In neutrophils and eosinophils, GM-CSF stimulates surface expression of CD11b/CD18 (55); these adhesion-promoting glycoproteins probably cause the transient margination of neutrophils and monocytes, mainly within the lungs, upon in vivo application of

GM-CSF. Additional direct effects include the secretion of other cytokines (56, 57), degranulation (58, 59), as well as inhibition of random mobility (5).

The inhibition of neutrophil migration was recently confirmed by the inability of granulocytes to migrate to a peripheral sterile inflammatory site using a standardized skin chamber assay (60). Thus these neutrophils recruited by GM-CSF, though highly activated, may not be available for migration to tissue infection. However, in clinical trials an increased incidence of infections has not been observed so far, and possibly the sterile skin chamber assay is not representative for bacterial or fungal invasion.

Many more effects of GM-CSF on granulocytes are indirect ("priming effects"), observed only in the presence of a secondary stimulus (such as f-met-leu-phe [fMLP]), and possibly mediated in part by the production of leukotriene B_4 (LTB_4) (3). These activities include enhanced phagocytosis and cytotoxic activity against bacteria and yeast (61, 62), increased respiratory burst (63–65), antibody-dependent cellular cytotoxicity (66, 67), and release of arachidonic acid (AA), LTB_4, and platelet-activating factor (PAF) (68–70). Several activators of neutrophil function have been shown to downregulate the GM-CSF receptors (71), which implies that they exert their biologic effects by downregulating GM-CSF receptors.

GRANULOCYTE-MONOCYTE COLONY-STIMULATING FACTOR IN CLINICAL TRIALS

Granulocyte-Monocyte Colony-Stimulating Factor in Phase I/II Trials

Dose escalation trials in patients with advanced malignancies have been conducted with both *E. coli*-derived nonglycosylated and with glycosylated yeast or mammalian-cell-derived GM-CSF (Table 18.1)

These studies have clearly defined a broad spectrum of dose- and schedule-dependent hematopoietic effects. Application of GM-CSF resulted in an increase of circulating neutrophils, eosinophils, and monocytes, and an increase in bone marrow cellularity irrespective of the route of administration. There was no consistent effect on lymphocytes, platelets, basophils, and reticulocytes. A transient fall in circulating neutrophils, eosinophils, and monocytes immediately after GM-CSF application, followed by leukocytosis, was described (72, 73, 75).

It seems apparent from the phase I studies listed in Table 18.1 that continuous intravenous and particularly subcutaneous application of GM-CSF are more potent and show less adverse effects than short intravenous infusions. Depending on the route of administration, the studies identified a maximal tolerated dosage (MTD) up to 32 μg/kg (1000 μg/m^2); much lower doses, however, were effective, and doses in the range of about 250–500 μg/m^2 given subcutaneously were considered optimal for further studies.

Other observations of the initial clinical studies include an activation of idiopathic thrombocytopenic purpura in one patient (75), lowering of serum cholesterol (76), an increase of bone marrow burst-forming units, erythrocyte (BFU-E) and colony-forming units, granulocyte-macrophage (CFU-GM) in S-phase (79), an enhanced expression of adhesion molecules (72, 77), and, surprisingly, a multilineage response in one study (78).

Although in vitro findings suggest a possible role for indirect and direct antitumor effects, no such effects of GM-CSF have been observed as yet in any of the clinical studies. Induction of in vivo cytotoxicity might be achieved by combining GM-CSF with other macrophage-activating cytokines, such as interferon gamma.

GM-CSF is generally well tolerated when given at doses required for the hematopoietic effects desired (cf. references listed in Tables 18.1, 18.2). Whether there are differences in the spectrum of side effects of glycosylated and nonglycosylated GM-CSF is unclear at this point.

Table 18.1. Summary of Published Data on GM-CSF in Clinical Trials: Phase I/II Trials/GM-CSF Following Standard Chemotherapy[a]

	Ref.	No. of Patients	Tumors	Chemoth.	Dose/Route	Remarks
			GM-CSF Phase I/II			
Herrmann	72	30	Adv. malign.	—	125–1000 µg/m² ivp., civ 5 days	MTD 1000 µg/m²
Philips	73	10	Adv. malign.	—	5–25 µg/m² d1 ivp 100–500 µg/m² d2–14 civ	
Steward	74	30	Misc. solid tumors	—	0.1–60 µg/kg ivp d1–10/d21–30	MTD 30 µg/kg 1 PR (liposarc.)
Lieschke	75	21	Adv. Malign.	—	0.3–30 µg/kg sc d1–10	MTD 30 µg/kg
Lieschke	76	21	Adv. Malign.	—	0.3–3 µg/kg ivp 3–20 µg/kg civ d1–10	Cholesterol
Steis	77	11	Adv.malign.	—	1–50 µg/kg civ d1–21	
Vadhan-Raj	78	25	Malign., incl. MDS	—	15–500 µg/m² civ d1–14	Multilineage responses
Aglietta	79	9	Misc. solid tumors	—	8 µg/kg d1–3	
			GM-CSF Following Standard Chemotherapy			
Antman	80	16	Sarcoma	MAID	4–64 µg/kg civ	MTD 32 µg/kg
Herrmann	81	22	Refract. neoplasms	Various	250 µg/m² sc d1–10	1. cycle − 2. cycle + GM-CSF
Gerhartz	82	40	Adv. malign.	Various	2–32 µg/kg civ d1–5	
Morstyn	83	46	SCLC	VP16 carboplat.	15 µg/kg sc d4–11/d8–15	

[a]Abbreviations: civ, continuous intravenous; ivp, intravenous push; MDS, myelodysplastic syndrome; PR, partial remission; sc, subcutaneously; VP16, etoposide.

Low-grade side effects seen in some patients include fever (<38.5°C), malaise, local thrombophlebitis, and bone pain. There may be an increase of alkaline phosphatase, γ-glutamyl transpeptidase (γ-GT), and lactic dehydrogenase levels and, with increasing dose, fluid retention, and temporary decrease of platelets may be observed. For doses >30 µg/kg pericarditis, vasculitis, thrombosis (around central lines), pulmonary emboli, thrombophlebitis, and a capillary leak syndrome have been reported. These dose-limiting adverse effects are most likely the result of induction of other cytokines such as IL-1 and TNF.

For *E. coli*-derived GM-CSF Lieschke et al. (75) described transient hypoxia and hy-potension following the first dose of GM-CSF in some patients; none of the patients who had first-dose reactions had similar symptoms with any of the following consecutive daily doses in the same treatment cycle. The reasons for these "first-dose effects" are unknown, though increased CD11b/18 expression resulting in neutrophil adhesion to pulmonary endothelial cells might be a significant contributing factor. The assessment of adverse effects has to consider not only the dose level of GM-CSF given but also the absolute level as well as the kinetics of circulating cells and the presence or absence of infection. As GM-CSF activates monocytes to release IL-1 and TNF (see above), particularly in the pres-

Table 18.2. Summary of Published Data on GM-CSF in Clinical Trials: GM-CSF Following High-Dose Chemotherapy and Bone Marrow Transplantation[a]

	Ref.	No. of Patients	Tumors	Chemoth.	Dose/Route	Remarks
			GM-CSF Following High-Dose Chemotherapy			
Stewart	84	9	Met. colorectal	Melphalan 120 μg/m²	3–10 μg/kg civ	
Gianni	85	15	Breast, NHL	Cyclophos. 7 g/m²	5.5 μg/kg civ days 1–14	
Logothetis	86	32	Urothelial tumors	hd M-VAC	120–500 μg/m² civ/sc days 3–13	Dose-finding study
Ho	87	23	Refract. NHL	Mitox hd ara-C	250 μg/m² civ	
Neidhart	88	8	Adv. malign.	Cyclophos. 5 g/m² Etoposide 1500 mg/m² Cisplatinum 150 mg/m²	?	Dose-finding study
			GM-CSF Following Bone Marrow Transplantation			
Brandt	89	19	Refr. breast Refr. melanoma	Comb. CTX	2–32 μg/kg civ 14 days	aBMT
Nemunaitis	90	15	Lymphoid malign.	Comb. CTX + TBI	15–240 μg/m² 2h iv 14 days	aBMT
Nemunaitis	91	37	Graft failure	Variable	60–1000 μg/m² 2h iv 14–21 days	
Devereux	92	31	Hodgkin's	BEAM	?	aBMT
Blazar	93	25	ALL	Variable	16–256 μg/m² 2h iv 14–21 days	aBMT, purged
Link	94	81	ALL/NHL	Variable	250–500 μg/m² civ	Double-blind placebo contr.
Rabinowe	95	23	NHL	Comb. CTX + TBI	250 μg/m² 2h iv 21 days	Double-blind placebo contr.
Nemunaitis	96	17	Lymphoid malign.	Comb. CTX + TBI	250 μg/m² 2h iv day 0–20	Phase III double-blind

[a]Abbreviations: aBMT, autologous bone marrow transplantation; ara-C, cytosine arabinoside; CTX, chemotherapy; hd, high-dose; TBI, total body irradiation.

ence of endotoxin, established or subclinical infection might initiate a cascade of biologic reactions (possibly "adverse events") when blood cell counts begin to rise in GM-CSF-treated patients following chemotherapy.

So far clinical studies do not indicate the development of antibodies to GM-CSF (97). However, recently the acquisition of antibodies to yeast-derived GM-CSF, directed against a portion of the molecule protected by O-glycosylation in the native growth factor, has been described (98). It remains to be determined whether this finding is of importance in cases of repeated administration of GM-CSF.

Tachyphylaxis to the proliferative effects of GM-CSF was generally not observed when this cytokine was given to patients over periods of days to weeks, and GM-CSF receptor downregulation appears to be a transient event (99). However, we have seen a patient with aplastic anemia treated with GM-CSF who became refractory to GM-CSF after 6 weeks of therapy; similar preliminary experience is reported by others (100). Because IL-3 treatment restored responsiveness to GM-CSF in our patient, it is likely that IL-3 replenished the bone marrow with progenitors sensitive to GM-CSF (101); GM-CSF receptor downregulation was unlikely since intermittent treatment with GM-CSF increased white blood cell counts only when preceded by IL-3 application in this patient.

Granulocyte-Monocyte Colony-Stimulating Factor Following Conventional-Dose Chemotherapy

Based on the observation of Bodey et al. (102) of a relationship between the degree and the duration of neutropenia and the incidence of fever and infection, trials with hematopoietic growth factors were initiated to try to reduce the period of dangerous neutropenia in tumor patients treated by cytotoxic agents. The GM-CSF trials listed in Table 18.1 all demonstrated a potent effect of this CSF in reducing chemotherapy-induced neutropenia. The study performed at our institution (81) also provided evidence for significant reduction of days with fever, days on antibiotics, and mucositis during a second cycle of chemotherapy, when GM-CSF was given.

The evaluation of febrile episodes in GM-CSF trials is frequently difficult, because it is not always obvious if febrile episodes are infectious in nature or related to GM-CSF application. Most studies have started CSFs the day after chemotherapy. Morstyn et al. (83) have shown that reduction in neutropenia could also be achieved if GM-CSF was started on day 4 after chemotherapy.

The most promising result of these studies was that GM-CSF might actually improve anticancer treatment by permitting safer administration of higher and/or more frequent doses of chemotherapy.

Presently it is a matter of debate whether the mature cells recruited in vivo by GM-CSF are functionally similar to their normal counterparts. Apart from the reduced migration mobility of GM-CSF-primed neutrophils (see above), there are indications of some concomitant loss of secondary granule contents (103). Jaswon et al. (104) have shown that mature neutrophils recruited in response to

GM-CSF in vivo are not as primed as neutrophils treated with GM-CSF in vitro. Whether this results in a loss of the maximal potential activity of neutrophils in clinical medicine is unknown. Prospective, blinded randomized trials will have to show to what extent GM-CSF therapy—by shortening the time and the extent of chemotherapy-induced myelosuppression—translates into reduced infections, reduced use of antibiotics, and shorter stays in hospitals.

Granulocyte-Monocyte Colony-Stimulating Factor Following High-Dose Combination Chemotherapy

High-dose chemotherapy either given alone or supported by hematopoietic stem cells is potentially curative in some chemosensitive tumors, and a relationship between dose intensity of most cytotoxic drugs and tumor response has been defined for several malignancies (for review see 105). Dose intensity should be adequate to overcome a threshold dose that produces response, and the average relative dose intensity received is probably a major factor determining outcome of chemotherapy (106).

Dose escalation, however, is mostly limited by myelosuppression as well as nonhematologic organ toxicity. To allow the use of dose-intensive regimens whose application is primarily limited by myelosuppression, and, at the same time, to eliminate the need for stem cell support, growth factor therapy is currently beginning to be studied by several investigators in conjunction with dose-intensive chemotherapy.

The studies summarized in Table 18.2 have convincingly shown that dose escalation is feasible and well tolerated when cytotoxic therapy is followed by GM-CSF application. The period of severe neutropenia was shortened in all studies; a surprising result of the study of Gianni (85) was the acceleration of platelet recovery. The relationship between dose and efficacy, however, is not clearly analyzed in these pioneering studies on high-dose chemotherapy.

The use of colony stimulating factors in dose escalation studies has to consider several problems:

1. Though GM-CSF allows the application of increased doses of chemotherapy and might reduce some organ toxicity of cytotoxic agents (89), the intensity of chemotherapy undoubtedly will be limited by nonhematopoietic adverse effects (107).
2. GM-CSF generally does not stimulate thrombopoietic recovery. Therefore, future trials should consider combinations of cytokines (e.g., IL-3 and GM-CSF, see beow). Other cytokines with thrombopoietic activity will, it is hoped, be available. IL-6 seems to be one of the most promising ones in this respect. Asano et al. (108) and Welte et al. (109) were the first to describe thrombopoietic activity of IL-6 in monkeys. Moreover, Welte et al. recently showed a similar increase in platelets when monkeys were given leukemia-inhibiting factor (LIF) (110). Our ongoing studies indicate that megakaryocytopoiesis is regulated by a specific CSF (Meg-CSF) (111); we have therefore initiated the biochemical characterization of this putative Meg-CSF.
3. The more intensive the regimen will be, the more the probability will increase that most of the committed progenitor cells are destroyed. This results in an increased input of progenitors from the pool of pluripotent cells. The question arises whether cytokines affect this process of recruitment and whether this might influence the probability of self-renewal and differentiation. This is of particular interest as myeloablative chemotherapy is known to induce high plasma levels of colony-stimulating activities; the additional exogenous supply of high levels of a cytokine following high-dose chemotherapy thus might result in combined or synergistic actions on primitive stem cells.
4. The kinetics of stem cell proliferation following intensive chemotherapy ± CSFs has not yet been studied in detail. Thus the duration of stem cell cycling—allowing the recovery of hematopoiesis—in this particular situation is unknown; this has to be kept in mind when repeated courses of high-dose cytotoxic chemotherapy are scheduled.

Use of Granulocyte-Monocyte Colony-Stimulating Factor Following Bone Marrow Transplantation

Based on the results of studies in primates undergoing autologous bone marrow transplantation, indicating that GM-CSF induces early neutrophil and platelet recovery (112, 113), a number of clinical trials with GM-CSF have been conducted to shorten the 3–4 weeks period of severe pancytopenia following bone marrow transplantation.

These studies (see Table 18.2) demonstrate that engraftment is accelerated. Neutrophil reconstitution was significantly hastened in all trials. Whether the time to the first granulocyte in the circulation can be reduced by GM-CSF is not yet clear; for example, Rabinowe et al. (95) and Brandt et al. (89) did not identify a difference in the time to reach 100 granulocytes betwen patients on placebo versus GM-CSF, although GM-CSF led to more rapid granulocyte recovery when the time to reach >500 and >1000 granulocytes per microliter was analyzed.

The effect of GM-CSF on platelet recovery is variable from study to study; early recovery was observed by the Seattle group (90, 96) and Blazar (93), whereas the other studies did not discern stimulation of thrombopoiesis. Possibly the results of ongoing randomized studies, using different schedules of administration of GM-CSF, will clarify this issue.

There are several indications from initial nonrandomized studies that GM-CSF reduces bacterial and fungal infections (89, 93) and the time of hospitalization (90). The data from randomized studies have shown that GM-CSF application results in a reduced incidence of infections (94, 96), in a shorter duration of intravenous antibiotic administration (95) and hospital stay (94–96), and less transplantation related toxicities (96) compared to placebo-treated patients. These studies suggest that GM-CSF will make autologous bone marrow transplantation safer and possibly applicable to more patients.

Studies of GM-CSF after allogeneic bone marrow transplantation only began after this cytokine was found to be safe and effective after autografting. The Seattle experience (45 patients with HLA-identical sibling donors) indicated that GM-CSF does not appear to influence either GVHD or graft rejection; however, engraftment appeared accelerated only in the group of patients that received cyclosporine/prednisone (114). In unrelated bone marrow transplantation GM-CSF may decrease the severity of early GVHD when compared to historical experience (114).

An important observation resulted from the use of GM-CSF in patients with graft failure following bone marrow transplantation. Fifty-seven percent of the patients responded to GM-CSF treatment; the overall survival rate was 59%, being significantly better than those of a historical control group. This is the first clinical study that documents improved survival in a group of patients treated with a hematopoietic growth factor (91).

Granulocyte-Monocyte Colony-Stimulating Factor-Induced Expansion of Peripheral Blood Stem Cells

Peripheral blood stem cell autografting has been used with increasing frequency following high-dose therapy for malignancy, as an alternative to the use of marrow stem cells. Successful transplantation with complete and sustained engraftment has been shown in various disorders, including acute nonlymphocytic leukemia (ANLL), lymphoma, neuroblastoma, breast cancer, and other solid tumors (115–124). When compared with autologous bone marrow transplantation, advantages of this modality—which can be done in an outpatient setting without the need for general anesthesia—include a more rapid restoration of neutrophils and platelets (116, 117, 122, 123), probably due to the high number of committed progenitor cells infused; the possibility of autografting when bone marrow aspiration is hampered by tumor cell infiltration, fibrosis, or hypoplasia following radio/chemotherapy; as well as the possibility of reduced contamination with malignant cells in disseminated cancer (125). The actual level of malignant cell contamination is a matter of debate (126, 127), as well as the exact dose of CFU-GM colonies and CD34-positive cells that have to be transplanted to allow a complete and sustained recovery (117, 128, 129).

Several ways to mobilize peripheral stem cells into circulation have been described. During rapid hematopoietic recovery following chemotherapy-induced myelosuppression, progenitor cells can be detected in the peripheral blood, particularly after cyclophosphamide treatment (130–137). GM-CSF given alone also expands the pool of circulating hematopoietic progenitors (72, 79, 138–140); this effect is increased by combining polychemotherapy with GM-CSF (138), and it is dramatically potentiated when GM-CSF is given following high-dose cyclophosphamide (141–143).

GM-CSF-exposed circulating progenitors apparently do provide rapid recovery and sustained hematopoiesis not only when both bone marrow and peripheral blood stem cells are reinfused (141) but also when given alone to patients following myeloablative therapy (139, 144).

As high-dose intensive chemotherapy either given alone or supported by hematopoietic stem cells is potentially curative in some tumors, we are currently performing a trial of recombinant human (rh) GM-CSF in polychemotherapy with synergistic agents that

Table 18.3. Summary of Published Studies as well as Our Unpublished Data on GM-CSF-Recruited Peripheral Blood Progenitor Cells[a,b]

Author	Growth Factor Dose/Route	Chemo-regimen	CD34/μl	CFU-GM/ml	BFU-E/ml	CFU-Meg/ml	CFU-GEMM/ml
Socinski (138)	—	—	nd	36	68	nd	nd
	GM-CSF 4–64 μg/kg/d	MAID	nd	70	75	nd	nd
	GM-CSF 4–64 μg/kg/d	MAID	nd	469	242	nd	nd
Herrmann (72)	GM-CSF <500 μg/m²	MAID	nd	2251	1117	nd	nd
	500 μg/m²	—	nd	30	nd	nd	nd
	1000 μg/m²	—	nd	120	nd	nd	nd
		—	nd	250	nd	nd	nd
Siena	—	—	0	50	nd	nd	nd
Gianni (141–143)	—	HD-CTX	6 (0–11)	1680	nd	nd	nd
	GM-CSF 5.5 μg/kg/d civ	HD-CTX	136 (0–1134)	14000 (5700–85,900)	nd	nd	nd
Haas (139)	GM-CSF 250 μg/m² civ, 10 days	—	nd	160	nd	nd	nd
	—	—	nd	1350	nd	nd	nd
Villeval (140)	GM-CSF 20 μg/kg/d sc/iv, 4 days	—	nd	105	nd	nd	nd
	—	—	nd	880	(3.3x)	(3.7x)	nd
Aglietta (79)	GM-CSF 8 μg/kg/d	—	nd	144	nd	nd	nd
	—	—	nd	638	nd	nd	nd
Our results	—	VCP/VIP	0.2 (0–3)	131 (0–785)	85 (0–659)	0	0
	—	VCP/VIP	46 (15–148)	3920 (330–5430)	3870 (540–6830)	0 (0–580)	0 (0–440)
	GM-CSF 250 μg/m² sc day 1–15	VCP/VIP	420 (190–1300)	6730 (2290–16,100)	800 (2000–13,930)	160 (0–610)	400 (0–2150)

[a] Abbreviations: See Tables 18.1 and 18.2. Nd, not determined; VCP, VP16 500 mg/m², cyclophosphamide 1600 mg/m², cisplatin 50 mg/m²; VIP, VP16 500 mg/m², ifosfamide 400 mg/m², cisplatin 50 mg/m².
[b] Data given as median including ranges (in parentheses).

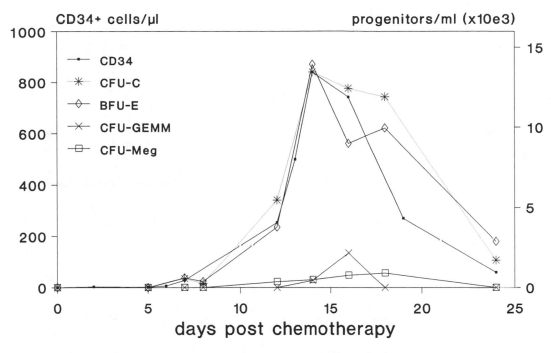

Figure 18.1. Circulating progenitor cells after chemotherapy + subcutaneous rhGM-CSF.

Table 18.4. CD34+ Cells/µl Blood after VIP or VCP Polychemotherapy with or without rhGM-CSF[a]

Prior Treatment	Growth Factor	CD34+/µl Blood	
		Median	Range
None	—	31	25–148
None	GM-CSF	738	636–839
Mild-moderate	—	52	46–121
Mild-moderate	GM-CSF	138	76–416
Intensive	—	13	10–15
Intensive	GM-CSF	10	1–19

[a]Abbreviations: VIP, VP16 500 mg/m^2, ifosfamide 4000 mg/m^2, cisplatin 50 mg/m^2; VCP, VP16 500 mg/m^2, cyclophosphamide 1600 mg/m^2, cisplatin 50 mg/m^2.

display few overlapping nonhematologic toxicities (etoposide 1500 mg/m^2, ifosfamide 12 g/m^2, and cisplatin 150 mg/m^2, administered intravenously over 3 days). This regimen was adapted from the studies of Neidhart et al. (145, 146), substituting ifosfamide for cyclophosphamide. Ifosfamide shows broad antitumor activity, particularly for sarcomas, germ cell tumors, lymphomas, lung cancer, and ovarian tumors (147). One can undergo considerable dose escalation over the usually prescribed doses (148). As studied so far in 12 patients, this approach is feasible and toxicity is acceptable (no grade III/IV organ toxicities), although severe myelosuppression occurs in all patients. Duration of neutropenia ($<$500/µl) and thrombocytopenia ($<$50,000/µl) following this regimen is 10–15 days.

To possibly shorten this period of profound pancytopenia, we are studying support of these patients with autologous peripheral blood stem cells. The concept is to first treat patients who are eligible for high-dose chemotherapy by the application of one-third of the cumulative doses as listed above, to offer them as soon as possible a highly effective treatment, and at the same time to try to mobilize peripheral blood stem cells, which might be collected by leukapheresis and retransfused to the patients after they have received the maximal dosage of chemotherapy (3-day cycle) in the subsequent cycle.

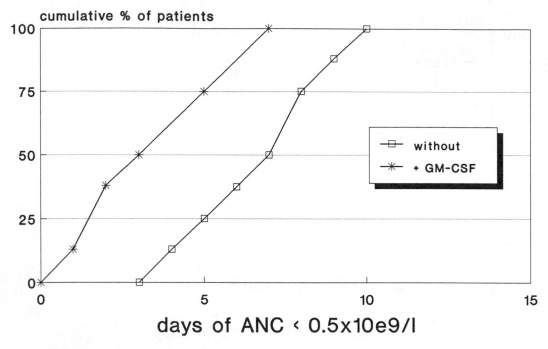

Figure 18.2.   Duration of neutropenia following polychemotherapy with or without rhGM-CSF.

So far 38 cycles of this 1-day chemo-therapy (etoposide 500 mg/m^2, ifosfamide 4 g/m^2, and cisplatin 50 mg/m^2, followed by subcutaneous GM-CSF on days 1–15) have been given to patients with miscellaneous solid tumors known to be chemosensitive. Be-tween days 12 and 16 after chemotherapy, peak numbers of CD34-positive cells of 300 per µl blood could be induced. Concomitant with the rise of CD34-positive cells, there was a dramatic increase of progenitors of the my-eloid (CFU-GM), erythroid (BFU-E), as well as megakaryocytic (CFU-Meg) and multipo-tential (colony-forming units for granulo-cytes, erythrocytes, monocytes, and mega-karyocytes [CFU-GEMM]) progenitor cells, with maximal colony numbers of 16,000/ml blood for CFU-GM and 2200/ml for CFU-GEMM re-spectively.

Table 18.3 summarizes our data and provides a comparison with published data on GM-CSF-induced peripheral blood stem cells. Figure 18.1 shows a representative time course of circulating CD34-positive cells as well as circulating colony-forming units after polychemotherapy in a patient treated with GM-CSF subcutaneously on days 1–15.

Based on the data of this preliminary series of patients studied, the absolute values for CD34-positive cells can be roughly di-vided into three groups, comprising patients with no prior radio/chemotherapy, patients with mild to moderate pretreatment, and heavily pretreated patients (Table 18.4). This heterogeneity probably reflects the degree of hematopoietic progenitor cell damage in the patients that have been pretreated differently. This regimen was well tolerated by all pa-tients studied so far; the median duration of neutrophils <500/µl was 8 days in patients treated without GM-CSF, whereas GM-CSF-application induced a significant reduction of the neutropenic period to a median of 3 days ($p < .01$) (Figure 18.2). There were no dif-ferences between GM-CSF-treated and non-treated patients in platelet recovery (data not shown).

Our data clearly indicate that combi-

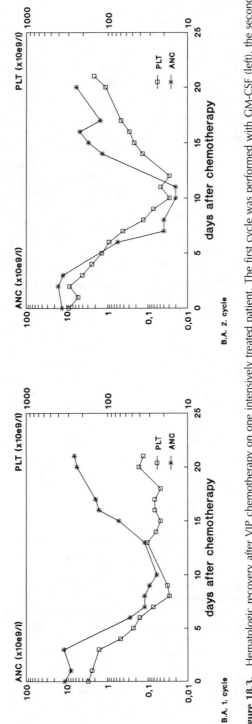

Figure 18.3. Hematologic recovery after VIP chemotherapy on one intensively treated patient. The first cycle was performed with GM-CSF (left), the second cycle with IL-3 plus GM-CSF (right). Neutrophil and platelet recovery are prevented. ANC, absolute neutrophil count.

nation chemotherapy followed by GM-CSF application allows successful expansion of the pool of circulating hematopoietic progenitors, comparable to the peripheral blood stem cell recruitment by single high-dose cyclophosphamide plus GM-CSF (141–143). Thus this approach combines successful peripheral blood stem recruitment with an effective combination chemotherapy that can be offered to patients with many different tumors (147, 149, 150).

We have now exploited the use of IL-3 plus GM-CSF in a sequential mode, combined with the same chemotherapy protocol, to evaluate if more progenitor cells can be induced to circulate by this combination. Our data (*Blood*, in press) indicate that IL-3 + GM-CSF is highly effective, with peak values of up to 1841/μl for CD34-positive cells, 23,340/ml blood for CFU-GM, 24,300/ml blood for BFU-E, 4450/ml blood for CFU-Meg, and 2070/ml blood for CFU-GEMM. Moreover, in heavily pretreated patients, the combination of IL-3 + GM-CSF might shorten the period of thrombocytopenia (<50,000/μl) up to 50% as compared to GM-CSF given alone, as exemplified in one patient (Figure 18.3).

These data document that after polychemotherapy-induced bone marrow hypoplasia, cytokines might be used to recruit peripheral blood stem cells to support hematopoietic recovery after subsequent high-dose intensification chemotherapy in chemosensitive malignancies.

REFERENCES

1. Huebner K, Isobe M, Croce XM, Golde DW, Kaufmann SE, Gasson JC. The human gene encoding GM-CSF is at 5q21–q32, the chromosome region deleted in the 5q- anomaly. Science 1985;230:1282.
2. Mijatake S, Otsuka T, Yokota T, Lee F, Arai K. Structure of the chromosomal gene for granulocyte macrophage colony stimulating factor: comparison of the mouse and human genes. EMBO J 1985;1:2561.
3. Gasson JC. Molecular physiology of granulocyte-macrophage colony-stimulating factor. Blood 1991; 77:1131-1145.
4. Arai K, Lee F, Miyajima, Miyatake S, Arai N, Yokota T. Cytokines: coordinators of immune and inflammatory responses. Ann Rev Biochem 1990;59:783–836.
5. Gasson JC, Eishart RH, Kaufman SE, et al. Purified human granulocyte-macrophage colony-stimulating factor: direct action on neutrophils. Science 1984; 226:1339.
6. Wong GG, Witek JS, Temple PA, et al. Molecular cloning of human and gibbon GM-CSF cDNAs and purification of the natural and recombinant human proteins. Cancer Cells 1985;3:235.
7. Moonen P, Mermod J-J, Ernst JF, Hirschi M, DeLamarter JF. Increased biological activity of deglycosylated recombinant human granulocyte/macrophage colony-stimulating factor produced by yeast or animal cells. Proc Natl Acad Sci USA 1987;84:4428.
8. Burgess AW, Begley CG, Johnson GR, et al. Purification and properties of bacterially synthesized human granulocyte-macrophage colony stimulating factor. Blood 1987;69:43.
9. Herrmann F, Oster W, Meuer SC, Lindemann A, Mertelsmann RH. Interleukin 1 stimulates T lymphocytes to produce granulocyte-monocyte colony-stimulating factor. J Clin Invest 1988;81:1415.
10. Wimperis JZ, Niemeyer CM, Sieff CA, Mathey-Prevot B, Nathan DG, Arceci RJ. Granulocyte-macrophage colony-stimulating factor and interleukin-3 mRNAs are produced by a small fraction of blood mononuclear cells. Blood 1989;74:1525.
11. Pluznik DH, Bickel M, Mergenhagen SE. B lymphocyte derived hematopoietic growth factors. Immunol Invest 1989;18:103.
12. Thorens B, Mermod JJ, Vassalli P. Phagocytosis and inflammatory stimuli induce GM-CSF mRNA in macrophages trough posttranscriptional regulation. Cell 1987;48:671.
13. Wodnar-Filipowicz A, Heusser CH, Moroni C. Production of the haemopoietic growth factors GM-CSF and interleukin-3 by mast cells in response to IgE receptor-mediated activation. Nature 1989;339:150.
14. Zucali JR, Dinarello CA, Oblon DJ, Gross MA, Anderson L, Weiner RS. Interleukin-1 stimulates fibroblasts to produce granulocyte-macrophage colony-stimulating activity and prostaglandin E_2. J Clin Invest 1986;77:1857.
15. Bagby GC Jr, Dinarello CA, Wallace P, Warner C. Hefeneider S, McCall E. Interleukin 1 stimulates granulocyte macrophage colony-stimulating activity release by vascular endothelial cells. J Clin Invest 1986;78:1316.
16. Rajavashisth TB, Andalbi A, Territo MC, Berliner JA, Navab M, Fogelman MA, Lusis AJ. Induction of endothelial cell expression of granulocyte and macrophage colony-stimulating factors by modified low-density lipoproteins. Nature 1990;344:254.
17. Demetri GD, Zenzie BW, Rheinwald JG, Griffin JD. Expression of colony-stimulating factor genes by normal human mesothelial cells and human malig-

nant mesothelioma cell lines in vitro. Blood 1989;74:940.

18. Horowitz MC, Coleman DL, Flood PM, Kupper TS, Jilka RL. Parathyroid hormone and lipopolysaccharide induce murine osteoblast-like cells to secrete a cytokine indistinguishable from granulocyte-macrophage colony-stimulating factor. J Clin Invest 1989;83:149.

19. DiPersio J, Billing P, Kaufman S, Eghtesady P, Williams RE, Gasson JC. Characterization of the human granulocyte-macrophage colony-stimulating factor receptor. J Biol Chem 1988;263:1834.

20. Bazan JF. Structural design and molecular evolution of a cytokine receptor superfamily. Proc Natl Acad Sci USA 1990;87:6934.

21. Gearing DP, King JA, Gough NM, Nicola NA. Expression cloning of a receptor for human granulocyte-macrophage colony-stimulating factor. EMBO J 1989;8:3667–3676.

22. Gough NM, Gearing DP, Nicola NA, Baker E, Pritchard M, Gallen DF, Sutherland GR. Localization of the human GM-CSF receptor gene to the X-Y pseudoautosomal region. Nature 1990;345:734.

23. Miyajima A, Kitamura T, Hayshida K, et al. Molecular analysis of the IL-3 and GM-CSF receptors. J Cell Biochem 1991; suppl 15F:37.

24. Gorman DM, Itoh N, Kitamura T, Schreurs J, Yonehara S, Yahara I, Arai K-i, Miyajima A. Cloning and expression of a gene encoding an interleukin 3 receptor-like protein: identification of another member of the cytokine receptor gene family. Proc Natl Acad Sci USA 1990;87:5459.

25. Itoh N, Yonehara S, Schreurs J, et al. Cloning of an interleukin-3 receptor gene: a member of a distinct receptor gene family. Science 1990;247:324.

26. Kanakura Y, Druker B, Cannistra SA, Furukawa Y, Torimoto Y, Griffin JD. Signal transduction of the human granulocyte-macrophage colony-stimulating factor and interleukin-3 receptors involves tyrosine phosphorylation of a common set of cytoplasmic proteins. Blood 1990;4:706–715.

27. Cannistra SA, Groshek P, Garlick R, Miller J, Griffin JD. Regulation of surface expression of the granulocyte-macrophage colony stimulating factor receptors in normal human myeloid cells. Proc Natl Acad Sci USA 1990;87:93.

28. Herrmann F, Ganser A, Lindemann A, Wieser M, Schulz G, Hoelzer D, Mertelsmann R. Stimulation of granulopoiesis in patients with malignancy by rhGM-CSF: assessment of two routes of administration. J Biol Response Mod 1989, in press.

29. Metcalf D. The consequences of excess levels of haemopoietic growth factors. Br J Haematol 1990;75:1–3.

30. Oster W, Mertelsmann R, Herrmann F. Role of colony-stimulating factors in the biology of acute/myelogenous leukemia. Int J Cell Cloning 1989;7:13–29.

31. Salmon S, Lui R. Effects of granulocyte-macrophage colony-stimulating factor on in vitro growth of human solid tumors. J Clin Oncol 1989;7:1346–1350.

32. Park LS, Friend D, Price V, et al. Heterogeneity in human interleukin-3 receptors. A subclass that binds human granulocyte/macrophage colony-stimulating factor. J Biol Chem 1989;264:5420.

33. Gesner TG, Mufson RA, Norton CR, Turner KJ, Yang YC, Clark SC. Specific binding internalization, and degradation of human recombinant interleukin-3 by cells of the acute myelogenous leukemia line, KG-1. J Cell Physiol 1988;136:493.

34. Park LS, Waldron PE, Friend D, et al. Interleukin-3, GM-CSF, and G-CSF receptor expression on cell lines and primary leukemia cells: receptor heterogeneity and relationship to growth factor responsiveness. Blood 1989;74:56.

35. Lopez AF, Eglinton JM, Gillis D, Park LS, Clark S, Vadas MA. Reciprocal inhibition of binding between interleukin 3 and granulocyte-macrophage colony-stimulating factor to human eosinophils. Proc Natl Acad Sci USA 1989;86:7022.

36. Raines M, Liu L, Quan S, DiPersio J, Golde DW. Molecular cloning of a soluble form of the human granulocyte-macrophage colony stimulating factor receptor (GM-CSF-R). J Cell Biochem 1991; suppl F:109.

37. Tomonaga M, Golde DW, Gasson JC. Biosynethetic (recombinant) human granulocyte-macrophage colony-stimulating factor: effect on normal bone marrow and leukemia cell lines. Blood 1986;67:31.

38. Metcalf D, Begley CG, Johnson GR, et al. Biologic properties in vitro of a recombinant human granulocyte-macrophage colony-stimulating factor. Blood 1986;67:37.

39. Donahue RE, Emerson SG, Wang EA, Wong GG, Clark SC, Nathan DG. Demonstration of burst-promoting activity of recombinant human GM-CSF on circulating erythroid progenitors using an assay involving the delayed addition of erythropoietin. Blood 1985;66:1479.

40. Bruno E, Briddell R, Hoffmann R. Effect of recombinant and purified hematopoietic growth factors on human megakaryocyte colony formation. Exp Hematol 1988;16:371.

41. Robinson BE, McGrath HE, Quesenberry PJ. Recombinant murine granulocyte macrophage colony stimulating factor has megakaryocyte colony stimulating activity and augments megakaryocyte colony stimulating by interleukin-3. J Clin Invest 1987;79:1648.

42. Quesenberry PJ, Ihle JN, McGrath E. The effect of interleukin-3 and GM-CSA-2 on megakaryocyte and myeloid clonal colony formation. Blood 1985;65:214.

43. Mazur EM, Cohen JE, Wong CG, Clark SC. Modest stimulating effect of recombinant human GM-CSF on colony growth from peripheral blood human

megakaryocyte progenitor cells. Exp Hematol 1987;15:1128.

44. Aglietta M, Monzeglio C, Sanavio F, et al. In vivo effect of human granulocyte-macrophage colony-stimulating factor on megakaryocytopoiesis. Blood 1991;6:1191–1194.

45. Kanz L, Löhr GW, Fauser AA. Examination of megakaryocytes and megakaryocytic progenitors (CFU-M) from human bone marrow for the expression of glycoprotein IIIa with use of flow cytometry. Exp Hematol 1985;13:438a.

46. Kanz L, Löhr GW, Fauser AA. Lymphokine(s) from isolated T lymphocyte subpopulations support multilineage hematopoietic colony (CFU-GEMM) and megakaryocytic colony (CFU-M) formation. Blood 1986;68:991–995.

47. Wing EJ, Magee DM, Whitside TL, Kaplan SS, Shadduck RK. Recombinant human granulocyte/macrophage colony-stimulating factor enhances monocyte cytotoxicity and secretion of tumor necrosis factor α and interferon in cancer patients. Blood 1989;73:643.

48. Rothenberg ME, Owen WF Jr, Silberstein DS, et al. Human eosinophils have prolonged survival, enhanced functional properties, and become hypodense when exposed to human interleukin 3. J Clin Invest 1988;81:1986–1992.

49. Oster W, Lindemann A, Mertelsmann R, Herrmann F. Granulocyte-macrophage colony-stimulating factor (CSF) and multilineage CSF recruit human monocytes to express granulocyte CSF. Blood 1989;73:64.

50. Hancock WW, Pleau ME, Kobzik L. Recombinant granulocyte-macrophage colony-stimulating factor down-regulates expression of IL-2 receptor on human mononuclear phagocytes by induction of prostaglandine. J Immunol 1988;140:3021.

51. Lindemann A, Riedel D, Oster W, Meuer SC, Blohm D, Mertelsmann R,. Herrmann F. GM-CSF induces secretion of interleukin-1 by polymorphonuclear neutrophils. J Immunol 1988;140:837–839.

52. Cannistra SA, Vellenga E, Groshek P, Rambaldi A, Griffin JD. Human granulocyte-monocyte colony-stimulating factor and interleukin-3 stimulate monocyte cytotoxicity through a tumor necrosis factor-dependent mechanism. Blood 1988;71:672–676.

53. Handman E, Burgess AW. Stimulation by granulocyte-macrophage colony-stimulating factor of Leishmania tropica killing by macrophages. J Immunol 1979;122:1134.

54. Bermudez LEM, Young LS. Recombinant granulocyte-macrophage colony-stimulating factor activates human macrophages to inhibit growth or kill Mycobacterium avium complex. J Leukocyte Biol 1990;48:67–73.

55. Arnaout MA, Wang EA, Clark SC, Sieff CA. Human recombinant granulocyte-macrophage colony-stimulating factor increases cell-to-cell adhesion and surface expression of adhesion-promoting surface glycoproteins on mature granulocytes. J. Clin Invest 1986;78:597.

56. Lindemann A, Riedel D, Oster W, Ziegler-Heitbrock WL, Mertelsmann R, Herrmann F. Granulocyte-macrophage colony-stimulating factor induces cytokine secretion by human polymorphonuclear leukocytes. J Clin Invest 1989;83:1308.

57. Lindemann A, Riedel D, Oster W, Meuer SC, Blohm D, Mertelsmann R, Herrmann F. Granulocyte/macrophage colony-stimulating factor induces interleukin 1 production by human polymorphonuclear neutrophils. J Immunol 1988;140:837.

58. Richter J, Andersson R, Olsson I. Effect of tumor necrosis factor and granulocyte/macrophage colony-stimulating factor on neutrophil degranulation. J Immunol 1989;142:3199.

59. Kaufmann S, DiPersio JF, Gasson JC. Effects of human GM-CSF on neutrophil degranulation in vitro. Exp Hematol 1989;17:800.

60. Peters WP, Stuart A, Affronti ML, Kim CS, Coleman RE. Neutrophil migration is defective during recombinant human granulocyte-macrophage colony-stimulating factor infusion after autologous bone marrow transplantation in humans. Blood 1988; 72:1310–1315.

61. Fleischmann J, Golde DW, Weisbart RH, Gasson JC. Granulocyte-macrophage colony-stimulation factor enhances phagocytosis of bacteria by human neutrophils. Blood 1986;68:708.

62. Villalta F, Kierszenbaum F. Effects of human colony-stimulating factor on the uptake and destruction of a pathogenic parasite (Trypanosoma cruzi) by human neutrophils. J Immunol 1986;137:1703.

63. Weisbart RH, Golde DW, Clark SC, Wong GG, Gasson JC. Human granulocyte-macrophage colony-stimulating factor is a neutrophil activator. Nature 1985;314:361.

64. Lopez AF, Williamson J, Gamble JR, et al. Recombinant human granulocyte-macrophage colony-stimulating factor stimulates in vitro mature neutrophil and eosinophil functions, surface receptor expression, and survival. J Clin Invest 1986;78:1220.

65. Nathan CF. Respiratory burst in adherent human neutrophils: triggering by colony-stimulating factors CSF-GM and SCF-G. Blood 1989;73:301.

66. Vadas MA, Nicola NA, Metcalf D. Activation of antibody-dependent cell-mediated cytotoxicity of the human neutrophils and eosinophils by separate colony-stimulating factors. J Immunol 1983;130:795.

67. Kushner BH, Cheung N-KV. GM-CSF enhances 3F8 monoclonal antibody-dependent cellular cytoxicity against human melanoma and neuroblastoma. Blood 1989;73:1936.

68. Dahinden CA, Zingg J, Maly FE, de Weck AL. Leu-

kotriene production in human neutrophils primed by recombinant human granulocyte/macrophage colony-stimulating factor and stimulated with the complement component C5A and FMLP as second signals. J Exp Med 1988;167:1281.

69. Wirthmueller U, De Weck AL, Dahinden CA. Platelet-activating factor production in human neutrophils by sequential stimulation with granulocyte-macrophage colony-stimulating factor and the chemotactic factors C5A or formyl-methionyl-leucyl-phenylalanine. J Immunol 1989;142:3213.

70. DiPersio JF, Billing P, Williams R, Gasson JC. Human granulocyte macrophage colony-stimulation factor (GM-CSF) and other cytokines prime neutrophils for enhanced arachidonic acid release and leukotriene B$_4$ sythesis. J Immunol 1988;140:4315.

71. Cannistra SA, Groshek P, Garlick R, Miller J, Griffin JD. Regulation of surface expression of granulocyte/macrophage colony stimulating factor receptor in normal human myeloid cells. Proc Natl Acad Sci USA 1990;87:93.

72. Herrmann F, Schulz G, Lindemann A, Meyerburg W, Oster W, Krumwieh D, Mertelsmann R. Hematopoietic responses in patients with advanced malignancy treated with recombinant human granulocyte-macrophage colony stimulating factor. J Clin Oncology, 1989;7:2.

73. Phillips N, Jacobs S, Stoller R, Earle M, Przepiorka D, Shadduck RK. Effect of recombinant human granulocyte-macrophage colony stimulating factor on myelopoiesis in patients with refractory metastatic carcinoma. Blood 1989;74:1.

74. Steward WP, Scarffe JH, Austin R, Bonnem E, Thatcher N, Morgenstein G, Crowther D. Recombinant human granulocyte macrophage colony-stimulating factor (rh GM-CSF) given as daily short infusions—a phase I dose-toxicity study. Br J Cancer 1989;59:142.

75. Lieschke GJ, Maher D, Cebon J, et al. Effects of bacterially synthesized recombinant human granulocyte-macrophage colony-stimulating factor in patients with advanced malignancy. Ann Int Med 1989;110:357.

76. Lieschke GJ, Maher D, O'Connor M, et al. Phase I study of intravenously administered bacterially synthesized granulocyte-macrophage colony-stimulating factor and comparison with subcutaneous administration. Cancer Res 1990;50:606.

77. Steis RG, VanderMolen LA, Longo DL, et al. Recombinant human granulocyte-macrophage colony-stimulating factor in patients with advanced malignancy: a phase Ib trial. J Natl Cancer Inst 1990;82:697.

78. Vadhan-raj S, Buscher S, LeMaistre A, et al. Stimulating of hematopoiesis in patients with bone marrow failure and in patients with malignancy by recombinant human granulocyte-macrophage colony-stimulating factor. Blood 1988;1:134–141.

79. Aglietta M, Piacibello W, Sanavio F, et al. Kinetics of human hemopoictic cells after in vivo administration of granulocyte-macrophage colony-stimulating factor. J Clin Invest 1989;83:551–557.

80. Antman KS, Griffin JD, Ellas A, et al. Effect of recombinant human granulocyte-macrophage colony-stimulating factor on chemotherapy-induced myelosuppression. N Engl J Med 1988;319:593–598.

81. Herrmann F, Schulz G, Wieser M, et al. Effect of granulocyte-macrophage colony-stimulating factor in neutropenia and related morbidity induced by myelotoxic chemotherapy. Am J Med 1990;88:619.

82. Gerhartz HH, Stern AC, Schmetzer H, Wolf-Hornung B, Wilmanns W. Placebo-controlled double blind study of granulocyte/macrophage colony-stimulating factor in chemotherapy-induced leukopenia. Blut 1989;59:339a.

83. Cebon J, Nicola N, Ward M, et al. Granulocyte macrophage colony stimulating factor (hGM-CSF) from human lymphocytes: the effect of glycosylation on receptor binding and biological activity. J Biol Chem 1990;265:4485–4491.

84. Steward WP, Scarffe JH, Dirix LY, et al. Granulocyte-macrophage colony stimulating factor (GM-CSF) after high-dose melphalan in patients with advanced colon cancer. Br J Cancer 1990;61:749–754.

85. Gianni AM, Bregni M, Siena S, Orazi A, Stern AC, Gandola L, Bonadonna G. Recombinant human granulocyte-macrophage colony-stimulating factor reduces hematologic toxicity and widens clinical applicability of high-dose cyclophosphamide treatment in breast cancer and non-Hodgkin's lymphoma. J Clin Oncol 1990;5:768–778.

86. Logothetis CJ, Dexeus FH, Sella A, Amato RJ, Kilbourn RG, Finn L, Gutterman JU. Escalated therapy for refractory urothelial tumors: methotrexate-vinblastine-doxorubicin-cisplatin plus unglycosylated recombinant human granulocyte-macrophage colony-stimulating factor. J Natl Cancer Inst 1990;82:667–672.

87. Ho AD, Del Valle F, Engelhard M, et al. Mitoxantrone/high-dose ara-C and recombinant human GM-CSF in the treatment of refractory non Hodgkin's lymphoma: a pilot study. Cancer 1990;66:423–430.

88. Stritt JA, Neidhart JA, Stidley C. Effects of radiation on patients receiving dose intensive chemotherapy with granulocyte-colony stimulating factor (G-CSF) and granulocyte-monocyte stimulating factor (GM-CSF). Proc ASCO 1990;9:284.

89. Brandt SJ, Peters WP, Atwater SK, et al. Effect of recombinant human granulocyte-macrophage colony-stimulating factor on hematopoietic reconstitution after high-dose chemotherapy and autologous bone marrow transplantation. New Engl J Med 1988;318:869–876.

90. Nemunaitis J, Singer JW, Buckner CD, Hill R, Storb R, Thomas ED, Appelbaum FR. Use of recombinant human granulocyte-macrophage colony-stimulating

factor in autologous marrow transplantation for lymphoid malignancies. Blood 1988;2:834–836.

91. Nemunaitis J, Singer JW, Buckner CD, et al. Use of recombinant human granulocyte-macrophage colony-stimulating factor in graft failure after bone marrow transplantation. Blood 1990;1:245–253.

92. Devereux S, Linch DC, Gribben JG, McMillan A, Patterson K, Goldstone AH. GM-CSF accelerates neutrophil recovery after autologous bone marrow transplantation for Hodgkin's disease. Bone Marrow Tranplant 1989;4:49–54.

93. Blazar BR, Kersey JH, McGlave PB, et al. In vivo administration of recombinant human granulocyte/macrophage colony-stimulating factor in acute lymphoblastic leukemia patients receiving purged autografts. Blood 1989;3:849–857.

94. Link H, Boogaerts M, Carella A, et al. Recombinant human granulocyte-macrophage colony-stimulating factor (RH-GM-CSF) after autologous bone marrow transplantation for acute lymphoblastic leukemia and non-Hodgkin's-lymphoma: a randomized double blind multicenter trial in Europe. Blood 1990;76:152a.

95. Rabinowe S, Freedman A, Demetrie G, et al. Randomized double blinded trial of rhGM-CSF in patients with B-cell non-Hodgkin's lymphoma (B-NHL) undergoing high dose chemoradiotherapy and monoclonal antibody purged autologous bone marrow transplantation (ABMT). Blood 1990;76:161a.

96. Nemunaitis J, Singe JW, Buckner CD, et al. Preliminary analysis of a randomized, placebo-controlled trial of rhGM-CSF in autologous bone marrow transplantation (ABMT). Proc ASCO 1990;9:10.

97. Urdal DL, Park LS. Studies on hematopoietic growth factor receptors using human recombinant IL-3, GM-CSF, G-CSF, M-CSF, IL-1, and IL-4. Behring Inst Mitt 1988;83:27–39.

98. Gribben JG, Devereux S, Thomas NSB, et al. Development of antibodies to unprotected glycosylation sites on recombinant human GM-CSF. Lancet 1990;335:434–437.

99. Cannistra SA, Groshek P, Garlick R, Miller J, Griffin JD. Regulation of surface expression of the granulocyte/macrophage colony-stimulating factor receptor in normal human myeloid cells. Proc Natl Acad Sci USA 1990;87:93–97.

100. Wallerstein Jr. R, Deisseroth A. Hematopoietic growth factors in cancer treatment. In: Principles and practice of oncology. PPO Updates, vol.4, no.9. Philadelphia: JB Lippincott, 1990:1–16.

101. Herrmann F, Lindemann A, Rhagavachar A, Heimpel H, Mertelsmann R. In vivo recruitment of GM-CSF-response myelopoietic progenitor cells by interleukin-3 in aplastic anemia: pilot study. Leukemia 1990;10:671–672.

102. Bodey GP, Buckley M, Sathe YS, Freireich EJ. Quantitative relationships between circulating leukocytes and infection in patients with acute leukemia. Ann Intern Med 1966;64:328–340.

103. Devereux S, Porter JB, Hyoes KP, Abeysinghe RD, Saib R, Linch CD. Secretion of neutrophil secondary granules occurs during granulocyte-macrophage colony-stimulating factor induced margination. Br J Haematol 1990;74:17–23.

104. Jaswon MS, Khwaja A, Roberts PJ, Jones HM, Linch DC. The effects of rhGM-CSF on the neutrophil respiratory burst when studied in whole blood. Br J Haematol 1990;75:181–187.

105. Devida VT. Principles of chemotherapy. In: Cancer, principles and practice of oncology. 3rd ed. Philadelphia: JB Lippincott, 1990.

106. Hryniuk WM. Average relative dose intensity and the impact on design of clinical trials. Semin Oncol 1987;1:66–74.

107. Bronchud MH, Howell A, Crowther D, Hopwood P, Souza L, Dexter TM. The use of granulocyte colony-stimulating factor to increase the intensity of treatment with doxorubicin in patients with advanced breast and ovarian cancer. Br J Cancer 1989;60:121–125.

108. Asano S, Okano A, Ozawa K. Nakahata T, Ishibashi T, et al. In vivo effects of rhIL-6 in primates: stimulated production of platelets. Blood 1990;75:1602–1605.

109. Zeidler C, Souza L, Welte K. In vivo effects of interleukin-6 on hematopoiesis in primates. Blood 1989;74:154a.

110. Zeidler C, Kanz L, Pietsch T, Boone T, Samal B, Welte K. Leukemia inhibitory factor (LIF) induces thrombocytosis in primates. Blood 1990;76(suppl 1):174a.

111. Kanz L, Kostielniak E, Welte K. Colony-stimulating activity unique for the megakaryocytic hemopoietic cell lineage, present in the plasma of a patient with the syndrome of thrombocytopenia with absent radii (TAR). Blood 1989;74:248a.

112. Monroy RL, Skelly RR, MacVittie TJ, et al. The effect of recombinant GM-CSF on the recovery of monkeys transplanted with autologous bone marrow. Blood 1987;70:1696–1699.

113. Nienhuis AW, Donahue RE, Karlsson S, et al. Recombinant human granulocyte-macrophage colony-stimulating factor (GM-CSF) shortens the period of neutropenia after autologous bone marrow transplantation in a primate model. J Clin Invest 1987;80:572–577.

114. Singer JW, Nemunaitis J, Bianco JC, et al. Rh-GM-CSF following allogeneic bone marrow transplantation from unrelated marrow donors: a phase II study. Blood 1990;10:566a.

115. Stiff PJ, Koester AR, Eagleton IE, Hindman T, Braud E. Autologous stem cell transplantation using peripheral blood stem cells. Transplantation 1987;44:585.

116. Reiffers J, Castaigne S, Tilly H, et al. Hematopoietic reconstitution after autologous blood stem cell transplantation: a report of 46 cases. Plasma Ther Transfus Technol 1987;8:360.

117. Juttner CA, To LB, Ho JQK, et al. Early lympho-hematopoietic recovery after autografting using peripheral blood stem cells in acute nonlymphoblastic leukemia. Transplant Proc 1988;20:40.
118. Cantin G, Marchand-Larache D, Bouchard MM, Leblond PF. Blood-derived stem cell collection in acute nonlymphoblastic leukemia: predictive factors for a good yield. Exp Hematol 1989;17:991.
119. Körbling M, Dörken B, Ho AD, Pezzutto A, Hunstein W, Fliedner TM. Autologous transplantation of blood-derived hemopoietic stem cells after myeloablative therapy in a patient with Burkitt's lymphoma. Blood 1986;2:529–532.
120. Körbling M, Holle R, Haas R, et al. Autologous blood stem-cell transplantation in patients with advanced Hodgkin's disease and prior radiation to the pelvic site. J Clin Oncol 1990;6:978–985.
121. Fermand J-P, Levy Y, Gerota J, et al. Treatment of aggressive multiple myeloma by high-dose chemotherapy and total body irradiation followed by blood stem cells autologous graft. Blood 1989;1:20–23.
122. Kessinger A, Armitage JO, Landmark JD, Smith DM, Weisenburger DD. Autologous peripheral hematopoietic stem cell transplantation restores hematopoietic function following marrow ablative therapy. Blood 1988;3:723–727.
123. Kessinger A, Armitage JO, Smith DM, Landman JD, Bierman PJ, Weisenburger DD. High-dose therapy and autologous peripheral blood stem cell transplantation for patients with lympha. Blood 1989;4:1260–1265.
124. Takaue Y, Watanabe T, Kawano Y, et al. Isolation and storage of peripheral blood hematopoietic stem cells for autotransplantation into children with cancer. Blood 1989;4:1245–1251.
125. To LB, Russel J, Moore S, Juttner CA. Residual leukemia cannot be detected in very early remission peripheral blood stem cell collections in acute nonlymphoblastic leukemia. Leuk Res 1987;11:327.
126. Moss TJ, Sanders DG, Lasky LC, Bostrom B. Contamination of peripheral blood stem cell harvests by circulating neuroblastoma cells. Blood 1990;9:1879–1883.
127. Mann SL, Deboer J, Kessinger DJ, Sharp JG. Culture of peripheral stem cell harvests. Proc Am Soc Oncol 1989;73:495.
128. Kessinger A, Armitage JO. The evolving role of autologous peripheral stem cell transplantation following high-dose therapy for malignancies. Blood 1991;2:211–213.
129. To LB, Dyson PG, Juttner CA. Cell-dose effect in circulating stem-cell autografting [Letter]. Lancet 1986;2:404–405.
130. Richman CM, Weiner RS, Yankee RA. Increase in circulating stem cells following chemotherapy in man. Blood 1976;47:1031–1039.
131. Lohrmann HP, Schreml W, Fliedner TM, Heimpel H. Reaction of human granulopoiesis to high-dose cyclophosphamide therapy. Blut 1979;38:9–16.
132. Abrams RA, McCormack K, Bowles C, Deisseroth AB. Cyclo-phosphamide treatment expands the circulating haemopoietic stem cell pools in dogs. J Clin Invest 1981;67:1392.
133. Korbling M, Burke P, Braine H, Eltenbein G, Sontos G, Kaizel H. Successful engraftment of blood-derived normal haemopoietic stem cells in chronic myelogenous leukaemia. Exp Hematol 1981;9:684.
134. Stiff PJ, Murgo AJ, Wittes RE, DeRisi MF, Clarkson BD. Quantification of the peripheral blood colony forming unit-culture rose following chemotherapy: could leukocytaphereses replace bone marrow for autologous transplantation? Transfusion 1983;23:500–503
135. Ruse-Riol F, Legros M, Bernard D, et al. Variations in committed stem cells (CFU-GM and CFU-TL) in the peripheral blood of cancer patients treated by sequential combination chemotherapy for breast cancer. Cancer Res 1984;44:2219–2224.
136. To LB, Haylock DN, Kimber RJ, Juttner CA. High levels of circulating haemopoietic stem cells in very early remission from acute non-lymphoblastic leukaemia and their collection and cryopreservation. Br J Haematol 1984;58:399–410.
137. To LB, Shepperd KM, Haylock DN, et al. Single high doses of cyclophosphamide enable the collection of high numbers of hemopoietic stem cells from the peripheral blood. Exp Hematol 1990;18:442–447.
138. Socinski MA, Cannistra SA, Elias A, Antman KH, Schnipper L, Griffin JD. Granulocyte-macrophage colony stimulating factor expands the circulating haemopoietic progenitor cell compartment in man. Lancet 1988;1:1194–1198.
139. Haas R, Ho AD, Bredthauer U, Cayeux S, Egerer G, Knauf W, Hunstein W. Successful autologous transplantation of blood stem cells mobilized with recombinant human granulocyte-macrophage colony-stimulating factor. Exp Hematol 1990;18:94.
140. Villeval J-L, Dührsen U, Morstyn G, Metcalf D. Effect of recombinant human granulocyte-macrophage colony stimulating factor on progenitor cells in patients with advanced malignancies. Br J Haematol 1990;74:36–44.
141. Gianni AM, Siena S, Bregni M, et al. Granulocyte-macrophage colony-stimulating factor to harvest circulating haemopoietic stem cells for autotransplantation. Lancet 1989;2:580–585.
142. Siena S, Bregni M, Brando B, Ravagnani F, Bonadonna G, Gianni AM. Circulation of CD34+ hematopoietic stem cells in the peripheral blood of high-dose cyclophosphamide-treated patients: enhancement by intravenous recombinant human granulocyte-macrophage colony-stimulating factor. Blood 1989;11:1905–1914.

143. Siena S, Bregni M, Brando B, et al. Flow cytometry for clinical estimation of circulating hematopoietic progenitors for autologous transplantation in cancer patients. Blood 1991;2:400–409.

144. Gianni AM, Tarella C, Siena S, et al. Durable and complete hematopoietic reconstitution after autografting or rhGM-CSF exposed peripheral blood progenitor cells. Bone Marrow Transplant 1990; 6:143–145.

145. Neidhart J, Mangalik A, Kohler W, et al. Granulocyte colony-stimulating factor stimulates recovery of granulocytes in patients receiving dose-intensive chemotherapy without bone marrow transplantation. J Clin Oncol 1989;11:1685–1692.

146. Neidhart J, Kohler W, Stidley C, et al. Phase I study of repeated cycles of high-dose cyclophosphamide, etoposide, and cisplatin administered without bone marrow transplantation. J Clin Oncol 1990;10:1728–1738.

147. Loehrer P. Current developments and future direction with ifosfamide. Semin Oncol 1989;16(suppl 3):1.

148. Elias AD, Eder JP, Shea T, Begg TS, Frei III E, Antman KH. High-dose ifosfamide with mesna uroprotection: a phase I study. J Clin Oncol 1990;8:170–178.

149. Pujol J-L, Rossi JF, Le Chevalier T, et al. Pilot study of neoadjuvant ifosfamide, cisplatin, and etoposide in locally advanced non-small cell lung cancer. Eur J Cancer 1990;7:798–801.

150. Coleman RE, Clarke JM, Slevin ML, et al. A phase II study of ifosfamide and cisplatin chemotherapy for metastatic or relapsed carcinoma of the cervix. Cancer Chemother Pharmacol 1990;27:52–54.

19

Delivery of High-Dose Chemotherapy with Recombinant Human Granulocyte Colony-Stimulating Factor Support

Sherri Brown, MaryAnn Foote, and George Morstyn

Human granulocyte colony-stimulating factor (HuG-CSF) is a hematopoietic growth factor that preferentially stimulates the production (1) and functional activity of neutrophils (2–7). HuG-CSF appears to be a part of the body's natural response to neutropenia (8).

The effects of HuG-CSF in elevating neutrophil counts are more rapid than the effects of other cytokines such as granulocyte-macrophage colony-stimulating factor (GM-CSF) and interleukin-3 (IL-3), because recombinant HuG-CSF (r-HuG-CSF) accelerates both the maturation and the marrow transit time of neutrophils (Fig. 19.1) (9).

Two forms of r-HuG-CSF have been used in clinical trials, an *E. coli*-derived product (Amgen, Thousand Oaks, CA and Kirin, Tokyo, Japan) and a Chinese-hamster-ovary (CHO)-cell-derived, glycosylated r-Hu-GSF (Chugai, Tokyo, Japan) (10–14). There have been no comparative clinical trials of these two products. Most published trials have used the *E. coli* product.

Recently, a review article concerning r-HuG-CSF was published that discusses the identification, cloning, regulation, production, and action of r-HuG-CSF, as well as results of clinical studies (15).

PHASE I AND II STUDIES WITH RECOMBINANT HUMAN GRANULOCYTE COLONY-STIMULATING FACTOR

Phase I/II trials established the specificity of r-HuG-CSF (16–18). Up to 12-fold increases occurred in peripheral blood neutrophil counts, with only small concurrent increases in monocytes and lymphocytes (less than 2-fold and usually within the normal range).

A dose-response relationship was established using r-HuG-CSF from 0.345 to 69 μg/kg/day. In phase I trials, the minimum doses that effectively elevated neutrophil values in all patients in the absence of chemotherapy were 1.15 μg/kg/day subcutaneously (SC) and 3.45 μg/kg/day intravenously (IV). The neutrophil count reached a plateau after 4–6 days of dosing at levels up to 11.5 μg/kg/day. In the absence of any dose-limiting toxicities, no maximum tolerated dose (MTD) has been established with clinical trials testing doses as high as 115 μg/kg/day.

Numerous laboratory studies have confirmed that the neutrophils produced in response to r-HuG-CSF are functional. This was further confirmed by two randomized, placebo-controlled phase III trials.

PHASE III STUDIES WITH RECOMBINANT HUMAN GRANULOCYTE COLONY-STIMULATING FACTOR

Phase III studies with r-HuG-CSF in combination with cancer chemotherapy have shown that the adjunctive use of r-HuG-CSF reduces the depth and the duration of chemotherapy-induced neutropenia. In a randomized, double-blind, placebo-controlled trial (19), 199 patients with small-cell lung cancer (SCLC) received r-HuG-CSF following conventional-dose chemotherapy (CAE [cyclophosphamide, doxorubicin, etoposide]). The primary end point of the trial was febrile neutropenia, which was defined as a body temperature $\geq 38.2°C$ associated with an absolute neutrophil count (ANC) $<1 \times 10^9$/liter. Double-blind treatment with the study drug was continued as long as the patient remained free of neutropenic fever. In both arms of the study, patients who experienced febrile neutropenia were allowed to receive open-label r-HuG-CSF.

The results of this study showed that the event rate for neutropenic fever across all cycles was 77% for placebo-treated patients and 40% for the r-HuG-CSF-treated patients ($P < .001$).

One-hundred thirty-five patients completed all six cycles of chemotherapy. Fifty-nine patients completed the study without experiencing febrile neutropenia, remaining on blinded study drug, 18 receiving placebo (17%), and 41 (43%) receiving GCS r-HuG-CSF. The median duration of grade-IV neutropenia (absolute neutrophil count [ANC] $<0.5 \times 10^9$/liter) was 6 days with placebo compared with 1 day with r-HuG-CSF (data from all cycles). During cycles of blinded study-drug treatment, the number of days of use of IV antibiotics, days of hospitalization, and incidence of culture-confirmed infections were reduced by approximately 50% when r-HuG-CSF was administered, as compared with placebo.

The major adverse effect associated with r-HuG-CSF was transient bone pain, presumably associated with bone marrow expansion, seen in 20% of patients, that occurred immediately before the increase in peripheral neutrophils. Based on its clinical benefit and safety profile, Crawford et al. (19) concluded that r-HuG-CSF was safe and efficacious. A criticism of the study was that the crossover design did not allow the impact of r-HuG-CSF support for chemotherapy on cancer outcome to be defined, because most patients received open-label r-HuG-CSF in both arms of the study.

A second phase III study was conducted by Trillet-Lenoir et al. (20). The study design was similar; however, following an episode of febrile neutropenia, patients maintained their original randomization rather than crossing over to open-label r-HuG-CSF.

The results of this study show that over all six cycles, 53% of the 64 placebo-treated patients but only 26% of the 65 r-HuG-CSF-treated patients had an episode of neutro-

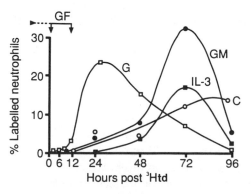

Figure 19.1. Time of appearance of labeled neutrophils in the circulation after injection of tritiated thymidine (^{3}HTd) in mice. C, controls; G, r-HuG-CSF; GM, recombinant murine GM-CSF; IL-3, recombinant mouse IL-3; G, growth factors. (Adapted from Lord BI, Molineaux G, Pojda Z, et al. Myeloid cell kinetics in mice treated with recombinant interleukin-3, granulocyte colony-stimulating factor [CSF] or granulocyte marrophage CSF in vivo. Blood 1991;77:2154–2159.)

penic fever. This, in turn, resulted in a statistically significant ($p < .002$) reduction in the use of parenteral antibiotics, with 58% of the placebo-treated patients and only 37% of the r-HuG-CSF-treated patients requiring such treatment. Additionally, 58% of the placebo-treated patients compared with 39% of the r-HuG-CSF-treated patients ($p < .04$) required hospitalization. The incidence of culture-confirmed bacterial infections was 33% of the placebo-treated patients and 20% of the r-HuG-CSF-treated patients ($p = .101$).

Over all six cycles, 61% of the placebo-treated patients required at least one reduction in their dose of chemotherapy compared with 29% of the r-HuG-CSF-treated patients ($p < .001$). As a result of differences in both dose delays and dose-reductions, r-HuG-CSF-treated patients received a greater dose intensity than did placebo-treated patients. However, this did not affect the overall survival. This may have been because the study was not designed to allow maximal dose intensification. Alternatively, SCLC may not be an optimal model in which to study dose intensification and its effects.

Preservation of intended dose intensity also was demonstrated in a randomized trial in non-Hodgkin's lymphoma conducted by Pettengell et al. (21). Eighty patients were randomized to treatment with or without r-HuG-CSF given as an adjunct to VAPEC-B chemotherapy.[a] R-HuG-CSF was given as a daily SC dose of 230 μg/m^2. There were 41 patients randomized to treatment with r-HuG-CSF and 39 to treatment without r-HuG-CSF. Febrile neutropenia occurred in 22% of the r-HuG-CSF-treated group versus 44% of the non-r-HuG-CSF-treated group, again demonstrating r-HuG-CSF's ability to decrease the incidence of febrile neutropenia. These differences were observed despite prophylactic ketoconazole and cotrimoxazole being given to both groups throughout the study. Doses were reduced in 10% of the group treated with r-HuG-CSF and 51% of the group treated without r-HuG-CSF. Fifty-nine percent of the r-HuG-CSF-treated group received over 95% of their intended dose of chemotherapy compared with 25% of the group treated without r-HuG-CSF. This trial, like the trial conducted by Trillet-Lenoir et al., demonstrated that chemotherapy dose-intensity can be preserved with r-HuG-CSF treatment, providing the groundwork for dose-escalation trials.

HIGH-DOSE CHEMOTHERAPY WITH RECOMBINANT HUMAN GRANULOCYTE COLONY-STIMULATING FACTOR SUPPORT

R-HuG-CSF has been used as an adjunct to high-dose chemotherapy, both with and without supportive hematopoietic cells given for marrow reconstitution.

Bronchud et al. (27) treated 17 patients with metastatic cancer with escalated doses of doxorubicin supported by r-HuG-CSF. There were four dose levels of doxorubicin ranging from 75 mg/m^2 to 150 mg/m^2. R-HuG-CSF was given by continuous IV infusion at a dose of 10 μg/kg. Additionally, 4 patients were treated with doxorubicin 75 mg/m^2 without r-HuG-CSF and served as the comparison group. For the comparison group, the median ANC count was greater than 2.5 $\times$ 10^9/ liter by day 19–21, making these patients eligible for retreatment with chemotherapy at 3-week intervals. In contrast, for the r-HuG-CSF-treated group, the ANC rose to normal or above normal levels by day 12–14 at all dose levels of doxorubicin. This allowed doxorubicin to be dosed at 2-week intervals (Fig. 19.2) and given at increased doses with r-HuG-CSF support for up to three cycles. R-HuG-CSF infusion was associated with a rapid

---

[a]VAPEC-B chemotherapy = doxorubicin 35 mg/ m^2, weeks 1, 3, 5, 7, 9, 11; cyclophosphamide, 350 mg/m^2, weeks 1, 5, and 9; etoposide, 100 mg/m^2 (orally daily for 5 days), weeks 3, 7, and 11; vincristine, 1.4 mg/m^2, weeks 2, 4, 6, 8, and 10; prednisolone, 50 mg orally daily, weeks 1 through 5, 25 mg orally daily, weeks 6 through 11, then tapered to 0 mg.

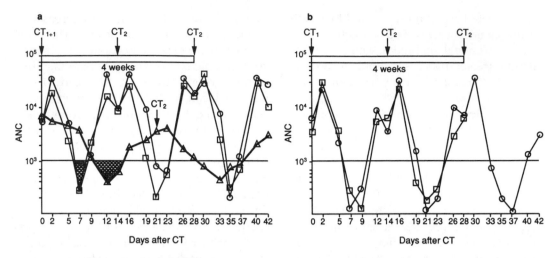

Figure 19.2. A, Median ANCs per cubic millimeter. *Open circles* = 75 mg/m^{-2} doxorubicin and 10 μg/kg r-HuG-CSF; *Open triangles* = 75 mg/m^{-2} doxorubicin. *Open squares* = 100 mg/m^{-2} doxorubicin and 10 μg/kg r-HuG-CSF. The shaded areas represent the total area of neutropenia (ANC < 1 × 10^9/liter) following the first doxorubicin dose at 75 mg/m^{-2}. **B**. Median ANC per cubic millimeter. *Open circles* = 125 mg/m^{-2} doxo-rubicin and 10 μg/kg r-HuG-CSF; *Open squares* = 150 mg/m^{-2} doxorubicin and 10 μg/kg r-HuG-CSF. (Adapted from Bronchud MH, Howell A, Crowther D, Hopwood P, Souza L, Dexter TM. The use of granulocyte colony-stimulating factor to increase the intensity of treatment with doxorubicin in patients with abnormal heart and ovarian cancer. Br J Cancer 1989;60:121–125.)

increase in peripheral neutrophil counts and an earlier nadir (day 7 with r-HuG-CSF compared with days 12–13 without r-HuG-CSF). In the two highest dose groups, platelet transfusions were required by 4/8 patients and the dose-limiting toxicity was mucositis, reported in 7/8 hospital admissions. Combining all doses of doxorubicin, 12/15 patients treated with r-HuG-CSF had a complete or partial response, with a median time to progression of disease of six months.

Several other dose-escalation studies are on-going using a variety of chemotherapy programs and r-HuG-CSF support. To date, Demetri et al. (23) have reported on 37 stage IIIB and IV breast cancer patients in a dose-escalation trial of CAF (cyclophosphamide, doxorubicin, and 5-fluorouracil) chemotherapy. Starting levels for the chemotherapy were cyclophosphamide 1000 mg/m^2, doxorubicin 60 mg/m^2, and 5-fluorouracil 600 mg/m^2. Both the cyclophosphamide and the doxorubicin were escalated, while the 5-fluorour-

acil was given at a constant dose. Patients were enrolled in sequential cohorts for four planned 28-day cycles using r-HuG-CSF at a dose of 10 μg/kg starting on day 2. At dose-level 4, (cyclophosphamide 3000 mg/m^2, doxorubicin 90 mg/m^2, and 5-fluorouracil 600 mg/m^2), 6 patients received full doses of CAF without delay for hematologic toxicity. At level 5, (cyclophosphamide 3000 mg/m^2, doxorubicin 120 mg/m^2, and 5-fluorouracil 600 mg/m^2), 1/5 patients was delayed for hematologic toxicity and 3 patients had grade-4 mucositis after cycle 2. The overall objective response rate, complete response plus partial response, was 76% (28/37) in patients receiving r-HuG-CSF.

Demetri et al. (24) also conducted a dose-escalation study of mitoxantrone in patients with advanced breast cancer. Doses of mitoxantrone were given as split doses on days 1 and 2 of a 28-day cycle. Four patients received mitoxantrone at 16 mg/m^2 without r-HuG-CSF to serve as a comparison group;

patients in the treated group received r-HuG-CSF 5 µg/kg/day SC on day 3 through the time of neutrophil recovery. In the first cycle, the median days of ANC $\leq 1000 \times 10^9$/liter were 6.5 for the comparison group and 0 for the group receiving r-HuG-CSF. Additional dose-escalation trials are ongoing in patients with non-small-cell lung cancer (25), CHOP and CHOPE (cyclophosphamide/doxorubicin/vincristine/prednisone/etoposide) in patients with non-Hodgkin's lymphoma (26, 27) and CNF (cyclophosphamide/mitoxatrone/5-fluorouracil) in patients with breast cancer (28). Although these trials are at an early stage, dose escalation is proceeding in each, following a demonstration in an initial cohort of patients that r-HuG-CSF markedly decreased neutropenia associated with standard-dose chemotherapy.

R-HuG-CSF also has been included in studies of a new cytotoxic agent. Serosy et al. (29) have studied taxol in a phase I dose-escalation trial for women with previously treated advanced stage ovarian cancer. Taxol was administered every 3 weeks to cohorts of three patients at each dose level as a 24-hour continuous IV infusion. Once the dose-limiting toxicity (DLT) was defined, four patients were treated at the preceding dose level. Dose levels were 170 mg/m^2, 200 mg/m^2, 250 mg/m^2, and 300 mg/m^2. Previous phase I trials in this patient population had defined a MTD of 175 mg/m^2, with dose-limiting myelosuppression and severe mucositis at higher doses. In this study, r-HuG-CSF was given as an adjunct to chemotherapy at a dose of 10 µg/kg/day subcutaneously. Taxol could be given safely at a dose of 250 mg/m^2, an increase in dose intensity of 43%, without dose-limiting myelosuppression or mucositis. At taxol doses of 300 mg/m^2, peripheral neurotoxicity was dose limiting.

Since the treatment for leukemia requires that patients' bone marrow be rendered hypoplastic, high-dose chemotherapy is used, providing rationale for r-HuG-CSF trials in this patient population. Ohno et al. (30) conducted a randomized, controlled study in 108 patients with relapsed or refractory acute leukemia who were given a standard course of intensive chemotherapy (mitoxantrone 5 mg/m^2, days 1–3; etoposide 80 mg/m^2, as a 1-hour IV infusion, days 1–5; and cytosine arabinoside 170 mg/m^2, as a 2-hour IV infusion, days 8–12). Patients who were assigned randomly to the r-HuG-CSF-treatment group received 200 µg/m^2/day as a 30-minute IV infusion after the last day of chemotherapy when there were fewer than 5% blasts in the bone marrow. R-HuG-CSF was continued until the peripheral neutrophil count was $>1.5 \times 10^9$/liter, at which time the dose was tapered. The median day on which the neutrophil count was $>0.5 \times 10^9$/liter or $>1 \times 10^9$/liter was day 20 and day 22, respectively, in the r-HuG-CSF-treated group, and day 28 and day 34, respectively, in the comparison group (Fig. 19.3). The incidence of febrile episodes (i.e., body temperature $>38.2°C$) was similar in both groups, but the incidence of documented infections was significantly less frequent in the r-HuG-CSF-treated group ($p = .028$). The authors concluded that r-HuG-CSF accelerates neutrophil recovery and reduces the incidence of documented infection without promoting the regrowth of leukemic cells.

USE OF RECOMBINANT HUMAN GRANULOCYTE COLONY-STIMULATING FACTOR WITH BONE MARROW TRANSPLANTATION

R-HuG-CSF has been used to promote hematologic recovery following ablative chemotherapy and autologous bone marrow reinfusion. Taylor et al. (31) treated 18 patients with refractory, relapsed Hodgkin's disease. Following cryopreservation of bone marrow, patients were treated with cyclophosphamide 1.5 g/m^2, days $-6--3$; carmustine 300 mg/m^2, day -6; and etoposide 125 mg/m^2, every 12 hours, days $-6--4$. Autologous bone marrow reinfusion was on

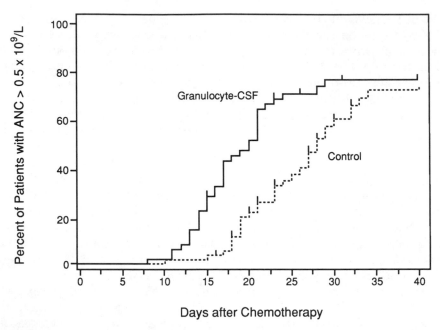

Days after Chemotherapy

Figure 19.3. Recovery of the neutrophil count to >500 per cubic millimeter after induction therapy. (Adapted from Ohno R, Tomonaga M, Kobayashi T, et al. Effect of granulocyte colony-stimulating factor after intensive radiation therapy in refrared or refractory acute leukemia. N Engl J Med 1990:3323:871–877.)

day 0, and patients were treated with r-HuG-CSF at 60 µg/kg/day beginning on day 1. Engraftment as measured by time to an absolute granulocyte count >0.5 × 10^9/liter was 13 days for the r-HuG-CSF group versus 22 days for historical controls. Platelet recovery was not significantly altered.

Peters et al. (32) also reported using r-HuG-CSF following autologous bone marrow transplantation (ABMT). The ablative chemotherapy regimen included cyclophosphamide 5625 mg/m^2 and carmustine 600 mg/m^2. Following reinfusion of autologous bone marrow cells, r-HuG-CSF was given IV in dose groups of 16, 32, and 64 µg/kg/day. Patients were compared with a historical-control group of 24 patients. Leukocyte counts at day 15 in r-HuG-CSF-treated patients were 6407 × 10^9/liter ± 17727 × 10^9/liter compared with 863 × 10^9/liter ± 645 × 10^9/liter for the historical-control group. Granulocyte phagocytosis was enhanced during r-HuG-CSF infusion; hydrogen peroxide production was un-

changed, as was granulocyte migration. R-HuG-CSF accelerated hematopoietic recovery while preserving or enhancing granulocyte function.

Sheridan et al. (33) treated 15 patients with nonmyeloid malignancies with oral busulphan (4 mg/kg) on day −7 through day −4 and with IV cyclophosphamide (60 mg/kg) on days −3 and −2. Autologous bone marrow was reinfused on day 0, and continuous SC infusions of r-HuG-CSF (20 µg/kg) were initiated 24 hours after the marrow infusion. The historical-comparison group for this study was a group of 18 patients treated at the same institution with the identical chemotherapy regimen and autologous bone marrow reinfusion, but without r-HuG-CSF support. The mean time to an ANC of 0.5 × 10^9/liter was 11 days in the r-HuG-CSF-treated group and 20 days in the historical-comparison group ($p < .0005$). The rate of rise of the circulating neutrophil count was exponential, in the range of 0.1–4.0 × 10^9/liter in patients receiving r-HuG-CSF, which was in stark contrast to the slow, approximately linear rise in the comparison group who did not receive r-HuG-CSF treatment (Fig. 19.4). Most peripheral blood neutrophils released with r-HuG-CSF treatment were mature segmented and band neutrophils, but some metamyelocytes, myelocytes, and promyelocytes also were noted. R-HuG-CSF did not effect red blood cell or platelet recovery. Although the incidence of fever was the same in both groups, the mean duration of care in reverse isolation, the duration of parental nutrition, the duration of IV antibiotic treatment, and the duration of hospital stay (for those r-HuG-CSF patients treated at the same hospital as the historical-comparison group) were significantly less in the r-HuG-CSF group than the comparison group (Table 19.1).

R-HuG-CSF also has been used in the setting of allogeneic bone marrow transplan-

tation. Masaoka et al. (34) reported a randomized, placebo-controlled study using r-HuG-CSF following ablative chemotherapy. Thirty-two patients were in the r-HuG-CSF-treated group and 34 patients were in the placebo group. The researchers reported that there was no significant difference between these two treatment groups in either the incidence of graft-versus-host disease or the rate of leukemic relapse during the first 90 days. However, the r-HuG-CSF-treated group recovered to an ANC $> 0.5 \times 10^9$/liter in a significantly shorter period of time.

USE OF RECOMBINANT HUMAN GRANULOCYTE COLONY-STIMULATING FACTOR WITH MOBILIZED PERIPHERAL BLOOD PROGENITOR CELLS

R-HuG-CSF has been used to mobilize peripheral blood progenitor cells (PBPC), which were then utilized to augment autologous bone marrow rescue following high-dose chemotherapy. Sheridan et al. (35) treated 14 patients with nonmyeloid malignancies. R-HuG-CSF was administered (after a leuka-

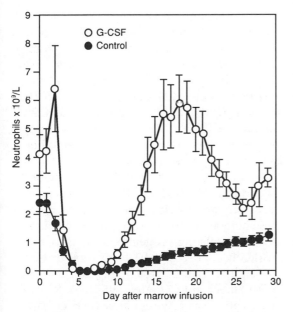

Figure 19.4. Mean (SEM) neutrophil count. *Open circles*, 15 patients treated with G-CSF; *filled circles*, 18 historical controls. (From Sheridan WP, Morstyn G, Wolf M, et al. Granulocyte colony-stimulating factor and neutrophil recovery after high-dose chemotherapy and autologous bone marrow transplantation. Lancet 1989;14:891–895.)

Table 19.1. Hematologic and Clinical Values[a]

Days (Ranges)[b]	r-HuG-CSF-treated patients	Controls
To neutrophil count above 0.5 × 10⁹/L	11 (2 to 4)	20 (5 to 5)[c]
Parenteral antibiotics (days)	11 (5 to 3)	18 (6 to 7)[d]
Isolation (days)	10 (2 to 7)	18 (4 to 2)[c]
Parenteral nutrition (days)	10 (7 to 4)	16 (5 to 6)
Time in hospital (days)	23 (11)	30 (11)

[a]Adapted from Sheridan WP, Morstyn G, Wolf M, et al. Granulocyte colony-stimulating factor and neutrophil recovery after high-dose chemotherapy and autologous bone marrow transplantation. Lancet 1989;14:891–895.
[b]After bone marrow infusion.
[c]$p < .0005$.
[d]$p = .002$.

pheresis for baseline values) at 12 μg/kg/day as a continuous infusion for 6 days. A leukapheresis procedure to collect mobilized PBPCs was performed on days 5, 6, and 7. Cells were cryopreserved, as was the harvested bone marrow. High-dose chemotherapy with busulphan and cyclophosphamide was given (33). Bone marrow and PBPCs were infused on day 0, and r-HuG-CSF at a dose of 12 μg/kg/day was administered 24 hours after the completion of chemotherapy. Patients receiving identical chemotherapy, bone marrow, and r-HuG-CSF without PBPCs served as a comparison group. Prior to treatment with r-HuG-CSF, the level of progenitor cells in the peripheral blood was $0.04 \pm 0.01 \times 10^3$ granulocyte-macrophage colony-forming unit (CFU-GM)/ml. After 5 days of treatment with r-HuG-CSF, progenitor levels increased fivefold over baseline, to a value of $1.7 \pm 0.3 \times 10^3$/ml ($p < .001$). A similar pattern of response was seen for erythroid progenitors. Although neutrophilia was induced by r-HuG-CSF treatment, the leukapheresis product was predominantly mononuclear cells. Importantly, the median time to platelet recovery ($>50 \times 10^9$/liter) was 25 days earlier than in controls (Fig. 19.5). The median number of units of platelets transfused was 47 units less than controls.

In addition to its use as a stand-alone agent, r-HuG-CSF also has been used in combination with cytotoxic chemotherapy to mobilize PBPC by Pettengell et al. (36, 37). Patients were treated with 7 weeks of VAPEC-B chemotherapy followed by r-HuG-CSF to mobilize PBPCs. R-HuG-CSF was given at a dose of 200 μg/m² for 7–9 days. Blood samples were taken and clonogenic assays performed to measure peak number of colonies per milliliter of blood (reported as mean ±SEM), specially noting CFU-GM, blast-forming units, erythroid (BFU-E); and colony-forming units, mixed (CFU-Mix). Twenty-two patients with newly diagnosed non-Hodgkin's lymphoma served as a comparison group, and their pre-VAPEC-B values were compared with those

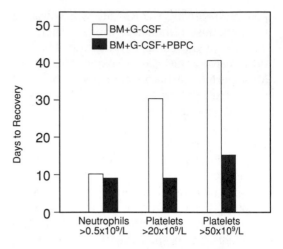

Figure 19.5. Neutrophil and platelet recovery in patients treated with bone marrow (BM) plus rHuG-CSF or bone marrow plus PBPC plus rHuG-CSF. (Based on Sheridan WP, Begley CG, Juttner CA, et al. Effect of peripheral-blood progenitor cells mobilised by filgrastin (GCSF) on platelet recovery after high-dose chemotherapy. Lancet 1992;339:640–644.)

obtained after chemotherapy mobilization (5 patients) and those obtained after chemotherapy plus r-HuG-CSF mobilization (5 patients). Pretreatment blood samples contained limited numbers of circulating progenitor cells (CFU-GM, $35 \pm 8 \times 10^9$/liter; BFU-E, $181 \pm 35 \times 10^9$/liter; and CFU-Mix, $0.9 + 0.5 \times 10^9$/liter), and these numbers were increased in the postchemotherapy-recovery phase (CFU-GM, $429 \pm 240 \times 10^9$/liter; BFU-E, $2200 \pm 703 \times 10^9$/liter; and CFU-Mix, 6×10^9/liter $\pm 6.2 \times 10^9$/liter). However, when r-HuG-CSF was given in the postchemotherapy-recovery phase, the number of circulating progenitors was increased markedly (CFU-GM, 9603×10^9/liter $\pm 1355 \times 10^9$/liter; BFU-E, 5169×10^9/liter $\pm 2036 \times 10^9$/liter; and CFU-Mix, $195 \pm 71 \times 10^9$/liter. There was a 59-fold increase over baseline in the total number of colonies.

To collect PBPCs, patients treated with r-HuG-CSF had a single 4-hour leukapheresis, processing approximately 15 liters of blood, and the harvested cells were cryopreserved. Following three cycles of consolidation and ablative chemotherapy, PBPCs were reinfused and r-HuG-CSF was restarted at a dose of 200 $\mu g/m^2$. Median time to a neutrophil count >500 × 10^9/liter was 9 days in the r-HuG-CSF plus PBPC group, 13 days in the r-HuG-CSF plus bone marrow group, and 19 days in a historical comparison group. Median time to platelet recovery to >20 × 10^9/liter was 13 days in the r-HuG-CSF plus PBPC group, 24 days in the r-HuG-CSF plus bone marrow group, and 20 days in a historical comparison group, once again supporting the use of cytokines and PBPCs to hasten hematopoietic engraftment.

CONCLUSIONS

R-HuG-CSF stimulates the production of functional neutrophils, decreasing the days of neutropenia normally associated with high-dose chemotherapy and resulting in clinical benefits, including decreased days of antibiotic usage, decreased numbers of culture-confirmed infections, and decreased days of hospitalization. It is clear that the reduction in neutropenia and infection allows the delivery of full-dose chemotherapy on time, as well as dose escalation. The contribution of dose-escalated chemotherapy programs to tumor response and patient survival has yet to be determined. As doses are increased, other adverse effects of chemotherapy, besides neutropenia, become dose limiting. These other dose-limiting toxicities can be both hematologic (e.g., thrombocytopenia, which may be overcome by the use of PBPCs) or nonhematologic (e.g., cardiomyopathy, which may be ameliorated by the new cardioprotective agents). A new direction for clinical research in oncology will involve the use of multiple cycles of high-dose chemotherapy, supported each time by an infusion of PBPCs. Cytokines alone or in combination will play an important role in this area.

REFERENCES

1. Metcalf D, Nicola NA. Proliferation effects of purified granulocyte colony-stimulating factor (G-CSF) on normal mouse haematopoietic cells. J Cell Physiol 1983;116:198–206.
2. Sullivan R, Griffin JD, Simons ER, et al. Effects of recombinant human granulocyte and macrophage colony-stimulating factors on signal transduction pathways in human granulocytes. J Immunol 1987; 139:3422–3430.
3. Lopez AF, Nicola NA, Burgess AW, et al. Activation of granulocyte cytotoxic function by purified mouse colony-stimulating factors. J Immunol 1983;131:2983–2988.
4. Vadas MA, Nicola NA, Metcalf D. Activation of antibody-dependent cell-mediated cytotoxicity of human neutrophils and eosinophils by separate colony-stimulating factors. J Immunol 1983;130:795–799.
5. Platzer E, Welte K, Gabrilove JL, Lu L, Harris, Mertelsmann R, Moore MA. Biological activities of a human pluripotent hemopoietic colony stimulating factor on normal and leukemic cells. J Exp Med 1985; 162:1788–1801.
6. Platzer E, Oez S, Welte K, et al. Human pluripotent hemopoietic colony stimulating factor: activities on human and murine cells. Immunobiology 1986; 172:185–193.
7. Yuo A, Kitagawa S, Okabe T, Urabe A, Komatsu Y, Itoh S, Takaku F. Recombinant human granulocyte colony-stimulating factor repairs the abnormalities of neutrophils in patients with myelodysplastic syndromes and chronic myelogenous leukemia. Blood 1987;70:404–411.
8. Cebon J, Layton J, Pavlovic R, Iaria J, Dyer W, Morstyn G. Endogenous cytokine production in response to sepsis in neutropenic and non-neutropenic patients. Proc ASH, 1991, in press.
9. Lord BI, Molineaux G, Pojda Z, et al. Myeloid cell kinetics in mice treated with recombinant interleukin-3, granulocyte colony-stimulating factor (CSF) or granulocyte macrophage CSF in vivo. Blood 1991; 77:2154–2159.
10. Dodwell D, Ferguson J, Howell A, Testa N, Campbell A. Intensification of Adriamycin and cyclophosphamide treatment for advanced breast cancer with subcutaneous G-CSF: identification of optimal time to collect peripheral blood stem cells. Proc ASCO, 1991, in press.
11. Asano S, Masaoka T, Takaku F. Multicenter phase II–III clinical studies of recombinant human granulo-

cyte colony-stimulating factor in bone marrow transplantation. Exp Hematol 1990;18:705.

12. Takada M, Fukuoka M, Furuse K, Ariyoshi Y, Nitani H, Ota K. Recombinant human G-CSF in patients with non-small cell lung cancer treated with combination chemotherapy of mitomycin, vindesine, and cisplatin (MVP). Proc Am Assoc Clin Oncol, 1990.

13. Takahashi S, Shirafuji, Shimane M, et al. Human granulocyte colony-stimulating factor combined conditioning regimen for bone marrow transplantation in high-risk myelogenous leukemias. Exp Hematol 1990;18:720.

14. Kodo H, Tajika K, Takahashi S, Ozawa K, Asano S, Takaku F. Acceleration of neutrophilic granulocyte recovery after bone-marrow transplantation by administration of recombinant human granulocyte colony-stimulating factor. Lancet 1988;2:38–39.

15. Demetri GD, Griffin JD. Granulocyte colony-stimulating factor and its receptor. Blood 1991;78:2791–2802.

16. Bronchud MH, Scarffe JH, Thatcher N, et al. Phase I/II study of recombinant human granulocyte colony-stimulating factor in patients receiving intensive chemotherapy for small cell lung cancer. Br J Cancer 1987;56:809–813.

17. Gabrilove JL, Jakubowski A, Scher H, et al. Effect of granulocyte colony-stimulating factor on neutropenia and associated morbidity due to chemotherapy for transitional-cell carcinoma of the urothelium. New Engl J Med 1988;318:1414–1422.

18. Morstyn G, Campbell L, Souze LM, et al. Effect of granulocyte colony stimulating factor on neutropenia induced by cytotoxic chemotherapy. Lancet 1988;26:667–672.

19. Crawford J, Ozer H, Stoller R, et al. Reduction by granulocyte colony-stimulating factor of fever and neutropenia induced by chemotherapy in patients with small-cell lung cancer. New Engl J Med 1991;315:164–170.

20. Trillet-Lenoir V, Green J, Manegold C, et al. Recombinant granulocyte colony stimulating factor reduces the infectious complications of cytotoxic chemotherapy. (manuscript submitted)

21. Pettengell R, Gurney H, Radford J, et al. A randomised trial of recombinant human granulocyte colony-stimulating factor to preserve dose intensity in non-Hodgkin's lymphoma (NHL). Proc ASCO 1989;8:A702.

22. Bronchud MH, Howell A, Crowther D, Hopwood P, Souza L, Dexter TM. The use of granulocyte colony-stimulating factor to increase the intensity of treatment with doxorubicin in patients with advanced breast and ovarian cancer. Br J Cancer 1989;60:121–125.

23. Demetri GD, Younger J, McGuire BW, Douville L, Armstrong S, Henderson IC. Dose escalation of cyclophosphamide/doxorubicin/5-FU(CAE) with ad-

junctive recombinant methionyl G-CSF (r-metG-CSF) in patients with advanced breast cancer. Proceedings Annual San Antonio Breast Cancer Symposium, 1991, in press.

24. Demetri GD, Horowitz J, McGuire GW, Merica EA, Howard G, Henderson JC. Pre-intensification of mitoxantrone with adjunctive G-CSF (r-metHuG-CSF) in patients with advanced breast cancer: a phase I trial. Proc ASCO, 1992, in press.

25. Johnson D, Belani C, Mason B, et al. A phase II trial of recombinant human granulocyte colony-stimulating factor (Neupogen, G-CSF) as an adjunct to cisplatin and etoposide chemotherapy in locally advanced or metastatic non-small cell lung carcinoma [Abstract]. Proc ASCO, 1992, in press.

26. Blayney DW, Williams S, Mortimer J, et al. Neupogen (r-metHuG-CSF) ameliorates neutropenia during CHOP therapy. Proc ASCO, 1992, in press.

27. Parker BA, Anderson JR, Canellos GP, Gockerman JP, Gottlieb AJ, Peterson BA. Dose escalation study of CHOP plus etoposide (CHOPE) without and with rh-G-CSF in untreated non-Hodgkin's lumphoma (NHL). Proc ASCO, 1991, in press.

28. Budd GT, Silver RT, Wile AC, Harkins B, Cruickshank C, McGuire B. Neupogen (recombinant met-human G-CSF) as an adjunct to CNF chemotherapy (cyclophosphamide, mitoxantrone, 5-fluorouracil) in advanced breast cancer. Proc ASCO, 1992, in press.

29. Sarosy G, Kohn E, Stone D, Rothenberg M, Jacob J, Adamo O. Phase I study of taxol and G-CSF in patients with refractory ovarian cancer. Submitted.

30. Ohno R, Tomonaga M, Kobayashi T, et al. Effect of granulocyte colony-stimulating factor after intensive radiation therapy in relapsed or refractory acute leukemia. N Engl J Med 1990;3323:871–877.

31. Taylor KMcD, Jagannath S, Spitzer G, et al. Recombinant human granulocyte colony-stimulating factor hastens granulocyte recovery after high-dose chemotherapy and autologous bone marrow transplantation in Hodgkin's disease. Clin Oncol 1989;7:1791–1799.

32. Peters WP, Kurtzberg J, Atwater S, et al. Comparative effects of rhuG-CSF and rhuGM-CSF on hematopoietic reconstitution and granulocyte function following high dose chemotherapy and autologous bone marrow transplantation (ABMT). Proc ASCO 1989;8:A709.

33. Sheridan WP, Morstyn G, Wolf M, et al. Granulocyte colony-stimulating factor and neutrophil recovery after high-dose chemotherapy and autologous bone marrow transplantation. Lancet 1989;14:891–895.

34. Masaoka T, Takaku F, Kato S, et al. Recombinant human granulocyte colony-stimulating factor for allogeneic bone marrow transplantation. Proc Annu Meet Am Assoc Cancer Res 1990;31:A1028.

35. Sheridan WP, Begley CG, Juttner CA, et al. Effect of peripheral blood progenitor cells mobilised by fil-

grastin (G-CSF) on platelet recovery after high-dose chemotherapy. Lancet 1992;339:640–644.

36. Pettengell R, Radford J, Scarffe H, Deakin D, Testa N, Crowther D. Peripheral blood progenitor cells (PBPC) for hematopoietic rescue for poor prognosis high grade NHL. Proc AACR, 1992, in press.

37. Pettengell R, Demuynck H, Testa NG, Dexter TM. The engraftment capacity of peripheral blood stem cells (PBSC) mobilized with chemotherapy ± GCSF. Proceedings Second International Symposium on Peripheral Blood Stem Cell Autografts, 1991, in press.

20

MACROPHAGE COLONY-STIMULATING FACTOR: BIOLOGY AND CLINICAL APPLICATIONS

John Nemunaitis and Jack W. Singer

Macrophage colony-stimulating factor (M-CSF) is a glycoprotein that stimulates the survival, proliferation, differentiation, and function of mononuclear phagocytes (1–4). These cells are critical to the body's defense against microbial invasion (5–11). Their role is to ingest and digest foreign matter, including microorganisms, particulate material, and tissue debris. When activated, mononuclear phagocytes secrete mediators of the inflammatory response, including lysozyme, neutral proteases (plasminogen activation, collagenase, elastase), acid hydrolases (proteases, lipases, phosphotases, deoxyribonucleases), complement components (C_1, C_2, C_3, C_4, C_5), enzyme inhibitors (plasmin inhibitors, α_2 macroglobulin), binding proteins (Fc receptors, fibronectin), endogenous pyrogens (interleukin-1 [IL-1], tumor necrosis factor [TNF]), prostaglandins, chemotactic factors for neutrophils, reactive metabolites of oxygen (superoxide, hydrogen peroxide, hydroxyradical), interferon, and cytokines that promote the proliferation and differentiation of myeloid (granulocyte colony-stimulating factor [G-CSF], granulocyte-monocyte colony-stimulating factor [GM-CSF]) and lymphoid cells (IL-1 and TNF) cells (8, 12–17). Mononuclear phagocytes originate in the marrow (promonocyte), circulate in the blood (mono-

cyte), and differentiate into transient and resident populations in various organs and tissues (tissue macrophages) (6). The number of circulating monocytes in the adult is approximately 10×10^9 cells. The total number of tissue macrophages is unknown; however, 0.4×10^9 monocytes enter tissues each day. Tissue macrophages are long-lived and retain self-renewal capacity, and are not dependent on incoming monocytes for compartment pool maintenance (18–21). In contrast, the pool of circulating neutrophils is 10–15 times greater than the number of circulating monocytes; however, the survival time of neutrophils is short. Neutrophils circulate for 6 hours before entering tissues, where they only survive for 48–72 hours. Studies using sex chromosome markers following allogeneic marrow transplantation reveal that hepatic Kupffer cells, alveolar macrophages, dermal Langerhans cells, microglial cells of the brain, and peritoneal, pleural, synovial, and lymph node macrophages are derived from monocyte precursors from donor bone marrow (20–24). Thus even though the number of circulating monocytes is less than the number of circulating neutrophils, the overall number of functioning monocytes and macrophages in the body may be equal to or greater than the number of neutrophils. Furthermore, following myeloablative chemotherapy, the number of circulating neutrophils and monocytes is significantly reduced; however, tissue macrophages are generally not affected and survive the myeloablative therapy. Tissue macrophages may be the sole defense against microorganism invasion in patients without circulating white blood cells. The purpose of this chapter is to review the biology and potential clinical applications of M-CSF.

IDENTIFICATION AND cDNA CLONING OF MACROPHAGE COLONY-STIMULATING FACTOR

The existence of hematopoietic colony-stimulating factors (CSF) was surmised in 1965 when clonal growth of hematopoietic cells in semisolid culture medium was found to be dependent on factors produced by feeder layers of adherent cells (25, 26). Recognition that hematopoietic cells are intrinsically incapable of unstimulated cell division and that cell division is dependent on continuous stimulation by appropriate specific regulatory molecules led to the use of colony formation as the method used to detect and characterize colony-stimulating factors (27). Over the subsequent years, techniques to purify these factors were developed (see Table 20.1). In 1969 CSF activity was described in human urine (28). Later, Metcalf showed that human urine stimulated the formation of monocyte colonies, colony-forming units, monocyte (CFU-M) (29). M-CSF was the first myeloid CSF to be purified (27, 30, 31), hence the initial name colony-stimulating factor-1 (CSF-1) (28, 29). However, complete identification of the cDNA sequence of M-CSF did not occur until after GM-CSF was sequenced (32, 33). M-CSF was purified to homogeneity, and the resultant amino acid sequence information was used to produce partial nucleotide sequences (27, 30, 31, 34). Synthetic oligonucleotides were used as hybridization probes to identify the M-CSF cDNA (35, 36). The recombinant product had identical biologic activity as highly purified native human

Table 20.1. Molecular Development of M-CSF: Historical Overview

Year	Event	Reference
1966	Discovery of myeloid cell colony formation in semisolid culture medium	25, 26
1969	Hematopoietic colony-stimulating activity (CSA) detected in human urine	28
1974	Monocyte colony formation induced by human urine	29
1975	Initial purification of a factor with monocyte CSA	27
1978	Further purification of human (h) M-CSF	30, 31
1981	NH_2 terminal sequence of purified hM-CSF determined	34
1985	1.8 kb cDNA sequence of hM-CSF cloned and expressed in mammalian cells	35
1987	4.0 kb cDNA sequence of hM-CSF cloned and expressed in mammalian cells	36
1989	Truncated form of the 4.0 kb cDNA sequence of hM-CSF cloned and expressed in E. coli	37

(h)M-CSF (35–37). There are multiple species of M-CSF mRNA derived from a single copy gene due to differential processing of the primary M-CSF transcript (35–39). Native M-CSF isolated from human urine is a heavily glycosylated homodimer. The two homologous subunits of the M-CSF molecule each contain nine cysteines and are linked together by one or more interchain disulfide bonds. The M-CSF maps at band q 33.1 on the left arm of chromosome 5 (40, 41). Alternative splicing of the primary M-CSF transcript generates multiple mRNAs ranging in size from 1.5 to 4.5 kilobases (kb) (42). The most abundant form of M-CSF yielded a 4.0-kb cDNA sequence (36). It encodes a 554 amino acid that is 91% homologous to the murine M-CSF (36). A second major form of the protein is encoded by a 1.6-kb mRNA and is 256 amino acids long (35). The amino acid sequences deduced from the nucleotide sequences of the cDNA clones suggest that the primary and transfected product is an integral membrane protein. M-CSF is assembled in 68-kD dimers and transported to the cell surface for secretion. The soluble portion is released from the cell surface by proteolytic cleavage (40, 43). In order to facilitate the production of large amounts of rhM-CSF, a truncated form of hM-CSF was produced in *E. coli.* This recombinant product had identical biologic activity as purified native hM-CSF and other recombinant human (rh) M-CSF molecules (37). Both in vitro and in vivo studies described in the rest of this chapter involved the use of purified native hM-CSF and/or rhM-CSF expressed in Chinese hamster ovary cells or *E. coli.*

Macrophage Colony-Stimulating Factor Receptor

The biologic effects of M-CSF are mediated through its binding to a single class of high-affinity receptors expressed on cells of monocyte lineage, placental cells, human choriocarcinoma cells, and some blasts from patients with myeloid leukemia (44–46). This receptor was found to be the human homologue of the transforming viral oncogene v-fms (47, 48). Exposure of saturating quantities of M-CSF to its receptor activates a receptor kinase and leads to autophosphorylation of the receptor on tyrosine within 1 minute. Nearly complete receptor downmodulation occurs within 15 minutes (48, 49). Only the mature cell surface form of the receptor is phosphorylated on tyrosine in response to M-CSF. The activation of the receptor kinase initiates a cascade of intracellular events that affect the proliferation and functional activities of receptor-bearing cells.

Expression of the receptor can be modulated by other cytokines (50). GM-CSF, IL-3, TNFα, and high concentrations of G-CSF downmodulate expression of the M-CSF receptor (50). Consistent with this, when FDCP-I/MAC cells, a myeloid precursor cell line that expresses IL-3, GM-CSF, and M-CSF receptors, is incubated with IL-3 or GM-CSF, the M-CSF receptor protein and mRNA are dramat-

ically reduced (51). When normal marrow cells are incubated with M-CSF and other cytokines such as IL-3, GM-CSF, or high concentrations of G-CSF, the biologic effect of M-CSF is significantly reduced (51). Response to M-CSF appears to be dependent on the particular cells expressing the M-CSF receptor and is affected by factors that may modulate the expression of the receptor. Furthermore, more than 90% of the clearance of circulating M-CSF is regulated by macrophages via M-CSF receptor endocytosis and intracellular degradation (52). Mature macrophages contain the largest number of M-CSF receptors, suggesting that the rate of macrophage production may be at least in part controlled by the number of mature macrophages. Receptors of M-CSF and other myeloid-stimulating factors have been identified on myeloid leukemia cells (53, 54). Blast cells from 7 of 15 patients with acute myelogenous leukemia (AML) were found to express M-CSF receptors (c-fms mRNA) (53). M-CSF also stimulates tritiated thymidine (^{3}H-TdR) uptake in a low percentage of patients with AML (see Table 20.2) (43, 55); however, it did not stimulate proliferation of a monocyte leukemia cell line (AML 193) or a myelomonocytic leukemia cell line (MV4-11) (56). Others suggest that M-CSF has been associated with differentiation of myeloblasts from patients with AML in vitro (55, 57, 58). M-CSF receptors have also been detected on malignant lymphoma and on solid tumor cells (59–61). A potential concern with the clinical application of M-CSF is that it will stimulate myeloid leukemia cells in some patients. However, in vitro studies suggest that M-CSF is less likely to be associated with this complication than other myeloid-stimulating factors (55, 56, 62).

Basal serum levels of M-CSF in normal mice range from 800 to 1200 u/ml. These levels rise sharply after antigeneic and infectious challenge, during an acute graft-versus-host reaction following allogeneic bone marrow transplant, with infection, with pregnancy, and following administration of chorionic gonadotropin (45, 63, 64). The obser-

Table 20.2.   Leukemia Cell Proliferation in Response to Cytokine Administration In Vitro[a]

Cell Lines	Stimulatory Cytokines	Nonstimulatory Cytokines	Reference
TALL-101	GM-CSF, IL-3	M-CSF, G-CSF, IL-1	56
AML-193	G-CSF, GM-CSF, IL-3	M-CSF, IL-1	56
MV4-11	G-CSF, GM-CSF, IL-3	M-CSF, IL-1	56
Leukemia Type (Number of Patients)	Stimulatory Cytokines In Vitro (Number of Patients)	Nonstimulatory Cytokines In Vitro	
AML (25)	IL-3 (19), GM-CSF (15), G-CSF (13), M-CSF (4)	None	55
AML (9)	GM-CSF (6), G-CSF (4)	M-CSF	62
ALL (6)	None	M-CSF, GM-CSF, G-CSF	62

[a]Abbreviations: ALL, acute lymphocytic leukemia.

vations that M-CSF receptors are located on human choriocarcinoma cell lines, M-CSF elevation during pregnancy, and its regulation by chorionic gonadotropin suggest that M-CSF may play a role in placental development (45).

BIOLOGIC EFFECTS OF MACROPHAGE COLONY-STIMULATING FACTOR ON PROLIFERATION OF MONOCYTES IN VITRO

M-CSF stimulates the survival, proliferation, and differentiation of monocytes and macrophages (1, 2, 4). IL-3 and GM-CSF stimulate proliferation of multipotent progenitors, including precursors of monocytes and macrophages, and also support the growth of human monocytes in culture (11, 32, 38). However, the monocytes stimulated by M-CSF differ from those grown in GM-CSF or IL-3 (11, 32, 38). Monocytes supported by M-CSF are elongated and spindle shaped in culture, and a greater percent of cells express CD14 and CD16. Monocytes supported by GM-CSF or IL-3 are round and less strongly adherent (65–67). M-CSF appears to be lineage restricted and has no activity in stimulating the growth of erythrocytes, lymphocytes, or megakaryocytes. It is a stimulator for monocyte colony formation (65, 68–71), although small numbers of granulocyte colonies are stimulated by M-CSF, but this may be an indirect

effect. For unknown reasons, the number of CFU-M produced in response to hM-CSF is 10- to 100-fold greater in mouse than in human marrow cells (72). This may be an in vitro artifact. If human marrow cells are cultured at low oxygen tension (5%) and in semisolid agarose, rather than agar, the effect of hM-CSF is more potent in human marrow cells (73), suggesting that the CFU-M assay is less than optimal.

Another determinant of monocyte growth in response to M-CSF is the presence of other cytokines. M-CSF stimulates monocyte production of many factors (Table 20.3). A number of these factors, such as G-CSF, GM-CSF, TNF-α, IL-1, and interferon (INF) α/β, act synergistically with M-CSF, not only enhancing monocyte colony formation but also enhancing multipotential colony formation (6, 56, 65, 69, 73–80). The synergistic effect of

Table 20.3.   Factors Produced by M-CSF-Stimulated Monocytes

Factor	Reference
G-CSF	130
GM-CSF	130
IL-1	131
TNFα	39, 84, 101
INF α/β	39, 86, 100, 101
Prostaglandin E	132
Neurotrophic factor	83
Thromboplastin	133
Plasminogen activator	134

other growth factors in combination with M-CSF was initially described with IL-1 (80). Subsequently, G-CSF, GM-CSF, TNFα, IL-3, and interferon have been shown to be synergistic with M-CSF in a dose-dependent manner in vitro. M-CSF is produced by many cells (see Table 20.4), and the rate of synthesis is influenced by several exogenous and endogenous factors (see Table 20.5).

Since multiple growth factors are present in vivo, in vitro studies with combinations of growth factors may be more accurate as a biologic model. Studies with combinations of cytokines reveal that TNFα inhibits

Table 20.4.   Cellular Source of M-CSF

Cell	Reference
Monocyte	135–137
B cells	138
T cells	139–142
Carcinoma	143
Mesangial cells	144
Fibroblasts	145
Osteoblasts	146
Endothelial cells	147
Bone marrow stromal cells	148–151
Preadipocyte cells	152
Keratinocytes	153
Astrocytes	154
Placental cells	45

Table 20.5.   Factors That Induce M-CSF Secretion

Factors	Reference
IL-1	148, 150, 155
IL-3	156
IL-4	155
TNFα	137
GM-CSF	136, 156
INF-γ	135
Lipopolysaccharide (LPS)	153, 157, 158
Chorionic gonadotropin	45
Staphylococcus	138
12-0-tetradecanoylphorbol-13-acetate (TPA)	136, 159
Phorbol myristic acid (PMA)	135, 156
Adherence to plastic	157, 158
Irradiation	151

monocyte colony growth when combined with GM-CSF but enhances growth with M-CSF (74, 75). M-CSF stimulated the growth of significantly more monocyte colonies from normal murine bone marrow than IL-3 (68). However, when marrow cells of 5-fluorouracil (5FU)-treated mice were stimulated with the same doses of M-CSF and IL-3, IL-3 induced the formation of significantly more monocyte colonies (68). 5FU-treated marrow contains a higher proportion of early progenitor cells than does normal marrow. Cells that appear to respond to IL-3 are more primitive than cells that respond to M-CSF (68). When M-CSF is combined with TNF, monocyte growth is enhanced; however, when it is combined with G-CSF, neutrophil growth is enhanced (81). Furthermore, when M-CSF is combined with growth factors, such as G-CSF, GM-CSF, IL-3, IL-1, and TNFα, at concentrations below which biologic activity can be detected using single factors, increased colony formation is observed (82). These studies suggest that monocyte proliferation and differentiation are influenced by a multiplicity of hematopoietic growth factors. It is likely that M-CSF acts predominantly on more mature cells (committed to monocyte differentiation) in the hematopoietic lineage. However, the proliferative response to M-CSF in vivo is dependent on the presence and concentration of other growth factors, as well as the proliferative status of the progenitor cells.

M-CSF stimulates the production of other hematopoietic growth factors (see Table 20.3), which have proliferative and antiproliferative effects of their own. It also stimulates production of other nonhematopoietic factors that may have clinical effects (Table 20.3). For instance, M-CSF stimulates monocyte secretion of neurotrophic factor, which promotes the growth of neurons in culture (83). Human immunodeficiency virus (HIV)-infected monocytes do not produce neurotrophic factor in response to M-CSF but instead secrete a factor that is toxic to neurons (83).

BIOLOGIC EFFECTS OF MACROPHAGE COLONY-STIMULATING FACTOR ON MONOCYTE FUNCTION IN VITRO

Monocytes and macrophages have many biologic functions and are key cells in the mammalian host defense systems. Monocytes are necessary to process and present antigens to lymphocytes and thus have a major role in the immune response. Drugs that increase the functional activity of monocytes such as M-CSF, therefore, can enhance response to antigens as well as increase other antimicrobial functions (Table 20.6). M-CSF appears to have greater function-enhancing activity than other growth factors (16, 84–86).

M-CSF increases monocyte/macrophage antibody-independent and antibody-dependent cell cytotoxicity (ADCC) against malignant cells (84, 85, 87–90). The mechanism of killing is poorly understood but is suspected to involve release of tumor cytotoxic agents such as TNF and/or oxygen metabolites. In the presence of monoclonal antibodies, M-CSF-treated monocytes and macrophages showed an increased capacity to selectively kill colon cancer, neuroblastoma, and melanoma cells (16, 84, 89). ADCC by monocytes has been shown to be mediated by specific receptors on the cell surface that bind to the Fc portion of IgG. The mechanisms of enhanced ADCC may in part be mediated by enhanced CD16 (FcRIII) expression (16). CD16 is a low-affinity receptor for IgG and has been shown to be important for ADCC (16). Other growth factors, such as GM-CSF, IL-3, and IL-1, also enhance monocyte ADCC; however, the effects of M-CSF are significantly greater (16, 84, 85).

When macrophages interact with microorganisms, such as bacteria or fungi, they respond by secretion of respiratory burst products: hydrogen peroxide, superoxide anion, and other reactive oxygen intermediates (17). These toxic oxygen metabolites mediate macrophage resistance to intracellular pathogens and have been identified as major effectors of *Candida* killing (17, 18, 91–93). M-CSF primes macrophages for enhanced production of oxygen reduction products when stimulated by microorganisms (91–94). As a result, M-CSF–treated monocytes have increased capability for intracellular killing of microorganisms, such as schistosomes, *Candida* species, bacterial species, *Mycobacterium,* and *Leishmania* (91–93, 95–97). M-CSF also enhances monocyte/macrophage migration, chemotaxis, and phagocytosis, as well as mannose receptor expression (91, 93, 98, 99) (Table 20.6). M-CSF stimulates the production of INF α/β. INF α/β further enhances the functional activities of M-CSF (39, 86, 100, 101). Functional effects of M-CSF are independent of INF and are enhanced when the two factors are combined (93, 95).

Antiviral activity of M-CSF has been shown in vitro using a vesicular stomatitis virus model (86). Macrophages infected with stomatitis virus after incubation with M-CSF had improved survival and reduced viral rep-

Table 20.6. Functional Activities Enhanced by M-CSF in Mononuclear Phagocytes

Activity	Reference
Direct tumor cell cytotoxicity	87, 88, 90, 160
Antibody-dependent cell cytotoxicity	84, 85, 89
Production of oxygen reduction products	94
Inhibition of stimulated lymphocyte proliferation	161
Inhibition of stimulated IL-2 production	161
Chemotaxis	91
Migration	98
Phagocytosis	93, 99
Fc receptor expression	4, 16
CD14, CD16, Ia expression	4, 16, 110
Mannose receptor expression	93
Antiviral activity	86
Replication of HIV (AIDS virus)	102, 103
Intracellular killing of microorganisms	91–93, 95, 97

lication in culture. However, the effect could be blocked by anti-INF antibody, indicating that the antiviral activity of M-CSF was indirect and mediated by INF (86). G-CSF, GM-CSF, and IL-3 had virtually no evidence of antiviral activity (86). Administration of M-CSF, GM-CSF, and IL-3 before infection of monocytes by HIV enhances monocyte HIV replication (102–104). However, when M-CSF is given on the day of or 7 days after HIV infection, there is no effect on HIV replication, suggesting that the predominant effect of M-CSF is on the monocyte and not the HIV virus. G-CSF did not affect HIV replication and INF α/β and γ decreased HIV replication (103, 104). Interestingly, preliminary results indicate that when GM-CSF is administered in combination with azidothymidime (AZT) (a potent inhibitor of HIV replication), the antiviral effects of AZT are potentiated. Similar studies with M-CSF have not been done.

PRECLINICAL IN VIVO TRIALS WITH MACROPHAGE COLONY-STIMULATING FACTOR

Pharmokinetic studies in mice indicate that 95% of injected M-CSF is cleared by liver and splenic macrophages (52, 105). Less than 2% of the injected M-CSF was recovered from any other organ. The plasma half-life of M-CSF after bolus injection was 6.4 hours in nonhuman primates and 2.4 hours in rats. Its clearance was dose dependent (105, 106). When rats were injected with a single dose of M-CSF at 5 μg/kg, the serum half-life was 23 minutes; however, at a dose of 1000 μg/kg, the serum half-life was 578 minutes (105, 106).

Administration of low doses of M-CSF (4 μg/kg/day) to normal mice for 8 days did not result in any change in neutrophil, monocyte, or lymphocyte levels (107). However, binding studies revealed that only 15% of the M-CSF receptors were occupied (107). In other studies, higher daily doses of M-CSF (≥250 μg/kg) were administered to normal mice and Lewis rats (81, 108) by intravenous

bolus injection for up to 4 days. Dose-dependent monocytosis and neutrophilia were observed in addition to transient lymphopenia (see Table 20.7). The monocytosis was partially inhibited by coadministration of dexamethasone (81). Dose-related monocytosis and reversible thrombocytopenia were observed at a dose of ≥500 μg/kg/day after 14 days of administration of M-CSF to Sprague-Dawley rats (105). No apparent toxicity was observed, and no abnormal histologic findings were observed at necropsy.

Consistent with in vitro studies, when myeloid CSFs, including M-CSF, are administered as single agents at low doses in vivo, no biologic activity is detectable; however, dual administration of cytokines such as M-CSF and GM-CSF at the same low doses to normal mice results in an increased number of committed granulocyte-macròphage progenitors (CFU-GM), multipotent progenitors (CFU-GEMM), late proliferative potential colony-forming cells (LPP-CFC), and high proliferative potential colony-forming cells (HPP-CFC) (82, 109). M-CSF appears to be synergistic with other myeloid CSFs in the murine system.

M-CSF has been administered subcutaneously, by an intravenous bolus injection, or by continuous infusion to nonhuman primates (105, 110). It was nontoxic and was associated with dose-related monocytosis, although in one trial, when 100–1000 μg/kg/day were administered over 14 days, peak monocyte levels occurred within 7 days of starting M-CSF and declined during continued M-CSF administration over the 7 subsequent days (105). Monocyte counts did not continue to decline after discontinuation of M-CSF. The most remarkable hematologic effect observed in this trial was a dose-related decline in platelet counts. At a dose of 50 μg/kg/day, platelet counts decreased by almost 50% from baseline. Primates receiving M-CSF at doses ≥175 μg/kg/day were unable to continue therapy with M-CSF due to severe thrombocytopenia. When the M-CSF was discontinued, platelet counts returned to baseline. Bone marrow analysis revealed in-

Table 20.7. Results of Preclinical Trials with M-CSF In Vivo

(Hematologic Status) Animal Model	Response to M-CSF	Reference
Mouse (normal)	No toxicity; monocytosis, lymphocytopenia, variable platelet and neutrophil effect, no change in red blood cell count	82, 108, 162, 163
Lewis rat (normal)	No toxicity; monocytosis, neutrophilia, lymphopenia, thrombocytopenia	81
B16 melanoma mouse (normal)	No toxicity; monocytosis induced, metastatic tumor spread reduced; monocyte ADCC enhanced	105, 111
Infected mouse (normal)	No toxicity; prophylactic administration significantly improved survival after Candida or E. coli infusion; improved monocyte function and anticandidal activity	42, 113
Mouse (osteopetrotic)	No toxicity; correction of defect related to lack of osteoclasts	118, 119
Mouse (neutropenic)	No toxicity; increased numbers of multipotent and granulocyte-macrophage–forming progenitors; enhanced neutrophil recovery, no effect on monocyte, lymphocyte, platelet, or red blood cell recovery; reduced bacteremia, improved early survival	114, 164
Infected mouse (neutropenic)	No toxicity; prophylactic administration improved survival after live Candida or E. coli infusion; improved monocyte function	112
Rabbit (normal)	No toxicity; decrease in plasma cholesterol level	105, 115, 116
Nonhuman primate (normal)	No toxicity; neutrophilia, moncytosis, thrombocytopenia	105, 110, 117

creased megakaryocytes, suggesting peripheral destruction of platelets rather than decreased production. The functional activities of monocytes from these primates were significantly enhanced, and expression of CD16, CD14 and HLA-DR was increased.

Potential antitumor activity of M-CSF was evaluated using a mouse B16 melanoma model (105, 111). Twenty-one days after injection of live melanoma cells into mice, M-CSF (n = 12) or placebo (n = 12) was administered over the subsequent 11 days. The animals were sacrificed 6 weeks later, and at necropsy the number of pulmonary metastases was then determined. The median number of pulmonary metastases in the control group was 65, compared to 1 in the M-CSF treated group. Six (50%) of the animals who received M-CSF did not have any pulmonary metastases, compared to only 1 (8%) of the control animals. Monocyte ADCC to the mel-

anoma cells was also enhanced in mice who received M-CSF.

In vitro studies indicated that M-CSF enhanced monocyte and macrophage functions necessary for destruction of invading microorganisms. To evaluate clinical potential and antimicrobial activities, M-CSF was administered to neutropenic and infected mice (42, 112, 113). In one series of studies, M-CSF was administered to mice before infusion of bacterial or fungal microorganisms. In the first study, a single infusion of M-CSF or placebo was administered 24 hours before E. coli (5 × 10^7 CFU/mouse). Survival was significantly improved in mice, who received M-CSF compared to placebo (80% versus 0%, p <.01) (112). The same effect was noted in neutropenic mice, suggesting that M-CSF directly enhanced host resistance to bacterial infection by functionally activating monocytes. In a subsequent study, M-CSF or placebo was administered before infusion of *Candida albicans*. The median survival of the placebo group was 3 days, compared to 15 days in the M-CSF group ($p < .01$), suggesting that M-CSF enhanced host resistance against *Candida albicans* infection (42). Others have also found that M-CSF could potentiate resistance to *Candida albicans* challenge, as shown by increased survival (median survival day 10 versus 19, $p < .01$) and significantly reduced recovery of viable *Candida* (113). Trials with administration of M-CSF during or after infusion of infectious microorganisms are currently in progress. When M-CSF is administered to mice rendered neutropenic with cyclophosphamide, a significant increase in numbers of CFU-GM and CFU-GEMM compared to placebo controls is observed. Similar effects were observed with lethal doses of radiation (7.8 Gy). M-CSF was administered (64 µg/kg/day) for 5 consecutive days, and neutrophil and CFU-GM recovery was enhanced (114). There were no differences in monocyte, lymphocyte, red blood cell, or platelet recovery, and survival was significantly improved. Animals in the control group primarily died of bacterial sepsis, suggesting that M-CSF may have prevented mortal infections.

In addition to antitumor and antiinfection activity predicted by in vitro studies, studies in animals reveal that M-CSF lowers serum cholesterol and low-density lipoprotein levels (115–117). It also corrects the congenital osteoclast deficiency in osteopetrotic (op/op) mice (118, 119).

CLINICAL TRIALS WITH MACROPHAGE COLONY-STIMULATING FACTOR

The first trial with M-CSF was begun in 1982 using a partially purified product. Eight patients with acute leukemia in remission following consolidation therapy were each administered seven doses of hM-CSF (120) (see Table 20.8). Toxicity was minimal. Granulocyte counts appeared increased in seven patients, and there was no significant change in monocyte, lymphocyte, or platelet counts. Serum colony stimulatory activity was increased following administration of M-CSF. Six normal volunteers also received hM-CSF, and toxicity included fever, pruritus, diaphoresis, and mild hypotension (121, 122).

In phase I–II trials with a more highly purified hM-CSF, toxicity was decreased and consisted of low-grade fever and chills in a small proportion of the patients (Table 19.8). In the first trial, 38 patients with a variety of malignancies were entered to receive five daily doses of hM-CSF following the same intensive chemotherapy regimen (123). This was a crossover randomized study in which all evaluable patients (n = 24) received two courses of chemotherapy and one course of hM-CSF or human serum albumin. No change in granulocyte recovery to 500 per cubic millimeter or 1000 per cubic millimeter was observed, although the number of days the absolute neutrophil count (ANC) was less than 2000 per cubic millimeter was 2 days less in the patients who received hM-CSF (123). There were no changes in monocyte, lymphocyte, red blood cell, or platelet counts. In the next trial, a similar design was used. Thirty-three patients with urogenital malignancy received seven daily doses of hM-CSF or human serum albumin after chemotherapy (122). Toxicity was minimal, and the period of neutrophil counts < 500 per cubic millimeter or < 1000 per cubic millimeter was not different, although the nadir of neutrophils was higher in the patients who received hM-CSF (850 ± 855 per cubic millimeter versus 468 ± 332 per cubic millimeter). In the third trial, 98 patients with gynecologic malignancy received seven daily doses of hM-CSF or nothing following chemotherapy (122). The mean number of days the ANC was <500 per cubic millimeter was 1 day less in the hM-CSF treated group (3.4 ± 3.3 versus 2.1 ± 2.8). The number of days the platelet count was less than 100,000 per cubic millimeter was also reported as being significantly less in the patients who received hM-CSF; however, these

Table 20.8. Clinical Use of Human M-CSF

Number of Patients (Disorder)	Response to M-CSF	Reference
6 (normal)	Moderate toxicity consisting of fever, itching, diaphoresis, hypotension (partially purified product)	120
8 (myelosuppression following cancer therapy)	Minimal toxicity; no significant change in granulocyte, monocyte, lymphocyte, or platelet counts (partially purified product)	121
24 (myelosuppression following cancer therapy)	Minimal toxicity (fever); compared to prospective controls the time to ANC > 500/mm^3, 1000/mm^3 was not different; the number of days the neutrophil count was less than 2000/mm^3 was 2 days less in the treated group ($p < .02$); no change in monocyte, lymphocyte, platelet counts (purified counts)	123
33 (urogenital malignancy)	Minimal toxicity (fever, chills); higher neutrophil nadir; no difference in days of neutropenia, lymphocytopenia, thrombocytopenia, and red blood cell counts (purified product)	122
9 (chronic neutropenia)	Minimal toxicity; transient increase in neutrophil counts; no change in monocyte, neutrophil counts; no change in monocyte, lymphocyte, platelet, red blood cell, and eosinophil counts; no description of infection (purified product)	165
51 (hematologic malignancy/BMT)	Minimal toxicity (low-grade fever, rash); day ANC > 500/mm^3 was 3 days earlier in M-CSF group compared to prospective controls ($p < .05$). No effect on monocyte, lymphocyte, or platelet recovery *observed*; no effect on recurrent disease, marrow rejection, on graft-versus-host disease; improved short-term survival (purified product)	122, 124, 125
98 (Myelosuppression following chemotherapy for gynecologic malignancy)	No toxicity; number of days ANC < 500/mm^3 was 3.4 ± 3.3 in M-CSF group compared to 2.1 ± 2.8 in prospective control group (purified product)	122
13 (lymphoma)	No toxicity; transient neutropenia, monocytopenia, and thrombocytopenia; significantly improved monocyte function (see Table 19.9) (purified product)	128
33 (fungal infection)	No toxicity; transient thrombocytopenia; no change in monocyte, neutrophil, lymphocyte counts; improved resolution of fungal infection in some patients (recombinant product); enhanced monocyte function; decreased cholesterol level	127

data are difficult to interpret since less than a quarter of the patients were evaluable for platelet recovery.

HM-CSF has also been administered to 51 patients following allogeneic (n = 37) or autologous (n = 14) bone marrow transplantation (BMT). Results were compared to concurrent nonrandomized controls. Two patients developed fever in association with

hM-CSF infusion; otherwise there was no toxicity. The incidence and severity of graft-versus-host disease (GVHD), the rate of graft failure, the rate of recurrent disease, and survival were not altered. Patients who received hM-CSF for 14 daily doses achieved an ANC of 500 per cubic millimeter 4 days earlier ($p < .05$) and an ANC of 1000 per cubic millimeter (122, 124, 125) 8 days earlier than the control patients. Subsequently, 119 patients receiving either allogeneic or syngeneic BMT received hM-CSF (n = 60) or placebo (n = 59). Neutrophil recovery to ≥500 per cubic millimeter was 3 days earlier (day 24 versus 27, p = .011), and survival at day 120 post BMT was significantly better (83 versus 66%, p = .031) for patients who received hM-CSF. Toxicity to hM-CSF was not detected, and platelet recovery, GVHD, rate of graft failure, and rate of recurrent disease was not different between the two groups (125). Since M-CSF directly augments G-CSF and GM-CSF production from peripheral blood monocytes, the enhanced neutrophil recovery observed may be indirectly related to M-CSF (126).

Monocyte function in patients receiving M-CSF was recently described (see Tables 20.8, 20.9). Thirteen patients with lymphoma with normal peripheral blood counts and bone marrow were given a single injection of M-CSF. Functions of monocytes before hM-CSF were compared to the functions of monocytes from the same patients shortly after hM-CSF infusion. After infusion of hM-CSF, monocytes had an enhanced respiratory burst activity in response to FMLP, enhanced migration as assessed by skin window assay (an artificially created inflammatory site), enhanced phagocytosis, and enhanced intracellular destruction of *Candida* organisms. No toxicity was seen except for transient decreases in neutrophil, monocyte, red blood cell, and platlet counts 2–4 hours after injection of hM-CSF. Lymphocyte counts were not altered. The investigations suggested that the thrombocytopenia may have been related to increased phagocytic clearance by activated splenic macrophages.

A phase I dose escalation trial of rhM-CSF was performed in which rhM-CSF was administered with amphotericin B 1–7 weeks to 24 patients with invasive fungal infection either before or after BMT (127). Daily doses of rhM-CSF ranged from 100–2000 $\mu g/m^2/$day. RhM-CSF at a dose of 2000 $\mu g/m^2/$day was associated with significant thrombocytopenia. Patients who received 2000 $\mu g/m^2/$day of rhM-CSF had a reversible mean reduction in platelet count of 61,000 per cubic millimeter while receiving rhM-CSF. The severity of GVHD in patients who had received allografts did not appear to be significantly affected. Neutrophil, monocyte, and lymphocyte counts were not altered. Six patients had histologic or radiologic resolution of fungal infection. Twelve patients were not evaluable for response, primarily because of refusal or inability to do diagnostic surgical procedures, and 6 patients did not respond to rhM-CSF. Two of the 6 patients who did not respond to rhM-CSF received less than 7 days of therapy, and 1 had an ANC of 0 and was unable to tolerate granulocyte transfusions. Overall, 10 of the 24 (42%) patients survived 100 days after initiation of therapy with rhM-CSF. No patient (10 with myeloid malignancy) developed recurrent disease during this time. Six patients with progressive fungal infection despite therapy with amphotericin received rhM-CSF before BMT. Five of these patients subsequently underwent BMT, and 4 were alive 100 days after therapy with M-CSF.

Survival appeared to be associated with performance status at the time of initiation of rhM-CSF. Only 1 of 8 patients with Karnofsky scores ≤20% survived more than 30 days after initiation of rhM-CSF, whereas 14 of 16 patients with Karnofsky scores ≥30% survived more than 30 days. Encouraged by these

Table 20.9. Effect of Single Dose of rM-CSF on Monocyte Function In Vivo (13 patients)[a]

Function	Result
Respiratory burst activity in response to FMLP	Significantly enhanced
Migration as assessed by skin window assay	Significantly enhanced
Phagocytosis of *Candida* organisms	Significantly enhanced
Intracellular destruction of *Candida* organisms	Significantly enhanced

[a]Data from Khwaja A, Johnson B, Addison IE, et al. In vivo effects of macrophage colony-stimulating factor on human monocyte function. Br J Haematol 1991;77:25–31.

phase I data, 9 additional patients have received rhM-CSF at a dose of 2000 μg/m²/day (unpublished data). The disease-free survival of the 33 patients who received rhM-CSF at day 100 after initiation of therapy is 44% compared to 19% in a recent historical control group (n = 58; p = .05). If patients with Karnofsky scores ≤20% are removed from both groups, the survival to day 100 of patients who received rhM-CSF (n = 21) was 65% compared to 26% of the historical controls (n = 38; p = .006) (unpublished data). A placebo-controlled, randomized trial is required to confirm this suggestion of efficacy.

These results are consistent with prior in vitro and animal studies and suggest that hM-CSF may be efficacious in patients with fungal infection due to its capacity to enhance monocyte functions associated with phagocytosis and killing of fungi. M-CSF's enhancement of monocyte migration suggests that it may increase monocyte and tissue macrophage migration to sites of deep-seated infection to a greater degree than G-CSF or GM-CSF (128). G-CSF does not directly affect monocyte migration, and GM-CSF inhibits monocyte migration by skin window assay.

Serum levels of hM-CSF are detectable in normal patients. There is no difference in serum levels of hM-CSF between males or females using radioimmune assays. Resting levels of hM-CSF are between 100 and 700 U/ml, and the predominant detectable hM-CSF molecule is the 85-kD protein (72). In animals during pregnancy, infection, and periods of neutropenia (ANC < 1000 per cubic millimeter), M-CSF serum levels increase to >1000 U/ml (45, 63, 129). Patients with myeloproliferative disorders and severe burns also have significant elevation of serum hM-CSF levels (117, 121). Elevated levels of M-CSF may be etiologic in tumor-associated monocytosis (76).

In summary, studies with M-CSF in vitro indicate that it stimulates monocyte growth and enhances monocyte/macrophage function. Potential clinical applications for therapy with M-CSF include its use for enhancement of hematopoietic reconstitution following myelosuppressive therapy, antitumor therapy, and antiinfection therapy. In comparison to rhGM-CSF, rhIL-3, and rhG-CSF, M-CSF appears to have a weaker effect on enhancement hematopoietic reconstitution. Although no trials with rhM-CSF for this use have been described, the results with purified M-CSF are not impressive. M-CSF enhances direct and antibody-dependent monocyte cytotoxicity against tumor cells. In vitro, the effect was significantly greater than observed with GM-CSF, G-CSF, and IL-3. Phase I/II trials with rhM-CSF in patients with metastatic malignancy are preliminary but suggest it will have limited, if any, efficacy when used alone. It may, however, be useful in conjunction with monoclonal antibodies to tumor-restricted antigens. M-CSF has been shown in vitro and in vivo to enhance monocyte and macrophage functions involved in defense against infectious microorganisms. Preliminary data from phase I/II clinical trials in patients with fungal infections appear encouraging. Phase III trials are in development to determine efficacy of rhM-CSF in fungal infections.

Exploration of the use of rhM-CSF in immune-compromised patients with chronic intracellular infections with organisms or conditions such as tuberculosis, atypical mycobacterium, brucellosis, rickettsia, and *Leishmania* and in patients with thermal injury, in combination with appropriate antibiotics, is of interest. Since M-CSF appears to be relatively nontoxic, further studies evaluating the cholesterol-lowering effects in patients with congenital hypercholesterolemia may also be worthwhile. Future trials will also need to evaluate the combination of M-CSF with other hematopoietic growth factors to evaluate its possible synergistic effects, especially in combination with growth factors that have minimal functional enhancing effect on monocytes.

REFERENCES

1. Metcalf D. Studies on colony formation in vitro by mouse bone marrow cells. J Cell Physiol 1970;76:89–100.

2. Stanley ER, Guilbert LJ, Tushimaki RJ. CSF-a, a mononuclear phagocyte lineage-specific hemopoietic growth factor. J Cell Biochem 1991;21:151–159.

3. Das SK, Stanley ER. Structure function studies of a colony stimulating factor (CSF-1). J Biol Chem 1982;257:13679–13684.

4. Becker S, Warren MK, Haskill S. Colony-stimulating factor-induced monocyte survival and differentiation into macrophages in serum-free cultures. J Immunol 1987;139:3703–3709.

5. Rosenthal AS. Regulation of the immune response: role of the macrophage. New Engl J Med 1980; 303:1153–1156.

6. Van Furth R, Raeburn JA, van Zwet TL. Characteristics of human mononuclear phagocytes. Blood 1979;54:485.

7. Territo MC, Cline MJ. Mononuclear phagocyte proliferation, maturation and function. Clin Haematol 1975;4:685–703.

8. Nathan CF, Murray HW, Cohn ZA. The macrophage as an effector cell. New Engl J Med 1980;303:622–626.

9. Stossel TP. Phagocytosis. New Engl J Med 1974; 290:717–723, 774–780, 833–839.

10. Babior BM. Oxygen-dependent microbial killing by phagocytes. New Engl J Med 1978;298:659–668, 721–725.

11. Weisbart RH, Gasson JC, Golde DW. Colony-stimulating factors and host defense. Ann Intern Med 1989;110:297–303.

12. North RJ. The concept of the activated macrophage. J Immunol 1978;121:806–809.

13. Karnovsky ML, Lazdins JK. Biochemical criteria for activated macrophages. J Immunol 1978;121:809–813.

14. Bianco C, Griffin FM Jr, Silverstein SC. Studies of the macrophage complement receptor. Alteration of receptor function upon macrophage activation. J Exp Med 1975;141:1278–1290.

15. Unanue ER. The regulation of lymphocyte functions by the macrophage. Immunol Rev 1978;40:227–255.

16. Young DA, Lowe LD, Clark SC. Comparison of the effects of IL-3, granulocyte-macrophage colony-stimulating factor, and macrophage colony-stimulating factor in supporting monocyte differentiation in culture. Analysis of macrophage antibody-dependent cellular cytotoxicity. J Immunol 1990;145:607–615.

17. Sasada M, Johnston RB Jr. Macrophage microbicidal activity. J Exp Med 1980;152:85–98.

18. Hocking WG, Golde DW. The pulmonary-alveolar macrophage. New Engl J Med 1979;301:580–587, 639–645.

19. Hobbs JR, Barrett AJ, Chambers D, et al. Reversal of clinical features of Hurler's disease and biochemical improvement after treatment by bone-marrow transplantation. Lancet 1981(Oct 3):709–712.

20. Gale RP, Sparkes RS, Golde DW. Bone marrow origin of hepatic macrophages (Kupffer cells) in humans. Science 1978;201:937–938.

21. Katz SI, Tamaki K, Sachs DH. Epidermal Langerhans cells are derived from cells originating in bone marrow. Nature 1979;282:324–326.

22. Wilson FD, Greenberg BR, Konrad PN, et al. Cytogenetic studies on bone marrow fibroblasts from a male-female hematopoietic chimera: evidence that stromal elements in human transplantation recipients are of host type. Transplantation 1978;25:87–88.

23. Golde DW, Hocking WG, Quan SG, et al. Origin of human bone marrow fibroblasts. Br J Haematol 1980;44:183–187.

24. Moore MAS, Metcalf D. Ontogeny of the haemopoietic system: yolk sac origin of in vivo and in vitro colony forming cells in the developing mouse embryo. Br J Haematol 1970;18:279–296.

25. Ichikawa Y, Pluznik DH, Sachs L. In vitro control of the development of macrophage and granulocyte colonies. Proc Natl Acad Sci 1966;56:488–495.

26. Bradley TR, Metcalf D. The growth of mouse bone marrow cells in vitro. Aust J Exp Biol Med Sci 1966;44:287–299.

27. Stanley ER, Hansen G, Woodcock J, et al. Colony stimulating factor and regulation of granulopoiesis and macrophage production. Fed Proc 1975;34:2272–2278.

28. Robinson WA, Stanley ER, Metcalf D. Stimulation of bone marrow colony growth in vitro by human urine. Blood 1969;33:396–399.

29. Metcalf D. Stimulation by human urine on plasma of granulepoiesis by human marrow cells in organ. Exp Hematol 1974;2:157–173.

30. Laukel H, Gassel WD, Dosch HM, et al. Preparation of colony stimulating activity from large batches of human urine and production of antisera against it. J Cell Physiol 1978;94:21–30.

31. Motoyoshi K, Takaku F, Mizoguchi H, et al. Purification and some properties of colony stimulating factor from normal human urine. Blood 1978;52:1012–1020.

32. Metcalf D. The granulocyte-macrophage colony stimulating factors. Science 1985;229:16–22.

33. Golde DW, Gasson JC. Hormones that stimulate the growth of blood cells. Sci Am 1988;259:62–70.

34. Hewick RM, Hunkapiller ME, Hood LE, et al. A gas liquid phase peptide and protein sequenator. J Biol Chem 1981;256:7990–7997.

35. Kawasaki ES, Ladner MB, Wang AM, et al. Molecular cloning of a complementary DNA encoding human macrophage-specific colony-stimulating factor (CSF-1). Science 1985;230:291–296.

36. Wong GG, Temple PA, Leary AC, et al. Human CSF-1: molecular cloning and expression of 4-kb cDNA encoding the human urinary protein. Science 1987;235:1504–1508.

37. Halenbeck R, Kawasaki E, Wrin J, et al. Renaturation and purification of biologically active recombinant human macrophage colony-stimulating factor expressed in E. coli. Biotechnology 1989;7:710–715.
38. Ralph P, Warren MK. Molecular biology, cell biology and clinical future of myeloid growth factors. Year Immunol 1989;5:103–125.
39. Ralph P, Warren MK, Nakoinz I, et al. Biological properties and molecular biology of the human macrophage growth factor, CSF-1. Immunobiology 1986;172:194–204.
40. Rettenmier CW, Roussel MF. Differential processing of colony-stimulating factor-1 precursors encoded by two human cDNAs. Mol Cell Biol 1988;8:5026–5034.
41. Pettenati MJ, LeBeav MM, Lemons RS, et al. Assignment of CSF-1 to 5q 33.1: evidence for clustering of genes regulating hematopoiesis and for their involvement in the deletion of the long arm of chromosome 5 in myeloid disorders. Proc Natl Acad Sci 1987;84:2970–2974.
42. Aukerman SC, Middleton J, Sampson-Johanes A, et al. Biological and preclinical activity of macrophage colony stimulating factor, M-CSF. In: Symann M, Quesenberry P, eds. Hematopoietic growth factors: from the basic to the clinical applications. Cheshire, England: Gardiner-Caldwell Communications, 1991, in press.
43. Manos MM. Expression and processing of a recombinant human macrophage colony stimulating factor in mouse cells. Mol Cell Biol 1988;8:5035–5039.
44. Bicknell DC, Williams DE, Broxmeyer HE. Correlation between CSF-1 responsiveness and expression of (CSF-1 receptor) c-fms in purified murine granulocyte-macrophage progenitor cells (CFU-GM). Exp Hematol 1988;16:88–91.
45. Bartocci A, Pollard JW, Stanley ER. Regulation of colony-stimulating factor-1 during pregnancy. J Exp Med 1986;164:956–961.
46. Guilbert LJ, Stanely ER. Specific interaction of murine colony-stimulating factor with mononuclear phagocytic cells. J Cell Biol 1980;85:153–159.
47. Sherr CJ. Regulation of mononuclear phagocyte proliferation by colony-stimulating factor-1. Int J Cell Cloning 1990;8:46–62.
48. Sherr CJ, Roussel MR, Rettenmier CW. Colony-stimulating factor-1 receptor (c-fms). J Cell Biochem 1988;38:179–187.
49. Downing JR, Rettenmier CW, Sherr CJ. Ligand-induced tyrosine kinase activity of the colony-stimulating factor-1 receptor in a murine macrophage cell line. Mol Cell Biol 1988;8:1795–1799.
50. Walker F, Nicola NA, Metcalf D, et al. Hierarchical down-modulation of hemopoietic growth factor receptors. Cell 1985;43:269–276.
51. Gliniak BC, Rohrschneider RL. Expression of the M-CSF receptor is controlled posttranscriptionally by the dominant actions of GM-CSF or multi-CSF. Cell 1990;63:1073–1083.
52. Bartocci A, Mastrogiannis DS, Migliorati G, et al. Macrophages specifically regulate the concentration of their own growth factor in the circulation. Proc Natl Acad Sci USA 1987;84:6197–6183.
53. Rambaldi A, Wakamiya N, Vallenga E, et al. Expression of the macrophage colony-stimulating factor and c-fms genes in human acute myeloblastic leukemia cells. J Clin Invest 1988;81:1030–1035.
54. Parwaresch MR, Kreipe H, Felgner J, et al. M-CSF and M-CSF receptor gene expression in acute myelomonocytic leukemias. Leuk Res 1990;14:27–37.
55. Salem M, Delwel R, Mahmoud LA, et al. Maturation of human acute myeloid leukaemia in vitro: the response to five recombinant haematopoietic factors in a serum-free system. Br J Haematol 1989;71:363–370.
56. Santoli D, Yang Y-C, Clark SC, et al. Synergistic and antagonistic effects of recombinant human interleukin (IL) 3, IL-1α, granulocyte and macrophage colony-stimulating factors (G-CSF and M-CSF) on the growth of GM-CSF-dependent leukemic cell lines. J Immunol 1987;139:3348–3354.
57. Myiauchi J, Wang C, Kelleher CA, et al. The effect of recombinant CSF-1 on the blast cells of acute myeloblastic leukemia in suspension culture. J Cell Physiol 1988;135:55–62.
58. Miyauchi J, Kelleher CA, Wong GG, et al. The effects of combinations of the recombinant growth factors GM-CSF, G-CSF, IL-3, and CSF-1 on leukemic blast cells in suspension culture. Leukemia 1988;2:382–387.
59. Horiguchi J, Sherman ML, Sampson-Johanes A, et al. CSF-1 and C-fms gene expression in human carcinoma cell lines. Biochem Biophys Res Commun 1988;157(1):395–401.
60. Paietta E, Raceuskis J, Stanley ER, et al. Expression of the macrophage growth factor, CSF-1 and its receptor C-fms by a Hodgkin's disease-derived cell line and its variants. Cancer Res 1990;50:2049–2055.
61. Kacinski GM, Carter D, Mittal K, et al. Ovarian adenocarcinomas express fms-complementary transcripts and fms antigen, often with coexpression of CSF-1. Am J Pathol 1990;137(1):135–147.
62. Pebusque M-J, Lopez M, Torres H, et al. Growth response of human myeloid leukemia cells to colony-stimulating factors. Exp Hematol 1988;16:360–366.
63. Praloran V, Raventos-Suarez C, Bartocci A, et al. Alterations in the expression of colony-stimulating factor-1 and its receptor during an acute graft-vs-host reaction in mice. J Immunol 1990;145:3256–3261.
64. Cheers C, Haigh AM, Kelso A, et al. Production of colony-stimulating factors (CSFs) during infection: separate determinations of macrophage-, granulocyte-, granulocyte-macrophage-, and multi-CSFs. Infect Immun 1988;56:247–251.

65. Bot FJ, van Eijk L, Schipper P, et al. Synergistic effects between GM-CSF and G-CSF or M-CSF on highly enriched human marrow progenitor cells. Leukemia 1990;4:325–328.

66. Chen BD, Mueller M, Chou TH. Role of granulocyte/macrophage colony stimulating factor in the regulation of murine alveolar macrophage proliferation and differentiation. J Immunol 1988;141:139–144.

67. Ohki K, Nogayama A. Establishment and characterization of factor-dependent macrophage cell lines. J Leuk Biol 1988;44:465–476.

68. Koike K, Stanley ER, Ihle JN, et al. Macrophage colony formation supported by purified CSF-1 and/or interleukin-3 in serum-free culture: evidence for hierarchical difference in macrophage colony-forming cells. Blood 1986;67:859–865.

69. Chen BD-M, Clark CR, Chou T-H. Granulocyte/macrophage colony-stimulating factor stimulates monocyte and tissue macrophage proliferation and enhances their responsiveness to macrophage colony-stimulating factor. Blood 1988;71:997–1002.

70. Rohtsein G, Rhondeau SM, Peters CA, et al. Stimulation of neutrophil production in CSF-1 response clones. Blood 1988;72:898–902.

71. Metcalf D. The molecular biology and functions of the granulocyte-macrophage colony-stimulating factors. J Am Soc Hematol 1986;67:257–267.

72. Hanamura T, Motoyoshi K, Yoshida K, et al. Quantitation and identification of human monocytic colony-stimulating factor in human serum by enzyme-linked immunosorbent assay. Blood 1988;72:886–892.

73. Broxmeyer HE, Copper S, Lu L, et al. Enhanced stimulation of human bone marrow macrophage colony formation in vitro by recombinant human macrophage colony-stimulating factor in agarose medium and at low oxygen tension. Blood 1990;76:323–329.

74. Branch D, Turner AR, Guilbert LJ. Synergistic stimulation of macrophage proliferation by the monokines tumor necrosis factor-alpha and colony-stimulating factor-1. Blood 1989;73:307–311.

75. Chen BD-M, Mueller M. Recombinant tumor necrosis factor enhances the proliferative responsiveness of murine peripheral macrophages to macrophage colony-stimulating factor but inhibits their proliferative responsiveness to granulocyte-macrophage colony-stimulating factor. Blood 1990;75:1627–1632.

76. Lee MY, Kaushansky K, Judkins SA, et al. Mechanisms of tumor-induced neutrophilia: constitutive production of colony-stimulating factors and their synergistic actions. Blood 1989;74:115–122.

77. Stanely ER, Bartocci A, Patinkin D, et al. Regulation of very primitive, multipotent, hemopoietic cells by hemopoietic-1. Cell 1988;45:667–674.

78. McNiece IK, Stewart FM, Deacon DM. Synergistic interactions between hematopoietic growth factors as detected by in vitro mouse bone marrow colony formation. Exp Hematol 1988;16:383–388.

79. Zhou Y-Q, Stanely ER, Clark SC, et al. Interleukin-3 and interleukin-1α allow earlier bone marrow progenitors to respond to human colony-stimulating factor 1. Blood 1988;72:1870–1874.

80. Jubinsky PT, Stanley ER. Purification of hemopoietin-1: a multilineage hemopoietic growth factor. Proc Natl Acad Sci USA 1985;82:2764–2768.

81. Ulich TR, del Castillo J, Watson LR, et al. In vivo hematologic effects of recombinant human macrophage colony-stimulating factor. Blood 1990;4:846–950.

82. Williams DE, Hangoc G, Cooper S, et al. The effects of purified recombinant murine interleukin-3 and/or purified natural murine CSF-1 in vivo on the proliferation of murine high- and low-proliferative potential colony-forming cells: demonstration of in vivo synergism. blood 1987;70:401–403.

83. Meltzer MS, Gendelman HE. Effects of colony-stimulating factors on the interaction of monocytes and the human immunodeficiency virus. Immunol Lett 1988;19:193–198.

84. Mufson RA, Aghajanian J, Wong G, et al. Macrophage colony-stimulating factor enhances monocyte and macrophage antibody-dependent cell-mediated cytotoxicity. Cell Immunol 1989;119:182–192.

85. Sampson-Johannes A, Carlino JA. Enhancement of human monocyte tumoricidal activity by recombinant M-CSF. J Immunol 1988;141:3680–3686.

86. Lee M-T, Warren MK. CSF-1 induced resistance to viral infection in murine macrophages. J Immunol 1987;138:3019–3022.

87. Wing EJ, Waheed A, Shadduck RK, et al. Effect of colony stimulating factor on murine macrophages. J Clin Invest 1982;69:270–276.

88. Ralph P, Nakoinz I. Stimulation of macrophage tumoricidal activity by the growth and differentiation factor CSF-1. Cell Immunol 1987;105:270–279.

89. Munn DH, Cheung NV. Phagocytosis of tumor cells by human monocytes cultured in recombinant macrophage colony stimulating factor. J Exp Med 1990;172:231–237.

90. Thomassen MJ, Barna BP, Wiedermann HP, et al. Modulation of human alveolar macrophage tumoricidal activity by recombinant macrophage colony stimulating factor. J Biol Resp Med 1990;9:87–91.

91. Wang M, Friedman H, Djeu JY. Enhancement of human monocyte function against Candida albicans by the colony-stimulating factors (CSF): IL-3, granulocyte-macrophage-CSF, and macrophage-CSF. J Immunol 1989;143:671–677.

92. Nozawa RT, Sekiguchi R, Yokota T. Stimulation by conditioned medium of L-929 fibroblasts, E. Coli lipopolysaccharide, and muramyl peptide of candidacidal activity of mouse macrophages. Cell Immunol 1980;53:116–124.

93. Karbassi A, Mecker JM, Foster JS, et al. Enhanced killing of Candida albicans by murine macrophages treated with macrophage colony-stimulating factor: evidence for augmented expression of mannose receptors. J Immunol 1987;139:417–421.

94. Wing EJ, Ampel NM, Waheed A, et al. Macrophage colony-stimulating factor (M-CSF) enhances the capacity of murine macrophages to secrete oxygen reduction products. J Immunol 1985;135:2052–2056.

95. Ho JL, Reed SG, Wick EA, et al. Granulocyte-macrophage and macrophage colony-stimulating factors activate intramacrophage killing of Leishmania mexicana amazonesis. J Infect Dis 1990;162:224–230.

96. Cheers C, Stanely ER. Macrophage production during murine listeriosis: colony-stimulating factor 1 (CSF-1) and CSF-1 binding cells in genetically resistant and susceptible mice. Infect Immun 1988; 56:2972–2978.

97. James SL, Woods Cook K, Lazdins JK. Activation of human monocyte-derived macrophages to kill schistosomula of Schistosoma mansoni in vitro. J Immunol 1990;145:2686–2690.

98. Wang JM, Girrfin JD, Rambaldi A, et al. Induction of monocyte migration by recombinant macrophage colony-stimulating factor. J Immunol 1988;141:575–579.

99. Munn DH, Cheung NV. Phagocytosis of tumor cells by human monocytes cultured in recombinant macrophage colony stimulating factor. J Exp Med 1990;172:231–237.

100. Moore RN, Hoffeld JT, Farrar JJ, et al. Role of colony stimulating factors as primary regulators of macrophage functions. In: Pick E, ed. Lymphokinesis. New York: Academic Press, 1991:119–129.

101. Warren MK, Ralph P. Macrophage growth factor CSF-1 stimulates human monocyte production of interferon, tumor necrosis factor, and colony stimulating activity. J Immunol 1986;137:2281–2285.

102. Grandlemar HE, Orenstein JM, Martin MA, et al. Efficient isolation of propagation of human immunodeficiency virus on recombinant colony stimulating factor-1-treated monocytes. J Exp Med 1988; 167:1428–1441.

103. Kalter DC, Nakamura M, Turpin JA, et al. Enhanced HIV replication in macrophage colony-stimulating factor-treated monocytes. J Immunol 1991;146:298–306.

104. Koyanagi Y, O'Brien WA, Zhao JQ, et al. Cytokines alter production of HIV-1 from primary mononuclear phagocytes. Science 1988;241:1673–1675.

105. Garnick MB, Stoudemire JB. Preclinical and clinical evaluation of recombinant human macrophage colony-stimulating factor (rhM-CSF). Int J Cell Cloning 1990;8:356–373.

106. Stoudemire J, Metzger M, Timony G, et al. Pharmokinetics of recombinant human macrophage colony stimulating factor (rhM-CSF) in primates and rodents. Cancer Res 1989;30:538.

107. Shadduck RK, Waheed A, Boegel F, et al. The effect of colony stimulating factor-1 in vivo. Blood Cells 1987;13:49–63.

108. Hume DA, Pavli P, Donahue RE, et al. The effect of human recombinant macrophage colony-stimulating factor (CSF-1) on the murine mononuclear phagocyte system in vivo. J Immunol 1988;141:3405–3409.

109. Broxmeyer HE, Williams DE, Hangoc G, et al. Synergistic myelopoietic actions in vivo after administration to mice of combinations of purified natural murine colony-stimulating factor-1, recombinant murine interleukin-3, and recombinant murine granulocyte/macrophage colony-stimulating factor. Proc Natl Acad Sci USA 1987;84:3871–3875.

110. Munn DH, Garnick MB, Cheung N-KV. Effects of parenteral recombinant human macrophage colony-stimulating factor on monocyte number, phenotype, and antitumor cytotoxicity in nonhuman primates. Blood 1990;75:2042–2048.

111. Hume DA, Donahue RE, Fidler JJ. The therapeutic effect of human recombinant macrophage colony stimulating factor (CSF-1) in experimental murine metastatic melanoma. Lymph Res 1989;8:69.

112. Chong KT, Langlois L. Enhancing effect of macrophage colony-stimulating factor (M-CSF) in leukocytes and host defense in normal and immunosuppressed mice. FASEB J 1988;2:1474.

113. Cenci E, Bartocci A, Puccetti P et al. Macrophage colony stimulating factor in murine candidiasis: serum and tissue levels during infection and protective effect of exogenous administration. Infect Immunol 1991;59:868–872.

114. Yanai N, Yamada M, Motoyoshi K, et al. Effect of human macrophage colony-stimulating factor on granulopoiesis and survival in bone-marrow-transplanted mice. Jpn J Cancer Res 1990;81:355–362.

115. Stoudemire J, Garnick MB. Cholesterol (CHL) lowering effects of recombinant human macrophage colony stimulating factor (rhM-CSF). Blood 1989; 74:332.

116. Shimano H, Yamada N, Motohoshi K, et al. Plasma cholesterol-lowering activity of monocyte colony stimulating factor (M-CSF). Ann NY Acad Sci 1990;587:362–370.

117. Granick MB, Stoudemire J. Marked serum cholesterol (c) and low density lipoprotein C (LDLC) lowering activity induced by human macrophage colony stimulating factor (rhM-CSF) and other hematopoietic growth factors (HGF) in primates. Clin Res 1989;37:260.

118. Felix R, Cecchini MG, Fleisch H. Macrophage colony stimulating factor restores in vivo bone resorption in the op/op osteopetrotic mouse. Endocrinology 1990;127:2592–2594.

119. Kodama H, Yamasaki A, Nose M, et al. Congenital osteoclast deficiency in osteopetrotic (op/op) mice

is cured by injections of macrophage colony stimulating factor. J Exp Med 1991;173:269–272.

120. Motoyoshi K, Takaku F, Kusumoto K, et al. Phase I and early phase II studies on human urinary colony stimulating factor. Jap J Med 1982;21:187.

121. Motoyoshi K, Takaku F, Miura Y. High serum colony-stimulating activity of leukocytopenic patients after intravenous infusions of human urinary colony-stimulating factor. Blood 1983;62:685–688.

122. Motoyoshi K, Takaku F. Human monocytic colony-stimulating factor (hM-CSF), Phase I/II clinical studies. In: Mertelsmann R, Herrmann F, eds. Hematopoietic growth factors in clinical applications. New York: Marcel Dekker, 1990:161–175.

123. Motoyoshi K, Takaku F, Maekawa T, et al. Protective effect of partially purified human urinary colony-stimulating factor on granulocytopenia after antitumor chemotherapy. Exp Hematol 1986;14:1069–1075.

124. Masaoka T, Motohoshi K, Takaku F, et al. Administration of human urinary colony stimulating factor after bone marrow transplantation. Bone Marrow Transplantation 1988;3:121–127.

125. Masaoka T, Shibata H, Ohno R, et al. Double blind test of human urinary macrophage colony stimulating factor for allogeneic and syngeneic bone marrow transplantation: effectiveness of treatment and 2 year follow up for relapse of leukemia. Brit J Haematol 1990;76:501–505.

126. Motoyoshi K, Yoshida K, Hatake K, et al. Recombinant and native human urinary colony-stimulating factor directly augments granulocyte and granulocyte-macrophage colony-stimulating factor production of human peripheral blood monocytes. Exp Hematol 1989;17:68–71.

127. Nemunaitis J, Meyers JD, Buckner CD, et al. Phase I trial of recombinant human macrophage colony stimulating factor (rhM-CSF) in patients with invasive fungal infections. Blood 1991;78:907–913.

128. Khwaja A, Johnson B, Addison IE, et al. In vivo effects of macrophage colony-stimulating factor on human monocyte function. Br J Haematol 1991;77:25–31.

129. Peterson V, Ralph P, Kaushansky K, et al. Impact of sepsis on the macrophage colony stimulating factor (M-CSF) response to inflammation following thermal injury. Blood 1988;72:433.

130. Motoyoshi K, Yoshida K, Hatoke K, et al. Recombinant and mature human urinary colony stimulating factor directly augments granulocytic and granulocyte-macrophage colony stimulating factor production of human peripheral blood monocytes. Exp Hematol 1989;17:68–71.

131. Moore RN, Oppenheim JJ, Farrar JJ, et al. Production of lymphocyte-activating factor (Interleukin-1) by macrophages activated with colony-stimulating factors. J Immunol 1980;125:1302–1305.

132. Kurland J, Buckman RS, Broxmeyer HE, et al. Limitation of excessive myelopoiesis by the intrinsic modulation of macrophage derived prostaglandin E. Science 1978;199:552–555.

133. Lyberg T, Stanley ER, Prydz H. Colony-stimulating factor-1 induces thromboplastin activity in murine macrophages and human monocytes. J Cell Physiol 1987;132:367–370.

134. Lin HS, Gaden S. Secretion of plasminogen activator by bone marrow derived mononuclear phagocytes and its enhancement by colony stimulating factor. J Exp Med 1979;150:231–245.

135. Rambaldi A, Young DC, Griffin JD. Expression of the M-CSF (CSF-1) gene by human monocytes. Blood 1987;69:1409–1415.

136. Horiguchi J, Warren MK, Kufe D. Expression of the macrophage-specific colony-stimulating factor in human monocytes treated with granulocyte macrophage colony-stimulating factor. Blood 1987;69:1259–1261.

137. Oster W, Lindermann A, Horn S, et al. Tumor necrosis factor (TNF)-alpha but not TNF-beta induces secretion of colony-stimulating factor for macrophages (CSF-1) by human monocytes. Blood 1987;70:1700–1703.

138. Pistoia V, Ghio R, Roncella S, et al. Production of colony-stimulating activity by normal and neoplastic human B lymphocytes. Blood 1987;69:1340–1347.

139. Reisbach G, Hultner L, Kranz B, et al. Macrophage colony-stimulating activity is produced by three different EBV-transformed lymphoblastoid cell lines. Cell Immunol 1987;109:246–254.

140. Otsuka Pharm. Macrophage colony-stimulating factor-preparation using human leukemia T-cell culture. Japanese patent J6 2169-799:22.01.86 [Abstract]. Derwent Biotech 1987;6:48.

141. Kawasaki C, Okamura S, Omori F, et al. Both granulocyte-macrophage colony-stimulating factor and monocytic colony-stimulating factor are produced by the human T-cell line, HUT 102. Exp Hematol 1990;18:1090–1093.

142. Kelso A, Glasebrook AL, Kanagawa O, et al. Production of macrophage-activating factor by T lymphocyte clones and correlation with other lymphokine activities. J Immunol 1982;129:550–556.

143. Ralph P, Warren MK, Lee MT, et al. Inducible production of human macrophage growth factor, CSF-1. Blood 1986;68:633–639.

144. Mori T, Bartocci A, Satriano J, et al. Mouse mesangial cells produce colony stimulating factor-1 (CSF-1) and express CSF-1 receptor. J Immunol 1990;144(12):4697–4702.

145. Fibbe WE, van Damme J. Human fibroblasts produce G-, M- and GM-CSF following stimulation by IL-1 and poly JC. Blood 1991, in press.

146. Elford PR, Felix R, Cacchini M, et al. Murine osteoblast-like cells and the osteogenic cell MC3T3-

E1 release a macrophage colony-stimulating activity in culture. Calcif Tissue Int 1987;41:151–156.

147. Sieff CA, Tsai S, Faller DV. Interleukin-1 induces cultured human endothelial cell production of granulocyte-macrophage colony-stimulating factor. J Clin Invest 1987;79:48–51.

148. Fibbe WE, Damme J, van Billiau A, et al. Interleukin-1 induces human marrow stromal cells in long-term culture to produce G-CSF and M-CSF. Blood 1988;71:430–435.

149. Nemunaitis J, Andrews DF, Crittenden C, et al. Response of simian virus 40 (SV40)-transformed, cultured human marrow stromal cells to hematopoietic growth factors. J Clin Invest 1989;83:593–601.

150. Fibbe WE, van Damme J, Billiau A, et al. Interleukin-1 induces human marrow stromal cells in long-term culture to produce granulocyte colony-stimulating factor and macrophage colony-stimulating factor. Blood 1988;71:430–435.

151. Naparstek E, Donnelly T, Shadduck RK, et al. Persistent production of colony-stimulating factor (CSF-1) by cloned bone marrow stromal cell line D2XRII after X-irradiation. J Cell Physiol 1986;126:407–413.

152. Lanotte M, Metcalf D, Dexter TM. Production of monocyte/macrophage colony-stimulating factor by preadipocyte cell lines derived from murine marrow stroma. J Cell Physiol 1982;112:123–127.

153. Chodakewitz JA, Lacy J, Edwards SE, et al. Macrophage colony-stimulating factor production by murine and human keratinocytes. Enhancement by bacterial lipopolysaccharide. J Immunol 1990; 144:2190–2196.

154. Thery C, Hetier E, Evrard C, et al. Expression of macrophage colony stimulating factor gene in mouse brain development. J Neurosci Res 1990;26:129–133.

155. Henschler R, Mantovani L, Oster W, et al. Interleukin-4 regulates mRNA accumulation of macrophage-colony stimulating factor by fibroblasts: synergism with interleukin-1β. Br J Haematol 1990; 76:7–11.

156. Vallenga E, Rambaldi A, Ernst TJ, et al. Independent regulation of M-CSF and G-CSF gene expression in human monocytes. Blood 1988;71:1529–1532.

157. Haskill S, Johnson C, Ellmer D, et al. Adherence induces selective mRNA expression of monocyte mediators and proto-oncogenes. J Immunol 1988; 140:1690–1694.

158. Lee M-T, Kaushansky K, Ralph P, et al. Differential expression of M-CSF, G-CSF, and GM-CSF by human monocytes. J Leukoc Biol 1990;47:275–282.

159. Horiguchi J, Sariban E, Kufe D. Transcriptional and posttranscriptional regulation of CSF-1 gene expression in human monocytes. Mol Cell Biol 1988;8:3951–3954.

160. Curley SA, Roh MS, Kleinerman E, et al. Human recombinant macrophage colony stimulating factor activates murine Kupffer cells to a cytotoxic state. Leuk Res 1990;9:355–363.

161. Wing EJ, Magee DM, Pearson AC, et al. Peritoneal macrophages exposed to purified macrophage colony-stimulating factor (M-CSF) suppress mitogen- and antigen-stimulated lymphocyte proliferation. J Immunol 1986;137:2768–2773.

162. Broxmeyer HE, Geissler K, Cooper S, et al. Influence of purified recombinant human macrophage colony stimulating factor in mice. Biotech Ther 1989;1:43–54.

163. Broxmeyer HE, Williams DE, Cooper S, et al. Comparative effects in vivo of recombinant murine interleukin-3, natural murine colony-stimulating factor-1, and recombinant murine granulocyte-macrophage colony-stimulating factor on myelopoiesis in mice. J Clin Invest 1987;79:721–730.

164. Broxmeyer HE, Williams DE, Copper S, et al. The influence in vivo of murine colony-stimulating factor-1 on myeloid progenitor cells in mice recovering from sublethal dosages of cyclophosphamide. Blood 1987;69:913–918.

165. Komiyama A, Ishiguro A, Kubo T, et al. Increases in neutrophil counts by purified human urinary colony-stimulating factor in chronic neutropenia of childhood. Blood 1988;71:41–45.

21

INTERLEUKIN-3: GENERAL BIOLOGY, PRECLINICAL AND CLINICAL STUDIES

Michel Symann

Originally, the murine lymphokine interleukin-3 (IL-3), identified by its ability to induce the enzyme 20-α-hydroxysteroid dehydrogenase in spleen cells from athymic nu/nu mice, was erroneously defined as a regulator of T cell differentiation. Eventually, more careful analysis demonstrated that IL-3 possesses a variety of activities that were previously attributed to other factors, including T-cell-stimulating factor, stem cell-activating factor, mast cell growth factor, eosinophilic colony-stimulating factor (CSF), megakaryocyte CSF, burst-promoting activity, etc. (1–3).

Multi-CSF (a synonym for IL-3) is potentially the most appropriate cytokine for clinical applications. This cytokine can interact with and has many properties common to other CSFs and can act on cells from all of the erythroid and myeloid lineages as well as on mast cells (4) (Fig. 21.1).

Murine IL-3 was the first hematopoietic growth factor to be cloned (5), and the availability of recombinant human multi-CSF has permitted the confirmation of earlier work in mice. Although cloning of the human IL-3 gene proved elusive, eventually the genes for gibbon and human IL-3 were found by expression cloning (6). The ability to express the cloned genes for mouse and human IL-3 providing the recombinant protein permitted major advances in our knowledge of this cytokine and its biologic processes. Preliminary tests of the effectiveness of IL-3 treatment for human patients are currently in progress. Therefore, this review will focus primarily on studies performed with purified or recombinant multi-CSF, and on the properties of IL-3 that are interesting in the clinical setting.

MOLECULAR BIOLOGY

The first description of cDNA clones coding for murine IL-3 were published in 1984 (7, 8); however, the corresponding human sequence was not identified until 1986 when an IL-3 cDNA clone was isolated from a gibbon T cell line (6). This gibbon cDNA was then used as a probe for the human gene. Because the murine probe did not efficiently hybridize to human DNA, it was concluded that there was only minor homology between the human and the mouse molecules, suggesting an early evolutionary divergence of these genes. There is, in fact, only 29% homology between the human and mouse proteins, and thus murine IL-3 is not biologically active in assays for human IL-3 and vice versa.

Mouse IL-3 is composed of 166 amino acids containing four cysteine residues and a signal sequence of approximately 26 amino acids (5). The human gene for IL-3 (Fig. 21.2) is 152 amino acids with a signal sequence of

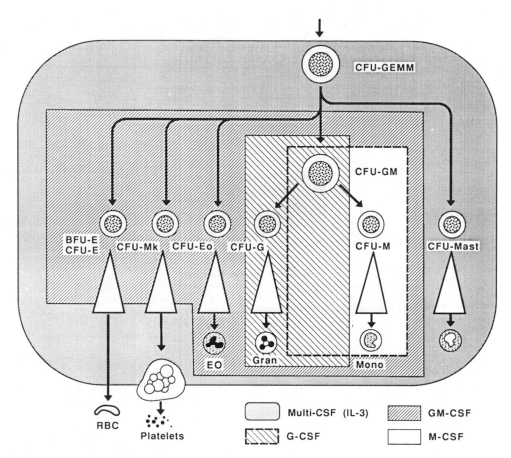

Figure 21.1. Biologic activity of the different CFSs. Cells enclosed by each CSF boundary respond to that CSF by proliferation or augmented function. Abbreviations: CFU, colony-forming unit; CU-GEMM, granulocyte, erythrocyte, macrophage, megakaryocyte; CFU-Mega, megakaryocyte; BFU-E: burst-forming unit erythroid; CFU-GM, granulocyte, monocyte-macrophage; CFU-mast, mastocyte. (Adapted with permission from Griffin JD. Clinical applications of colony stimulating factors. Oncology 1988;2:15–21.)

19 amino acids. It has two potential glycosylation sites and two cysteine residues linked by a disulfide bond. The observation that both recombinant IL-3 produced in bacteria as well as the naturally produced IL-3 exhibit similar activities suggests the carbohydrate component present on the molecule is not required for biologic activity either in vitro or in vivo (9, 10).

The structure of the mouse and human genes is very similar, each containing five exons and four introns (Table 21.1). In mice, the IL-3 gene is located on chromosome 11 and is closely linked to the granulocyte-monocyte colony-stimulating factor (GM-CSF) gene (11). In humans, the IL-3 gene is located on the long arm of chromosome 5, between bands q23–q31 (12); it is separated from the GM-CSF gene by approximately 9 kb of DNA (13) and is also close to the IL-4 and IL-5 genes (14). Other genes that have been mapped to this same general locus include macrophage colony-stimulating factor (M-CSF) (15), the M-CSF receptor (16), endothelial cell growth factor ECGF (17), and the platelet-derived growth factor (PDGF) receptor (18). It is possible that IL-3, GM-CSF, M-CSF, IL-4, and IL-5 have all evolved from a common ances-

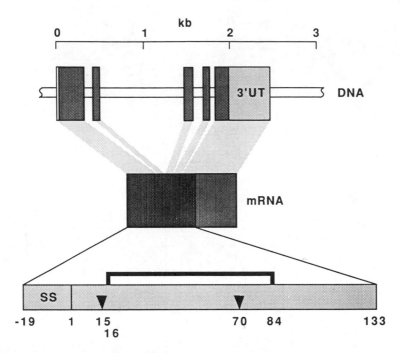

Figure 21.2. Human IL-3 structure. The IL-3 gene consists of five exons with 5′ and 3′ untranslated segments. The polypeptide contains a 19 amino acid signal sequence to be cleared from the mature protein. There is one disulfide bond between cysteine residues 16 and 84. N-glycosylation sites are present at residues 15 and 70. (Adapted with permission from Hamblin AS. Lymphokines. Washington, D.C.: IRL Press, 1988.) (By permission of Oxford University Press.)

Table 21.1.   Molecular Characteristics of Human and Mouse IL-3

	Mouse	Human
Chromosome location	11	5
Gene size	3 kb	3 kb
Gene structure	5 exons	5 exons
mRNA size	0.9 kb	0.9 kb
Protein weight	20–30 k	15–25 K
Signal sequence	27 amino acids	19 amino acids
Potential glycosylation site	4	2
Essential disulfide bond	1	1

tor gene through gene duplication and divergence. The molecular events involved in the transcriptional regulation of the different cytokine genes by external signals is an unknown and currently intense area of research.

CELLULAR SOURCE

Expression of the IL-3 gene (Table 21.2), as detected by Northern blot analysis, was thought to be restricted to activated T cells and T cell tumor lines (19), with the exception of activated natural killer (NK) cells (20, 21), murine mast cell lines (4), and the murine leukemia cell line, WEHI3B (22). In several studies, Northern blot analysis did not detect IL-3 transcripts in murine and human Dexter stromal cells. This suggested that IL-3 is not involved in constitutive hematopoiesis but is instead a mechanism whereby the immune system induces hematopoiesis (23, 24). More recent experiments using the polymerase chain reaction (PCR) suggest that IL-3 mRNA is present in normal human bone marrow stroma (25) and in human monocytes stimulated by the calcium ionophore

Table 21.2. Cells Expressing IL-3ᵃ

Cell Type	Stimuli	Reference
Nonmalignant sources		
T lymphocytes	PHA/PMA	19
Monocytes	Calcium ionophore A23187	26
NK cells	PDBu—A23187	20, 21
Mast cells	IgE—A23187	3
Bone marrow stroma cells		25
Thymic epithelial cells		27
Keratinocytes		28
Astrocytes		29
Tumor cell lines		
T cell tumor lines		19
Myeloid leukemia WEH13B		22

ᵃAbbreviations: PDBu, phosphodibutyrate; PHA, phytohemag-glutinin; PMA, phorbol myristate acetate.

A23187, but not in resting monocytes (26). In both instances biologically active IL-3 was detectable as well. Clearly, a role for IL-3 in steady-state hematopoiesis is not completely ruled out. In addition, human thymic epithelial cells (27), murine but not human skin keratinocytes (28), and murine astrocytes or neuronal cells (29) were found to express an mRNA that is homologous to the T cell IL-3 cDNA.

INTERLEUKIN-3 RECEPTOR AND SIGNAL TRANSDUCTION

The mechanism by which colony-stimulating factors (CSFs) stimulate cells to proliferate and differentiate is poorly understood; however it is widely accepted that the first event is the binding of the growth factor to its specific membrane receptor. IL-3 receptors are present on both murine and human bone marrow cells, although they have not yet been fully characterized. Successful iodination of murine IL-3 (mIL-3) was used to estimate the IL-3 receptor density at between 2000 and 5000 molecules per cell on different factor-dependent cell lines (30).

Clearly, the molecular characterization of cytokine receptors is hampered by their low abundance on cells. A number of different estimates of the mIL-3 receptor's molecular weight have been reported. Sorensen et al. identified a 67-kd protein as the receptor (31), and May and Ihle reported a single mIL-3 receptor of 65–70 kd (32). Nicola and Peterson reported two different sizes for the mIL-3 receptor, 60 and 70 kd (33), while Park et al. found also two receptors but reported their sizes as 70 and 115 kd (34).

A binding component of the mouse IL-3 receptor has been recently cloned (35). This protein, when expressed in transfected fibroblasts, bound IL-3 with low affinity, did not possess a kinase sequence, and was nonfunctional, which indicates that additional components must be required for functional high-affinity IL-3 receptors. Comparative sequence analysis indicates that significant similarity is present in the external domains of the receptors for IL-2, IL-3, IL-4, IL-6, IL-7, GM-CSF, granulocyte colony-stimulating factor (G-CSF), and erythropoietin (for a review see 36). The human IL-3 receptor has not yet been cloned.

Studies on KG-1 cells using radiolabeled recombinant human IL-3 identified a 69-kd IL-3 binding protein distinct from the 93-kd GM-CSF receptor (37). Although these two binding proteins are distinct, GM-CSF and IL-3 competed for binding to KGI cells at 4° C, a temperature that blocks cell metabolism and receptor downmodulation. Other authors have also observed binding of IL-3 and GM-CSF to KG-1 cells, primary monocytes (38–40), leukemic myeloblasts (41), and to normal eosinophils (42). On the other hand, another team studying human myeloblasts and monocytes suggested that a common binding structure between GM-CSF and IL-3 is the reason for GM-CSF and IL-3 cross competition (43). Clearly, the interaction between IL-3 and GM-CSF receptors remains to be clarified, but data suggest there is heterogeneity in the binding sites for IL-3 and GM-CSF, where a subset of the receptor can bind IL-3 only, a subset GM-CSF only, while another subset binds both. Molecular cloning of the human IL-3 receptor and the β chain of the GM-CSF receptor is necessary to further understand the interaction of both ligands with their receptors.

After binding, murine IL-3 is rapidly internalized and specifically cleaved before its complete degradation in the lysosome, and the internalized receptors are apparently recycled back to the cell surface (44). Murine IL-3 appears to induce the downregulation of its own receptor, proportional to the concentration of mIL-3 present in the culture medium. In the mouse, receptor-receptor interactions have been demonstrated, and occupancy of the IL-3 receptor downmodulating the other CSF receptor occurs in a hierarchical sequence (45). It has been proposed that this phenomenon is part of the mechanism that controls hematopoietic cell differentiation (46).

The second messenger mediating IL-3 activity has not yet been unequivocally determined. Three major biochemical pathways have been implicated in growth-factor-mediated cell proliferation. For some growth factors, stimulation of their cell surface receptor initiates phospholipase C hydrolysis of a membrane-bound inositol lipid, producing two second messengers, diacylglycerol (DAG) and inositol 1,4,5-triphosphate (IP3). The regulation of phospholipase C activation is mediated by guanine nucleotide binding proteins (G proteins). DAG acts by stimulating protein kinase C, whereas IP3 releases calcium from internal stores. The other two pathways include activation of receptor-associated tyrosine kinases and the accumulation of cAMP in response to ligands that activate adenylate cyclase. mIL-3 has been shown to activate protein kinase C (PKC, a serine-threonine kinase) by cytosol-to-membrane translocation (47) and to induce the threonine phosphorylation of a 68-kd protein in an IL-3-dependent cell line (48). However, there are some data to suggest that IL-3 activates protein kinase C without hydrolysis of inositol phospholipids (49), while other data

indicate an inhibition of IL-3 stimulated proliferation by pertussis toxin, a known G protein inhibitor that perhaps reflects activation of alternate signaling systems (50). For the moment, the picture is far from clear. Recent evidence suggests that mouse IL-3 stimulation of growth-factor-dependent cell lines rapidly induces thyrosine phosphorylation and the appearance of a 140-kd phosphotyrosine-containing membrane protein (51–53). However, the mechanisms of signal transduction by the tyrosine kinases are still poorly understood. Recently, it has been reported that human IL-3 and GM-CSF induce rapid tyrosine phosphorylation of the same substrate in the cytosol (54).

Since GM-CSF and IL-3 share many biologic activities, it may not be surprising that they share similar surface binding sites and signal transduction pathways.

BIOLOGIC ACTIVITIES OF MURINE INTERLEUKIN-3 IN VITRO

The effects of purified and recombinant murine (m) IL-3 have been studied on bone marrow, spleen, and fetal liver cells as well as on continuous cell lines of hematopoietic origin. Altogether, these studies demonstrate that IL-3 has a broad spectrum of activities (Table 21.3), including proliferative and differentiation effects, interaction with other hematopoietic growth factors, survival effects, and activation of effector cell function. In addition, there is evidence that IL-3 increases the level of hematopoietic progenitor homing receptors.

Proliferative and Differentiation Effects

Initial studies demonstrated that purified or recombinant IL-3 in soft agar induces bone marrow colony formation, and thus IL-3 was classified as a CSF (2, 55–56). These studies indicate that IL-3 specifically supports the maintenance and stimulates the proliferation and differentiation of granulocyte-mac-

Table 21.3. Biologic Activities of IL-3[a]

	References	
	rm IL-3	rh IL-3
In Vitro		
Stimulation of proliferation and differentiation		
CFU-S	55, 56, 57	
All myeloid progenitor cells	55, 57, 62, 63, 65, 66	99–103, 127
Pulmonary alveolar macrophages	60	
Bone marrow mast cells	83	
Survival		
Hematopoietic cell lines, CFU-G	86, 89	115
Monocytes, macrophages		116
Eosinophils		117
Connective mast cells	85	
Enhancement of effector cell function		
Monocytes-macrophages		
Antibody-independent tumoricidal activity		122
Cytokine secretion		40, 122, 123
Phagocytosis	90, 91	
Eosinophils		
Antibody-dependent cell-mediated cytotoxicity		97
Basophils		
Histamine release		128, 129
Adhesiveness for endothelium		130
Responsiveness to C3a		131
Mast cells	92	
Chemotaxis		132
Upregulation of homing receptors	96, 97	
In Vivo		
Proliferation of CFU-S day 8 and day 14	137	
Increase in all myeloid progenitor cells	10, 133, 134, 135	149, 150
Increase in eosinophils, granulocytes, monocytes	10, 133, 134, 135	145, 150
platelets	135	
Potentiation of subsequent administration of		144–152
GM-CSF, erythropoietin, or G-CSF		144–152
Reduction of neutropenia and thrombopenia		
after myelosuppressive therapy		153, 154

[a]Abbreviations: h, human; m, murine; r, recombinant.

rophages, eosinophils, megakaryocytes, and, in presence of erythropoietin, erythroid and multipotential colony-forming cells.

A direct effect of IL-3 on progenitors of neutrophils and macrophages has been established by experiments on individual cells (57). The ability of IL-3 to directly support the differentiation of granulocytes and monocytes from bone marrow progenitors has been demonstrated in dose-response studies using pure IL-3 in serum-free cultures (57, 58). Peritoneal exudate macrophages and blood monocytes do not undergo clonal growth, in vitro, in response to IL-3 as they do with M-CSF (59), while pulmonary alveolar macrophages can be induced by IL-3 to proliferate in vitro (60).

Production of eosinophils from bone marrow precursors in vitro is supported by IL-3, although to a lesser extent than by IL-5 (61). In primary suspension cultures of bone marrow from normal or parasitized mice, IL-3 stimulates a lower eosinophil production than IL-5. However, IL-3 was sevenfold more effective than IL-5 in generating eosinophil colony-forming units and increasing the number of IL-5-responsive progenitors.

IL-3 stimulates megakaryocyte colony formation and promotes the differentiation of individual megakaryocytes in vitro (62, 63). In addition, IL-3 plus IL-6 has a demonstrated additive effect on megakaryocyte development, presumably due to the ability of IL-3 to expand the population of IL-6-responsive cells (64).

IL-3 cannot support full erythroid differentiation in the absence of erythropoietin, but increases the number of progenitors that can become committed to the erythroid lineage (55, 56, 65, 66). Thus it has been suggested that IL-3 supports the proliferation of early stem cells that are capable of commitment to the myeloid lineages. A direct effect of IL-3 on late day 12 colony-forming unit-spleen (CFU-S) in simple suspension has been demonstrated (67). In these experiments, IL-3 stimulated CFU-S proliferation in vitro by increasing the proportion of CFU-S in S-phase. The in vitro counterparts of late-day 12 CFU-S are thought to be multipotential blast cell colonies (68). In this assay, regenerated bone marrow and spleens from 5-fluorouracil (5-FU) treated mice, enriched for immature progenitors, were used to study regulatory factors involved in early stem cell development. Blast cell colonies arise from progenitors that are not in cell cycle and do not require exogenously added growth factor for maintenance and viability (69). IL-3 does not initiate the proliferation of stem cells in G_0, but once the cells begin to proliferate and differentiate, their continued growth is dependent upon the addition of IL-3 and to a lesser extent on GM-CSF (70, 71). Dose-response analysis indicates the sensitivity of stem cells to IL-3 may decline as they slowly differentiate (72).

There is ample evidence that hematopoietic growth factors act synergistically, with combinations of two or more capable of inducing proliferation and differentiation more efficiently than they can individually (Table 21.4). At the present time, at least six growth factors have been shown to act in synergy with IL-3 on a variety of target cells, including M-CSF (58, 59), G-CSF (73), erythropoietin (6, 74), IL-1 (75), IL-4 (76, 77), IL-6 (64, 78, 79), and IL-11 (80). The observation that G-CSF or IL-6 works synergistically with IL-3 to support the blast colony formation of day 4 post-5-FU spleen cells is interesting because it apparently results from shortening the average period of G_0 residence for stem cells (73, 78, 79). Furthermore, G-CSF or IL-6 can act synergistically with IL-3 to support the proliferation of multipotential progenitors derived from day 2 post-5-FU bone marrow. This combination of G-CSF or IL-6 with IL-3 is synergistic for both the course of colony development, the absolute number of colonies, and the number of multilineage colonies (73, 78). Studies on the interaction of growth factors with nonhematopoietic target cell populations (81, 82) have led to a two-signal model where a competence factor and a progression factor interact to mediate the transition of cells from G_0 to a cycling state. Perhaps IL-6 and G-CSF act as competence factors, shortening the G_0 period of hematopoietic stem

Table 21.4. Synergistic Activities of Murine IL-3 In Vitro[a]

IL-3 Source	Factor Synergized	Cell Target	Ref.
nmIL-3	nM-CSF	CFU-M	58
nmIL-3	nM-CSF	Blood monocyte; peritoneal macrophage	59
rmIL-3	rhG-CSF	Blast cell colonies, CFU-MIX	73
nmIL-3	nhEPO	day 12 CFU-S, CFU-MIX, BFU-E	74
rmIL-3	rhIL-1	Pluripotential stem cells	75
rmIL-3	rmIL-4	CFU-mast, connective tissue type	76, 77
nmIL-3	rhIL-6	day 14–CFU-S	78
		Blast cell colonies CFU-MIX	79
rmIL-3	rmIL-6	CFU-GM CFU-Mk	64
rmIL-3	rhIL-11	CFU-Mk	80

[a]Abbreviations: CFU-Mk, colony-forming unit-megakaryocyte; h, human m, murine; n, natural; r, recombinant.

cells while IL-3 functions as the progression factor necessary for continuous proliferation. However, the molecular basis for these synergistic effects is still poorly understood.

Mast cells that reside near the blood vessels in connective tissue contain large quantities of heparin and histamine and can be distinguished from mucosal mast cells in the digestive tract because these cells contain little histamine but have chondroitin sulfate granules. IL-3 possesses much of the activity previously attributed to mast-cell growth factor or P-cell-stimulating factor (2, 55, 56). Recent evidence indicates that IL-3 can support the proliferation of mucosal mast cells while IL-4 induces proliferation of connective tissue mast cells (83–85).

A potential role for IL-3 in the regulation of diffentiation in the lymphoid lineage currently remains unclear and controversial.

Cell Survival

Experiments using continuous cell lines uniquely responsive to multi-CSF have underscored the need for IL-3 in the survival of hematopoietic cells (86). Following withdrawal of multi-CSF, cell death may occur due to the failure of membrane glucose transport and the maintenance of intracellular ATP levels (87, 88). Death of hematopoietic precursors upon withdrawal of IL-3 (or other relevant CSF) in vitro occurs through an active process of self-destruction, referred to as apoptosis (89). The absence of specific signals results in apoptosis depending upon protein synthesis in the dying cells. Suppression of apoptosis by IL-3 or other CSF may be important for regulating the volume of hematopoietic precursors in the bone marrow.

Functional Activation

IL-3 is also a potent activator of end cells in some lineages and supports their development. Two studies found an augmentation of phagocytosis in marrow or peritoneal macrophages exposed to IL-3 in vitro (90, 91) although no effect was observed on mature neutrophils (10). In addition, the stimulation of connective tissue mast cell migration by IL-3, but not by IL-4, has been reported (92). In this study, IL-4 was unable to potentiate the chemoattractant activity of IL-3.

UpRegulation of the Homing Receptor

Recognition and selective homing to the marrow, by intravenously transplanted hematopoietic stem cells, is thought to be mediated by homing receptors on hematopoietic progenitor cell membranes containing specific galactosyl and mannosyl sites (93). A brief in vitro exposure of marrow cells to IL-3 significantly increases their ability to reconstitute the hematopoietic organs of lethally irradiated recipients (94). Further work has shown that IL-3 increases the homing receptors on marrow cells by 200%–300%, the seeding efficiency of CFU-S, and the survival of transplanted mice (95, 96), and these data may be clinically relevant for bone marrow transplantation. Thus in vivo pretreatment of the donor with IL-3 or brief ex vivo incubation of donor cells might improve the efficiency of seeding and mitigate postgrafting cytopenia.

GIBBON RHESUS AND HUMAN INTERLEUKIN-3 BIOLOGIC ACTIVITIES IN VITRO

Gibbon and human IL-3 are 93% homologous and exhibit similar biologic properties (97). The nucleotide sequence of the rhesus IL-3 gene displays 92.9% homology with that of the human IL-3 gene. In vitro, both rhesus and human IL-3 have comparable stimulatory activity on normal and malignant human hematopoietic cells, although human IL-3 appears to be 100-fold less effective in stimulating rhesus hematopoietic progenitors (98).

Proliferative and Differentiation Effects

The biologic activity of human IL-3 (Table 21.3) is similar to murine IL-3 in that it can stimulate the in vitro production of primitive blast cell colonies, as well as granulocyte-macrophages, megakaryocytes, eosinophils, basophils, and, in the presence of erythropoietin, multilineage, early, and late erythroid colonies (99–103). By comparison to GM-CSF, IL-3 is more effective in supporting primitive blast cell, erythroid, and megakaryocytic colony formation. By comparison to G-CSF, IL-3 is less effective in supporting granulocyte colonies. These studies were done with unfractionated progenitor cells in the presence of serum or plasma. The induced production of CSF's by a variety of accessory cells and the presence of growth factors and cofactors in serum and plasma make it very difficult to attribute one specific activity to an individual CSF. In serum-free cultures of highly enriched progenitor cells, plated at low densities, IL-3 alone is a poor stimulus for the proliferation of progenitor cells, although when combined with G-CSF, M-CSF, or erythropoietin, these factors can yield a full range of neutrophil colonies, monocyte colonies, or erythroid bursts, respectively (104–107). These results suggest that the best hematopoietic response in therapeutic trials might result from a combination of an early-acting broad-spectrum factor such as IL-3 with lineage-specific late-acting factors.

A combination of GM-CSF and IL-3 was shown to be synergistic for burst-forming unit-erythroid (BFU-E) in one study (105) but had no additive effect in another (107). In liquid cultures of purified CD34+ cells isolated from the umbilical cord, preculturing the cells with IL-3 enhanced their proliferative responses to GM-CSF in secondary cultures, while the inverse had no effect (108). Similarly IL-6, which does not stimulate blast cell colony formation, accelerated the formation of IL-3–supported blast cell colonies (109). Furthermore, in a plasma clot megakaryocyte colony-forming assay, IL-11 in combination with IL-3 increased the number of colonies (80), and in cultures of low-density, nonadherent antibody-depleted CD34+ cells, recombinant human stem cell factor was synergistic with IL-3, resulting in an increase in colony numbers and size (110). Again, these observations may be clinically relevant for hematologic reconstitution using a combination CSF therapy.

In addition to serving as a growth factor for normal hematopoietic cells, IL-3 has been shown to support the formation of acute myeloid blast cell colonies in a significant number of patients (111, 112). In one study, IL-3 high-afffinity receptors were found on leukemic cells in 13 out of 15 primary acute myelocytic leukemia (AML) cases (113). In view of the potential clinical usefulness of IL-3 in AML patients, this creates a substantial concern.

Cell Survival

Human hematopoietic stem cells in the G_0 phase can survive in culture for more than 2 weeks in the absence of early hematopoietic regulators, such as IL-3 (114). Some evidence suggests that in methylcellulose cultures, when granulocyte colony-forming units (CFU-G) disappear in cultures depleted of G-CSF for 21 weeks, IL-3 can promote the survival of CFU-G without recruitment of less mature progenitor cells (115). Similarly, IL-3 can induce the in vitro maintenance of eosinophils and monocytes/macrophages by affecting their survival (116, 117).

Functional Activation

Human IL-3 is a demonstrated potent activator of most mature effector cell functions, except for neutrophils, in agreement with the theory that IL-3 responsiveness is lost during the later stages of neutrophil development (97, 118). The expression of high-affinity IL-3 binding sites has been detected on human monocytes, (119) eosinophils, and basophils (120, 121).

IL-3 has also been found to significantly enhance antibody-independent tumoricidal activity in the monocyte response to a secondary stimulus (endotoxin) (122). This effect is most likely mediated through an increased release of tumor necrosis factor (TNF) and activation of TNF transcription. Similarly, recombinant human (Rh) IL-3 induces the expression of M-CSF mRNA as well as the secretion of M-CSF and G-CSF by monocytes (40, 123).

Eosinophils have been shown to respond to IL-3 in vitro. Gibbon IL-3 (gIL-3) is a powerful stimulus of mature human eosinophil functions, including the enhancement of antibody-dependent cell-mediated cytotoxicity, phagocytosis, and superoxide anion production (97). Eosinophil infiltration in carcinomas of the lung, colon, and uterine cervix has been associated with increased patient survival (124–126), perhaps making it desirable to induce eosinophilia and enhance eosinophil cytotoxic function in these patients.

rhIL-3 fails to induce histamine release by basophils from normal donors (127) but is active on IgE$^+$ basophils from atopic donors (128, 129). Although IL-3 alone cannot induce the release of histamine, preincubation of cells with IL-3 enhances histamine degranulation and the release of leukotriene in response to C5a (130, 131). In addition, IL-3 can also act as a chemotactic factor for mast cells (132).

IN VIVO EFFECTS OF MURINE INTERLEUKIN-3

The broad proliferative effects of recombinant IL-3 found in vitro have also been observed in a number of in vivo studies (10, 133, 134). Intraperitoneal or subcutaneous administration of IL-3 in normal mice induces a 10-fold increase in blood eosinophils and a 2- to 3-fold increase in granulocytes and monocytes. In one study, IL-3 given subcu-

taneously three times daily for 54 hours increased platelet levels by 20% (135). In addition, there were dose related increases in CFU-G, macrophage colony-forming units (CFU-M), granulocyte-monocyte colony-forming units (CFU-GM); colony-forming unit, mixed (CFU-MIX), BFU-E, and erythroid colony-forming units (CFU-E) and mast cell numbers in the spleen, although there was little effect on bone marrow cellularity or progenitor cell frequency. IL-3 treatment of lethally irradiated bone marrow transplanted mice induced rapid increases in both bone marrow and spleen cellularity and progenitor cell content when compared to the same treatment in normal mice (136). Chronic infusion of IL-3 into normal mice stimulated the proliferation of both day 8 and day 11 CFU-S in the bone marrow and the spleen (137). In lactoferrin-suppressed animals, a lower dose of IL-3 is sufficient to enhance the cycling status and absolute numbers of all bone marrow and splenic progenitors (138, 139). Furthermore, the concentration of IL-3 required to produce a stimulatory effect in vivo can be reduced if it is administered with concentrations of M-CSF or GM-CSF that are not active in vivo (139, 140). In contrast to the effects described for myeloid cell lineages, no positive or negative changes were observed on lymphoid cell lineages (141). In a recent study, the simultaneous administration of IL-3 and IL-6 induced a platelet increase that was only slightly greater than the sum of the effects of IL-3 alone and IL-6 alone; however suboptimal doses of IL-3 or IL-6 were not tested (135). In 5-FU-treated mice, neither IL-3 nor IL-6 affects platelet recovery. In contrast, a combination of IL-3 and IL-6 given either immediately or 2 days following 5-FU decreased the platelet nadir and diminished the time required for recovery to normal platelet levels (142). This suggests that the stimulation of megakaryocytopoiesis by IL-3 and IL-6 may be clinically beneficial (Table 21.5).

Iodine-125-labeled IL-3 was used to determine the serum half-life, organ distribution, and fate of in vivo administration of IL-

Table 21.5. Synergistic Activities of Murine IL-3 in Vivo[a]

IL-3 Source	Factor Synergized	Cell Target	Ref.
rmIL-3	rmGM-CSF	CFU-MIX CFU-GMN BFU-E	140
rmIL-3	nmM-CSF	CFU-MIX CFU-GM BFU-E	140
rmIL-3	rhIL-6	CFU-Mk and megakaryocytes	142

[a]Abbreviations: CFU-Mk, colony-forming units h = human; m = murine; n = natural; r = recombinant.

3 (143). IL-3 has an initial half-life of 3–5 minutes, followed by a second phase of 50 minutes. Hematopoietic cells in the bone marrow and spleens of intravenously injected mice were clearly labeled. A high proportion of the labeled IL-3 is localized in the liver, while the kidney appears to be an active site of IL-3 degradation based on the rapid appearance of labeled material in the urine.

PRECLINICAL STUDIES WITH HUMAN INTERLEUKIN-3 IN HEALTHY PRIMATES

Interleukin-3 Alone

The first simian studies employing the continuous intravenous infusion of rhIL-3 (20 μg/kg/day) elicited a modest and delayed leukocytosis in normal macaques (Table 21.6). The white blood cell (WBC) counts extended from a baseline mean of 7750 cells/μl to a maximum mean of 17,000, largely attributed to neutrophils, eosinophils, lymphocytes, and atypical basophils, which appeared 1–3 days after termination of continuous intravenous infusion of IL-3 for 1 week (144). A consistent increase in reticulocytes and an occasional increase in platelets was also observed, and more recent studies have confirmed these findings (145–149). In addition, increases in the peripheral blood levels of CFU-E, BFU-E, CFU-GM, CFU-M, and CFU-MIX have also been

reported (149, 150). Recently, studies on nonhuman primates using homologous recombinant rhesus IL-3 revealed the dose dependence of stimulating production in all myeloid lineages compared to the response obtained after administration of murine recombinant IL-3 in mice (150). These data underscore the species specificity of IL-3 and indicate that in vitro studies using human IL-3 in nonhuman primates do not reveal its maximum potential.

Simultaneous Administration of Interleukin-3 and Granulocyte-Monocyte Colony-Stimulating Factor

The simultaneous administration of rhIL-3 (100 μg/kg/day × 14 subcutaneously) with rhGM-CSF (5.5 μg/kg/day × 14 subcutaneously) induced an elevation of WBCs similar to that observed in monkeys treated with rhGM-CSF alone (146).

Recombinant Human Interleukin-3 Followed by Recombinant Human Granulocyte-Monocyte Colony-Stimulating Factor, Granulocyte Colony-Stimulating Factor, or Erythropoietin

The relatively low magnitude of IL-3-induced leukocytosis and the corresponding delay in its response time, compared to either G-CSF or GM-CSF, are consistent with the conclusion that IL-3 is predominantly a stimulator of early progenitors and insufficient alone to support end-stage blood cell maturation. Several studies have investigated sequential administration of IL-3 followed by GM-CSF in monkeys (144, 146, 147, 149–152), giving rhIL-3 for 7–14 days followed by low doses of rhGM-CSF (Table 21.7). This suboptimal dose of GM-CSF on its own only supports a moderate increase in leukocytosis (a two- to three-fold increase above the baseline). In IL-3 pretreated monkeys, low-dose

Table 21.6.   Recombinant Human IL-3 In Vivo[a]

Recipients	Express System-Specific Activity	Dose/Route	Hematopoietic Effects	Toxicity	Ref.
Cynomolgus macaques	*E. coli* 3–5.10⁶ U/mg	20 µg/kg/d × 7 continuous IV	Modest delayed increase in neutrophils, eosinophils, lymphocytes, eosinophils, basophils. Consistent increase in reticulocytes, occasional increase in platelets.	None from 5–50 µg/kg/d	144
Cynomolgus macaques	Yeast 5×10^7 U/mg	100 µg/kg/d × 8 IV bolus	No change	—	145, 147, 151
Rhesus monkeys	*E. coli* 4.6×10^6 U/mg	11, 33, 100 µg/kg/d × 14 SC doses	Two- to threefold increase in WBC dose-dependent elevation of eosinophils and basophils (up to 40% of WBCs).	With 100 µg/kg increase in plasma histamine levels and urticaria	146
Baboons and macaques	*E. coli* 1.2×10^7 U/mg	20 µg/kg/d × 5 in 3 SC per day	As in ref. 118; increase in bone marrow CFU-E and BFU-c + reticulocytes at posttreatment days 5 and 9, respectively	—	148
Rhesus monkeys	*E. coli* 4.6×10^6 U/mg	33 µg/kg/d × 11–14 SC	As in ref 120. At the end of treatment increased PB level of CFU-GM (12×), BFU-E (9×) CFU-MIX (12×), CFU-Mk (13×). No change in bone marrow progenitor cells.	—	149

[a]Abbreviations: CFU-Mk, colony-forming units, megakaryocyte; IV, intravenously; PB, peripheral blood; SC, subcutaneously.

Table 21.7. rhIL-3 In Vivo Followed by rhGM-CSF

Recipients	Express System Specific Activity	Dose	Hematopoietic Effects	Ref.
Cynomolgus macaques	IL-3: *E. coli* $3-5 \times 10^6$ U/mg GM-CSF: *E. coli* 1.2×10^7 U/mg	20 µg/kg/d × 7 followed by 2 ug/kg/d × 4	Dramatic increase in the level of PB neutrophils, eosinophils, monocytes, basophils, reticulocytes, platelets, and lymphocytes, within 2 days of the GM-CSF start. WBC reached 50 to 60,000 cells/µl.	144
Cynomolgus macaques	IL-3: Yeast 5×10^7 U/mg GM-CSF: *E. coli* 5×10^7 U/mg	10 or 100 µg/kg/ d × 8 followed by 10 µg/kg/d ×5	Dramatic increase in the levels of WBC of all lineages and platelets following GM-CSF.	145, 147, 151
Rhesus monkeys	IL-3: *E. coli* 4.6×10^6 U/mg GM-CSF: CHO 3.5×10^6 U/mg	11, 33 or 100 µg/ kg/d × 14 followed by 5.5 µg/kg/d × 14	Independent of IL-3 doses prompt rise in WBC by days 4–6 of GM-CSF. Neutrophils increased 4–14×, eosinophils × 14–80×, basophils declined during rhGM-CSF. After 33 µg/kg of IL-3, GM-CSF expanded PB CFU-GM (63×); in BM consistent decrease of progenitors of all types.	146, 149

*a*Abbreviations: BM, bone marrow; BP, peripheral blood; CHO, Chinese hamster ovary cells.

GM-CSF treatment markedly increased peripheral blood white cells of all myeloid lineages, and occasionally in some animals platelets and reticulocytes as well, exemplifying the synergy between rhIL-3 and rhGM-CSF. Interestingly, GM-CSF administration in IL-3-primed monkeys expanded their pool of circulating stem cells (149, 152), a phenomenon that can be clinically exploited to facilitate the collection of a sufficient number of stem cells for autografting. Similarly, the sequential administration of IL-3 followed by substimulating doses of G-CSF induced a significant rise in peripheral blood granulocytes (151).

Administration of rh erythropoietin (Epo) to rhIL-3 pretreated monkeys expanded all bone marrow erythroid progenitor classes and increased reticulocytes beyond the levels observed when animals are treated with Epo alone (148). Again, these results support the concept that IL-3 acts synergistically with lineage-restricted growth factors to produce an expansion of different committed progenitors. Finally, these studies highlight the potential benefit that can be derived by using combinations of hematopoietic growth factors in the clinic.

ADMINISTRATION OF HUMAN INTERLEUKIN-3 TO MYELOSUPPRESSED PRIMATES

Cyclophosphamide Trials

The treatment of three healthy cynomolgus macaques with 60 mg/kg/day × 2 of cyclophosphamide followed 24 hours later, or not, by a 14-day course of IL-3 (20 µg/kg/day continuous intravenous infusion) was analyzed by Gillio et al. (153). The cyclophosphamide treatment and subsequent IL-3 were repeated at 35-day intervals. The degree of neutropenia and leukopenia was markedly diminished in the single IL-3 treated animal. In the two control animals, the absolute neutrophil count nadir following cycles 1 and 2 was 400 and 100 neutrophils per microliter, respectively. It is interesting to note that the IL-3-treated animal did not drop its absolute neutrophil count to less than 1000 per microliter. While no basophilia or eosinophilia developed in the control animals, WBC recovery in the rhIL-3-treated monkey was predominantly in neutrophils, eosinophils, and basophils. In another study (154), two monkeys receiving cyclophosphamide (60 mg/kg/day × 2) were treated with rhGM-CSF (10 µg/kg/day) from day 6–day 20, postcyclophosphamide. One monkey received additional rhIL-3 (10 µg/kg/day subcutaneously) from day 1–day 24, postcyclophosphamide. Under these conditions, the combination of rhIL-3 with rhGM-CSF was not superior to rhGM-CSF alone.

5-Fluorouracil Trial

Six cynomolgus primates were treated with 5-FU (75 mg/kg/day × 2) followed by the treatment of two animals with a 14-day course of rhIL-3 (20 µg/kg/day subcutaneously) (153). Control animals post 5-FU experienced an absolute neutrophil count (ANC) nadir of 0 cells per microliter while IL-3 treated primates developed an ANC nadir above 400 cells and exhibited significant acceleration in their recovery of both total WBC and neutrophil counts. In addition, animals receiving IL-3 experienced a more prompt recovery of platelets.

Busulfan Trial

Two monkeys were treated with two cycles of busulfan (4 mg/kg/day on days 1–4 and 6 mg/kg/day on days 42–45) (154). One of them received rhIL-3 (100 µg/kg/day subcutaneously) from day 7–24 after the first course of busulfan, while the other was treated from day 48–54 after the second course of busulfan. rhIL-3 had no effect on the regeneration of neutrophils postbusulfan, but the absolute number of basophils and eosinophils was significantly higher in the rhIL-3–treated animals compared to controls.

Preclinical studies on normal healthy primates have shown that while IL-3 alone can induce only a modest leukocytosis, it can prime the animals for sustaining a heightened response to the subsequent administration of late-acting factors such as GM-CSF and Epo. This suggests that the optimal clinical regimens may be combinations of hematopoietic growth factors. Following chemotherapy, IL-3 appears to be a potent stimulator of hematopoiesis, and to a certain extent, it can abrogate chemotherapeutically induced cytopenias. No organ toxicity has been reported in IL-3-treated animals. Taken altogether, these studies suggest a promising future for IL-3 treatment of patients at risk for infections resulting from neutropenia or bleeding due to thrombocytopenia.

CLINICAL APPLICATIONS

IL-3 has already progressed from the molecular clone to clinical treatment as phase I–II studies are currently in progress. Three different sources of rhIL-3 are being studied in humans. Yeast-derived IL-3 has been used to treat cancer patients with normal hematopoiesis who were not receiving chemotherapy (155–158), for patients with secondary bone marrow failure (155) with aplastic anemia (159–161), and in myelodysplastic syndromes (162–164). *B. licheniformis* (165) and *E. coli* (166) derived IL-3 have been studied in patients receiving myelosuppressive therapy.

Cancer Patients with Normal Hematopoiesis (Not Receiving Chemotherapy)

Ganser et al. (155) treated patients that had preserved bone marrow function for 15 days with IL-3 at doses ranging from 30 µg/m² to 500 µg/m² (daily subcutaneous bolus injection). During the second week of its administration, dose-dependent increases in platelet counts as well as in WBC and absolute neutrophil counts, monocytes, eosinophils, lymphocytes, and reticulocytes were observed. Basophils increased moderately without reaching pathologic levels. Interestingly, platelet counts continued to rise for an additional week after discontinuing IL-3 treatment, and only returned to baseline levels during the following 2–3 weeks. Treatment with IL-3 led to an overall increase in bone marrow cellularity with trilinear stimulation of hematopoietic cells (155, 156). Significant eosinophilia and in some instances bone marrow fibrosis developed. Administration of IL-3 also effectively increased the percentage of actively cycling granulocyte-erythrocyte-monocyte-megakaryocyte colony-forming units (CFU-GEMM), BFU-E, and CFU-GM at day 14 and CFU-GM at day 7 (158). Moderate increases in circulating GFU-GEMM and GFU-GM at day 14 were seen after 7 days of rhIL-3, but not at the end of treatment (157).

The authors elected to use a dose of 250 $\mu g/m^2$/day in further clinical trials due to its good tolerability and biologic activity even though they did not reach the maximum tolerated dose in their preliminary phase I-II studies. Sequential application of IL-3 for 5 days followed by a 10-day course of GM-CSF increased circulating hematopoietic progenitors more effectively than IL-3 alone (158). Again, this supports the concept that IL-3 primes bone marrow hematopoietic progenitors to proliferate in response to GM-CSF.

Patients with Secondary Bone Marrow Failure

In patients with secondary hematopoietic failure due to previous chemo- or radiotherapy, a multiple lineage response was also observed. Platelet counts increased from 1.3-fold to 14.3-fold in five of eight evaluable patients. Their response was delayed when compared to patients with normal hematopoiesis (155), although the same bone marrow changes were observed in the latter patients (155, 156).

Patients with Aplastic Anemia

Ganser et al. treated nine aplastic anemia patients with IL-3 at doses ranging from 250–500 $\mu g/m^2$/day (given as subcutaneous bolus injection daily) for 15 days (159). In these patients a slight increase in neutrophils, eosinophils, lymphocytes, and monocytes was observed. Increases in platelet numbers appeared in one patient only. There was no correlation between the increase in reticulocyte counts that appears in some patients and an increase in mature erythrocytes. Only 3 of 9 patients with aplastic anemia had increased cellularity of their bone marrow (156, 159), and stimulatory effects of IL-3 were only transient in these patients. Similar results have been reported by Kurzrock et al. (160) and Gillio et al. (161).

Patients with Myelodysplastic Syndromes

In four studies (160–163), stimulation of hematopoiesis in all cell lineages was found in a proportion of patients with myelodysplastic syndromes. IL-3 treatment of a patient with refractory anemia resulted in complete restoration of a nonclonal pattern of peripheral blood cells, while the bone marrow was monoclonal as determined by restriction fragment length polymorphism analysis of the X chromosome genes, phosphoglycerate kinase, and hypoxanthine phosphoribotyl transferase (164). Administration of IL-3 led to an increase in the bone marrow cellularity of all patients, although there was also an increase in the degree of fibrosis (156, 162). In one patient, the percent of blast cells in the bone marrow increased from 2% to 26% (162).

Patients Receiving Myelosuppressive Therapy

Preliminary results of ongoing phase I-II studies have been reported at several meetings. Postmus et al. investigated the effectiveness of IL-3 (*B. licheniformis* derived) in preventing chemotherapy-induced myelo-suppression in patients with relapsed small cell lung cancer undergoing treatment with vincristine, ifosfamide, mesna, and carbopla-tin or cyclophosphamide, doxorubicin, and etoposide (165). They administered IL-3 sub-cutaneously in a daily dose of 1–16 g/kg × 14 days during the first but not the second cycle of chemotherapy. Treatment with IL-3 in the 8–16 μg/kg/day dose significantly ac-celerates the recovery of WBCs, neutrophils, and platelets on day 15 after chemotherapy. de Vries et al. treated 11 ovarian cancer pa-tients with IL-3 (*E. coli* derived) after 1, 3, and 5 cycles of carboplatin and cyclophospha-mide. The patients did not receive IL-3 in cycles 2, 4, and 6 (166). Again, at the 5 μg/kg dose WBC, neutrophil, and platelet recov-ery appeared to be significantly faster in the IL-3-treated patients.

Side Effects

Side effects were mild (155–166), with the most frequent being World Health Or-ganization (WHO) grade II fever often asso-ciated with a flu-like syndrome. Other side effects included flush, local erythema, bone pain, nausea, and vomiting. Patients receiving higher doses (250–500 μg/m^2/day or 8–16 μg/kg) also developed persistent headaches and itching, pleural effusions (160), and atrial fibrillation (160).

CONCLUSIONS AND FUTURE PROSPECTS

The promise of IL-3 treatment shown in preclinical studies appears to be supported by the early clinical trial data reported thus far. The use of IL-3 either as a single agent or combined with other cytokines including G-CSF or IL-6 for the treatment of cancer pa-tients has two potential major benefits: It may reduce the period of neutropenia and throm-bocytopenia, and thus significantly decrease the morbidity associated with conventional chemotherapy, and perhaps improve the re-sponse rate and survival by allowing more intensive chemotherapy regimens with or without bone marrow transplantation. Never-theless, in the setting of autologous bone marrow transplantation, two major limita-tions must be considered. First is the limi-tation on the number and the quality of he-matopoietic stem cells capable of responding to growth factors. Initial clinical studies have already demonstrated that the response to GM-CSF is dramatically reduced in patients pre-treated with intensive chemotherapy or, where the graft was purged in vitro, with 4-hydro-cyclophosphamide (167). It is unlikely that the cytokines will alleviate the problem of insuf-ficient stem cell numbers, of radiochemo-therapy-induced stem cell defects, or of dam-age to the bone marrow microenvironment. The second limitation is the nonhemato-poietic toxicities caused by a majority of in-tensification drugs, which will require a re-definition of the maximum tolerated dose, which currently is only related to myelo-suppression.

Finally, there are two other questions of major concern. Does IL-3 influence the growth of human cancer cells? Since leu-kemic myeloblasts express IL-3 receptors (43, 113, 168), it must be anticipated that in some instances the leukemic cells will be stimu-lated to proliferate. Indeed, IL-3 induces the growth of clonogenic blastic cells from acute nonlymphocytic leukemia patients and in-creases the uptake of thymidine by leukemic myeloblasts (43, 168–170). However, there is not a simple relationship between the pres-ence of the IL-3 receptor and the prolifera-tive response of leukemic cells (41, 43, 168). IL-3 also stimulates the growth of colon (171) and small cell (172, 173) tumor cell lines. Whether these in vitro findings apply to the in vivo situation and whether treatment with IL-3 can render cancer cells more susceptible to cytotoxic chemotherapy remains to be an-swered by forthcoming trials.

The second question concerns the tox-icity of long-term administration of IL-3. Pos-sible complications arising from the excessive production and activation of mature cells and exhaustion of the stem cell compartment should be considered. Although we do not have information concerning this problem in humans, overexpression of IL-3 in murine bone marrow cells transfected with a retrovirus carrying the murine IL-3 gene results in a fatal but nonneoplastic myeloproliferative syndrome (174, 175). This does not exclude the possibility that enhanced proliferation is a preliminary event that can lead to rapid accumulation of other genetic abnormalities. Thus far, depletion of progenitor cells appears unlikely based on the present data from experimental studies in mice and clinical trials with GM-CSF (176).

REFERENCES

1. Ihle JN, Pepersack L, Rebar L. Regulation of T cell differentiation: in vitro induction of 20 alpha hydroxysteroid dehydrogenase in splenic lymphocytes from athymic mice by a unique lymphokine. J Immunol 1981;126:2184–2189.
2. Ihle JN, Keller J, Oroszlan S, et al. Biological properties of homogenous interleukin-3. I: Demonstration of WEHI-3 growth factor activity, mast cell growth factor activity, P-cell stimulating factor activity, colony stimulating factor activity and histamine producing cell stimulating factor activity. J Immunol 1983;131:282–287.
3. Ihle JN. The molecular and cellular biology of interleukin-3. In: Cruse JM, Lewis RE Jr, eds. The year in immunology. New York: Karger, 1989.
4. Plaut M, Pierce JH, Watson CJ, Hanley-Hyde J, Nordan RP, Paul WE. Mast cell lines produce lymphokines in response to cross-linkage of Fc and RI or to calcium ionophores. Nature 1989;339:64–67.
5. Fung MC, Hapel AJ, Ymer S, et al. Molecular cloning of cDNA for murine interleukin-3. Nature 1984; 307:233–237.
6. Yang YC, Ciarletta AB, Temple PA, et al. Human IL-3 (multi-CSF): identification by expression cloning of a novel hematopoietic growth factor related to murine IL-3. Cell 1986;47:3–10.
7. Griffin JD. Clinical applications of colony stimulating factors. Oncology 1988;2:15–21.
8. Yokota T, Lee F, Rennick D, et al. Isolation and characterization of a mouse cDNA clone that expresses mast-cell growth-factor activity in monkey cells. Proc Natl Acad Sci USA 1984;81:1070–1074.
9. Kindler V, Thorens B, de Kossodo S, et al. Stimulation of hematopoiesis in vivo by recombinant bacterial murine interleukin-3. Proc Natl Acad Sci USA 1986;83:1001–1005.
10. Metcalf D, Begley CG, Johnson GR, Nicola NA, Lopez AF, Williamson DJ. Effects of purified bacterially synthesized murine multi-CSF (IL-3) on hematopoiesis in normal adult mice. Blood 1986;68:46–57.
11. Barlow DP, Bucan M, Lehrach H, Hogan BLM, Cough NM. Close genetic and physical linkage between the murine haemopoietic growth factor genes GM-CSF and multi-CSF (IL-3). EMBO J 1987;6:617–623.
12. Le Beau MM, Epstein ND, O'Brien SJ, et al. The interleukin 3 gene is located on human chromosome 5 and is deleted in myeloid leukemias with a deletion of 5q. Proc Natl Acad Sci USA 1987;84:5913–5917.
13. Yang Y-C, Kovacic S, Kriz R, et al. The human genes for GM-CSF and IL3 are closely linked in tandem on chromosome 5. Blood 1988;71:958–961.
14. Van Leeuwen BH, Martinson ME, Webb GC, Young IG. Molecular organization of the cytokine gene cluster, involving the human IL-3, IL-4, IL-5 and GM-CSF genes, on human chromosome 5. Blood 1989; 73:1142–1148.
15. Pettenati MJ, Le Beau MM, Lemons RS, et al. Assignment of CSF-1 to 5q33.1: Evidence for clustering of genes regulating hematopoiesis and for their involvement in the deletion of the long arm of chromosome 5 in myeloid disorders. Proc Natl Acad Sci USA 1987;84:2970–2974.
16. Le Beau MM, Westbrook CA, Diaz MO, et al. Evidence for the involvement of GM-CSF and FMS in the deletion (5q) in myeloid disorders. Science 1986;231:984–987.
17. Jaye M, Howk R, Burgess W, et al. Human endothelial cell growth factor: cloning, nucleotide sequence and chromosome localization. Science 1986;233:541–545.
18. Yarden Y, Escobedo JA, Kuang WJ, et al. Structure of the receptor for platelet-derived growth factor helps define a family of closely related growth factor receptors. Nature 1986;323:226–232.
19. Niemeyer CM, Sieff CA, Mathey-Prevot B, et al. Expression of human interleukin-3 (multi-CSF) is restricted to human lymphocytes and T-cell tumor lines. Blood 1989;73:945–951.
20. Cuturi MC, Anegon I, Sherman F, et al. Production of hematopoietic colony-stimulating factors by human natural killer cells. J Exp Med 1989;169:569–583.
21. Wimperis JZ, Niemeyer CM, Sieff CA, Mathey-Prevot B, Nathan DG, Arceco RJ. Granulocyte-macrophage colony-stimulating factor and interleukin-3 mRNAs are produced by a small fraction of blood mononuclear cells. Blood 1989;74:1525–1530.
22. Ymer SW, Tulker WQ, Saudersou GS, Hapel AJ, Campbell HD, Young IG. Constitutive synthesis of interleukin-3 by leukaemia cell line WEHI-3B is due to retroviral insertion near the gene. Nature 1985;317:255–258.

23. Temeles DS, McGrath HE, Shadduck RK, Quesenberry PJ. Growth factor production by murine Dexter stromal cells. Blood 1989;74(suppl 1):116a.
24. Humphries RK, Kay RJ, Dougherty GJ, et al. Growth factor mRNA in long-term human marrow cultures before and after addition of agents that induce cycling of primitive hemopoietic progenitors. Blood 1988;72(suppl 1):396a.
25. Barge AJ, Johnson GA, Simmons P, Torok-Storb B. Interleukin 3 transcript, bioactivity and protein is detectable in normal bone marrow stroma in the absence of mature T-lymphocytes. Blood 1989; 74(suppl 1):115a.
26. Ernst TJ, Ritchie AR, Stopak KS, Griffin JD. Human monocytes produce IL-3 in response to stimulation with the calcium ionophore A231987. Blood 1989;74(suppl 1):116a.
27. Dalloul AH, Arock M, Fourcade C, et al. Human thymic epithelial cells produce interleukin-3. Blood 1991;77:69–74.
28. Luger TA, Kock A, Kernbauer R, Schwarz T, Ansel JC. Keratinocyte-derived interleukin 3. Ann NY Acad Sci 1988;548:253–261.
29. Farrar WL, Vinocour M, Hill JM. In situ hybridization histochemistry localization of interleukin-3 mRNA in mouse brain. Blood 1989;73:137–140.
30. Palaszynski EW, Ihle JN. Evidence for specific receptors for interleukin-3 on lymphokine-dependent cell lines established from long term bone marrow cultures. J Immunol 1984;132:1872–1879.
31. Sorensen P, Farber NM, Krystal G. Identification of the interleukin-3 receptor using an iodinatable, cleanable, photoreactive cross-linking agent. J Biol Chem 1986;261:9094–9097.
32. May WS, Ihle JN. Affinity isolation of the interleukin-3 surface receptor. Biochem Biophys Res Commun 1986;135:870–879.
33. Nicola NA, Peterson L. Identification of distinct receptors for two hemopoietic growth factors (granulocyte colony-stimulating factor and multipotential colony-stimulating factor) by chemical cross-linking. J Biol Chem 1986;261:12384–12389.
34. Park LS, Friend D, Gillis S, Urdat DL. Characterization of the cell surface receptor for a multi-lineage colony-stimulating factor (CSF-2alpha). J Biol Chem 1986;261:205–210.
35. Itoh N, Yonehara S, Schreurs J, et al. Cloning of an interleukin-3 receptor gene: a member of a distinct receptor gene family. Science 1990;247:324–327.
36. Cosman D, Lyman SD, Idzerda RL, et al. A new cytokine receptor super-family. Trends Biochem Sci 1990;15:265–270.
37. Gesner T, Mufson RA, Turner KJ, Clark SC. Identification through chemical cross-linking of distinct granulocyte-macrophage colony-stimulating factor and interleukin 3 receptors on myeloid leukemic cells, KG-1. Blood 1989;74:2652–2656.
38. Park LS, Friend D, Price V, et al. Heterogeneity in human interleukin-3 receptors. A subclass that binds human granulocyte/macrophage colony stimulating factor. J Biol Chem 1989;264:5420–5427.
39. Taketazu F, Chiba S, Shibuya K, et al. IL-3 specifically inhibits GM-CSF binding to the higher affinity receptor. J Cell Physiol 1991;146:251–257.
40. Oster W, Lindemann A, Mertelsmann R, Herrmann F. Granulocyte-macrophage colony-stimulating factor (CSF) and multilineage CSF recruit human monocytes to express granulocyte CSF. Blood 1989;73:64–68.
41. Onetto-Pothier N, Aumont N, Haman A, Park L, Clark SC, De La Hoang T. IL-3 inhibits the binding of GM-CSF to AML blasts, but the two cytokines act synergistically in supporting blast proliferation. Leukemia 1990;4:329–336.
42. Lopez, AF, Eglington JM, Gillis D, Park LS, Clark S, Vadas MA. Reciprocal inhibition of binding between IL-3 and GM-CSF to human eosinophils. Proc Natl Acad Sci USA 1989;86:7022–7026.
43. Budel EM, Elbaz O, Hoogerbrugge H, et al. Common binding structure for granulocyte-macrophage colony-stimulating factor and interleukin-3 on human acute myeloid leukemia cells and monocytes. Blood 1990;75:1439–1445.
44. Murthy SC, Sorensen PHB, Mui ALF, Krystal G. Interleukin-3 down-regulates its own receptor. Blood 1989;73:1180–1187.
45. Walker, F, Nicola NA, Metcalf D, Burgess AW. Hierarchical down-modulation of hemopoietic growth factor receptors. Cell 1985;43:269–276.
46. Nicola NA. Why do hemopoietic growth factor receptors interact with each other? Immunol Today 1987;8:134–140.
47. Farrar WL, Thomas TP, Anderson WB. Altered cytosol/membrane enzyme redistribution on interleukin-3 activation of protein kinase C. Nature 1985;315:235–237.
48. Evans S, Remick D, Farrar WL. The multilineage haemopoietic growth factor IL-3 and activation of protein kinase C stimulate phosphorylation of common substrates. Blood 1986;68:906–913.
49. Whetton AD, Monk PN, Consalvey SD, Huang SJ, Dexter TM, Downes CP. Interleukin 3 stimulates proliferation via protein kinase C activation without increasing inositol lipid turnover. Proc Natl Acad Sci USA 1988;85:3284–3288.
50. Kelvin DJ, Shreeve M, McCauley C, Mcleod DL, Simard G, Connolly JA. Interleukin-3 stimulated proliferation is sensitive to pertussis toxin: evidence for a guanyl nucleotide regulatory protein-mediated signal transduction mechanism. J Cell Physiol 1989;138:273–280.
51. Isfort RJ, Stevens D, May WS, Ihle JN. Interleukin 3 binds to a 140 kDa phosphotyrosine containing cell surface protein. Proc Natl Acad Sci USA 1988;85:7982–7986.

52. Ferris DK, Willette-Brown J, Martensen T, Farrar WL. Interleukin 3 and phorbol ester stimulate tyrosine phosphorylation of overlapping substrate proteins. FEBS Lett 1989;246:153–158.

53. Schreurs J, Sugawara M, Arai K-I, Ohta Y, Miyajima A. A Monoclonal antibody with IL-3 like activity blocks IL-3 binding and stimulates tyrosine phosphorylation. J Immunol 1989;142:819–825.

54. Kanakura Y, Druker B, Cannistra SA, Furukawa Y, Torimoto Y, Griffin JD. Signal transduction of the human granulocyte-macrophage colony-stimulating factor and interleukin-3 receptors involves tyrosine phosphorylation of a common set of cytoplasmic proteins. Blood 1990;76:706–715.

55. Rennick DM, Lee FD, Yokota T, Arai KI, Cantor H, Nabel GJ. A cloned MCGF cDNA encodes a multilineage hematopoietic growth factor: multiple activites of interleukin-3. J Immunol 1985;134:910–914.

56. Hapel AJ, Fung MC, Johnson RM, Yougn IG, Johnson G, Metcalf D. Biologic properties of molecularly cloned and expressed murine interleukin-3. Blood 1985;65:1453–1459.

57. Clark-Lewis I, Schrader JW. Molecular structure and biological activities of P cell stimulating-factor (interleukin-3) In: Schrader JW, ed. Lymphokines. Vol. 15. San Diego: Academic Press, 1988:1–37.

58. Koike K, Ihle JN, Ogawa M. Macrophage colony formation supported by purified CSF-1 and/or interleukin 3 in serum-free culture: evidence for hierarchical difference in macrophage colony-forming cells. Blood 1986;67:859–864.

59. Chen BD, Clarck CR. Interleukin-3 regulates the in vitro proliferation of both blood monocytes and peritoneal exudate macrophages: synergism between CSF-1 and IL-3. J Immunol 1986;137:563–570.

60. Chen BD-M, Mueller M, Olencki T. Interleukin-3 (IL-3) stimulates the clonal growth of pulmonary alveolar macrophage of the mouse: role of IL-3 in the regulation of macrophage production outside the bone marrow. Blood 1988;72:685–690.

61. Warren DJ, Moore MA. Synergism among interleukin-1, interleukin-3 and interleukin-5 in the production of eosinophils from primitive hemopoietic stem cells. J Immunol 1988;140:94–99.

62. Quesenberry PJ, Ihle JN, McGrath E. The effects of interleukin 3 and GM-CSF on megakaryocyte and myeloid clonal colony formation. Blood 1985;65:214–217.

63. Ishibashi T, Burnstein SA. Interleukin 3 promotes the differentiation of isolated single megakaryocyte. Blood 1986;67:1512–1514.

64. Rennick D, Jackson J, Yang G, Wideman J, Lee F, Hudak S. Interleukin 6 interacts with interleukin 4 and other hematopoietic growth factors to selectively enhance the growth of megakaryocytic, erythroid, myeloid, and multipotential progenitor cells. Blood 1989;73:1828–1835.

65. Lotem J, Shabo Y, Sachs L. Regulation of megakarcyocyte development by interleukin 6. Blood 1989; 74:1545–1551.

66. Suda J, Suda T, Kubota K, Ihle JN, Saito M, Miura Y. Purified interleukin-3 and erythropoietin support the terminal differentiation of hemopoietic progenitors in serum-free culture. Blood 1986; 67:1002–1006.

67. Spivak JL, Smith RR, Ihle JN. Interleukin-3 promotes the in vitro proliferation of murine pluripotent hematopoietic stem cells. J Clin Invest 1985;76:1613–1621.

68. Nakata T, Ogawa M. Identification in culture of a class of hemopoietic colony-forming units with extensive capability to self-renew and generate multipotential hemopoietic colonies. Proc Natl Acad Sci USA 1982;3843–3847.

69. Suda T, Suda J, Ogawa M. Proliferative kinetics and differentiation of murine blast cell colonies in culture: evidence for variable G_0 periods and constant doubling rates of early pluripotent hemopoietic progenitors. J Cell Physiol 1983;117:308–318.

70. Suda T, Suda J, Ogawa M, Ihle JN. Permissive role of interleukin 3 (IL-3) in proliferation and differentiation of multipotential hemopoietic progenitors in culture. J Cell Physiol 1985;124:182–190.

71. Koike K, Ogawa M, Ihle JN, Miyake T, Shimizu T, Miyajima A, Yokota T, Arai KI. Recombinant murine granulocyte-macrophage (GM) colony-stimulating factor supports formation of GM and multipotential blast cell colonies in culture: comparison with the effects of interleukin-3. J Cell Physiol 1987;131:458–464.

72. Koike K, Ihle JN, Ogawa M. Declining sensitivity to interleukin 3 of murine multipotential hemopoietic progenitors during their development. Application to a culture system that favors blast cell colony formation. J Clin Invest 1986;77:894–899.

73. Ikebuchi K, Clark SC, Ihle JN, Souza LM, Ogawa M. Granulocyte colony-stimulating factor enhances interleukin-3 dependent proliferation of multipotential hemopoietic progenitors. Proc Natl Acad Sci USA 1988;85:3445–3449.

74. Migliaccio G, Migliaccio AR, Visser JWM. Synergism between erythropoietin and interleukin-3 in the induction of hematopoietic stem cell proliferation and erythroid burst colony formation. Blood 1988;72:944–951.

75. Iscove NN, Shaw AR, Keller G. Net increase of pluripotent hematopoietic precursors in suspension culture in response to IL-1 and IL-3. J Immunol 1989;142:2332–2337.

76. Rennick D, Yang G, Muller-Sieburg C, Smith C, Arai N, Takabe Y, Gemmell L. Interleukin 4 (B-cell stimulatory factor 1) can enhance or antagonize the factor-dependent growth of hemopoietic progenitor cells. Proc Natl Acad Sci USA 1987;84:6889–6893.

77. Tsuji K, Nakahata T, Takagi M, Kobayashi T, Ishiguro A, Kikuchi T, Naganuma K, Koike K, Miyajima A, Arai K-I, Akabane T. Effects of interleukin-3 and interleukin-4 on the development of "connective tissue-type" mast cells: interleukin-3 supports their proliferation synergistically with interleukin-3. Blood 1990;75:421–427.

78. Ikebuchi K, Wong GG, Clark SC, Ihle JN, Hirai Y, Ogawa M. Interleukin 6 enhancement of interleukin-3 dependent proliferation of multipotential hemopoietic progenitors. Proc Natl Acad Sci USA 1987;84:9035–9039.

79. Bodine DM, Karlsson S, Nienhuis AW. Combination of interleukins 3 and 6 preserves stem cell function in culture and enhances retrovirus-mediated gene transfer into hematopoietic stem cells. Proc Natl Acad Sci USA 1989;86:8897–8901.

80. Larson D, Leary A, Hahn-Cordes L, et al. Interleukin-11 (IL-11) synergizes with IL-3 in promoting human and murine megakaryocyte colony formation in vitro. Blood 1990;76(suppl 1):464a.

81. Stiles GD, Capone GT, Scher CD, Antoniades HN, Van Wyk JJ, Pledger WJ. Dual control of cell growth by somatomedins and platelet-derived growth factor. Proc Natl Acad Sci USA 1979;76:1279–1283.

82. Wharton W. Hormonal regulation of discrete portions of the cell cycle: commitment to DNA synthesis is commitment to cellular division. J Cell Physiol 1983;117:423–429.

83. Razin E, Ihle JN, Seldin D, et al. Interleukin-3: a differentiation and growth factor for the mouse mast cell that contains chondroitin sulfate E proteoglycan. J Immunol. 1984;132:1479–1486.

84. Hamaguchi Y, Kanakura Y, Fujita J, et al. Interleukin 4 as an essential factor for in vitro clonal growth of murine connective tissue type mast cells. J Exp Med 1987;165:268–273.

85. Nakamata T, Kobayashi T, Ishiguro A, et al. Extensive proliferation of mature connective-tissue type mast cells in vitro. Nature 1986;324:65–67.

86. Metcalf D. Multi-CSF dependent colony formation by cells of a murine hematopoietic cell line: specificity and action of multi-CSF. Blood 1985;65:357–362.

87. Whetton AD, Dexter TM. Effect of haematopoietic cell growth factor on intracellular ATP levels. Nature 1983;303:629–631.

88. Whetton AD, Bazil GW, Dexter TM. Haematopoietic cell growth factor mediates cell survival via its action on glucose transport. EMBO J 1984;3:409–413.

89. Williams GT, Smith CA, Spooncer E, Dexter TM, Taylor DR. Haemopoietic colony stimulating factors promote cell survival by suppressing apoptosis. Nature 1990;343:76–79.

90. Crapper RM, Vairon G, Hamilton JA, Clark-Lewis I, Schrader JW. Stimulation of bone marrow-derived and peritoneal macrophages by a T lymphocyte-derived hemopoietic growth factor, persisting cell-stimulating factor. Blood 1985;66:859–866.

91. Bleiberg I, Kletter Y, Riklis I, Fabian I. Induction of murine macrophage fungal killing by interleukin 3. Exp Hematol 1989;17:895–897.

92. Matsuura N, Zetter BR. Stimulation of mast cell chemotaxis by interleukin 3. J Exp Med 1989;170:1421–1426.

93. Aizawa S, Tavassoli M. Marrow uptake of galactosyl-containing neoglycoproteins: implications in stem cell homing. Exp Hematol 1988;16:811–813.

94. Fabian I, Bleiberg I, Riklis I, Kletter Y. Enhanced reconstitution of hematopoietic organs in irradiated mice, following their transplantation with bone marrow cells pretreated with recombinant interleukin 3. Exp Hematol 1987;15:1140–1144.

95. Tavassoli M, Omoto E, Konno M. Up modulation of homing receptors and improvement in grafting efficiency of marrow cells induced by preincubation with IL-3 and GM-CFS. Blood 1989;74(suppl 1):117a.

96. Tavassoli M, Konno M, Shiota Y, Omoto E, Minguell JJ, Zanjani ED. Enhancement of the grafting efficiency of transplanted marrow cells by preincubation with interleukin-3 and granuloycte-macrophage colony-stimulating factor. Blood 1991;77:1599–1606.

97. Lopez AF, To LB, Yang YC, et al. Stimulation of proliferation, differentiation, and function of human cells by primate interleukin 3. Proc Natl Acad Sci USA 1987;84:2761–2765.

98. Burger H, van Leen RW, Dorssers CJ, Persoon NLM, Lemson PJ, Wagemaker G. Species specificity of human interleukin-3 demonstrated by cloning and expression of the homologous rhesus monkey (Macaca mulatta) gene. Blood 1990;76:2229–2234.

99. Sieff CA, Neimeyer CM, Nathan DG, et al. Stimulation of human hematopoietic colony formation by recombinant gibbon multi-colony-stimulating factor of interleukin-3. J Clin Invest 1987;80:818–823.

100. Leary AG, Yang YC, Clark SC, Gasson JC, Golde DW, Ogawa M. Recombinant gibbon interleukin 3 supports formation of human multilineage colonies and blast cell colonies in culture: comparison with recombinant human granulocyte-macrophage colony stimulating factor. Blood 1987;70:1343–1348.

101. Messner HA, Yamasaki K, Jamal N, et al. Growth of human hemopoietic colonies in response to recombinant gibbon interleukin 3: comparison with human recombinant granulocyte and granulocyte-macrophage colony-stimulating factor. Proc Natl Acad Sci USA 1987;84:6765–6769.

102. Emerson SG, Yang YC, Clark SC, Long MW. Human recombinant granulocyte-macrophage colony stimulating factor and interleukin-3 have overlapping but distinct hematopoietic activities. J Clin Invest 1988;82:1282–1287.

103. Sonoda Y, Yang YC, Wong GG, Clark SC, Ogawa M.

Erythroid burst-promoting activity of purified recombinant human GM-CSF and interleukin-3 with anti-GM-CSF and anti-IL3 sera and studies in serum free cultures. Blood 1988;72:1381–1386.

104. Sonoda Y, Yang YC, Wong GG, Clark SC, Ogawa M. Analysis in serum-free culture of the target of recombinant human hemopoietic growth factors: interleukin 3 and granulocyte/macrophage-colony-stimulating factor are specific for early developmental stages. Proc Natl Acad Sci USA 1988;85:4360–4364.

105. Sieff CA, Ekern SC, Nathan DG, Anderson JW. Combinations of recombinant colony-stimulating factors are required for optiimal hematopoietic differentiation in serum-deprived culture. Blood 1989;73:688–693.

106. Migliaccio G, Migliaccio AR, Adamson JW. In vitro differentiation of human granulocyte/macrophage and erythroid progenitors: comparative analysis of the influence of recombinant human erythropoietin, G-CSF, GM-CSF, and IL-3 in serum-supplemented and serum-deprived cultures. Blood 1988; 72:248–256.

107. Mitjavila MT, Natazawa M, Brignaschi P, Debili N, Breton-Gorius J, Vainchenker W. Effects of five recombinant hematopoietic growth factors on enriched human erythroid progenitors in serum-replaced cultures. J Cell Physiol 1989;138:617–623.

108. Saeland S, Caux C, Favre C, et al. Combined and sequential effects of human IL-3 and GM-CSF on the proliferation of CD34+ hematopoietic cells from cord blood. Blood 1989;73:1195–1201.

109. Leary AG, Ikebuchi K, Hirai Y, et al. Synergism between interleukin-6 and interleukin-3 supporting proliferation of human hematopoietic stem cells: comparison with interleukin-1alpha. Blood 1988; 71:1759–1763.

110. McNiece IK, Langley KE, Zsebo KM. Recombinant human stem cell factor synergises with GM-CSF, G-CSF, IL-3 and Epo to stimulate human progenitor cells of the myeloid and erythroid lineages. Exp Hematol 1991;19:226–231.

111. Delwel R, Dorssers L, Touw I, Wagemaker G, Löwenberg B. Human recombinant multilineage colony stimulating factor (interleukin-3): stimulator of acute myelocytic leukemia progenitor cells in vitro. Blood 1987;70:333–336.

112. Saeland S, Caux C, Favre C, et al. Effects of recombinant human interleukin-3 on CD34-enriched normal hematopoietic progenitors and on myeloblastic leukemia cells. Blood 1988;72:1580–1588.

113. Budel LM, Touw IP, Delwel R, Clark SC, Löwenberg B. Interleukin-3 and granulocyte-monocyte colony-stimulating factor receptors on human aute myelocytic leukemia cells and relationship to the proliferative response. Blood 1989;74:565–571.

114. Leary AG, Hirai Y, Kishimoto T, Clark SC, Ogawa M.

Survival of hemopoietic progenitors in the G_0 period of the cell cycle does not require early hemopoietic regulators. Proc Natl Acad Sci USA 1989;86:4535–4538.

115. Bot FJ, van Eijk L, Schipper P, Löwenberg B. Effects of human interleukin-3 on granulocytic colony forming cells in human bone marrow. Blood 1989;73:1157–1160.

116. Elliott MJ, Vadas MA, Eglinton JM, et al. Recombinant human interleukin-3 and granulocyte-macrophage colony-stimulating factor show common biological effects and binding characteristics on human monocytes. Blood 1989;74:2349–2359.

117. Rothenburg ME, Owen WF, Silberstein DA, et al. Human eosinophils have prolonged survival, enhanced functional properties and became hypodense when exposed to human interleukin-3. J Clin Invest 1988;81:1986–1992.

118. Lopez AF, Dyson PG, To LB, et al. Recombinant human interleukin-3 stimulation of hematopoiesis in humans: loss of responsiveness with differentiation in the neutrophilic myeloid series. Blood 1988; 72:1797–1804.

119. Urdal DL, Price V, Sassenfeld HM, Cosman D, Gillis S, Park LS. Molecular characterization of colony-stimulating factors and their receptors: human interleukin-3. Ann NY Acad Sci 1989;554:167–176.

120. Valent P, Besemer J, Liehl E, Stockinger H, Bettelheim P. Expression of interleukin receptors on human eosinophils, basophils and mast cells. Molecular Biotherapy 1989;1(suppl 1):42.

121. Lopez AF, Lyons AB, Eglinton JM, et al. Specific binding of human interleukin-3 and granulocyte-macrophage colony-stimulating factor to human basophils. J Allergy Clin Immunol 1990;85:99–102.

122. Cannistra SA, Vellenga E, Groshek P, Rambaldi A, Griffin JD. Human granulocyte-monocyte colony-stimulating factor and interleukin-3 stimulate monocyte cytotoxicity through a tumor necrosis factor-dependent mechanism. Blood 1988;71:672–676.

123. Vellenga E, Rambaldi A, Ernst TJ, Ostapovicz D, Griffin JD. Independent regulation of M-CSF and G-CSF gene expression in human monocytes. Blood 1988; 71:1529–1532.

124. Kolb E, Muller EM. Local responses in primary and secondary human lung cancers. II: Clinical correlations. Br J Cancer 1979;40:410–416.

125. Pastrnak A, Jansa P. Local eosinophilia in stroma of tumors related to prognosis. Neoplasma 1984;31:323–326.

126. Pretlow TP, Keith EF, Cryar AK, et al. Eosinophil infiltration of human colonic carcinomas as a prognostic indicator Cancer Res 1983;43:2997–3000.

127. Valent P, Schmidt G, Besemer J, et al. Interleukin-3 is a differentiation factor for human basophils. Blood 1989;73:1763–1769.

128. MacDonald SM, Schleimer RP, Kagey-Sobotka A, Gillis S, Lichtenstein LM. Recombinant IL-3 induces histamine release from human basophils. J Immunol 1989;142:3527–3532.

129. Alam R, Welter JB, Forsythe PA, Lett-Brown MA, Grant JA. Comparative effect of recombinant IL-1,2,3,4 and 6, IFN-gamma, granulocyte-macrophage-colony-stimulating factor, tumor necrosis factor-alpha and histamine-releasing factors on the secretion of histamine from basophils. J Immunol 1989;142:3431–3435.

130. Bischoff SC, de Weck AL, Dahinden CA. Interleukin-3 and granulocyte/macrophage-colony-stimulating factor render human basophils responsive to low concentrations of complement component C3a. Proc Natl Acad Sci USA 1990;87:6813–6817.

131. Kurimoto Y, De Weck AL, Dahinden CA. Interleukin-3 dependent mediator release in basophils triggered by C5a. J Exp Med 1989;170:467–479.

132. Matsuura N, Zetter BR. Stimulation of mast cell chemotaxis by interleukin 3. J Exp Med 1989; 170:1421–1426.

133. Kindler V, Thorens B, De Kossodo S, et al. Stimulation of hematopoiesis in vivo by recombinant bacterial murine interleukin-3. Proc Natl Acad Sci USA 1986;83:1001–1005.

134. Metcalf D, Glenn Begley C, Nicola NA, Johnson GR. Quantitative responsiveness of murine hemopoietic populations in vitro and in vivo to recombinant multi-CSF (IL-3). Exp Hematol 1987;15:288–295.

135. Carrington PA, Hill RJ, Stenberg PE, et al. Multiple in vivo effects of interleukin-3 and interleukin-6 on murine megakaryocytopoiesis. Blood 1991;77:34–41.

136. Metcalf D, Begley CG, Johnson GR. Hemopoietic effects of purified bacterially synthesized multi-CSF in normal and marrow-transplanted mice. Immunobiology 1986;172:158–164.

137. Lord BR, Molineux B, Testa NG, Kelly M, Spoonler E, Dexter TM. The kinetic response of haemopoietic precursor cells in vivo, to highly purified, recombinant interleukin-3. Lymphokine Res 1986; 5:97–104.

138. Broxmeyer HE, Williams DE, Cooper S, et al. Comparative effects in vivo of recombinant murine interleukin 3, natural murine colony-stimulating factor-1 and recombinant murine granulocyte-macrophage colony-stimulating factor on myelopoiesis in mice. J Clin Invest 1987;79:721–730.

139. Williams DE, Hangoc G, Cooper S, et al. The effects of purified recombinant murine interleukin-3 and/or purified natural murine CSF-1 in vivo on the proliferation of murine high- and low- proliferative potential colony-forming cells: demonstration of in vivo synergism. Blood 1987;70:401–403.

140. Broxmeyer HE, Williams DE, Hangoc G, Cooper S, Gillis S, Shadduck RK, Bicknell DC. Synergistic myelopoietic actions in vivo after administration to mice of combinations of purified natural murine colony-stimulating factor 1, recombinant murine interleukin 3, and recombinant murine granulocyte/macrophage colony-stimulating factor. Proc Natl Acad Sci USA 1987;84:3871–3875.

141. Kimoto M, Kindler V, Higaki M, Ody C, Izui S, Vassalli P. Recombinant murine IL-3 fails to stimulate T or B lymphopoiesis in vivo but enhances immune responses to T cell-dependent antigens. J Immunol 1988;140:1889–1894.

142. Carrington PA, Hill RJ, Levin J, Verotta D. Effects of interleukin-3 and interleukin-6 on platelet recovery in mice treated with 5-fluorouracil. Blood 1990; 76(suppl 1), 451a.

143. Metcalf D, Nicola NA. Tissue localization and fate in mice of injected multipotential colony-stimulating factor. Proc Natl Acad Sci USA 1988;85:3160–3164.

144. Donahue RE, Seehra J, Metzger M, et al. Human IL-3 and GM-CSF act synergistically in stimulating hematopoiesis in primates. Science 1988;241:1820–1823.

145. Krumwieh D, Seiler FR. In vivo effects of recombinant colony stimulating factors on hematopoiesis in cynomolgus monkeys. Transplant Proc 1989; 21:2964–2967.

146. Mayer P, Valent P, Schmidt G, Liehl E, Bettelheim P. The in vivo effects of recombinant human interleukin-3: demonstration of basophil differentiation factor, histamine-producing activity, and priming of GM-CSF-responsive progenitors in nonhuman primates. Blood 1989;74:613–621.

147. Krumwieh D, Weinmann E, Seiler FR. Human recombinant derived IL-3 and GM-CSF in hematopoiesis of normal cynomolgus monkeys. Behring Inst Mitt 1988;83:250–257.

148. Umemura T, Al-Khatti A, Donahue RE, Papayannopoulou Th, Stamatoyannopoulos G. Effects of interleukin-3 and erythropoietin on in vivo erythropoiesis and F-cell formation in primates. Blood 1989;74:1571–1576.

149. Geissler K, Valent P, Mayer P, et al. Recombinant human interleukin-3 expands the pool of circulating hemopoietic progenitor cells in primates—synergism with recombinant human granulocyte/macrophage colony-stimulating factor. Blood 1990; 75:2305–2310.

150. Wagemaker G, van Gils F CJM, Burger H, et al. Highly increased production of bone marrow-derived blood cells by administration of homologous interleukin-3 to rhesus monkeys. Blood 1990;76:2235–2241.

151. Krumwieh D, Weinmann E, Siebold B, Seiler FR. Preclinical studies on synergistic effects of IL-1, IL-3, G-CSF and GM-CSF in cynomolgus monkeys. Int J Cell Cloning 1990;8:229–248.

152. Winton EF, Rozmiarek SK, Jacobs PC, et al. Marked increase in marrow and peripheral blood multi-lin-

eage and megakaryocyte progenitor cells induced by short-course sequential recombinant human IL-3/GM-CSF in a non-human primate. Blood 1990; 76(suppl 1):172a.

153. Gillio AP, Gasparetto C, Laver J, Abboud M, Bonilla MA, Garnick MB, O'Reilly RJ. Effects of interleukin-3 on hematopoietic recovery after 5-fluorouracil or cyclophosphamide treatment of cynomolgus primates. J Clin Invest 1990;85:1560–1565.

154. Zeidler C, Krumwieh D, Seiler F, Welte K. Effects of recombinant human interleukin-3 (rhIL-3) in chemotherapy induced myelosuppression in primates. Blood 1988;72(suppl 1):140a.

155. Ganser A, Lindemann A, Seipelt G, et al. Effect of recombinant human interleukin-3 in patients with normal hematopoiesis and in patients with bone marrow failure. Blood 1990;76:666–676.

156. Falk S, Seipelt G, Ganser A, Ottmann OG, Hoelzer D, Stutte HJ, Hubner K. Bone marrow findings after treatment with recombinant human interleukin-3. Am J Clin Pathol 1991;95:355–362.

157. Ottmann OG, Ganser A, Seipelt G, Eder M, Schulz G, Hoelzer D. Effects of recombinant human interleukin-3 on human hematopoietic progenitor and precursor cells in vivo. Blood 1990;76:1494–1502.

158. Ganser A, Lindemann A, Seipelt G, et al. Synergistic effects of sequential IL-3/GM-CSF treatment in comparison to IL-3 alone in vivo. Blood 1990; 76(suppl 1):145a.

159. Ganser A, Lindemann A, Seipelt G, et al. Effects of recombinant human interleukin-3 in aplastic anemia. Blood 1990;76:1287–1292.

160. Kurzrock R, Talpaz M, Salewski E, Gutterman JU. Phase I study of recombinant human interleukin-3 in patients with bone marrow failure. Blood 1989;74(suppl 1):154a.

161. Gillio AP, Castro-Malaspina H, Gasparetto C, et al. A phase I trial of recombinant human interleukin-3 in patients with myelodysplastic syndrome and aplastic anemia [Abstract]. Blood 1990;76(suppl 1):145a.

162. Ganser A, Seipelt G, Lindemann A, et al. Effects of recombinant human interleukin-3 in patients with myelodysplastic syndromes. Blood 1990;76:455–462.

163. Dunbar CE, Smith D, Kimball J, Garrison L, Nienhuis AW, Young NS. Sequential treatment with recombinant human growth factors to compare activity of GM-CSF and IL-3 in the treatment of primary myelodysplasia [Abstract]. Blood 1990;76(suppl 1): 141a.

164. Ganser A, Bartram CR, Ottmann OG, et al. Stimulation of non-clonal hematopoiesis in patients with hematological disorders by recombinant human GM-CSF or interleukin-3. Blood 1990;76(suppl 1):144a.

165. Postmus PE, Gietema JA, Damsma O, Willemse PHB,

de Vries EGE, Vellenga E. Phase I trial of rh-interleukin-3 (IL-3) s.c. in patients (PTS) with relapse of small cell lung cancer (SCLC) treated with chemotherapy (CT). Proc Am Soc Clin Oncol 1991; 10:248.

166. de Vries EGE, Biesma B, Willemse PHB, et al. Efficacy, tolerability and pharmacokinetics of rhIL-3 for patients (PTS) with chemotherapy (CT). Proc Am Soc Clin Oncol 1991;10:194.

167. Blazar BR, Kersey JH, McGlave PB, et al. In vivo administration of recombinant human granulocyte/macrophage colony-stimulating factor in acute lymphoblastic leukemia patients receiving purged autografts. Blood 1989;73:849–857.

168. Park LS, Waldron PE, Friend D, et al. Interleukin-3, GM-CSF, and G-CSF receptor expression on cell lines and primary leukemia cells: receptor heterogeneity and relationship to growth factor responsiveness. Blood 1989;74:56–65.

169. Miryauchi J, Kelleher CA, Yang YC, et al. The effects of three recombinant growth factors, IL-3, GM-CSF and G-CSF on the blast cells of acute myeloblastic leukemia maintained in short-term suspension culture. Blood 1987;70:657–663.

170. Vellenga E, Ostapovicz, O'Rourke B, Griffin JD. Effects of recombinant IL-3, GM-CSF and G-CSF on proliferation of leukemic clonogenic cells in short-term and long-term cultures. Leukemia 1987;1:584–589.

171. Berdel WE, Danhause-Riedl S, Steinhauser G, Winton EF. Various human hematopoietic growth factors (interleukin-3, GM-CSF, G-CSF) stimulate clonal growth of nonhematopoietic tumor cells. Blood 1989;73:80–83.

172. Vellenga E, Biesma B, Meyer C, Wagteveld L, Esselink M, de Vries EGE. The effects of five hematopoietic growth factors on human small cell lung carcinoma cell lines: interleukin-3 enhances the proliferation in one of the eleven cell lines. Cancer Res 1991;51:73–76.

173. Pedrazzoli P, Zibera C, Gibelli N, Bacciocchi G, della Cuna GR, Cazzola M. GM-CSF and IL-3 stimulate proliferation of small cell lung cancer (SCLC) cells [Abstract]. Blood 1990;76(suppl 1):160a.

174. Chang JM, Metcalf D, Lang RA, Gonda TJ, Johnson GR. Nonneoplastic hematopoietic myeloproliferative syndrome induced by dysregulated multi-CSF (IL-3) expression. Blood 1989;73:1487–1497.

175. Wong PMC, Chung SW, Dunbar CE, Bodine DM, Ruscetti S, Nienhuis AW. Retrovirus-mediated transfer and expression of the interleukin-3 gene in mouse hematopoietic cells result in a myeloproliferative disorder. Mol Cell Biol 1989;9:798–808.

176. Lord BI, Dexter TL. Will treatment with haematopoietic growth factors deplete progenitors cells? Focus Growth Factor 1990;1(3):1–2.

22

ERYTHROPOIETIN IN HIGH-DOSE CHEMOTHERAPY

Carole B. Miller

Erythropoietin is a single-chain glyco-protein hormone produced mainly by the peritubular cells of the kidneys in response to hypoxia (1–3). A small amount of erythropoietin is produced in the adult liver. Erythropoietin has a very restricted range of target cell activity. It stimulates the growth and differentiation of both primitive erythroid progenitors (burst-forming units-erythroid [BFU-E]) and committed erythroid progenitors (colony-forming units-erythroid [CFU-E]) (3, 4). In contrast to other circulating mature blood cells that require interaction with their growth factors for function, mature red blood cells lack receptors for erythropoietin, and the hormone cannot affect the mature progeny of stimulated erythroid progenitors (3).

In patients with iron deficiency anemia or hemolytic anemia (5, 6), there is an inverse relationship between the erythropoietin level measured in the serum by a sensitive immunoassay and the degree of anemia (Fig. 22.1). In patients with end stage renal disease, this relationship between erythropoietin level and anemia is lost when the serum creatinine rises above 1.5 mg/dl (7). However, even in anephric patients, erythropoietin is never absent from plasma.

CHEMOTHERAPY-INDUCED ANEMIA

Anemia is common in patients with cancer (8) and often worsens with chemo-therapy. The anemia associated with malignancy and chemotherapy is a normochromic, normocytic anemia associated with an inadequate reticulocyte response (9). The hematologic picture is similar to that of the anemia of chronic renal failure. Similarly to patients with chronic renal failure (7), patients with cancer have an inadequate erythropoietin response to anemia (10). When patients with cancer were compared to iron-deficient controls, for any degree of anemia, the erythropoietin response in the cancer patients was significantly lower than the controls. This decreased erythropoietin response to anemia was more pronounced in the 45 patients who were treated with chemotherapy; however, there was no difference in patients treated with or without a regimen containing cisplatin. The observed decreased erythropoietin response to anemia was not related to clinical evidence of nephrotoxicity. The etiology for the decreased erythropoietin response to anemia is unknown but may be related to direct inhibition by chemotherapy (11) or by cytokine release.

Anemias associated with an inadequate erythropoietin response similar to the anemia of cancer and chemotherapy have responded to treatment with recombinant human erythropoietin (rHuEPO). Both the anemia of chronic renal failure (12, 13) and the anemia associated with human immuno-

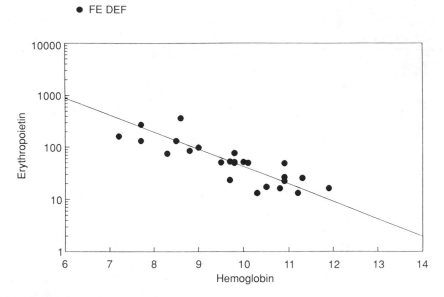

Figure 22.1.   Erythropoietin-hemoglobin relationship in 27 uncomplicated deficiency anemia patients.

deficiency virus and zidovudine therapy (14) have shown decreased transfusion requirement with rHuEPO therapy. Similarly, the anemia associated with cancer appears to be responsive to rHuEPO. Oster et al. (15) reported on 6 patients with neoplastic bone marrow infiltration related to low-grade lymphoma (5) or multiple myeloma (1) who were transfusion dependent prior to rHuEPO treatment. Four of 6 patients did not require transfusion during rHuEPO therapy, and there was a significant increase in hemoglobin over baseline during the study period (P = .03). Ludwig et al. (16) described the treatment with rHuEPO of 13 patients with anemia related to multiple myeloma. rHuEPO was given at a dose of 150 units/kg three times a week subcutaneously with dose escalation by 50 units/kg every 3 weeks. Eleven patients responded with at least a 2 g/dl increase in hemoglobin at a median of 5 weeks of treatment. Both reticulocyte count and erythroid progenitor population in the bone marrow increased significantly; however, there was no significant change in the granulocyte progenitors

in the marrow. These studies suggest that rHuEPO may be useful in patients with anemia associated with cancer and neoplastic bone marrow infiltration.

Patients with chemotherapy-induced anemia have shown responses to treatment with rHuEPO. Henry et al. (17) reported on a multicenter trial of rHuEPO given three times a week subcutaneously at a dose of 150 units/kg for 8 weeks compared to placebo in the treatment of chemotherapy-induced anemia. A total of 135 patients treated with cisplatin-containing regimens and 159 patients treated with regimens not containing cisplatin were randomized. Preliminary analysis shows an increase in hematocrit and decreased transfusion requirement in the rHuEPO-treated patients.

We participated in a phase I/II trial of rHuEPO in chemotherapy-induced anemia (18–20). Forty-nine patients were treated with escalating doses (25, 50, 100, 200, and 300 units/kg) of rHuEPO given intravenously five times a week for 4 weeks. Patients were grouped into patients with or without cisplatin as part of their chemotherapeutic regimen. Maximal responses were seen in both arms at the 100 and 200 units/kg dose levels, with 70% of the patients treated at these dose levels responding with increase in hemoglobin of greater than 1 g/dl over the 4 weeks without transfusion. Hemoglobin change from baseline is shown in Figure 22.2. These patients continued on their chemotherapeutic regimens during the rHuEPO therapy, and the increase in the hemoglobin seen in the responders was not related to normal marrow recovery from chemotherapy. Time course of hemoglobin response to rHuEPO in two patients is shown in Figure 22.3. Patients tolerated rHuEPO well without significant toxicity. There was not a clinically significant effect of rHuEPO seen on blood pressure in the patients with chemotherapy-induced anemia (Fig. 22.4), as had been seen in patients with end stage renal disease treated with rHuEPO. These

data suggest that rHuEPO is a safe, effective therapy for chemotherapy-induced anemia.

ERYTHROPOIETIN AFTER BONE MARROW TRANSPLANT

High-dose chemotherapy with bone marrow transplantation can successfully treat high-risk patients with leukemia (21–24) and lymphoma (25, 26). Anemia is universal after both autologous and allogeneic bone marrow transplantation, and red blood cell transfusion is common in the posttransplant period. The etiology of the anemia after bone marrow transplantation is multifactorial, with both increased utilization and inadequate production of red blood cells playing roles.

Increased utilization of red blood cells occurs as a result of toxicities of the chemotherapy and immunosuppression. Bleeding is common after bone marrow transplan-

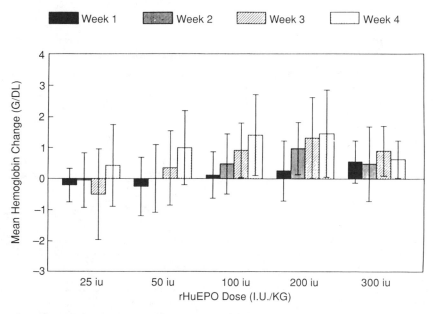

Figure 22.2. Hemoglobin change from pretreatment (mean ± standard deviation) in 49 chemotherapy patients receiving rHuEPO five times a week for 4 weeks at doses of 25, 50, 100, 200, or 300 units/kg intravenously. Patients who required red blood cell transfusion were censored at time of transfusion. There was a significant hemoglobin increase from baseline at the 100-unit/kg dose level after 4 weeks and at the 200-unit/kg dose level after 3 and 4 weeks of treatment.

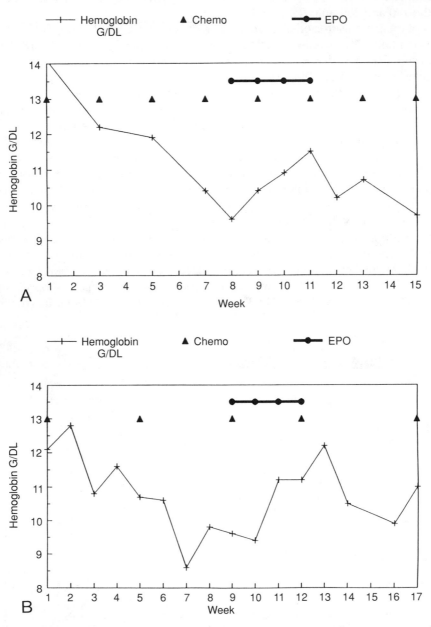

Figure 22.3. Hemoglobin response of two individual patients to intravenous rHuEPO five times a week for 4 weeks. Chemotherapy cycles are represented by *triangles,* rHuEPO administration by *closed circles.* Progressive anemia is shown in both patients in association with chemotherapeutic cycles preceding rHuEPO. An increase in hemoglobin is seen in association with rHuEPO treatment despite continued chemotherapy. **A,** rHuEPO dose 200 units/kg, cisplatin-based chemotherapeutic regimen. **B,** rHuEPO dose 100 units/kg, chemotherapeutic regimen that did not contain cisplatin.

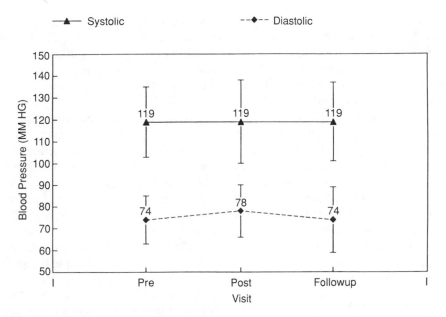

Figure 22.4. Mean ± standard deviation blood pressure measurements in 49 patients treated with rHuEPO pretreatment, at the completion of 4 weeks of rHuEPO and at follow-up 4 weeks after last dose of rHuEPO.

tation both as a result of thrombocytopenia and of direct organ toxicities. Hemorrhagic cystitis (27–31) is a common complication seen after bone marrow transplantation, caused by a metabolite of cyclophosphamide (acrolein) (27) that is directly toxic to the bladder mucosa and viral infections including adenovirus (32) and BK virus (30). Hemorrhagic cystitis occurs in 10% to 40% of patients after bone marrow transplant and when severe in approximately 25% of the cases can cause massive hemorrhage with marked increase in transfusion requirements. Gastrointestinal blood loss related to graft-versus-host disease, viral infections, and gastritis is an important source of blood loss in these patients (33, 34). Thrombocytopenia contributes to excess blood loss and may be related to decreased production, which may be protracted in patients after autologous bone marrow transplant with chemically purged marrow grafts (23, 35), immune mechanisms (36–38), or idiopathic refractoriness related to venoocclusive disease of the liver (39).

Another cause of anemia in this popu-lation is increased destruction of red blood cells by hemolysis related to blood group incompatibility (40, 41), microangiopathy associated with drugs (cyclosporine A) (42), or idiopathic hemolytic uremic syndrome (43).

Inadequate production of red blood cells is a primary cause of anemia after bone marrow transplant. After the marrow graft is infused, there is a period of time when the marrow stem cell reserve is decreased (44, 45) and the erythroid producing cells are repopulating the marrow (46). This is demonstrated by a period of reticulocytopenia (46), which is dependent on the type of marrow graft. In patients after autologous bone marrow transplant with marrow purged with 4-hydroperoxycyclophosphamide (4HC), time to recovery of reticulocytes to greater than 2% is 36.4 ± 7.3 days (47) and is correlated with hematopoietic progenitor recovery in vitro after treatment with 4HC (47). The time to reticulocyte recovery is generally earlier (24–28 days) in patients who receive unmanipulated autologous marrow grafts (48). After allogeneic bone marrow transplant, the recovery of granulocytes is generally within 3 to 4 weeks after marrow infusion (21, 24); however, erythroid recovery is often delayed despite adequate erythroid progenitors present in the marrow as early as 2 weeks after marrow reinfusion (45, 49). The median time to a reticulocyte count of greater than 2% in 50 consecutive patients after allogeneic bone marrow transplant at Johns Hopkins was 31 days, whereas the median time to 500 neutrophils in the same patients was 17.5 days. The number of red blood cell transfusions administered after bone marrow transplants is variable. Tables 22.1 and 22.2 demonstrate transfusion requirements in different centers for allogeneic and autologous transplants. For each type of transplant, a number of factors may influence the transfusion requirement, including treatment and incidence of graft-versus-host disease, preparative and purging regimens, and viral infections. Also, recipient-donor blood group compatibility is an important predictor of the red blood cell transfusion requirement. In a study of 81 patients with aplastic anemia receiving allografts (50), the median number of red blood cell units transfused after transplant was 4.5, 12, and 17.5 units in ABO compatible, minor incompatible, and major incompatible transplants, respectively. In this cohort of patients, the only other predictor of an increased red blood cell transfusion requirement was older recipient age.

While many factors influence erythroid recovery after bone marrow transplantation, the prolonged reticulocytopenia and resultant large transfusion requirement after bone marrow transplantation is in part related to a relative erythropoietin deficiency at a time of marrow recovery. Birgegard et al. (51) described an increased erythropoietin response without anemia immediately after cytotoxic therapy; however, the levels fell over subsequent weeks despite the patient's developing anemia. Others have reported similar findings of increased erythropoietin levels immediately following high-dose chemotherapy, which peak approximately 1 week after bone marrow reinfusion (52–55). The etiology for this early rise in erythropoietin level without anemia is unknown but appears to be consistent between centers and regimens.

The erythropoietin response to anemia later after bone marrow transplantation is less consistent between reports. Schapira et al. (53) reported on the erythropoietin response in 31 patients after autologous bone marrow transplantation (n = 14) or allogeneic bone marrow transplantation (n = 17) compared to a reference population of 11 people with normal hematocrits and 16 patients with aplastic anemia or myelodysplastic syndrome. By 4 weeks after cytotoxic therapy, the erythropoietin response to anemia was markedly depressed in patients compared to con-

Table 22.1. Red Blood Cell Transfusion after Autologous Bone Marrow Transplantation[a]

Reference	No. Patients	Disease	Units RBC
Davis (64)	20	AML	30 ± 29
	20	LY	14 ± 8
Benson (65)	10	BR	12.7 (8–17)
	9	ST, AL, LY	21.7 (8–43)
Ireland (55)	6	ST, AL, LY	9
Schapira (53)	14	ST, LY, ST, BR	12 ± (8–19)
Blazer (66)	50	AL	8 (3–16)
Carey (25)	34	LY	4 (0–21)

[a]Abbreviations: AL, acute Leukemia; BR, breast; LY, lymphoma; RBC, red blood cell; ST, solid tumor.

Table 22.2. Red Blood Cell Transfusion after Allogeneic Bone Marrow Transplantation[a]

Reference	No. Patients	Disease	Units RBC
Johns Hopkins	50	Al, CML	21
Storb (67)	20	AA	15 (3–37)
	20	AL	10.5 (3–25)
	12	CML	18.2 (7–42)
Ireland (55)	11	CML, AL	12.6
Schapira (53)	17	CML, AL, LY	8 ± 4 (0–17)
Abedi (54)	36	CML, AL	13 (2–52) TCD 4 (0–14)
Petz (68)	125	AL, CML	6.6

[a]Abbreviations: AA, aplastic anemia; AL, acute leukemia; CML, chronic myelogenous leukemia; LY, lymphoma; RBC, red blood cell; TCD, T cell depleted.

trols. Renal insufficiency was only seen in 1 patient in this group. They did not describe any difference in the erythropoietin response of patients after allogeneic bone marrow transplant versus that of patients after autologous bone marrow transplant or in association with amphotericin use or liver function test abnormalities. Beguin et al. (49) described the erythropoietin response in 24 patients after bone marrow transplantation (14 allogeneic and 10 autologous). They found that the erythropoietin response to anemia in patients undergoing autologous bone marrow transplant was not different than in controls; however, in the allogeneic bone marrow transplant group, there was an inadequate erythropoietin response to anemia that persisted up to a year after transplant. While there was greater evidence of nephrotoxicity in the allogeneic bone marrow transplant patients compared to the autologous bone marrow transplant patients, there was not a significant correlation between renal function and impairment in the erythropoietin response to anemia. The erythropoietin response to anemia was lower in patients with acute graft-versus-host disease, but chronic graft-versus-host disease did not appear to effect erythropoietin responses. Cytomegalovirus infection was an independent predictor of an impaired erythropoietin response to anemia. They did not find a correlation between cyclosporine A levels or duration of therapy with cyclosporine A and the erythropoietin response to anemia.

Abedi et al. (54) did find that erythropoietin levels were lower in patients who had received cyclosporine as prophylaxis for graft-versus-host disease compared to patients receiving T cell depletion. However, they did not find a correlation between acute graft-versus-host disease and a decreased erythropoietin level. While patients with nephrotoxicity had lower erythropoietin levels than patients without nephrotoxicity, the decreased erythropoietin levels in the cyclosporine A treated patients was seen in patients with and without renal impairment. We

studied the erythropoietin response in 70 patients after bone marrow transplantation compared with the erythropoietin response to anemia in iron-deficient controls (56). Patient characteristics are summarized in Table 22.3. The typical patterns of erythropoietin response after bone marrow transplant in two patients are shown in Figure 22.5. Patient A underwent autologous bone marrow transplantation for acute myelogenous leukemia. The typical early erythropoietin elevation without significant anemia is demonstrated. The erythropoietin levels fell over the subsequent weeks without a significant change in hemoglobin levels. In patient B, who underwent an allogeneic transplant for chronic myelogenous leukemia, a similar pattern is seen early after transplant. In the later posttransplant course, severe liver dysfunction in association with acute graft-versus-host disease developed. The markedly increased erythropoietin level is related to a rise in bilirubin, as will be discussed later.

When the whole group of transplant patients is considered, erythropoietin levels were appropriate for hemoglobin pretransplant. At the time of bone marrow reinfusion after the cytotoxic therapy, erythropoietin levels were markedly elevated even without anemia, and there was no correlation between erythro-

Table 22.3. Patient Characteristics[a]

BMT Type	Allogeneic	42
	Autologous	28
Sex	Male	40
	Female	30
Disease	Acute myelogenous leukemia	22
	Chronic myelogenous leukemia	23
	Acute lymphocytic leukemia	9
	Non-Hodgkin's lymphoma	13
	Hodgkin's lymphoma	2
Prep	BU-CY	28
	CY-TBI	31
	BU-CY-VP16	11

[a]Abbreviations: BU- CY, busulfan 4 mg/kg/day for 4 days, cyclophosphamide 40 mg/kg/day for 4 days; BU-CY-VP16, busulfan 4 mg/k/day for 4 days, cytoxan 50 mg/kg/day for 3 days overlapping with etoposide 10 mg/kg/day for 3 days; CY-TBI, cyclophosphamide 50 mg/kg/day for 4 days, total body irradiation (300 rad/day for 4 days).

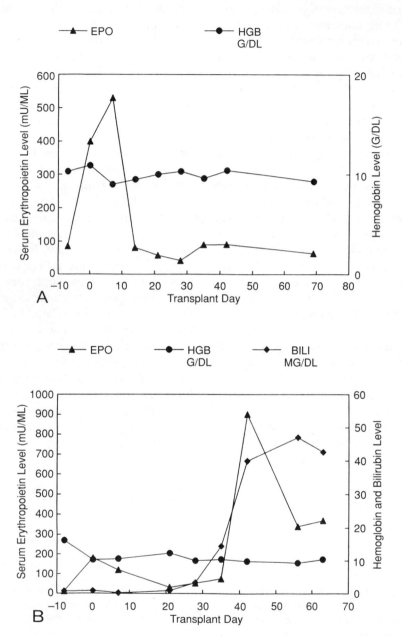

Figure 22.5. Erythropoietin and hemoglobin levels in two patients after bone marrow transplantation. **A**, Patient with acute myelogenous leukemia after autologous transplant. **B**, Patient with chronic myelogenous leu- kemia after allogeneic transplant. She developed severe liver disease and bilirubin elevation in association with refractory acute graft-versus-host disease.

poietin and hemoglobin levels. The marked erythropoietin elevation was independent of the transplant-conditioning regimen, use of radiation therapy, of type of transplant (allogeneic versus autologous) and persisted for approximately 2 weeks after conclusion of the high-dose cytotoxic chemotherapy. The etiology for this increase is unknown and appears unrelated to hepatotoxicity.

Over the next 2 weeks, erythropoietin levels in most patients decreased. At weeks 4 and 5 after transplant, the expected inverse relationship between hemoglobin and erythropoietin levels controls was again not seen. Instead, erythropoietin levels were only correlated with bilirubin levels, and patients with elevated bilirubin showed a marked increase in erythropoietin levels ($P = .001$). The increased erythropoietin levels in association with hepatic dysfunction after bone marrow transplant is similar to the extreme elevations in erythropoietin levels that is seen in anephric renal failure patients who develop hepatitis (57, 58). When bone marrow transplant patients with hyperbilirubinemia were excluded (serum bilirubin greater than 2 mg/dl), at the time of projected marrow recovery, for any given degree of anemia, erythropoietin levels were depressed in both allogeneic and autologous bone marrow transplant patients compared to those of iron-deficient controls. This depressed erythropoietin response to anemia was not related to clinical nephrotoxicity. In contrast to others as described above, we did not find any difference in the erythropoietin response to anemia in allogeneic versus autologous transplants at our center. Within the allogeneic bone marrow transplant patients, the erythropoietin response to anemia was more severely depressed in patients with acute graft-versus-host disease compared to patients without acute graft-versus-host disease.

This depressed erythropoietin response to anemia persisted up to 1 year after bone marrow transplant. Sixty percent of the patients seen at the 6-month follow-up visit remained anemic (hemoglobin < 11 g/dl).

Allogeneic bone marrow transplant patients were more likely to be anemic at the 6-month visit than autologous bone marrow transplant patients (20 of 28 versus 4 of 13, $P = .01$). The erythropoietin response to anemia in the anemic patients remained markedly depressed compared to that of iron-deficient controls. While only a small percentage of patients were anemic at the 12-month visit, anemic patients continued to respond with an inappropriately low erythropoietin response for the degree of anemia.

These data in conjunction with others suggest that at the time of erythroid recovery, there is inadequate stimulation of erythroid progenitors due to inappropriately low endogenous erythropoietin levels. The etiology for the inadequate erythropoietin response to anemia is not known but may be related to toxic effect on erythropoietin-producing cells due to drugs or infections or may be related to direct suppression of erythropoietin production by cytokines. Tumor necrosis factor levels are often elevated after bone marrow transplant (59). Cytokines, including tumor necrosis factor, can suppress erythropoietin production in Hep3B cell lines (60). Regardless of the etiology, the inadequate erythropoietin response to anemia after bone marrow transplant suggests that exogenous rHuEPO treatment may be beneficial in patients after bone marrow transplant.

USE OF RECOMBINANT HUMAN ERYTHROPOIETIN AFTER BONE MARROW TRANSPLANTATION

The use of rHuEPO after bone marrow transplantation is still in the very early stages of investigation. Link et al. (61) reported preliminary data showing an increased reticulocyte count and decreased time of red blood cell transfusion support in 12 patients treated with rHuEPO after allogeneic bone marrow transplant compared to 44 historical controls. Two dose schedules were used in this trial: 150 units/kg two times a week and 100 units/kg by continuous infusion.

We have now completed treatment of 10 adult patients after HLA-matched related allogeneic bone marrow transplant for chronic myelogenous leukemia, acute lymphocytic leukemia, and acute myelogenous leukemia in an ongoing pilot trial (62). We compared transfusion requirements in patients treated with rHuEPO to the 50 consecutive adult allogeneic bone marrow transplant patients transplanted for the same diseases in the preceding 18 months. rHuEPO was given intravenously five times a week at a dose of 100 units/kg starting day 5 after bone marrow transplant. Dosing was changed to 150 units/kg three times a week after 4 weeks and was continued for a maximum of 10 weeks or until the hematocrit was greater than 35% for a week without blood transfusion. rHuEPO was restarted if the hematocrit fell below 30%. Study patients were transfused according to the same guidelines used in the historical controls by an independent transfusion service. Generally, patients were transfused to maintain a hematocrit of approximately 30% while aplastic and 25% after white blood cell recovery. Using these transfusion guidelines, the median number of red blood cell transfusions in the historical controls during the study period (day 5 to day 82 posttransplant) was 18 units.

Patient characteristics are summarized in Table 22.4. One patient died on day 18 related to severe venoocclusive disease of the liver after only 12 days of rHuEPO therapy and was considered inevaluable for efficacy. Nine patients completed at least 4 weeks of therapy and were considered evaluable for efficacy.

Two additional patients died while on study. Patient 8 died of interstitial pneumonitis day 74 after transplant. He had been off rHuEPO for 11 days because of clinical response. Patient 9 died of hepatic failure in the setting of refractory graft-versus-host disease on day 55 after transplant. No suspected rHuEPO-related toxicity was seen in any of the patients described here.

All patients engrafted promptly (Table

Table 22.4. Patient Characteristics rHuEPO after Allogeneic Bone Marrow Transplantation[a]

	Age	Disease	Prep	ABO[b]	Status
1	42	CML-CP	CY-TBI	Comp	Alive/CR
2	34	CML-CP	BU-CY	Comp	Alive/CR
3	18	AML-CR1	BU-CY	Comp	Alive/CR
4	29	AML-CR1	BU-CY	Comp	Alive/CR
5	44	CML-CP	CY-TBI	Minor	Alive/CR
6	46	CML-CP	BU-CY	Comp	Alive/CR
7	36	ALL-CR1	CY-TBI	Minor	Died D18-VOD
8	55	ALL-CR2	CY-TBI	Major	Died D74-IP
9	54	CML-CP	BU-CY	Comp	Died D55-GVHD
10	45	CML-CP	BU-CY	Comp	Alive/CR

[a]ALL-CR#, acute lymphocytic anemia, complete remission number; AML-CR#, acute myelogenous leukemia, complete remission number; BU-CY, busulfan 4 mg/kg/day for 4 days, cyclophosphamide 40 mg/kg/day for 4 days; CML-CP, chronic myelogenous leukemia, chronic phase; CR, complete remission; CY-TBI, cyclophosphamide 50 mg/kg/day for 4 days, total body irradiation (300 rads/day for 4 days); GVHD, graft-versus-host disease; IP, interstitial pneumonitis; VOD, venoocclusive disease.
[b]ABO compatibility: Comp, compatible; Major, major ABO incompatibility; Minor, minor ABO incompatibility.

22.5). The median time to 500 granulocytes was not different in the treated group versus the controls (17 days versus 17.5 days, $P = .43$, Wilcoxon Rank Sum test). Interestingly, the median time to 1000 leukocytes was less in the rHuEPO patients compared to controls (13.5 days versus 17 days, $P = .03$).

The time course of corrected reticulocyte recovery is shown for all patients compared to historical controls in Figure 22.6. The median time to corrected reticulocyte count of greater than 2% was 19 days in the rHuEPO-treated group compared to 31 days in the control group ($P = .005$, Wilcoxon Rank Sum test). Erythroid activity as measured by the corrected reticulocyte count was highly rHuEPO-dependent as seen in two individual patients' reticulocyte time course (Fig. 22.7). Patient 1 became red blood cell transfusion independent on day 26 after transplant, and rHuEPO was discontinued per protocol after 5 weeks of treatment (day 33 after bone marrow transplant). Her corrected reticulocyte count fell to 0 2 weeks after stopping rHuEPO (day 44 after bone marrow transplant), with a progressive fall in her hematocrit requiring

Table 22.5.   Hematopoietic Parameters[a]

Pt	1 Duration of rHuEPO	EPO Level	2 RET >2% (Day)	3 No. RBC	4 ANC >500 (Day)	5 WBC >1000 (Day)	6 PLT >20 (Day)
1	5	12	17	8	18	19	16
2	8	73	24	14	24	18	14
3	10	27	14	6	13	12	45
4	5 (3)	0	17	18	17	12	8
5	10	5	31	19	14	13	>82
6	7	ND	19	12	17	14	27
7	2	81	NE	NE	NE	NE	NE
8	8	3	31	10	21	17	22
9	7	30	14	19	12	12	>54
10	5 (4)	174	21	37	15	14	27

[a]Abbreviations: ND, not done; NE, not evaluable.
1. Duration of rHuEPO treatment to attain hematocrit of greater than 35 for a week without red blood cell (RBC) transfusion; number in parentheses indicates number of weeks after rHuEPO restarted.
2. Day to corrected reticulocyte (RET) count >2%.
3. Number of RBC transfusions from rHuEPO start (day 5) to day 82.
4. Day to absolute neutrophil count (ANC) greater than 500/mm.
5. Day to WBC greater than 1000/mm.
6. Day to platelet (PLT) count greater than 20,000/mm without transfusion.

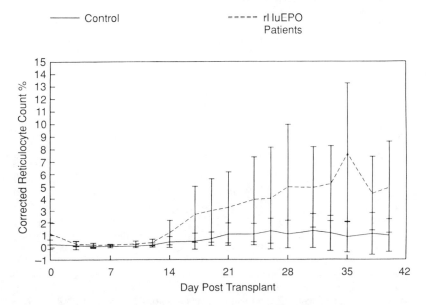

Figure 22.6.   Mean ± standard deviation corrected reticulocyte count for the first 40 days after bone marrow transplantation in rHuEPO-treated allogeneic bone marrow transplant patients (9) compared to non-rHuEPO-treated historical controls (50).

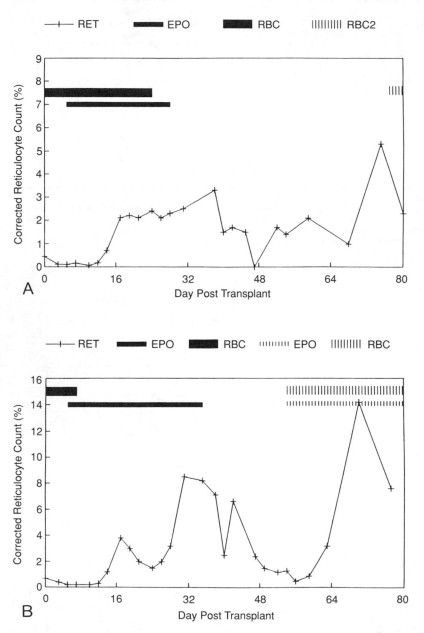

Figure 22.7.   Corrected reticulocyte response to rHuEPO in two patients ———. The *thick solid line* (RBC) represents time of initial red blood cell transfusion support; long *vertical lines* (RBC 2) represent resumption of red blood cell transfusion requirement. The *thinner solid line* (EPO) represents initial period of rHuEPO treatment at dose of 100 units/kg, five times a week for 4 weeks followed by 150 units/kg three times a week until the hematocrit was greater than 35% for a week without red blood cell transfusion. The *short vertical lines* (EPO2) represent the restart of rHuEPO treatment when hematocrit fell below 30%. **A**, Patient 1, with chronic myelogenous leukemia. **B**, Patient 4, with acute myelogenous leukemia in first complete remission.

transfusion on day 80 after transplant. Patient 4 became red blood cell transfusion independent on day 8 after bone marrow transplant, and rHuEPO was discontinued per protocol after 5 weeks of treatment (day 36 after bone marrow transplant). Her corrected reticulocyte count fell to 0.48% on day 56 after bone marrow transplant (20 days after stopping rHuEPO), despite the development of a gastrointestinal hemorrhage related to cytomegalovirus enteritis with a resultant hematocrit fall to 26.3%. rHuEPO was restarted on day 56 after bone marrow transplant with a corrected reticulocyte peak of 14.2% on day 70 (2 weeks after restarting rHuEPO) despite ganciclovir therapy.

The mean number of red blood cell transfusions over time in patients compared to historical controls is shown in Figure 22.8. While lower for the treatment group, there were no significant differences in either the mean (15.8 versus 18.7, $P = .42$, Student's T test) or median (14 versus 18, $P = .22$, Wilcoxon Rank Sum test) red blood cell transfusion requirement for day 5 to day 82 after transplant (study period) between the rHuEPO-treated patients and controls.

Despite a significant increase in reticulocyte count compared to historical controls, a significant decrease in transfusion requirement compared to historical controls was not observed, and dose escalation is planned.

Ayash et al. (63) have reported preliminary results of a trial of rHuEPO in high-dose chemotherapy with autologous marrow rescue. Ten patients with solid tumors have completed treatment at this time. Patients were treated with rHuEPO at a dose of 200 units/kg daily intravenously beginning day 1 after transplant with iron supplementation. rHuEPO was continued for 28 days or until the hematocrit was greater than 35% without transfusion. Red blood cells were given for a hematocrit of less than 25%. Preparative regimens were either ifosfamide, etoposide, and carboplatin (n = 5); cyclophosphamide, carmustine (BCNU), and cisplatin (n = 3); or cyclophosphamide, thiotepa, and carboplatin (n = 2) (Table 22.6). The median number of

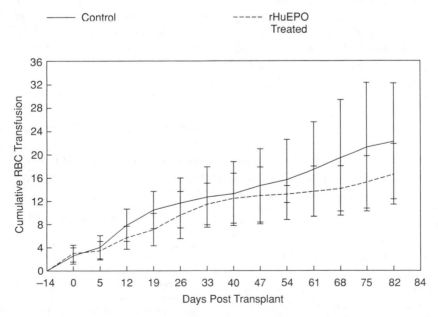

Figure 22.8. Cumulative red blood cell transfusion (mean ± standard deviation) in 9 rHuEPO-treated patients compared to 50 historical controls.

Table 22.6.   rHuEPO after Autologous Transplantation[a]

		1			
Pt	Prep	No. RBC	2 ANC >500	3 HCT >30	4 PLT >20
1	I, E, CB	4	12	17	9
2	I, E, CB	9	13	17	17
3	I, E, CB	10	13	14	11
4	C, BC, CP	6	21	24	26
5	C, T, CB	10	26	32	30
6	C, BC, CP	5	25	N.A.	31
7	I, E, CB	12	25	24	22
8	C, T, CB	8	22	24	22
9	I, E, CB	6	14	16	14
10	C, BC, CP	6	21	N.A.	19

[a]Abbreviations: BC, BCNU; CB, carboplatin; CP, cisplatin; E, etoposide; I, ifosfamide; T, thistepa.
1. Number of red blood cell (RBC) transfusions from rHuEPO start.
2. Day to absolute neutrophil count (ANC) greater than 500/mm.
3. Day to hematocrit (HCT) greater than 30% without transfusion.
4. Day to platelet (PLT) count greater than 20,000/mm without transfusion.

prior chemotherapy regimens in these patients was 4.5.

Hematologic data for the 10 patients are shown in Table 22.6. The median number of red blood cell units transfused during the study period in the rHuEPO patients was seven (range 4 to 12), which did not differ significantly from the number of units required by historical controls on the same intensification regimens (median nine units, range four to two). In the subset of patients treated with the cyclophosphamide, BCNU, cisplatin regimen, there was a trend toward reduction in red blood cell requirements (six versus nine units). Eight of 10 patients reached a hematocrit of greater than 30% independent of blood transfusion during the study period, compared to only 3 of 12 historical controls. In these 8 responders, examination of the peripheral blood revealed nucleated red blood cells (median day 14 after bone marrow infusion), followed by a reticulocytosis (median peak reticulocyte count 8.5%, range 2.2% to 16%). The median day to hematocrit greater than 30 in all patients was 24, with a median

duration of rHuEPO treatment of 26 days (range 14 to 31).

Engraftment was prompt, with a median day to greater than 500 granulocytes of 24 in all patients (historical controls median day to 500 granulocytes was 22 days), and the median day to a platelet count of greater than 20,000 per cubic milliliter was day 21. Interestingly, in the five patients treated with the ifosfamide-based regimen, there was evidence of quicker neutrophil engraftment (13 days to absolute neutrophil count of greater than 500, compared to 25 days in the historical controls treated with the same regimen) and platelet engraftment (21 versus 27 days). In these patients a decrease in platelet utilization was also seen (median 23 versus 59 units in historical controls).

These data suggest a trend toward earlier erythroid recovery but failed to show a statistically significant decrease in red blood cell transfusion requirement after autologous bone marrow transplants.

CONCLUSIONS

Bone marrow transplantation, both allogeneic and autologous, is associated with a significant need for red blood cell transfusions. The anemia after transplantation is complicated by a relative erythropoietin deficiency for the degree of anemia. Preliminary studies suggest that rHuEPO is safe after bone marrow transplantation and may speed erythroid recovery after bone marrow transplantation. Further studies are in progress to determine whether rHuEPO can decrease the transfusion requirement after bone marrow transplantation.

REFERENCES

1. Koury ST, Bondurant MC, Koury MJ. Localization of erythropoietin synthesizing cells in murine kidneys by in situ hydridization. Blood 1988;71:524–527.
2. Schuster SJ, Wilson JH, Erslev AJ, Caro J. Physiologic regulation and tissue localization of renal erythropoietin messenger RNA. Blood 1987;70:316–318.
3. Spivak JL. Erythropoietin: a brief review. Nephron 1989;52:289–294.

4. Dessypris EN, Graber SE, Krantz SB, Stone WJ. Effects of recombinant erythropoietin on the concentration and cycling status of human marrow hematopoietic progenitor cells in vivo. Blood 1988;72:2060–2062.

5. Adamson JW. The erythropoietin/hematocrit relationship in normal and polycythemic man: implications of marrow regulation. Blood 1968;32:597–609.

6. Garcia JF, Ebbe SN, Hollander L. Radioimmunoassay of erythropoietin: circulating levels in normal and polycythemic human beings. J Lab Clin Med 1982; 90:624–635.

7. Chandra M, Clemons GK, McVicar MI. Relation of serum erythropoietin levels to renal excretory function: evidence for lowered set point for erythropoietin production in chronic renal failure. J Pediatr 1988;113:1015–1021.

8. Cartwright GE. The anemia of chronic disorders. Semin Hematol 1966;3:351–375.

9. Dainiak N, Kulkarni V, Howard D, Kalmanti M, Dewey M, Hoffman R. Mechanisms of abnormal erythropoiesis in malignancy. Cancer 1983;51:1101–1106.

10. Miller CB, Jones RJ, Piantadosi S, Abeloff MD, Spivak JL. Decreased erythropoietin response in patients with the anemia of cancer. N Engl J Med 1990;322:1689–1691.

11. Fisher JW, Roh BL. Influence of alkylating agents on kidney erythropoietin production. Cancer Res 1964;24:983–988.

12. Eschbach JW, Kelly MR, Haley NR, Abels RI, Adamson JW. Treatment of the anemia of progressive renal failure with recombinant human erythropoietin. N Engl J Med 1989;321:158–161.

13. Casati S, Passerini P, Campise MR, et al. Benefits and risks of protracted treatment with human recombinant erythropoietin in patients having haemodialysis. Br Med J 1987;295:1017–1020.

14. Fischl M, Galpin JE, Levine JD, et al. Recombinant human erythropoietin for patients with AIDS treated with zidovudine. N Engl J Med 1990;322:1488–1493.

15. Oster W, Herrmann F, Gamm H, et al. Erythropoietin for the treatment of anemia of malignancy associated with neoplastic bone marrow infiltration. J Clin Oncol 1990;8:956–961.

16. Ludwig H, Fritz E, Kotzmann H, Hocker P, Gisslinger H, Barnas U. Erythropoietin treatment of anemia associated with multiple myeloma. N Engl J Med 1990;322:1693–1699.

17. Henry DH, Rudnick SA, Bryant E. Preliminary report of two double blind, placebo controlled studies using recombinant human erythropoietin in the anemia associated with cancer. Blood 1989;73(suppl):6.

18. Plantanias LC, Miller CB, Mick R, et al. Treatment of chemotherapy-induced anemia in cancer patients with recombinant human erythropoietin. J Clin Oncol 1991;9:2021–2026.

19. Miller CB, Platania LC, Ratain MJ, et al. A phase I/II trial of erythropoietin in the treatment of asplatin-associated anemia. JNCI, 1992, in press.

20. Miller CB. Chemotherapy-induced anemia. In: Gurland HJ, Moran J, Samtleben W, Scigalla P, Wieczorek L, eds. Erythropoietin in renal and non-renal anemias. Contributions to Nephrology. Basel: Karger, 1991:248–251.

21. Santos GW, Tutschka PJ, Brookmeyer R, et al. Marrow transplantation for acute nonlymphocytic leukemia after treatment with busulfan and cyclophosphamide. Marrow Transplant 1983;309:1347–1352.

22. Gorin NC, Aegerter P, Bauvert B, et al. Autologous bone marrow transplantation for acute myelocytic leukemia in first remission: a European survey of the role of marrow purging. Blood 1990;75:1606–1614.

23. Yeager AM, Kaizer H, Santos GW, et al. Autologous bone marrow transplantation in patients with acute nonlymphocytic leukemia, using ex vivo marrow treatment with 4-hydroperoxycyclophosphamide. New Engl J Med 1986;315:141–147.

24. Geller RB, Saral R, Piantadosi S, et al. Allogeneic bone marrow transplantation after high-dose busulfan and cyclophosphamide in patients with acute nonlymphocytic leukemia. Blood 1989;73:2209–2218.

25. Carey PJ, Proctor SJ, Taylor P, et al. Autologous bone marrow transplantation for high-grade lymphoid malignancy using melphalan/irradiation conditioning without marrow purging or cryopreservation. Blood 1991;77:1593–1598.

26. Jones RJ, Piantadosi S, Mann RB, et al. High-dose cytotoxic therapy and bone marrow transplantation for relapsed Hodgkin's disease. J Clin Oncol 1990;8:527–537.

27. Levine LA, Richie JP. Urological complications of cyclophosphamide. J Urol 1990;141:1063–1069.

28. Stillwell TJ, Benson RC. Cyclophosphamide-induced hemorrhagic cystitis. Cancer 1988;61:451–457.

29. Droller MJ, Saral R, Santos G. Prevention of cyclophosphamide-induced hemorrhagic cystitis. Urology 1982;20:256–258.

30. Arthur RR, Keerti VS, Baust SJ, Santos GW, Saral R. Association of BK viruria with hemorrhagic cystitis in recipients of bone marrow transplants. N Engl J Med 1986;315:230–234.

31. Brugieres L, Hartmann O, Travagli JP, et al. Hemorrhagic cystitis following high-dose chemotherapy and bone marrow transplantation in children with malignancies: incidence, clinical course, and outcome. J Clin Oncol 1989;7(2):194–199.

32. Ambinder RF, Burns W, Forman M, et al. Hemorrhagic cystitis associated with adenovirus infection in bone marrow transplantation. Arch Intern Med 1986;146:1400–1401.

33. Holland HK, Wingard JR, Saral R. Herpesvirus and enteric viral infections in bone marrow transplantation clinical presentations, pathogenesis, and therapeutic strategies. Cancer Invest 1990;8:507–519.

34. McDonald GB, Shulman HM, Sullivan KM, Spencer GD. Intestinal and hepatic complications of human bone marrow transplantation. Part I. Gastroenterology. 1986;90:460–477.

35. Rowley SD, Zuehisdorf M, Braine HG, et al. CFU-GM content of bone marrow graft correlates with time to hematologic reconstitution following autologous bone marrow transplantation with 4-hydroperoxy-cyclophosphamide-purged bone marrow. Blood 1987;70:271–275.

36. Banaji M, Bearman S, Buckner CD. The effects of splenectomy on engraftment and platelet transfusion requirements in patients with CML undergoing marrow transplantation. Am J Hematol 1986;22:275–283.

37. First LR, Smith BR, Lipton J. Isolated thrombybcytopenia after allogeneic bone marrow transplantation: existence of transient and chronic thrombocytopenic syndrome. Blood 1985;65:368–374.

38. Anasetti C, Rybka W, Sullivan KM. Graft-versus-host disease is associated with autoimmune-like thrombocytopenia. Blood 1989;73:1054–1058.

39. Jones RJ, Lee KSK, Beschorner WE, et al. Venoocclusive disease of the liver following bone marrow transplantation. Transplantation 1987;44:778–783.

40. Blacklock HA, Prentice HG, Evans JPM. ABO-incompatible bone marrow transplantation: removal of red blood cells from donor marrow avoiding recipient antibody depletion. Lancet 1982;2:1061–1064.

41. Braine HG, Sensenbrenner LL, Wright SK. Bone marrow transplantation with major ABO blood group incompatibility using erythrocyte depletion of marrow prior to infusion. Blood 1982;60:420–425.

42. Holler E, Kolb HJ, Mraz HW, et al. Microangiopathy in patients on cyclosporine prophylaxis who developed acute graft-versus-host disease after HLA-identical bone marrow transplantation. Blood 1989;73:2018–2024.

43. Rabinowe SN, Soiffer RJ, Tarbell NJ, et al. Hemolytic-uremic syndrome following bone marrow transplantation in adults for hematologic malignancies. Blood 1991;77:1837–1844.

44. Ma DDF, Varga DE, Biggs JC. Haemopoietic reconstitution after allogeneic bone marrow transplantation in man: recovery of haemopoietic progenitors (CFU-Mix, BFU-E and CFU-Gm). Br J Haematol 1987;65:5.

45. Vellenga E, Sizoo W, Hagenbeek A, Lowenberg B. Different repopulation kinetics of erythroid (BFU-E), myeloid (CFU-GM) and T lymphocyte (TL-CFU) progenitor cells after autologous and allogeneic bone marrow transplantation. Br J Haematol 1987;65:137.

46. Arnold R, Schmeiser T, Wolfgang H, et al. Hemopoietic reconstitution after bone marrow transplantation. Exp Hematol 1986;14:271–277.

47. Rowley SD, Piantadosi S, Santos GW. Correlation of hematologic recovery with CFU-GM content of autologous bone marrow grafts treated with 4-hydro-

peroxycyclophosphamide. Culture after cryopreservation. Bone Marrow Transplant 1989;4:553–558.

48. Lu Calvin, Braine HG, Kaizer H, Saral R, Tutschka PJ, Santos GW. Preliminary results of high-dose busulfan and cyclophosphamide with syngeneic or autologous bone marrow rescue. Cancer Treat Rep 1984;68:711–717.

49. Beguin Y, Clemons GK, Oris R, Fillet G. Circulating erythropoietin levels after bone marrow transplantations: inappropriate response to anemia in allogeneic transplants. Blood 1991;77:868–873.

50. Wulff JC, Santner TJ, Storb R. Transfusion requirements after HLA-identical marrow transplantation in 82 patients with aplastic anemia. Vox Sang 1983;44:366–374.

51. Birgegard G, Wide L, Simonsson B. Marked erythropoietin increase before fall in Hb after treatment with cytostatic drugs suggests mechanism other than anaemia for stimulation. Br J Haematol 1989;72:462–466.

52. Piroso E, Erslev AJ, Caro J. Inappropriate increase in erythropoietin titers during chemotherapy. Am J Hematol 1989;32:248–254.

53. Schapira L, Antin JH, Ransil BJ, et al. Serum erythropoietin levels in patients receiving intensive chemotherapy and radiotherapy. Blood 1990;76:2354–2359.

54. Abedi MR, Backman L, Bostrom L, Lindback B, Ringden O. Markedly increased serum erythropoietin levels following conditioning for allogeneic bone marrow transplantation. Bone Marrow Transplant 1990;6:121–126.

55. Ireland RM, Atkinson K, Concannon A, Dodds A, Downs K, Biggs JC. Serum erythropoietin changes in autologous and allogeneic bone marrow transplant patients. Br J Haematol 1990;76:128–134.

56. Miller CB, Jones RJ, Burns WH, Zahurak M, Santos GW, Spivak JL. Impaired erythropoietin (EPO) response after bone marrow transplantation (BMT). Exp Hematol 1990;18:700.

57. Klassen DK, Spivak JL. Hepatitis related hepatic erythropoietin production. Am J Med 1990;89:684–686.

58. Brown S, Caro J, Erslve AJ, Murray TG. Spontaneous increase in erythropoietin and hematocrit value associated with transient liver enzyme abnormalities in an anephric patient undergoing hemodialysis. Am J Med 1980;68:280–284.

59. Holler E, Kolb HJ, Moeller A, et al. Increased serum levels of tumor necrosis factor precede major complications of bone marrow transplantation. Blood 1990;75(4):1011.

60. Faquin WC, Schneider TJ, Goldberg MA. Effects of inflammatory cytokines on erythropoietin production in Hep3B Cells. Blood 1990;6:142a.

61. Link H, Diedrich H, Ebell W, et al. Recombinant human erythropoietin after allogeneic bone marrow

transplantation. Bone Marrow Transplant 1990;5(Suppl 2):219a.

62. Miller CB, Huelskamp AM, Mills SR, Jones RJ. A pilot trial of recombinant human erythropoietin (rhEPO) after allogeneic bone marrow transplantation (alloBMT). Exp Hematol 1991;19:577.

63. Ayash L, Elias A, Demetri G, et al. Recombinant human erythropoietin (EPO) in anemia associated with autologous bone marrow transplantation (ABMT). Blood 1990;76:131a.

64. Davis J, Fuller A, Braine H, Rowley S. Blood component use in autologous bone marrow transplantation [Abstract]. Transfusion 1989;29:605.

65. Benson K, Noll L, Shively J, Saleh R, Fields K. Transfusion requirements in autologous bone marrow transplant (ABMT) patients [Abstract]. Blood 1990;395.

66. Blazar BR, Kersey JH, McGlave PB, et al. In vivo administration of recombinant human granulocyte/macrophage colony-stimulating factor in acute lymphoblastic leukemia patients receiving purged autografts. Blood 1989;73:849–857.

67. Storb R, Weiden PL. Transfusion problems associated with transplantation. Semin Hematol 1981;18:163–176.

68. Petz LD, Scott EP. Supportive care. In: Blume KG, Petz LD, eds. Clinical bone marrow transplantation, New York: Churchill Livingstone, 1983:177–213.

Section III

Laboratory and Clinical Support for Dose-Intensive Therapy

23

NURSING FOR PATIENTS RECEIVING HIGH-DOSE CHEMOTHERAPY WITH HEMATOPOIETIC RESCUE

Elizabeth C. Reed and Theresa Franco

The number of allogeneic and autologous bone marrow transplants and the number of centers performing these procedures have increased dramatically over the last few years (1, 2). This growth, in part, can be attributed to advancements in supportive care that have decreased transplant-associated mortality. Supportive care administered by skilled personnel continues to be a central issue in marrow transplantation. Increases in marrow transplant activity coupled with the shortages of nurses have highlighted the essential role nursing plays in marrow transplant (3). A successful marrow transplant program is dependent on the ability to recruit, educate, and maintain a quality nursing staff. Such a staff has skills that include the ability to assess and manage pediatric and adult patients with oncologic and critical care problems along with the expertise to provide the supportive care needed during marrow transplantation.

This chapter is intended for the physician, nursing director, or hospital administrator who is developing or reorganizing a marrow transplant unit. We will not provide detailed information on actual nursing practices but rather a comprehensive view of the roles and responsibilities nursing staff assume while caring for a marrow transplant patient. Additionally, the various transplant environments, care policies, staffing, education, and support needs of a transplant unit will be discussed.

NURSING TASKS DURING BONE MARROW TRANSPLANTION

Outpatient, Pretransplant Phase

During the pretransplant phase, a patient is evaluated to determine if he or she is a suitable candidate for high-dose therapy and marrow support. To be eligible for transplant the patient must have an appropriate indication for high-dose therapy and be free of conditions that would substantially increase the risks of high-dose therapy. Patients must also have an appropriate source of hematopoietic stem cells, adequate venous access, an understanding of the procedure that allows informed consent, and financial resources sufficient to pay for the procedure.

Medicine, nursing, and other disciplines including social services, dentistry, and physical therapy collaborate to accomplish a comprehensive pretransplant evaluation. Nurses often coordinate the activities of the various health care disciplines during this phase and frequently are the first members of the transplant team to greet the patient.

The nurse/coordinator obtains the patient's past medical records, pathology slides, and radiologic studies. Arrangements for shipping blood samples from the patient and potential marrow donors are made. The nurse/coordinator also obtains insurance and financial information and, with the hospital business office, begins to obtain preliminary financial approval for the marrow transplant.

When the patient arrives at the transplant center, the nurse orients the patient and his or her family to the clinic and hospital and arranges for any living accommodations they may need. The nurse/coordinator assesses the patient and presents the findings to the physician. She or he also assists physicians and supports the patient during diagnostic procedures, including bone marrow aspiration and biopsy and lumbar puncture. Laboratory tests and consults from other disciplines are scheduled to complete the pretransplant evaluation.

The nurse/coordinator takes responsibility for the education of the patient, the donor, and the family. The patient, family, and donor must have a clear idea of what the transplant process entails as well as the possible associated risks and benefits. The nursing staff must be well informed, relaying information that is consistent both with what has been discussed and what will be discussed in the future. This is achieved through a variety of teaching aides including informational pamphlets, videos, and slide-tape presentations.

The nurse/coordinator must be prepared to field questions regarding every aspect of marrow transplant, including those investigational protocols that the patient has been asked to consider. To improve the education level regarding investigational protocols, the medical staff and nursing staff discuss new studies that accrue marrow transplant patients. Descriptions of the protocols with the investigators' telephone numbers must be readily available to the nursing staff.

The nurse/coordinator is actively involved in the informed consent process. The nurse, acting as a patient advocate, must be confident that the patient has an adequate understanding of the risks and benefits of the treatments being offered (4). The out- and inpatient nurses may both participate in patient education, or the outpatient nurse/coordinator may communicate to the inpatient nursing staff a summary of the important points discussed during the informed consent process. Knowledge of an adequate informed consent process and the reasoning behind the decision for marrow transplantation allows better understanding and cooperation from both the inpatient and outpatient nursing staffs during the patient's treatment.

Once a patient is considered eligible for high-dose therapy and informed consent has been obtained, the stem cell product must be collected. If the patient is going to receive autologous stem cells, the nurse will arrange for a preoperative evaluation, reserve the operating room, and notify the marrow processing and freezing laboratory. Collection of autologous stem cells from the peripheral blood requires several apheresis procedures (5). The nurse arranges for apheresis, monitors blood counts, and obtains orders for any blood or platelet transfusion that is needed.

Responsibility for the education, emotional support, and arranging of medical evaluation of the allogeneic marrow donor also belongs to the outpatient nurse/coordinator. The nurse/coordinator contacts all potential donors and arranges to obtain blood for HLA typing, mixed lymphocyte culture, and serologic testing. Suitable donors are evaluated for medical problems that may cause complications during marrow harvest (6, 7). The nurse also evaluates the donor's understanding of the harvest and transplant process and ensures that proper informed consent has been given.

Careful exploration of the social and psychologic issues present between the donor-recipient pair takes place before marrow donation. As many as 10%–20% of adult marrow donors suffer psychologic difficulties related to marrow donation (8). Many donors likely have received inadequate psychologic and educational preparation before marrow donation. Better preharvest preparation may prevent future difficulties. The child donor often offers ethical, social, and educational challenges to the transplant team (9). The outpatient nurse should spend sufficient time with the child donor and have access to resources such as play therapists, child psychiatry, and ethics consultants. Regardless of the age of the donor, the transplant team should make special efforts to support the donor throughout the entire transplant process.

Inpatient Transplant Phase

The inpatient phase can be divided into four steps: the administration of chemotherapy and radiation, the infusion of the hematopoietic rescue products, support during marrow aplasia, and postengraftment management. After admission to the marrow transplant setting, the patient's primary nurse performs a thorough assessment of the patient. The patient's past medical history and the information gathered in the pretransplant evaluation are reviewed, and a physical assessment is done. The nurse explores the patient's coping strategies, family dynamics, and social background. Establishing the amount of transplant information the patient has retained from the outpatient setting is another high priority during the first admission day. Once these assessments are complete, the nurse can orient the patient and family to the environment, the care routines, and the various medical personnel on the unit. The inpatient primary nurse is responsible for formulating and initiating an individualized care plan (10). To prepare a comprehensive care plan, tailored to the individual, there must be strong communication lines among the inpatient and outpatient nursing staff personnel and the consultants involved with the patient.

Chemotherapy and radiation are usually begun within the first 24–48 hours of hospitalization, a time that is stressful to both patient and nurse. Expectations of changes in appearance, recollection of previous chemotherapy, a feeling of reaching the point of no return, as well as side effects of the therapy are among the many difficulties that patients must confront (11). The rigorous schedules for administering chemotherapy, infusion of large volumes of fluid, management of side effects, and the need for close monitoring of the patient create a busy and challenging situation for even the most experienced nurse.

After the completion of high-dose therapy the stem cell product is infused. Infusion of bone marrow or peripheral stem cells requires aggressive hydration, a system that double-checks the identity of the patient and the source of the graft, and standardized thawing and infusion of stem cells or marrow over a limited period of time with frequent patient assessments. In addition to experiencing continued side effects of the chemotherapy and radiation, the patient may have adverse reactions to the infusion of bone marrow or peripheral stem cells (12). Side effects can include changes in vital signs, dyspnea, chest tightness, nausea and vomiting, abdominal cramping, fall in urinary output, and hemoglobinuria. Close monitoring of patients during the stem cell infusion and timely nursing intervention are necessary for the optimal management of infusion complications.

Many of the activities of a marrow transplant team are aimed at successful supportive care during the period of marrow aplasia. Assigning the same nurses to the patient improves continuity of care and rapport with the patients and their families. Most important, when nurses care for the same patient throughout the hospitalization, they are aware of the patient's baseline condition and can detect subtle changes that may allow early treatment intervention.

Complications caused by infection or hemorrhage that occur during marrow aplasia account for significant mortality during the

1st 100 days after transplant. The nursing staff are closely involved in preventing infections by adhering to infection control policies and meticulously caring for catheters and the perirectal area. Encouraging patient compliance with routine mouth care, oral antibiotics for gastrointestinal decontamination, incentive spirometry, and daily exercise also decreases infection.

Failure to recognize and treat infections in neutropenic patients often results in sepsis and death (13). Every nurse must understand the implications of the first neutropenic fever, and the policies that ensure prompt medical evaluation and institution of treatment. The staff must know the signs of sepsis as well as mechanisms of hemodynamic monitoring, and the antibiotic, fluid, and pressor therapy administration necessary for the management of sepsis. The proper administration of antimicrobial agents such as aminoglycosides, vancomycin, and amphotericin as well as monitoring for side effects of these agents consumes a great deal of nursing time during this intensive period.

Transfusions of irradiated packed red blood cells and platelets are necessary in virtually every patient. White blood cells are less frequently transfused. Because of the complications associated with white cell transfusions, clear guidelines for administering this blood product must be available to all nurses (14, 15). Platelet refractoriness and bleeding frequently occur during transplant. Many approaches to the prevention and treatment of platelet refractoriness are appropriate (16). Whichever approach is chosen, it should be applied systematically to enhance patient management.

Formal nutritional assessments are done by consulting dieticians. However, the nursing staff are responsible for recording the patient's oral intake, infusing hyperalimentation solutions and lipids, and monitoring for and treating hyperalimentation-induced hyperglycemia. The nurse is also instrumental in encouraging patients to begin eating after recovery from mucositis.

Despite aggressive measures for the prevention of infection, appropriate blood product support, and adequate nutrition, some patients have serious complications during the period of marrow aplasia. In addition to sepsis and bleeding the transplant nurse often manages renal failure that requires hemodialysis, hepatic veno-occlusive disease with hepatorenal failure, respiratory failure requiring mechanical ventilation, and severe mucositis and skin toxicity (17).

Although fevers and mucositis often resolve with the appearance of granulocytes, late complications may occur after white cell engraftment. These late complications include graft-versus-host disease, cytomegalovirus disease, and fungal infections (18, 19). Nurses in the hospital and clinic areas must be able to recognize the earliest signs and symptoms of each of these serious complications.

The patient who has recovered neutrophils, has adequate oral intake, and is free of infection is ready for hospital discharge. One of the most rewarding tasks of the inpatient bone marrow transplant nurse is to provide discharge instructions to patients and their families. Printed discharge booklets can ensure consistent instruction and provide a reference for the patient and family at home. Table 23.1 summarizes the major areas that should be addressed during discharge education. A smooth transition from inpatient to

Table 23.1. Topics for Discharge Teaching

Catheter care
Oral care
Skin care
Diet/food preparation
Environmental considerations
Physical activity
Sexual activity
Psychosocial concerns
Conditions that require physician attention
Medications
Outpatient follow-up
Contact numbers
    (outpatient nurse/coordinator, primary nurse,
    physician)

outpatient care helps to alleviate feelings of insecurity that occur when the intensity of care and monitoring is decreased. Continuity of care is maintained by providing a summary of the patient's medical and educational needs for the outpatient team.

Outpatient Posttransplant Phase

The outpatient nurse/coordinator again assumes responsibility for the patient and focuses on continued education and coordinating communication between the transplant team and the referring physician. During this phase the outpatient nurse closely monitors blood counts and other laboratory data, coordinates outpatient therapy that may be necessary, and arranges diagnostic studies needed for restaging of the malignancy or the detection of chronic graft-versus-host disease. Frequent office visits during the early discharge period are necessary for detection and treatment of late complications. The nurse coordinator continues to be the contact and resource person for the patient, family, and often the referring physician after the patient returns home.

THE IMPACT OF THE TRANSPLANT ENVIRONMENT ON NURSING

The type of protective environment provided for marrow transplant patients is a basic consideration when planning or reorganizing a marrow transplant care area. Although some transplant programs care for two patients in one room, one patient per room with protective isolation during times of profound neutropenia is more common. Isolation measures vary from simple handwashing before entering a conventional room to the use of laminar airflow rooms with sterile food and supplies along with skin and gut decontamination. Many factors, including the types of transplants performed, the length of neutropenia, and the incidence of *Aspergillus* infection, will influence the choice of the en-

vironmental system (20). Three systems currently available are conventional air supply systems, high-efficiency particulate air (HEPA) filtration systems, and laminar airflow units. Each system varies in its impact on nursing practices and staffing needs.

Conventional Air Supply

This plan for air handling presents no special demands on the nursing staff. However, to accommodate all levels of nursing care that a marrow transplant patient may need, the rooms should be equipped with wiring for cardiac monitoring, dialysis hookup, dual oxygen, air and suction outlets, several (10–12) electrical outlets, and a private shower. There must be adequate space for several intravenous pumps, a ventilator, a dialysis machine, commode, exercise bike, and the patient's personal belongings. If there are pediatric patients, accommodations should be provided for a parent to stay in the room. The walls, floors, and fixtures should be of materials that can be easily and thoroughly disinfected.

High-Efficiency Particulate Air Filtration System

This system delivers air at a high rate through at least two filters and has the capability of filtering fungal spores from the air. Most HEPA filtration systems also create increased air pressure in the areas supplied, relative to the rest of the hospital. Some marrow transplant units may have all areas, including hallways and nursing support areas, supplied by a HEPA filtration system, while others only supply the patient's rooms. The efficacy of the system is compromised by leaving doors or windows open. The environment should be monitored through periodic room pressure checks as well as volumetric air sampling or settling plates for the detection of air-borne mold species. This system makes few demands on nursing time, but nursing usually coordinates personnel from infection control, housekeeping, and building maintenance for proper monitoring and upkeep of the system.

Laminar Airflow

Laminar airflow units have one entire wall composed of HEPA filters. Air is forced through the filters at a high rate in a unidirectional pattern with an air exchange rate that is 10 times greater than in environments with HEPA filtration using smaller filters. The air filtration and air exchange rate in laminar airflow units clear air of fungal spores and bacteria, essentially sterilizing the air. Laminar airflow with sterilization of the room, supplies, and food in concert with decontamination of the patient's skin and gut has been shown to decrease the number of infections and days of fever during neutropenia. However, this approach did not improve the overall survival of marrow transplant patients treated for leukemia and aplastic anemia (21). Aplastic anemia patients nursed in laminar airflow units were reported to have a lower incidence of graft-versus-host disease (22). Laminar airflow is expensive in terms of the system itself, supplies, storage space and nursing time. Storage areas, located in patient care areas, for the sterile masks, gowns, and other supplies must be available. Rapid restocking must also be possible. Two drawbacks to the laminar airflow environment are the added time needed to enter and care for patients and the restrictions the system places on interactions between the patient and the nursing staff, medical staff, and family. If laminar airflow is to be used effectively and uniformly with good patient compliance, the nursing staff must thoroughly understand the rationale and procedures behind its use. Resources must be available to help the staff deal with the work and stress of isolation that the patient, family, and they themselves may experience in a laminar airflow environment.

STANDARDIZED CARE POLICIES AND ORDERS

Standardized nursing management of conditions and complications that are frequently encountered during high-dose cancer therapy can facilitate quality patient care and control variables that may impact on clinical research. We believe that all units need guidelines that standardize the management of central venous catheters, oral mucositis, first neutropenic fever, and infusion of bone marrow and peripheral stem cells. Depending on the treatment regimens used in the unit, standardized guidelines for the prophylaxis of hemorrhagic cystitis might be useful.

Central Venous Catheters

Silastic catheters that remain in the vein for long periods of time were developed for patients who required long-term intravenous hyperalimentation. With minor alterations these catheters can be used for the infusion of intravenous fluids, medications, blood products, and for the withdrawal of blood samples (23). The need for reliable venous access as well as multiple daily blood draws have made these catheters an essential part of marrow transplant in virtually all transplant centers.

The nursing guidelines for central venous catheter care should outline the daily care needed for the catheter entrance and exit sites and the procedures for accessing the line for infusion therapy and blood draws, as well as the routines for heparinization and cap changes (24). There should also be an educational program in place that provides uniform instructions on catheter care for the patients and their families.

The nurses must feel comfortable with all aspects of catheter care and be aware of the possible complications associated with central venous catheters. The nursing staff also needs to know techniques for solving frequently encountered catheter-related complications. The complications of central venous catheters in marrow transplant patients have been reviewed by several authors (25, 26). The most common complications are infections, clots that occlude the end of the catheter, and catheter displacement. Any of these complications can result in premature removal of the catheter. Careful catheter insertion followed by scrupulous nursing care may decrease the number of complications. A standardized approach to the complications that do occur may salvage some catheters. Thirty-two percent of catheters function after a single bolus of urokinase, and 95% of all catheters are salvaged after a continuous infusion of urokinase (27, 28).

Mucositis

Mucositis caused by chemotherapy and radiation is a common complication during marrow transplant (29). The severity may range from mild mouth and throat soreness to severe tissue necrosis with swelling, bleeding, and ulceration that obstruct the upper airway. Nurses routinely assess the condition of the oropharynx, institute the prophylaxis and treatment of bacterial and fungal superinfections of the oral cavity, and treat chemotherapy-induced mucositis.

Prophylaxis for oral mucositis should include measures that keep the oral cavity and teeth clean while minimizing the risks for bleeding and bacteremia. Prophylactic treatment should be aimed at preventing or reducing colonization with *candida* and preventing activation of herpes simplex (30, 31).

Consistent monitoring of the oral cavity is an important aspect of transplant nursing. The nursing staff at the University of Nebraska developed an oral mucositis scoring system (presented in Table 23.2) that allows uniform scoring and documentation of mucositis (32). This tool facilitates objective comparisons of mouth care techniques and is also useful when scoring treatment regimens for their toxic side effects.

The nurse monitors the patient's level of mouth comfort and adjusts the treatment for mucositis accordingly. Comfort may be improved with topical anesthetics such as Lidocaine or Benadryl. Patients who experience pain and difficulty with swallowing find it useful to have a suction catheter at the bedside for handling secretions. Many patients may require a constant intravenous infusion of morphine for adequate pain control. Nurses must be thoroughly acquainted with continuous infusion pumps and able to adjust doses of morphine to optimize pain control while avoiding confusion, somnolence, and respiratory depression in the patient.

First Neutropenic Fever

During marrow transplant, prompt recognition, evaluation, and treatment of the first neutropenic fever is critical to a successful outcome. All nurses on the transplant team must understand the dire consequences of untreated sepsis in neutropenic patients. Nursing must accept the responsibility for coordinating the medical staff and pharmacy to ensure that all neutropenic patients are medically evaluated and receive appropriate treatment within an hour of first fever.

In addition to education, written guidelines that include a clear definition of fever, the frequency and methods for measuring the body temperature, and a policy for antipyretic use are helpful. Guidelines should also address the routine diagnostic procedures for detection of infection and the standard drugs and doses for the treatment of neutropenic fever.

Stem Cell Infusions

Although nurses may not infuse the stem cell products in all centers, they are involved in preparing the patient and equipment as well as monitoring for complications of the infusion. Safeguards must be established to ensure that the correct rescue product is thawed and given to the appropriate patient (33). Such safeguards include a procedure for identifying the patient and identification of the stem

Table 23.2   Oral Assessment Guide[a]

Category	Tools for Assessment	Methods of Measurement	Numerical and Descriptive Ratings[b]		
			1	2	3
Voice	Auditory	Converse with patient	Normal	Deeper or raspy	Difficulty talking or painful
Swallow	Observation	Ask patient to swallow. To test gag reflex, gently place blade on back of tongue and depress	Normal swallow	Some pain on swallow	Unable to swallow
Lips	Visual/palpatory	Observe and feel tissue	Smooth and pink and moist	Dry or cracked	Ulcerated or bleeding
Tongue	Visual/palpatory	Feel and observe appearance of tissue	Pink and moist and papillae present	Coated or loss of papillae with a shiny appearance with or without redness	Blistered or cracked
Saliva	Tongue blade	Insert blade into mouth, touching the center of the tongue and the floor of the mouth	Watery	Thick or ropy	Absent
Mucous membranes	Visual	Observe appearance of tissue	Pink and moist	Reddened or coated (increased whiteness) without ulcerations	Ulcerations with or without bleeding
Gingiva	Tongue blade or visual	Gently press tissue with tip of blade	Pink and stippled and firm	Edematous with or without redness	Spontaneous bleeding or bleeding with pressure
Teeth or dentures (or denture bearing area)	Visual	Observe appearance of teeth or denture bearing area	Clean and no debris	Plaque or debris in localized areas (between teeth if present)	Plaque or debris generalized along gum line or denture bearing area.

[a]From J. Eilers, copyright 1983.
[b]Scoring: Based on observation, assign a number value to each category.
   1 = healthy normal conditions
   2 = deterioration
   3 = serious problems

   Tally the score—range is 8–24.
   Score of 8 = healthy oral cavity.
   Score of 24 = severe problems with oral cavity.

cell product that traces the product from collection to infusion. Infusion policies defining patient premedication, hydration fluids, thawing conditions, infusion set-up, infusion time, and monitoring routine are also needed. Nurses are educated as to the possible technical difficulties encountered during stem cell infusions as well as the medical complications that may occur during and after infusion. Finally, the nurse documents the thawing and infusion process and the rescue product that was infused for the purposes of quality control and evaluation of engraftment.

Prophylaxis of Hemorrhagic Cystitis

There are several measures that help protect the bladder from acrolein, the metabolite of cyclophosphamide and ifosfamide that is thought to cause hemorrhagic cystitis. Aggressive hydration with frequent urination or hydration and bladder irrigation have been the traditional methods used for preventing cystitis (34). The availability of mesna, a drug that binds acrolein and reduces its toxicity to bladder urothelium, has also been used (35). Trials in marrow transplant patients receiving high doses of cyclophosphamide comparing mesna to hydration and mesna to hydration and bladder irrigation have found that mesna was equal to hydration and irrigation in the prevention of cystitis (36, 37). The latter trial, however, found fewer urinary tract infections in the mesna group when compared to patients treated with bladder irrigation.

Outside of a comparative trial, bladder-protective measures that are standardized for all patients avoids confusion and facilitates nursing. These standards should state the hydration fluid and rate, frequency of urination, and the times for hydration initiation. Criteria for stopping, continuing, or restarting hydration for this purpose should be outlined. Similar guidelines should be specified for bladder irrigation as well as any for monitoring for urinary tract infection that may be necessary.

NURSING MANAGEMENT FOR MARROW TRANSPLANTATION

The nurse manager in marrow transplantation has broad responsibilities that require in-depth skills and knowledge of marrow transplantation. Equally important is the ability to understand and communicate the purpose and philosophy of the transplant team. The nurse-manager's success depends heavily on open communication and collaboration with the medical team, especially the medical director of the unit. Interactions between the medical and nursing directors set the stage for the transplant team's motivation and morale and the delivery of care.

Personnel Planning

Providing adequate personnel and effective education for the nursing staff not only enhances the daily operation of the transplant unit but also is an important key to the transplant program's future growth and development. Staffing needs are determined by the number and types of high-dose therapies, the age ranges of the patients, the research activity in the area, and the level of critical care support. Many transplant programs have chosen to provide comprehensive critical care to maintain patient continuity in an environment with high-efficiency air filtration. However, managing marrow transplant patients that require cardiac and hemodynamic monitoring, mechanical ventilation, and hemodialysis greatly increases the personnel and educational needs of the area.

The average number of hours nurses spend in marrow transplant units directly caring for the patient is much greater than the nursing care hours spent in medical-surgical areas (38). In fact, the number of care hours in some transplant units is no different from that in intensive care units. One transplant unit that was providing comprehensive critical care and a laminar airflow environment reported that an average of 18–20 hours of bedside care was spent per patient per day (39).

Most units require an average nurse to patient ratio of 1:2 to 1:4. Because of the rapid changes that can occur in patients' conditions, the acuity of care should be assessed every shift and staffing adjusted accordingly. Frequent changes in staffing require flexibility in scheduling that can be achieved through variations in the number of hours per shift and days per week the staff nurses work. For instance, offering 4-, 8-, 10-, and 12-hour shifts allows an overlap of personnel that can meet unexpected care demands. Implementing partnerships between staff nurses and nursing technicians can enhance productivity (40).

Staff Recruitment and Retention

The nursing care of marrow transplant patients is demanding, requiring excellent judgment and training. Many nurses are attracted to the area because they want to broaden the scope of their practice and are seeking increased challenges and responsibilities. However, to recruit adequate staff, community and state-wide attention should be focused on the marrow transplant team. Publicity and educational programs that emphasize the positive aspects of cancer treatment, research, and multidisciplinary teamwork help to attract motivated nurses to the area.

When selecting nurses for the transplant team, diversity in experience and background is important. Nurses with experience in oncology are often recruited. However, hiring nurses with backgrounds in critical care, pediatrics, emergency medicine, and general medicine and surgery creates a versatile staff that contains resources for most care needs. Selected new graduates, given the proper support and orientation, can also be effective members of the transplant team. Individuals with qualities such as self-direction, assertiveness, flexibility, and comfort in a change-oriented environment should be actively recruited.

Retention of nurses in the transplant area is the first priority of the nurse manager. High nurse turnover is devastating to the transplant team's morale, experience level, and collaborative efforts with the medical staff. Table 23.3 lists several strategies that promote staff stability.

Staff retention may be improved when the professional growth of the marrow transplantation nurses is fostered. Involving nurses in research can provide professional opportunity and improve job satisfaction. Nursing involvement in research occurs on several levels (41). The nursing staff is often asked to participate in medicine-initiated research by performing phlebotomies, administering study drugs, recording side effects, etc. Nursing participation should be requested, not assumed, and nursing's contribution to the project must be recognized. When designing a study that requires participation from nurses, staff representatives should be asked to evaluate the study's impact on nursing time and overall feasibility (42). After study initiation, interim and final results of the studies should be presented to the nursing staff. Including nurses in such discussions improves understanding of the project, stimulates interest in future research, and acknowledges the important role nurses play in clinical studies.

Nurse-initiated research should be encouraged and supported by nursing management and the medical staff (43). Interest in primary investigation can be stimulated by providing time and support for research projects, journal clubs, and conferences. Attending national meetings will allow nurses to present their investigations and exchange ideas with other investigators. Resources for such projects should be included in the transplant unit's budget.

Education for the Nurses

Quality marrow transplant care is accomplished through a comprehensive educational program for nurses. All of the disciplines involved in marrow transplantation

Table 23.3. Strategies and Their Implementation for Retaining Marrow Transplant Nurses

Strategies	Implementation
1. Communication of bone marrow transplant program philosophy	• Educational programs stating transplant team objectives • Forum multidisciplinary team meetings • Participation of nurse in preadmission interview through discharge
2. Educational program	• Didactic core curriculum • Orientation with clinical facilitator • Continuing education for experienced nurses • Participation in regional, national, international conferences
3. Physician-nurse collaboration	• Rounds with physicians • Weekly team meetings • Joint projects • Patient care conferences • Social activities
4. Financial issues	• Bonuses/stipends • Oncology differential • Selective reimbursements • Paid membership to professional organization
5. Participation in research	• Introduction to the research process • Nurse liaison group to medical research group • Forums for presentation of transplant team research • Resources for nurse-initiated research (study design, statistics, funding, etc.)
6. Psychosocial support	• Informal/formal support groups • Ethics committee • Social worker liaison • Bereavement program • Psychiatry • Time off
7. Opportunites for professional growth	• Instructor at educational offerings • Presentations at Nursing Grand Rounds • Consultant to new marrow transplant programs • Nurse-initiated research • Participation in conferences • Contribution to the literature
8. Opportunities for alternate experiences	• Rotation to outpatient setting, med./surg., general oncology, pediatrics, intensive care. • Exchange program with another transplant center

should contribute to the orientation curriculum and should also update education through inservices and lectures. Didactic teaching is most effective when reinforced with clinical practice (44). Table 23.4 is a plan for the education of marrow transplant nurses that combines didactic education with clinical experience. The nurse manager should design a flexible orientation and educational program that can be tailored to the nurse's back-

ground and experience. Special educational opportunities should be available for nurses throughout their careers on the unit.

CONCLUSIONS

Successful high-dose therapy and stem cell rescue can only be accomplished with a multidisciplinary team. Nurses are valuable and versatile members of the team. They have

Table 23.4   Education Plan for Bone Marrow Transplant Nurses[a]

Didactic Components	Clinical Components
Basic bone marrow transplant	6–9 months' experience
• Basic immunology	• Orient to unit routines/standards
• History of transplant	• Become familiar with treatment protocols
• Transplant process	• Care for transplant patient
• Nursing care of transplant patient	• Attend multidisciplinary team meeting
• Primary drug therapy	• Work with outpatient coordinator
• Acute complications	• Observe harvest, apheresis, stem cell infusion,
• Patient discharge information	catheter placement
• Introduction to clinical research	• Participate in research data collection
Basic critical care	12–18 months' experience
• Assessment of the critically ill transplant patient	• Rotation to intensive care setting
• Pulmonary complications/ventilator management	• Care for critically ill transplant patient with
• Basic arrhythmia recognition and treatment	facilitator
• Impaired renal function/supportive measures	• Participation in skill labs (ventilator management,
• Ethical/legal considerations	hemodynamic monitoring, dialysis equipment)
	• Participate in research rounds
Intermediate bone marrow transplantation	18–24 months' experience
• Transplant drug therapies	• Rotation to intensive care setting
—growth factors	• Care for critically ill patient with facilitator
—immune globulin	• Participation in skill labs (ventilator management,
—cyclosporine	hemodynamic monitoring, dialysis equipment)
• Management of viral and fungal infections	• Participate in research rounds
• Nursing implications of clinical research	
Advanced bone marrow transplantation	24 to 36 months' experience
• Advanced trends in transplant	• Collaborate with physicians in case study analysis
• Hemorrhagic complications (DIC/DAH)	• Assist in development of research studies
• Veno-occlusive disease	• Facilitate orientee caring for transplant patient
• Acute and chronic GVHD	
• Long-term complications	
• CMV prophylaxis and treatment	
• Current research in transplant	
Advanced critical care	24 to 36 months' experience
• Detection and treatment of sepsis/multisystem organ failure	• Collaborate with physician in case study analysis
• Advanced arrhythmia recognition/drug therapy	• Assist in development of research studies
• Hemodynamic parameters in clinical decision making	• Facilitate orientee critically ill transplant patient
	• Obtain ACLS certification

[a]Abbreviations: ACLS, Advanced Cardiac Life Support; CMV, cytomegalovirus; DAH, diffuse alveolar hemorrhage; DIC, disseminated intravascular coagulation; GVHD, graft-versus-host disease.

responsibilities that may range from coordination of patients' initial evaluation and education to primary inpatient supportive care. Providing an environment appropriate for the transplant population and existing resources will enhance supportive care. Care guidelines for common conditions and complications that occur during high-dose therapy standardize care and facilitate education. The medical and nursing directors are responsible for fostering collaboration and cooperation between the two disciplines that results in a quality marrow transplantation program. Finally, managers from medicine and nursing must strive to provide opportunities in education and research that will attract and maintain a skilled and innovative marrow transplant nursing team.

REFERENCES

1. Bortin MM, Rimm AA. Increasing utilization of bone marrow transplantation. Transplantation 1986;42:229–234.
2. Advisory Committee of the International Autologous Bone Marrow Transplant Registry (ABMTR). Autologous bone marrow transplants: different indications in Europe and North America. Lancet 1989;(August 5):317–318.
3. Secretary's Commission on Nursing, DHHS, Washington, DC, 1988, Vol. I-III.
4. Bujorian GA. Clinical trials: patient issues in the decision-making process. Oncol Nurs Forum 1988; 15:779–783.
5. Heal JM, West BL, Brightman A. Harvesting of committed hematopoietic progenitor cells (CFU-GM) by hemapheresis. Transfusion 1986;26:136–140.
6. Bortin MM, Buckner CD. Major complications of marrow harvesting for transplantation. Exp Hematol 1983;11:916–921.
7. Buckner CD, Clift RA, Sanders JE, et al. Marrow harvesting from normal donors. Blood 1984;64:630–634.
8. Wolcott DL, Wellisch DK, Fawzy FI, et al. Psychological adjustment of adult bone marrow transplant donors whose recipient survives. Transplantation 1986; 41:484–488.
9. Williams TE. Ethical and psychosocial issues in bone marrow transplantation in children. In: Johnson FL, Pochedly C, eds. Bone Marrow Transplantation in Children. New York: Raven Press, 1990:497–504.
10. Manthey M. Primary care management. In: The Practice of primary care nursing. Boston: Blackwell Scientific 1980:47–64.
11. Brown H, Kelly M. Stages of bone marrow transplantation. In: Coping with physical illness 2: new perspectives. New York: Plenum Press, 1984:241–252.
12. Kessinger A, Schmit-Pokorny K, Smith D, et al. Cryopreservation and infusion of autologous peripheral blood stem cells. Bone Marrow Transplant 1990; 5(suppl 1):25–27.
13. Schimpff SC, Satterlee W, Young VM, et al. Empiric therapy with carbenicillin and gentamicin for febrile patients with cancer and granulocytopenia. N Engl J Med 1971;284:1061–1065.
14. Wright DG, Robichaud KJ, Pizzo PA, et al. Lethal pulmonary reactions associated with the combined use of amphotericin B and leukocyte transfusions. New Engl J Med 1981;304:1185–1189.
15. Winston DJ, Ho WG, Howell CL, et al. Cytomegalovirus infections associated with leukocyte transfusions. Ann Intern Med 1980;93:671–675.
16. Storb R, Weiden PL. Transfusion problems associated with transplantation. Semin Hematol 1981;18:163–176.
17. McDonald GB, Shulman HM, Sullivan KM, et al. Intestinal and hepatic complications of human bone marrow transplantation. Part I. Gastroenterology 1986;90:460–477.
18. Meyers JD, Flournoy N, Thomas ED. Nonbacterial pneumonia after allogeneic marrow transplantation: a review of ten years' experience. Rev Infect Dis 1982;4:1119–1132.
19. Talbot GH, Provencher M, Cassileth PA. Persistent fever after recovery from granulocytopenia in acute leukemia. Arch Intern Med 1988;148:129–135.
20. Sherertz RJ, Belani A, Kramer BS, et al. Impact of air filtration on nosocomial aspergillus infections: unique risk of bone marrow transplant recipients. Am J Med 1987;83:709–718.
21. Buckner CD, Clift RA, Sanders JE, et al. Protective environment for marrow transplant recipients. Ann Intern Med 1978;89:893–901.
22. Storb R, Prentice RL, Buckner CD, et al. Graft-versus-host disease and survival in patients with aplastic anemia treated by marrow grafts from HLA-identical siblings. New Engl J Med 1983;308:302–307.
23. Hickman RO, Buckner CD, Clift RA, et al. A modified right atrial catheter for access to the venous system in marrow transplant recipients. Surg Gynecol Obstet 1979;148:871–875.
24. Camp-Sorrell D. Advanced central venous access: selection, catheters, devices and nursing management. J Intravenous Nurs 1990;13:361–370.
25. Press OW, Ramsey PG, Larson EB, et al. Hickman catheter infections in patients with malignancies. Medicine 1984;63:189.
26. Ulz L, Petersen FB, Ford R, et al. A prospective study of complications in Hickman right-atrial catheters in marrow transplant patients. J Parenter Enter Nutr 1990;14:27–30.
27. Monturo CA, Dickerson RN, Mullen JL. Efficacy of thrombolytic therapy for occlusion of long-term catheters. J Parenter Enter Nutr 1990;14:312–314.
28. Haire WD, Lieberman RP, Lund GB, et al. Obstructed central venous catheters: restoring function with a 12-hour infusion of low-dose urokinase. Cancer 1990;66:2279–2285.
29. Weisdorf DJ, Bostrom B, Raether D, et al. Oropharyngeal mucositis complicating bone marrow transplantation: prognostic factors and the effect of chlorhexidine mouth rinse. Bone Marrow Transplant 1989;4:89–95.
30. Cuttner J, Troy KM, Funaro L, et al. Clotrimazole treatment for prevention of oral candidiasis in patients with acute leukemia undergoing chemotherapy. Results of a double-blind study. Am J Med 1986;81:771–774.
31. Saral R, Burns WH, Laskin OL, et al. Acyclovir prophylaxis of herpes-simplex-virus infections. N Engl J Med 1981;305:63–67.
32. Eilers J, Berger AM, Petersen MC. Development, testing and application of the oral assessment guide. Oncol Nurs Forum 1988;15:325–330.

33. Rowley SD, Davis JM. Standards for bone marrow processing laboratories. Transfusion 1990;30:55–56.
34. Watson NA, Notley RG. Urologic complications of cyclophosphamide. Br J Urol 1973;45:609.
35. Ehrlich RM, Freedman A, Goldsobel AB, et al. The use of sodium 2-mercaptoethane sulfonate to prevent cyclophosphamide cystitis. J Urol 1984;131:960–962.
36. Shepherd JD, Pringle LE, Barnett MJ, et al. 2-Mercaptoethane sulfonate (Mesna) vs hyperhydration (HH) for the prevention of cyclophosphamide induced hemorrhagic cystitis in bone marrow transplantation [Abstract]. Proc Am Soc Clin Oncol 1990;9:12.
37. Vose JM. Personal communication to author, 1991.
38. Tillman MC. A comparison of nursing care requirements of patients on general medical-surgical units and on an oncology unit in a community hospital. Oncol Nurs Forum 1984;11:42–45.
39. Kelleher J, Jennings M. Nursing management of a marrow transplant unit: a framework for practice. Semin Oncol Nurs 1988;4:60–68.
40. Manthey M. Practice partnerships: the newest concept in care delivery. J Nurs Admin 1989;19:33–35.
41. Engelking C. Facilitating clinical trials. Cancer 1991;67:1793–1797.
42. Smith D. Collaboration in nursing research: a multidisciplinary approach. Int J Nurs Studies 1988;25:73–78.
43. Ellett ML. Clinical nursing research: recipe for success. Gastroenterol Nurs 1990;13:18–23.
44. Alspach J. The education of critical care nurses: assessing who cares. In: The educational process in critical care. St. Louis: Mosby, 1982:3–15.

24

HICKMAN LINE MANAGEMENT

William D. Haire

Catheters providing access to the venous circulation are used in most, if not all, patients undergoing high dose antineoplastic therapy. These devices, while necessary for patient care, are subject to a host of malfunctions and can be a source of both morbidity and mortality. Understanding catheters and catheter-related complications is important for individuals providing high-dose cancer therapy.

High-dose therapy implies the acceptance of significant toxicity. The degree of toxicity to many systems, especially the bone marrow and intestinal tract, is lethal unless the function of these organs is temporarily assisted. Infections must be treated with antibiotics, oxygen-carrying capacity must be maintained by red cell transfusions, bleeding must be prevented and treated by transfusions of platelets and plasma products, and nutrition must be provided parenterally. This type and intensity of supportive care requires reliable access to the vascular space for prolonged periods of time. Vascular access via the subcutaneous veins of the arm is inadequate for patients undergoing high-dose cancer therapy (1) for two basic reasons: (*a*) These patients are frequently unable to meet their oral nutritional needs because of nausea, vomiting, mucositis, diarrhea, and malabsorption and often must be provided with parenteral nutrition (2). Parenteral nutrition solutions cannot be given via peripheral veins because of their sclerotic effects (3). (*b*) These

patients need multiple infusions of medications and blood products as well as repeated phlebotomies for diagnostic testing (4). Frequent venipuncture results in physical and emotional trauma to many patients (5) and often achieving vascular access repeatedly is impossible.

Alternative means of achieving venous access have been devised for patients undergoing high-dose cancer therapy. Central venous catheterization via the subclavian vein was proposed in 1969 for administration of total parenteral nutrition (TPN) (6). Broviac and coworkers subsequently developed a silicone rubber catheter for TPN (7). Silicone rubber was used to minimize thrombosis. This catheter was inserted into the subclavian vein via a subcutaneous tunnel in the anterior chest wall and held in place by a novel Dacron cuff on the subcutaneous portion of the catheter. In addition to forming a stable anchor to the chest wall, the subcutaneous tunnel and Dacron cuff were a barrier to infections. Hickman and colleagues modified Broviac's catheter by increasing the internal diameter and wall thickness to allow for more rapid infusion and removal of blood products. They found the new catheter to be well suited to use by allogeneic marrow transplant recipients (1). Since that time, subcutaneously tunneled silicone rubber central venous catheters have been routinely used in marrow transplant patients (2, 8). The use of these catheters has made possible high-dose therapy as we know it today. However, like most other therapeutic interventions, central venous catheters provide a potential for many complications as well as benefits.

CATHETER TYPES AND PLACEMENT TECHNIQUES

Among patients undergoing high-dose antineoplastic therapy, catheters are used for two basic purposes: (*a*) venous access for diagnostic phlebotomy and administration of blood products, medications, and parenteral nutrition; and (*b*) venous access for peripheral stem cell (PSC) harvest by apheresis for those patients undergoing PSC transplantation.

Catheters for Routine Venous Access

Catheters designed for nonapheresis venous access can be divided into totally and partially implantable systems. Totally implantable systems consist of a subcutaneous infusion chamber connected to a length of silicone rubber tubing. Because these catheter systems are subcutaneous, venous access requires inserting a small, specially designed needle through the skin and diaphragm atop of the chamber (9). Partially implantable systems have a length of catheter outside the body at all times. Both systems are available in single- and double-lumen configurations. Potential advantages of the totally implantable systems are a reduced risk of infection, absence of body image alteration, and reduced maintenance requirement (9). These potential advantages are most helpful in outpatients needing venous access infrequently and are less applicable to high-dose therapy patients requiring frequent or continual venous access. No studies comparing the two types of catheters in patients receiving high-dose therapy have been done. Consequently, the decision to use one system instead of the other must be made on data comparing the two systems in other clinical settings.

In standard-dose chemotherapy, the totally implantable systems have a number of limitations (5). The potential for extravasation of drugs into the subcutaneous space due to unrecognized needle malposition is one. Limits on the type and volume of infusate through the small needle bore and the need for specially trained nurses are also recognized drawbacks to the totally implanted devices (5). In pediatric patients, the infection rate was lower in a group with totally implanted systems (10). This difference, however, only became apparent in catheters left in place for over 100 days and may have been accentuated by institutional policy limiting phlebotomy from these systems. This advantage may be lost in patients undergoing high-dose therapy, who have catheters in almost constant use and have them removed prior to 100 days (11, 12). Because partially implanted systems have a well-documented record in high-dose therapy (4, 11–13) while totally implanted systems have not been studied in this patient population, totally implanted systems are seldom used as the sole method of venous access in this setting.

Among partially implantable catheter systems, there are two basic catheter designs: (*a*) the open-ended Hickman type and (*b*) the valve-ended Groshong type (Fig. 24.1). The valve of the Groshong catheter is closed except during infusion and withdrawal, preventing backflow of blood into the catheter and thus possibly minimizing the number of "flushes" required to maintain catheter patency and thrombotic occlusion rates (14, 15). As with totally implantable catheter systems, this theoretical advantage would most benefit outpatients requiring infrequent venous access. The theoretical advantages of this catheter system over the classical open-ended systems have not been widely tested. The only study directly comparing the two catheter types, done in a group of high-dose therapy patients (16), showed that there was no difference in the rates of venographically documented subclavian vein thrombosis between the two types of catheters (Table 24.1).

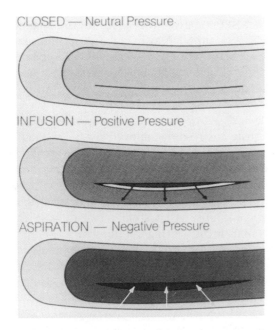

CLOSED — Neutral Pressure

INFUSION — Positive Pressure

ASPIRATION — Negative Pressure

Figure 24.1. The pressure-sensitive two-way valve on the end of a Groshong catheter. When there is neutral pressure inside the catheter, the valve remains closed, preventing backflow of blood into the catheter lumen. (From Camp LD. Care of the Groshong catheter. Oncol Nurs Forum 1988;15:745–749.)

Table 24.1. The Venographic Appearance of the Sub-clavian Vein after Cannulation by Various Catheter Types[a]

Venogram	Double Lumen		Single Lumen	
	Groshong	Hickman	Groshong	Hickman
Total Obstruction	5	4	0	1
Partial Obstruction	2	5	1	4
Normal	4	3	5	1
Total 35	11	12	6	6

[a]From Haire WD, Lieberman RP, Lund GB, Edney JA, Kessinger A, Armitage JO. Thrombotic complications of silicone rubber catheters during autologous marrow and peripheral stem cell transplantation: prospective comparison of Hickman and Groshong catheters. Bone Marrow Transplant 1991;7:57–59.

Additionally, there was a trend for the valve-ended catheters to become occluded by thrombi more frequently than open-ended catheters. In patients receiving high-dose therapy, therefore, the valve-ended catheters offer no advantage over open-ended catheters. In our institution, the 10.8F Hickman catheter (Davol, Inc., Cranston, RI) has become the standard venous access device used during high-dose therapy.

Subclavian venous access catheters are generally tunneled through the subcutaneous tissue of the anterior chest wall. The subcutaneous tunnel anchors the catheter's Dacron cuff, allowing the catheter to be firmly held in place without sutures. The tunnel also provides a physical barrier to infection (7).

Catheters can be placed via a venotomy in the surgically exposed subclavian, cephalic, or internal jugular vein (1, 7) or percutaneously using an introducer and "peel-away sheath" (17). The percutaneous approach is faster (18), but catheter placement under direct vision avoids multiple attempts at subclavian puncture and may minimize bleeding complications in thrombocytopenic patients (19). The relative ease of the percutaneous technique has led us to make it our standard, in both the operating room and the radiology special procedures suite (20).

The percutaneous placement technique is, however, not without drawbacks. Because this technique does not allow direct visualization of the subclavian vein, patients with unusual anatomy or occult subclavian vein occlusion may not be able to be catheterized using this technique alone. This problem is common in patients undergoing high-dose therapy. Many such patients have had subclavian catheters placed earlier in their course of therapy and subsequently removed. Subclavian vein thrombosis, often asymptomatic, occurs in as many as 38% of such patients (21). While the natural history of these thrombi is not well defined, evidence suggests that recanalization of the thrombosed vein is rare (22). Chronic, asymptomatic occlusion of the subclavian vein prevents percutaneous catheter placement in 18% of patients presenting for high-dose therapy (23). Preoperative duplex ultrasound scanning of the subclavian vein can often identify occluded veins that cannot be successfully catheterized (23).

Clavicular shadowing and other variables hinder evaluation of the proximal portion of the subclavian vein (24, 25). Focal stenoses in this area that prevent catheter placement can be missed by surveillance duplex ultrasound (26) (Fig. 24.2). In such cases, intraoperative venography and fluoroscopic guidance (27) can generally allow a catheter to be placed or alternative sources of venous access to be found.

Catheters for Peripheral Stem Cell Apheresis

Peripheral blood stem cells for transplantation are collected by repeated apheresis procedures. Each procedure requires withdrawal and reinfusion of blood at 60 ml/min for as long as 4 hours. The apheresis procedures are usually repeated 8 times to harvest enough stem cells for transplantation (28, 29), although as many as 20 procedures have been required. Most candidates for peripheral stem cell transplantation do not have adequate peripheral veins for repeated collections (28, 29) and require venous access devices. As might be expected, catheters adequate for routine supportive care are inadequate for stem cell apheresis. An ideal venous access device for stem cell collection should meet four criteria: (*a*) It should be usable repeatedly for apheresis for up to several months, (*b*) it should be available for venous access during the transplantation procedure, (*c*) it should cause no more apheresis-related complications than peripheral veins, and, (*d*) it should cause no complications itself.

Attempts to fulfill these criteria were begun with commercial apheresis/hemodi-

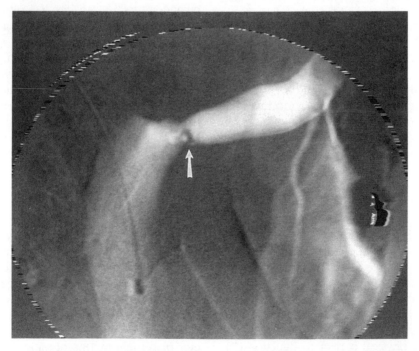

Figure 24.2. An arm venogram demonstrating a proximal stenosis of the subclavian vein (*arrow*). This stenotic lesion is probably the result of a subclavian vein thrombus from a catheter previously placed for chemotherapy and subsequently removed. The patient had neither a history of symptomatic subclavian vein thrombosis nor current symptoms of subclavian vein occlusion. This lesion was not seen on preoperative duplex scan of the subclavian vein, and it prevented percutaneous catheter placement.

alysis catheters inserted into the subclavian vein (30). The subclavian route has classically been avoided due to initial reports of arrhythmias during therapeutic apheresis (31). These complications were attributed to reinfusion of room temperature, citrate-anticoagulated blood too close to the heart. Later experience showed that granulocyte harvest from normal blood donors could be performed via right atrial catheters (32) without causing arrhythmias. The subclavian central approach, therefore, was felt to be a reasonable avenue for peripheral stem cell collection. Even so, subclavian apheresis catheters were carefully placed so that their tips were at the junction of the innominate veins and the superior vena cava, well away from the heart. With this approach, stem cell collection apheresis could be done repeatedly over protracted periods of time. Apheresis via this route was not associated with symptomatic arrhythmias and gave no more citrate reactions (nausea, dysesthesias, presyncope) than were reported with apheresis via peripheral veins. These catheters could also be left for venous access during transplantation. Thus these catheters fulfilled the first three requirements for an ideal venous access device for peripheral stem cell harvest. However, the final criterion, that they cause no problems themselves, was not met. These catheters had a high frequency of thrombotic complications: symptomatic subclavian vein thrombosis (2 of 17 patients) and thrombotic occlusion of the catheter preventing apheresis (11 of 17 catheters). These thrombi could be prevented with a continuous heparin infusion at 1000 units/hour through the catheter (Table 24.2). Heparin prophylaxis of this magnitude, however, added expense and risk. In addition to thrombotic complications, 3 of 18 subclavian apheresis catheters spontaneously withdrew from the vein, possibly due to the short intravascular segment necessitated by the high placement of the catheter tip. These mechanical (withdrawal) and thrombotic problems led us to pursue an entirely different approach to venous access for peripheral stem cell collection.

Table 24.2. Effect of Prophylactic Heparin Therapy on Thrombosis-Related Access Failure[a]

Primary Heparin Prophylaxis	Total	Access Failure
No	17[b]	11
Yes	5	0
p (Fisher's exact test)		0.01

[a]From Haire WD, Edney JA, Landmark JD, Kessinger A. Thrombotic complications of subclavian apheresis catheters in cancer patients: prevention with heparin infusion. J Clin Apheresis 1990;5:188–191. Copyright © 1990 *Journal of Clinical Apheresis*. Reprinted by permission of Wiley-Liss, a division of John Wiley and Sons, Inc.
[b]Includes one patient in whom heparin prophylaxis was prematurely discontinued.

The percutaneous, translumbar approach to the abdominal aorta is a traditional route for arteriography (33). Modifying this technique, Denny and coworkers inserted catheters into the inferior vena cava for TPN in two patients (34). We postulated that this approach to the central venous circulation might reduce the thrombotic complications during peripheral stem cell collection by placing the catheter in a larger vein and reduce mechanical problems by providing a longer intravascular segment of catheter.

Percutaneous inferior vena cava placement of apheresis catheters is accomplished by initially tunneling subcutaneously from an incision in the right flank to a point just cephalad to the posterior superior iliac crest (Fig. 24.3) (35). The catheters then are placed through the paraspinous musculature into the inferior vena cava (Fig. 24.4) and advanced to a point just below the renal veins (Fig. 24.5).

Bleeding complications of catheter placement were not seen. Complications of apheresis—especially citrate reactions—were rare (Table 24.3). Indeed, citrate reactions were much less common with inferior vena cava catheters than with subclavian apheresis catheters using the same collection protocol. Infectious complications were also infrequent and generally responded to antibiotics. Venous access failure, due to thrombotic and mechanical catheter obstruction, continued to be a problem, though not as great as with

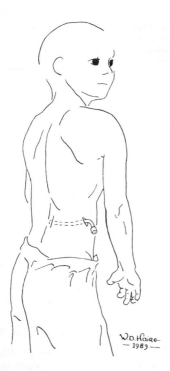

Figure 24.3. A diagram of the position of a percutaneously placed inferior vena cava apheresis catheter. The catheter enters the subcutaneous space through an incision in the flank and is tunneled subcutaneously (*dashed lines*) to an incision just cephalad to the posterior superior iliac crest, where it goes deep to enter the inferior vena cava.

subclavian catheters. These catheters also functioned well for venous access during peripheral stem cell transplantation. As more experience with inferior vena cava catheter placement was gained, the rate of mechanical complications dropped, presumably reflecting greater technical facility in placement technique (29). The rate of thrombotic complications, especially thrombotic catheter occlusion preventing apheresis, remained constant. This suggested that thrombosis was inherent with either the catheter, its location, or the patient population.

Experience with subclavian catheters in high-dose therapy patients showed that symptomatic subclavian vein thrombosis was less common in patients who were thrombocytopenic at time of catheter placement (13).

This observation suggested that platelets are involved in the pathogenesis of catheter-related thrombosis. Consequently, attempts were made to reduce the incidence of thrombotic occlusion of inferior vena cava apheresis catheters by inhibiting platelet function with oral aspirin during stem cell collection. A dose of 325 mg daily was begun the day after catheter placement (36). This regimen was safe and resulted in fewer thrombotic catheter occlusions. More important, aspirin use resulted in a greater number of thrombosis-free apheresis procedures than historical controls (Fig. 24.6). With aspirin prophylaxis, percutaneously placed translumbar silicone rubber apheresis catheters come very close to satisfying all criteria for an ideal venous access device for peripheral stem cell harvest.

COMPLICATIONS OF CATHETERIZATION DURING THERAPY

Complications of catheterization can be divided into infectious and noninfectious types. Noninfectious complications generally involve failure of venous access due to occlusion of the catheter lumen but do not directly threaten the patient's health. Infectious complications influence venous access because they occasionally require catheter removal, but more often threaten the overall health of the patient. These two types of complications will be considered separately.

Noninfectious Complications

Noninfectious complications of catheterization include either mechanical failure of the catheter or thrombotic complications caused by the catheter (37, 38). Mechanical failure can result from simple misplacement of the catheter in the subcutaneous or intravascular space, resulting in lumenal obstruction, or can be due to migration, with or without fracture of the catheter. The presenting symptom of most mechanical catheter complications is acquired venous access

```

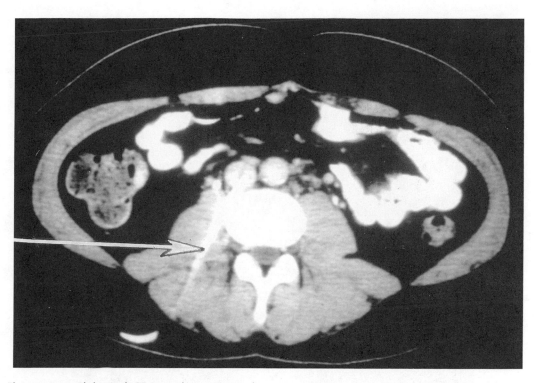

**Figure 24.4.** Abdominal CT scan demonstrating the course of an inferior vena cava apheresis catheter (*arrow*) from the subcutaneous tissue of the back to the vena cava. (From Lund GB, Lieberman RP, Haire WD. Central venous catheters. Semin Intervent Radiol 1989;6:162–175.)

failure, defined as inability to withdraw from or infuse through (under normal pressure) the catheter after having successfully done so on at least one occasion. Rarely, pain on infusion is the only sign of catheter failure.

Fracture of the external portion of the catheter is often signaled by visible leakage and can be detected by examination of the catheter. Internal catheter fracture will occasionally be detected by x-ray as a discontinuity in the radiopaque line on the catheter. Often, however, injection of radiographic contrast medium through the catheter with fluoroscopic observation of its flow pattern is necessary to detect a fracture (37, 38). Fractures external to the body can often be repaired with commercial kits and generally do not require catheter removal. Fractures in the subcutaneous space require catheter removal. Complete separation of the distal portion of the catheter with intravascular migra-

tion generally requires removal of both the fixed and migrated portions of the catheter (39).

Mechanical complications include constriction by anchoring sutures (38), but migration of the catheter in either the intravascular or subcutaneous space (38) is more common. Migration of the subcutaneous portion of the catheter results in access failure by either pulling the intravascular portion of the catheter back to where the tip abuts the vein wall or by pulling it entirely out of the vascular space. Removal is the only option available in the latter situation (38). Spontaneous migration of the catheter tip into the jugular, contralateral subclavian, or intercostal veins can occur, both at the time of catheter placement (38) and after it has been in place and functioning normally for extended periods of time (40, 41). Venous access failure due to intravascular malposition can often
```

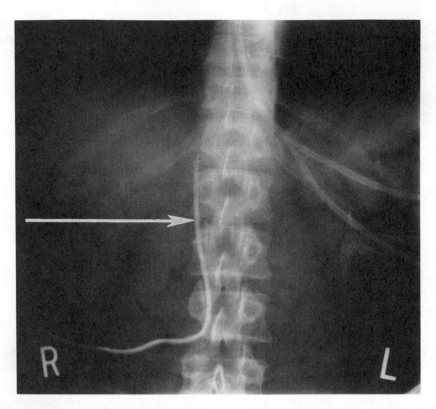

Figure 24.5. Abdominal radiograph taken after percutaneous translumbar placement of a silicone rubber apheresis catheter (*arrow*) into the vena cava. (From Haire WD, Lieberman RP, Lund GB, Boyle BM, Armitage JO, Kessinger A. Translumbar inferior vena cava catheters: safety and efficacy in peripheral stem cell transplantation. Transfusion 1990;30:511–515.)

be corrected with a tip-deflector or J-wire (42). Repositioning via guidewires introduced through the dysfunctional catheter is generally successful and is acceptable in pancytopenic patients undergoing high-dose therapy. However, alternative methods of catheter repositioning using techniques currently available for percutaneous foreign body removal (snaring the catheter via a separate femoral, jugular, or basilic vein puncture) are occasionally required (40). These more invasive approaches present greater risk to the pancytopenic patient. The decision to use these techniques requires risk/benefit analysis. For instance, in a case of withdrawal occlusion due to migration of the catheter tip against the wall of an patent vein, no therapeutic intervention way be required. However, if a mal-

positioned catheter is directing flow into the thyroid plexus and administration of chemotherapy is planned, repositioning of the catheter to redirect the flow may be necessary to prevent complications (43).

Thrombotic complications of central venous catheters cause three distinct clinical problems: (*a*) venous access failure due to thrombotic occlusion of the catheter tip, (*b*) symptomatic subclavian/innominate vein thrombosis, and (*c*) asymptomatic subclavian/innominate vein thrombosis. These syndromes all have different implications for care of the patient undergoing high-dose therapy.

Thrombotic occlusion of the catheter tip is the most common cause of acquired venous access failure, accounting for 57% of such episodes (38). This percentage rises if in-

Table 24.3. Subjective Complications of Apheresis via Peripheral Veins and Catheters Placed either in the Subclavian Vein or the Inferior Vena Cava

	Via Subclavian Catheter	Via IVC[a] Catheter	Via Peripheral Veins (30)
No. of procedures	182	469	887
Hypotension	4 (2%)	1 (0.2%)	6.5%
Dysesthesias	15 (8.2%)	7 (1.5%)	5.5–8.5%
Lightheadedness	10 (5.5%)	2 (0.4%)	—
Nausea	6 (3.3%)	7 (1.5%)	7.2–15%
Total	35 (19.2%)	17 (3.6%)	—

[a]IVC, inferior vena cava.

ability to withdraw through the catheter is the only problem (44). The only adverse outcome of this type of thrombosis is loss of venous access. However, this represents a significant impediment to the care of high-dose therapy patients. Prevention would be the best solution to the problem. Methods of prophylaxis shown to work in other patient populations, such as heparin (30, 45–47), aspirin (36), or warfarin administration (48) have not been studied in patients undergoing high-dose therapy. The relative magnitude of changes

in the protein C anticoagulant system between patients undergoing conventional-dose (49) and high-dose (50, 51) therapy, as well as other potential qualitative and quantitative differences in the procoagulant, anticoagulant, and fibrinolytic systems (52), may prevent these medications from working (or may cause unexpected toxicity) in the setting of high-dose therapy. Consequently, beyond meticulous nursing care including periodic flushing of the catheter with 5 ml of 10 unit/ml heparinized saline (53, 54), there is no effective method of preventing thrombotic catheter occlusion in these patients. Further study is definitely needed in this area.

The only method of diagnosing thrombosis-related venous access failure is with radiographic contrast medium injection of the dysfunctional catheter. Power injection techniques may enhance the sensitivity of the study but run the risk of catheter rupture (55). Hand injection with serial filming is recommended for clinical use.

The 5000-unit bolus of urokinase has gained widespread acceptance as the initial, empiric therapy of dysfunctional catheters because of its success in initial reports (56,

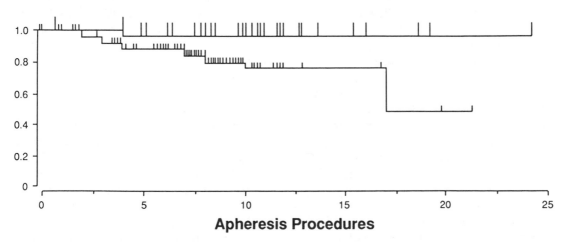

Figure 24.6. Kaplan:Meier survival curves comparing the thrombus-free apheresis procedures performed on patients given aspirin (*upper line*) and those not given any antithrombotic prophylaxis (*lower line*). The difference between the two groups is statistically significant (p = .024, log rank analysis). (From Haire WD, Lieberman RP, Lund GB, Kessinger A. Translumbar inferior vena cava catheters: Bone Marrow Transplantation 1991;7:389–392.)

57). Unfortunately, these early studies failed to objectively diagnose the type of catheter obstruction by contrast injection. A recent study of catheters radiographically proven to be obstructed by thrombus showed that three separate 5000-unit boluses of urokinase did not restore function in 68% of the catheters (58). This treatment is benign and has a modest success rate. Consequently, it is reasonable to use as initial, empiric therapy of dysfunctional catheters. If this is not successful in restoring catheter function, radiographic contrast injection is required before proceeding therapeutically.

Published treatments for thrombosed catheters refractory to bolus urokinase are (a) surgical repositioning in the operating room (5) or (b) urokinase infusion (59). The first approach is invasive and has an unknown success rate. The second approach is noninvasive, has a high success rate, and is generally recommended. A 250,000-unit vial of urokinase is infused at a rate of 40,000 units/hour for 6 hours. This infusion protocol has resulted in dissolution of thrombi in 17 of 19 catheters (Fig. 24.7) (60). If catheter function is not restored after the initial infusion, an additional 6-hour infusion can safely be used. A 12-hour, 500,000-unit infusion of urokinase has a success rate of 95% (59). Follow-up of catheters salvaged with urokinase infusion has shown that many of these catheters can be used until they are no longer required (Table 24.4). Changes in plasma coagulation parameters are slight (Table 24.5) and are limited to clinically insignificant decreases in α-2-antiplasmin and plasminogen activator inhibitor levels. No bleeding complications have been seen. Catheters whose function has not been restored by a 12-hour infusion of urokinase should be restudied by contrast injection. Occasionally, the urokinase infusion will dissolve the pericatheter thrombus, demonstrating a coexistent malposition of the tip responsible for the persistent occlusion (60). Tissue plasminogen activator can restore function in thrombotically occluded catheters resistant to bolus urokinase therapy (61),

but its role in treatment of thrombotic catheter occlusion is unclear.

Symptomatic subclavian vein thrombosis occurs with a high frequency in some groups of patients undergoing high-dose therapy. This complication occurs in less than 1% of patients undergoing allogeneic and syngeneic transplantation (12) but occurs in over 20% of autologous marrow transplants (13).

The reasons behind the heterogeneity in reported thrombosis rates are not completely understood. While abnormalities of the naturally occurring anticoagulant and fibrinolytic systems are common in patients presenting for autologous marrow transplantation (62), they are not helpful in predicting catheter-related thrombosis (63). The type of malignancy may have some bearing on these complications. Patients undergoing stem cell transplantation for Hodgkin's disease have a higher thrombosis rate than patients treated for non-Hodgkin's lymphoma (63). The finding of high levels of monocyte tissue factor on peripheral blood monocytes in patients with untreated (64) and relapsed Hodgkin's disease presenting for stem cell transplantation (65) may explain some of these differences in thrombotic complication rates.

Patients undergoing placement of bilateral subclavian catheters on the day of autologous marrow harvest have a higher likelihood of thrombosis than other patient populations (13). This suggests that changes in the procoagulant, anticoagulant, and fibrinolytic system that occur after major surgery may contribute to the development of catheter-related thrombosis in autologous marrow transplantation.

Platelets also appear to be involved in the pathogenesis of catheter-related thrombosis. Data supporting this contention come from two observations; (a) that thrombocytopenic patients have a lower rate of subclavian vein thrombosis after catheter placement (13) and (b) that aspirin reduces the rate of thrombotic catheter occlusion in some populations (36). Marked changes in the pro-

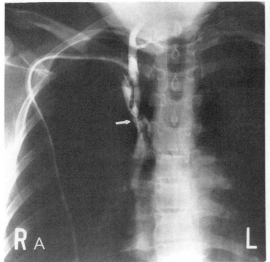
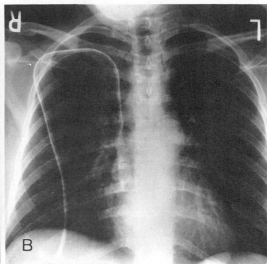

Figure 24.7. **A**, Contrast injection of a catheter showing a partially obstructive thrombus with retrograde flow into the jugular vein (*arrow*). **B**, After a 12-hour infusion of urokinase, the contrast injection shows complete dissolution of the obstructive thrombus. (From Haire WD, Lieberman RP, Lund GB, Edney J, Wieczorek BM. Obstructed central venous catheters: restoring function with a 12-hour infusion of low-dose urokinase. Cancer 1990;66:2279–2285.)

tein C anticoagulant system occur after high-dose therapy (50) and may also play a role in the pathogenesis of catheter-related thrombosis.

As with thrombotic catheter occlusion, no pharmacologic maneuver effective in preventing catheter-induced subclavian vein thrombosis in patients receiving conventional doses of antineoplastic therapy has been evaluated in patients undergoing high-dose therapy. At this time, avoiding simultaneous bilateral subclavian catheter placement and marrow harvest (particularly in patients with Hodgkin's disease) is the only current recommendation to limit subclavian vein thrombosis in these patients. Further study of pathogenic mechanisms and methods of prophylaxis of thrombosis in these patients is needed.

Diagnosis of subclavian vein thrombosis requires a high degree of clinical suspicion. The symptoms and signs of thrombosis (shoulder, arm, or neck pain; a feeling of "tightness" in the arm or hand; swelling of the arm or hand; prominence of the subcutaneous veins of the shoulder or chest) are nonspecific and can be quite subtle.

Once suspected, the diagnosis should be objectively confirmed. Contrast injection of the catheter will image the venous system only distal to the catheter tip and may miss thrombi limited to the subclavian/innominate systems. Computed tomography can detect thrombi in this area (66) but has not been sufficiently studied to allow statements of its sensitivity and specificity in this anatomic location. Duplex ultrasound and magnetic resonance imaging (MRI) are very specific in their ability to image these thrombi, but their sensitivity is low (Tables 24.6 and 24.7) (24, 25), especially if the thrombi are limited to the central portions of the subclavian and innominate veins (Fig. 24.8). In suspected subclavian thrombosis, screening with one of these modalities is helpful if thrombosis is found. However, if the MRI study or duplex scan is normal, radiographic contrast venography via a vein of the arm or hand must be done to

Table 24.4. Catheter Follow-up after Successful Urokinase Infusion[a]

Day Post-Urokinase	Event
1 through 6	1 Catheter removed electively
	2 Catheters removed due to infection
	3 Catheters dismissed from institutional follow-up
7 through 13	1 Catheter removed electively
	1 Patient died with catheter in place
14 through 20	2 Catheters removed for rethrombosis
	1 Catheter removed for infection
	3 Catheters dismissed from institutional follow-up
21 through 27	1 Catheter removed electively
	1 Catheter rethrombosed, responded to subsequent urokinase infusion
	1 Patient died with catheter in place
28 on	3 Catheters rethrombosed, responded to subsequent urokinase infusion
	4 Catheters removed electively
	1 Catheter removed due to infection
	4 Patients died with catheter in place
	1 Catheter dismissed from institutional follow-up
Total	29 Successful catheter infusions

[a]From Haire WD, Lieberman RP, Lund GB, Edney J, Wieczorek BM. Obstructed central venous catheters: restoring function with a 12-hour infusion of low-dose urokinase. Cancer 1990;66:2279–2285.

objectively confirm or rule out the diagnosis.

Therapy of catheter-related subclavian vein thrombosis is controversial. The acute consequences of catheter-induced subclavian vein thrombosis are pain and swelling of the arm/shoulder and pulmonary embolization (67). The frequency of pulmonary embolism (as suspected clinically) in patients receiving conventional chemotherapy is estimated to be 12% (68, 69). The frequency of pulmonary embolism may be higher if lung scans are done in all patients with symptomatic catheter-induced thrombosis, not just those with symptoms suggestive of embolism (70). The

risk of pulmonary embolism in high-dose therapy patients is not known. Long-term consequences of catheter-induced subclavian vein thrombosis could be postulated to be (a) symptoms of venous insufficiency, similar to those seen after spontaneous subclavian vein thrombosis (71–73), and (b) prevention of subsequent subclavian vein catheterization. The frequency with which any form of therapy prevents these sequelae will determine its role in treatment of symptomatic subclavian vein thrombosis.

Anticoagulation is aimed at preventing thrombus extension and pulmonary embolization. While it is effective in venous thrombosis in the leg (74), heparin anticoagulation does not appear to routinely prevent pulmonary embolization with subclavian vein thrombi (69). Fibrinolytic therapy of catheter-induced subclavian vein thrombosis has been advocated to relieve the pain and swelling and prevent symptoms of chronic venous insufficiency (75, 76). This approach can dissolve thrombi (at least acutely), and the patients quickly become asymptomatic and have a low likelihood of chronic venous insufficiency (75). However, fibrinolytic therapy is invasive (limiting its utility in patients with profound cytopenias and mucositis from high-dose therapy) and expensive (75). Additionally, acute pulmonary embolism and long-term venous patency rates with fibrinolytic therapy are not known. Recent studies using more conservative therapy, such as anticoagulation or no active intervention, have shown rapid resolution of pain and swelling and almost no chronic venous insufficiency (13, 69, 77). Both conservative management and fibrinolytic therapy result in rapid resolution of the acute symptoms of venous obstruction, have a low likelihood of chronic venous insufficiency, and have unknown rates of pulmonary embolism and long-term asymptomatic subclavian vein occlusion. Consequently, anticoagulant therapy (in an attempt to minimize the likelihood of pulmonary embolization) is the preferred treatment of symptomatic subclavian vein thrombosis. When anticoag-

Table 24.5. Coagulation and Fibrinolytic Parameters Before and After Urokinase Infusion[a]

	Pre-treatment[b]	Post-treatment[b]	p[c]
Protime (seconds)	12.6 ± 1.5	12.9 ± 2.2	n.s.
PTT (seconds)	28.6 ± 5.6	32.2 ± 9.5	0.02
Fibrinogen (mg/dl)	473 ± 143	479 ± 126	n.s.
Plasminogen (% normal)	104.5 ± 15.6	86.9 ± 21	0.002
Alpha-2-antiplasmin (% normal)	92 ± 11	74 ± 15	0.01
Plasminogen activator inhibitor (IU/ml)	6.8 ± 6.3	2.2 ± 2.4	0.01

[a]From Haire WD, Lieberman RP, Lund GB, Edney J, Wieczorek BM. Obstructed central venous catheters: restoring function with a 12-hour infusion of low-dose urokinase. Cancer 1990;66:2279–2285.
[b]Mean ± standard deviation.
[c]Mann-Whitney U test.
[d]Partial thromboplastin time.

Table 24.6. Results of Phlebography[a]

		Normal	Partial Occlusion	Complete Occlusion
	Normal	18	6	5[b]
Duplex scan	Partial occlusion	—	8	—
	Complete occlusion	—	—	6
Total: 43		18	14	11

[a]From Haire WD, Lynch TG, Lund GB, Lieberman RP, Edney JA. Limitations of magnetic resonance imaging and ultrasound-directed (duplex) scans in the diagnosis of subclavian vein thrombosis. J Vasc Surg 1991;13:391–397.
[b]Occlusion of proximal portion of left subclavian vein.

Table 24.7. Results of Phlebography[a]

		Normal	Partial Occlusion	Complete Occlusion
	Normal	15	6	1
MRI scan	Partial occlusion	—	2	—
	Complete occlusion	—	—	4
Total: 28		15	8	5

[a]From Haire WD, Lynch TG, Lund GB, Lieberman RP, Edney JA. Limitations of magnetic resonance imaging and ultrasound-directed (duplex) scans in the diagnosis of subclavian vein thrombosis. J Vasc Surg 1991;13:391–397.

ulant therapy is relatively contraindicated due to mucositis or thrombocytopenia, withholding anticoagulation until the catheter is no longer needed or the contraindication resolves is a reasonable therapeutic option. In patients who have suffered pulmonary embolism, anticoagulation is strongly recommended. If this cannot be done due to clinical contraindications, the catheter should be removed. If embolization occurs despite anticoagulation (69), placement of a Greenfield filter in the superior vena cava can be performed (78) once the catheter has been removed.

The third thrombotic complication of subclavian catheterization, asymptomatic subclavian/innominate vein thrombosis, has only recently been recognized in patients receiving high-dose antineoplastic therapy. One-fourth of patients undergoing autologous marrow transplantation develop totally occlusive asymptomatic subclavian vein thrombosis, while another 34% develop partially occlusive thrombi (16). The clinical significance of these thrombi is unknown. Consequently, the risk/benefit analysis of potential therapy cannot be estimated. However, the presence of these thrombi as a source of pulmonary

Figure 24.8. Arm venogram showing a short segmental occlusion of the proximal portion of the subclavian vein (*arrow*) that was not seen with either duplex scanning or MRI (From Haire WD, Lynch TG, Lund GB, Lieberman RP, Edney JA. Limitations of magnetic resonance imaging and ultrasound-directed (duplex) scans in the diagnosis of subclavian vein thrombosis. J Vasc Surg 1991;13:391–97.)

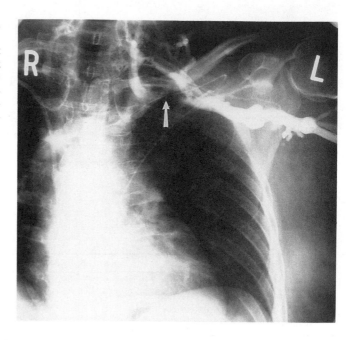

emboli should be kept in mind in patients with unexplained pulmonary symptoms. As with symptomatic thrombi, duplex ultrasound has low sensitivity but a high degree of specificity in diagnosis of asymptomatic subclavian vein thrombosis (26).

Infectious Complications

Infectious complications are an inherent risk of central venous catheters (79). Infectious complications lead to the removal of 1.5%–13% of all subclavian catheters placed in patients undergoing marrow transplantation (4, 11, 12). Three of 39 (7%) inferior vena cava apheresis catheters used for venous access during transplantation were removed due to infections (29). These complications take two forms: (*a*) infection of the skin entry site and subcutaneous tunnel and (*b*) bacteremia. The former generally precedes the latter (80), though it may not always be clinically apparent. Organisms present at the skin entry site can be rapidly transported along the length of the subcutaneous portion of the catheter and into the vascular space (81). Conse-

quently, preventing colonization/infection of the skin entry site and passage of organisms along the subcutaneous tunnel are keys to preventing catheter-related bacteremia (80). Prophylactic antibiotics given prior to catheter placement do not prevent subsequent catheter-related infection (82, 83). While care of the insertion site is obviously important, there are few studies objectively evaluating the various forms of local incision care (80). Leaving the entry site uncovered may be as effective as the transparent film or gauze dressings that are currently widely employed (84). The Dacron cuff used to anchor the catheter in the subcutaneous space provides a physical barrier to passage of organisms along the subcutaneous tunnel. This may, in part, account for the lower infection rate seen with Hickman-type catheters (85). Silver-impregnated collagen cuffs attached to the catheter are also an effective barrier to organism transport. While these cuffs are commercially available for use with long-term central venous catheters and can be used in patients undergoing high-dose antineoplastic therapy, their use in this setting has not been studied.

In other patient populations, however, this antimicrobial barrier reduced the rate of subcutaneous infection and lowered bacteremia rates from up to 13.8% to less than 1% (86, 87). Until data are available to suggest otherwise, their use in high-dose therapy patients is logical and recommended.

Multilumen catheters are reported to have a higher infection rate than single-lumen catheters (88, 89). Unfortunately, to date it has been impossible to determine if these differences in infection rates are related entirely to differences in catheter design (80). Prospective, randomized trials will be necessary to answer this question. Nevertheless, use of double-lumen catheters is widely accepted in high-dose therapy patients.

Diagnosis of catheter-related infectious complications is a difficult clinical task (90). Diagnosis of overt entry site and subcutaneous tunnel infection is relatively straightforward, with widely accepted criteria for diagnosis (82, 90). Entry site infection is defined as erythema, induration, and/or tenderness within 2 cm of the catheter entry site. The same constellation of signs more than 2 cm above the entry site is classified as infection of the subcutaneous tract. Proving that the catheter is the source of fever or bacteremia without clinically evident entry site or tunnel infection is more difficult. Quantitative cultures of blood drawn through the catheter (90) or of material obtained from the inside of the catheter by a specially designed brush (91) can give information without removing the catheter. Unfortunately, these techniques are not widely available, limiting their clinical application. Quantitative culture of the tip after removal of the catheter can also be helpful (92) but necessitates sacrificing the catheter. Fortunately, more than 50% of the catheter-related infections are caused by *Staphylococcus epidermidis* and can generally be successfully treated with antibiotics without resorting to catheter removal (90). Exceptions to this rule include infections due to *Staphylococcus aureus* (93), *Pseudomonas* species (94) and *Candida* species (95). These are generally unresponsive to antibiotic therapy alone and require catheter removal.

SUMMARY AND CONCLUSIONS

Despite the problems encountered with central venous catheters, high-dose antineoplastic therapy would be impossible without them. Even though they have been a widely used for over a decade, many catheter management areas remain undefined. The areas of prediction, prophylaxis, and diagnosis of catheter-related complications are in particular need of further study. Patients undergoing high-dose therapy constitute a special subset of central venous catheter users. The most effective method of dealing with catheter-related complications in these patients may not be identical to the approach in other patient populations. Further investigation of complications of currently available venous access devices and novel approaches to the problem of venous access in high-dose therapy patients is warranted. Only by objective study of this group of patients can we find ways of prediction, prevention, diagnosis, and treatment of catheter-related complications that are safe and effective in the growing number of patients eligible for high-dose antineoplastic therapy. However, with the use of techniques proven effective in other groups of patients, many of the catheter-related complications in high-dose therapy patients can be effectively managed. This is especially true of noninfectious complications leading to venous access failure.

REFERENCES

1. Hickman RO, Buckner CD, Clift RA, Sanders JE, Stewart P, Thomas ED. A modified right atrial catheter for access to the venous system in marrow transplant recipients. Surg Gynecol Obstet 1979;148:871–875.
2. Petz LD, Scott EP. Supportive care. In: Blume KG, Petz LD, eds. Clinical bone marrow transplantation. New York: Churchill Livingstone, 1983:201–202.
3. Grant JP. Catheter access. In: Rombeau JL, Caldwell MD, eds. Parenteral nutrition. Philadelphia: WB Saunders, 1986:306.
4. Sanders JE, Hickman RO, Aker S, Hersman J, Buckner CD, Thomas ED. Experience with double lumen

right atrial catheters. J Parenter Enter Nutr 1982;6:95–99.

5. Raaf JH. Results from use of 826 vascular access devices in cancer patients. Cancer 1985;55:1312–1321.

6. Dudrick SJ, Wilmore DW, Vars HM, Rhoads HJ. Can intravenous feeding as the sole means of nutrition support growth in the child and restore weight loss in the adult? An affirmative answer. Ann Surg 1969;169:974–984.

7. Broviac JW, Cole JJ, Schribner BH. A silicone rubber atrial catheter for prolonged parenteral alimentation. Surg Gynecol Obstet 1973;136:602–606.

8. Spruce WE. Supportive care in bone marrow transplantation. In: Johnson FL, Pochedly C, eds. Bone marrow transplantation in children. New York: Raven Press, 1990:72.

9. Lokich JJ, Bothe AJ, Benotti P, Moore C. Complications and management of implanted venous access catheters. J Clin Oncol 1985;3:1710–1717.

10. Mirro J, Rao BN, Stokes DC, et al. A prospective study of Hickman/Broviac catheters and implantable ports in pediatric oncology patients. J Clin Oncol 1989; 7:214–222.

11. Ulz L, Petersen FB, Ford R, et al. A prospective study of complications in Hickman right atrial catheters in marrow transplant patients. J Parenter Enter Nutr 1990;14:27–30.

12. Petersen FB, Clift RA, Hickman RO, et al. Hickman catheter complications in marrow transplant recipients. J Parenter Enter Nutr 1986;10:58–62.

13. Haire WD, Lieberman RP, Edney JA, et al. Hickman catheter-induced thoracic vein thrombosis: frequency and long-term sequelae in patients receiving high-dose chemotherapy and marrow transplantation. Cancer 1990;66:900–908.

14. Camp LD. Care of the Groshong catheter. Oncol Nurs Forum 1988;15:745–749.

15. Maliviya VK, Deppe G, Gove N, Malone JM. Vascular access in gynecologic cancer using the Groshong catheter. Gynecol Oncol 1989;33:313–316.

16. Haire WD, Lieberman RP, Lund GB, Edney JA, Kessinger A, Armitage JO. Thrombotic complications of silicone rubber catheters during autologous marrow and peripheral stem cell transplantation: prospective comparison of Hickman and Groshong catheters. Bone Marrow Transplant 1991;7:57–59.

17. Kirkemo A, Johnson MR. Percutaneous subclavian vein placement of the Hickman catheter. Surgery 1982; 91:349–351.

18. Jansen RFM, Wiggers T, van Geel BN, van Putten WLJ. Assessment of insertion techniques and complication rates of dual lumen central venous catheters in patients with hematological malignancies. World J Surg 1990;14:101–106.

19. Coit DG, Turnbull ADM. A safe technique for the placement of implantable vascular access devices in patients with thrombocytopenia. Surg Gynecol Obstet 1988;167:429–431.

20. Robertson LJ, Mauro MA, Jaques PF, Radiologic placement of Hickman catheters. Radiology 1989;170:1007–1009.

21. Bern MM, Lokich JJ, Wallach SR, et al. Very low doses of warfarin can prevent thrombosis in central venous catheters. Ann Intern Med 1990;112:423–428.

22. Axelsson K, Effson F. Phlebograpy in long-term catheterization of the subclavian vein. Scand J Gastroenterol 1978;13:933–938.

23. Haire WD, Lynch TG, Lieberman RP, Edney JA. Clinical utility of preoperative duplex ultrasound before subclavian vein catheterization in cancer patients who have undergone prior subclavian vein catheter placement. Arch Surg, in press.

24. Haire WD, Lynch TG, Lund GB, Lieberman RP, Edney JA. Limitations of magnetic resonance imaging and ultrasound-directed (duplex) scans in the diagnosis of subclavian vein thrombosis. J Vasc Surg 1991; 13:391–397.

25. Knudson GJ, Weidmeyer DA, Erickson SJ, et al. Color doppler sonographic imaging in the assessment of upper extremity deep venous thrombosis. AJR 1990; 154:399–403.

26. Haire WD, Lynch TG, Lieberman RP, Lund GB, Edney JA. Utility of duplex ultrasound in the diagnosis of asymptomatic catheter-induced subclavian vein thrombosis. J Ultrasound Med, 1991;10:493–496.

27. Selby JB, Tegtmeyer CJ, Amodeo C, Bittner L, Atuk NO. Insertion of subclavian hemodialysis catheters in difficult cases: value of fluoroscopy and angiographic techniques. AJR 1989;152:641–643.

28. Haire WD, Lieberman RP, Lund GB, Boyle BM, Armitage JO, Kessinger A. Translumbar inferior vena cava catheters: safety and efficacy in peripheral stem cell transplantation. Transfusion 1990;30:511–515.

29. Haire WD, Lieberman RP, Lund GB, Wieczorek BM, Armitage JO, Kessinger A. Translumbar inferior vena cava catheters: experience with 58 catheters in peripheral stem cell collection and transplantation. Transfusion Sci 1990;11:195–200.

30. Haire WD, Edney JA, Landmark JD, Kessinger A. Thrombotic complications of subclavian apheresis catheters in cancer patients: prevention with heparin infusion. J. Clin Apheresis 1990;5:188–191.

31. Sutton DMC, Cardella CJ, Uldall PR, Deveber GA. Complications of intensive plasma exchange. Plasma Ther 1981;2:19–23.

32. Williams BM, Sanders JE, Clift RA, et al. Use of arteriovenous shunts and right atrial catheters for daily granulocyte collection. J Clin Apheresis 1987;3:171–173.

33. Lipchick EO, Rogoff SM. Abdominal aortography: translumbar, femoral, and axillary artery catheterization techniques. In: Abrams HL, ed. Abrams angiography. Boston: Little, Brown 1983:1032.

34. Denny DF, Dorfman GS, Greenwood LH, Horowitz NR, Morse SS. Translumbar inferior vena cava Hick-

man catheter placement for total parenteral nutrition. AJR 1987;148:621–622.

35. Lund GB, Lieberman RP, Haire WD, Martin V, Kessinger A, Armitage JO. Translumbar inferior vena cava catheters for long-term venous access. Radiology 1990;174:31–35.

36. Haire WD, Lieberman RP, Lund GB, Kessinger A. Translumbar inferior vena cava catheters. Bone Marrow Transplant 1991;7:389–392.

37. Lund GB, Lieberman RP, Haire WD. Central venous catheters. Semin Intervent Radiol 1989;6:162–175.

38. Cassidy FP Jr, Zajko AB, Bron KM, Reilly JJ, Peitzman AB, Steed DL. Non-infectious complications of long-term central venous catheters: radiologic evaluation and management. AJR 1987;149:671–675.

39. Cho SR, Tisnado J, Beachley MC, Vines FS, Alford WL. Percutaneous unknotting of intravascular catheters and retrieval of catheter fragments. AJR 1983;141:397–402.

40. Mullen JL, Oleaga J, Ring EJ. Catheter migration during home hyperalimentation. JAMA 1977;238:1946–1947.

41. Ouriel K, Brennan JK, Desch C, Lyons JM, Schloerb PR. Migration of a permanent central venous catheter. J Parenter Enter Nutr 1983;7:410–411.

42. Lois JF, Gomes AS, Pusey E. Nonsurgical repositioning of central venous catheters. Radiology 1987;165:329–333.

43. Falchuk SC, Ahlgren JD, Holt RW. Acute thyroiditis as a complication of chemotherapy administration through a Hickman catheter. Cancer Treat Rep 1987;7–8:788–790.

44. Tschirhart JM, Rao MK. Mechanism and management of persistent withdrawal occlusion. Am Surg 1988;54:326–328.

45. Brismar B, Hardstedt C, Jacobson S, Kagar L, Malmborg AS. Reduction of catheter-associated thrombosis in parenteral nutrition by intravenous heparin therapy. Arch Surg 1982;117:1196–1199.

46. Fabri PJ, Mirtallo KM, Ruberg RL, et al. Incidence and prevention of thrombosis of the subclavian vein during total parenteral nutrition. Surg Gynecol Obstet 1982;155:238–240.

47. Imperial J, Bistrian BR, Bothe A, Bern M, Blackburn GL. Limitation of central vein thrombosis in total parenteral nutrition by continuous infusion of low-dose heparin. J Am Coll Nutr 1983;2:63–73.

48. Bern MM, Lokich JJ, Wallach SR, et al. Very low doses of warfarin can prevent thrombosis in central venous catheters. Ann Intern Med 1990;112:423–428.

49. Rogers JS, Murgo JA, Fontana JA, Raich PC. Chemotherapy for breast cancer decreases plasma protein C and protein S. J Clin Oncol 1988;6:276–281.

50. Harper PL, Jarvis J, Jennings I, Luddington R, Marcus RE. Changes in the natural anticoagulants following bone marrow transplantation. Bone Marrow Transplant 1990;5:39–42.

51. Haire WD, Kessinger A, Armitage JO. Protein C and antithrombin III deficiencies occur during autologous marrow transplantation [Abstract]. J Cell Biochem 1990;44(suppl 14a):319.

52. Ruiz MA, Marugan I, Estelles A, et al. The influence of chemotherapy on plasma coagulation and fibrinolytic systems in lung cancer patients. Cancer 1989;63:643–648.

53. Hadaway LC. Evaluation and use of advanced IV technology part 1: central venous access devices. J Intravenous Nurs 1989;12:73–82.

54. Brown JK, Stoner MH, Barley ZA. Tunneled catheter thrombosis: factors related to incidence. Oncol Nurs Forum 1990;17:543–549.

55. Johnson RL, Lieberman RP, Kaplan PA, Haire WD. Silicone rubber catheter venography using standard angiographic techniques. Cardiovasc Intervent Radiol 1988;11:45–49.

56. Lawson M, Bottino JC, Hurtibise MR, et al. The use of urokinase to restore the patency of occluded central venous catheters. Am J Intravenous Ther Clin Nutr 1982;9:29–32.

57. Hurtibise MR, Bottino JC, Lawson M, et al. Restoring patency of occluded central venous catheters. Arch Surg 1980;115:212–213.

58. Monturo CA, Dickerson RN, Mullen JL. Efficacy of thrombolytic therapy for occlusion of long-term catheters. J Parenter Enter Nutr 1990;14:312–314.

59. Haire WD, Lieberman RP, Lund GB, Edney J, Wieczorek BM. Obstructed central venous catheters: restoring function with a 12-hour infusion of low-dose urokinase. Cancer 1990;66:2279–2285.

60. Haire WD, Lieberman RP, Kessinger A, Bierman PB, Armitage JO. Six hour infusion of urokinase restores function of thrombotically occluded central venous catheters that have not responded to standard therapy [Abstract]. Blood 1990;76(suppl 1):509.

61. Atkinson JB, Bagnall HA, Gomperts E. Investigational use of tissue plasminogen activator (t-PA) for occluded central venous catheters. J Parenter Enter Nutr 1990;14:310–311.

62. Conlan MG, Haire WD, Armitage JO, Kessinger A. Prothrombotic hemostatic abnormalities in patients with refractory malignant lymphoma. Bone Marrow Transplant 1991;7:475–479.

63. Conlan MG, Haire WD, Lieberman RP, Lund GB, Kessinger A, Armitage JO. Catheter-related thrombosis in patients with refractory lymphoma undergoing autologous stem cell transplantation. Bone Marrow Transplant 1991;7:235–240.

64. Viero P, Cortellazo S, Cassarato C, Barbui T, Colluci M, Semararo M. Increased production of mononuclear cell procoagulant activity in Hodgkin's disease. Eur J Cancer Clin Oncol 1983;11:1539–1543.

65. Haire WD, Pirruccello SJ, Armitage JO, Carson SD. Increased monocyte tissue factor in Hodgkin's disease [Abstract]. Clin Res 1990;38:841.

66. Kaufman J, Demas C, Stark K, Flancbaum L. Catheter-related septic central venous thrombosis: current therapeutic options. West J Med 1986;145:200–2003.
67. Leiby JM, Purcell H, DeMaria JJ, Kraut EH, Sagone AL, Metz EN. Pulmonary embolism as a result of Hickman catheter-related thrombosis. Am J Med 1989; 86:228–231.
68. Horattas MC, Wright DJ, Fenton AH, et al. Changing concepts of deep venous thrombosis of the upper extremity: report of a series and review of the literature. Surgery 1988;104:561–567.
69. Donayre CE, White GH, Mehringer SM, Wilson SE. Pathogenesis determines late morbidity of axillosubclavian vein thrombosis. Am J Surg 1986;152:179–184.
70. Monreal M, Lafoz E, Ruiz J, Valls R, Alastrue A. Upper-extremity deep venous thrombosis and pulmonary embolism: a prospective study. Chest 1991;99:280–283.
71. Inahara T. Surgical treatment of "effort" thrombosis of the axillary and subclavian veins. Am Surg 1968;34:479–483.
72. Swinton NW, Edgett JW, Hall RJ. Primary subclavian-axillary vein thrombosis. Circulation 1968;38:737–745.
73. Adams JT. McEvoy RK, DeWeese JA. Primary deep venous thrombosis of the upper extremity. Arch Surg 1965;91:29–42.
74. Hull RD, Raskob GE, Hirsch J, et al. Continuous intravenous heparin compared with subcutaneous heparin in the initial treatment of proximal-vein thrombosis. N Engl J Med 1986;315:1109–1114.
75. Fraschini G, Jadeja J, Lawson M, Holmes FA, Carrasco HC, Wallace S. Local infusion of urokinase for the lysis of thrombosis associated with permanent central venous catheters in cancer patients. J Clin Oncol 1987;5:672–678.
76. Rubenstein M, Creger W. Successful streptokinase therapy for catheter-induced subclavian vein thrombosis. Arch Intern Med 1980;140:1370–1371.
77. Smith VC, Hallet JW. Subclavian vein thrombosis during prolonged catheterization for parenteral nutrition: early management and long-term follow-up. South Med J 1983;76:603–606.
78. Pais SO, DeOrchis DF, Mirvis SE. Superior vena cava placement of a Kimray-Greenfield filter. Radiology 1987;165:385–386.
79. van Hoff J, Berg AT, Seashore JH. The effort of right atrial catheters on infectious complications of chemotherapy in children. J Clin Oncol 1990;8:1255–1262.
80. Toltzis P, Goldman DA. Current issues in central venous catheter infection. Annu Rev Med 1990;41:169–176.
81. Cooper GL, Schiller AL, Hopkins CC. Possible role of capillary action in pathogenesis of experimental catheter-associated dermal tunnel infections. J Clin Microbiol 1988;26:8–12.
82. Press OW, Ramsey PG, Larson EB, Fefer A, Hickman RO. Hickman catheter infections in patients with malignancies. Medicine 1984;63:189–200.
83. McKee R, Dunsmuir R, Whitby M, Garden OJ. Does antibiotic prophylaxis at the time of catheter insertion reduce the incidence of sepsis in intravenous nutrition? J Hosp Infect 1985;10:77–82.
84. Petrosino B, Becker H, Christian B. Infection rates in central venous catheter dressings. Oncol Nurs Forum 1988;15:709–717.
85. Mitchel A, Atkins S, Royle GT, Kettlewell MGW. Reduced catheter sepsis and prolonged catheter life using a tunnelled silicone rubber catheter for total parenteral nutrition. Br J Surg 1982;69:420–422.
86. Maki DG, Cobb L, Garman JK, et al. An attachable silver-impregnated cuff for prevention of infection with central venous catheters: a prospective randomized multicentered trial. Am J Med 1988;85:307–314.
87. Flowers RH, Schwenzer KJ, Kopel RF, et al. Efficacy of an attachable subcutaneous cuff for the prevention of intravascular catheter-related infection. JAMA 1989;261:878–883.
88. Early TF, Gregory RT, Wheeler JR, Snyder SO, Gayle RG. Increased infection rate in double-lumen versus single-lumen Hickman catheters in cancer patients. South Med J 1990;69:420–422.
89. Hilton E, Haslett TM, Borenstein MT, Tucci V, Isenberg HD, Singer C. Central catheter infections: single versus triple lumen catheters. Am J Med 1988;84:667–672.
90. Clarke DE, Raffin TA. Infectious complications of indwelling long-term central venous catheters. Chest 1990;97:966–972.
91. Markus S. Buday S. Culturing indwelling central venous catheters in situ. Infect Surg 1989;157–162.
92. Jones PG, Hopfer RL, Elting L, Jackson JA, Fainstein V, Bodey GP. Semiquantitative cultures of intravascular catheters from cancer patients. Diagn Microbiol Infect Dis 1986;4:299–306.
93. Dugdale DC, Ramsey PG. Staphylococcus aureus bacteremia in patients with Hickman catheters. Am J Med 1990;89:137–141.
94. Benezra D, Kiehn TE, Gold JWM, Brown AE, Turnbull ADM, Armstrong D. Prospective study of infections in indwelling central venous catheters using quantitative blood cultures. Am J Med 1988;84:495–498.
95. Dato VM, Dajani AS. Candidemia in children with central venous catheters: role of catheter removal and amphotericin B therapy. Pediatr Infect Dis J 1990; 9:309–314.

25

BLOOD BANK SUPPORT IN PATIENTS UNDERGOING HIGH-DOSE CANCER THERAPY

Kenneth C. Anderson

The therapeutic advances made using high-dose combination chemotherapeutic approaches in the past (i.e., curative therapies for childhood acute lymphoblastic leukemias) would not have been possible without the parallel development of transfusion medicine expertise to support patients through the hematologic complications of therapy. Similarly, the current use of high-dose chemoradiotherapy to treat a broad spectrum of malignant diseases has been possible due to advances in the technology of hematopoietic stem cell support. Specifically, refinements in testing for HLA compatibility, coupled with new approaches to both prevent and treat graft-versus-host disease (GVHD), have resulted in widespread utilization of allogeneic bone marrow transplantation (BMT) (1–3). Since only 40% of patients have HLA-matched related donors, allogeneic BMT using unrelated HLA-matched donors has also been tested, with promising preliminary results (4, 5). Moreover, there is increased use of high-dose therapy followed by autologous BMT, with or without purging of marrow tumor cells, to treat both hematologic cancers and solid tumors (6). Finally, use of autologous peripheral blood stem cell (PBSC) transplantation is also increasing to restore hematologic and immune function after high-dose ablative therapies.

The role of the blood component laboratory in treatment with high-dose chemotherapy is central and multifaceted. This chapter will focus specifically on the following aspects: provision of appropriate red blood cell (RBC), platelet (plt), and blood component support both before and after high-dose therapies to avoid transfusion-related alloimmunization, GVHD, and cytomegalovirus (CMV) infection; processing and cryopreservation of stem cells from bone marrow and peripheral blood; ABO compatibility in allogeneic BMT; as well as future directions including the use of PBSC transplantation, recombinant growth factors, and leukopoor blood components to hasten engraftment, lessen toxicity, and decrease blood component needs after these high-dose ablative treatments.

BLOOD COMPONENT SUPPORT

The blood component laboratory plays a critical role by providing appropriate RBC, plt, and blood component support to patients both before and after high-dose therapy. Several patient factors may influence hematologic recovery and immune reconstitution and therefore the magnitude of blood product support required in patients who undergo

437

high-dose therapies (7–12). In all BMT recipients, hematologic engraftment may be compromised due to disease and/or treatment-related effects on the marrow microenvironment. Reconstitution after allogeneic BMT may be relatively enhanced since the donor marrow is healthy; however, engraftment may be adversely affected by regimens employed in the recipient to either prevent or treat GVHD. Moreover, in vitro T cell depletion of donor marrow, which can effectively abrogate GVHD, has in some patients resulted in failure to engraft and graft rejection. Autologous marrow may be intrinsically compromised due to the patient's underlying disease and cytotoxic therapy received prior to marrow harvesting, due to in vitro techniques utilized for removal of tumor cells, or due to cryopreservation. In syngeneic BMT, donor marrow is histocompatible and healthy and neither manipulated nor cryopreserved. However, the underlying disease and prior treatment of the recipient may, as is true in other types of BMT, compromise the marrow microenvironment and thereby adversely affect engraftment.

After high-dose chemoradiotherapy and BMT, there is a period of pancytopenia lasting at least 2–4 weeks when patients require multiple RBC and plt transfusions (9–15). For example, patients with aplastic anemia undergoing allogeneic BMT received a median of 9 (range, 1–82) and 44 (range, 6–468) units of RBCs and plts, respectively, primarily during the first 4 weeks postgrafting (13). Bensinger and colleagues have examined various clinical parameters that predict for increased transfusion requirements in 303 patients with acute nonlymphocytic leukemia in first remission who underwent allogeneic BMT (15). Method of prophylaxis against GVHD, the development of acute GVHD, method of prophylaxis against infection, and donor-recipient ABO compatibility all influenced the need for transfusion support. For example, patients with grades 3–4 acute GVHD required more blood product support than those with grades 1–2 acute GVHD: a median

of 217 units of plts and 27.5 units of RBCs in the former group, compared to 91 units of plts and 14 units of RBCs in the latter patients.

There are few studies comparing similar patients who have received allogeneic BMT and autologous BMT in terms of engraftment, required blood product support, and outcome. Kersey and colleagues have examined patients with non T-cell acute lymphoblastic leukemia, 46 of whom underwent monoclonal antibody (MoAb)-purged autologous BMT and 45 of whom received allogeneic marrow grafts (16). Autologous marrow recipients engrafted more quickly, had shorter hospital stays, had fewer early deaths, and although unreported, presumably had less transfusion requirements than allogeneic BMT recipients. The latter group took longer to engraft, had longer hospital stays, and had more early deaths related to GVHD and infection. However, due to a higher relapse rate in the autologous graft recipients than in the allogeneic recipients, long-term disease-free survival was equivalent in autologous and allogeneic BMT recipients. The time to hematologic engraftment and transfusion needs for patients undergoing high-dose therapies followed by BMT and PBSC transplantation for hematologic cancers and solid tumors at our institute are delineated in Table 25.1 (17–22). As can be seen, the volume of transfusion support required is great, regardless of the source of stem cells or underlying disease.

TRANSFUSION STRATEGY

Any patients who are potential candidates for high-dose therapies must be identified early in order to avoid transfusion-related effects that might adversely influence outcome after subsequent high-dose therapy. Specifically, transfusion strategy must avoid alloimmunization, exposure, and transfusion-associated (TA) GVHD in patients who may subsequently receive high-dose therapy.

Table 25.1.   Hematologic Engraftment and Transfusion Requirements after Hematopoietic Stem Cell Transplantation[a]

| Disease | Number of Patients | Source of Hematopoietic Stem Cells | Days from Reinfusion to | | Units of Red Cells Transfused | Units of Platelets Transfused[c] | Ref. |
			Granulocytes $>5 \times 10^2/mm^{3b}$	Platelets $>2 \times 10^4/mm^{3b}$			
Breast cancer	29	ABM	21(10–44)	23(10–81)	13(4–101)	105(11–1350)	17
Breast cancer	12	APB	14(10–26)	12(8–15)	8(2–19)	23(10–277)	17, 18
T-cell lymphoma and leukemia	14	ABM	23(13–48)	26(15–43)	12(5–20)	69(20–131)	20
B cell lymphoma	100	ABM	27(10–99)	29(10–137)	11(2–75)	66(11–604)	19
Multiple myeloma	11	ABM	21(12–46)	23(12–53)	10(4–30)	41(4–139)	21
Hematologic malignancies	69	ALBM	18(13–53)	24	9(2–89)	72(8–736)	22

[a]Abbreviations: ABM, autologous bone marrow; ALBM, allogeneic bone marrow; APB, autologous peripheral blood.
[b]Median (range) day posttransplant.
[c]Each unit contains 5.5×10^{10} platelets. Each transfusion contains 6–8 units.

Alloimmunization

The likelihood of transfusion-related sensitization to HLA antigens varies in different patient populations and, in some studies, appears to correlate with the number of donor exposures (23). Since many patients undergoing BMT have received previous transfusions, sensitization to HLA antigens may have occurred. The effect of HLA sensitization on marrow engraftment is most evident in the setting of aplastic anemia: Reported graft rejection rates range from 25%–60% in multiply transfused patients with aplastic anemia given HLA-identical sibling marrow grafts (24–26). A recent analysis of 625 patients with aplastic anemia who received allografts from HLA-identical donors demonstrated either no or transient engraftment in 68 (11%) patients (27). Of a variety of clinical parameters analyzed, post-BMT treatment with cyclosporine and avoidance of pre-BMT blood transfusions were associated with improved survival.

Although graft failure post-BMT associated with histocompatibility differences between donor and recipients is often attributed to rejection by host T lymphocytes, persistent host antibodies specific for donor antigen may also mediate graft failure. This can occur either by antibody dependent cell-mediated cytotoxicity or complement-mediated cytotoxicity. Specifically, host anti-HLA class I antibodies have been associated with graft failure and death, and host anti-ABO antibodies have persisted for up to 18 months post-BMT and resulted in erythroid hypoplasia (28). Therefore, the need for transfusions should be critically evaluated in patients who are eligible for subsequent allogeneic marrow grafting. Transfusions from family members, and especially those from the potential marrow donor, should be avoided due to the risk of sensitization of the patient to both HLA and non-HLA antigens.

Patients undergoing BMT also require large numbers of cellular blood product transfusions after BMT and therefore experience multiple homologous blood donor exposures (Table 25.1). Since sensitization to HLA antigens has in some series increased with number of transfusions and related donor exposures (29), one might expect that patients would therefore be at high risk to develop alloimmunization after marrow grafting. A retrospective analysis of 264 patients with severe aplastic anemia who underwent allogeneic BMT did in fact document the development of refractoriness to transfusion of random donor platelets in 71 (34%) patients; both number of platelets transfused (if ≥ 40 units) and development of lymphocytotoxic antibodies correlated with refractoriness to transfusion (23). This ability to form anti-HLA antibodies post-high-dose therapy is somewhat surprising, given the known in vitro immune deficiency noted in such patients for the first year post-BMT (7, 8).

TRANSFUSION GUIDELINES

Since patients undergoing BMT are likely to require large numbers of blood components both before and after marrow grafting, they would be an appropriate group in which to employ strategies to avoid alloimmunization, i.e., use of single donor products, ultraviolet (UV) irradiation, or leukodepletion of components before transfusion. Leukodepletion of blood components prior to transfusion to patients with leukemia has been best studied: Techniques that result in 10^6 or fewer residual leukocytes in transfused products correlate with delay or avoidance of alloimmunization in transfusion recipients (30–35), whereas components with $>10^8$ contaminating leukocytes do not abrogate sensitization (36). Although some reports suggest that the use of single-donor platelets can minimize alloimmunization (37, 38), this remains an area of active study. At present, leukodepleted blood products can be readily obtained either by filtration or apheresis technology and should be utilized from the outset to avoid sensitization to HLA and other antigens and related clinical sequelae.

Cytomegalovirus Infection

Cellular blood components transfused from CMV-seropositive donors to CMV-seronegative transplant recipients can cause CMV seroconversion and infection (39–53). In allogeneic BMT, it has long been known that the serologic status of the patient pre-BMT is the most important predictor of CMV infection post-BMT and that transfusions from CMV-seropositive donors to CMV-seronegative recipients can cause CMV seroconversion and infection (39–41, 45, 46, 50, 53). In an early study of prophylactic granulocytes in recipients in allogeneic BMT, for example, lack of

infection was documented only in the setting of seronegative recipients who received granulocytes from seronegative donors (43). Either transfusion with seronegative blood products or treatment with immune globulin appears to lessen CMV infection after allogeneic BMT when both donor and patient are seronegative, but not when either are seropositive (45, 46); utilizing both immune globulin and CMV-seronegative blood products appears to confer no additional benefit. CMV infection, strongly associated with acute GVHD (40, 50) may become less frequent due to the development of effective prophylaxis for GVHD. In addition, acyclovir therapy can lessen the incidence of CMV infection and related morbidity, thereby improving survival of seropositive allogeneic BMT recipients (54). Finally, recent reports document successful therapy of CMV pneumonia after BMT with ganciclovir and either intravenous immune globulin or CMV immune globulin (55, 56). Based upon these and other studies, methods of CMV prophylaxis have to date been reserved for allogeneic BMT when both donor and recipient are seronegative.

CMV infection in autologous BMT recipients is less common, perhaps related to the rarity of GVHD in autologous BMT recipients. Although equivalent numbers of autologous and allogeneic BMT recipients either seroconvert to or excrete CMV, this has clinical sequelae only in allogeneic BMT recipients who have GVHD (40). Methods for CMV prophylaxis such as immune globulin, seronegative blood products, or posttransplant acyclovir therapy have therefore not been utilized in autologous BMT recipients. However, pretransplant CMV serology also predicts for CMV infection post autologous BMT (41), and engraftment may be delayed post autologous BMT in patients with CMV infection (57). Moreover, a recent analysis of 159 autologous BMT recipients, all of whom received CMV-unscreened blood products, documented a probability of CMV infection of 22.5% in CMV-seronegative patients and 61.1% in seropositive recipients (51). In this series, CMV pneumonia developed in 11 patients at a median of 100 days post-BMT and was fatal in 9 cases. At our institute we have provided frozen deglycerolized RBCs and plts from CMV-seronegative donors to 400 patients undergoing autologous BMT and noted no seroconversion or clinical evidence of CMV infection. Thus preventative measures against CMV, similar to those used in allogeneic BMT, may also be warranted in autologous BMT.

TRANSFUSION GUIDELINES

The traditional CMV-seronegative cellular blood products have been frozen deglycerolized RBCs and plts harvested from CMV-seronegative donors. Recently, however, filtration to deplete leukocytes from RBCs prior to transfusion has been shown to decrease transfusion-acquired CMV infection in infants (47). Leukocyte-poor blood components have also been shown to decrease CMV seroconversion in patients undergoing treatment for acute leukemia (48, 52). Preliminary data from Seattle suggest that provision of filtered RBCs and plt transfusions from unscreened donors to CMV-seronegative patients undergoing autologous BMT may prevent seroconversion or infection in the recipient (49). Finally, De Witte and colleagues have recently shown that leukocyte depletion of blood products and acyclovir prophylaxis may also prevent primary CMV infection in CMV-seronegative allogeneic BMT recipients (58). Although needing further confirmation in larger studies, the ability to utilize filtered blood products as CMV seronegative would markedly expand the donor pool and thereby the supply of noninfectious components.

Transfusion-Associated Graft-Versus-Host Disease

Recipients of allogeneic BMT are profoundly immunosuppressed and at risk for opportunistic infections and GVHD (7, 8). Recipients of autologous grafts have also received high-dose ablative therapy and are similarly immunocompromised and at risk, albeit perhaps to a lesser extent, for GVHD and infection (7, 8, 14). All such patients undergoing high-dose chemotherapy are at risk for the development of TA-GVHD after receiving cellular blood products (59). The most commonly reported manifestations are skin rash, abnormal results on liver function tests, and severe pancytopenia. The degree of pancytopenia has generally been profound, perhaps related to the HLA disparity evident between donor and recipient in TA-GVHD. In contrast, GVHD occurs post allogeneic BMT when marrow and donor have been chosen by virtue of histocompatibility. TA-GVHD results in an overall 84% mortality rate after a median of 21 days (range, 8–1050 days) (59).

TA-GVHD can be effectively prevented by gamma irradiation of the blood product prior to transfusion. Recent studies suggest that irradiation at 1500–2000 rads can reduce mitogen-responsive lymphocytes by 5–6 logs compared to unirradiated controls (60). It has previously been recommended that the lowest dose of gamma irradiation capable of inhibiting lymphocyte proliferation (1500–2500 cGy) be utilized to irradiate blood components prior to transfusion (61). However, the observation that a small percentage of lymphocytes survive irradiation at these doses, coupled with a single reported case of apparent TA-GVHD in a BMT recipient who received only components irradiated at 2000 rad (60), suggests that existing blood product irradiation guidelines may require reassessment.

A potential alternative method to prevent TA-GVHD would be to deplete lymphocytes from blood products prior to transfusion. T lymphocytes mediate GVHD and the incidence and severity of GVHD post allogeneic BMT can be reduced if T cells are eliminated from the donor marrow prior to grafting by a variety of techniques (62). While it may not be either possible or practical to treat blood components in a similar fashion, techniques are presently available for the depletion of leukocytes to produce leukopoor RBCs and plts that contain 10^6 lymphocytes (63, 64). However, since the number and precise T cells required to mediate TA-GVHD remain undefined, it is unknown whether depletion of leukocytes using these currently available techniques would decrease the risk of TA-GVHD. Recently a canine model has been used to demonstrate that UV rather than gamma irradiation of transfused leukocytes can abrogate GVHD in recipient animals (65). Preliminary studies in man have utilized UV irradiation of blood components to minimize alloimmunization (66), but future studies are needed to determine whether UV light can avoid TA-GVHD in transfusion recipients without adverse effects on in vitro function or in vivo recovery of UV-treated RBCs or plts.

TRANSFUSION GUIDELINES

A recently completed survey of blood component irradiation practices in the United States found that 88% and 81.4% of allogeneic and autologous BMT recipients, respectively, received irradiated cellular components (67). Although it is reassuring that the overwhelming majority of patients do receive irradiated components, it is disturbing that not all patients receive them. A recent documentation of several cases of fatal TA-GVHD in recipients of autologous BMT (68) further suggests that irradiation of cellular components transfused to BMT recipients is not yet uniform practice. It is essential that all patients undergoing high-dose cancer chemotherapy be supported solely with blood components treated with at least 1500 rad prior to their transfusion.

BONE MARROW PROCESSING

Quality Control

As the use of BMT has increased as a treatment strategy, the blood component laboratory has become increasingly involved in marrow processing. However, at present bone marrow is not a licensed blood product, and

no federal regulations concerning its collection, transportation, processing, storage, or transfusion exist. The rapid expansion of BMT centers and increasingly complicated processing techniques suggest that standards should now be developed to ensure recipient safety and laboratory quality control. It has recently been suggested that bone marrow processing laboratories should adopt the laboratory standards already existing for blood banks, i.e., regulations concerning storage, freezing, transfusion, etc., thereby treating marrow as any other blood product (69).

Automated Processing in the Blood Bank

Bone marrow processing may consist of several steps: concentration and washing; sedimentation with hydroxyethyl starch, Ficoll-Hypaque, or Percoll; purging and washing; cryopreservation and storage; and thawing and reinfusion. The goal of marrow processing is depletion of RBCs, plasma, and fat with minimal loss of progenitor cells. Although originally done manually by simple centrifugation, cell separators are now utilized for preferential concentration of progenitor cells with increased elimination of other hematopoietic cells. A variety of automated procedures have now been published for marrow processing using various cell separators, and engraftment has been documented after infusion of such marrow (70–78). For example, Angelini and colleagues have recently found the COBE 2991 (COBE Corp., Denver, CO) and Fenwal CS3000 (Fenwal Corp., Deerfield, IL) cell separators to be equivalent (Table 25.2) (78).

The blood component laboratory may also carry out depletion (purging) of tumor cells from autologous marrow prior to grafting or removal of T cells from allogeneic marrow prior to BMT as prophylaxis against GVHD. Purging of tumor cells from autologous marrow is being evaluated to (*a*) allow patients with overt tumor involvement to undergo autologous BMT and (*b*) deplete

Table 25.2. Efficiency of Automated Bone Marrow Stem Cell Processing

	Cell Separator Utilized	
	COBE 2991[a]	Fenwal CS 3000[a]
Number of marrows processed	70	20
Percent recovery of mononuclear cells	89 ± 5	86 ± 9
Percent red cell removal	98 ± 1	85 ± 10
Percent granulocyte removal	97 ± 4.5	90 ± 1.1
Percent recovery of colony-forming units—granulocytes/macrophages	80	75

[a]Ficoll-Hypaque gradient was used.

subclinical residual marrow cells when tumor is not evident on cytopathologic examination. There can be up to 10^8 tumor cells in marrow when histopathologic examination is normal. Three lines of evidence suggest that this may be the case: (a) the ability to derive tumor cell lines from marrows that appear to be pathologically normal (79); (b) the observed time to relapse and known tumor doubling times in patients with hematologic cancers, which suggest that tumor cells were present when not pathologically evident; and (c) the use of more sensitive techniques, such as gene rearrangement or polymerase chain reaction technology (80), which can confirm the presence of a single malignant cell within 10^6 marrow cells.

Purging of tumor cells from grafts prior to autologous BMT has permitted this approach to be utilized for patients with up to 20% histopathologic involvement with tumor (19); to date, however, no study has proven the need for purging. It is of note that Gorin and colleagues (81) have recently examined 263 patients with standard risk acute myelocytic leukemia in first complete remission autografted after total body irradiation and noted a higher leukemia-free survival rate (63%) and lower relapse rate (23%) in recipients of mafosfamide-purged marrows than in recipients of nonpurged marrows (34% leukemia-free survival and 55% relapse rate). In allogeneic BMT, T cell depletion of donor marrow prior

to grafting has decreased the incidence of GVHD; however, increased graft failure, graft rejection, and relapse rates have lessened enthusiasm for this approach to abrogating GVHD (62). Although purging is therefore not proven to be essential in either setting, it is nonetheless under active study, particularly in autologous BMT. The conditions for pharmacologic purging of autologous marrow tumor cells on a cell separator, i.e., marrow RBC and drug concentration, have been established (82–84). Moreover, when using cell separator technology for MoAb-based purging of autologous marrow tumor cells, a 4–5 log depletion can be achieved using only 50% of the MoAb and complement in 50% of the time required for manual techniques (76).

Cryopreservation

Autologous marrow cells depleted of erythrocytes, granulocytes, and plasma are usually frozen, often in the blood component laboratory, in 10% dimethylsulfoxide (DMSO) in a rate-controlled freezer, set to cool at a constant 1° C per minute, and are then stored until the time of infusion in either liquid or vapor phase of liquid nitrogen. However, recovery of colony-forming units—granulocytes/macrophages (CFU-GMs) from unfractionated bone marrow stored in vapor-phase liquid nitrogen was higher in 5% DMSO and 6% hydroxyethyl starch than that from marrow stored in 10% DMSO alone (85). Moreover, marrows frozen by simple immersion in a −80° C freezer, without controlled rate freezing, and stored at this temperature have resulted in satisfactory engraftment after autotransplantation. As is true in the preparation of other blood components, it is also critical to develop techniques, similar to those used for the handling of other blood components, to avoid bacterial contamination during marrow collection and processing (86).

Autologous Red Cell Salvage

The RBCs that are separated from donated marrow can be transfused to the marrow donor, either the patient undergoing autologous BMT or the allogeneic marrow donor, after the marrow harvest. Homologous transfusions can thereby be avoided. For example, no homologous transfusions were needed in 16 patients who received their own marrow-residual RBCs after bone marrow harvest, with a mean drop in hemoglobin level from preoperative levels of only 1 ± 0.2 mg/dl (87).

THE IMPORTANCE OF ABO COMPATIBILITY IN ALLOGENEIC BONE MARROW TRANSPLANTATION

ABO incompatibility between marrow donor and recipient may be either major, with isohemagglutinin in the recipient directed against donor RBC antigens, or minor, with isohemagglutinin in the donor directed against recipient RBC antigens.

Major ABO Incompatibility

Major ABO incompatibility has the potential risk of severe hemolytic reactions, graft rejection, or delayed engraftment (9, 10, 12, 88–94). Attempts to overcome major ABO incompatibility have included depletion of RBCs from the bone marrow graft prior to BMT (95, 96) and/or removal of isohemagglutinin from the recipient by large-volume plasma exchanges or immunoadsorption (Table 25.3) (97). In addition, some investigators have

supplemented these techniques with pre-BMT transfusions of donor-type blood or purified A or B substance to completely absorb recipient isohemagglutinins (98, 99). Although studies suggest that major ABO-incompatible HLA-matched transplants have resulted in no increase in patient mortality, incidence of rejection, delayed engraftment, or GVHD compared with ABO-compatible controls (88, 91, 100), some reports suggest that RBC engraftment can be delayed in this setting (9, 10, 12, 96). Current practice in major ABO-incompatible HLA-matched BMT is to deplete RBCs from marrow before BMT, to anticipate possible delayed erythropoiesis and hemolysis after BMT, and to utilize methods to deplete recipient isohemagglutinin only when it is present in high (≥1:128) titer.

Minor ABO Incompatibility

Potential adverse outcomes of minor ABO incompatibility between marrow donor and recipient include rapid immune hemolysis at the time of infusion of donor marrow due to passive transfer of isohemagglutinin in the marrow plasma and delayed immune hemolysis caused by anti-RBC antibodies produced by the donor marrow (9, 10, 12). There is no effect of minor ABO incompatibility on graft rejection, the incidence or severity of GVHD, or patient survival (88–91). Although exchange transfusion of the recipient before BMT using RBCs of the donor's blood group has been utilized to pre-

Table 25.3. ABO-Incompatible Allogeneic Bone Marrow Transplantation

Type of ABO Incompatibility	
Major	Minor
1. Deplete erythrocytes from marrow graft	1. Remove marrow plasma
2. Remove isohemagglutinins from recipient (if ≥1:128 titer)	2. Transfuse O or donor-type red cells
a. Plasma exchange	
b. Extracorporeal immuno-adsorption	3. Monitor closely for hemolysis, especially in patients on cyclosporine, patients receiving T-cell-depleted marrow, or patients receiving marrow from unrelated donor
c. In vivo adsorption by transfusion of donor-type red cells, A or B substance	4. Exchange transfusion (rarely necessary)

vent hemolysis caused by passive transfer of isohemagglutinin in the marrow product, this is rarely a clinically significant problem and can more easily be avoided by removing plasma from the marrow prior to infusion. Minor ABO incompatibility can result in adverse reactions due to the production of anti-A and/or anti-B antibodies by donor marrow lymphocytes early (1–3 weeks) posttransplant, particularly in patients on cyclosporine therapy or those receiving T-cell-depleted allografts (93, 94). This may be particularly severe and associated with reactive hemolysis in the setting of minor ABO-incompatible HLA-matched BMT using unrelated donors (101). The rapidity of engraftment and related production of isohemagglutinins is somewhat surprising, given the delay in humoral reconstitution noted after BMT (7, 8). In this setting, transfusions of either group O or donor group RBCs are utilized to dilute the recipient red cells, and patients are closely monitored for evidence of hemolysis; in some cases, exchange transfusion has been required due to very rapid engraftment of donor lymphocytes and production of anti-RBC antibodies (Table 25.3). An example of hemolysis noted 11 days after transplantation of type O marrow to type A recipient necessitating exchange transfusion is displayed in Table 25.4.

When differences in RBC antigens exist between donor and recipient, they can be useful in documenting and assessing the timing and extent of engraftment; special care is then taken to avoid patient exposure to antigen via transfusion. For example, we have recently utilized RBC typing, coupled with DNA fragment length polymorphism and cytogenetic analyses, to document 22 cases of mixed chimerism and 21 cases with complete donor hematopoiesis in recipients of HLA-matched allogeneic BMT (102). Interestingly, Kaplan-Meier estimates of survival and disease-free survival for patients with mixed chimerism and complete donor hematopoiesis were equivalent.

Table 25.4. Clinical Course of Patient Undergoing HLA-matched ABO Minor Incompatible Allogeneic Bone Marrow Transplantation[a]

Day of Hospitalization	Clinical Course
1 and 2	Cyclophosphamide (60 mg/kg/day) ablative therapy
3–6	Total body irradiation (200 cGy twice daily, total 1400 cGy)
6	Infusion of marrow (type O) to patient (type A)
13	Broad-spectrum antibiotics begun, due to leukopenia and fever
16	Donor lymphocytes produce anti-A and hemolysis: Hct falls 29.1% to 21.2%; LDH 950 IU, total bilirubin 1.8 mg/dl, direct bilirubin 0.6 mg/dl, direct antiglobulin test positive
16–18	Phlebotomy of 6 units and transfusion of 12 units type O frozen deglycerolized red cells, Hct stable at 30%
22	Discharged with Hct stable at 30% and granulocytes >500/mm^3, normal liver function tests, negative direct antiglobulin test

[a]Abbreviations: Hct, hematocrit; LDH, lactic dehydrogenase.

FUTURE DIRECTIONS

Leukopoor and/or Single-Donor Blood Components

Known adverse consequences in recipients of transfusion that are due to residual leukocytes within the transfused cellular products include alloimmunization, transmission of CMV infection, and febrile transfusion reactions (FTRs). The only potential beneficial effect of leukocytes within transfused blood products is a purported white cell-mediated graft-versus-leukemia effect, but this remains controversial (103, 104). As noted above, leukodepletion prior to transfusion for the prevention of alloimmunization has been best studied; techniques that result in 10^6 residual leukocytes in transfused patients delay or avoid alloimmunization in transfusion recipients (30–35), whereas leukopoor components with >10^8 contaminating leukocytes do not abrogate sensitization (36). Several investigators have also demonstrated that provision of leukodepleted cellular blood products may be useful for the avoidance of transfusion-associated CMV infection in neonates, patients with hematologic malignancies, or transplant recipients (47–49, 51, 52, 58). These studies utilized leukodepleted products from the outset in all transfusions and suggest that all potential marrow recipients may be appropriate candidates for this approach.

Additional adverse consequences of contaminating leukocytes within transfused cellular blood products include FTRs, TA-GVHD, and immunomodulation (59, 105). FTRs are associated with antibodies to HLA and other leukocyte antigens (106–109) and can be avoided, even in patients with a history of prior FTRs, by removal of leukocytes prior to transfusion (109–112); however, the extent of depletion required is not well defined. Studies to date have not examined the utility of using exclusively leukopoor blood products, as described above to avoid alloimmunization and CMV infection, to avoid FTRs. Studies in animals demonstrate that 10^7 leukocytes per kilogram transfusion recipient weight are necessary to mediate transfusion-related GVHD, suggesting that leukodepletion prior to transfusion may therefore be useful to avoid TA-GVHD. In human, however, the precise number and type of T cells that mediate TA-GVHD are not defined; thus the potential utility of blood product leukodepletion to avoid TA-GVHD is also unknown. Finally, while it is clear that transplant recipients are already immunocompromised and would be at potential risk from any additional transfusion-associated immunosuppression, the extent of this complication of transfusion and its mechanism of action are under evaluation. At present, avoidance of FTRs, TA-GVHD, and immunomodulation remains a potential but unproven benefit of providing exclusively leukopoor cellular blood components.

Leukodepletion studies have previously examined washing, centrifugation and, most recently, filtration techniques to remove leukocytes from cellular blood components. Currently, filters are able to deplete either RBCs and plts to a level of $\leq 10^6$ residual leukocytes (63, 64). Importantly, examination of leukocytes using a hemocytometer has a limit of detection of $\geq 10^6$ leukocytes per product. The number of residual leukocytes within transfused components necessary to mediate alloimmunization, CMV infection, FTRs, TA-GVHD, and immunomodulation is uncertain but likely differs for each effect. The continued evaluation of more efficient depletion techniques, coupled with the recently described cytofluorometric techniques that reproducibly count leukocyte concentrations as low as 0.1 white blood cell per microliter (113, 114), will define the scientific basis, clinical utility, and cost-effectiveness of transfusing exclusively leukopoor cellular components.

Single-Donor Platelets

Several potential advantages have been reported for the transfusion of plts obtained from a single donor. First, some investigators have either suggested or reported that a decreased incidence of sensitization of the recipient may be noted after transfusion of single-donor plts (115, 116). Gmur et al., for example, conducted a prospective randomized study of 54 patients who had not been previously transfused and demonstrated that alloimmunization occurred less frequently, after a longer time, and after a higher number of transfusions of single-donor compared to multiple-donor plts (115). Sintnicolaas and coworkers also conducted a randomized study of this effect of single-donor and multiple-donor plt transfusions in 23 cancer patients with severe thrombocytopenia and hemorrhage (116). Although plt recovery in both groups was similar after the first transfusion, plt recoveries after the second transfusion were significantly better in those receiving single-donor transfusion. This was primarily due to a gradual decline in plt recovery values with subsequent multiple-donor transfusions.

The above studies suggest that alloimmunization can occur early in patients receiving multiple-donor platelets, that multiple donor transfusions are then ineffective, and that restriction of the number of donors per transfusion may postpone the development of refractoriness to random-donor plt transfusions in thrombocytopenic patients. A second potential advantage of single-donor plts stems from the decreased risk of infection when exposed to fewer donors. For example, the need to provide plts from CMV-seronegative donors or from HLA-matched donors can most easily be achieved by pheresis of several units of plts from an individual donor rather than pooling random donor concentrates from 8–10 CMV-seronegative or HLA-matched donors, respectively. Thus the major advantages of single-donor plts are the exposure of recipient patients to fewer donors and a potential decreased risk of infectious complications or alloimmunization.

Recent data indicate that the use of single-donor apheresis plts is increasing (117). Moreover, technology is now available for the collection of leukopoor apheresis plts. It is important to point out, however, that there is as yet no definitive evidence that single-donor plts are more useful in minimizing alloimmunization or infection than pooled random donor concentrates. Indeed, if filtration to produce leukopoor blood components prior to transfusion can minimize both alloimmunization and risk of CMV infection, then the only absolute indication for the use of single-donor plts would be in sensitized patients who need HLA-matched plt transfusions.

The Role of Recombinant Hematopoietic Growth Factors

The hematopoietic growth factors are glycoprotein hormones that regulate the proliferation and differentiation of hematopoietic progenitor cells and function of mature blood cells (118). Erythropoietin (EPO), a glycoprotein produced in response to hypoxia in the kidney, induces RBC production by stimulating the mitotic activity of erythroid progenitor cells, burst-forming units—erythroid (BFU-Es) and colony-forming units—erythroid (CFU-Es) and early erythroid precursor cells in the bone marrow. The gene for EPO has been cloned, and a recombinant human EPO (rHuEPO) indistinguishable from the natural hormone on the basis of protein sequencing and biologic and immunologic activity has been produced (119, 120). Moreover, cloning, expression, and biologic characterization of the human EPO receptor have recently been reported (121). Recombinant EPO is already of proven efficacy in treatment of the anemia of chronic renal failure (122, 123) and anemia in patients with AIDS treated with zidovudine (124). It may also be useful to treat the anemia of cancer, since endogenous EPO levels may be inappropriately low (125–127). Specifically, levels of endogenous EPO are low in the first month after BMT, during which time transfusion needs are greatest (127). Supplemental rHuEPO may therefore also be useful to hasten RBC engraftment and to decrease RBC transfusion requirements (128).

Interestingly, in a rat model, EPO caused a dose-dependent increase in both reticulocyte and plt numbers (129). Consistent with this observation are studies in humans demonstrating that rHuEPO increases both bone marrow (130) and peripheral blood circulating hematopoietic progenitor cells (131, 132). Thus rHuEPO may also alter engraftment and transfusion requirements of cells of other than erythroid lineage.

Recombinant human granulocyte-macrophage colony-stimulating factor (rHuGM-CSF) may also be useful post-BMT. It has been shown to accelerate hematopoietic recovery in primates undergoing autologous BMT (133, 134). Administration of rHuGM-CSF post autologous BMT in man led to accelerated total leukocyte and granulocyte recovery and reduced morbidity and mortality compared to historical controls (135, 136). However, a temporary reduction of granulocytes occurred upon discontinuation of growth factor, emphasizing the need to determine whether engraftment is not only enhanced but also sustained by growth factor stimulation. It does appear, in some studies, to shorten hospital stays post-BMT (137). A recent study of rHuGM-CSF on hematopoietic recovery in patients who underwent autologous BMT demonstrated enhanced engraftment only in patients who received adequate CFU-GMs in the marrow grafts (138). Finally, it has recently been demonstrated that rHuGM-CSF can be effectively used to treat patients with graft failure after BMT (139).

A variety of other growth factors may also be useful post-BMT. Recombinant interleukin-3 (rHuIL-3), for example, promotes the survival, proliferation, and development of multipotential hematopoietic stem cells and of committed progenitor cells of the granulocyte/macrophage, erythroid, eosinophil, megakaryocyte, mast cell, and basophilic lineages (140–142). Its range of activities appears to be broader than that of other colony-stimulating factors, and in particular, it appears to be a more potent stimulator of megakaryocytopoiesis (143–145). Preliminary studies suggest that it may also be a multilineage hematopoietin in vivo in patients with normal bone marrow function and in patients with secondary bone marrow failure (146). Moreover, recent evidence demonstrates that rHuIL-3 can enhance the effect of EPO on erythropoiesis (147), suggesting that combinations of growth factors may be beneficial post-BMT.

Peripheral Blood Stem Cell Autotransplantation

Hematopoietic stem cells can be collected from the peripheral blood of laboratory animals by cytapheresis and successfully reconstitute myelopoiesis following marrow-lethal treatment (148). In man, autologous PBSCs have been collected from patients dur-ing the chronic phase of chronic myelogenous leukemia and subsequently reinfused after the patient has received high-dose therapy for accelerated or blastic phase disease (149). These cells engraft, as evidenced by return to the chronic phase. Other investigators have also utilized reinfusion of PBSCs to achieve hematopoietic reconstitution after high-dose chemotherapy and total body irradiation (150, 151). The potential advantages of PBSCs are several: Leukapheresis is an outpatient procedure similar to plt donation and avoids the need for hospitalization, general anesthesia, and bone marrow harvest; adequate numbers of stem cells can be collected from patients with hemipelvectomies or tumor involving the pelvic bones, or after pelvic irradiation; and it may be possible to harvest adequate numbers of PBSCs from patients with tumor-involved marrow. In multiple myeloma, for example, studies have demonstrated that the relative number of malignant stem cells is markedly reduced in peripheral blood relative to bone marrow, suggesting a potential benefit for PBSC grafting (152). It should be noted, however, that even patients with solid tumors may have tumor cells contaminating PBSC collections (153).

There are two major disadvantages of PBSC transplantation, namely, the need for multiple (8–10) phereses to achieve adequate numbers of stem cells and the concern whether PBSCs can result in long-term engraftment of all lineages. The number of phereses can be decreased if leukapheresis is done at the time of recovery from high-dose chemotherapy, especially with the additional stimulus of rHuGM-CSF. A variety of chemotherapy regimens for patients with both hematologic and solid tumors increase the peripheral blood CFU-GMs up to 20-fold over the baseline level at the time of leukocyte recovery (154–159). Moreover, Antman and colleagues have demonstrated that the number of CFU-GMs were increased by the combination of postchemotherapy rebound plus rHuGM-CSF: a 9- to 14-fold and 30-fold increase relative to the number of CFU-GMs noted after rHuGM-CSF or chemotherapy alone, respectively (160). Thus augmentation of PBSCs by rHuGM-CSF, especially during the period of leukocyte recovery after chemotherapy, may facilitate collection of adequate numbers of PBSCs with fewer leukaphereses, thereby enhancing the feasibility of autografting.

In patients with lymphomas and breast cancer, Gianni and coworkers have recently achieved more rapid engraftment when both autologous BMT and PBSC transplantation were used together, markedly reducing the number of transfusions (RBCs and plts) and infectious complications, as well as shortening the hospital stay (161). Siena and colleagues have further shown that CD34-antigen-bearing (CD34+) cells in the circulation are fivefold increased by rHuGM-CSF after high-dose cyclophosphamide, and that these cells possess qualitatively normal hematopoietic colony growth and high cloning efficiency compared to bone marrow CD34+ cells (162). We have recently utilized PBSCs to reconstitute hematopoiesis in 12 women who underwent high-dose ablative therapy for breast cancer (18). PBSCs were harvested (four leukaphereses) at the time of recovery from chemotherapy and while on rHuGM-CSF. Granulocytes >500 per cubic millimeter and plts >20,000 per cubic millimeter were noted at a median of 14 and 12 days post infusion of PBSCs. A median of 8 units of RBCs and 23 units of plts were utilized, and hospital stay was a median of 24 days. In 29 comparable women with breast cancer who underwent autologous BMT, granulocytes >500 per cubic millimeter and plts >20,000 per cubic millimeter were observed at 21 and 23 days post-BMT, respectively. They required a median of 13 units of RBCs and 105 units of plts during a median hospital stay of 38 days. The ease of harvesting PBSCs, coupled with such complete and prompt hematologic recovery, will permit investigation of more intensive cytoreductive therapy as initial treatment of selected tumors with curative intent.

Finally, recent studies in monkeys demonstrated that administration of rHuIL-3 led to a dose-dependent increase in peripheral blood progenitors of basophilic, eosinophilic, and neutrophilic granulocytes, monocytes, erythrocyte, and platelet lineages (163). Treatment with this interleukin may therefore also facilitate PBSC collection and autotransplantation. Moreover, rHuIL-3 synergizes with rHuGM-CSF in expanding the pool of circulating hematopoietic cells in primates (164), suggesting that combinations of growth factors may further facilitate PBSC collection. The role of the blood component laboratory in provision of hematopoietic stem cells may therefore expand in the future and permit rapid engraftment of all cell lineages after high-dose, potentially curative chemotherapy programs.

SUMMARY AND CONCLUSIONS

The provision of appropriate blood component support has in the past been critical for the development of curative treatment programs, i.e., aggressive combination chemotherapy in childhood leukemias. The blood component laboratory will continue to play a central and broadening role in the treatment of cancer, specifically in the harvesting, processing, and transfusion of hematopoietic stem cells from marrow and peripheral blood sources to restore hematologic and immune function after high-dose ablative therapies. The use of recombinant growth factors appears to both facilitate the harvesting of hematopoietic stem cells from peripheral blood and to hasten engraftment after transplantation. Innovative treatment strategies including intensive myeloablative therapies may now be used for a broad spectrum of patients with presently incurable cancers. Transfusion medicine expertise will be essential to ensure that appropriate blood components are provided before and after hematopoietic stem cell transplantation, to collect hematopoietic stem cells, and to avoid immune and infectious complications in patients treated in this fashion.

REFERENCES

1. Atkinson K, Horowitz MN, Gale RP, et al. Risk factors for chronic graft-versus-host disease after HLA-identical sibling bone marrow transplantation. Blood 1990;75:2459–2464.
2. Storb R, Deeg HD, Whitehead J, et al. Methotrexate and cyclosporine compared with cyclosporine alone for prophylaxis of acute graft versus host disease after marrow transplantation for leukemia. N Engl J Med 1986;314:729–735.
3. Martin PJ, Schoch G, Fisher L, et al. A retrospective analysis of therapy for acute graft-versus-host disease: initial treatment. Blood 1990;76:1464–1472.
4. Beatty PG, Clift RA, Mickelson EM, et al. Marrow transplantation from related donors other than HLA-identical siblings. N Engl J Med 1985;313:765–771.
5. McGlave P, Scott E, Ramsey N, et al. Unrelated donor bone marrow transplantation therapy for patients with chronic myelogenous leukemia. Blood 1987;70:877–881.
6. Armitage JO, Gale RP. Bone marrow autotransplantation in man: report of an international cooperative study. Lancet 1986;2:960–962.
7. Witherspoon RP, Lum LG, Storb R. Immunologic reconstitution after human marrow grafting. Semin Hematol 1984;21:2–10.
8. Lum LG. The kinetics of immune reconstitution after human marrow transplantation. Blood 1987;69:369–380.
9. Anderson KC. The role of the blood bank in hematopoietic stem cell transplantation. Transfusion, 1992, in press.
10. Anderson KC, Dzik W. Blood bank support in bone marrow and organ transplantation. In: Benz EJ, Cohen HJ, Furie B, Hoffman R, Shattil SJ, eds. Hematology: basic principles and practice. New York: Churchill Livingstone, 1990:1670–1678.
11. Brand A, Class HJ, Falkenburg JHF, et al. Blood component therapy in bone marrow transplantation. Semin Hematol 1984;21:141–155.
12. Petz LD. Immunohematologic problems associated with bone marrow transplantation. Transf Med Rev 1987;1:85–100.
13. Wulff JC, Santner TJ, Storb R, et al. Transfusion requirements after HLA identical marrow transplantation in 82 patients with aplastic anemia. Vox Sang 1983;44:366–374.
14. Anderson KC, Ritz J, Takvorian T, et al. Hematologic engraftment and immune reconstitution post-transplantation with anti-B1 purged autologous bone marrow. Blood 1987;69:597–604.
15. Bensinger W, Peterson FB, Banaji M, et al. Engraftment and transfusion requirements after allogeneic marrow transplantation for patients with acute non-lymphocytic leukemia in first complete remission. Bone Marrow Transplant 1989;4:409–414.
16. Kersey JH, Weisdorf D, Nesbit ME, et al. Comparison of autologous and allogeneic bone marrow transplantation for treatment of high-risk refractory acute lymphoblastic leukemia. N Engl J Med 1987;317:461–467.
17. Antman K, Eder JP, Elias A, et al. High dose combination alkylating agent preparative regimen with autologous bone marrow support: the Dana-Farber Cancer Institute/Beth Israel Hospital experience. Cancer Treat Rep 1987;71:119–125.
18. Elias A, Mazanet R, Wheeler C, et al. Peripheral blood progenitor cells (PBSC): two protocols using GM-CSF potentiated progenitor cell collection. In: Dicke KA, Armitage J, eds. Autologous bone marrow transplantation. Proceeding of the Fifth International Symposium. Omaha, NE: University of Nebraska Free Press, 1991:875–880.
19. Freedman AS, Takvorian T, Anderson KC, et al. Autologous bone marrow transplantation in B-cell non-Hodgkin's lymphoma: very low treatment-related mortality in 100 patients in sensitive relapse. J Clin Oncol 1990;8:784–791.
20. Anderson KC, Soiffer R, DeLage R, et al. T cell depleted autologous bone marrow transplantation therapy: analysis of immune deficiency and late complications. Blood 1990;76:235–244.
21. Anderson KC, Barut BA, Ritz J, et al. Monoclonal antibody purged autologous marrow transplantation therapy for multiple myeloma. Blood 1991;77:712–720.
22. Soiffer RJ, Canning C, Mauch P, et al. Prevention of graft-versus-host disease by selective depletion of CD6-positive T lymphocytes from donor bone marrow. Blood, 1991, Submitted.
23. Klingemann HG, Self S, Banaji M, et al. Refractoriness to random donor platelet transfusions in patients with aplastic anemia: a multivariate analysis of data from 264 cases. Br J Haematol 1987;66:115–121.
24. Storb R, Weiden PL. Transfusion problems associated with transplantation. Semin Hematol 1981;18:163–176.
25. Elfenbein GJ, Anderson PN, Klein DL, et al. Difficulties in predicting bone marrow rejection in patients with aplastic anemia. Transplant Proc 1978;10:441–445.
26. Storb R, Prentice RL, Thomas ED. Marrow transplantation for treatment of aplastic anemia. An analysis of factors associated with graft rejection. N Engl J Med 1977;296:61–66.
27. Champlin RE, Horowitz MM, van Bekkum DW, et al. Graft failure following bone marrow transplantation for severe aplastic anemia: risk factors and treatment results. Blood 1989;73:606–613.
28. Barge AJ, Johnson G, Witherspoon R, et al. Antibody-mediated marrow failure after allogeneic bone marrow transplantation. Blood 1989;74:1477–1480.

29. Shulman NR. Immunologic considerations attending platelet transfusion. Transfusion 1966;6:39–49.
30. Fisher M, Chapman JR, Tung A, et al. Alloimmunization to HLA antigens following transfusion with leukocyte-poor and purified platelet suspensions. Vox Sang 1985;49:331–335.
31. Murphy MF, Metcalf P, Thomas H, et al. Use of leukocyte-poor blood components and HLA-matched platelet donors to prevent HLA alloimmunization. Br J Haematol 1986;62:529–534.
32. Brand A, Claas FHJ, Voogt PJ, et al. Alloimmunization after leukocyte depleted multiple random donor platelet transfusions. Vox Sang 1988;54:160–166.
33. Andreu G, Dewailly J, Leberre C, et al. Prevention of HLA immunizations with leukocyte-poor packed red cells and platelet concentrates obtained by filtration. Blood 1988;72:964–969.
34. Sniecinski I, O'Donnell MR, Nowicki B, et al. Prevention of refractoriness and HLA alloimmunization using filtered blood products. Blood 1988; 71:1402–1407.
35. Saarinen UM, Kekomaki R, Siimes MA, et al. Effective prophylaxis against platelet refractoriness in multitransfused patients by use of leukocyte-free blood components. Blood 1990;75:512–517.
36. Schiffer CA, Dutcher JP, Aisner J, et al. A randomized trial of leukocyte depleted platelet transfusion to modify alloimmunization in patients with leukemia. Blood 1983;62:815–820.
37. Gmur J, von Felton A, Osterwalder B, et al. Delayed alloimmunization using random single donor platelet transfusions: a prospective study in thrombocytopenic patients with acute leukemia. Blood 1983; 2:473–479.
38. Sintnicolaas K, Vriesendorp HM, Sizoo W, et al. Delayed alloimmunization by random single donor platelet transfusions. A randomized study to compare single donor and multiple donor platelet transfusions in cancer patients with severe thrombocytopenia. Lancet 1981;1:750–754.
39. Paulin T, Ringden O, Lonnqvist B, et al. The importance of pre bone marrow transplantation serology in determining subsequent cytomegalovirus infection. Scand J Infect Dis 1986;18:199–209.
40. Wingard JR, Chen DYH, Burns WH, et al. Cytomegalovirus infection after autologous bone marrow transplantation with comparison to infection after allogeneic bone marrow transplantation. Blood 1988;71:1432–1437.
41. Reusser P, Schoch HG, Fisher L, et al. Cytomegalovirus (CMV) infection after autologous bone marrow transplantation (ABMT): occurrence of disease and impact on engraftment [Abstract]. Blood 1988;72(suppl):402a.
42. Winston DJ, Ho WG, Howell CL, et al. Cytomegalovirus infections associated with leukocyte transfusions. Ann Intern Med 1980;93:671–675.
43. Hersman J, Meyers JD, Thomas ED, et al. The effect of granulocyte transfusions upon the incidence of cytomegalovirus infection after allogeneic marrow transplantation. Ann Intern Med 1982;96:149–152.
44. Adler SP, Lawrence LT, Baggett J, et al. Prevention of transfusion associated cytomegalovirus infection in very low birth weight infants using frozen blood and donors seronegative for cytomegalovirus. Transfusion 1984;24:333–335.
45. Winston DJ, Ho WG, Lin CH, et al. Intravenous immune globulin for prevention of cytomegalovirus infection and interstitial pneumonia after bone marrow transplantation. Ann Intern Med 1987; 106:12–18.
46. Bowden RA, Sayers M, Fluornoy N, et al. Cytomegalovirus immune globulin and seronegative blood products to prevent primary cytomegalovirus infection after marrow transplantation. N Engl J Med 1986;314:1006–1010.
47. Gilbert GL, Hayes K, Hudson IL, et al. Prevention of transfusion-acquired cytomegalovirus infection in infants by blood filtration to remove leukocytes. Lancet 1989;1:1228–1231.
48. Murphy MF, Grint PCA, Hardiman AE, et al. Use of leukocyte-poor blood components to prevent primary cytomegalovirus (CMV) infections in patients with acute leukaemia. Br J Haematol 1988;70:253–255.
49. Bowden RA, Sayers M, Cays M, et al. The role of blood product filtration in the prevention of transfusion associated cytomegalovirus (CMV) infection after marrow transplant [Abstract]. Transfusion 1989; 29:595.
50. Miller W, Flynn P, McCullough J, et al. Cytomegalovirus infection after bone marrow transplantation: an association with acute graft-versus-host disease. Blood 1986;67:1162–1167.
51. Reusser P, Fisher LD, Buckner CD, et al. Cytomegalovirus infection after autologous bone marrow transplantation: occurrence of cytomegalovirus disease and effect on engraftment. Blood 1990;75:1888–1894.
52. de Graan-Hentzen YCE, Gratama JW, Mudde GC, et al. Prevention of primary cytomegalovirus infection in patients with hematologic malignancies by intensive white cell depletion of blood products. Transfusion 1989;29:757–760.
53. Hillyer CD, Snydman DR, Berkman EM. The risk of cytomegalovirus infection in solid organ and bone marrow transplant recipients: transfusion of blood products. Transfusion 1990;30:659–666.
54. Meyers JD, Reed EC, Shepp DH, et al. Acyclovir for prevention of cytomegalovirus infection and disease after allogeneic marrow transplantation. N Engl J Med 1988;318:70–75.
55. Reed EC, Bowden RA, Dindliker PS, et al. Treatment of cytomegalovirus pneumonia with ganciclovir and

intravenous cytomegalovirus immunoglobulin in patients with bone marrow transplants. Ann Intern Med 1988;109:783–788.

56. Emmanuel D, Cunningham I, Jules-Elysse K, et al. Cytomegalovirus pneumonia after bone marrow transplantation successfully treated with the combination of ganciclovir and high-dose immune globulin. Ann Intern Med 1988;109:777–782.

57. Verdonck LF, van der Linden JA, Bast BJEG, et al. Influence of cytomegalovirus infection on the recovery of humoral immunity after autologous bone marrow transplantation. Exp Hematol 1987;15:864–868.

58. De Witte T, Schattenberg A, Van Djik BA, et al. Prevention of primary cytomegalovirus infection after allogeneic bone marrow transplantation by using leukocyte-poor random donor blood products from cytomegalovirus-unscreened blood bank donors. Transplantation 1990;50:964–968.

59. Anderson KC, Weinstein HJ. Transfusion-associated graft versus host disease. N Engl J Med 1990;323:315–321.

60. Drobyski W, Thibodeau S, Truitt RL, et al. Third party mediated graft rejection and graft-versus-host disease after T cell depleted bone marrow transplantation, as demonstrated by hypervariable DNA probes and HLA-DR polymorphism. Blood 1989;74:2285–2294.

61. Leitman SF, Holland PV. Irradiation of blood products: indications and guidelines. Transfusion 1985; 25:293–300.

62. Anderson KC, Nadler LM, Takvorian T, et al. Monoclonal antibodies: their use in bone marrow transplantation. In: Brown E, ed. Progress in hematology. Orlando: Grune & Stratton, 1987:137–181.

63. Wenz B. Leukocyte-free red cells: the evolution of a safer blood product. In: McCarthy LJ, Baldwin ML, eds. Controversies of leukocyte-poor blood and components. Arlington, VA: American Association of Blood Banks, 1989:27–48.

64. Dzik WH. Leukocyte-poor platelet products. In: McCarthy LJ, Baldwin ML, eds. Controversies of leukocyte-poor blood and platelet components. Arlington, VA: American Association of Blood Banks, 1989:49–80.

65. Deeg HJ, Graham TC, Gerhard Miller L, et al. Prevention of transfusion-induced graft-versus-host disease in dogs by ultraviolet irradiation. Blood 1989;74:2592–2595.

66. Brand A, Claas FHJ, van Rood JJ. UV-irradiated platelets: ready to use? Transfusion 1989;29:377–378.

67. Anderson KC, Goodnough LT, Pisciotto P, et al. Variation in blood component irradiation practice: implications for prevention of transfusion associated graft versus host disease. Blood 1991;77:2096–2102.

68. Postmus PE, Mulder NH, Elema JD. Graft versus host

disease after transfusions of non-irradiated blood cells in patients having received autologous marrow. Eur J Cancer Clin Oncol 1988;24:889–894.

69. Rowley SD, Davis JM. Standards for bone marrow processing laboratories, Transfusion 1990;30:571–572.

70. Weiner RS, Tobias JS, Yankee RA. The processing of human bone marrow for cryopreservation and reinfusion. Biomedicine 1976;24:226–231.

71. Linch DC, Knott LJ, Patterson KG, et al. Bone marrow processing and cryopreservation. J Clin Pathol 1982;35:186–190.

72. Gilmore MJML, Prentice HG, Corringham RE, et al. A technique for the concentration of nucleated bone marrow for in vitro manipulation or cryopreservation using the IBM 2991 blood cell processor. Vox Sang 1983;45:294–302.

73. Gilmore MJML, Prentice HG. Standardization of the processing of human bone marrow for allogeneic transplantation. Vox Sang 1986;51:202–206.

74. Faradji A, Andreu G, Pillier-Loriette C, et al. Separation of mononuclear bone marrow cells using the COBE 2997 blood cell separator. Vox Sang 1988; 55:133–138.

75. English D, Lamberson R, Graves V, et al. Semiautomated processing of bone marrow grafts for transplantation. Transfusion 1989;29(1):12-16.

76. Leach MF, Howell AL, Ball ED, et al. Automated elimination of leukemic cells using antibody and complement [Abstract]. Transfusion 1987;27(6):526.

77. Areman EM, Cullis H, Sacher RA, et al. Automated isolation of mononuclear cells using the Fenwal CS3000 blood cell separator. Prog Clin Biol Res 1990;333:379–385.

78. Angelini A, Dragani A, Iacone A, et al. Human bone marrow processing using the COBE 2991 and CS 3000 blood cell separators for further ex vivo manipulation. Haematologica 1990;75(suppl 1):43–47.

79. Benjamin D, Magrath IT, Douglas EC, et al. Derivation of lymphoma cell lines from microscopically normal bone marrow in patients with undifferentiated lymphomas: Evidence of occult bone marrow involvement. Blood 1983;61:1017–1019.

80. Eisenstein BI. The polymerase chain reaction. N Engl J Med 1990;332:178–183.

81. Gorin NC, Aegerter P, Auvert B, et al. Autologous bone marrow transplantation for acute myelocytic leukemia in first remission: a European survey of the role of marrow purging. Blood 1990;75:1606–1614.

82. Rowley SD, Zuehlsdorf M, Braine HG, et al. CFU-GM content of bone marrow graft correlates with time to hematologic reconstitution following autologous bone marrow transplantation with 4-hydroperoxycyclophosphamide-purged bone marrow. Blood 1987;70:271–275.

83. Jones RJ, Zuehlsdorf M, Rowley SD, et al. Variability

in 4-hydroperoxycyclophosphamide activity during clinical purging for autologous bone marrow transplantation. Blood 1987;70:1490–1494.

84. Rowley SD, Jones RJ, Piantadosi S. Efficacy of ex vivo purging for autologous bone marrow transplantation in the treatment of acute nonlymphoblastic leukemia. Blood 1989;74:501–506.

85. Stiff PJ, Koester AR, Weidner MK, et al. Autologous bone marrow transplantation using unfractionated cells cryopreserved in dimethylsulfoxide and hydroxyethyl starch without controlled-rate freezing. Blood 1987;70:974–978.

86. Rowley SD, Davis J, Dick J, et al. Bacterial contamination of bone marrow grafts intended for autologous and allogeneic bone marrow transplantation. Transfusion 1988;28:109–121.

87. Sonneveld P, deLeeuw CA, Schipperus M, et al. Transfusion of red cells after autologous bone marrow harvest in patients with acute leukemia and malignant lymphoma. Transfusion 1990;30:310–313.

88. Buckner CD, Clift RA, Sanders JE. ABO-incompatible marrow transplants. Transplantation 1978;26:233–238.

89. Gale RP, Feig S, Ho W, et al. ABO blood group system and bone marrow transplantation. Blood 1977;50:185–194.

90. Biggs JC, Concannon J, Dodds A. Allogeneic bone marrow transplantation across the ABO barrier. Med J Aust 1979;2:173–175.

91. Lasky LC, Warkentin PI, Kersey JH, et al. Hemotherapy in patients undergoing blood group incompatible bone marrow transplantation. Transfusion 1983;23:277–285.

92. Rowley S, Braine H. Probable hemolysis following minor and incompatible marrow transplantation (IMT). Blood 1982 60(suppl):171a.

93. Hows J, Beddow K, Gordon-Smith E. Donor-derived red blood cell antibodies and immune hemolysis after allogeneic bone marrow transplantation. Blood 1986;67:177–181.

94. Hazelhurst GR, Brenner MK, Wimperis JZ. Hemolysis after T-cell depleted bone marrow transplantation. Scand J Haematol 1986;37:1–3.

95. Braine HG, Sensenbrenner L, Wright SK, et al. Bone marrow transplantation with major ABO blood group incompatibility using erythrocyte depletion of marrow prior to infusion. Blood 1982;60:420–425.

96. Blacklock HA, Prentice HG, Evans JPM, et al. ABO-incompatible bone marrow transplantation: removal of red blood cells from donor marrow avoiding recipient antibody depletion. Lancet 1982;2:1061–1064.

97. Bensinger WI, Buckner CD, Thomas ED, et al. ABO-incompatible marrow transplants. Transplantation 1982;33:427–429.

98. Bleyer WA, Blaese RM, Bujak JS. Long term remission from acute myelogenous leukemia after bone marrow transplantation and recovery from acute graft-versus-host reaction and prolonged immunocompetence. Blood 1975;45:171–181.

99. Gorgone BC, Ritz J, Anderson KC. In vivo neutralization of isohemagglutinin (IH) prior to HLA matched ABO incompatible bone marrow transplantation. Blood 1985;66:267a.

100. Marmont AM, Domasio EE, Bacigalupo A, et al. A to O bone marrow transplantation in severe aplastic anemia: dynamics of blood group conversion of early dyserythropoiesis in the engrafted marrow. Br J Haematol 1978;36:511–518.

101. Gajewski JL, Petz LD, Calhoun L, et al. Immune mediated hemolysis followed by massive reactive hemolysis associated with minor ABO incompatible bone marrow transplants from unrelated donors. Blood 1990;76(suppl):1584.

102. Roy DC, Tantravahi R, Murray C, et al. Natural history of mixed chimerism after bone marrow transplantation with CD6-depleted allogeneic marrow: a stable equilibrium. Blood 1990;75:296–304.

103. Tucker J, Murphy MF, Gregory W, et al. Removal of graft-versus-leukemia effect by the use of leukocyte-poor blood components in patients with acute myeloblastic leukemia [Letter]. Br J Haematol 1988; 69:118.

104. Lopez J, Fernandez-Villalta MJ, Gomez-Reino F, et al. Absence of graft-versus-leukemia effect of standard hemotherapy in patients with acute myeloblastic leukemia [Letter]. Transfusion 1990;30:191.

105. Blumberg N, Heal JM. Transfusion and host defenses against cancer recurrence and infection. Transfusion 1989;29:236–245.

106. De Rie MA, van der Plas-van Dalen CM, Engelfriet CP, et al. The serology of febrile transfusion reactions. Vox Sang 1985;49:126–134.

107. Heinrich D, Meuller-Eckhardt C, Stier W. The specificity of leukocyte and platelet alloantibodies in sera of patients with nonhemolytic transfusion reactions. Absorption and elution studies. Vox Sang 1973;25:442–456.

108. Payne R. The association of febrile transfusion reactions with leuko-agglutinins. Vox Sang 1957;2:233–241.

109. Brubaker DB. Clinical significance of white cell antibodies in febrile non-hemolytic transfusion reactions. Transfusion 1990;30:733–737.

110. Menitove JE, McElligott MC, Aster RC. Febrile transfusion reaction: what blood component should be given next? Vox Sang 1982;42:318–321.

111. Chambers LA, Kruskall MS, Pacini DG, et al. Febrile reactions after platelet transfusion: the effect of single versus multiple donors. Transfusion 1990;30:219–221.

112. Anderson KC, Gorgone BC, Wahlers E, et al. Preparation and utilization of leukocyte poor apheresis platelets. Transf Sci 1991;12:163–170.

113. Bodensteiner DC. A flow cytometric technique to accurately measure post-filtration white blood cell counts. Transfusion 1989;29:651–653.

114. Dzik WH, Ragosta A, Cusack WF. Flow-cytometric method for counting very low numbers of leukocytes in platelet products. Vox Sang 1990;59:153–159.

115. Gmur J, von Felton A, Osterwalder B, Honnegger H, et al. Delayed alloimmunization using random single donor platelet transfusions: a prospective study in thrombocytopenic patients with acute leukemia. Blood 1983;2:473–479.

116. Sintnicolaas K, Vriesendorp HM, Sizoo W, et al. Delayed alloimmunization by random single donor platelet transfusions. A randomized study to compare single donor and multiple donor platelet transfusions in cancer patients with severe thrombocytopenia. Lancet 1981;1:750–754.

117. Mac N, Surgenor D, Walker EL, Hao SS, et al. Collection and transfusion of blood in the United States 1982–1988. N Engl J Med 1990;322:1646–51.

118. Groopman JE, Molina JM, Scadden DT. Hematopoietic growth factors: biology and clinical applications. N Engl J Med 1990;321:1449–1459.

119. Erslev A. Erythropoietin coming of age. N Engl J Med 1987;316:101–103.

120. Zanjani ED, Ascensao JL. Erythropoietin. Transfusion 1989;29:46–57.

121. Jones JJ, D'Andrea AD, Haines LL, et al. Human erythropoietin receptor: cloning, expression, and biological characterization. Blood 1990;76:31–35.

122. Eschbach JW, Egrie JC, Downing MR, et al. Correction of the anemia of end-stage renal disease with recombinant human erythropoietin. Results of a phase I and II clinical trial. N Engl J Med 1987;316:73–78.

123. Eschbach JW, Kelly MR, Halley NR, et al. Treatment of the anemia of progressive renal failure with recombinant human erythropoietin. N Engl J Med 1989;321:158–163.

124. Fischl M, Galpin JE, Levine JD, et al. Recombinant human erythropoietin for patients with AIDS treated with zidovudine. N Engl J Med 1990;322:1488–1493.

125. Ludwig H, Fritz E. Kotzmann H, et al. Erythropoietin treatment of anemia associated with multiple myeloma. N Engl J Med 1990;322:1693–1699.

126. Miller CB, Jonla RJ, Piantadosi S, et al. Decreased erythropoietin response in patients with the anemia of cancer. N Engl J Med 1990;322:1689–1692.

127. Schapira L, Antin JH, Ransil BJ, et al. Serum erythropoietin levels in patients receiving intensive chemotherapy and radiotherapy. Blood 1990;76:2354–2359.

128. Ayash L, Elias A, Demetri G, et al. Recombinant human erythropoietin (EPO) in anemia associated with autologous bone marrow transplantation (ABMT) [Abstract]. Blood 1990;76(suppl 1):131a.

129. Berridge MV, Fraser JK, Carter JM, et al. Effects of recombinant human erythropoietin on megakaryocytes and on platelet production in the rat. Blood 1988;72:970–977.

130. Dessypris EN, Graber SE, Krantz SB, et al. Effects of recombinant erythropoietin on the concentration and cycling status of human marrow hematopoietic progenitor cells in vivo. Blood 1988;72:2060–2062.

131. Ganser A, Bergmann M, Volkers B, et al. In vivo effects of recombinant human erythropoietin on circulating human hemopoietic progenitor cells. Exp Hematol 1989;17:433–435.

132. Geissler K, Stockenhuber F, Kabrna E, et al. Recombinant human erythropoietin and hematopoietic progenitor cells in vivo [Abstract]. Blood 1990;73:222a.

133. Nienhius AW, Donahue RE, Karisson S, et al. Recombinant human granulocyte-macrophage colony stimulating factor (GM-CSF) shortens the period of neutropenia after autologous marrow transplantation in a primate model. J Clin Invest 1987;80:573–577.

134. Monroy RL, Skelly RR, MacVittie TJ, et al. The effect of recombinant GM-CSF on the recovery of monkeys transplanted with autologous marrow. Blood 1987;70:1696–1699.

135. Brandt SJ, Peters WP, Atwater SK, et al. Effects of recombinant human granulocyte-macrophage colony-stimulating factor on hematopoietic reconstitution after high-dose chemotherapy and autologous bone marrow transplantation. N Engl J Med 1988;318:869–876.

136. Nemunaitis J, Singer JW, Buckner CD, et al. Use of recombinant human granulocyte-macrophage colony-stimulating factor in autologous marrow transplantation for lymphoid malignancies. Blood 1988;72:834–836.

137. Rabinowe SN, Freedman A, Demetri G, et al. Randomized double blinded trial of rhGM-CSF in patients with B-cell non-Hodgkin's lymphoma (B-NHL) undergoing high dose chemoradiotherapy and monoclonal antibody purged autologous bone marrow transplantation (ABMT) [Abstract]. Blood 1990;76(suppl):161a.

138. Blazar BR, Kersey JH, McGlave PB, et al. In vivo administration of recombinant human granulocyte-macrophage colony-stimulating factor in acute lymphoblastic leukemia patients receiving purged autografts. Blood 1989;73:849–857.

139. Nemunaitis J, Singer JW, Buckner CD, et al. Use of recombinant human granulocyte-macrophage colony-stimulating factor in graft failure after bone marrow transplantation. Blood 1990;76:245–253.

140. Leary AG, Yang YC, Clark SC, et al. Recombinant gibbon interleukin 3 supports formation of human multilineage colonies and blast cell colonies in culture: comparison with recombinant human granu-

locyte-macrophage colony-stimulating factor. Blood 1987;70:1343–1348.

141. Saeland S, Caux C, Favre C, et al. Effects of recombinant human interleukin 3 an CD34-enriched normal hematopoietic progenitors and on myeloblastic leukemia cells. Blood 1988;72:1580–1588.

142. Sonoda Y, Yang YC, Wong GG, et al. Analysis in serum-free culture of the targets of recombinant human hematopoietic growth factors: interleukin 3 and granulocyte-macrophage colony-stimulating factor are specific for early development stages. Proc Natl Acad Sci USA 1988;85:4360–4364.

143. Bruno R, Briddell R, Hoffman R. Effect of recombinant and purified hematopoietic growth factors on human megakaryocyte colony formation. Exp Hematol 1988;16:371–377.

144. Lu L, Briddell RA, Graham CD, et al. Effect of recombinant and purified haematopoietic growth factors on in vitro colony formation by enriched populations of human megakaryocytic progenitor cells. Br J Haematol 1988;70:149–156.

145. Teramura M, Katahira J, Hoshino S, et al. Clonal growth of human megakaryocyte progenitors in serum-free cultures: effect of recombinant human interleukin-3. Exp Hematol 1988;16:843–848.

146. Ganser A, Lindemann A, Seipe HG, et al. Effects of recombinant interleukin-3 in patients with normal hematopoiesis and in patients with bone marrow failure. Blood 1990;76:666–676.

147. Umemura T, Al-Khatti A, Donahue RE, et al. Effects of interleukin-3 and erythropoietin on in vivo erythropoiesis and F. cell formation in primates. Blood 1989;74:1571–1576.

148. Sarpel SC, Axel Z, Harvath L, et al. The collection, preservation and function of peripheral blood hematopoietic cells in dogs. Exp Hematol 1979;7:113–118.

149. Goldman JR, Catovsky D, Galton DAG. Reversal of blast cell crisis in CGL by transfusion of stored autologous buffy-coat cells. Lancet 1978;1:437–438.

150. Lasky LC. Hematopoietic reconstitution using progenitors recovered from blood. Transfusion 1989;29:552–557.

151. Kessinger A, Armitage JO. The evolving role of autologous peripheral stem cell transplantation following high dose therapy for malignancies. Blood 1991;77:211–213.

152. Griepp PR, Ahmann G, Katzman JA, et al. Peripheral blood as a source of stem cells in myeloma. Blood 1988;72(suppl):243a.

153. Moss TJ, Sanders DG, Lasky LC, et al. Contamination of peripheral blood stem cell harvests by circulat-

ing neuroblastoma cells. Blood 1990;76:1879–1883.

154. Richman CM, Weiner RS, Yankee RA. Increase in circulating stem cells following chemotherapy in man. Blood 1976;47:1031–1039.

155. Lohrmann HP, Schreml W, Lang M, et al. Changes of granulopoiesis during and after adjuvant chemotherapy of breast cancer. Br J Haematol 1978;40:369–381.

156. Abrams RA, Johnston-Early A, Kramer C, et al. Amplification of circulating granulocyte-monocyte stem cell numbers following chemotherapy in patients with extensive small cell carcinoma of the lung. Cancer Res 1981;41:35–41.

157. Stiff PJ, Murgo AJ, Wittes RE, et al. Quantification of the peripheral blood colony forming unit-culture rise following chemotherapy: could leukocytapheresis replace bone marrow for autologous transplantation? Transfusion 1983;23:500–503.

158. Ruse-Riol F, Legros M, Bernard D, et al. Variations in committed stem cells (CFU-GM & CFU-TL) in the peripheral blood of cancer patients treated by sequential combination chemotherapy for breast cancer. Cancer Res 1984;44:2219–2224.

159. To LB, Haylock DN, Kimber RJ, et al. High levels of circulating hematopoietic stem cells in very early remission from acute non-lymphocytic leukaemia and their collection and cryopreservation. Br J Haematol 1984;58:399–410.

160. Antman KS, Griffin JD, Elias AS, et al. Effect of recombinant human granulocyte-macrophage colony-stimulating factor on chemotherapy-induced myelosuppression. N Engl J Med 1988;319:593–598.

161. Gianni AM, Bregni M, Siena S, et al. Rapid and complete hematopoietic reconstitution followed by combined transplantation of autologous blood and bone marrow cells. A changing role for high dose chemo-radiotherapy? Hematol Oncol 1989;7:139–148.

162. Siena S, Bregni M, Brando B, et al. Circulation of CD34+ hematopoietic stem cells in the peripheral blood of high dose cyclophosphamide-treated patients: enhancement by intravenous recombinant human granulocyte-macrophage colony-stimulating factor. Blood 1989;74:1905–1914.

163. Wagemaker G, van Gils CJM, Burger H, et al. Highly increased production of bone marrow-derived blood cells by administration of homologous interleukin-3 to rhesus monkeys. Blood 1990;76:2235–2241.

164. Geissler K, Valent P, Mayer P, et al. Recombinant human interleukin-3 expands the pool of circulating hematopoietic progenitor cells in primates—synergism with recombinant human granulocyte/macrophage colony-stimulating factor. Blood 1990;75:2305–2310.

26

INFECTIOUS DISEASES

Rein Saral

Infections are major causes of morbidity and mortality following high-dose chemotherapy with or without bone marrow transplantation. There are multiple reasons why patients receiving such therapy are susceptible to life-threatening infections. An appreciation of these reasons and the types of infections encountered has led to the development of therapeutic maneuvers that have decreased morbidity and mortality from these infections.

Treatment with high-dose chemotherapy is limited by organ system toxicity. The bone marrow is a major organ damaged by intensive chemotherapy. The damage may cause only suppression, so that in time regeneration of marrow function occurs, or it may be ablative, requiring the use of bone marrow transplantation to restore bone marrow functions. Granulocytopenia occurring secondary to intensive chemotherapy is a major risk factor that predisposes patients to develop severe life-threatening infections. The level of granulocytopenia observed determines the risk of these infections. Several levels of granulocytopenia have been defined as placing patients at risk. The risk rises as the count drops to below 500 granulocytes per cubic millimeter and increases dramatically as the count drops below 100 granulocytes per cubic millimeter. Damage to other organs secondary to the disease or its treatment with intensive therapy in conjunction with granulocytopenia results in sites where bacterial and fungal pathogens can not only cause localized infection but also create portals of entry into the bloodstream for these organisms, leading to bacteremia and/or fungemia. With the absence of granulocytes and without appropriate antibiotic therapy, bacteremia and/or fungemia lead to septic shock and death.

RISK FACTORS

There are three major areas where infection develops in the granulocytopenic patients: the gastrointestinal tract, including the oral cavity; the respiratory tract; and the skin. Patients who receive intensive therapy should be examined by a dentist or oral surgeon prior to the initiation of treatment. Periodontal disease, which occurs in the vast majority of patients over the age of 35 and which develops earlier in many patients, causes damage to tissues that may be sites of infection when granulocytopenia develops. Many compounds used in the treatment of cancer have mucosal toxicity, which in many instances may be dose limiting. The development of drug-related mucositis causes disruption in the normal barriers to infection and results in sites of infection. Mucositis may be potentiated by reactivation of herpes simplex virus, as discussed later in this chapter.

This direct toxicity against cells also occurs in the gastrointestinal tract. Since many of these cells are highly proliferative, it is common for significant damage to occur after treatment with chemotherapeutic agents. This damage leads to symptoms such as chest pain with esophagitis and diarrhea and abdominal cramps with small and large bowel damage. The timing of this damage occurs parallel with damage to the bone marrow. Therefore, destruction of normal anatomic barriers to infection occurs at the same time profound granulocytopenia develops, leading to a high risk for developing serious infection. The perianal area is frequently a site of infection. Diarrhea secondary to treatment may cause local irritation, exacerbated by the presence of structural abnormalities such as hemorrhoids. Damage to the skin may create potential sites for infection.

Virtually all patients receiving intensive chemotherapy with or without bone marrow transplantation have placement of long-term venous access devices such as Hickman, Broviac, or Groschong catheters. These devices facilitate administration of chemotherapy, antibiotics, blood products, fluids, and other therapies important in the treatment of patients. In addition, they make blood drawing more convenient and reduce the number of venipunctures required, which diminishes the risk of infection from another skin site. However, these devices create potential sites of infections. Tenderness and erythema at the exit site or tunnel may be clues to an infected line. Line-associated bacteremias may occur independent of exit site or tunnel infection but are difficult to diagnose. Bone marrow aspiration and/or biopsy sites, venipuncture sites, paracentesis or thoracentesis sites, and the axillary and groin areas are other sites of potential infection.

The respiratory tract may be a site of infection. Sinusitis is not uncommon in patients. We have found a significant number of patients with sinus abnormalities, particularly in patients who have a history of receiving chemotherapy that resulted in significant bone marrow suppression and granulocytopenia. We routinely evaluate sinuses prior to bone marrow transplantation with computerized axial tomography (CAT) to determine whether the area may be a site of infection in the posttransplant period. The other respiratory area at risk for infection is the lungs. Alterations in ciliary functions and mucus production secondary to treatment increase the risk of pathogens' establishing infections.

Patients receiving intensive chemotherapy are at risk for infection not only because of bone marrow suppression and granulocytopenia but also because of abnormalities in cellular and humoral immune defense mechanisms. These abnormalities may occur because of underlying disease or the intensive chemotherapy used to treat the disease. For example, patients who receive autologous bone marrow transplantation may experience combined immunodeficiency in the posttransplant period, placing them at risk for infections until immunologic reconstitution occurs. Finally, patients treated for a malignant disease may be at increased risk secondary to involvement or impingement of the disease on vital passageways such as a bronchus, ureter, etc.

BACTERIAL INFECTIONS— GENERAL

Bacterial pathogens are the most common cause of the initial infection in granulocytopenic patients. Over the past decade there has been an appreciable change in the type of bacterial organisms documented to cause the initial infection in granulocytopenic patients. Historically, aerobic gram-negative rods were the most frequently isolated organisms causing infection. While many such organisms were isolated, three organisms—*Pseudomonas aeruginosa*, *Klebsiella pneumoniae*, and *Escherichia coli*—were the most frequently documented to cause bacteremia. The high rate of septic shock and death in untreated or inadequately treated granulocytopenic patients with sepsis from these organisms has been important in designing treatment strategies for febrile granulocytopenic patients, as discussed later in this chapter. More recently gram-positive organisms have become more common as the initial organism causing infection in the granulocytopenic patient. In our last antibiotic therapy trial at Johns Hopkins involving bone marrow transplant recipients, 70% of documented initial infections in granulocytopenia were caused by gram-positive organisms.

Staphylococcus epidermidis, Streptococcus viridans, Staphylococcus aureus, and *Streptococcus pneumoniae* are the most frequently documented gram-positive organisms causing bacteremia. While these organisms are generally less pathogenic than gram-negative organisms in granulocytopenic patients, there are exceptions. *Streptococcus mitis* (a subspecies of *Streptococcus viridans*) sepsis has been associated with fulminant septic shock leading to patients' demise. Initially, this organism was seen in pediatric patients undergoing bone marrow transplantation. However, at Johns Hopkins we have observed septic shock secondary to bacteremia with this organism in adults and in patients receiving intensive chemotherapy without bone marrow transplantation. One common feature in the majority of cases has been the presence of severe mucositis.

Fungal organisms are rarely the cause of the initial infection in granulocytopenic patients but will be discussed later as a significant cause of subsequent infection.

BACTERIAL INFECTIONS— EMPIRIC THERAPY

Perhaps the most important principle of managing the initial infection in the granulocytopenic patient is the use of empiric antibiotic therapy for presumed infection. Fever is the most important sign of infection and at times the only sign of infection in this patient population. The development of fever (temperature ≥101° F on one occasion or ≥100.5° F on three separate occasions in 24 hours) in a granulocytopenic patient prompts a careful history and physical examination.

Cultures of blood should be obtained (minimum of two separate cultures), and any suspected site of infection should be cultured. Antibiotics are then initiated empirically to treat presumed infection. The choice of antibiotics as initial coverage has been the basis of multiple studies to establish an optimal regimen. There are several considerations that need to be considered prior to making specific recommendations.

It is important to recognize that infection in granulocytopenia is a life-threatening event and is a medical emergency requiring rapid evaluation and prompt initiation of systemic antibiotic therapy. One needs to be familiar with the types of organisms that have been observed in one's institution and their potential susceptibility patterns. It is important to select antibiotics that are broad spectrum and bactericidal and have minimal toxicity. Most institutions use combination antibiotic therapy for granulocytopenic patients with suspected infection, although studies using monotherapy have been reported to be successful as well.

The specific choice of antibiotics has been the object of multiple studies over the years. While an ideal combination has not yet been developed, the use of a variety of different approaches has reduced mortality from infection as the sole cause of death to less than 5%. Effective combinations studied have involved the use of an aminoglycoside plus a broad-spectrum penicillin with antipseudomonal activity or a broad-spectrum cephalosporin. Gentamycin, tobramycin, and amikacin are the aminoglycosides most commonly used. At Johns Hopkins gentamycin was used as the initial aminoglycoside since the bacterial flora in our patient population had not developed significant resistance to this agent. However, because of the emergence of resistant organisms, other institutions have used amikacin or tobramycin. Ticarcillin, mezlocillin, azlocillin, and piperacillin are effective antipseudomonal penicillins that have been used in combination with an aminoglycoside and broad-spectrum cephalosporins such as ceftazidime and have also been evaluated as therapy in combination with an aminoglycoside. Because of potential toxicity (ototoxicity and nephrotoxicity) and the expense of monitoring blood levels, combination regimens not including aminoglycosides have been used as initial empiric therapy. These combinations have included double β-lactam (i.e., ceftazidime plus piperacillin) combinations. In addition studies are currently being performed evaluating the combination of a β-lactam and quinoline (azlocillin-ciprofloxacin), and there are in vitro data suggesting the efficacy of imipenem and quinoline against both gram-negative and gram-positive organisms. The use of double β-lactam combinations is not recommended because of concerns regarding the likelihood of drug antagonism, the concern about effective activity against *Pseudomonas aeruginosa*, and the potential for emergence of resistance. However, with the availability of new broad-spectrum antibiotics, further studies evaluating combinations of antibiotics not containing an aminoglycoside will be important.

The use of combination antibiotic therapy has been shown in multiple studies to be associated with an improvement in response rates. These studies have also shown that synergy between antibiotics and high bactericidal activity is important in the management of profoundly granulocytopenic (<100 granulocytes per cubic millimeter) patients with gram-negative bacteremia.

In recent years, studies have been performed using monotherapy in granulocytopenic patients with presumed infection. Pizzo and his colleagues studied the use of ceftazidime only as therapy for febrile granulocytopenic patients. The control group in this study included patients who received gentamycin, cephalothin, and carbenicillin. This trial demonstrated that ceftazidime alone was adequate initial therapy. The trial has generated some criticism from other investigators. Using death as an end point, ceftazidime was found to be effective. However, the results are less impressive if failure of therapy includes not only death secondary to infection but also no clinical improvement or antimicrobial modification. Concerns have also been raised about the large type II error in a trial attempting to show equivalence between two regimens. Finally, the population studied was heterogeneous, and many patients had relatively short durations of granulocytopenia.

At Johns Hopkins we conducted a randomized, double-blind trial comparing ceftazidime alone to our standard regimen of gentamycin and ticarcillin in bone marrow transplant recipients. One hundred thirty-five evaluable patients were enrolled in the study. Seventy patients received gentamycin and ticarcillin, and 65 received ceftazidime. Seventy-six patients received allogeneic transplant, 57 received autologous transplants, and 2 received syngeneic transplant. The median duration of granulocytopenia was 22 days in each group. Treatment was initiated at time of first fever (38.2° C) in granulocytopenia (<500 granulocytes per cubic millimeter). Infection was documented in 32 of the 70 patients receiving gentamycin and ticarcillin and 27 of the 65 patients receiving ceftazidime. Gram-positive organisms accounted for 71% of the documented infections, and gram-negative organism for only 29% of the documented infections. Complete responses were similar in both groups of patients, 38 of 70 (54%) in the gentamycin-ticarcillin group and 32 of 65 (49%) in the ceftazidime group. Bacteriologic response rates among those in whom an infection was documented occurred in 36 of 37 (97%) patients receiving gentamycin and ticarcillin and 27 of 29 (93%) patients receiving ceftazidime. Of note is the bacteriologic response rate of 90% (18 of 20) in patients with gram-positive infections who received ceftazidime, although the compound has only modest activity against gram-positive organisms and the majority of these patients were subsequently treated with vancomycin. We found no difference between the groups in colonization with resistant bacterial pathogens or fungi, and no difference in superinfection. There was no difference in organ toxicity in the two groups, including nephrotoxicity. We concluded from this small clinical trial that in our institution ceftazidime was an acceptable alternative to an aminoglycoside-containing regimen in managing the initial infection in bone marrow transplant recipients with severe granulocytopenia.

Recently, investigators at the University of Maryland Cancer Center have performed a study comparing monotherapy with imipenem to treatment with amikacin plus piperacillin, in a prospective randomized double-blind clinical trial. In this trial, equivalence between the two regimens was established. The use of monotherapy has been tested in clinical trials; however, further studies are necessary before a categorical recommendation can be made endorsing such an approach as initial therapy for presumed infection in profoundly granulocytopenic patients.

Because of the marked increase in the number of gram-positive organisms causing the initial infection in the granulocytopenic patient, the role of expanding the initial antibiotic coverage to include more effective gram-positive coverage has been raised. *Staphylococcus epidermidis* has been noted with increasing frequency as a significant cause of gram-positive bacteremias. This organism is highly resistant, and vancomycin is currently the only effective agent. The sites of origin of these organisms are multiple, and while bacteremia is a cause of morbidity, in general, mortality from these infections is quite low. At Johns Hopkins a review of 78 documented cases of *Staphylococcus epidermidis* sepsis, only 2 deaths were attributable to the infection. In these two cases the patients died 8 and 9 days after the first positive culture, and vancomycin therapy was not used in either case. Wade and colleagues reported a large series of patients with *Staphylococcus epidermidis* bacteremia with moderate morbidity and no mortality. In a trial performed at Johns Hopkins, Karp and colleagues randomized 60 patients with profound granulocytopenia to receive vancomycin or placebo in addition to broad-spectrum gram-negative coverage with their initial fever. The use of empiric vancomycin resulted in more rapid disappearance of fever, reduced the overall days of fever, and prevented the development of later gram-positive infection, compared to the placebo-controlled recipients. Other investigators have suggested that empiric therapy is not necessary. In a large series from the National Cancer Institute, the authors noted a high success rate with vancomycin in treating gram-positive infections after the organism was identified as causing infection. They concluded that empiric therapy with vancomycin was not necessary but should be administered when a documented infection occurs. In a series of 55 patients with documented *Staphylococcus epidermidis* sepsis treated with vancomycin, a complete response was observed within 96 hours in 90% of patients who received vancomycin, with no overall treatment failures or death from the infection.

The high incidence of gram-positive organisms causing initial infection and the recent awareness that α-hemolytic *Streptococcus* bacteremia (*Streptococcus mitis*) may cause a shock syndrome with high mortality in contrast to the relatively benign course associated with *Staphylococcus epidermidis* bacteremia has affected our recommendation for gram-positive coverage in profoundly granulocytopenic patients. At Emory we currently recommend the empiric use of vancomycin in our patients who receive intensive chemotherapy with or without bone marrow transplantation. However, each institution has to review its experience with infections before this recommendation is routinely applied to its patient population.

BACTERIAL INFECTION— PROPHYLAXIS

Other strategies to reduce infection in granulocytopenic patients include the use of prophylactic antibiotics and a protective environment. Multiple studies have been performed to evaluate these approaches. Historically, the use of laminar airflow rooms to provide isolation from nosocomial pathogens was popular for patients who received intensive chemotherapy. Unfortunately, except for isolated studies this approach does not seem to have a beneficial effect on increased survival. Currently most patients treated with intensive therapy are placed in single rooms equipped with nonlaminar airflow, generating approximately 25 to 30 air exchanges per hour. Thorough handwashing is perhaps the most important element in reducing spread of infection on a unit. Attempts should be made to reduce invasive procedures and traumatic procedures. For example, temperatures are never taken rectally on granulocytopenic patients. While food may be a source of potential pathogens, sterilized food is extremely unpalatable, and there is generally a good correlation between the patient's caloric intake and the patient's circulating granulocyte count. However, we do recommend that patients avoid fresh vegetables and fresh fruit. Careful attention to good patient hygiene is important and is reinforced by educating the patient.

The rationale for using prophylactic antibiotics is reduction or elimination of potential pathogens from the alimentary tract since the gram-negative organisms residing there may cause the most severe infections in the granulocytopenic patient. A number of different regimens have been evaluated that appear to reduce but not eliminate the risk of infection. Both oral nonabsorbable and absorbable and intravenous antibiotics have been used to decrease the risk of infection and have been studied in controlled clinical trials. The use of gentamycin, vancomycin, and nystatin given orally demonstrated the value of nonabsorbable antibiotics in reducing the incidence of severe infection in granulocytopenic patients. Unfortunately, at Johns Hopkins we were unable to demonstrate universal compliance on the part of patients given these agents. Compliance rates with oral nonabsorbable antibiotics in our studies at Johns Hopkins varied from as low as 30%–40% to

80%–90%. Several trials have demonstrated that trimethoprim-sulfamethoxazole given as prophylaxis reduced infections in granulocytopenic patients compared to placebo recipients. However, after a number of positive studies, several investigators have failed to demonstrate the benefit from trimethoprim-sulfamethoxazole prophylaxis.

Compliance has also been an issue that has influenced the efficacy of this form of antibacterial prophylaxis. In the past few years several studies have evaluated the use of the quinolones as prophylaxis. These studies have been performed with placebo controls or treatment with oral nonabsorbable antibiotics or trimethoprim-sulfamethoxazole. The quinolones studied included norfloxacin, ofloxacin, enoxacin, pefloxacin, and ciprofloxacin. The published studies have demonstrated a decrease in the number of gram-negative infections and a reduction in morbidity. However, the use of quinolones has not obviated the need for systemically administered broad-spectrum antibiotics, and several studies have suggested that an increase in the incidence of gram-positive infections occurs in these patients. To date there is no compelling evidence to suggest the use of one quinolone as the best method to prevent infection in patients experiencing severe, prolonged (>14 days) granulocytopenia, and further comparative studies are necessary.

At Johns Hopkins we have had the greatest experience with the use of norfloxacin. Karp and colleagues demonstrated the efficacy of norfloxacin in acute leukemia patients who experienced prolonged granulocytopenia in a prospective, randomized, placebo-controlled trial. As in other studies evaluating the quinolones, there was a reduction in gram-negative infections, and in this trial a delay in time to initiation of systemic antibiotic therapy. We have now had well over a 5-year experience using norfloxacin at Johns Hopkins. We confirmed the ease with which the compound was accepted by patients, resulting in a high compliance rate, and have noted a marked reduction in gram-negative bacteremia consistent with the results obtained in the controlled study. Sepsis caused by *Pseudomonas aeruginosa*, the most devastating gram-negative organism, virtually disappeared in this time frame. Over the years patients at Johns Hopkins were monitored to detect the emergence of antibiotic-resistant gram-negative organisms in the gastrointestinal tract. Over the 5-year period of time we were unable to detect the emergence of quinolone resistant organisms in patients given norfloxacin prophylaxis.

BACTERIAL AND FUNGAL SUPERINFECTION

Granulocytopenic patients who are placed on prophylactic antibiotics and/or empiric antibiotic therapy for presumed infections are at risk for developing superinfection, defined as an infection with an organism that is resistant to or not covered by the systemic antibiotics being used to treat the patient.

The risk of developing superinfection is dependent on the duration of granulocytopenia. Based on experience, investigators have placed patients into two categories to define their risk for developing superinfection. Patients with a granulocyte count of less than 1000 granulocytes for less than 14 days are defined as having "short-term" granulocytopenia and generally have a low risk of developing superinfection. In contrast, patients with long-term granulocytopenia (greater than 14 days) are at significant risk for developing superinfection. The organisms that cause superinfection include antibiotic-resistant gram-negative bacteria, gram-positive bacteria (especially if the patient is receiving initial empiric therapy; e.g., vancomycin is not directed at treating these organisms), and fungi. The clinical picture in which superinfection should be suspected is (*a*) failure to respond to empiric antibiotics, manifest as persistent fever with or without clinical deterioration; (*b*) new infection at a clinical site; (*c*) response to initial empiric therapy followed by relapse with new fever; or (*d*) documented sepsis.

Superinfection with antibiotic-resistant gram-negative bacteria is a potentially fatal complication in granulocytopenic patients. While the value of surveillance cultures has been debated, we have used surveillance cultures to monitor the emergence of antibiotic-resistant gram-negative bacteria in patients who develop "long-term" granulocytopenia secondary to intensive chemotherapy. Twice weekly throat and stool swabbings are obtained and placed on media containing the antibiotics we use as initial empiric therapy for patients with fever in granulocytopenia. This allows us to identify colonization with bacteria resistant to the antibiotics the patient is receiving. The organisms are speciated, and susceptibility information is generated. This information is useful in determining the use of alternative antibiotics if the clinical situation suggests that these colonizing organisms are causing superinfection. While persistent fever may be a clue to superinfection, it is important not to switch or add antibacterial antibiotic coverage on the basis of fever alone. If a patient is stable with no change in clinical status and no increase or progression of fever, the patient should be examined, cultured, and maintained on the original antibiotics prescribed. However, if there is clinical deterioration, progressive fever, or new fever after a complete febrile response, the antibacterial antibiotic regimen may be changed.

Clearly, if a positive blood or body site culture for gram-negative bacteria is obtained, the antibiotic regimen needs to be changed. The antibiotics recommended to treat suspected superinfection with resistant gram-negative bacteria depend on the initial antibiotics used and the institutional experience with such organisms. If there is a proven superinfection, antibiotic susceptibility data on the organism isolated dictates the specific antibiotics recommended. If the clinical picture is suggestive of septic shock, secondary to a resistant gram-negative organism, we treat the patient with amikacin and piperacillin or imipenem since we do not use these agents as initial empiric therapy. It is important not to add antibiotics but to substitute antibiotics to prevent patients from being on up to six or seven different antibiotics for the same purpose. In fact, at Emory we review the care of all patients on more than three antibacterial antibiotics to determine the rationale for their use.

Gram-positive organisms are a frequent cause of superinfection if empiric therapy with vancomycin is not used with initial antibiotic therapy. In general, these infections are not as serious as those caused by resistant gram-negative organisms. However, they cause significant morbidity. The major cause of gram-positive infection has been *Staphylococcus epidermidis*. A major site of gram-positive infection is the long-term venous access catheter used in the vast majority of patients treated with intensive chemotherapy. Clinical findings consistent with catheter infection are tenderness and erythemia at the exit site (most common) or over the tunnel. If catheter infection is suspected or proven and caused by a gram-positive organism, vancomycin treatment should be sufficient to control the infection without removing the line. However, some investigators would remove the line in addition to using antimicrobial therapy if a tunnel infection was observed. At Emory we also preserve the line if a gram-positive bacteremia is documented and treat with vancomycin. Vancomycin remains the treatment of choice for gram-positive superinfection. We have found that the use of 500 mg of vancomycin every 12 hours is equivalent to 500 mg given every 6 hours and 1 gram given every 12 hours in patients with documented gram-positive infection, and this has reduced the cost of vancomycin therapy if it is given empirically with the first fever or later when suspected or documented gram-positive infections are treated.

A major infection complication in patients experiencing "long-term" granulocytopenia is the development of systemic fungal infection. Fungi are rarely the cause of initial infection in granulocytopenic patients, but both yeast and filamentous fungi are a significant cause of superinfection. *Candida* and *Aspergillus* species are the most common fungal pathogens documented to cause infection. However, the list of other fungi that cause disseminated infection increases each year and includes *Fusarium*, *Trichosporon* species, and *Torulopsis glabrata*.

Candida species cause localized infection in the oral cavity, the genital area, and the gastrointestinal tract. In granulocytopenic patients dissemination of *Candida* may occur, leading to potentially fatal infection. A number of *Candida* strains have been shown to be significant pathogens in this patient population. *Candida albicans* is the most common strain, but investigators at Johns Hopkins demonstrated several years ago that *Candida tropicalis* is also a significant pathogen in granulocytopenic patients. In a study evaluating the role of fungal surveillance cultures as predictors of disseminated fungal infection, we found that 80% of our patients were colonized with *Candida albicans* but that only 5% of these patients developed disseminated infection. In contrast, only 30% of patients were colonized by *Candida tropicalis* but 56% of these patients with long-term granulocytopenia developed disseminated infection. Other institutions have confirmed our observations that *Candida tropicalis* is a major fungal pathogen in granulocytopenic patients.

Other *Candida* species have also emerged as significant pathogens. Prior to 1981, we observed only one case of disseminated infection with *Candida krusei*. By 1990 *Candida krusei* had emerged as a major fungal pathogen causing disseminated infections in bone marrow transplant patients at Johns Hopkins. The use of fluconazole prophylaxis reduced infection with *Candida albicans* and *Candida tropicalis* but increased colonization in surveillance cultures by *Candida krusei* from approximately 15% to 40%. This increased colonization translated into disseminated infection with *Candida krusei*. In fact, 10–20 documented disseminated *Candida* infections at Johns Hopkins in 1990 in long-term granulocytopenic patients were caused by *Candida krusei*. *Candida parapsilosis*, *Candida lusitaniae*, *Candida guillermondii*, and *Torulopsis glabrata* are other yeasts that cause disseminated infection.

Diagnosis of disseminated *Candida* remains an unresolved problem. Techniques such as lysis centrifugation may increase our ability to diagnose *Candida* sepsis, and a recently reported antigen detection method may provide adequate sensitivity and specificity to be useful. However, clinical suspicion is important. Clues to disseminated infections include refractory or new fever while on antibacterial antibiotics. The mean interval to documented *Candida* sepsis is between 9 and 11 days following onset of profound granulocytopenia. Embolic skin lesions, particularly caused by *Candida tropicalis*, may be the first evidence of disseminated infection. New-onset renal failure may not be due to nephrotoxicity but secondary to invasion of the kidney with *Candida*, and myalgias may be caused by muscle invasion by *Candida*.

One specific type of *Candida* infection is important to recognize in patients who receive several treatments with high-dose granulocytopenia producing therapy. Originally described as hepatosplenic candidiasis, it might be better termed chronic disseminated candidiasis. Patients who receive intensive chemotherapy develop persistent fever, abdominal discomfort, and liver function abnormalities when their granulocytopenia resolves. These patients develop deep-seated *Candida* abscesses in the liver, spleen, kidneys, and lungs as their bone marrow recovers and granulocytopenia resolves. If unrecognized, it may lead to the patient's demise, or it may preclude the initiation of further intensive therapy until adequately treated. If unsuspected, further treatment of these patients with intensive chemotherapy leads to granulocytopenia and acute dissemination of *Candida* and death. If suspected, a CAT scan and ultrasound should be performed, but final confirmation requires biopsy.

Management of *Candida* infections consists of prophylaxis, empiric therapy, and treatment of established infections. The use of local agents such as nystatin and clotrimazole, while effective compared to placebo controls in the prevention or treatment of localized *Candida* infection, has no role in the prevention or treatment of disseminated *Candida* infections.

Attempts have been made to define strategies to prevent *Candida* infections from occurring. The use of prophylactic systemic antifungal agents has not completely reduced *Candida* infections in granulocytopenic patients. Several years ago our group at Johns Hopkins demonstrated that intravenous miconazole when administered with empiric antibacterial therapy at the time of the first fever reduced the incidence of fungemia compared to placebo controls in a prospective, randomized clinical trial. However, that approach did not obviate the need to use intravenous amphotericin B for suspected cases of fungal sepsis. Recently fluconazole, a triazole with an excellent spectrum of activity against *Candida* and with little toxicity, has been shown to provide effective prophylaxis against *Candida* when administered at the same time empiric antibacterial antibiotics are initiated. Our group substituted fluconazole for miconazole as antifungal prophylaxis in early 1990 in bone marrow transplant patients at Johns Hopkins. While we observed a significant reduction in disseminated *Candida albicans* and *Candida tropicalis* infection, we noted an increase in disseminated infection with *Candida krusei*, as noted earlier. This is not totally unexpected since in vitro studies demonstrate resistance of *Candida krusei* to fluconazole. We and others have also observed increased colonization with *Torulopsis glabrata* in patients receiving fluconazole. In addition, fluconazole and miconazole lack activity against *Aspergillus*. While the development of fluconazole represents a significant advance in antifungal chemotherapy, no completely effective and nontoxic agent has yet been shown to date to prevent disseminated yeast infections.

Perhaps the most beneficial way to prevent disseminated *Candida* infections is by use of empiric antifungal therapy for presumed *Candida* infection. Amphotericin B has been administered in controlled trials as empiric and antifungal therapy in granulocytopenic patients. In one study febrile patients were randomized to receive amphotericin B or no antifungal therapy after 7 days of antibacterial therapy. Benefit was observed in patients receiving amphotericin B therapy. The European Organization for Research in Treatment of Cancer (EORTC) conducted a trial where febrile granulocytopenic patients were randomized to receive amphotericin B or no antifungal therapy 4 days after initiating bacterial therapy. The results of this trial also demonstrated benefits to patients receiving amphotericin B. At Emory we currently recommend amphotericin B therapy in persistently febrile granulocytopenic patients 6 days after initiating antibacterial antibiotics. Clearly, therapy with amphotericin B is initiated earlier if there are clinical signs of *Candida* sepsis.

In granulocytopenic patients with documented disseminated infection with *Candida*, amphotericin B is the treatment of choice. While fluconazole is a promising agent and is effective in patients with granulocytes, the use of this agent to treat disseminated *Candida* infections in granulocytopenic patients requires further study. The dose of amphotericin B used in our institution at Emory to treat proven infection is 0.5 mg–1.0 mg/kg. Addition of flucytosine has demonstrated synergy in vitro against certain *Candida* species and is recommended in selected clinical situations, although controlled clinical trials supporting this approach are not available. In using flucytosine in combination with amphotericin, we aim for peak serum levels of 30–60 μg/ml to reduce potential toxicity from this combination.

The exact duration of treatment in pa-tients with disseminated *Candida* infection is not clear. Resolution of granulocytopenia is an important determinant in overall outcome. Therapy can be discontinued when the patient reconstitutes bone marrow and granulocytopenia and fever resolve. However, if significant visceral involvement is detected after resolution of granulocytopenia, extended therapy is necessary. If amphotericin alone or in combination with flucytosine is not effective in treating deep-seated *Candida* infections in these patients, a trial of fluconazole is indicated.

Aspergillus infections are a cause of significant life-threatening infection in granulocytopenic patients. *Aspergillus fumigatus* and *Aspergillus flavus*, the most common species causing infection in humans, are ubiquitous in nature and acquired primarily through the respiratory tract. One use of air filtration in rooms is to prevent acquisition of *Aspergillus* spores by highly susceptible patients. The institutional variation in prevalence of these infections is explained by the importance of environmental exposure to the organism. Other factors are important in determining the risk of developing *Aspergillus* infection. One clear-cut risk factor is duration of granulocytopenia. Studies at the University of Pennsylvania demonstrated a risk of developing pulmonary aspergillus of 1% per day by the 22nd day of granulocytopenia. However, this risk increased to 4.5% per day between the 22nd and 36th day of granulocytopenia. At Johns Hopkins we found that the risk of developing invasive aspergillosis was only 0.3% in patients with a median duration of granulocytopenia of 17 days, 3.5% in patients with a median duration of granulocytopenia of 24 days, and 14% in patients with a median duration of granulocytopenia of 32 days.

Patients who experience multiple chemotherapy treatments resulting in significant granulocytopenia may have subclinical or unappreciated pulmonary infection caused by *Aspergillus*. These patients are at risk for reactivation infection of endogenous organisms when treated again with chemotherapy that produces long-term granulocytopenia.

Pulmonary signs or symptoms that develop in granulocytopenic patients may be caused by many medical factors. However, pulmonary signs and symptoms may be a clinical indication that a patient has invasive pulmonary aspergillosis. In patients with documented invasive aspergillosis, over 70% present with sudden onset of pleuritic chest pain, hypoxemia, cough, or hemoptysis. The presence of these symptoms in conjunction with new fever or increased fever late in granulocytopenia is very suggestive of invasive pulmonary aspergillosis. In the Johns Hopkins experience median time to development of pulmonary aspergillosis was 19 days after onset of granulocytopenia. While a chest x-ray may reveal infiltrates consistent with aspergillosis, a negative chest x-ray does not rule out the disease. Pulmonary CAT scans have been extremely useful in defining lesions and are indicated if aspergillosis is suspected. Features on CAT scans highly suggestive of pulmonary aspergillosis have been defined by radiologists. Tests to diagnose aspergillosis short of biopsy are currently not available. However, an ELISA technique used to detect carbohydrate components of *Aspergillus* antigen in serum is promising and is currently being evaluated as a tool for early diagnosis.

Treatment of established invasive pulmonary *Aspergillus* has yielded extremely poor results in the past. Survival rates of zero have been reported by many investigators. In recent years the prompt initiation of high-dose amphotericin B alone or in combination with flucytosine early in the course of invasive pulmonary aspergillosis may be effective in controlling the disease until resolution of granulocytopenia. Burch and colleagues reported that 13 of 14 patients with pulmonary aspergillosis survived after treatment with high-dose amphotericin B (1.0–1.5 mg/kg) alone or in combination with flucytosine given to achieve peak serum levels between 30 and 60 μg/ml. Patients were treated within 2 days

of onset of respiratory symptoms. The only patient who died failed to recover marrow. At Emory our current policy is to institute early high-dose amphotericin B in a dose of 1.0– 1.5 mg/kg along with flucytosine for patients with suspected or proven invasive pulmonary aspergillosis. Patients with documented disease continue to receive treatment after discharge from the hospital, receiving amphotericin at least three times per week for an average of 1 month following discharge. Recently, studies have suggested that the use of growth factors such as recombinant human macrophage colony-stimulating factor (rhM-CSF) may facilitate recovery from deep-seated fungal infections. Further clinical studies are necessary to validate this observation.

In patients who have had a previous episode of aspergillosis, the use of high-dose amphotericin B (1.0 mg/kg) and flucytosine proved effective when used as prophylaxis to prevent the disease in a small group of patients who received high-dose chemotherapy for their disease. Treatment was initiated 2 days prior to chemotherapy and continued until resolution of granulocytopenia. A total of nine patients received 13 courses of treatment, resulting in profound, prolonged granulocytopenia. No deaths were reported. This study involved a small number of patients and was uncontrolled; however, it is the only study suggesting that the use of antifungal agents in high doses may prevent aspergillosis from causing significant disease in patients at high risk. Because of the small numbers, these observations need to be confirmed in additional studies. While treatment for *Aspergillus* has rarely improved the overall success rate in controlling the infection, more active and less toxic compounds need to be developed to treat or prevent these infections.

In spite of the hurdles presented by infection with bacterial and fungal organisms in patients experiencing prolonged granulocytopenia, mortality rates from these infections has been markedly reduced. While a cookbook approach to managing these patients does not cover all of the permutations of infection in the granulocytopenic patient, each institution should generate an algorithm for management of bacterial and fungal infection, recognizing that it offers only broad guidelines. Our current algorithm is illustrated in Tables 26.1 and 26.2 and Figure 26.1. A systematic approach leads to orderly and consistent therapy. If possible, clinical trials are encouraged to challenge conventional wisdom and to determine whether infection management can be performed in a more effective and less toxic manner. The introduction of hematopoietic growth factors alone or in combination has and will continue to reduce the risks of infection by shortening the period of bone marrow failure following intensive chemotherapy; but until we can reduce the period of granulocytopenia further, organized preventive and treatment strategies will be necessary to prevent morbidity and mortality from bacterial and fungal infections.

VIRAL INFECTION

Patients receiving intensive chemotherapy may have alterations in their cellular or humoral immune system because of their basic disease and or therapy. These patients are susceptible to viral pathogens that may cause morbidity and mortality. The herpesvirus group have been well studied, and therapeutic and preventative strategies have been developed to deal with these infections.

Herpes simplex virus infections occur in a high percentage of patients receiving intensive chemotherapy. In studies done in allogeneic bone marrow, patients who were seropositive (antibody to herpes simplex virus) for the virus had a 70%–80% reactivation of herpes simplex virus following intensive preparation with chemotherapy alone or with radiation therapy. All patients who reactivated virus developed severe lesions. The incidence of reactivation in seropositive patients receiving autologous bone marrow transplantation is 70%–80% as well. Patients receiving intensive therapy for acute leukemia and lymphoma have a reactivation rate of between 50% and 70%, and the vast majority develop clinically significant lesions with this reactivation. Solid tumor patients have been less well studied, but there are reports of clinically significant reactivation in this patient population. Reactivated herpes simplex virus causes severe mucocutaneous lesions in the oral and genital areas. In untreated patients healing may not occur for 4–6 weeks after onset of infection. These lesions may be atypical and confused with therapy-induced mucositis. Herpes simplex virus may cause esophagitis and, less commonly, pneumonia or disseminated infection.

These infections occur predictably after

Table 26.1. Antibiotic Prophylaxis[a]

Patient Type	Start Day	Drug	Dose/Route/Freq	Stop Day
All pts.	Admission	Norfloxacin	400 mg PO BID	ANC > 500 × 1–2 days
All pts.	Admission	Fluconazole	400 mg PO QD (convert to IV if unable to take PO)	ANC > 500 × 1 day or when amphotericin started
All pts.	0	Vancomycin	500 mg IV q12h	ANC > 500 × 1–3 days
All pts.	Prior to discharge	Trimethoprim Sulfamethoxazole	1 DS tab PO BID twice weekly	Day 180
HSV + pts.	0	Acyclovir	200 mg/m^2 IV q8H	Day 35
Pts. with CMV + blood culture	Day of CMV + culture	Ganciclovir[b]	5 mg/kg q12h × 2 wks. then 5 mg/kg 5 times per week	Day 120

[a]Abbreviations: ANC, absolute neutrophil count; CMU, cytomegalovirus; DS, double strength; HSV, herpes simplex virus.
[b]For allogeneic transplant recipients only.

Table 26.2. Dosage Guidelines for Renal Insufficiency[a]

Drug	Creatinine Clearance (ml/min)[b]			
	≥80	50–79	10–49	<10
Ceftazidine	1 gm q8h	1 gm q8h	1 gm q12h	1 gm q24h
Piperacillin	5 gm q8h	5 gm q8h	5 gm q12h	5 gm q24h
Acyclovir	200 mg/m² q8h	200 mg/m² q8h	200 mg/m² q12h	100 mg/m² q24h
Fluconazole	400 mg q24h	400 mg q24h	400 mg q24h	400 mg q48h
Norfloxacin	400 mg q12h	400 mg q12h	400 mg q24h	400 mg q24h
Vancomycin	500 mg q12h[c]	500 mg q24h[c]	—[d]	—[d]
Amikacin[e]	7 mg/kg q8h[c]	7 mg/kg q12h[c]	—[d]	—[d]

[a]Data from Medical Letter. Handbook of Antimicrobial Therapy. New Rochelle, NY: Medical Letter, 1988.
[b]Males:

$$CrCl = \frac{(140 - age) \times Ideal\ body\ weight}{72 \times serum\ creatinine}$$

females: above × 0.85
(For patients over 60 years of age, if creatinine < 1.0, use 1.0 in above formula.)
[c]Obtain peak and trough levels after third dose. Pharmacokinetic team will evaluate levels and make recommendations for further dosing regimens.
[d]Dose based on drug levels. Give single dose (vanco 1 gm and amikacin 7 mg/kg). Consult pharmacokinetic team for recommendations regarding timing of drug levels and further dosing recommendations.
[e]Round doses off to the nearest 25 mg.

treatment. Median time to onset of lesions is 8 days after allogeneic or autologous bone marrow transplantation or 17 days after initiation of preparative chemotherapy. Median time to onset of lesions in the acute leukemia population is also 17 days following initiation of intensive therapy. The reactivation of herpes simplex virus occurs at the time that therapy-induced mucositis develops. Studies have demonstrated that mucositis is more severe if herpes simplex virus reactivation occurs. Disruption of mucous membranes secondary to reactivation of the virus creates damage to the anatomic barriers protecting these patients from bacterial and fungal pathogens and provides portals of entry for these organisms.

Acyclovir has been shown to be an effective anti-herpes-simplex agent in multiple prospective, randomized, double-blind, placebo-controlled trials. At Johns Hopkins our group demonstrated in allogeneic and autologous bone marrow transplant recipients and leukemia patients that acyclovir could prevent herpes simplex virus reactivation and infection if given during the period of risk. Others have confirmed these results in the same and other patient populations. Acyclovir may also be used to treat established

herpes simplex virus infection. In patients with a high incidence and predictable pattern of reactivation, we recommend acyclovir prophylaxis to prevent reactivation. In well over 1000 patients, this approach has prevented reactivation in over 99% of patients treated. We prefer to use intravenous acyclovir for hospitalized patients, although oral acyclovir provides equivalent results if patients are compliant. The exact dose and dose schedule to provide effective prophylaxis has not yet been determined. Currently we use 125 mg/m² given intravenously every 6 hours or oral acyclovir 400 mg given five times per day. If prophylaxis is not administered, treatment should be initiated quickly after diagnosis using a schedule similar to the one proposed for prophylaxis.

With the introduction of acyclovir into clinical practice, a concern was raised about the emergence of acyclovir-resistant strains of herpes simplex virus. While these strains have been observed, especially after treatment of established lesions in immunocompromised patients, very few pathogenic acyclovir-resistant strains causing clinically significant disease have been reported. However, patients containing such virus in clini-

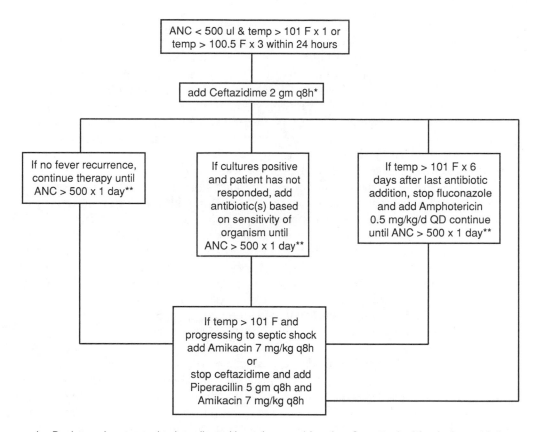

Figure 26.1.   Algorithm for febrile neutropenic patient.

* Dosing regimens need to be adjusted based on renal function. See attached for dosing guidelines.

** When ANC > 500, discontinue antibiotics sequentially as follows
   ANC > 500 x 1 day -- discontinue antifungal
   ANC > 500 x 2 days -- discontinue gram negative coverage
                        (ceftazidime, amikacin, imipenem)
   ANC > 500 x 3 days -- discontinue vancomycin

cally significant lesions have responded to foscarnet (phosphonoformic acid), so alternative therapy exists if such a clinical presentation is encountered.

Cytomegalovirus is the major viral pathogen causing morbidity and mortality in severely immunocompromised patients. Historically, the virus has been the most common infectious cause of death in allogeneic bone marrow transplantation recipients. Cytomegalovirus pneumonia in allogeneic bone marrow transplant recipients had an 85% mortality before the advent of effective therapy or prophylaxis of the disease. Cytomegalovirus infection occurs secondary to reactivation of the virus in patients who are seropositive (serum antibody to cytomegalovirus). Patients who are seronegative generally acquire the virus through blood transfusion (red blood cell or platelet transfusion) given as supportive care to manage patients following intensive therapy. The type of illness caused by cytomegalovirus depends on the degree of immunosuppression in the patient population at risk. Cytomegalovirus may cause unexplained fever or a mononucleosis-like illness, suppress bone marrow function, and cause enteritis, retinitis, and pneumonitis. Analysis of the clinical syndromes observed in patients receiving autologous rather than allogeneic bone marrow transplantation suggests that severe life-threatening disease is less frequently observed in autologous bone marrow transplant recipients. At Johns Hopkins we observed that while the infection rate in autologous and allogeneic bone marrow transplant patients were similar, patients receiving allogeneic marrow transplantation were more likely to develop severe disease such as cytomegalovirus pneumonia. In a study of over 700 patients, the likelihood of developing cytomegalovirus pneumonia was 2% in autologous bone marrow transplant recipients and 10% in allogeneic bone marrow transplant recipients ($p = .001$). Other centers have reported a slightly higher incidence of cytomegalovirus pneumonia in their autologous marrow transplant patients. Studies suggest that cytomegalovirus infection in autologous bone marrow transplant patients may suppress bone marrow function and recovery following autologous bone marrow transplantation. Wingard at Johns Hopkins has confirmed these results, but other studies have not. Investigators at the University of Maryland have demonstrated that cytomegalovirus is a significant pathogen in acute leukemia patients.

Further studies are necessary to establish the role of cytomegalovirus as a pathogen in patients receiving intensive chemotherapy. These studies should be facilitated by sensitive and specific diagnostic tests for the virus that have been established in the past few years. Cultures for cytomegalovirus require days to weeks to interpret. The use of rapid diagnostic techniques with the use of accelerated culture or antigen detection have improved our ability to detect infection with the virus. Since therapy is now available for severe life-threatening disease and prophylaxis has demonstrated efficacy in allo-

geneic bone marrow transplant recipients, rapid diagnosis becomes exceedingly important for management purposes.

With the use of ganciclovir and passively administered antibody, mortality from cytomegalovirus pneumonia has been reduced from 85% to 40%–50%. Although the studies evaluating this therapy were uncontrolled, the results are impressive and represent the first therapeutic approach affecting mortality from this devastating disease. Studies evaluating the use of ganciclovir as a way to prevent cytomegalovirus infection in allogeneic bone marrow transplant recipients have yielded positive results. Allogeneic bone marrow transplant patients at the City of Hope and Stanford University hospitals had bronchoalveolar lavage performed at day 35 posttransplant. If cytomegalovirus was demonstrated in the lavage specimen, patients were randomized to receive prophylactic ganciclovir or to observation. Patients receiving ganciclovir had a statistically significant reduction in the development of cytomegalovirus pneumonia. Other studies done in a similar patient population confirm that ganciclovir is effective prophylaxis against serious cytomegalovirus infection in allogeneic bone marrow transplantation recipients who develop asymptomatic shedding of the virus. No studies have been performed evaluating ganciclovir in the prophylaxis of serious cytomegalovirus infections in autologous bone marrow transplant patients or in patients receiving intensive chemotherapy without transplantation, and this approach is not recommended unless it is part of a well-defined prospective study.

A convenient way to prevent cytomegalovirus infection in patients seronegative for the virus is the use of seronegative blood products. This approach has become the standard of care in seronegative patients undergoing allogeneic bone marrow transplantation from a seronegative donor. In seronegative autologous bone marrow transplant patients and seronegative patients who receive other forms of intensive therapy, attempts should be made to provide seronegative blood product support. If this is not possible, the use of filters for blood products may reduce the risk of transmitting the virus.

In addition, passively administered immunoglobulin has reduced the risks of severe cytomegalovirus infection in seronegative allogeneic bone marrow transplantation and may be useful if cytomegalovirus-negative blood products cannot be provided. The use of immunoglobulin for the prophylaxis of severe cytomegalovirus in seropositive patients (allogeneic or autologous) has not been demonstrated to be effective in prospective controlled clinical trials and cannot be recommended for this purpose at the present time.

Varicella-zoster virus infections may be a cause of significant morbidity and mortality. Primary infections with the virus in immunocompromised patients may be life-threatening. This is generally a problem in pediatric patients since most adults have had primary infection with the virus. For immunocompromised patients at risk for primary infection with varicella because of exposure to the disease, passively administered antibody may reduce severity of disease from the virus. Varicella-zoster virus vaccine has been shown to be effective in immunocompromised children. If patients develop varicella infections intravenous acyclovir is indicated as therapy.

The most common manifestation of varicella-zoster virus infection in immunocompromised adult patients is herpes zoster. Reactivation of the virus results in dermatomal herpes zoster that is far more serious in the immunocompromised patient than in normal patients. The major risk to this population is cutaneous dissemination and visceral involvement with the virus, although acute pain, extensive dermatomal lesions, and postherpetic pain are frequently observed. The risk of developing herpes zoster is 50% in allogeneic bone marrow transplant recipients. In autologous bone marrow transplant patients the risk for developing herpes zoster

depends on the patient's underlying disease. In patients with lymphoma and Hodgkin's disease, the risk is greater than 40%; in acute leukemia it is approximately 25%, and in solid tumors it is 10%–15%. Patients who develop dermatomal zoster are at risk for developing disseminated disease. The risk of cutaneous dissemination may be as high as 50%, and in the pre-antiviral era patients with cutaneous dissemination frequently developed visceral complications that led to mortality rates between 10% and 20%. Acyclovir, vidarabine, and interferon all proved to be effective therapy in prospective, randomized controlled clinical trials with placebo controls. In a direct comparative study intravenous acyclovir proved to be superior to vidarabine in the treatment of herpes zoster in severely immunocompromised patients and is currently the treatment of choice. Early therapy is most effective (less than 72 hours after onset of lesions). Intravenous acyclovir is recommended for therapy of varicella-zoster infections in severely immunocompromised patients (500 mg/m^2 given every 8 hours). Oral therapy (800 mg five times a day) has been shown to be effective in normal patients with herpes zoster if given early in the disease but deserves further study in immunocompromised patients.

Less than 10 years ago there were no effective and nontoxic therapies for herpesvirus infections. Today we have therapeutic approaches that can prevent and treat herpes simplex virus, cytomegalovirus, and varicella-zoster virus infections. These therapies have lessened morbidity and mortality following intensive treatment, and fortunately, many of the consequences of these infections can now be placed in historical texts.

Suggested Reading

Anaissie E, Bodey GP, Kantarjian H, et al. New spectrum of fungal infections in patients with cancer. Rev Infect Dis 11:369–378, 1989;11:369–378.

Consensus Panel, Immunocompromised Host Society. The design, analysis and reporting of clinical trials on the empirical antibiotic management of the neutropenic patient. J Infect Dis 1990;161:397–401.

Denning DW, Stevens DA. Antifungal and surgical treatment of invasive aspergillosis. Rev Infect Dis 1990; 12:1147.

EORTC International Antimicrobial Therapy Cooperative Group. Empiric antifungal therapy in febrile granulocytopenic patients. Am J Med 1989;86:668–672.

EORTC International Antimicrobial Therapy Cooperative Group and the National Cancer Institute of Canada—Clinical Trials Group. Vancomycin added to empirical combination antibiotic therapy for fever in granulocytopenic cancer patients. J Infect Dis 1991;163:951–958.

Holland HK, Wingard JR, Saral R. Viral infections in bone marrow transplantation: clinical presentations, pathogenesis, and therapeutic strategies. Cancer Invest 1990;8:507–519.

Hughes WT, Armstrong D, Bodey GP, et al. Guidelines for the use of antimicrobial agents in neutropenic patients with unexplained fever. J Infect Dis 1990;161:381–396.

Karp JE, Dick JD, Angelopulos C, et al. Empiric use of vancomycin during prolonged treatment-induced granulocytopenia. AM J Med 1986;81:237–242.

Klastersky J, Zinner SH, Calandra T, et al. Empiric antimicrobial therapy for febrile granulocytopenic cancer patients: lesson from four EORTC trials. Eur J Cancer Clin Oncol 1988;24(suppl 1):S35–S45.

Levin MJ, Zaia JA, Spector SA, Bowden RA, Meyers JD,

Emanuel D. Current approaches to the prevention and treatment of cytomegalovirus disease after bone marrow transplantation (symposium). Semin Hematol 1990;27:1–28.

Pater JL, Weir L. Reporting the results of randomized trials of empiric antibiotics in febrile neutropenic patients—a critical survey. J Clin Oncol 1986;4:346–352.

Rubin RH, Young LS. Clinical approaches to infection in the compromised host. 2nd ed. New York: Plenum, 1988.

Saral R. Candida and Aspergillus infections in immunocompromised patients: an overview. Rev Infect Dis 1991;13:487–492.

Saral R. Management of mucocutaneous herpes simplex virus infections in immunocompromised patients. Am J Med 1988;29:85:57–60.

Saral R, Burns WH, Prentice HG. Herpes virus infections: clinical manifestations and therapeutic strategies in immunocompromised patients. Clin Hematol 1984; 13(3):645–660.

Straus S, Ostrove J, Inchauspe G, et al. Varicella-zoster virus infections. Ann Intern Med 1988;108:221–237.

Walsh TJ, Lee JW, Lecciones J, et al. Empirical amphotericin B in febrile granulocytopenic patients. Rev Infect Dis 1991;13:496–503.

Zaia JA, Hooper JA. Pathogenesis of cytomegalovirus-associated diseases (symposium). Transplant Proc 1991; 23:1–181.

27

Pulmonary Complications of Bone Marrow Transplantation

*Richard A. Robbins, Elizabeth C. Reed, Joseph H. Sisson, John R. Spurzem,
William P. Vaughan, and Stephen I. Rennard*

Pulmonary complications represent a major cause of morbidity and mortality in patients who receive marrow transplantation (1, 2). Both infectious and noninfectious complications contribute significantly to the morbidity and mortality (1, 2). These two major categories can be further subdivided into complications that occur prior to transplantation, complications that occur early after transplantation (i.e., during the initial 100 days after bone marrow transplantation), and complications that occur late after transplantation (i.e., after the initial 100 days). Because the diagnostic considerations vary considerably with the time relative to transplantation, this subdivision has been useful clinically (1, 2).

The type of marrow transplant also affects the incidence of pulmonary complications (1, 2). The frequent development of graft-versus-host disease in the allogeneic bone marrow transplant patient and the subsequent need for prolonged immunosuppressive therapy to control the graft-versus-host disease leads to an increase in pulmonary complications, especially late complications.

PULMONARY COMPLICATIONS PRIOR TO TRANSPLANTATION

Patients may present with a compromised respiratory status at the time of marrow transplantation. This is not surprising for several reasons: (*a*) These patients have often received prior chemotherapy and/or radiation therapy, which can damage the lung; (*b*) patients may have metastatic disease to the lung and (*c*) patients are often immunocompromised because of previous therapy or because of their underlying disease.

Infectious Complications

The incidence of infectious complications occurring immediately prior to transplantation is unclear. However, in a small series of 55 patients, 20 asymptomatic patients underwent bronchoscopy and bronchoalveolar lavage prior to bone marrow transplantation. Three of 20 patients had diffuse *Candida* colonization of the airways, and one patient had *Pneumocystis carinii* identified in the bronchoalveolar lavage fluid (3). These data suggest that infections prior to transplantation may be relatively frequent, even in asymptomatic patients.

Noninfectious Complications

Patients may present for bone marrow transplantation with a variety of noninfectious pulmonary complications. These include the mechanical effects of tumor, which can result in upper airway obstruction; lower airway obstruction from diffuse malignant disease in the airways; or development of pleural effusions, which decrease lung volumes by compression. In addition, the effects of prior chemotherapy or radiation therapy can result in restrictive lung disease.

Bronchitis characterized by bronchial erythema, edema, and friability and the presence of increased numbers of neutrophils within the bronchial lumens occurs in up to 30% of patients prior to bone marrow transplantation (3). Although the pathogenesis is unclear, no infectious organisms have been identified in the majority of subjects, suggesting that the bronchitis is usually noninfectious in origin. Interestingly, the presence of bronchitis appears to predict the occurrence of later pulmonary complications (3).

EARLY PULMONARY COMPLICATIONS

Infectious Pulmonary Complications

VIRAL

Cytomegalovirus (CMV) is the most common cause of viral pneumonia in the early transplantation period. An incidence as high as 50% has been reported (1, 2, 4–6). Two clinical presentations of CMV pneumonia have been described (5, 6). One is characterized by the sudden onset of respiratory failure 1–2 months after bone marrow transplantation, with a miliary pattern on chest x-ray. This presentation is presumed to result from hematogenous dissemination of CMV to the lungs from an extrapulmonary source in patients lacking antibody directed against CMV. The second presentation appears as a more typical pneumonia clinically and radiographically and is often seen 3–4 months after transplantation. It has been postulated that this latter pattern results from reactivation of CMV that the patient had previously acquired. Interestingly, it appears to take a prolonged period of immunosuppression to permit development of CMV pneumonia because it is rare in autologous transplant recipients as opposed to allogeneic recipients receiving treatment for graft-versus-host disease.

Identification of CMV as a cause of pneumonia can be difficult. The virus tends to grow slowly in culture, and the development of effective therapy has generated a need for more rapid diagnosis. Open lung biopsy has frequently been used, but it is invasive and may have serious morbidity and mortality in this patient population. Because of the potential complications of open lung biopsy, many physicians have been hesitant to use open lung biopsy at early stages of an infection when the patient appears clinically well. This has led to the frequent use of bronchoscopy with bronchoalveolar lavage. However, the presence of the typical cytoplasmic or intranuclear inclusions in cells obtained by bronchoalveolar lavage, indicative of CMV pneumonia, occurs in <70% of CMV-infected patients (7–11). Therefore, a variety of techniques to improve the sensitivity of bronchoscopy and bronchoalveolar lavage have been used. These include CMV culture with centrifugation, CMV culture by the shell vial technique, CMV detection by monoclonal antibodies directed against cell surface antigens, and in situ hybridization (11–17). These techniques have led to more rapid and more sensitive detection of CMV pneumonia, allowing early therapy while awaiting culture confirmation.

The use of ganciclovir and immune globulin has significantly reduced the mortality rate of CMV pneumonia, which can be as high as 90% if untreated (18–22). Although ganciclovir in combination with immune globulin is effective in the treatment of CMV, the use of ganciclovir as a prophylactic agent during transplantation has been limited due to toxicity (2). Recently, bronchoscopy and bronchoalveolar lavage, performed at 35 days after bone marrow transplantation, have been used to identify CMV in the lungs of asymptomatic allogeneic bone marrow transplant recipients (23). Prophylactic administration of ganciclovir to these asymptomatic patients significantly reduced the incidence of subsequent CMV pneumonia. Passive immunization with human immunoglobulin against CMV has also been advocated and may be effective in reducing the incidence of CMV pneumonia (24, 25). Some centers utilize immunoglobulin therapy prophylactically for patients with a negative CMV serology.

Other viral causes of pneumonia occur considerably less frequently than CMV. Other herpes-viruses probably account for the majority of the remaining viral infections but account for <10% of all pneumonias after marrow transplantation (1). Of these, herpes simplex appears to account for the majority of other early viral pneumonias (27, 28). Herpes simplex pneumonia usually occurs within the first 3 weeks after transplantation (26, 27). In addition, herpes simplex can also produce a severe tracheobronchitis, which is responsive to acyclovir (28). *Varicella-zoster,* another herpesvirus that is an infrequent cause of pneumonia, usually appears after the first 100 days after bone marrow transplantation (29). The use of prophylactic acyclovir has reduced the incidence of both herpes simplex and varicella-zoster pneumonia (2). Other viruses have only been sporadically reported (30).

FUNGAL

Fungi are frequent causes of pneumonia in the first 100 days after transplantation (1, 2). Two species of fungi, *Candida* and *Aspergillus,* appear to account for the majority of the fungal pneumonias, with an incidence of 18%–55% (2, 26). Both species can present diagnostic and therapeutic challenges.

The diagnosis of *Candida* pneumonia is often problematic due to frequent colonization of the upper airway and/or bronchi with this organism (2). Therefore, the isolation or identification of *Candida* from either the sputum or bronchial washings is not by itself diagnostic or pneumonia. Attempts have

been made to circumvent this problem by several techniques. First, a protected brush specimen may help exclude colonization of the upper airway or bronchi (2). Second, the detection of a *Candida* antigen in bronchoalveolar lavage fluid may be more indicative of pneumonia than colonization (31). Third, the fluids recovered from the first aliquot of saline infused during bronchoalveolar lavage can be processed separately from the fluids recovered from the later aliquots. The fluid recovered from the first 20-ml aliquot infused into the lung during bronchoalveolar lavage is enriched for bronchial material, while the fluids recovered from the later aliquots are enriched for alveolar material (32). Therefore, the detection of *Candida* predominantly in the fluid recovered from the first aliquot may indicate colonization, while the detection of *Candida* predominantely in the fluid recovered from the later aliquots may indicate pneumonia.

The definitive diagnosis of *Candida* pneumonia traditionally has required the demonstration of tissue invasion. Transbronchial biopsy is often contraindicated in these patients due to thrombocytopenia, and open lung biopsy may result in significant morbidity and mortality. Therefore, when *Candida* pneumonia is suspected, we currently perform bronchoscopy with bronchoalveolar lavage with separate processing of the fluids recovered from the first aliquot of infused saline and the fluids recovered from the later aliquots. If *Candida* is identified by silver staining or culture predominantly in the later aliquots and there are no other pathogens identified, a presumptive diagnosis of *Candida* pneumonia is made. Therapy is then initiated with amphotericin B or 5-flucytosine, because the organism is usually sensitive to these drugs (33).

Infection secondary to *Aspergillus* species can represent a major cause of morbidity and mortality in marrow transplant recipients. The incidence of *Aspergillus* pneumonia can be reduced by laminar flow isolation (34). Nevertheless, in most transplant centers, the organism continues to be a relatively frequent cause of pulmonary infection (34). *Aspergillus* infection often presents very early after marrow transplantation, even while the patient is aplastic from chemotherapy and/or radiation therapy. On chest x-ray or CT scans single and multiple nodules can be seen, which may cavitate (35). However, *Aspergillus* infection can also present radiographically as a lobar or multilobar pneumonia (36). The presence of multiple nodules suggests hematogenous dissemination. Careful inspection for skin or CNS infection is required. Skin biopsy is often diagnostic. The organism tends to be invasive, penetrating the interstitial and vascular structures when the lung is involved, and therefore, the patient may have hemoptysis, or there may be bloody fluid recovered by bronchoalveolar lavage (37, 38). Although *Aspergillus* can be detected by bronchoalveolar lavage, it is clear that bronchoalveolar lavage may have a significant false-negative rate (34). Currently, if bronchoalveolar lavage is nondiagnostic and *Aspergillus* pneumonia is suspected, open lung biopsy is indicated to make a definitive diagnosis.

The treatment of *Aspergillus* pneumonia can be difficult. In contrast to *Candida* pneumonia, treatment of *Aspergillus* usually requires high doses of amphotericin B for prolonged periods (39). For this reason some have advocated surgical resection of localized disease. However, patients with localized disease have been cured by amphotericin B alone. One study has suggested that prophylactic administration of amphotericin B as an aerosol may prevent subsequent *Aspergillus* pneumonia (40). Studies attempting to confirm this approach or to assess the use of low-dose systemic amphotericin B for prophylaxis are underway (2).

PROTOZOAL

Pneumocystis carinii pneumonia is an infrequent cause of pneumonia in the autologous marrow transplant recipient. The incidence of *Pneumocystis* pneumonia in allogeneic transplant recipients has been dramatically reduced by the prophylactic use of trimethoprim-sulfamethoxazole (1, 34). However, if prophylaxis is contraindicated or has been discontinued, *Pneumocystis* pneumonia may occur. Inhaled pentamidine has been successfully used as prophylactic therapy for *Pneumocystis* in patients with the acquired immunodeficiency syndrome (41). It seems likely that inhaled pentamidine could also be successfully used in the allogeneic marrow transplant recipient for prophylaxis.

The other reported cause of protozoal pneumonia is *Toxoplasma gondii* (1, 2). It can lead to fatal pneumonia, but fortunately, appears rarely.

BACTERIAL

Pneumonia secondary to bacterial infections is now less common than previously reported, and the isolation and identification of a bacterial source as a cause of pneumonia occur in the minority of patients (1, 2). As pointed out by Krowka et al. (1), reasons for this include the use of Hickman catheters, the early use of prophylactic antibiotics, and the use of trimethoprim-sulfamethoxazole for *Pneumocystis* prophylaxis, which is also likely beneficial as a prophylactic agent against bacterial pneumonia.

When bacteria are identified, the organisms appear similar to the usual organisms that cause hospital-acquired pneumonias (1, 2, 34). *Legionella* species appear to be a rare cause of pneumonia in most centers, but outbreaks have occurred when a contaminated common source is present—for example, a water supply containing *Legionella* (42). *Legionella* pneumonia has a high mortality rate in marrow transplant recipients, and its early diagnosis is probably best established by direct fluorescent staining of bronchoalveolar lavage fluid (2, 42).

Noninfectious Pulmonary Complications

DIFFUSE ALVEOLAR HEMORRHAGE

Diffuse alveolar hemorrhage (DAH) is a frequent cause of morbidity and mortality in the marrow transplant population and in one series was the most common cause of death (43). DAH is recognized on bronchoalveolar lavage when sequential instillation and aspiration of normal saline results in recovered lavage fluid that becomes progressively bloodier with each recovered aliquot. DAH is often seen in older patients and often presents with dyspnea, diffuse consolidation on chest x-ray, high fevers, severe mucositis, and renal insufficiency. Interestingly, the onset of DAH seems to correlate with the onset of white blood cell recovery, usually at 1–3 weeks after transplantation. Untreated DAH is associated with progressive pulmonary insufficiency, with the majority of patients eventually requiring ventilatory support; it proceeds to death in >75% of patients.

The pathogenesis of DAH is unknown. However, no organisms to explain the syndrome have been identified. The correlation of the onset of DAH with the onset of white blood cell recovery suggests a possible pathogenic relationship (43, 44). In some patients neutrophils have been identified in the bronchoalveolar lavage fluid despite agranulocytosis in the blood (43, 44). It has been suggested that progressive lung injury by neutrophils already damaged by chemotherapy and/or radiation therapy may lead to the onset of this syndrome (43).

Recently, the use of high-dose corticosteroids has been reported to be potentially beneficial in DAH (45). These observations have been confirmed in a larger series of patients (46). It appears that high doses ($\geq$100 mg/day of methylprednisolone or its equivalent) are required because lower doses ($\leq$30 mg/day) demonstrate no differences in survival compared to untreated historical controls.

Other causes of alveolar hemorrhage occur in transplant patients. Severe thrombocytopenia, which frequently occurs in these patients, may result in alveolar hemorrhage (47). Aspergillus pneumonia can also result in alveolar hemorrhage (38). These two entities can be separated from DAH by administering platelet transfusions, which should resolve the alveolar hemorrhage when it is secondary to profound thrombocytopenia, or by identification of Aspergillus by bronchoalveolar lavage or open lung biopsy, in patients with Aspergillus pneumonia (38, 47).

ADULT RESPIRATORY DISTRESS SYNDROME

Adult respiratory distress syndrome (ARDS) is an acute lung injury resulting from a variety of causes including sepsis, aspiration, pancreatitis, and multiple transfusions (48). All of these would be expected to occur more frequently in marrow transplant recipients, and therefore, marrow transplant patients would be expected to have a high incidence of ARDS. In this context, ARDS is clinically indistinguishable from DAH because both are acute lung injuries that result in progressive respiratory failure, diffuse consolidation on chest x-ray, decreased pulmonary compliance, and a high mortality rate (43, 48). Although DAH may well be a subset of patients with ARDS, two important differences exist. First, DAH is associated with bloody returns on bronchoalveolar lavage, which may occur but is not characteristic of ARDS (48, 49). Second, and more important, DAH appears to be responsive to corticosteroid therapy while ARDS is not (45, 46, 50, 51).

IDIOPATHIC INTERSTITIAL PNEUMONITIS

Idiopathic interstitial pneumonitis is a term used to explain diffuse lung disease occurring after marrow transplantation in which no infectious etiology can be found. The incidence is relatively high, with 29% of marrow transplant patients developing diffuse pulmonary infiltrates in the first 6 months after transplantation where no infectious etiology can be found (4). Like DAH, idiopathic interstitial pneumonitis is associated with a peak incidence at about 2 weeks after marrow transplantation, increased age, total body irradiation, and a high mortality rate (4, 43,

52–55). Therefore, it seems likely that DAH represents a significant subset of the patients with idiopathic interstitial pneumonitis (43).

PULMONARY EDEMA

Diffuse pulmonary infiltrates are frequently encountered early after marrow transplantation. One important cause of these infiltrates is pulmonary edema, with an incidence approaching 50% (56). Dickout et al. (57) have demonstrated that the institution of diuretics and the reduction of the administered volume of parenteral hyperalimentation at the first clinical sign of fluid overload can help eliminate this problem.

DRUG AND TRANSFUSION-ASSOCIATED COMPLICATIONS

The incidence of drug- or transfusion-related events that occur after marrow transplantation is unknown but is probably underestimated (1, 2). Both transfusions and drugs have been associated with diffuse pulmonary consolidation, and given the frequency with which both are used during the course of marrow transplantation, it would be surprising if a significant incidence was not present. There appear to be no specific pathologic criteria for the diagnosis of drug or transfusion-associated lung disease (1). Therefore, given the multitude of diagnostic possibilities in these often severely ill patients, separation from other causes of diffuse consolidation is difficult.

PULMONARY EMBOLISM

During the infusion of bone marrow, it is common for patients to develop some degree of dyspnea. In an autopsy series, calcific marrow fragments have been identified in the lungs of some bone marrow transient recipients and may explain, at least in part, the transplant dyspnea that often occurs with marrow infusion (58). Pulmonary emboli secondary to clots formed in the vasculature that subsequently dislodge and embolize to the lung are rare (1). Interestingly, blood clots

can form on an indwelling Hickman catheter, suggesting that when pulmonary embolism is suspected, consideration should be given to this source of emboli (W. Haire, personal communication).

DISEASE RECURRENCE

An important diagnostic consideration in the investigation of either a localized or diffuse lung disorder is the recurrence of the patient's underlying malignancy. The incidence is unknown, but 6% of bone marrow transplant patients had a leukemic recurrence at the time of autopsy (59). Bronchoalveolar lavage may identify malignant cells, or an open lung biopsy may be required to demonstrate malignant disease in the lung.

LYMPHOCYTIC BRONCHITIS

Graft-versus-host disease is a frequent occurrence in patients with allogenic transplantation. Organs often affected include the skin, liver, and large and small bowels. Beschorner et al. (60) have suggested that lymphocytic bronchitis may represent acute graft-versus-host disease in the lung. Patients with lymphocytic bronchitis develop nonproductive cough and dyspnea soon after transplantation but have no evidence of pneumonia on chest x-ray. At autopsy these patients had lymphocytes infiltrating the bronchial submucosa and the epithelium, with a loss of cilia and damage to the submucosal glands and goblet cells. The degree of lymphocyte infiltration seemed to correlate with the clinicopathologic grade of graft-versus-host disease. In support of this concept, Chan et al. (2) have described the frequent occurrence of bronchial inflammation in patients with graft-versus-host disease that improves with therapy directed at the graft-versus-host disease. However, it is controversial whether lymphocytic bronchitis is the bronchial manifestation of graft-versus-host disease or if other causes such as infectious bronchitis account for the symptoms and the presence of the increased numbers of lymphocytes and histologic changes within the airways (2).

PLEURAL EFFUSION

Pleural effusions with or without pleural rubs occur relatively commonly during the early period after bone marrow transplantation (56). These may occasionally cause minor pain or become large enough to interfere with the patient's ventilation. Although the etiology is clear in some patients, such as those with hepatic vein thrombosis, in the majority of patients the etiology is unknown (56). Diagnostic possibilities include serositis secondary to chemotherapy and/or radiation therapy, tumor lysis, and lymphatic obstruction secondary to mediastinal tumor. Rarely infections, spontaneous hemorrhage, laceration of a mediastinal vessel, or disease recurrence are identified as a cause. In the majority of patients, the pleural effusions will eventually resolve. Therefore, unless infection or recurrence of the patients' underlying malignancy is suspected, or effusions are large enough to compromise the patients' ventilation, we observe the effusions rather than performing thoracentesis. When effusions become a problem because of their size, repeated thoracentesis has been used in preference to chest tube placement because of the risk of infection in the presence of aplasia.

LATE PULMONARY COMPLICATIONS

Late pulmonary complications are defined as those that occur >100 days after bone marrow transplantation (1). The majority of complications occur within the 1st year and usually within the 1st 6 months after transplantation (1, 2). Although complications may occur in patients who receive autologous bone marrow transplantation, the majority of complications occur in those who have received allogeneic transplantation and are receiving immonosuppressive therapy for graft-versus-host disease (1, 2).

Infectious Pulmonary Complications

VIRAL

The major late viral cause of pneumonia is CMV (1, 2). There is little to clinically indicate CMV pneumonia compared to other pneumonias (4–6). However, patients may present with a prolonged prodrome of malaise and fever without or with only minor pulmonary symptomatology and a negative chest x-ray (61–63). Shedding of CMV in bronchoalveolar lavage fluid has been demonstrated to occur frequently in this situation (62, 63). Activation of the inflammatory cells in the lower respiratory tract to produce cytokines such as tumor necrosis factor or interleukin-1 may be responsible for this prodrome (61).

Varicella-zoster was formerly a frequent viral cause of late pulmonary complications. However, the use of prophylactic acyclovir has dramatically reduced the incidence of this viral pneumonia (1, 2, 64). When the patient does not receive prophylactic acyclovir, the initial manifestation of varicella-zoster is usually a cutaneous infection, and pneumonia results from dissemination (2, 64). The use of acyclovir during the initial cutaneous infection has dramatically decreased the incidence of varicella-zoster dissemination and pneumonia (64).

FUNGAL

Compared to early pulmonary complications, the occurrence of fungal pneumonia as a late pulmonary complication after bone marrow transplantation is much less frequently reported (1, 2).

PROTOZOAL

Prophylactic therapy with trimethoprim-sulfamethoxazole has dramatically reduced the incidence of *Pneumocystis* pneumonia. However, it is still occasionally seen and tends to be severe when present (2). As previously discussed, inhaled pentamidine may be an effective alternative prophylactic therapy.

BACTERIAL

In contrast to the early pulmonary complications after bone marrow transplantation, bacterial infections are frequently identified as the cause of late pulmonary complications (1, 2, 64). Gram-positive cocci, particularly *Streptococcus pneumoniae* and *Staphylococcus aureus,* are frequently responsible for pneumonia, septicemia, or sinus infections (1, 2, 28, 64, 65). These infections appear to be more prevalent in patients with chronic graft-versus-host disease and those patients transplanted with incompletely HLA-matched bone marrow (1, 2, 64). Obstructive lung disease may occur late after transplantation (see below). Bacterial infections, particularly with the gram-negative organisms *Haemophilus* or *Pseudomonas aeurginosa,* may be present and are a frequent cause of death in patients with obstructive lung disease (1, 2, 66).

NONINFECTIOUS LATE PULMONARY COMPLICATIONS

Three major causes of noninfectious late pulmonary complications occur late after bone marrow transplantation: (*a*) obstructive lung disease secondary to bronchiolitis obliterans, (*b*) restrictive lung disease secondary to pulmonary fibrosis, and (*c*) recurrent malignancy (1, 2).

Obstructive Lung Disease

Obstructive lung disease secondary to bronchiolitis obliterans occurs relatively frequently, usually at about 6–12 months after allogeneic bone marrow transplantation (1, 2, 67–71). The patients usually present with symptoms of a nonproductive cough and dyspnea on exertion. Chest x-rays often reveal hyperinflation, but either localized or diffuse consolidations may be present. Pulmonary function tests demonstrate nonreversible airflow obstruction, hyperinflation (elevated total lung capacity), air trapping (elevated residual volume), and a reduced diffusing capacity for carbon monoxide (DLCO). The major risk factor appears to be graft-versus-host disease, with the diagnosis of bronchiolitis obliterans unusual in its absence.

The optimal methods for the diagnosis of bronchiolitis obliterans are controversial. Bronchoscopy with bronchoalveolar lavage may help to exclude an infectious process (67). Bronchoalveolar lavage often demonstrates the presence of increased lymphocytes in the recovered lavage fluid, which is in contrast to the usual observation of elevated neutrophils in the lavage fluid recovered from patients with bronchiolitis obliterans due to other causes (2, 72). Transbronchial biopsy is usually nondiagnostic, and definitive diagnosis often requires an open lung biopsy (2). However, some centers currently make the diagnosis on clinical grounds in a patient with compatible symptoms, radiographic, and pulmonary function tests when bronchoscopy and bronchoalveolar lavage demonstrate an elevated number of lymphocytes and an absence of pathogens in the bronchoalveolar lavage fluid (2).

Therapy for bronchiolitis obliterans is increased immunosuppression, usually accomplished by increasing the dosage of corticosteroids (2). Generally, initial doses of 50–100 mg of prednisone (or its equivalent) are advocated with adjustment of dosage, depending on the patient's response. Most patients stabilize but do not significantly improve their airflow obstruction, although air trapping and dyspnea may improve. Experience with other immunosuppressive agents such as cyclosporine A or azathioprine is less extensive.

Restrictive Lung Disease

Restrictive lung disease is frequent after transplantation, with 20% of patients having mild to moderate restrictive disease 1 year after transplantation (1, 2, 64, 73). The causes for this restriction and presumed fibrosis probably include chemotherapy and/or radiation therapy, previous pulmonary infections, or possibly recurrent aspiration of gastric contents (1, 2, 64, 73). Chan et al. (2) have pointed out that patients at risk for this complication include patients treated with more cytotoxic agents for their primary malignancy, patients with severe graft-versus-host disease, and patients with pulmonary complications early after bone marrow transplantation. However, most patients with restrictive lung disease have a stable course and may actually have a small improvement over 2–3 years after transplantation (74). Those who succumb with restrictive lung disease usually die as a result of bacterial pneumonia, septicemia, or recurrence of their malignancy.

Disease Recurrence

The lung is a frequent site for recurrence of malignancy. Presentation can be varied, with the patient entirely asymptomatic or severely dyspneic and coughing. Chest x-rays can also be varied, with single or multiple nodules, localized or diffuse consolidation, localized or extensive atelectasis, or pleural effusions. In general, most cases can be diagnosed by the usual clinical methods, including bronchoscopy with bronchoalveolar lavage and/or transbronchial biopsy, transthoracic needle biopsy, thoracentesis, or pleural biopsy. However, open lung biopsy is occasionally required.

DIAGNOSTIC APPROACH

Prior to Transplantation

The clinical approach to the diagnosis of pulmonary disease prior to transplantation is dictated by the clinical circumstances. An aggressive approach is often taken because of the supposition that an asymptomatic or minimally symptomatic infectious process may become clinically manifest during the period of aplasia or that restrictive disease secondary to chemotherapy or radiation therapy may be compounded by additional therapy (3).

An appropriate approach for suspected infectious pneumonias is to perform bronchoscopy and bronchoalveolar lavage with silver staining and Papanicolaou staining along with cultures for bacteria, fungi, and viruses. If the initial bronchoalveolar lavage proves to be nondiagnostic, the lavage procedure is repeated or the patient is observed with administration of empiric antibiotics. If the second bronchoalveolar lavage is nondiagnostic or the patient clinically deteriorates, open lung biopsy is considered.

It seems reasonable to treat pneumonias or other reversible pulmonary dysfunctions identified prior to transplantation. We favor treating any pathogens or severe bronchitis present and delaying chemotherapy and bone marrow transplantation until after resolution has been demonstrated by bronchoscopy and bronchoalveolar lavage or other methods.

The role of pulmonary function testing in pretransplantation assessment is unclear, but it seems reasonable to perform pulmonary function testing on those patients who might potentially have pulmonary disorders. This would include patients with prior chemotherapy and/or radiation therapy to the thorax or patients with a significant smoking history. However, the use of pulmonary function testing in predicting the outcome of transplantation is unknown. In a small series, patients with only mildly or moderately abnormal pulmonary function tests did not have a significant increase in morbidity or mortality compared to patients with normal pulmonary function testing (3). This observation will require confirmation in a larger series of patients with longer periods of observation after transplantation. The degree of pulmonary function testing abnormalities that should preclude transplantation is also unclear. However, the addition of chemotherapy and/or radiation therapy to a patient with severe respiratory compromise would seem likely to result in worsening of any pulmonary dysfunction.

Early Complications

The diagnostic approach to the bone marrow transplant patient with the onset of a pulmonary complication must be dictated by the clinical context of the situation (1, 2). In those patients who develop fever but do not have signs or symptoms indicative of pneumonia and have no consolidation on chest x-ray, perform routine cultures and begin empiric antibiotic coverage while carefully observing the patient. In contrast, if signs and symptoms of a possible pneumonia are present or consolidation is seen on chest x-ray, first evaluate the patient for any signs of fluid overload, and if absent, proceed with bronchoscopy and bronchoalveolar lavage. Transbronchial biopsy is not performed because it appears to add only to the morbidity of the procedure (especially in the presence of thrombocytopenia) and not to the diagnostic yield (75). Empiric antibiotic coverage is begun, and the results of the bronchoalveolar lavage are awaited. If the bronchoscopy with bronchoalveolar lavage is nondiagnostic, observe, repeat the procedure, or proceed to open lung biopsy, depending on the apparent speed of progression of the process or the suspicion of *Aspergillus* infection. Open lung biopsy is controversial and is used sparingly in our institution unless *Aspergillus* infection is suspected. Because of potential bleeding complications, we do not perform needle biopsies if the platelet count is <100,000 per cubic millimeter or if *Aspergillus* is suspected. However, others have successfully utilized needle biopsy with platelet counts as low as 30,000 per cubic millimeter for the diagnosis of *Aspergillus* infection (56).

Late Complications

In general, the diagnostic approach used by most centers is similar to that for early pulmonary complications. A patient presenting with pulmonary symptomatology is evaluated by history and physical examination and

appropriate laboratory testing, usually including chest x-ray or computerized tomography (CT) scanning and pulmonary function testing. Many proceed to bronchoscopy with bronchoalveolar lavage or to transbronchial biopsy if a diffuse process is identified or transthoracic needle biopsy for a localized lesion. If these are nondiagnostic, consideration is given to an open lung biopsy.

SURVEILLANCE

Prior to Transplantation

Although definite recommendations for surveillance prior to transplantation cannot be given, some general guidelines can be made. A careful history and physical exam should be performed, with particular attention to any respiratory complaints and percussion and auscultation of the lungs. A chest x-ray and/or CT scan of the chest screens for occult pulmonary disease. Routine pulmonary function testing gives important baseline information.

The role of bronchoscopy with bronchoalveolar lavage in pulmonary surveillance prior to transplantation is controversial. In a small series of patients pretransplantation bronchoscopy and bronchoalveolar lavage revealed abnormalities in 75% of the patients, and abnormal bronchoscopic findings were observed in 63% of those patients who were asymptomatic and had normal lung physical examinations, chest x-rays, and pulmonary function tests (3). The observed abnormalities most often consisted of diffuse bronchial inflammation associated with an increased percentage of neutrophils recovered by bronchoalveolar lavage. Interestingly, the presence of an abnormal pretransplantation bronchoscopy was associated with an increase in pulmonary complications during the transplant (3). The observation that increased neutrophils in the pretransplantation bronchoalveolar lavage fluid predict pulmonary complications during the transplant has recently been confirmed in a larger series of patients (JH Sisson, unpublished data).

Early Pulmonary Complications

It is convenient to divide the acute period of bone marrow transplantation into the time of hospitalization and the immediate posthospitalization period. The majority of pulmonary complications occur within the hospitalization period, and therefore, careful observation and pulmonary surveillance are indicated. In addition to the usual daily auscultation of the lungs, weights, and fluid assessments, most centers also perform sputum, nasal, and/or throat cultures on a routine basis. Chest x-rays on a routine schedule are also usual in most centers. The roles of routine spirometry, CT scanning of the chest, gallium lung scanning, arterial blood gas and pulse oximetry measurements, and measurement of diffusing capacities for carbon monoxide as pulmonary surveillance procedures are unknown, but these are performed at some centers.

The role of bronchoscopy and bronchoalveolar lavage as a surveillance procedure is controversial. Bronchoscopy with bronchoalveolar lavage immediately prior to transplantation has been disappointing in its capacity to detect occult pulmonary disease (3). It is unclear if routine bronchoscopy with bronchoalveolar lavage at later times after transplantation is useful. Bronchoscopy with bronchoalveolar lavage at a time approximating the peak incidence of DAH may be useful because early diagnosis followed by corticosteroids seems to improve survival. However, whether the very early diagnosis of DAH in an asymptomatic patient will improve the outcome of therapy is unknown.

Bronchoscopy with bronchoalveolar lavage at about the time of discharge from the hospital may be useful in allogeneic bone marrow recipients because it approximates the time of the first peak of CMV pneumonia (5). The use of bronchoscopy and bronchoalveolar lavage in this situation is supported by the data of Schmidt et al. (23). Routine bronchoscopy with bronchoalveolar lavage were performed on asymptomatic allogeneic bone marrow transplant recipients 35 days after bone marrow transplantation. CMV was detected in nearly 40% of the patients. Importantly, therapy with ganciclovir significantly reduced the subsequent development of CMV pneumonia.

After discharge from the hospital, the patient remains at an increased risk for pulmonary complications. For this reason chest x-rays and pulmonary function testing are often performed on a routine basis. Bronchoscopy with bronchoalveolar lavage to detect CMV pneumonia at about its second peak of incidence (100 days) may be useful, and trials are currently ongoing to assess the effectiveness of this approach.

Late Pulmonary Complications

Few studies are available regarding surveillance for late pulmonary complications. Periodic chest x-rays or CT scans seem reasonable to detect recurrent malignancy in asymptomatic patients. Early detection of bronchiolitis obliterans would seem desirable because the patients have either no or minimal improvement when treated with corticosteroids (2). Therefore, periodic pulmonary function testing also appears reasonable. The role of other methods that might detect bronchiolitis obliterans earlier in its course, such as pulmonary exercise stress testing or the demonstration of elevated lymphocytes in bronchoalveolar lavage fluid, is unknown.

SUMMARY AND CONCLUSIONS

Considerable progress has been made in the diagnosis and therapy of pulmonary complications after bone marrow transplantation. Reduction in the incidence, morbidity, and mortality of pulmonary complications has been achieved by the use of prophylactic antibiotic therapy, the development of effective drugs for some viruses, and the application of bronchoscopy and bronchoalveolar lavage to allow earlier and less invasive diagnosis of pulmonary complications compared to open lung biopsy. However, pulmonary complications are still frequent. It seems likely that as doses of chemotherapy and radiation therapy are increased in an attempt to cure less responsive and more extensive malignant disease, toxicity to the lung may be dose limiting. New techniques in transplantation, diagnosis, and surveillance, or the determination of the optimal application of existing techniques, will likely continue to improve outcomes. Furthermore, more effective drugs with less toxicity are continually being introduced into clinical practice, which should also reduce the morbidity and mortality of pulmonary complications associated with bone marrow transplantation.

REFERENCES

1. Krowka MJ, Rosenow EC III, Hoagland HC. Pulmonary complications of bone marrow transplantation. Chest 1985;87:237.
2. Chan CK, Hyland RH, Hutcheon MA. Pulmonary complications following bone marrow transplantation. Clin Chest Med 1990;2:323.
3. Vaughan WP, Linder J, Robbins R, Arneson A, Rennard SI. Pulmonary surveillance using bronchoscopy and bronchoalveolar lavage during high-dose antineoplastic therapy. Chest 1991;99:105.
4. Meyers JD, Flournoy N, Thomas ED. Nonbacterial pneumonia after allogenic marrow transplantation: A review of ten years' experience. Rev Infect Dis 1982;4:1119.
5. Beshorner WE, Hutchins GM, Burns WE. Cytomegalovirus pneumonia in bone marrow transplant recipients. Miliary and diffuse patterns. Am Rev Respir Dis 1980;122:107.
6. Smith CB. Cytomegalovirus pneumonia. State of the art. Chest 1986;95:1825.
7. Springmeyer SC, Hackman RC, Holle R, et al. Use of bronchoalveolar lavage to diagnose acute diffuse pneumonia in the immunocompromised host. J Infect Dis 1986;154:605.
8. Crawford SW, Bowden RA, Hackman RC, Gleaves CA, Myers JD, Clark JG. Rapid detection of cytomegalovirus pulmonary infection by bronchoalveolar lavage and centrifugation culture. Ann Intern Med 1988;108:180.
9. Paradis IL, Grgurich WF, Drummer JS, Dekker A, Dauber JH. Rapid detection of cytomegalovirus pneumonia from lung lavage cells. Am Rev Respir Dis 1988;138:697.
10. Woods GL, Thompson AB, Rennard SI, Linder J. De-

tection of cytomegalovirus in bronchoalveolar lavage specimens. Chest 1990;98:568.
11. Emmanuel D, Peppard J, Stover D, Gold J, Armstrong D, Hammerling U. Rapid immuno diagnosis of cytomegalovirus pneumonia by broncheoalveolar lavage using human and murine monoclonal antibodies. Ann Intern Med 1986;104:476.
12. Cordonnier C, Escudier E, Nicolas J, et al. Evaluation of three assays on alveolar lavage fluid in the diagnosis of cytomegalovirus pneumonitis after bone marrow transplantation. J Infect Dis 1987;155:495.
13. Hackman RC, Myerson D, Meyers JD, et al. Rapid diagnosis of cytomegalovirus pneumonia by tissue immunofluorescence with a murine monoclonal antibody. J Infect Dis 1983;151:325.
14. Martin WJ, Smith TF. Rapid detection of cytomegalovirus in bronchoalveolar lavage specimens by a monoclonal antibody. J Infect Dis 1983;151:325.
15. Woods GL, Young A, Johnson A, Thiele G. Detection of cytomegalovirus by 24-well plate centrifugation assay using a monoclonal antibody to an early nuclear antigen and by conventional cell culture. J Virol Methods 1987;18:207.
16. Churchill MA, Zaia JA, Forman SJ, Sheibani K, Azumi N, Blume KG. Quantification of human cytomegalovirus DNA in lungs from bone marrow transplant recipients with interstitial pneumonia. J Infect Dis 1987;155:501.
17. Hilborne LH, Nieberg RK, Cheng L, Lewin KL. Direct in situ hybridization for rapid detection of cytomegalovirus in bronchoalveolar lavage. Am J Clin Pathol 1987;87:766.
18. Collaborative DHPG treatment study group. Treatment of serious cytomegalovirus infections with 9-(1,2 dihydroxy-2-propoxymethyl) guanine in patients with AIDS and other immunodeficiencies. N Engl J Med 1986;314:801.
19. Shepp DH, Dandliker DS, de Miranda P, et al. Activity of 9-[2-hydroxy-1-(hydroxy-methyl) ethoxymethyl] guanine in the treatment of cytomegalovirus pneumonia. Ann Intern Med 1985;103:368.
20. Emanuel D, Cunningham J, Jules-Eysee K, et al. Cytomegalovirus pneumonia after bone marrow transplantation successfully treated with the combination of ganciclovir and high-dose intravenous immune globulin. Ann Intern Med 1988;109:777.
21. Reed EC, Bowden RA, Dandliker PS, Lilleby KE, Meyers JD. Treatment of cytomegalovirus pneumonia and intravenous cytomegalovirus immunoglobulin in patients with bone marrow transplants. Ann Intern Med 1988;109:783.
22. Schmidt GM, Kovacs A, Zaia JA, et al. Ganciclovir/immunoglobulin combination therapy for the treatment of human cytomegalovirus-associated interstitial pneumonia in bone marrow allograft recipients. Transplantation 1988;46:905.
23. Schmidt GM, Horak DA, Niland JC, et al. A random-

ized, controlled trial of prophylactic ganciclovir for cytomegalovirus pulmonary infection in recipients of allogenic bone marrow transplants. N Engl J Med 1991;324:1005.

24. O'Reilly RJ, Reich L, Gold J, et al. A randomized trial of intravenous hyperimmune globulin for the prevention of cytomegalovirus (CMV) infections following marrow transplantation: preliminary results. Transplant Proc 1983;15:1405.

25. Reed EC, Bowden RA, Dandliker PS, Gleaves CA, Meyers JD. Efficacy of cytomegalovirus immunoglobulin in marrow transplant recipients with cytomegalovirus pneumonia. J Infect Dis 1987;156:641.

26. Ramsey PG, Fife KH, Hackman RC, Meyers JD, Corey L. Herpes simplex virus pneumonia: clinical, virologic, and pathologic features in 20 patients. Ann Intern Med 1982;97:813.

27. Meyers JD, Atkinson K. Infection in bone marrow transplantation. Clin Haematol 1983;12:791.

28. Legge RH, Thompson AB, Linder J, et al. Acyclovir responsive herpetic tracheobronchitis. Am J Med 1988;85:561.

29. Watson JG. Problems of infection after bone marrow transplantation. J Clin Pathol 1983;36:683.

30. Englund JA, Sullivan CJ, Jordan MC, et al. Respiratory syncytial virus infection in immunocompromised adults. Ann Intern Med 1988;109:203.

31. Ness M, Rennard SI, Vaughan WP, Ghafouri MA, Linder J. Detection of Candida antigen in bronchoalveolar lavage fluid. Acta Cytolegica 1988;32:347.

32. Rennard SI, Ghafouri M, Thompson AB, et al. Fractional processing of sequential bronchoalveolar lavage to separate bronchial and alveolar samples. Am Rev Respir Dis 1990;141:208.

33. Edwards JE, Lehrer RI, Stiehm ER, Fischer TJ, Young LS. Severe Candidal infections. Ann Intern Med 1978;89:91.

34. Cordonnier C, Bernaudin J-F, Fleury J, et al. Pulmonary complications occurring after allogenic bone marrow transplantation. A study of 130 consecutive transplant patients. Cancer 1986;58:1047.

35. Kuhlman JE, Fishman EK, Burch PA, Karp JE, Zenhouni EA, Siegelman SS. Invasive pulmonary aspergillosis in acute leukemia. The contribution of CT to early diagnosis and aggressive management. Chest 1987;92:95.

36. Tucker AK, Pennington J, Guyer PB. Pulmonary fungal infection complicating treated malignant disease. Clin Radiol 975;26:129.

37. Williams D, Krick J, Remington J. Pulmonary infection in the compromised host. Part 1. Am Rev Respir Dis 1976;114:359.

38. Kahn FW, Jones JM, England DM. Diagnosis of pulmonary hemorrhage in the immunocompromised host. Am Rev Respir Dis 1987;136:155.

39. Aisner J, Schimpft SC, Wiernik PH. Treatment of invasive aspergillosis; relation of early diagnosis and treatment to response. Ann Intern Med 1977;86:539.

40. Conneally E, Cafferkey MT, Daly PA, Keune CT, McCann SR. Nebulized amphotericin B as prophylaxis against invasive aspergillosis in granulocytopenic patients. Bone Marrow Transplant 1990;5:403.

41. Centers for Disease Control. Guidelines for prophylaxis against Pneumocystis carinii pneumonia for persons with human immuno deficiency virus. JAMA 1989;262:335.

42. Kugler JW, Armitage JO, Helms CM, et al. Nosocomial legionnaire's disease. Occurrence in recipients of bone marrow transplants. Am J Med 1983;74:281.

43. Robbins RA, Linder J, Stahl MG, et al. Diffuse alveolar hemorrhage in autologous bone marrow transplant recipients. Am J Med 1989;87:511.

44. Robbins R, Thompson AB, Rennard S, et al. Association of neutrophils with diffuse alveolar hemorrhage in autologous bone marrow transplantation. Clin Res 1988;36:373A.

45. Chao NJ, Duncan SR, Long GD, Horning SJ, Blume KG. Corticosteroid therapy for diffuse alveolar hemorrhage in autologous bone marrow transplant recipients. Ann Intern Med 1991;114:145.

46. Metcalf JM, Armitage J, Arneson M, et al. The effect of glucocorticoids on survival and development of subsequent opportunistic infections in bone marrow transplant patients with diffuse alveolar hemorrhage. Am Rev Respir Dis 1991;143:A474.

47 Drew WL, Finley TN, Golde DW. Diagnostic lavage and occult pulmonary hemorrhage in thrombocytopenic immunocompromised patients. Am Rev Respir Dis 1977;116:215.

48. Ashbaugh DG, Bigelow DB, Petty TL, et al. Acute respiratory distress in adults. Lancet 1967;2:319.

49. Robbins RA, Russ WD, Rasmussen JK, Clayton MM. Activation of the complement system in the adult respiratory distress syndrome. Am Rev Respir Dis 1987;135:651.

50. Bernard GR, Luce JM, Sprung CL, et al. High-dose corticosteroids in patients with the adult respiratory distress syndrome. N Engl J Med 1987;317:1565.

51. Bone RC, Fisher CJ, Clemmer TP, et al. Early methylprednisolone treatment for the septic syndrome and the adult respiratory distress syndrome. Chest 1987;92:1032.

52. Neiman PE, Reeves W, Ray G, et al. A prospective analysis of interstitial pneumonia and opportunistic viral infection among recipients of allogenic bone marrow grafts. J Infect Dis 1977;136:754.

53. Curdozo BL, Hagenbeck A. Interstitial pneumonitis following bone marrow transplantation: pathogenesis and therapeutic considerations. Eur J Cancer Clin Oncol 1985;21:43.

54. Applebaum FR, Meyers JD, Fefer A, et al. Nonbacterial nonfungal pneumonia following bone marrow transplantation in 100 identical twins. Transplantation 1982;33:265.

55. Pecago R, Hill R, Applebaum FR, et al. Interstitial pneumonitis following autologous bone marrow transplantation. Transplantation 1986;42:515.
56. Clark JG, Crawford SW. Diagnostic approaches to pulmonary complications of marrow transplantation. Chest 1987;91:477.
57. Dickout WJ, Chan CK, Hyland RH, et al. Prevention of acute pulmonary edema after bone marrow transplantation. Chest 1987;92:303.
58. Arbrahams C, Catchatourian R. Bone fragment emboli in the lungs of patients undergoing bone marrow transplantation. Am J Clin Pathol 1983;79:360.
59. Sloane JP, Depledge MH, Powles RL, Morgenstern GR, Trickey BS, Dudy PJ. Histopathology of the lung after bone marrow transplantation. J Clin Pathol 1983; 36:546–554.
60. Beshorner WE, Saral R, Hutchins GM, et al. Lymphocytic bronchitis associated with graft-versus-host disease in recipients of bone marrow transplants. N Engl J Med 1978;299:1030.
61. Grundy JE, Shanley JD, Griffiths PD. Is cytomegalovirus interstitial pneumonitis in transplant recipients an immunopathological condition? Lancet 1987;2:996.
62. Chan CK, Kasupski GJ, Fyles G, et al. Clinical significance of cytomegalovirus pulmonary infection detected by monoclonal antibodies in allogenic bone marrow transplant recipients. Chest 1988;94:575.
63. Chan CK, Kasupski GJ, Steale, et al. Rapid immunodiagnosis of cytomegalovirus pulmonary complications by bronchoalveolar lavage after allogenic bone marrow transplantation. Chest 1988;94:57s.
64. Sullivan KM, Deeg HJ, Sanders JE, et al. Late complications after bone marrow transplantation. Semin Hematol 1984;21:53.
65. Winston DJ, Schiftman G, Wang DC, et al. Pneumococcal infections after bone-marrow transplantation. Ann Intern Med 1979;91:835–841.
66. Ralph DD, Springmeyer SC, Sullivan KM, Hackman RC, Starb R, Thomas ED. Rapidly progressive air-flow obstruction in marrow transplant recipients: possible association between obliterative bronchiolitis and chronic graft-versus-host disease. Am Rev Respir Dis 1984;129:641.
67. Chan CK, Hyland RH, Hutcheon MA, et al. Small airways disease in recipients of allogenic bone marrow transplants. Medicine (Baltimore) 1987;66:327.
68. Roca J, Grañeña A, Rodriguez-Roisin R, Alvarez P, Ayusti-Vidal A, Rozman C. Fatal airway disease in an adult with chronic graft-versus-host disease. Thorax 1982;37:77.
69. Kurzrock R, Zander A, Kanojia M, et al. Obstructive lung disease after allogenic bone marrow transplantation. Transplantation 1984;37:156.
70. Link H, Reinhard U, Niethammer D, Kruger GRF, Waller HD, Wilms K. Obstructive ventilation disorder as a severe complication of chronic graft-versus-host disease after bone-marrow transplantation. Exp Hematol 1982 10(suppl):92.
71. Chan CK, Hyland RH, Hutcheon MA, et al. Risk factors for obstructive airways disease after allogenic bone marrow transplantation. Am Rev Respir Dis 1988;137(suppl):111.
72. Kindt GC, Weiland JE, Davis WB, Gadek JE, Dorinsky PM. Bronchiolitis in adults: a reversible cause of airway obstruction associated with airway neutrophils and neutrophil products. Am Rev Respir Dis 1989;140:483.
73. Suteida TG, Apperley JF, Hughes JMB, et al. Pulmonary function after bone marrow transplantation for chronic myeloid leukemia. Thorax 1988;43:163.
74. Fyles G, Chan CK, Hyland RH, et al. Restrictive ventilatory defect after allogenic bone marrow transplantation. Am Rev Respir Dis 1988;137(suppl):313.
75. Springmeyer SC, Silvestri RC, Sale GE, et al. The role of transbronchial biopsy for the diagnosis of diffuse pneumonias in immuno compromised marrow transplant recipients. Am Rev Respir Dis 1982;126:763.

28

HEPATIC COMPLICATIONS OF BONE MARROW TRANSPLANTATION

Lois J. Ayash

To understand the pathogenesis of the liver injury that occurs as a result of complications from a bone marrow transplant procedure requires a modicum of knowledge of anatomy. The normal liver, weighing 1400–1600 gms, consists of two major and two rudimentary lobes (1). Simplistically, these lobes are subdivided into ill-defined lobules. In the centers of the lobules are hepatic veins, and at their periphery are portal triads, consisting of hepatic artery, portal vein, and bile duct. Throughout the lobule and abutting the hepatocytes run sinusoids, which are lined by endothelial and reticuloendothelial (Kupffer) cells. These sinusoids receive the tributaries of the portal vein and hepatic artery. On the opposite side of the hepatocyte are the bile canaliculi, which extend from the central vein to the portal triad. There they meet and form larger ductules. Because of its dual blood supply (portal vein and hepatic artery), the nutritional needs of the liver are easily met under normal conditions. With excessive metabolic demands, however, hepatocytes furthest removed from the portal region succumb to the effects of acute hypoxia.

Bone marrow transplantation (BMT) can affect the normal functioning of the liver in a variety of ways. Chemotherapy, total body irradiation (TBI), and medications can directly produce effects ranging from asymptomatic elevation of liver function tests to hepatitis and venoocclusive disease (VOD). Immune mechanisms are implicated in the pathogenesis of acute and chronic graft-versus-host disease (GVHD), resulting in a variably severe loss of liver function. Finally the hepatic sequelae of infectious disseminations include cholestasis, hepatitis, abscess, and infarct.

The etiology of the liver injury can generally be predicted in the context of other ongoing multisystem processes and the timing of the insult (Table 28.1). Within 30 days after bone marrow reinfusion (day 0), the acute effects of the preparative regimen may result in cholestasis, hepatitis, or VOD. The duration and depth of neutropenia predispose to bacterial, fungus, or viral (herpes simplex) infections. Total parenteral nutrition contributes to cholestasis. From days +30–+100, the presence and treatment or prophylaxis of acute GVHD becomes an important contributor to the morbidity and mortality of BMT. The profound immunosuppression and erosion of normal mucosal barriers give rise to local and disseminated viral (cytomegalovirus, varicella-zoster, Epstein-Barr), bacterial, and fungal infections. From day +100, the development of chronic GVHD with suppression of humoral and cell-mediated immunity leads to sinopulmonary bacterial infections. Viral infections (including hepatitis C) and drug-induced hepatic in-

Table 28.1.   Timing of Hepatic Complications of Bone Marrow Transplantation

Day	0–+30	+30–+100	>100
	Chemotherapy	Acute GVHD	Chronic GVHD
	Radiotherapy	Bacteria	Bacteria
	VOD	Fungi	Virus: hepatitis C,
	Bacteria	Virus: cytomegalovirus,	cytomegalovirus,
	Fungi	varicella-zoster,	varicella-zoster,
	Virus: herpes simplex	Epstein-Barr	Epstein-Barr
	Total parenteral nutrition	Immunosuppressants	Immunosuppressants
	Drug	Drug	Drug

jury are not infrequent. With this introduction, the pathogenesis and sequelae of hepatic
VOD, GVHD, and infections will be discussed
in greater detail.

VENOOCCLUSIVE DISEASE

Introduction

VOD of the liver is a well-recognized
complication of high-dose chemoradiotherapy administration, accounting for significant
morbidity and mortality in the BMT setting.
Hepatic VOD is a specific clinical entity with
pathologic correlation, diagnosed only in the
absence of other obvious causes of liver dysfunction. VOD was first described in 1954 after Bras, Jelliffe, and Stuart demonstrated the
role of an obliterating process in hepatic vein
radicals in the morphogenesis of childhood
cirrhosis in Jamaica (2). The ingestion of Ja-
maican bush teas, which are known to contain pyrrolizidine alkaloids toxic to the liver,
led to clinical manifestations of tender hepatomegaly, ascites, and jaundice (3). Since
those early reports, VOD has been associated
with the administration of hepatic irradiation
and single and combination chemotherapy,
both at standard doses and at dosages requiring stem cell support (4–15).

Pathology and Pathogenesis

Bras et al. coined the term "venooclu-
sive disease" to describe a predominantly obliterative process in the hepatic radicals of
children developing cirrhosis after ingestion
of herbal teas (2, 16). Acutely, subendothelial
intimal thickening with partial occlusion of
the lumen in small and medium-sized
branches of the hepatic vein is associated with
centrilobular congestion. If the process becomes chronic, necrosis of pericentral
hepatocytes followed by centrilobular fibrosis will ensue. After examining 204 autopsies
of patients who had undergone high-dose
chemotherapy with bone marrow transplantation, Shulman et al. considered VOD present if the terminal hepatic venules (<75 μm)
or small sublobular veins (75–300 μm) had
concentric subintimal thickening and luminal
narrowing by either edematous reticulum fibers or collagen (17). Venous thrombi were
not present.

The pathogenesis of the lesions of VOD
is incompletely understood. There has been
controversy over whether the inciting lesions
cause a primarily vascular (endothelial) or
hepatocellular injury or both concurrently.
Animal models have reproduced histologic
lesions identical to human VOD. Rats fed escalating single oral doses of *Crotalaria fulva*
developed VOD lesions in 8–12 days after
administration (3, 18). However, the dosage
of the extract appeared crucial to the histologic development of typical VOD lesions. A
single large dose (approximating the LD_{50})
was most effective in producing VOD; repeated small doses did not lead to occlusive
lesions but to a portal-type cirrhosis. The histologic sequence of events revealed a non-
uniform centrilobular loss of glycogen (3–12
hours after dosage), centrilobular congestion

(at 24 hours), and then centrilobular hemorrhagic necrosis (at 48 hours). With more substantive insults, the central hepatic veins developed thickening of the endothelium by collagen fibers (at 3–4 days), often causing partial occlusion of the lumen (at 7–12 days). With significant occlusion of the hepatic vessels, collateral channels then appeared.

Further investigations have pointed to a prominent role for a primary endothelial injury. McLean observed that signs of hepatic outflow obstruction (portal hypertension, ascites, hepatomegaly) appeared prior to histologic evidence of venous occlusion in rats. Performing transillumination studies with dimethylnitrosamine in rat livers, she found patchy sinusoidal obstruction (between 16–24 hours after a dose of *C. fulva*) by red blood cells with resultant decrease in portal blood flow, increase in portal hypertension, and development of collateral flow (19). Electron micrographic studies done in monkeys treated with monocrotaline revealed that, from 6 hours after a single dose, endothelial cells of the sinusoids and hepatic central veins developed necrosis (20, 21). The increased permeability of the vessel walls by red blood cells and debris resulted in vascular swelling and progressive outflow obstruction.

The role of cytokines as mediators of endothelial cell injury is accruing considerable interest in the pathogenesis of treatment-related complications. Pretransplant conditioning regimens, by causing mucosal disruption, might stimulate host macrophages (in liver, Kupffer cells) to release factors such as tumor necrosis factor α (TNF α) and interleukin-1 (IL-1). TNF, by virtue of its myriad effects on endothelium, including promoting the expression of adhesion molecules of effector cells, may initiate and/or exacerbate tissue injury. Heslop et al. found that lymphocytes, cultured from autologous BMT recipients, spontaneously secreted gamma interferon within the first 10 weeks after BMT at levels significantly higher than those of patients receiving standard chemotherapy alone (22). Low levels of TNF were also produced. They theorized that in vivo activation of regenerating lymphocytes could facilitate cytokine production. Holler et al. found a strong relationship between major treatment-related complications during the 1st 6 months after BMT and elevations of TNF α levels (23). They retrospectively analyzed serial TNF serum levels obtained between day −8 and day +100 in 56 predominantly allogeneic patients receiving cyclophosphamide/ TBI or cyclophosphamide/busulfan. In 22 patients developing complications (including one with VOD), mean TNF levels were sixfold greater than in patients with uneventful courses ($p < .0001$). Elevated TNF levels predated the clinical appearance of interstitial pneumonitis, microangiopathy, and severe GVHD. The clinical appearance of endothelial leakage syndrome and VOD were closely associated with elevations of TNF α levels.

Clinical Definition of Venoocclusive Disease

The manifestations of VOD in association with childhood cirrhosis were summarized by Jelliffe et al. as occurring in three stages (2, 16). An acute syndrome of hepatomegaly, often with ascites, developed within 5–10 days of an upper respiratory infection treated with herbal teas. The syndrome usually resolved within 4–6 weeks. A subacute stage manifested by persistent hepatomegaly, often with recurrent ascites, can resolve spontaneously or pass into a chronic stage with development of cirrhosis.

The clinical manifestations of VOD in association with BMT have confirmed an acute and often terminal stage in survivors of the initial insult. There is no definitive evidence, however, that a subacute or chronic stage with cirrhosis exists. McDonald et al. from the Fred Hutchinson Cancer Research Center (FHCRC) classified patients with VOD if at least two of the following features were present within 30 days of marrow reinfusion: (*a*) jaundice, (*b*) hepatomegaly and right upper quadrant (RUQ) pain, and (c) ascites and/or unexplained weight gain (24). This clinical definition of VOD has been utilized by other BMT centers in subsequent clinical studies (14, 15). Because the clinical manifestations are not unique to the diagnosis of VOD, all other suspected causes of liver dysfunction must be excluded.

Drug Therapy: Standard Dose

PYRROLIZIDINE ALKALOIDS

Pyrrolizidine alkaloids are esters of the amino-alcohols derived from the pyrrolizidine nucleus and are found in such toxic plant species as *Crotalaria, Senecio* (ragwort), and *Heliotropium* (3). After metabolic conversion in the liver, these compounds are capable of producing alkylating groups at both ester linkage sites and thus act as bifunctional alkylating agents.

The diagnosis of childhood VOD secondary to consumption of herbal tea containing these compounds was presumptive at best in the early studies (2, 16). The spontaneous resolution of clinical symptoms, often before adequate histologic material could be obtained, and the difficulty in excluding other causes of hepatomegaly (kwashiorkor, malaria, infectious hepatitis, syphilis) common in third-world nations led to presumptive but not confirmatory evidence of the association of pyrrolizidine alkaloid ingestion and VOD. Animal models (cows, goats, rats) were then developed whereby escalating oral doses of *Crotalaria* were administered, and histologic evaluation proved the association between alkaloid ingestion and VOD (3, 18) (see "Pathogenesis").

The natural history of Jamaicans developing pyrrolizidine alkaloid–induced VOD revealed an approximately 50% complete recovery from the acute insult, a 30% development of subacute illness, and a 20% hepatic failure resulting in death (25). Approximately one-third of those with subacute disease eventually progressed to nonportal cirrhosis, resulting in a 30% overall mortality.

Pyrrolizidine alkaloid ingestion is not limited to underdeveloped countries, however. Two United States reports confirmed VOD induced by a herbal tea (comfrey or *Symphytum officinale*) bought at a health food store and a herb (*Senecio longilobus*) used as a garlic and cough medicine (26, 27).

SINGLE AND COMBINATION CHEMOTHERAPY

The first reported cases of modern-day chemotherapy causing VOD occurred in 1976 in two patients with acute leukemia receiving the antimetabolite 6-thioguanine (28). Although both patients had received recent intensive induction therapy, the symptoms of VOD occurred while each was receiving maintenance therapy with chronic oral 6-thioguanine. The role of cytosine arabinoside in the pathogenesis of those two cases could not be excluded as a contributing factor. Since then, other antineoplastic drugs (dacarbazine, azathioprine) used as single agents have also been implicated in the development of VOD (29–31). Further reports of VOD developing in patients receiving multiagent chemotherapy have led investigators to question whether the interaction of antineoplastic drugs might lead to a greater than expected risk of developing VOD (32, 33).

Drug Therapy: Bone Marrow Transplantation Studies

HIGH-DOSE SINGLE-AGENT CHEMOTHERAPY WITH BONE MARROW TRANSPLANTATION

Single-agent alkylating agents, when prescribed in doses high enough to require stem cell support, have been known to cause VOD. For agents such as carmustine (BCNU), busulfan, and mitomycin C, hepatic dysfunction and/or VOD have become dose-limiting toxicities (34–38).

HIGH-DOSE COMBINATION CHEMOTHERAPY WITH BONE MARROW TRANSPLANTATION

The following features were a composite drawn from three large series in the literature (13–15). One hundred seventeen of 781 patients (14%) who underwent BMT for a hematologic or solid tumor malignancy developed VOD within 30 days of bone marrow reinfusion. A variety of preparative regimens, with or without TBI, were administered in these studies.

Incidence and Predisposing Factors

McDonald et al. from FHCRC documented 53 cases of VOD in 255 consecutive patients (incidence 21%) undergoing allogeneic or autologous transplantation (13, 24) (Table 28.2). Preparative regimens included predominantly cyclophosphamide with three TBI dosage schemas or cyclophosphamide and busulfan. Age greater than 15 years, a diagnosis other than acute lymphocytic leukemia, and an elevated serum glutamic-oxaloacetic transaminase (SGOT) prior to BMT all were predictive for subsequent development of VOD. They surmised that the elevated SGOT was secondary to a chronic non-A, non-B viral hepatitis acquired from multiple blood transfusions in a largely leukemic patient population. Jones et al. from Johns Hopkins documented 52 cases in 235 patients (incidence 22%) undergoing allogeneic or autologous transplantation (14). Preparative regimens included either cyclophosphamide/TBI or cyclophosphamide/busulfan. An elevated SGOT pretransplant was predictive for VOD, while a diagnosis of acute leukemia in first remission was associated with a decreased risk. Ayash et al. from Dana-Farber Cancer Institute/Beth Israel Hospital (DFCI/BIH) noted a much lower incidence of VOD (12 of 291; 4.1%) in solid tumor and lymphoma patients undergoing autologous BMT (15). Patients received either a single alkylating agent (BCNU), triple alkylating agent chemotherapy, or cyclophosphamide with fractionated TBI. The only pretransplant characteristic predictive for the subsequent development of VOD was metastatic liver involvement. Only the DFCI/BIH series found any association between preparative regimen and VOD. No individual preparative drug had a significant effect on the development of VOD. However, schedule and combination of agents showed an important association. A single 2 hour infusion of BCNU in a dosage equal to or greater than 450 mg/

Table 28.2. Significant Pretransplant Characteristics in Patients with VOD

	Seattle	J. Hopkins	Boston
Reference	24	14	15
No. of patients	255	235	291
No. with VOD	53 (21%)	52 (22%)	12 (4.1%)
Age	Yes: >15 yrs. (increased risk)	No	No
Diagnosis	Yes: other than ALL[a] (increased risk)	Yes: acute leukemia in 1st remission (decreased risk)	No
Liver metastases	No	No	Yes: presence increases risk
Preparative regime	No	No	Yes: single-bolus BCNU w/other alkylators (increased risk)
Elevation of liver function tests	Yes: SGOT (increased risk)	Yes: SGOT (increased risk)	No

[a]ALL, acute lymphoblastic leukemia.

m^2 led to an increased incidence of VOD when compared with the same dose administered in a fractionated schedule ($p = .02$) in combination with two other chemotherapeutic agents. All three series failed to find an association with sex of recipient, hepatitis B serology, or type of graft (allogeneic or autologous).

Clinical Features

Unexplained weight gain with salt and water retention was the first sign of VOD that appeared (mean day +7.4) in over 90% of patients. Virtually all patients (99%) developed jaundice (mean day +10) with or without RUQ pain and/or hepatomegaly (mean day +12). A lesser percentage of patients developed either ascites (73%) or hepatic encephalopathy (48%) approximately 3 days later.

Hyperbilirubinemia was a constant feature, appearing around day +7–+12. Mean peak values of bilirubin averaged 15.0 mg/dl (range 1.6–69.0). Those patients who were destined to have severe and often fatal VOD had consistently higher peak values of bilirubin than did those with less serious VOD. An elevated SGOT (mean peak 441 IU/dl; range 20–7600) developed in the majority of patients, appearing from day +7 to approximately day +16. Alkaline phosphatase was often elevated in those patients with an elevated SGOT. Onset of alkaline phosphatase elevation (mean peak 380 IU/dl; range 100–1860) varied from day +8 to +11.

VOD was the cause or a major contributing factor in 56 of 117 (47%) patient deaths occurring a mean of 34 days after marrow reinfusion, or about 22 days after the onset of VOD. The majority of patients had multiorgan failure, often associated with sepsis and hemorrhage. Patients who were destined to die of VOD had significantly higher peak bilirubin levels, often had developed hepatic encephalopathy, and either had yet to become platelet-transfusion independent or had

become refractory to platelet transfusions. For those patients with nonfatal VOD, virtually all had complete clinical resolution of hepatic symptomatology and liver function abnormalities.

Observations from Other Studies

Hepatic irradiation has long been known to cause VOD when administered either as a single large dose or as multiple small fractionated doses (39). Investigators at Seattle observed that life-threatening or fatal regimen-related liver toxicity was more likely in allogeneic patients receiving higher-dose TBI (15.75 Gy versus 12.0 Gy, $p = .02$) (40). Fractionation and lower total dose of TBI appear to decrease the incidence of VOD. A closer look at the dose rate of TBI may also merit further investigation.

Pharmacokinetics of chemotherapeutic agents have the potential to aid in predicting patients at risk to develop VOD as well as to allow for modulation of chemotherapeutic dosage based on early pharmacokinetic measurements. Henner et al. studied the pharmacokinetics of BCNU in patients receiving a high-dose combination of cyclophosphamide, BCNU, and cisplatin (41). There was substantial variability of BCNU clearance in patients receiving 300–750 mg/m² as a single 2-hour infusion. There was a trend for patients with a high bioavailability (lower clearance) of BCNU to have a higher incidence of hepatotoxicity, including VOD. Grochow et al. studied busulfan pharmacokinetics in patients receiving oral busulfan (1 mg/kg every 6 hours for 16 doses) followed by intravenous cyclophosphamide (50 mg/kg for 4 days) (42). A tenfold variability in busulfan area-under-the-curve (AUC) was observed, with a significant incidence of VOD noted in patients with a high AUC.

Preventive measures to decrease the occurrence of GVHD have led to interactions increasing the risk of VOD. The potent immunosuppressant cyclosporine, when given concurrently with high-dose cyclophosphamide in aplastic anemia patients undergoing BMT, was shown to cause severe hepatotoxicity and VOD (43). A combination of cyclosporine and methotrexate prophylaxis in a cohort of patients receiving busulfan (4 mg/kg × 4 days) and cyclophosphamide (60 mg/kg intravenously × 2 days) led to a substantially increased incidence (14 of 20 patients; 70%) of VOD in one series (44).

Treatment

Treatment of established VOD has largely been supportive in nature. Treatment of hepatic insufficiency includes plasma expanders to maintain intravascular volume, spironolactone to decrease extravascular fluid accumulation, lactulose with protein restriction to treat encephalopathy, and avoidance of sedatives and opiates. Steroids have been tried with mixed success in hopes of decreasing the fibrotic component of VOD. More aggressive forms of treatment have included portocaval shunting and liver transplantation (45).

More enterprising clinical trials have recently been conducted in hopes of preventing VOD. A trial of anticoagulation to overcome a primary endothelial injury with resultant deposition of coagulation factors in the subendothelium of affected sinusoids and venules has been undertaken by Bearman et al. (46). Heparin was administered to 28 patients from the day preparative therapy was begun through day +14 (range 20–26 days of heparin). Seven received full-course therapy, and 21 stopped treatment early because of bleeding or anticipated bleeding. Heparin was deemed ineffective in preventing VOD (incidence rate 70%). Gluckman et al. administered prostaglandin E1 (PGE1) from the beginning of preparative therapy through day +30 in 50 patients undergoing allogeneic BMT (47). PGE1 may have protective effects on vascular endothelium by means of vasodilatation, inhibition of platelet aggregation, ac-

tivation of the fibrinolytic system, and acceleration of thrombolysis by tissue plasminogen activator. The incidence of VOD was less in patients treated with PGE1 (12.2% versus 25.5%) when compared with a control population. Bianco et al. used the agent pentoxyfylline (PTX) to diminish regimen-related toxicity (48). Pentoxyfylline stimulates vascular endothelium to produce prostaglandins I2 and E2 and inhibits monocyte/macrophage production of TNF α, theoretically ameliorating toxicity. Eight allograft recipients, prepared with cyclophosphamide and fractionated TBI, were given prophylactic oral PTX (400 mg four times daily) until day 100 post-BMT. Pentoxyfylline significantly reduced the incidence (25% versus 65%) and severity of VOD when compared with matched controls.

Further investigation in the manipulation of mediators of endothelial injury appears warranted. Baglin et al. treated a single patient with established VOD with recombinant tissue plasminogen activator (rt-PA) (49). rt-PA has a high affinity for fibrin-bound plasminogen, resulting in activation of plasmin on fibrin clots without excessive systemic defibrination. This patient was treated with a 3-hour 50-mg infusion of rt-PA daily for 4 days with rapid resolution of ascites, encephalopathy, liver function, and coagulation abnormalities. Further trials of rt-PA, PGE1, and PTX either alone or in combination to prevent and treat VOD are clearly necessary to confirm the initial observations. One possible therapeutic approach to prevent VOD is derived from preclinical studies performed by Teicher et al. in mice (50). Mice pretreated with glutathione monoethyl ester (GSHet) were effectively protected from the lethal effects of monocrotaline, BCNU, or cyclophosphamide. GSHet is rapidly transported into cells, leading to increased levels of glutathione, a thiol cellular defense known to protect against hepatotoxins. GSHet appeared to protect critical normal tissues without protecting tumor cells.

GRAFT-VERSUS-HOST DISEASE OF THE LIVER

Introduction

GVHD is the leading factor contributing to the morbidity and mortality associated with allogeneic BMT. Billingham defined the requirements for the development of GVHD: (*a*) immunocompetent cells (i.e., mature T cells) must be present in the graft; (*b*) the host must be antigenically different from the donor; and (*c*) the host must be incapable of rejecting the graft (51). HLA antigens, the protein products of the major histocompatibility complex (MHC) present on the surfaces of nucleated cells, are recognized by donor T cells. Antigenic differences between donor and recipient result in activation of T cells with development of GVHD.

Acute GVHD (aGVHD) clinically manifests itself as an immune-mediated attack against skin, liver, and gastrointestinal epithelium. Although hepatic aGVHD has been noted rarely to arise de novo, it usually occurs with or after skin involvement has appeared. Chronic GVHD (cGVHD), on the other hand, presents with clinical features suggestive of collagen-vascular disease. An autoimmune phenomenon has been implicated in the setting of both humoral and cell-mediated dysfunction.

Acute Graft-versus-Host Disease

Pathology and Pathogenesis

Early pathologic diagnosis of aGVHD may be difficult due to contributing toxic effects of the conditioning regimen on rapidly dividing normal tissues. Skin biopsy, usually the first diagnostic test performed, may be equivocal or difficult to distinguish from a toxic drug reaction and may require rectal or hepatic tissue to confirm the diagnosis.

Epithelial degenerative changes in interlobular bile ducts with cholestasis are the characteristic features of aGVHD present on liver biopsy (52–57). Mild lobular hepatocel-

lular injury and portal lymphocytic infiltration are present within 2 weeks of disease onset. With disease progression, atypia or destruction of bile ducts with filling of ductal lumens by cellular debris or epithelial ingrowths is seen. With severe GVHD, hepatocytes show ballooning degeneration, bile pigmentation, and dropout. There may be Kupffer cell hyperplasia, bridging and piecemeal necrosis, and dilated cholangioles filled with bile.

Alloimmune reactions are directed against disparate major and minor histocompatibility or other alloantigens present on the epithelium of bile ducts, skin, and gut (57). These "foreign" antigens stimulate mature T cell (helper and/or suppressor cell) activation, cytokine release, and T cell proliferation (58). Clonal expansion and differentiation of effector cells ensue. It is not clear whether cytotoxic T cells directly induce injury or whether cytokines (e.g., TNF α) released by these effector cells mediate the damage. Holler et al. found that elevation of TNF α serum levels preceded the clinical appearance of significant GVHD (23). TNF levels were obtained between day −8 and day +100 in 52 patients undergoing allogeneic bone marrow transplantation. In 4 patients who later developed grades II–IV GVHD, maximal elevations of TNF levels preceded maximal clinical symptoms by 24–54 days, suggesting early cytokine release was necessary to later effect clinical manifestations. In a mouse model, Piguet showed that prophylactic use of an antibody neutralizing TNF α could prevent histologic changes of aGVHD, again implying an important role for TNF in the pathogenesis of GVHD (59).

CLINICAL MANIFESTATIONS OF ACUTE GRAFT-VERSUS-HOST DISEASE

Incidence and Predisposing Factors

aGVHD occurs in approximately 40%–50% of patients undergoing allogeneic BMT, with reported mortality rates generally between 30% and 40% (or about half of all affected individuals). Factors associated with increasing the risk of developing aGVHD include (*a*) increasing genetic disparity at the MHC locus, (*b*) increasing number of T cells infused, (*c*) ABO incompatibility, (*d*) increasing age of the recipient, (*e*) sex of the donor (opposite-sex donors in Seattle and Johns Hopkins series; female donors in International Bone Marrow Transplant Registry [IBMTR] studies), (*f*) intensity of the preparatory regimen, and (*g*) prophylaxis administered to prevent GVHD (60–62).

Clinical Features

aGVHD can appear at any time up to day +100 post marrow reinfusion, but appears most commonly by week 3 or 4. Many of the early signs or symptoms, especially those related to hepatic disease, are nonspecific and may be overshadowed by other transplant-related complications. A clinical system grading the severity of GVHD and incorporating individual organ involvement is presented in Table 28.3 (62).

Skin is the earliest and most frequently affected site of disease (63). Palms, soles, and ears followed by trunk, face, and extremities develop an erythematous pruritic maculopapular rash. The rash can become confluent, progress to erythroderma with bullae, then to toxic epidermal necrolysis. Liver disease may occur several days after skin lesions have appeared, although it can rarely precede the

rash. Elevation of liver function tests, without clinical symptoms of hepatitis, is the most common hepatic abnormality. Elevations of conjugated bilirubin (up to 40 × normal) and alkaline phosphatase (up to 20 × normal), with less extreme elevations of transaminases (up to 10 × normal) are characteristic. Patients commonly develop jaundice, less commonly ascites, and only in severe cases progress to fulminant hepatic failure. It is uncommon to develop hepatic metabolic dysfunction; low levels of serum albumin are usually secondary to gastrointestinal loss rather than a true decrease in hepatic synthesis capability. Gastrointestinal symptoms of crampy abdominal pain and profuse bloody diarrhea usually occur with or after skin and liver disease have appeared.

Clinical Course and Treatment

The poor outcome associated with moderate to severe aGVHD is primarily related to the mortality resulting from opportunistic infections developing in the setting of prolonged immunodeficiency. Patients in whom GVHD develops already are immune deficient from either or both the underlying disease and the TBI-containing preparative regimen. GVHD lesions allow entry of infectious organisms through disruption of normal mucosal barriers in skin and gut. GVHD is also associated with an increased incidence (? reactivation) of cytomegalovirus infections.

Table 28.3. Severity of Individual Organ Involvement in Acute GVHD[a]

Severity	Skin	Liver (Bilirubin level)	Gastrointestinal (Diarrhea)
+1	Maculopapular rash <25% body surface	2–2.9 mg/dl	500–999 ml stool/day
+2	Maculopapular rash 25%–50% body surface	3–5.9 mg/dl	1000–1499 ml stool/day
+3	Generalized erythroderma	6–14.9 mg/dl	1500–2000 ml stool/day
+4	Generalized erythroderma w/bullous formation and desquamation	≥15 mg/dl	>2000 ml stool/day

[a]Adapted from Glucksberg H, Storb R, Fefer A, et al. Clinical manifestation, of graft-versus-host disease in human recipients of marrow from HLA-matched sibling donors. Transplantation 1974;18:295–304.

And finally, the treatment of GVHD itself involves immunosuppressive agents.

Mild (grade I) GVHD usually resolves successfully without treatment. The mainstay of treatment for more extensive aGVHD is glucocorticoids, although cyclosporine, antithymocyte globulin (ATG), and monoclonal antibody (OKT3) are frequently employed. Although the clinical symptoms of GVHD may improve with treatment, survival overall has not significantly improved. Resolution of liver function abnormalities may take weeks to months, and the metabolism of drugs (e.g., cyclosporine) used to treat GVHD may itself be compromised by the liver dysfunction.

Martin et al. performed a retrospective analysis of treatment in 740 patients (incidence 37%) developing grade II–IV aGVHD after allogeneic BMT. Initial treatment (number of patients) included glucocorticoids (531), cyclosporine (170), ATG (156), or monoclonal antibody (3), either alone (633) or in combination (107) (64). Because of the presence of other transplant-related complications, treatment outcome could not be evaluated in 58% of patients with liver dysfunction and 24% of patients with gastrointestinal symptoms. In evaluable patients, 43% of those with skin, 35% with liver, and 50% with gastrointestinal symptoms improved with treatment. Among the 75 patients with moderate to severe hepatic dysfunction from other transplant-related complications, 26% showed improvement after treatment for GVHD. The overall complete (18%) and partial response to treatment for aGVHD was 44%. Factors associated with a favorable outcome included GVHD prophylaxis with the combination cyclosporine/methotrexate and treatment of aGVHD with glucocorticoids or cyclosporine (rather than ATG). Factors associated with an unfavorable outcome included HLA disparity of recipient and donor, other hepatic regimen-related complications, and early-onset GVHD.

Chronic Graft-versus-Host Disease

PATHOLOGY AND PATHOGENESIS

The histologic appearance of chronic GVHD (cGVHD) lesions suggest a collagen-vascular disease etiology. Early skin manifestations of hyperkeratosis, mononuclear cell infiltration at the dermoepidermal junction and around eccrine units, proceed to an atrophic epidermis and dense dermal fibrosis (52, 63, 65). Liver biopsy performed on de novo cGVHD reveals a chronic lobular, chronic persistent, or chronic active hepatitis with a lobular, portal, or periportal inflammatory reaction, respectively (52, 57). Centrilobular cholestasis and focal hepatocellular necrosis can be found. With disease progression, there is more evident portal inflammation and fibrosis and a significant reduction or absence of small interlobular bile ducts. Concentric periductal fibrosis can mimic the changes seen with primary sclerosing cholangitis (66).

Immunologic analysis supports an autoimmune phenomenon active in cGVHD. There is abundant evidence for both humoral and cell-mediated dysregulation. Humoral abnormalities include immunoglobulin and complement deposition along dermal basement membranes, hypergammaglobulinemia, and increased autoantibody production (58, 65, 67, 68). Cellular immune abnormalities commonly seen are involution of the thymic epithelium, increased nonspecific T suppressor cell activity, impaired proliferation of B cells and antibody production, and defects in T helper cell function (58, 68–70). Hypotheses for the pathogenesis of cGVHD have questioned the role of thymic injury resulting in the development of nontolerant T cells as well as cytotoxic T cells provoking increased cytokine production with subsequent collagen formation by fibroblasts.

CLINICAL MANIFESTATIONS OF CHRONIC GRAFT-VERSUS-HOST DISEASE

Incidence and Predisposing Factors

cGVHD will develop in approximately 10% of all patients who undergo allogeneic BMT, or in 30% of all long-term (>150 days) survivors. Although the classical definition of cGVHD has its appearance from day +100 onward, presentations as early as day +40–+50 have been recorded. And while the majority of cases have appeared by 3–6 months, onset or persistence of disease as late as 1 year after BMT may occur. cGVHD most commonly develops as a direct continuation from acute GVHD; however, de novo (incidence 20%–30%) disease and disease developing after acute GVHD has resolved also occur. Chronic GVHD is most likely to appear in older patients and in those with a history of moderate to severe acute GVHD (71).

Clinical Features

Chronic GVHD has two manifestations: a localized disease (skin and/or liver; incidence 10%) with a favorable prognosis without treatment, and a generalized multisystem disease with a less favorable prognosis even with treatment (65, 71). Features reminiscent of collagen-vascular disease (e.g., Sjögren's syndrome, scleroderma, dermatomyositis) dominate the clinical presentation.

Skin lesions, often activated by sun exposure, begin as erythematous rashes with areas of hyper- or hypopigmentation. Lesions are often described as lichen planus-like and, if untreated, may become sclerotic, with joint contractures. A sicca-like syndrome results in xerostomia, keratoconjunctivitis, pulmonary fibrosis, and esophageal strictures with dysphagia. Liver involvement manifests primarily as elevation of liver function tests in a setting of multisystem GVHD. Elevation of alkaline phosphatase (5–10 × normal) is characteristic, often accompanied by mild transaminase (3–6 × normal) and intermittent bilirubin elevations. A minority of patients have clinical jaundice; cirrhosis or hepatic failure is exceedingly rare. Anemia, thrombocytopenia, eosinophilia, and circulating auto-antibodies are common laboratory findings.

Clinical Course and Treatment

The marked immune dysregulation present with cGVHD results in an impaired response to infection. Bacterial organisms (especially *Pneumococcus* and encapsulated organisms), varicella-zoster, and cytomegalovirus are major factors contributing to the morbidity and mortality associated with cGVHD.

Prognosis is excellent for patients with localized disease, which rarely requires treatment. The clinical course is more complex and less favorable with generalized disease. In general, survival is greatest with de novo presentation and least with continuance of aGVHD. Wingard et al. listed factors associated with an unfavorable outcome: (*a*) progressive onset from aGVHD, (*b*) lichenoid skin changes, (*c*) elevated serum bilirubin, (*d*) persistent thrombocytopenia, and (*e*) failure to respond to 9 months of treatment (72). If there were two or more risk factors present, there was a less than 20% chance of prolonged survival. Sullivan, in his analysis of 52 cGVHD patients followed for 2–7 years after BMT, felt that Karnofsky performance score was the best overall measure of the severity of the disease (71).

Treatment consists of a prolonged course of immunosuppressive agents, supportive measures such as artificial tears and sun block, and prophylactic oral antibiotics. Sullivan found the combination of prednisone (1 mg/kg every other day) and either azathioprine or cyclophosphamide (each at 1.5 mg/kg/day) was more effective than prednisone alone for extensive disease (71). Liver function abnormalities usually improve with therapy but may remain elevated for a prolonged period of time. After discontinuation of therapy, recurrence of cGVHD is not uncommon and may be documented by rising alkaline phosphatase levels. Despite therapeutic measures, the mortality attributable to cGVHD remains formidable.

INFECTIONS

There are many factors in influencing the type and severity of infections that arise during and following a bone marrow transplant. Transplant-related factors include type of graft (allogeneic versus autologous), purging of T cells from the graft, and prophylaxis to prevent GVHD. Host-related factors include regimen-related toxicity of the preparative treatment, duration and depth of neutopenia, and the intensity of cellular and immune dysfunction caused by the preparative regimen or the development of GVHD (73–76).

The immediate posttransplant period, until complete recovery from the acute toxic effects of the preparative regimen and the period of aplasia, may give rise to bacterial, fungal, or herpes simplex viral infections. From day +30 to day +100, with the development of aGVHD or continuation of immunosuppressants to prevent GVHD, cytomegalovirus assumes a prominent role along with bacterial and fungal organisms in causing infection. After day +100, especially with the combined immunodeficiency seen with cGVHD, encapsulated bacteria, varicella-zoster, and organisms causing chronic viral hepatitis become important.

Bacteria

Historically, gram-negative bacterial infections (especially *Pseudomonas* and *Enterbacteriaceae*), arising from disruption of normal mucosal barriers, were the major causes of acute mortality in the early aplastic period. With the advent of indwelling intravenous catheters and oral antibiotic prophylaxis, gram-positive organisms (*Staphylococcus* and *Streptococcus*) now have assumed a new importance. α Streptococcus (usually *S. mitus*) has been implicated in an acute "shock" syndrome that has resulted in death in 21% of symptomatic patients in one series (77). Encapsulated bacteria remain a prominent cause of pulmonary and sinus infections occurring with cGVHD.

Liver function abnormalities occurring during the course of bacterial infection or sepsis vary widely in clinical significance. Asymptomatic elevations in alkaline phosphatase and/or bilirubin reflect intrahepatic cholestasis. Microabscesses, symptomatic macroabscesses, and cholangitis may result in more prolonged and persistent liver function abnormalities.

Fungi

Symptomatic fungal infections arise in the setting of T-cell-depleted grafts, mucosal barrier disruption from chemoradiotherapy, prolonged neutropenia, and/or aGVHD. The high mortality is a reflection of the difficulty of making a diagnosis of fungal dissemination antemortem. Persistent fevers may be the only manifestation of disease; surveillance cultures have a very low predictive value; fungal cultures and radiologic examinations lack high sensitivity for detection; and liver biopsy is hazardous to perform in the face of thrombocytopenia. Because of these difficulties, empiric antifungal therapy is instituted in the appropriate setting when the probability of fungal infection is high.

CANDIDA

Candida albicans infection has been reported in 10%–20% of patients undergoing BMT. Meyers et al., in a retrospective study of 1510 patients undergoing BMT in Seattle from 1980–1986, found a 11.3% incidence of infection (78). Median onset of detection of fungus by blood cultures was 2 weeks and by tissue diagnosis 3 weeks after marrow reinfusion. There was a significant increase in invasive candidiasis from 1984 to 1986, with an overall fatality rate of 73% (higher in patients with tissue involvement than with fungemia alone).

Fever of unknown origin in a patient whose white blood cell count is recovering is the most common presentation of hepatosplenic involvement (79). Unfortunately, hepatic dissemination is rarely diagnosed before autopsy. Liver disease usually occurs in the setting of multiorgan involvement but may occur without overt fungemia. Abdominal pain is more frequently reported than is true hepatomegaly. A "shock-like" syndrome associated with widespread fungal disease and hepatic failure has been observed. A persistent elevation of alkaline phosphatase is characteristic (median duration 130 days in one study); SGOT and bilirubin levels rarely remain high. However, progressive elevation of liver function tests occurs with worsening of disease status.

Radiologic tests (ultrasound and computerized tomography [CT] scan) are neither highly specific nor sensitive in detecting liver abscesses. "Bull's eye" lesions, with hypoechogenic or low-attenuation contour and hyperechogenic or contrast-enhanced central areas, are sought but may not appear until neutrophil recovery has occurred. If a liver image shows a lesion(s) suggestive of fungus, a needle-directed biopsy should be obtained.

Pathologic tissue is necessary to confirm the presence of yeast and pseudohyphae. Fungal organisms are often present in the center of microabscesses, requiring serial sections and special stains for detection. Obstruction of hepatic veins or biliary ducts by fungus may be seen. Although serial liver biopsies are employed to determine success of antifungal therapy, the absence of organisms is not proof that the infection has resolved (79).

ASPERGILLUS

In a retrospective analysis of 1658 patients undergoing BMT from 1980 through 1987, Meyers et al. recorded an incidence of *Aspergillus* infections of 4.5% (78). Median onset of detection of disease was 6 weeks after BMT, and overall mortality was 84%. Respiratory tract infections (sinus and lung) predominate and are always present in cases of dissemination. Hepatic failure has been reported (80).

Antemortem diagnosis is extremely difficult to confirm. Blood cultures are positive in less than 30% of cases. Chest x-rays may reveal nodular infiltrates or a wedge-shaped silhouette consistent with pulmonary infarction. The hallmark of invasive aspergillosis is invasion of blood vessel walls by hyphae with formation of thrombus and subsequent tissue infarction (including liver).

Virus

Viral infections in the BMT setting can arise from acquisition of a new virus, reactivation of a latent virus, or reinfection of a viral species to which the patient has previously been exposed. The acute toxicity of the preparative regimen, the use of TBI, the transfusion of infected blood products, the presence of GVHD, and the means of preventing GVHD influence the timing and severity of the viral infection.

HERPES SIMPLEX

Herpes simplex virus (HSV) serology obtained before BMT can identify patients at risk for reactivation of latent virus. The use of prophylactic acyclovir until immune reconstitution is complete has significantly decreased the incidence of active infection. When disease does occur, it may present with oral or genital ulcers (during the period of aplasia) or with widespread cutaneous and/or visceral dissemination (within the 1st year after BMT). Liver infection is usually one manifestation of a systemic dissemination. Hepatitis, with marked elevation in transaminases and bilirubin levels, can progress to hepatic necrosis and failure in rare instances (57, 81).

Immunofluorescent staining with monoclonal antiviral antibodies, the demonstration of multinucleated giant cells by Tzanck prep, and a cytopathic effect on tissue biopsy will aid in diagnosis.

CYTOMEGALOVIRUS

Cytomegalovirus (CMV) infection can arise via the allograft of a seropositive donor, via transfusion of blood products from seropositive donors, by reactivation of latent virus, or by reinfection of a new strain of virus (82). Approximately 50% of patients undergoing primarily allogeneic BMT develop active CMV infection, and 15%–20% succumb to the disease. The risk factors associated with an increased risk of developing CMV infection in seronegative recipients include use of seropositive donor marrow, use of seropositive blood products, and the presence of aGVHD (83).

The onset of symptomatic infection is usually between day +30 and day +100. Clinical manifestations are varied and include fever, pneumonitis (the most severe presentation; incidence 10% in allogeneic BMT), hepatitis, enteritis, and graft failure. At autopsy, liver involvement is not uncommon, even in previously asymptomatic patients.

Tissue biopsy confirms the presence of large cytomegalic cells. CMV inclusions may be variably present in hepatocytes, bile duct epithelium, and Kupffer cells during active infection (57). Immunocytochemistry can directly localize CMV-specific antigens using labeled antibody. In situ hybridization employs RNA or DNA probes to recognize CMV-specific nucleic acid sequences (84).

VARICELLA-ZOSTER VIRUS

Varicella-zoster virus (VZV) infections occur as reactivation of virus in a seropositive recipient, most commonly at a median of 5 months after BMT. The reported incidence varies from 16%–40%, with an overall mortality of 10%–15% (73, 85). Although most common in the allogeneic population, especially in association with GVHD, autologous patients are also at risk (incidence 10%–28%).

VZV can present as localized dermatomal disease or with widespread cutaneous and/or visceral dissemination. In those with visceral disease, a diagnosis of VZV is often not considered in the absence of cutaneous vesicular lesions. Although cutaneous disease can lead to scarring and neuralgia, a mortality rate up to 50% accompanies visceral dissemination. While pneumonitis is the most common and serious manifestation, liver disease can present in myriad ways, including asymptomatic transaminase elevation, mild symptomatic hepatitis, or fulminant hepatic failure (86).

A diagnosis of VZV infection can be made by immunofluorescence staining of vesicular contents with monoclonal antibodies, demonstration of intranuclear inclusions and multinucleated giant cells, and viral culture (87). Acyclovir should be instituted promptly and preferably before dissemination has been documented.

HEPATITIS C VIRUS

The natural history of hepatitis C virus (HCV) formerly non-A, non-B hepatitis, is unknown in the BMT setting. In developed countries, the epidemiology of HCV mimics that of hepatitis B in that the virus can be transmitted through blood and blood products and by intimate contact. HCV has been felt to be the causal agent responsible for the chronic hepatitis that develops more than 6–12 months after BMT. It usually manifests as an asymptomatic elevation of alanine aminotransferase (ALT), though clinical jaundice may occur in 25% of patients.

With the recent advances in the diagnosis of HCV, Alter et al. measured antibody to HCV by radioimmunoassay in prospectively followed transfusion recipients and donors (88). Antibody to HCV appeared a mean of 22 weeks after transfusion and 15 weeks after the onset of clinical hepatitis. Approximately 50% of infected patients had elevated ALT levels (mean duration of ALT elevation was 8 years). All 15 patients with chronic hepatitis by liver biopsy had seroconverted for the antibody, and 20% of those had evidence of cirrhosis. Measurement of anti-HCV in conjunction with liver biopsy may delineate the natural history of HCV in BMT patients and help differentiate the syndrome from GVHD or drug effect.

OTHER VIRAL SYNDROMES

Epstein-Barr Virus

A B cell lymphoproliferative syndrome associated with Epstein-Barr virus (EBV) has been recognized, especially in recipients of T-cell-depleted grafts (incidence <1%). The B cells, which contain multiple copies of the

EBV genome, may evolve from a reactive polyclonal to a monoclonal B cell lymphoma. Disease onset is usually between days +50 and +80 but may appear more than 1 year after BMT (89). Clinical features may mimic mononucleosis, including lymph node enlargement, hepatosplenomegaly, elevated liver function tests, anemia, and thrombocytopenia. Liver biopsy may reveal portal and sinusoidal infiltration by immunoblastic B cells (57). Treatment strategies have included removal of immunosuppressants, acyclovir, anti–B cell monoclonal antibodies, α interferon, and immunoglobulin (90).

Adenovirus

In one reported series, adenovirus was a source of BMT infection alone or coexisting with other viruses (51 of 1051 patients; incidence 4.8%) (91). Ten patients had invasive adenovirus (lung, liver, kidney) diagnosed by biopsy or autopsy. Four died of pneumonia; two died with focal or massive hepatic necrosis. The only identifiable risk factor was the presence of moderate to severe GVHD. Pathology revealed characteristic "smudge" cells and intranuclear inclusions.

SUMMARY AND CONCLUSIONS

Research efforts directed at ameliorating the toxicities associated with high-dose chemotherapy may ultimately decrease the morbidity and mortality associated with BMT. Prevention of hepatic injury has practical advantages and can be approached from many directions.

To modulate the toxicities associated with the preparative regimen, pharmacologic monitoring of drug levels (e.g., BCNU, busulfan) and early calculation of the projected AUC may allow for withholding of further drug dosages in those patients with expected slow clearance. Close attention to schedule of administration of particular agents (e.g., BCNU, cyclophosphamide, TBI) may reveal a greater therapeutic index with multiple dosing rather than one large bolus dose. Prophylactic administration of agents (e.g., pentoxyfylline, prostaglandins) that alleviate the effects of excessive cytokine release may limit the severity of hepatic injury, including VOD.

Efforts to prevent acute and chronic GVHD remain an active area of investigation. The combination of cyclosporine and methotrexate has been advantageous, and ongoing clinical trials with selective T cell depletion are promising.

Perhaps the most significant advance has been the surge of basic and clinical research in the use of hematopoietins and peripheral blood progenitor cells (PBPC). Colony-stimulating factors (granulocyte-macrophage, colony-stimulating factor [GM-CSF], granulocyte colony-stimulating factor [G-CSF]) have in most instances decreased the period of neutropenia, the usage of antibiotics, and the number of febrile days (92). The ability of colony-stimulating factors to augment PBPC collections has resulted in an even more pronounced lessening of the duration of aplasia (93, 94). These advances in stem cell support, coupled with the use of prophylactic oral antibiotics and antiviral medications, should lessen the incidence and severity of infections and allow for the administration of dose-intensive therapy needed for optimal cytoreduction.

REFERENCES

1. Robbins SL. Pathologic basis of disease. Philadelphia: WB Saunders, 1974:985–988.
2. Jelliffe DB, Bras G, Mukherjee KL. Veno-occlusive Disease of the liver and indian childhood cirrhosis. Arch Dis Child 1957;32:369–385.
3. McLean EK. The toxic actions of pyrrolizidine (Senecio) alkaloids. Pharm Rev 1970;2(4):429–483.
4. Jacobs P, Miller JL, Uys CJ, Dietrick BE. Fatal veno-occlusive disease of the liver after chemotherapy, whole-body irradiation and bone marrow transplantation for refractory acute leukemia. S Afr Med J 1979;55:5–10.
5. Woods WG, Dehner LP, Nesbit ME. Fatal veno-occlusive disease of the liver following high-dose chemotherapy, irradiation and bone marrow transplantation. Am J Med 1980;68:285–290.
6. Fajardo LF, Colby TV. Pathogenesis of veno-occlusive liver disease after radiation. Arch Pathol Lab Med 1980;104:584–588.

7. Asbury RF, Rosenthal SN, Descalzi ME. Hepatic veno-occlusive disease due to DTIC. Cancer 180;45:2670–2674.

8. McIntyre RE, Magidson JG, Austin GE, Gale RP. Fatal veno-occlusive disease of the liver following high dose BCNU and autologous bone marrow transplantation. Am Soc Clin Pathol 1981;75(4):614–617.

9. Gill RA, Onstad GR, Cardamone JM, et al. Hepatic veno-occlusive disease caused by 6-thioguanine. Ann Intern Med 1982;96:58–60.

10. Lazarus HM, Gottfried MR, Herzig RH, et al. Veno-occlusive disease of the liver after high-dose mitomycin C therapy and autologous bone marrow transplantation. Cancer 1982;49:1789–1795.

11. Atkinson K, Biggs J, Noble G, et al. Preparative regimens for marrow transplantation containing busulfan are associated with hemorrhagic cystitis and hepatic veno-occlusive disease but a short duration of leucopenia and little oro-pharyngeal mucositis. Bone Marrow Transplant 1987;2:385–394.

12. McClay E. Allergy-induced hepatic toxicity associated with dacarbazine. Cancer Treat Rep 1987;71(2):219–220.

13. McDonald GB, Sharma P, Matthews DE, et al. The clinical course of 53 patients with veno-occlusive disease of the liver after marrow transplantation. Transplantation 1985;39:603–608.

14. Jones RJ, Lee KS, Beschorner WE, et al. Veno-occlusive disease of the liver following bone marrow transplantation. Transplantation 1987;44(6):778–783.

15. Ayash LJ, Hunt M, Antman K, et al. Hepatic veno-occlusive disease in autologous bone marrow transplantation of solid tumors and lymphomas. J Clin Oncol 1990;8:1699–1706.

16. Bras G, Jeliffe DB, Stuart KL. Veno-occlusive disease of the liver with nonportal type of cirrhosis occurring in Jamaica. Arch Pathol 1954;57:285–300.

17. Shulman HM, McDonald GB, Matthews DE, et al. An analysis of hepatic veno-occlusive disease and centrilobular hepatic degeneration following bone marrow transplantation. Gastroenterology 1980;79:1178–1191.

18. McLean E, Bras G, Gyorgy P. Veno-occlusive lesions in livers of rats fed *Crotalaria fulva*. Br J Exp Pathol 1964;45:242–247.

19. McLean EK. The early sinusoidal lesion in experimental veno-occlusive disease. Br J Exp Pathol 1969;50:223–229.

20. Allen JR, Carstens LA. Sequential ultrastructural changes in hepatic vessels of monkeys with veno-occlusive disease. Am J Pathol 1968;52:13a.

21. Allen JR, Carstens LA, Katagiri G. Hepatic veins of monkeys with veno-occlusive disease. Sequential ultrastructural changes. Arch Pathol 1969;87:279–289.

22. Heslop H, Gottlieb D, Reittie J, et al. Spontaneous and interleukin 2 induced secretion of tumor necrosis factor and gamma interferon following autologous marrow transplantation or chemotherapy. Br J Hematol 1989;72:122–126.

23. Holler E, Kolb HJ, Kempeni J, et al. Increased serum levels of tumor necrosis factor alpha precede major complications of bone marrow transplantation. Blood 1990;75:1011–1016.

24. McDonald GB, Sharma P, Matthews DE, et al. Veno-occlusive disease of the liver after bone marrow transplantation: diagnosis, incidence and predisposing factors. Hepatology 1984;4(1):116–122.

25. Stuart KL, Bras G. Veno-occlusive disease of the liver. Q J Med 1957;26:291–315.

26. Bach N, Thung S, Schaffner F. Comfrey herb tea-induced veno-occlusive disease. Am J Med 1989;87:97–99.

27. Stillman AE, Huxtable R, Constroe P, et al. Hepatic veno-occlusive disease due to pyrrolizidine (*Senecio*) poisoning in Arizona. Gastroenterology 1977;73:349–352.

28. Griner P, Elbadawi A, Packman C. Veno-occlusive disease of the liver after chemotherapy of acute leukemia: a report of two cases. Ann Intern Med 1976;85:578–582.

29. Asbury R, Rosenthal S, Descalzi M, et al. Hepatic veno-occlusive disease due to DTIC. Cancer 1980;45:2670–2674.

30. McClay E. Allergy-induced hepatic toxicity associated with dacarbazine. Cancer Treat Rep 1987;71:219–220.

31. Read A, Wiesner R, LaBreque D. Hepatic veno-occlusive disease associated with renal transplantation and azathioprine therapy. Ann Intern Med 1986;104:651–655.

32. Gill R, Onstad G, Cardamone J, et al. Hepatic veno-occlusive disease caused by 6-thioguanine. Ann Intern Med 1982;96:58–60.

33. D'Cruz C, Wimmer R, Harcke T, et al. Veno-occlusive disease of the liver in children following chemotherapy for acute myelocytic leukemia. Cancer 1983;52:1803–1807.

34. McIntyre R, Magidson J, Austin G, Gale RP. Fatal veno-occlusive disease of the liver following high-dose 1,3-Bis (2-chloroethyl)-1-nitrosourea (BCNU) and autologous bone marrow transplantation. Am J Clin Pathol 1981;75:614–617.

35. Phillips GL, Fay JW, Herzig GP, et al. Intensive 1,3-Bis (2-chloroethyl)-1-nitrosourea (BCNU), NSC #4366650 and cryopreserved autologous marrow transplantation for refractory cancer: a phase I-II study. Cancer 1983;52:1792–1802.

36. Kanfer EJ, Petersen FB, Buckner CD, et al. Phase I study of high-dose dimethylbusulfan followed by autologous bone marrow transplantation in patients with advanced malignancy. Cancer Treat Rep 1987;71:101–102.

37. Gottfried MR, Sudilovsky O. Hepatic veno-occlusive disease after high-dose mitomycin C and autologous bone marrow transplantation therapy. Hum Pathol 1982;13:646–650.

38. Lazarus H, Gottfried MR, Herzig RH, et al. Veno-occlusive disease of the liver after high-dose mitomycin C therapy and autologous bone marrow transplantation. Cancer 1982;49:1789–1795.

39. Fajardo LF, Colby TV. Pathogenesis of veno-occlusive liver disease after radiation. Arch Pathol Lab Med 1980;104:584–588.

40. Bearman SI, Appelbaum FR, Buckner CD, et al. Regimen-related toxicity in patients undergoing bone marrow transplantation. J Clin Oncol 1988;6:1562–1568.

41. Henner WD, Peters WP, Eder JP, et al. Pharmacokinetics and immediate effects of BCNU in man. Cancer Treat Rep 1986;70:877–880.

42. Grochow LB, Jones RJ, Brundrett RB, et al. Pharmacokinetics of busulfan: correlation with veno-occlusive disease in patients undergoing bone marrow transplantation. Cancer Chemother Pharmacol 1989;25:55–61.

43. Deeg HJ, Shulman H, Schmidt E, et al. Marrow graft rejection and veno-occlusive disease of the liver in patients with aplastic anemia conditioned with cyclophosphamide and cyclosporin. Transplantation 1986;42:497–501.

44. Essell JH, Borst DL, Harman GS, et al. Marked increase in veno-occlusive disease of the liver (VOD) associated with methotrexate (MTX) graft versus host disease (GVHD) prophylaxis in patients receiving busulfan/cyclophosphamide [Abstract 2137]. Blood 1990;76(suppl 1):537a.

45. Nimer SD, Milewicz AL, Champlin RW, et al. Successful treatment of hepatic veno-occlusive disease in a bone marrow transplant patient with orthotopic liver transplantation. Transplantation 1990;49:819–821.

46. Bearman SI, Hinds MS, Wolford JL, et al. A pilot study of continuous infusion heparin for the prevention of hepatic veno-occlusive disease after bone marrow transplantation. Bone Marrow Transplant 1990;5:407–411.

47. Gluckman E, Jolivet I, Scrobohaci ML, et al. Use of prostaglandin E1 for prevention of liver veno-occlusive disease in leukemic patients treated by allogeneic bone marrow transplantation. Br J Hematol 1990;74:277–281.

48. Bianco J, Nemunaitis J, Almgren J, et al. Pentoxyfylline (PTX) diminishes regimen-related toxicity (RRT) in patients undergoing bone marrow transplantation (BMT) [Abstract 2103]. Blood 1990;76(suppl 1):528a.

49. Baglin TP, Harper P, Marcus RE. Veno-occlusive disease of the liver complicating ABMT successfully treated with recombinant tissue plasminogen activator (rt-PA). Bone Marrow Transplant 1990;5:439–441.

50. Teicher BA, Crawford JM, Holden SA, et al. Glutathione monoethyl ester can selectively protect liver from high dose BCNU or cyclophosphamide. Cancer 1988;62:1275–1281.

51. Billingham RE. The biology of graft-versus-host reactions. Harvey Lect 1966–67;62:21–78.

52. Wick MR, Moore SB, Gastineau DA, Hoagland HC. Immunologic, clinical, and pathologic aspects of human graft-versus-host disease. Mayo Clin Proc 1983;58:603–612.

53. Shulman HM, McDonald GB. Liver disease after marrow transplantation. In: Sale GE, Shulman HM, eds. The pathology of bone marrow transplantation. New York: Masson, 1984:104–135.

54. Snover DC, Weisdorf SA, Ramsay NK, et al. Hepatic graft-versus-host disease: a study of the predictive value of liver biopsy in diagnosis. Hepatology 1984;4:123–130.

55. Shulman HM, Sharma P, McDonald GB. Discriminant analysis of liver histology in graft-versus-host disease [Abstract]. Lab Invest 1985;52:61A.

56. Slavin RE, Woodruff JM. The pathology of bone marrow transplantation. Pathol Annu 1974;9:291–344.

57. McDonald GB, Shulman HM, Sullivan KM, Spencer GD. Intestinal and hepatic complications of human bone marrow transplantation. Gastroenterology 1986;90:460–477;770–784.

58. Ferrara JLM, Deeg HJ. Graft versus host disease. N Engl J Med 1991;324:667–674.

59. Piguet PF, Grau GE, Allet B, Vassalli P. Tumor necrosis factor/cachesin is an effector of skin and gut lesions of the acute phase of graft versus host disease. J Exp Med 1987;166:1280.

60. Vogelsang GB, Hess AD, Santos GW. Acute graft-versus-host disease: clinical characteristics in the cyclosporin era. Medicine 1988;67:163–174.

61. Gale RP. Graft-versus-host disease. Immunol Rev 1985;88:193–214.

62. Glucksberg H, Storb R, Fefer A, et al. Clinical manifestations of graft-versus-host disease in human recipients of marrow from HLA-matched sibling donors. Transplantation 1974;18:295–304.

63. James WD, Odom RB. Graft-versus-host disease. Arch Dermatol 1983;119:683–689.

64. Martin PJ, Schoch G, Fisher L, et al. A retrospective analysis of therapy for acute graft-versus-host disease: initial treatment. Blood 1990;76:1464–1472.

65. Shulman HM, Sullivan KM, Weiden PL, et al. Chronic graft-versus-host syndromes in man: a long-term clinicopathologic study of 20 Seattle patients. Am J Med 1980;69:204–217.

66. Epstein O, Sherlock S, Thomas HC. Primary biliary cirrhosis is a dry gland syndrome with features of chronic graft-versus-host disease. Lancet 1980;1:1166–1168.

67. Tsoi MS, Storb R, Jones E, et al. Deposition of IgM and complement at the dermo-epidermal junction in acute and chronic graft-versus-host disease in man. J Immunol 1978;120:1485–1492.

68. Sullivan KM, Deeg J, Sanders JE, et al. Late complications after marrow transplantation. Semin Hematol 1984;21:53–63.

69. Tsoi MS, Storb R, Dobb S, et al. Nonspecific suppressor cells in patients with chronic graft-versus-host disease after marrow purging. J Immunol 1979; 123:1970–1976.

70. Tsoi MS, Storb R, Dobb S, et al. Cell-mediated immunity to non-HLA antigens of the host by donor lymphocytes in patients with chronic graft-versus-host disease. J Immunol 1980;125:2258–2262.

71. Sullivan KM, Shulman HM, Storb R, et al. Chronic graft-versus-host disease in 52 patients: adverse natural course and successful treatment with combination immunosuppression. Blood 1981;57:267–276.

72. Wingard JR, Piantadosi S, Vogelsang GB, et al. Predictors of death from chronic graft-versus-host disease after bone marrow transplantation. Blood 1989;764:1428–1435.

73. Wingard JR. Advances in the management of infectious complications after bone marrow transplantation. Bone Marrow Transplant 1990;6:371–383.

74. Winston DJ, Gale RP, Meyer DV, Young LS. Infectious complications of human bone marrow transplantation. Medicine 1979;58:1–31.

75. Kahls P, Danzer S, Kletter K, et al. Functional asplenia after bone marrow transplantation: a late complication related to extensive chronic graft-versus-host disease. Ann Intern Med 1988;109:461–464.

76. Pirsch JD, Maki DG. Infectious complications in adults with bone marrow transplantation and T cell depletion of donor marrow: increased susceptibility to fungal infections. Ann Intern Med 1986;104:619–631.

77. Villablanca J, Steiner M, Kersey J, et al. Alpha streptococcal bacteremia in bone marrow transplantation patients [Abstract 46]. Proc ASCO 1989;8:13.

78. Meyers JD. Fungal infections in bone marrow transplantation patients. Semin Oncol 1990;3(suppl 6):10–13.

79. Thaler M, Pastakia B, Shawker T, et al. Hepatic candidiasis in cancer patients: the evolving picture of the syndrome. Ann Intern Med 1988;108:88–100.

80. Walsh TJ, Hamilton SR. Disseminated aspergillosis complicating hepatic failure. Arch Intern Med 1983;143:1189–1191.

81. Corey L, Spear P. Infections with herpes simplex virus. N Engl J Med 1986;314:749–758.

82. Gottsdiener KM. Transplanted infections: donor to host transmission with the allograft. Ann Intern Med 1989;110:1001–1016.

83. Meyers JD, Fluornoy N, Thomas ED. Risk factors for cytomegalovirus infections after bone marrow transplantation. J Infect Dis 1986;153:478–488.

84. Spector SA. Diagnosis of cytomegalovirus infection. Semin Hematol 1990;27(2 suppl 1):11–16.

85. Locksley RM, Fluornoy N, Sullivan KM, Meyers JD. Infection with varicella-zoster virus after marrow transplantation. J Infect Dis 1985;152:1172–1181.

86. Straus SE, Ostrove JM, Inchauspe G, et al. Varicella-zoster virus infections. Ann Intern Med 1988;108:221–237.

87. Weller TH. Varicella and herpes zoster. N. Engl J Med 1983;309:1362–1368.

88. Alter M. Non A non B hepatitis: sorting through a diagnosis of exclusion. Ann Intern Med 1989;110:583–585.

89. List AF, Greco FA, Vogler LB. Lymphoproliferative disease in immunocompromised hosts: the role of Epstein-Barr virus. J. Clin Oncol 1987;5:1673–1689.

90. Blanche S, LeDeist F, Veber F, et al. Treatment of severe Epstein-Barr virus-induced polyclonal B-lymphocyte proliferation by anti-B-cell monoclonal antibodies. Ann Intern Med 1988;108:199–203.

91. Shields AF, Hackman RC, Fife KH, et al. Adenovirus infections in patients undergoing bone marrow transplantation. N Engl J Med 1985;312:529–533.

92. Neminaitis J, Rabinowe SN, Singer JW, et al. Recombinant granulocyte-macrophage colony stimulating factor after autologous bone marrow transplantation for lymphoid cancer. N Engl J Med 1991;324:1773–1778.

93. Gianni AM, Bregni M, Siena S, et al. Rapid and complete hematopoietic reconstitution following combined transplantation of autologous blood and bone marrow cells. A changing role for high dose chemoradiotherapy. Hematol Oncol 1989;7:139–148.

94. Elias A, Ayash L, Anderson K, et al. Hematologic support during high dose intensification for breast cancer: recruitment of peripheral blood progenitor cells by GM-CSF and chemotherapy [Abstract 2135]. Blood 1990;76(suppl 1):536a.

29

THE CARDIOVASCULAR SYSTEM AND ANTICANCER THERAPY

Paul D. Lindower and David J. Skorton

The last several decades have witnessed increasingly successful outcomes in the treatment of malignancies with anticancer therapy. Complicating this success is the fact that a greater proportion of cancer patients are surviving longer and beginning to manifest some of the long-term side effects from radiation and chemotherapy. The cardiovascular system, formerly felt to be relatively radioresistant (1) and generally spared from the major side effects of most chemotherapy may be significantly affected by some anticancer therapies (2, 3). Most commonly implicated in cardiovascular adverse effects are high-dose radiation therapy for lymphomas (4, 5), anthracycline treatment for a variety of malignancies (6, 7), and high-dose cyclophosphamide used in preparation for bone marrow transplantation (8). In some instances, toxicity to the cardiovascular system may be the dose-limiting factor in determining the treatment regimen. At issue in treating the patient is providing the maximum beneficial dose of therapy to obtain a remission of disease without inducing serious side effects. It is therefore important for the oncologist and primary care practitioner to be informed regarding potentially serious toxicities of therapy and their management. The intent of this chapter is to provide an overview of the general features of cardiotoxic effects of anticancer therapy and to provide an

approach to their diagnosis, management, and prevention.

RADIATION-INDUCED HEART DISEASE

The heart had long been considered a relatively radioresistant organ, as evidenced from early experimental studies in rodents (1). Subsequently, in the mid-1960s it became recognized that patients who had undergone curative forms of radiation therapy to the chest for Hodgkin's and non-Hodgkin's lymphoma experienced the development of dose-related cardiovascular disease (9). It has been definitively shown that the heart is in fact subject to radiation-induced injury that may involve all cardiac tissues. Most commonly affected is the pericardium, but myocardium, endocardium, papillary muscles, valvular structures, and coronary arteries may also be adversely affected by radiation (Table 29.1).

Experimental Studies

The radiosensitivity of the heart has been demonstrated in several animal models. Unlike early studies in rodents (1), subsequent experiments in New Zealand white rabbits have provided insight into the pathologic changes that occur in the cardiovascular system with radiation; these findings appear to

Table 29.1. Classification of Radiation-Related Cardiac Disease[a]

1. Acute pericarditis caused by necrosis of tumor adjacent to the heart)
2. Delayed pericarditis
   a. Acute radiation-induced pericarditis, without effusion.
   b. Acute radiation-induced pericarditis, with effusion, with/without cardiac tamponade.
   c. Chronic effusive pericarditis
   d. Effusive-constrictive pericarditis
   e. Chronic pericardial constriction
   f. Occult constrictive pericarditis
3. Myocardial fibrosis
4. Occlusive coronary artery disease
5. Conduction abnormalities
6. Valvular regurgitation or stenosis

[a]From Rosenthal DS, Braunwald E. Hematological-oncological disorders and heart diseases. In: Braunwald E, ed. Heart disease. 3rd ed. Philadelphia: WB Saunders, 1988:1734–1757.

closely parallel those changes seen in humans. In rabbits treated with a single dose of 2000 rads of radiation to the chest, three phases of toxicity may be observed (Fig. 29.1) (10). An acute phase is noted in the first 48 hours after treatment. Histologically, an inflammatory exudate of granulocytes is seen involving all heart tissues. These changes resolve over the ensuing 3–5 days, and throughout this time period the animals appear clinically well. Subsequently an intermediate latent phase occurs during which there are no definite manifestations of disease either by clinical examination or by light microscopy of tissue. Electron microscopy, however, reveals lesions of the myocardial capillary endothelium. Lastly, a late phase develops after approximately 70 days where there is progressive thickening and fibrosis of the pericardium with or without accompanying effusion or tamponade. Additionally, at this phase the animals are found to have extensive myocardial fibrosis.

Studies in humans suggest sequelae of radiation similar to those seen in animals. One autopsy series evaluated 16 patients who had received greater than 3500 rads of radiation to the chest. This study revealed pericardial

and other cardiac damage in all patients (11). Ninety-four percent of patients had thickened pericardia, and one-third were noted to have evidence for cardiac tamponade. Fifty percent of the patients had interstitial myocardial fibrosis involving the right ventricle to a greater extent than the left, presumably since the right ventricle is a more anterior structure and less shielded from the anteriorly weighted radiation than are the underlying tissues. In addition, endocardial and valvular thickening were noted along with coronary artery narrowing.

Pathophysiology

The pathophysiologic changes seen in radiation-induced heart disease have been ascribed to several mechanisms, which may occur in combination (4). Radiation appears to damage capillary endothelium, resulting in microvascular obliteration, bringing about ischemia and ultimately pericardial and myocardial fibrosis. Alternatively, pericardial disease potentially may be a result of radiation-induced modifications of pericardial antigens with a subsequent autoimmune reaction. Further, pericardial effusions may develop simply as a result of fibrotic obstruction to cardiac lymphatic drainage.

Several risk factors have been identified that may contribute to the likelihood of developing radiation-induced heart disease (5). These include a large tumor mass or substantial mediastinal lymphadenopathy, concomitant use of chemotherapy, and elevation of the erythrocyte sedimentation rate. Lymphocytopenia has been found to be relatively protective against the development of radiation-induced heart disease.

Effects of Radiation on Specific Cardiac Tissues

PERICARDIUM

Radiation-induced heart disease is most commonly manifest as pericarditis. Acute pericarditis may rarely occur several days fol-

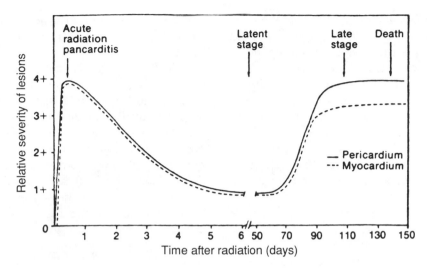

Figure 29.1. Temporal cause of radiation-induced cardiac abnormalities in an experimental model. Early acute radiation pancarditis is followed by a latent stage, during which severe lesions of the myocardial capillaries can be appreciated on electron microscopy. Following latent stage chronic pericardial and myocardial abnormalities are noted. (From Taymor-Luria H, Cohn K, Pasternak RC. Diagnostic challenge: how to identify radiation heart disease. J. Cardiovasc Med 1983;Jan:13–123.)

lowing treatment. This may represent an inflammatory response of the pericardium to necrosis of cancer tissue adjacent to the heart. Pericarditis more commonly is delayed and appears within the first 12 months of treatment, but may also occur up to 15 years later (12). Delayed pericarditis may be accompanied by a pericardial effusion with or without tamponade and may ultimately be manifest as constrictive disease. Delayed pericarditis is reported to occur in approximately 10%–15% of patients with Hodgkin's disease treated with greater than 4000 rads of radiation to the mediastinum (5).

MYOCARDIUM, ENDOCARDIUM, AND VALVES

Radiation-induced heart disease may also be manifest by involvement of myocardial, endocardial, or valvular structures. In one series of 21 women with breast cancer treated with radical mastectomy and postoperative radiation to the chest, a mild transient decrease in left ventricular systolic function was noted on echocardiography (13). This decrease in function resolved by 6 months following radiation treatment.

Endomyocardial fibrosis has been noted on histopathologic study of patients who have received radiation therapy to the chest. This may be manifest clinically as conduction abnormalities, restrictive cardiomyopathy, or valvular incompetence. Mitral regurgitation may result from radiation-induced papillary dysfunction, and aortic insufficiency may occur secondary to valvular thickening. One autopsy series found greater than three-fourths of patients treated with over 3500 rads of radiation therapy to the chest had evidence of myocardial fibrosis (12).

CORONARY ARTERIES

There is an association between radiation therapy and the development of occlusive disease of the coronary arteries. In one case report, a 15-year-old boy without any risk factors for premature atherosclerosis died from an acute myocardial infarction shortly after receiving 4000 rads of radiation therapy to the chest for Hodgkin's disease (9). Additional supportive evidence implicating radiation therapy as a cause of occlusive coronary artery disease is found in studies of experimental animals treated with radiation (14). Further, there are unique changes noted in the coronary arteries of patients treated with mediastinal radiation (11). In this setting there is severe fibrosis of the arterial wall media and adventitia in continuity with overlying epicardial fibrous tissue within the field of radiation. The proximal vessels appear to be more severely affected than the distal vessels, and involvement is also seen in other arteries that are irradiated. The plaque lesions seen in coronary arteries following radiation therapy are distinct from those typically seen in atherosclerotic cardiovascular disease. There is a relative lack of lipid material in the intima and a significant loss of smooth muscle tissue in the media, changes distinct from those of atherosclerosis.

Late Effects of Radiation

An increasing number of patients have been found to have radiation-induced heart disease up to 15 years following their treatment (12, 15). In one series of 81 patients, 11% (9 patients) were ultimately noted to have symptoms of dyspnea on exertion and evidence of elevated jugular venous pressure up to 10 years following radiation therapy (15). They underwent evaluation with right heart catheterization, and 67% were found to have frank constrictive pericarditis, while the remaining 33% were found to have an abnormal response to fluid challenge felt to represent occult constrictive disease. Another series of 25 patients who were treated with 4000 rads of radiation to the chest for Hodgkin's disease were found to have multiple cardiac abnormalities up to 15 years following treatment (12). These abnormalities were manifest as decreased ventricular systolic function, pericardial effusion, electrocardiographic changes, and clinical symptoms of

chest pain, palpitations, dyspnea on exertion, orthopnea, paroxysmal nocturnal dyspnea, and fatigue.

Techniques of radiation therapy have improved over the last several decades in an effort to reduce potential damage incurred by radiation. The cardiac silhouette is excluded as much as possible from the primary beam, and radiation is delivered through both anterior and posterior ports with judicious use of subcarinal blocks. It is hoped that these measures will reduce the subsequent incidence of radiation damage to the cardiovascular structures.

CARDIOTOXIC EFFECTS OF CANCER CHEMOTHERAPY

A number of chemotherapeutic agents have been shown to have toxic cardiac effects, ranging from nonspecific electrocardiographic changes to the development of frank congestive cardiomyopathy. The most notorious agents are the anthracyclines and their derivatives, which engender the chronic, dose-dependent development of congestive cardiomyopathy with systolic ventricular failure (6). In addition, high-dose cyclophosphamide is known to be cardiotoxic, although damage from this agent manifests more acutely with myocarditis and cardiomyopathy, with failure not dependent on cumulative dose (8).

Doxorubicin

Doxorubicin is an anthracycline antibiotic that has strong antitumor activity against a variety of cancers including acute leukemias; Hodgkin's and non-Hodgkin's lymphoma; breast, lung, and ovarian cancers; and sarcomas. The drug's tumoricidal effect is felt to be largely due to its ability to bind to DNA and thereby inhibit rapidly dividing cells (16).

CARDIAC EFFECTS

Doxorubicin has particular biochemical effects that may promote cardiac toxicity. These effects include its ability to form free radical species that may then bring about lipid and membrane peroxidation (17). Free radical formation has been documented in animal studies. For example, malondialdehyde, a breakdown product of lipid peroxides, has been demonstrated in the cardiac tissues of mice treated with doxorubicin (18). The effects of the free radicals may be potentiated in cardiac tissue as the myocardium appears to possess a relatively poor free radical scavenger enzyme system with low catalase and superoxide dismutase activities, and weak nicotinamide adenine dinucleotide phosphate (NADPH) reducing capacity (16).

Several clinical risk factors have been identified that are associated with the development of doxorubicin-induced congestive cardiomyopathy (Table 29.2) (19). Age extremes in both the pediatric population and those over the age of 70 years; prior cardiac disease including hypertension, coronary artery disease, and valvular disease; prior history of radiation therapy; prior history of cyclophosphamide administration; and increasing cumulative dose of doxorubicin, especially doses greater than 550 mg/m^2 (Fig. 29.2) (20) all seem to contribute to the risk of developing cardiotoxicity.

Doxorubicin-induced congestive heart failure has held a reputation for a particularly grim prognosis, with reported mortalities of up to 60% (3). One recent case series would indicate that patients who develop doxorubicin-induced heart failure may actually fare

somewhat better (21). Of 43 patients with cancer who were treated with doxorubicin and who developed congestive failure, 58% responded well to standard therapy with digoxin, diuretics, and afterload reduction. Of the remaining 42%, over half initially responded to treatment, while the remainder died with refractory failure. The overall mortality of doxorubicin-induced congestive failure alone in this series of patients was 28%.

The cardiac effects of doxorubicin may be divided temporally into early and late categories (3). Acutely, during the peri-infusion period, a variety of electrocardiographic changes have been described, including nonspecific ST and T wave changes, premature atrial and ventricular contractions, supraventricular tachyarrhythmia, and, rarely, sudden cardiac death. Transient early left ventricular dysfunction may also rarely occur, especially in patients with poor underlying cardiac function. Finally, an acute pericarditis and myocarditis syndrome has been occasionally noted.

Late effects of doxorubicin, which are of greater clinical importance, may develop weeks to months following therapy and are manifest as a degenerative cardiomyopathy with congestive heart failure. These chronic effects are dependent on the total cumulative dose, and their incidence ranges from 2%–20% depending on the presence of underlying risk factors.

HISTOPATHOLOGIC ABNORMALITIES

Doxorubicin induces characteristic lesions of the myocardial cells as seen on electron microscopy of biopsy specimens (Fig. 29.3) (22, 23). These changes include vacuolar degeneration of the sarcoplasmic reticulum and mitochondria, along with myofibrillar "drop out." A pathologic grading scale has been developed that rates the severity of morphologic damage on a scale from 0.0 (normal) to 3.0 (severe damage) (Table 29.3). A grade of 2.0 or greater denotes more than 25% probability that a patient will develop

Table 29.2. Risk Factors Associated with the Development of Doxorubicin Cardiotoxicity[a]

Cumulative dose (>550 mg/m^2)
Age extremes
Preexistent coronary artery disease
Hypertension
Metastatic pericardial or myocardial disease
Prior mediastinal irradiation
Coexistent chemotherapy with alkylating agents

[a]From Rosenthal DS, Braunwald E. Hematological-oncological disorders and heart diseases. In: Braunwald E, ed. Heart disease. 3rd ed. Philadelphia: WB Saunders, 1988:1734–1757.

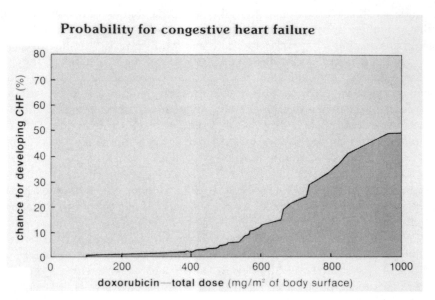

Figure 29.2.   Relationship between cumulative dose of doxorubicin and probability of developing congestive heart failure. At approximately 550 mg/m², the chance of developing congestive heart failure exceeds 5%; it rises steeply thereafter. (From Greene HL, Reich SD, Dalen JE. Drug therapy: how to minimize doxorubicin toxicity. J Cardiovasc Med 1982;Mar:306–321.)

congestive cardiomyopathy with further doxorubicin administration. The biopsy score correlates directly with the cumulative dose of doxorubicin. Myocardial function declines exponentially with increasing biopsy score. Initially, despite significant morphologic damage of the myocytes, myocardial function may remain relatively intact. However, with additional myocardial damage, there is an increasing decline in myocardial function. Dramatic worsening of ventricular function could potentially develop with subsequent doxorubicin dosages.

MONITORING TECHNIQUES

At issue in treating cancer patients with doxorubicin is providing the individual patient with a dose of the chemotherapeutic agent sufficient to produce a remission without inducing a severe cardiomyopathy or other toxicity. The arbitrary limitation of doxorubicin dosage to <550 mg/m² could potentially withhold further life-prolonging treatment and likewise could encourage further administration of drug in the face of significant toxicity. The best independent standard for monitoring cardiotoxicity due to doxorubicin is right heart catheterization with right ventricular endomyocardial biopsy (23). This procedure, however, is expensive, invasive, has known risks, and requires a catheterization laboratory and experienced cardiologist and cardiac pathologist. A number of noninvasive monitoring techniques have been employed in following the course of cardiac function in patients treated with doxorubicin. These include electrocardiography, phonocardiography, echocardiography, and radionuclide angiography. The latter technique is particularly useful in following patients serially while they are receiving therapy (24–27). The radionuclide angiogram provides functional assessment of the heart in the form of left and right ventricular ejection fractions, and its results correlate with those found on biopsy. Further, it is safe, relatively inexpensive, readily available, reasonably sensitive, and reproducible.

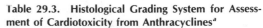

Table 29.3. Histological Grading System for Assessment of Cardiotoxicity from Anthracyclines[a]

Grade[b]	Morphology
0	Normal myocardial ultrastructural morphology
1	Isolated myocytes affected by distended sarcotubular system and/or early myofibrillar loss; damage to <5% of all cells in 10 plastic blocks
1.5	Changes similar to those in grade 1 but with damage to 6%–15% of all cells in 10 plastic blocks
2.0	Clusters of myocytes affected by myofibrillar loss and/or vacuolization, with damage to 16%–25% of all cells in 10 plastic blocks
2.5	Many myocytes, ≤26%–35% of all cells in 10 plastic blocks, affected by vacuolization and/or myofibrillar loss
3.0	Severe and diffuse myocyte damage (>35% of all cells in 10 plastic blocks) affected by vacuolization and/or myofibrillar loss

[a]From Billingham ME, Bristow MR. Evaluation of anthracycline cardiotoxicity: predictive ability and functional correlation of endomyocardial biopsy. Cancer Treat Symp 1984;3:71–76.
[b]At grade 2.5, only 1 more dose of anthracycline should be given without further evaluation. At grade 3.0, no more anthracycline should be given.

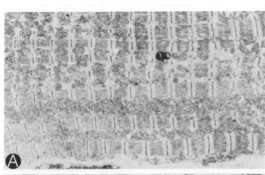

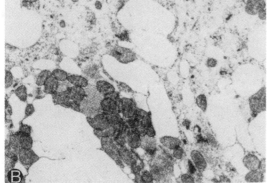

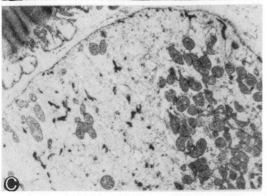

Figure 29.3. Electron microscopic abnormalities noted in endomyocardial biopsy specimens in doxorubicin cardiotoxicity. **A,** Normal cardiac muscle fiber (corresponding to histologic grade 0). **B,** vacuolization of cardiocytes. **C,** More severe damage leading to myofibrillar dropout. (From Ali MK, Ewer MS. Cancer and the cardiopulmonary system. New York: Raven Press, 1984: 62 and 63.)

Left ventricular systolic function as assessed by radionuclide angiography has been shown to correlate with the clinical status of the patient. In one study, serial radionuclide studies were obtained in 55 patients receiving doxorubicin (24). Even a decrease in left ventricular ejection fraction of <10% was found to precede the development of congestive heart failure and as such was a sensitive marker for declining cardiac function. In six patients with moderate dysfunction and left ventricular ejection fraction <45%, further therapy was withheld, and none of the patients developed congestive failure. The overall change in ejection fraction and lowest ejection fraction correlated with the cumulative dose of doxorubicin. Additional studies have demonstrated that combined rest and exercise radionuclide studies increase the sensitivity for detecting patients at risk for congestive failure but that this occurs at the expense of specificity. In one study, resting radionuclide angiography had a sensitivity of 53% with a specificity of 75%, and these changed to 89% and 41%, respectively, with the addition of an exercise study (26).

Although there is not unanimity of opinion, reasonable recommendations (Fig. 29.4) (26) for cardiac monitoring during the administration of doxorubicin might include empiric dose limitation to 450 mg/m^2 in patients without any cardiovascular risk factors. If additional therapy is to be given, then a baseline study of left ventricular ejection fraction should be obtained by radionuclide angiography and followed every other dose (or each 100 mg/m^2) until the ejection fraction is <45% or fails to rise >5% with exercise.

In such instance, right heart catheterization with endomyocardial biopsy should be performed. If the subsequent biopsy grade is 2.0 or less, the patient may safely receive further therapy. Otherwise, in patients with resting ejection fractions <30% or biopsy scores >2.0, further doxorubicin therapy should be withheld, as these patients are at significant risk for developing congestive cardiomyopathy. In patients with cardiovascular risk factors, a baseline radionuclide assessment should be performed prior to the third dose of doxorubicin and repeated every other dose (or each 100 mg/m^2) with application of the above principles.

It should be noted that a variety of factors may contribute to variability of ejection

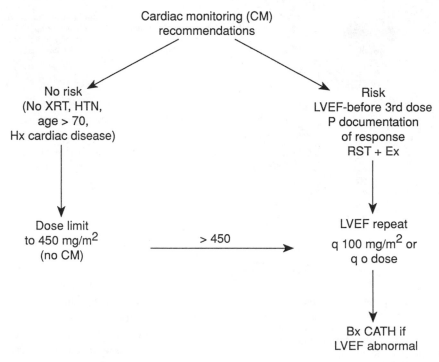

Figure 29.4. A suggested method of monitoring cardiac status during anthracycline therapy. In the absence of risk factors or history of cardiac disease, no cardiac monitoring is suggested until a cumulative dose of 450 mg/m^2 is reached. At that point, if further anthracycline is to be given, then serial assessment of left ventricular ejection fraction is suggested. This serial assessment of ejection fraction is suggested earlier in the course of anthracycline therapy if there is a history of risk factors for cardiac disease. (From McKillop JH, Bristow MR, Goris ML, Billingham ME, Bockemuehl K. Sensitivity and specificity of radionuclide ejection fractions in doxorubicin cardiotoxicity. Am Heart J 1983;106:1084–1086.)

fractions in serial studies of individual patients (28). Such factors include technical artifacts, variation in sympathetic tone, changes in cardiac loading conditions (particularly afterload), and the intrinsic inotropic effect of doxorubicin itself. Studies should be performed as possible in the absence of confounding clinical factors, and at least several weeks following the last dose of doxorubicin, in an effort to minimize acute inotropic effects of the drug.

PREVENTIVE MEASURES

Several clinical trials have been performed in which methods of administration have been altered in an attempt to attenuate the cardiotoxicity of doxorubicin without altering its antitumor effects. The administration of various concomitant agents has been attempted, including vitamin E, N-acetylcysteine, and verapamil, generally with disappointing results (6). Reduced toxicity, however, has been achieved in trials where the dosage schedule was altered to administer the drug by slow intravenous infusion over 96 hours rather than over 30 minutes (as it is usually given) (29). In one study, 21 patients receiving the slow infusion were compared to 30 control patients. Ten percent of those receiving the slow infusion, compared to 47% of those in the control group, were found to have severe morphologic changes on biopsy. Additionally, mean histologic scores were significantly different (0.9 and 1.6, respectively). The reduced toxicity was felt to be best explained on the basis of a significantly reduced peak plasma level of the drug in the slow infusion group as compared to the control group. There was no evidence for compromise of antitumor activity of the drug.

Similarly, another trial involved the administration of an ethylene diamine tetraacetic acid (EDTA)-like chelating agent, ICRF-187 (razoxane), concomitantly with doxorubicin in 92 women with breast cancer (30). Congestive heart failure developed in 4% of patients receiving ICRF-187 versus 24% in patients receiving placebo, and the biopsy score was >2.0 (severe) in 0% and 38% of the ICRF-187 and placebo groups, respectively. ICRF-187 apparently offers significant protection against cardiac toxicity without altering the antitumor effect of doxorubicin. The exact mechanism of this protection is unclear but is felt to be related to chelation of ferrous ion, which decreases doxorubicin's tendency to form an iron compound capable of generating free radicals.

Studies also have been done utilizing doxorubicin analogues in an attempt to identify a compound with retained antitumor activity but significantly less cardiotoxicity. One such analogue epirubicin, the 4' epimer of doxorubicin, has approximately 60% of the cardiotoxic effects of doxorubicin and similar anti-cancer effects (31). Epirubicin is continuing to undergo clinical trials. Another such agent is mitoxantrone, a synthetic anthraquinone similar to doxorubicin with retained antitumor activity and less cardiotoxicity (32).

Doxorubicin is a very efficacious antitumor agent whose usefulness is limited by dose-related cardiotoxicity. Substantial individual variability in susceptibility to the cardiotoxic effects precludes mere empiric dose limitation of the drug. Patients may be followed with serial radionuclide angiographic determination of left ventricular ejection fraction for early identification of the development of cardiotoxicity. Patients who develop doxorubicin-induced heart failure may respond to aggressive therapy with digoxin, diuretics, and afterload reduction. The cardiotoxic effects of doxorubicin may be further limited by administering it as a slow infusion, possibly with coadministration of protective agents (ICRF-187). Finally, related analogue compounds with retained antitumor effects and less cardiotoxicity are under evaluation.

Cyclophosphamide

Cyclophosphamide is an alkylating agent used both as an immunosuppressant and as an antitumor agent. At standard dosages it has several commonly recognized side effects, including myelosuppression, alopecia, interstitial pneumonitis, impaired water excretion, and hemorrhagic cystitis. At higher doses it has been associated with significant cardiotoxicity (8).

MECHANISM OF ADVERSE CARDIAC EFFECTS AND HISTOPATHOLOGIC CHANGES

Cyclophosphamide's toxic effects on the heart have been described as an "acute lethal carditis" (33). These effects generally occur within 3 weeks of treatment and are not due to cumulative doses of the drug. The appearance of cardiotoxicity may manifest itself clinically as acute or subacute onset of congestive failure with pulmonary congestion, weight gain, and oliguria. The electrocardiogram reveals a decrease in the QRS voltage, along with nonspecific ST and T wave changes, and prolongation of the QT interval, although these changes are not predictive of those patients who subsequently develop congestive failure (8). Those patients who do not develop heart failure appear to ultimately recover from these abnormal findings and return to their baseline status. Histopathologic changes of the myocardium due to cyclophosphamide toxicity appear to represent a toxic vasculitic process manifest as transmural cardiac hemorrhage and necrosis along with interstitial edema and separation of the muscle fibers (34).

PATHOPHYSIOLOGY

Cyclophosphamide is felt to exert its cardiotoxic effects through damage to vascular structures, particularly the myocardial capillary endothelium (34). This damage results in increased capillary permeability and microthromboses, ultimately producing extravasation of plasma and red blood cells into the myocardium. Further, this extravasated plasma itself contains cyclophosphamide, which may cause additional local damage.

CLINICAL STUDIES

The incidence, clinical characteristics, and prognosis of cyclophosphamide-induced cardiotoxicity were reviewed in a case series of patients undergoing bone marrow transplantation (8). Thirty-two patients received high-dose cyclophosphamide (180 mg/kg). Decreased left ventricular function was noted on echocardiogram 5–16 days after treatment. Thirty-three percent of the patients developed a pericardial effusion. The electrocardiogram revealed decreased QRS voltage, even in patients without pericardial effusions. Twenty-eight percent of the patients developed congestive heart failure, and 67% of those with failure died. Cardiac tamponade developed in 19%. The associated changes of decreased QRS voltage, decreased left ventricular systolic function, and presence of a pericardial effusion on echocardiogram seen in patients treated with high-dose cyclophosphamide did not appear to correlate with the development of heart failure. Those patients who did not develop failure ultimately had full reversal of these abnormal findings.

Another study evaluated a series of patients for cyclophosphamide-induced cardiotoxicity with respect to dose per body surface area (35). Eighty-four percent were treated with cyclophosphamide in preparation for bone marrow transplantation. Seventeen percent developed congestive heart failure felt to be secondary to cyclophosphamide, and 43% of those with heart failure died. The dose of cyclophosphamide was calculated with respect to the patient's body surface area, and 13 of 14 patients who developed heart failure had been given >1.55 gm/m^2. There was no significant difference in the outcome of the transplantation in patients given the higher versus lower dose of cyclophosphamide. Cyclophosphamide-induced heart failure was much more likely; however, if patients had received >1.55 gm/m^2 of the drug.

In another study of 17 patients with acute leukemias, the cardiotoxic effect of cyclophosphamide in combination with total body irradiation was evaluated with noninvasive studies of cardiac size and function (36). Serial measurements of left ventricular systolic function were obtained before and after preparation for bone marrow transplantation with cyclophosphamide given at 90 mg/kg and 900 cGy radiation therapy. As a group, the patients showed no statistically significant decline in left ventricular ejection fraction (58% to 56%). However, 7 patients had a decline in their ejection fraction from an average baseline of 60% to 50%. None of the patients developed clinical evidence of heart failure, and the results were felt to demonstrate that cyclophosphamide at this dose in this regimen was safely tolerated although associated with a mild decline in ventricular function in some patients. Thus patients should be followed long-term, since the natural history of their left ventricular function is unknown.

Cyclophosphamide is an alkylating agent with effective immunosuppressive and antitumor effects. When given at high doses (>180 mg/kg), it is associated with development of an acute cardiomyopathy that occurs in the clinical setting of severe heart failure and reduced QRS voltage on electrocardiogram and that is not dependent on the cumulative dose of the drug. Patients receiving greater than 1.55 gm/m^2 appear to be at greater risk for developing heart failure. Those who do not develop failure generally have full recovery of their clinical electrocardiographic abnormalities. It is unclear whether concomitant use of cyclophosphamide with radiation therapy or other chemotherapy significantly contributes to combined toxicity. At present, it is reasonable that patients receiving high-dose cyclophosphamide should be followed closely for the development of cardiac toxicity.

Other Agents

AMSACRINE

Amsacrine is an acridine derivative with antitumor activity against acute leukemias. Its mode of action is felt to be similar to that of the anthracyclines with DNA-binding prop-

erties. It is felt to have similar but less severe cardiotoxic effects than doxorubicin, with acute arrhythmias and chronic cardiomyopathy described in the literature. A recent review noted that of 6000 patients treated with amsacrine, only 1.4% were reported to have presumed cardiotoxicity ranging from electrocardiographic changes to development of congestive heart failure (37). There was no apparent cumulative effect of the drug, and a potential risk factor for the development of arrhythmia was hypokalemia.

5-FLUOROURACIL

5-Fluorouracil is an antimetabolite anticancer agent that acts by inhibiting thymidylate synthetase and synthesis of DNA. It has been noted to have cardiotoxic effects that mimic ischemia, manifest as electrocardiographic changes, acute myocardial infarction, cardiogenic shock, and sudden cardiac death (38). Although these findings were reproducible with readministration of the drug, they are otherwise poorly characterized. Use of 5-fluorouracil should probably be avoided in patients with known underlying ischemic heart disease, and it should be given in a monitored setting to those patients with prior known sensitivity.

CYTOSINE ARABINOSIDE

High-dose cytosine arabinoside treatment has been associated with the development of cardiac arrhythmias (39) and pericarditis (40). A case report described the development of pericarditis in a 25-year-old man with acute lymphocytic leukemia treated with intermittent high-dose cytosine arabinoside. The patient ultimately developed tamponade and underwent pericardiocentesis. Evaluation of the pericardial fluid was negative for malignant cells, gram stain, acid fast stain, antinuclear antibody, viral, fungal, or bacterial cultures.

CONCLUSIONS

The increasing success of treating malignancies with anticancer therapy has been complicated in that a larger proportion of patients are surviving longer and manifesting late toxic effects from radiation and chemotherapy. Specifically, potential cardiovascular toxicity may be the dose-limiting factor in determining cancer patients' treatment regimens. Improvements in radiation therapy techniques and noninvasive monitoring of cardiac function during chemotherapy have assisted the overall clinical management of patients. Further preventive measures include the development of less cardiotoxic anticancer drugs along with the coadministration of protective agents during therapy. It remains important for the oncologist and primary care practitioner to be informed regarding the potential toxic effects of anticancer therapies. It is hoped that through greater awareness and prevention, the incidence of cardiovascular toxicity from anticancer therapy will decline.

Acknowledgments

The authors thank Carolyn Frisbie for expert preparation of the manuscript.

References

1. Leach JE, Sugiura K. The effect of high voltage roentgen rays on heart of adult rats. Am J. Roentgenol Rad Therapy 1941;45:414–425.
2. Kantrowitz NE, Bristow MR. Cardiotoxicity of antitumor agents. Prog Cardiovasc Dis 1984;27:195–200.
3. Rosenthal DS, Braunwald E. Hematological-oncological disorders and heart disease. In: Braunwald E, ed. Heart disease. 3rd ed. Philadelphia: WB Saunders, 1988:1734–1757.
4. Stewart JR, Fajardo LF. Radiation-induced heart disease: an update. Prog Cardiovasc Dis 1984;27:173–194.
5. Taymor-Luria H, Cohn K, Pasternak RC. Diagnostic challenge: how to identify radiation heart disease. J Cardiovasc Med 1983;Jan:113–123.
6. Greene HL, Reich SD, Dalen JE. Drug therapy: how to minimize doxorubicin toxicity. J Cardiovasc Med 1982;Mar:306–321.
7. Unverferth DV, Magorien RD, Leier CV, Balcerzak SP. Doxorubicin cardiotoxicity. Cancer Treat Rev 1982;9:149–164.
8. Gottdiener JS, Appelbaum FR, Ferrans VJ, Deisseroth A, Ziegler J. Cardiotoxicity associated with high-dose cyclophosphamide therapy. Arch Intern Med 1981;141:758–763.
9. Cohn KE, Stewart JR, Fajardo LF, Hancock EW. Heart disease following radiation. Medicine 1967;46:281–298.
10. Stewart JR, Fajardo LF. Radiation-induced heart disease: clinical and experimental aspects. Radiol Clin North Am 1971;9:511–531.
11. Brosius FC, Waller BF, Roberts WC. Radiation heart disease: analysis of 16 young (aged 15 to 33 years) necropsy patients who received over 3,500 rads to the heart. Am J Med 1981;70:519–530.
12. Gottdiener JS, Katin MJ, Borer JS, Bacharach SL, Green MV. Late cardiac effects of therapeutic mediastinal irradiation: assessment by echocardiography and radionuclide angiography. N Engl J Med 1983;308:569–572.
13. Ikaheimo MJ, Niemela KO, Linnaluoto MM, Jakobsson MJT, Takkunen JT, Taskinen PJ. Early cardiac changes related to radiation therapy. Am J Cardiol 1985;56:943–946.
14. Amromin GD, Gildenhorn HL, Solomon RD, Nadkarni BB, Jacobs ML. The synergism of X-irradiation and cholesterol-fat feeding on the development of coronary artery lesions. J. Atherosclerosis Res 1964;4:325–334.
15. Applefeld MM, Cole JF, Pollock SH, et al. The late appearance of chronic pericardial disease in patients treated by radiotherapy for Hodgkin's disease. Ann Intern Med 1981;94:338–341.
16. Young RC, Ozols RF, Myers CE. The anthracycline antineoplastic drugs. N Engl J Med 1981;305:139–153.
17. Fu LX, Waagstein F, Hjalmarson A. A new insight into adriamycin-induced cardiotoxicity. Int J Cardiol 1990;29:15–20.
18. Myers CE, McGuire WP, Liss RH, Grotzinger K. Adriamycin: the role of lipid peroxidation in cardiac toxicity and tumor response. Science 1977;197:165–167.
19. Von Hoff DD, Layard MW, Basa P, et al. Risk factors for doxorubicin-induced congestive heart failure. Ann Intern Med 1979;91:710–717.
20. Lefrak EA, Pitha J, Rosenheim S, Gottlieb JA. A clinicopathologic analysis of adriamycin cardiotoxicity. Cancer 1973;32:302–314.
21. Haq MM, Legha SS, Choksi J, et al. Doxorubicin-induced congestive heart failure in adults. Cancer 1985;56:1361–1365.
22. Bristow MR, Mason JW, Billingham ME, Daniels JR. Doxorubicin cardiomyopathy: evaluation by phonocardiography, endomyocardial biopsy, and cardiac catheterization. Ann Intern Med 1978;88:168–175.
23. Billingham ME, Bristow MR. Evaluation of anthracycline cardiotoxicity: predictive ability and functional correlation of endomyocardial biopsy. Cancer Treat Symp 1984;3:71–76.
24. Alexander J, Dainiak N, Berger HJ, et al. Serial assessment of doxorubicin cardiotoxicity with quantitative radionuclide angiocardiography. N Engl J Med 1979;300:278–283.

25. Gottdiener JS, Mathisen DJ, Borer JS, et al. Doxo-rubicin cardiotoxicity: assessment of late left ven-tricular dysfunction by radionuclide cineangiogra-phy. Ann Intern Med 1981;94:430–435.
26. McKillop JH, Bristow MR, Goris ML, Billingham ME, Bockemuehl K. Sensitivity and specificity of radio-nuclide ejection fractions in doxorubicin cardiotox-icity. Am Heart J 1983;106:1048–1056.
27. Choi BW, Berger HJ, Schwartz PE, et al. Serial radio-nuclide assessment of doxorubicin cardiotoxicity in cancer patients with abnormal baseline resting left ventricular performance. Am Heart J 1983;106:638–643.
28. Dey HM, Kassamali H. Radionuclide evaluation of doxorubicin cardiotoxicity: the need for cautious interpretation. Clin Nucl Med 1988;13:565–568.
29. Legha SS, Benjamin RS, Mackay B, et al. Reduction of doxorubicin cardiotoxicity by prolonged contin-uous intravenous infusion. Ann Intern Med 1982; 96:133–139.
30. Speyer JL, Green MD, Kramer E, et al. Protective ef-fect of the bispiperazinedione ICRF-187 against doxorubicin-induced cardiac toxicity in women with advanced breast cancer. N Engl J Med 1988;319:745–752.
31. Torti FM, Bristow MM, Lum BL, et al. Cardiotoxicity of epirubicin and doxorubicin: assessment by en-domyocardial biopsy. Cancer Res 1986;46:3722–3727.
32. Unverferth DV, Unverferth BJ, Balcerzak SP, Bashore

TA, Neidhart JA. Cardiac evaluation of mitoxantrone. Cancer Treat Rep 1983;67:343–350.
33. Appelbaum FR, Strauchen JA, Graw RG Jr. Acute le-thal carditis caused by high-dose combination che-motherapy: a unique clinical and pathological entity. Lancet 1976;10:58–62.
34. Slavin RE, Millan JC, Mullins GM. Pathology of high dose intermittent cyclophosphamide therapy. Hum Pathol 1975;6:693–709.
35. Goldberg MA, Antin JH, Guinan EC, Rappeport JM. Cyclophosphamide cardiotoxicity: an analysis of dos-ing as a risk factor. Blood 1986;68:1114–1118.
36. Baello EB, Ensberg ME, Ferguson DW, et al. Effect of high-dose cyclophosphamide and total-body ir-radiation on left ventricular function in adult pa-tients with leukemia undergoing allogeneic bone marrow transplantation. Cancer Treat Rep 1986; 70:1187–1193.
37. Weiss RB, Grillo-Lopez AJ, Marsoni S, Posada JG Jr, Hess F, Ross BJ. Amsacrine-associated cardiotoxicity: an analysis of 82 cases. J Clin Oncol 1986;4:918–928.
38. Ensley JF, Patel B, Kloner R, Kish JA, Wynne J, Al-Sarraf M. The clinical syndrome of 5-fluorouracil car-diotoxicity. Invest New Drugs 1989;7:101–109.
39. Willemze R, Zwaan FE, Colpin G, Keuning JJ. High dose cytosine arabinoside in the management of re-fractory acute leukaemia. Scand J Haematol 1982; 29:141–146.
40. Vaickus L, Letendre L. Pericarditis induced by high-dose cytarabine therapy. Arch Intern Med 1984; 144:1868–1869.

30

DERMATOLOGY

Ellen Beth Rest and Thomas D. Horn

Patients receiving high-dose cancer therapy experience a diverse array of cutaneous sequelae. Certain cutaneous disorders occur almost exclusively in this population and afford a fertile source of investigation. Other eruptions develop commonly in the general population, yet proper identification is complicated by the necessity to remain vigilant for graft-versus-host disease (GVHD) in patients receiving a bone marrow transplant and for cutaneous signs of systemic infection in all aplastic patients. Drug hypersensitivity and toxicity, while rarely life-threatening, also develop commonly due to the myriad medications given to each person.

Certain cutaneous eruptions are quite distinct in their morphologies. Primary lesion types are described in Table 30.1. Other rashes are less clinically specific, requiring examination of skin tissue to help establish a diagnosis. The notion that one red rash looks like any other impedes our understanding of important biologic events. Successful clinicopathologic correlation and prospective study have resulted in a great expansion of our knowledge of the causes of cutaneous eruptions occurring in patients with profound marrow aplasia. In this chapter, we focus on common eruptions of vital significance to patient management as well as newly recognized and less common cutaneous findings. The clinical and histologic manifestations of lymphoma and leukemia cutis are not discussed here.

DRUG TOXICITY AND HYPERSENSITIVITY

Mucutaneous reactions to chemotherapeutic agents are varied and depend on the agent or agents in use (Table 30.2). The reactions have been grouped according to pathophysiologic mechanism and are presented below.

Cytotoxic Effects

Cytotoxic agents affect rapidly dividing cell populations such as those in the hair, nails, and oral mucosa, causing alopecia, Beau's lines, and stomatitis, respectively.

ALOPECIA

The anagen or growing hair contains a very rapidly proliferating cell population and therefore is a target for cytotoxic agents. Approximately 85% of the scalp hair follicles are in the anagen phase at any one time; thus a majority of the scalp hair is affected by cytotoxic drugs. There is inhibition of mitotic activity within the hair matrix, resulting in fragile or defective hair shafts that are subject to breakage with minimal trauma (anagen effluvium). There may be complete inhibition of hair shaft formation. Scalp hair is affected first (Fig. 30.1), but with repeating cycles of treatment, hair-bearing areas with lower percentages of anagen follicles, such as the beard, axilla, pubis, eyelash, and eyebrow, may be

Table 30.1. Primary Dermatologic Lesions

Lesion	Description	Example
Macule	Small, circumscribed area of color change; erythema, hypo- or hyperpigmentation; little to no surface change	Lentigo
Papule	Small (>1 CM) elevated lesion	Melanocytic nevus
Patch	Large circumscribed area of color change; hypo- or hyperpigmentation; little to no surface change	Café-au-lait spot
Plaque	Large (<1 CM) elevated lesion	Psoriatic lesions
Vesicle	Small (<0.5 CM) elevated, fluid-filled lesion; fluid is clear	Early herpes zoster
Bulla	Large (0.5 CM) elevated fluid-filled lesion; fluid is clear	Bullous pemphigoid
Nodule	Palpable solid lesion, below the epidermis	Lipoma
Pustule	Discrete elevated lesion containing purulent material	Folliculitis
Erosion	Discrete depressed lesion resulting from loss of a portion of epidermis; may result from rupture of vesicle or bulla; generally nonscarring	Bullous impetigo
Ulcer	Discrete depressed lesion resulting from loss of full thickness of epidermis and some portion of dermis; may result from rupture of vesicle or bulla; scarring	Pyoderma gangrenosum

affected. Hair loss is initially noted at 1–2 weeks after the initiation of therapy and is maximal at 1–2 months.

Drugs that are most commonly associated with alopecia are bleomycin, cyclophosphamide, dactinomycin, daunorubicin, doxorubicin, 5-fluorouracil, hydroxyurea, mechlorethamine, methotrexate, mitomycin, vinblastine, and vincristine (1). Combinations of agents such as cyclophosphamide and doxorubicin may be additive in effect and cause the most severe changes (2).

Hair generally regrows after discontinuation of chemotherapeutic agents, starting 4–6 weeks later, but complete regrowth may take 1–2 years. Some patients complain that the hair never regains its original color, texture, or thickness (3). Attempts to prevent alopecia after administation of chemotherapeutic agents have been variably successful. Scalp tourniquets and scalp hypothermia have been tried but generally only retard the development of alopecia and may not be used in hematologic malignancy (4, 5). A recent study (6) investigated the potential of Imuvert, a biologic response modifier derived from *Serratia marcescens*, to protect against chemotherapy-induced alopecia in rats. Imuvert offered complete protection against alopecia induced by cytarabine and doxorub-

icin and partial protection against cyclophosphamide-induced alopecia.

STOMATITIS

Stomatitis is a well-known cytotoxic effect of chemotherapeutic agents. Agents that are commonly associated with stomatitis include 5-fluorouracil, methotrexate, dactinomycin, doxorubicin, daunorubicin, bleomycin, cytarabine, and less frequently cyclophosphamide, 6-mercaptopurine, mithramycin, mitomycin C, vincristine, procarbazine, amsacrine, and interleukin-2. Symptoms, generally oral burning, begin within 1 week of drug administration, and stomatitis progresses rapidly with discrete and then confluent ulceration (Fig. 30.2). Common sites of involvement include buccal mucosa, tongue, and gingivae, although any oropharyngeal site may be involved (7). There is some evidence that poor oral hygiene prior to bone marrow transplantation (BMT) may predispose the patient to stomatitis. Involvement may be severe, preventing adequate oral intake of fluid and nutrition. Secondary infection by bacteria, viruses, or fungi, especially *Candida* sp., may complicate stomatitis.

Prevention of stomatitis is generally not successful. Allopurinol mouthwash was initially thought to be helpful in preventing mu-

Table 30.2. Mucocutaneous reactions to chemotherapeutic agents

Drug	Common Effects	Occasional Effects	Rare Effects
Alkylating agents			
Cyclophosphamide	Alopecia	Hyperpigmentation of skin or nails, stomatitis	Urticaria, anaphylaxis
Chlorambucil			Urticaria
Melphalan			Urticaria, angioedema, anaphylaxis, nail pigmentation
Busulfan	Diffuse hyperpigmentation		Bullae, porphyria cutanea tarda
Thiotepa			Alopecia, patterned hyperpigmentation, diffuse hyperpigmentation
Mechlorethamine (topical administration)	Contact dermatitis		Localized hyperpigmentation, urticaria
Dacarbazine		Flushing	Alopecia, inflammation of actinic keratoses, urticaria, photosensitivity
Carmustine		Flushing	Alopecia, stomatitis
Antimetabolites			
Methotrexate	Stomatitis	Alopecia, radiation recall	Erythematous macules and papules, photoreactivation, horizontal bands of hyperpigmentation in hair ("flag sign"), urticaria
5-fluorouracil	Stomatitis, alopecia	Photosensitivity	Diffuse or patterned hyperpigmentation, especially over veins used for drug infusion, hyperpigmentation of nails, nail cracking and brittleness, inflammation of actinic keratoses, acral erythema, urticaria
Cytarabine		Alopecia	Acral erythema, neutrophilic eccrine hidradenitis, inflammation of actinic keratoses
6-mercaptopurine			Stomatitis
6-thioguanine			Stomatitis, inflammation of actinic keratoses
Antibiotics			
Bleomycin	Stomatitis, alopecia	Generalized hyperpigmentation, pigmentation over pressure areas, flagellate hyperpigmentation	Generalized erythema, neutrophilic eccrine hidradenitis, radiation enhancement or recall, hypersensitivity reactions, acral sclerosis, Raynaud's phenomenon
Dactinomycin		Alopecia, stomatitis, acneiform eruption	Radiation recall or enhancement, inflammation of actinic keratoses, erythema multiforme

Drug			
Doxorubicin	Alopecia, Stomatitis	Hyperpigmentation of nails, acral areas, or buccal mucosa, radiation recall or enhancement	Urticaria, angioedema, inflammation of actinic keratoses, acral erythema
Daunorubicin	Stomatitis	Patterned pigmentation of skin, nails, or oral mucosa, alopecia	Urticaria
Mithramycin	Macular erythema of the head and trunk (flushing)	Erythematous papules on face, stomatitis, postinflammatory hyperpigmentation	Toxic epidermal necrolysis
Mitomycin C			Stomatitis, hyperpigmentation, photosensitivity, pruritic vesicular eruption
Vinca Alkyloids			
Vincristine	Stomatitis		Inflammation of actinic keratoses
Vinblastine	Stomatitis		Photosensitivity
Miscellaneous Agents			
L-Asparaginase	Urticaria, anaphylaxis, Serum sickness type reaction		Erythema, edema and pruritus of feet
Procarbazine			Alopecia, stomatitis, maculopapular rash, urticaria
Hydroxyurea	Alopecia, hyperpigmentation, nail dystrophy	Lichen planus-like skin lesions	Acral erythema, fixed drug eruption, radiation enhancement, dermatomyositis-like eruption
Amsacrine	Stomatitis, alopecia		Hypersensitivity reactions
Cisplatin			Inflammation of actinic keratoses, hypersensitivity reactions
Etoposide	Diffuse erythematous macules and papules		Alopecia, radiation recall, hypersensitivity
Cytokines			
Interleukin-2	Edema	Macular erythema	Stomatitis, telogen effluvium, punctate ulcerations, erythema nodosum, exacerbation of psoriasis
α-interferon	Alopecia, pruritus	Erythema	Exacerbation of psoriasis, increased growth of eyelashes, radiation enhancement
γ-interferon			
GM-CSF[a]			Maculopapular eruption

[a]GM-CSF, granulocyte-macrophage colony-stimulating factor.

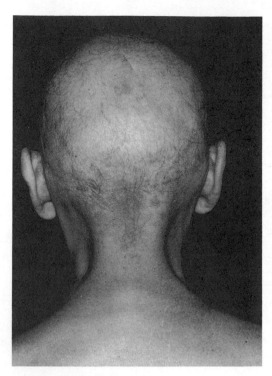

Figure 30.1. Alopecia. Chemotherapy-induced alopecia in a patient who received doxorubicin, cytoxan, and vincristine. (Reproduced with permission from Antoinette F. Hood, M.D.)

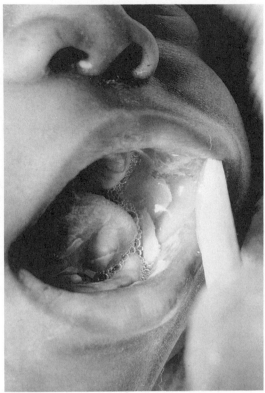

Figure 30.2. Stomatitis. Stomatitis in an infant treated with intrathecal methotrexate for acute lymphocytic leukemia. (From Bronner AK, Hood AF. Cutaneous complications of chemotherapeutic agents. J Am Acad Dermatol 1983;9:648.)

cositis induced by 5-fluorouracil; however, a randomized double-blind placebo-controlled study (8) showed no helpful effect. β-Carotene was helpful in reducing severity of mucositis in an uncontrolled study of 20 patients with oral squamous carcinoma who received a combination of radiotherapy and chemotherapy (vincristine, bleomycin, and methotrexate) (9). Investigational protocols include a cryotherapy-based scheme with 5-fluorouracil administration. Cooling of the oral mucosa (via sucking ice chips) during periods of peak 5-fluorouracil serum concentration after bolus administration causes vasoconstriction and decreased blood flow to the area, leading to a localized decrease in 5-fluorouracil concentration and lessening the severity of mucositis (10).

Supportive measures are essential. Diet should be bland, soft, and of neutral temperature. Topical anesthetics may be used, either focally or as rinses in combination with analgesics and mucosal coating agents. Lubricants such as petrolatum help keep lips moist and intact. Oral hygiene is performed with soft toothbrush and unwaxed dental floss as tolerated. Mouthwashes, generally quarter-strength hydrogen peroxide, saline, or sodium bicarbonate, given every 2 hours aid with removal of debris (11). High-calorie nutritional supplementation should be given, and parenteral nutrition may be required.

The mucosa generally begins to heal approximately 1 week after discontinuation of the chemotherapeutic agent. Production of stomatitis by a particular agent in an individual is generally reproducible and is avoided only by decreasing dosage or discontinuation of the offending agent.

BEAU'S LINES

The cytotoxic effects of chemotherapeutic agents on the nail matrix are reflected by Beau's lines, transverse depressions in the nail plate noted several weeks after administration of an agent (Fig. 30.3). The depressions move distally with growth of the nail plate and eventually disappear. Inhibition of mitotic activity within the nail matrix is the mechanism of formation of Beau's lines.

Hypersensitivity Reactions

Hypersensitivity reactions to antineoplastic agents occur, although less commonly than cytotoxic reactions. Because bone marrow transplantation patients receive multiple medications, identifying the cause for a hypersensitivity reaction may be difficult.

Type I (immediate hypersensitivity) reactions are IgE medidated and manifest as urticaria, angioedema, or anaphylaxis. The agent most commonly associated with type I reaction is L-asparaginase, affecting approximately two-thirds of patients receiving this medication (12). Acute urticaria is most commonly seen after administration of this agent, but anaphylaxis, chronic urticaria, and serum sickness-type reactions may also occur. Type I reactions occur with higher frequencies if L-asparaginase is administered as a sole agent, intravenously, at high doses, or with cumulative doses.

Cisplatin also may cause an immediate hypersensitivity reaction, including flushing, pruritus, urticaria, erythema, dyspnea, bronchospasm, diaphoresis, and hypotension (13). Reactions occur shortly after infusion of the agent and can be partially prevented by premedication with antihistamines and steroids. The frequency of the reaction is about 5% but is considerably higher when cisplatin is given in combination therapy.

Other agents causing documented hypersensitivity reactions include cyclophosphamide (14) and mechlorethamine. Agents causing urticaria through some unknown mechanism include chlorambucil, melphalan, thiotepa, methotrexate, bleomycin, daunorubicin, and doxorubicin (2, 15).

Type III reactions, immune complex-mediated reactions, are clinically manifest as urticaria, vasculitis, and possibly erythema multiforme (Fig. 30.4). Erythema multiforme-type reactions were reported after treatment with hydroxyurea and mechlorethamine (16).

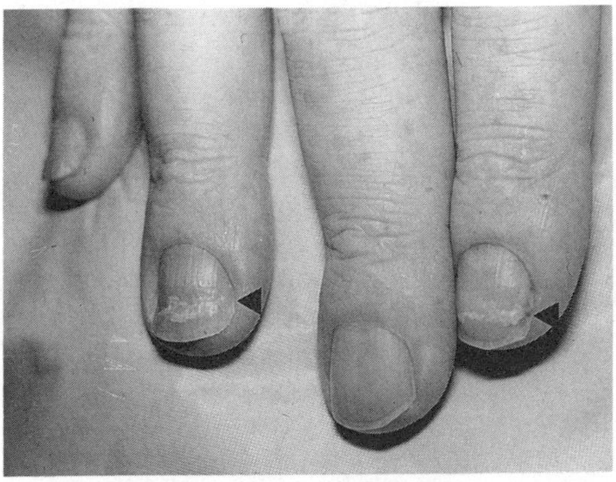

Figure 30.3.   Beau's lines. Transverse depressions (*arrows*) in the nail plate. (From Hood AF. Cutaneous complications of immunosuppressive agents. Dermatol Clin 1983;1:591–606.)

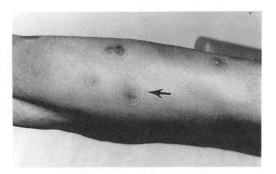

Figure 30.4.   Erythema multiforme. The hallmark of erythema multiforme is the target lesion (*arrow*). In this patient, there is a vesicular quality in the external ring of the "bull's eye." Lesions commonly involve the palms and soles.

Toxic epidermal necrolysis was reported following administration of mithramycin (17). Complement activation, urticaria, and angioedema were reported with procarbazine administration (18).

Type IV reactions are cell-mediated responses and are characterized by allergic contact dermatitis. The agent that is most often associated with development of allergic contact dermatitis is mechlorethamine, which occurs in greater than one-third of patients receiving topical therapy with this agent (19, 20).

Radiation Interactions

Interactions of chemotherapeutic agents with radiation, of both the ionizing and the ultraviolet types, are well documented. These reactions are grouped as follows. Radiation recall reactions are those in which tissues that have been irradiated months to years earlier become inflamed upon exposure to an antineoplastic medication (21) (Fig. 30.5). Implicated agents include dactinomycin (22), doxorubicin (23), etoposide, and bleomycin (24). Radiation enhancement refers to synergism between concurrent or nearly concurrent courses of x-irradiation and antineoplastic agent therapy. Implicated agents include dactinomycin (25), methotrexate (26), and doxorubicin (27).

Photosensitivity refers to the lowering of the dose of ultraviolet irradiation required to cause cutaneous erythema. Reports of increased photosensitivity are associated with dacarbazine (28), 5-fluorouracil (29), vinblastine (30), and mitomycin C (31). Photoreactivation is an uncommon reaction consisting of erythema in areas of prior ultraviolet B (UVB)-induced erythema (sunburn). This effect was reported with high-dose methotrexate (32).

Pigmentary Changes

Changes in skin pigmentation following administration of antineoplastic agents are generally poorly understood. The changes are

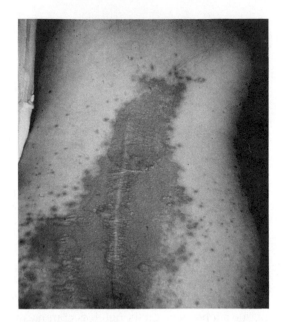

Figure 30.5. Radiation recall. Marked erythema appeared 3 days after systemic doxorubicin therapy. Erythema is largely limited to the previous radiation port. (From Adrian RM, Hood AF, Skaren AT. Mucocutaneous reactions to antineoplastic agents. CA 1980; 30:148.)

most commonly hyperpigmentation and may be diffuse or localized, involving skin, hair, or nails. Pigmentary changes are of cosmetic concern to the patient. The hyperpigmentation due to busulfan is of added significance as dyschromia correlates with systemic toxicity (33).

Diffuse hyperpigmentation is reported after therapy with busulfan, cyclophosphamide, 5-fluorouracil, high-dose thiotepa, and methotrexate. Hyperpigmentation following busulfan accompanies a syndrome that mimics Addison's disease but without biochemical evidence of that disorder (34). The pigmentation may resolve after discontinuation of therapy but may persist after prolonged treatment courses. The syndrome may be associated with the development of pulmonary fibrosis on busulfan.

Localized hyperpigmentation may take many forms (Fig. 30.6). Bleomycin is associated with a patterned hyperpigmentation sec-

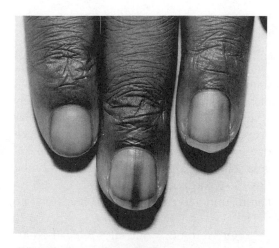

Figure 30.6. Localized hyperpigmentation. Longitudinal streaks of the nail plate and mild darkening of the proximal nail fold following hydroxyurea therapy. (Reproduced with permission from Antoinette F. Hood, M.D.)

ondary to trauma (generally scratching) during bleomycin administration (Fig. 30.7) (35). Patterned hyperpigmentation during therapy with thiotepa is attributed to excretion of thiotepa in sweat, causing localized toxicity under bandages and electrocardiogram pads (36) (Fig. 30.8).

Doxorubicin may cause darkening of the oral mucosa or the nails and skin over the metacarpophalangeal and interphalangeal joints. Oral hyperpigmentation may be seen with busulfan, cyclophosphamide, and 5-fluorouracil. Darkened horizontal bands within the hair are reported with high-dose methotrexate and have been referred to as the "flag sign" of chemotherapy (15). Depigmentation is reported following topical application of thiotepa to the eye.

Cutaneous Reactions to the Therapeutic Use of Cytokines

The availability of human recombinant immunomodulating agents has greatly influenced cancer therapy. Intravenous infusions of pharmacologic doses of cytokines results in a variety of cutaneous changes.

INTERLEUKIN-2

Interleukin-2 (IL-2) was given as a sole agent to 41 patients with a variety of neoplasms (37). Dosage varied from 2×10^2 to 3×10^4 U/kg given intravenously over 5 minutes to 24 hours. Cutaneous reactions included purpuric rashes, erythroderma, urticaria, and edema. A skin biopsy specimen from a patient with erythroderma and petechiae showed thrombosis of deep dermal vessels and a mixed superficial perivascular infiltrate of lymphocytes, neutrophils, and plasma cells. Patients who were receiving IL-2 and lymphokine-activated killer cells from tumor-in-

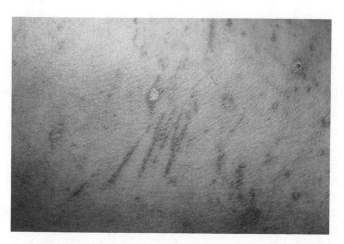

Figure 30.7. Flagellate hyperpigmentation. Linear hyperpigmentation following bleomycin administration. (Reproduced with permission from Antoinette F. Hood, M.D.)

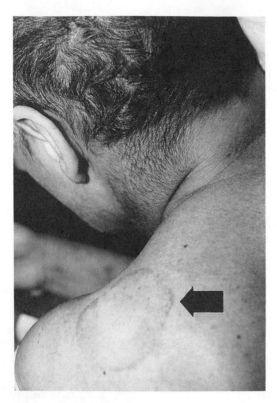

Figure 30.8. Thiotepa-induced hyperpigmentation. Annular hyperpigmentation (*arrow*) arose underneath an electrocardiogram pad after high-dose thiotepa therapy.

filtrating lymphocytes had persistent erythematous macules with pruritus and burning, located on the head and neck. Other reported complications include stomatitis and hair loss.

INTERFERONS

The interferons are a heterogeneous group of biologic response modifiers that have been used alone and in combination with antineoplastic agents against numerous types of tumors. Interferons α, β, and γ have all been used in a therapeutic manner.

Interferon α (IFN-α) caused the development of symptoms of connective tissue disorders mimicking rheumatoid arthritis and lupus erythematosus (38). One patient developed a cutaneous eruption resembling eosinophilic fasciitis. Dry, scaling skin occurred

in 10 to 13 patients receiving IFN-α for myeloproliferative disorders (39). Four patients developed hair loss, and two developed erythematous plaques. In a phase I trial of intramuscular IFN-α and intravenous IL-2, 58% of patients developed a mild to moderately severe erythematous pruritic maculopapular eruption. Nineteen percent of patients developed oral lesions, including stomatitis, angular cheilitis, ulcerations, and fissures of the lips (40). Local injection of IFN-α caused inflammation and pruritus at the injection site (41).

Interferon β serine (IFN-βs) caused erythema, tenderness, induration, or ulceration at injection sites when given subcutaneously for treatment of hairy cell leukemia (42). Nonspecific "rash" was also reported with IFN-βs use (43). Interferon γ (IFN-γ) caused "a cutaneous allergic reaction" when given for cutaneous T cell lymphoma (44). Lesions of psoriasis developed at injection sites of IFN-γ in patients with a history of psoriasis (45).

GRANULOCYTE-MACROPHAGE COLONY-STIMULATING FACTOR

Intravenous granulocyte-macrophage colony-stimulating factor (GM-CSF) is given to shorten the period of bone marrow aplasia after administration of high-dose chemotherapy, to obtain cell cycle synchrony prior to administration of cycle-specific chemotherapeutic agents, and to enhance neutrophil function in human immunodeficiency virus (HIV) infected persons. A cutaneous eruption consisting of erythematous macules and papules with confluence was reported (46). A skin biopsy specimen showed a superficial perivascular infiltrate of mononuclear cells, eosinophils, and neutrophils at a time of marrow aplasia. In another specimen, an increase in the number of macrophages present within the papillary dermis was observed. These histologic features are referable to the known effects of GM-CSF.

Miscellaneous Reactions

ACRAL ERYTHEMA

Patients receiving high-dose chemotherapy, especially with cytarabine, may develop painful erythematous macules on the hands and less commonly on the feet (47). The lesions are usually symmetric and appear within the 1st weeks after receiving cytarabine. The macules may progress to bullae, which may increase discomfort. Subsequent or concurrent cyclosporine administration reportedly increased the discomfort associated with this acral erythema (48). Resolution occurs over the next 1–2 weeks, with desquamation. Drug-induced acral erythema may occur alone or in conjunction with acute GVHD. Histologic features of non-GVHD-associated acral erythema include vacuolar alteration of the basal cell layer, mild to moderate atypia of epidermal cells, and numerous dyskeratotic keratinocytes throughout the epidermis (47). These features may be seen with a grade II cutaneous GVHR, and these disorders may only be distinguished by clinical correlation and/or by serial biopsies looking for progression of findings compatible with GVHD. In a series of 72 patients pretreated with lomustine (CCNU), cytarabine, and doxorubicin, 39% of patients experienced acral erythema, and the occurrence of acral erythema was predictive of achievement of clinical remission (49).

Cytarabine is most commonly associated with acral erythema, but other implicated agents include cyclophosphamide, methotrexate, 5-fluorouracil, and doxorubicin. The pathophysiologic basis for this reaction is not understood, but a direct toxic effect is the most likely cause. The reason for involvement of hands and feet only is not clear but may relate to the high concentration of eccrine glands in these sites.

NEUTROPHILIC ECCRINE HIDRADENITIS

Neutrophilic eccrine hidradenitis (NEH) was initially reported in 1981 in a man undergoing therapy for myelogenous leukemia (50). He developed erythematous, edematous plaques on the neck and shoulder on the 8th day of treatment with doxorubicin, cytarabine, vincristine, and prednisone. A skin biopsy specimen revealed striking infiltration of the eccrine coils by mature polymorphonuclear leukocytes, with necrosis of the eccrine glandular epithelium. The eruption resolved spontaneously over the next several days. A series of cases was reviewed in 1988 (51), and a more varied clinical presentation was revealed. Lesions may be erythematous, tender plaques or macules, pruritic nodules, or hyperpigmented plaques. They may be localized or widely scattered. The histologic picture is less variable, showing necrosis of the eccrine structures, mostly glandular epithelium, and a neutrophilic infiltrate (Fig. 30.9). Cytarabine was the agent initially described, but bleomycin has also recently been implicated (51). The mechanism of injury is unclear and may be related to the concentration of chemotherapeutic agent in sweat. However, this theory does not explain the localized occurrence of the phenomenon, since eccrine structures are widely distributed within the skin.

INFLAMMATION OF KERATOSES

Preexisting actinic keratoses may become erythematous and pruritic with systemic administration of chemotherapeutic agents (Fig. 30.10). This effect is best known with 5-fluorouracil but has been observed either alone or in combination with pentostatin, dactinomycin, vincristine, dacarbazine, doxorubicin, cisplatin, cytarabine, and 6-thioguanine (15). The mechanism is unknown but may be similar to a radiation recall phenomenon, since actinic keratoses are lesions caused by chronic ultraviolet damage to the skin (15).

FOLLICULITIS

Dactinomycin may cause a folliculitis resembling acne. Multiple pustular lesions are

Figure 30.9. Neutrophilic eccrine hidradenitis. Neutrophils surround and invade several eccrine coils in this photomicrograph. The eccrine glands are necrotic (*arrows*). Relatively unaffected eccrine epithelium is also present (*arrowhead*).

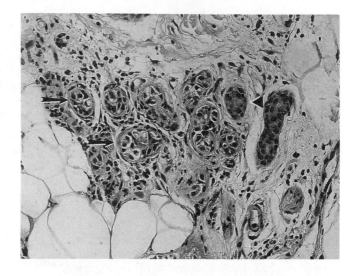

Figure 30.10. Inflammation of keratoses. Arrows delimit the area of erythema containing many confluent actinic keratoses. Erythema appeared after systemic 5-fluorouracil therapy. (Reproduced with permission from Russell L. Corio, D.D.S., M.S.D., M.A.)

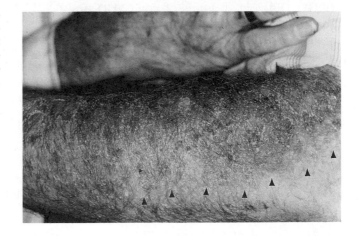

seen (52). Methotrexate given in high doses may cause a similar reaction.

PORPHYRIA CUTANEA TARDA

The development of porphyria cutanea tarda was reported in a patient treated with busulfan for chronic myelogenous leukemia (53). Another patient with chronic myelogenous leukemia treated with busulfan and hydroxyurea subsequently underwent BMT (54). Two years later the patient developed porphyria cutanea tarda, with elevated urinary uroporphyrin excretion and decreased erythrocyte uroporphyrinogen decarboxylase ac-

tivity. The patient's past medical history was further complicated by cytomegalovirus hepatitis and prior exposure to benzene; thus the relationship of the development of porphyria cutanea tarda to BMT is unproven.

BULLOUS DISORDERS

Miliaria Crystallina

Miliaria crystallina is a disorder of superficial eccrine duct obstruction. It consists of multiple, noninflammatory, superficial vesicles that generally appear on the chest and trunk after a febrile episode. The vesicles are delicate and easily broken. The eruption is asymptomatic. Tzanck smear is negative. Histologically, there is an intracorneal or subcorneal vesicle associated with the intraepidermal portion of the eccrine duct. The basis for the obstruction of the duct is not clear. The lesions resolve without treatment and are important because they may be mistaken for those of viral infection or other bullous disorder. A period of hypohidrosis in involved skin follows the eruption.

Toxic Epidermal Necrolysis

Toxic epidermal necrolysis (TEN) is a blistering disorder characterized by extensive epidermal necrosis and large flaccid bullae. The most common cause is a reaction to a drug, such as an anticonvulsant, nonsteroidal antiinflammatory agent, or antibiotic. TEN has been reported in BMT patients (55). The histologic features of TEN are a subepidermal bulla with full-thickness necrosis of the epidermis and a scant lymphocytic infiltrate. These features cannot be reliably distinguished from grade IV graft-versus-host reaction (GVHR). Indeed, TEN may not be a separate entity necessarily exclusive of a grade IV cutaneous GVHR. In five of nine patients with TEN following BMT (56), an acute GVHR appeared to be the cause of the TEN, with accompanying extracutaneous symptoms of GVHD and no suspect medications. In the remaining four, an adverse drug reaction appeared to be the cause. The occurrence of TEN, whatever the cause, was associated with a poor prognosis; all patients died, seven early in the course and two several months later. In this study, all patients were treated with high-dose corticosteroids.

Optimal therapy for TEN is controversial. Discontinuation of as many medicines as possible is mandatory. The benefit of high-dose corticosteroids is debated. Corticosteroid-induced immunosuppression may lead to a worsening of infectious complications. If corticosteroids are used, initiation of therapy should be within the first 24 hours of the onset of the eruption.

Staphylococcal Scalded Skin Syndrome

Staphylococci are responsible for an increasing number of infections in BMT patients. Staphylococcal scalded skin syndrome (SSSS) is a blistering disorder caused by toxin-producing staphylococci of phage group II. In the general population SSSS is a disease of young children. The toxin is excreted by the kidney, and renal immaturity allows accumulation of the toxin. Affected adults are generally those with compromised renal function. Clinically, the disorder is characterized by diffuse erythema, skin tenderness, and fever. Within 12–14 hours large flaccid bullae are present, which are easily broken. As with TEN, there may be large areas of denudation, and temperature maintenance and fluid balance may be problems. Histologically, this disorder shows a separation within the upper epidermis, usually in the granular layer, with the accumulation of edema fluid within the separation. Inflammation is mild.

There is one reported case of SSSS in an allogeneic bone marrow recipient (57). He developed acute GVHD 2 weeks after transplant as manifested by rash, diarrhea, and jaundice and confirmed by biopsy of the large intestine. He subsequently developed chronic GVHD. On day 90 after transplantation he developed a bullous eruption on the chest that spread to the back, chest, and face, which was thought to be TEN associated with grade IV GVHD. A skin biopsy revealed a separation within the granular layer of the epidermis, confirming the diagnosis of SSSS. Subsequent cultures of blood, catheter tip, and cutaneous crusts grew *Staphylococcus aureus*, one of which was phage group II. Skin biopsy was essential in this case to establish the diagnosis. The level of separation can be adequately assessed by frozen section histology and is useful in early differentiation of SSSS from grade IV GVHD and TEN. Therapy consists of appropriate antibiotics and supportive care.

Venoocclusive Disease

Hepatic venoocclusive disease is a serious complication of intensive chemotherapy administration. Affected patients develop hepatic dysfunction, with hepatomegaly, hepatic tenderness, hyperbilirubinemia, ascites, and weight gain. Hypoproteinemia may be severe, and edema associated with decreased oncotic pressure may lead to large bullae, especially in dependent areas. Bullae contain clear fluid that may become pustular. Secondary infection of denuded areas may be a problem.

Transient Acantholytic Dermatosis

Transient acantholytic dermatosis (TAD) manifests as pruritic, erythematous, often excoriated papules on the trunks of middle-aged men. The etiology of this eruption is felt to relate to heat exposure and sweating. TAD has been described in febrile patients receiving high-dose chemotherapy (58). Generalized erythematous papules develop, remain for several days to weeks, and resolve with defervescence. The clinical differential diagnosis includes septic emboli. Histologically, TAD consists of acantholytic (rounded and detached) keratinocytes forming an intraepidermal vesicle (Fig. 30.11). No therapy is warranted beyond oral antihistamines for pruritus.

CUTANEOUS ERUPTION OF LYMPHOCYTE RECOVERY

A cutaneous eruption develops at the time of earliest recovery of peripheral lymphocytes after chemotherapy-induced marrow aplasia in approximately 50% of patients who have not received BMT (59). This eruption is characterized by diffuse erythematous macules that resolve with desquamation upon complete hematologic recovery. Tempera-

ture elevation accompanies the eruption in nearly all cases. The macules do not have the preferential acral distribution of an acute GVHR but otherwise are clinically similar. Histologically, one finds a superficial perivascular lymphocytic infiltrate composed of CD4+ cells, mild dermal and epidermal edema, and rare dyskeratotic keratinocytes.

The etiology of this eruption may relate to homing of these T lymphocytes to the skin with subsequent production of cytokines capable of mediating the cutaneous changes observed. Whether a similar eruption occurs in BMT recipients is unknown. An acute cutaneous GVHR differs from the eruption of lymphocyte recovery principally by beginning acrally and by the histologic finding of significant numbers of dyskeratotic keratinocytes. It is possible that certain eruptions in BMT recipients that do not fulfill the criteria of a grade II GVHR actually arise due to the eruption of lymphocyte recovery or a similar process.

CUTANEOUS NEOPLASMS

An increased incidence of cutaneous neoplasms, mostly squamous cell carcinomas, is seen in organ transplant recipients (60). A study of 56 BMT patients who were followed for a minimum of 40 months following BMT revealed three mucocutaneous malignancies, two squamous cell carcinomas and one melanoma (61). The three patients all had chronic GVHD and were treated with immunosuppressive agents, including azathioprine, prednisone, cyclosporine A, and cyclophosphamide. In these cases, prolonged immunosuppression and local factors including damage by GVHD may have played a role in the development of mucocutaneous neoplasms.

INFECTION

Infections occurring in recipients of high-dose chemotherapy are many and varied. This section is not intended to exhaus-

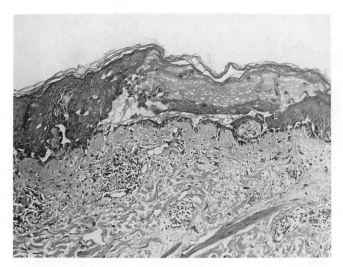

Figure 30.11. Photomicrograph of transient acantholytic dermatosis. An intraepidermal vesicle is present, containing rounded and detached keratinocytes (acantholysis). This papulovesicular eruption is associated with fevers and sweating. (From Arch Dermatol 1987;123:238–240. Copyright 1987, American Medical Association.)

tively discuss all of the possible infectious agents; rather, the focus will be on common pathogens causing primary and secondary cutaneous infection after high-dose chemotherapy administration. Careful examination of the skin is important, as primary infections may be identified before dissemination occurs and cutaneous septic lesions may be the earliest sign of systemic infection and a source of organism identification.

Bacterial Infection

Over the past several years there appears to have been a change in the spectrum of organisms responsible for septicemia in BMT patients, with higher incidences of gram-positive septicemias caused by *Staphylococcus* and *Streptococcus* (62). Normal skin flora such as *Staphylococcus epidermidis* have been implicated as a cause of septicemia in conjunction with indwelling catheters. Additionally, the α-streptococci from the oral cavity have been isolated in increased frequency (63). Cutaneous lesions of bacterial sepsis are typical of other septic emboli, characterized by erythematous macules, pustules, or nodules, possibly ulcerated (Figs. 30.12, 30.13). Histologic examination may reveal the organisms within dermal foci of neutrophils and

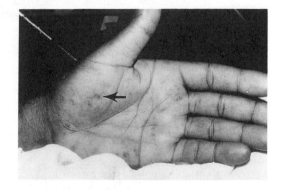

Figure 30.12. Septic emboli due to *Staphylococcus aureus*. Nonblanching, tender, erythematous to violaceous macules and papules (*arrow*) are present on the palm.

necrotic debris, usually within or associated with blood vessels.

A specific cutaneous manifestation of *Pseudomonas aeruginosa* sepsis is ecthyma gangrenosum. The lesions start as hemorrhagic bullae. Subsequently they appear as found, indurated, ulcerated plaques with surrounding erythema. There may be an overlying necrotic black eschar. *Pseudomonas* organisms can be cultured from aspirated material, skin biopsy specimens, or blood. Ecthyma gangrenosum was reported in a patient 2 years after BMT as a localized infec-

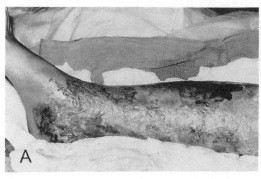
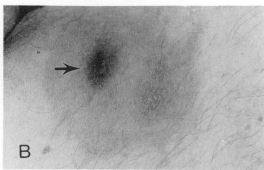

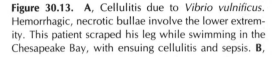

Figure 30.13. A, Cellulitis due to *Vibrio vulnificus.* Hemorrhagic, necrotic bullae involve the lower extremity. This patient scraped his leg while swimming in the Chesapeake Bay, with ensuing cellulitis and sepsis. **B,** This closer view of an early phase of *V. vulnificus* cellulitis displays an erythematous macule with central hemorrhage (*arrow*).

tion (64). A skin biopsy specimen of ecthyma gangrenosum shows a necrotizing vasculitis with mild neutrophilic infiltration and leukocytoclasis. Many gram-negative bacilli are seen in the perivascular areas.

Fungal Infection

Fungal infections are common following intensive chemotherapy treatment. *Candida* and *Aspergillus* are the organisms most often responsible for invasive infections (65), but the number of unusual fungi reported to cause infection is legion. Infections may be systemic or limited to mucocutaneous surfaces.

CANDIDIASIS

Infections with *Candida* sp. continue to be a major problem in patients who are leukopenic after intensive chemotherapy. Infections may be limited to mucous membranes or skin, or they may be systemic. In one study of 34 patients undergoing intensive cancer therapy and autologous BMT (66), 12 patients developed either oropharyngeal, cutaneous, or vaginal candidiasis. Most of the patients, including those experiencing mucocutaneous candidiasis, received oral, nonabsorbable antifungal prophylaxis. Clinically, oral candidiasis presents as friable white patches

on the buccal mucosa, tongue, palate, gingivae, or tonsillar region. The underlying mucosa is erythematous. Ulceration or necrosis may be present. A microscopic examination of a scraping of the whitish material will reveal masses of pseudohyphae and spore forms.

Primary cutaneous candidiasis presents as erythematous papules and pustules generally located in moist areas of the skin such as the gluteal or crural folds. Treatment is best accomplished with a topical antifungal cream and application of astringents.

Disseminated candidiasis occurred in 171 of 1510 patients undergoing BMT between 1980 and 1987 at the University of Washington (65). Fungemia alone occurred in 46 of the patients, whereas 56 patients had positive blood cultures plus tissue invasion. Recipients of allogeneic grafts had a higher incidence of candidiasis than did patients receiving autologous grafts. Among allogeneic recipients, those with T cell-depleted grafts had a higher incidence of disseminated candidiasis.

Skin lesions occur in 10%–13% of all patients with disseminated candidiasis. The lesions are usually on the trunk or extremities and may be few in number or numerous. Erythematous papulonodules that may become hemorrhagic are the classic lesions (Fig. 30.14). There may be necrosis, which causes the le-

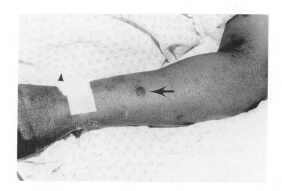

Figure 30.14. *Candida* sepsis. Hemorrhagic, erythematous nodules (*arrow*) are characteristic of fungal septic emboli.

sions to resemble ecthyma gangrenosum. Erythema and induration of the skin surrounding catheter sites may be caused by *Candida* infection. Histologic examination is variable, showing mild inflammation or microabscesses with leukocytoclastic vasculitis. Aggregates of hyphac and spores measuring 3–6 microns are found, which stain with periodic acid- Schiff or Gomori methenamine silver (Fig. 30.15). Organisms may be sparse, and step sectioning of the tissue may be required.

ASPERGILLOSIS

Aspergillus is a saprophytic fungus generally found in decaying vegetation. Human exposure to *Aspergillus* is common, and inoculation occurs primarily through the respiratory tract, although mucocutaneous surfaces may also serve as primary infection sites. The species most commonly associated with human infection is *Aspergillus fumigatus*, but other species such as *Aspergillus flavus*, *Aspergillus niger*, and *Aspergillus terreus* have been reported to cause infections in immunocompromised hosts.

Two forms of cutaneous aspergillosis are observed in patients undergoing intensive chemotherapy. Primary cutaneous aspergillosis occurs near the sites of intravenous catheters, especially under arm boards or anchoring devices. The lesions are papules, plaques, or hemorrhagic bullae that become necrotic. Dissemination may occur. Secondary cutaneous aspergillosis occurs after dissemination of infection from a pulmonary or other source. Lesions are tender, erythematous papules or nodules that may ulcerate (Fig. 30.16). Skin biopsy specimens from both the primary or secondary cutaneous forms show numerous septate hyphae measuring 2–4 microns in diameter that branch at acute angles. Vascular involvement is often prominent.

PITYROSPORUM FOLLICULITIS

Patients typically develop perifollicular, faintly erythematous macules and papulopus-

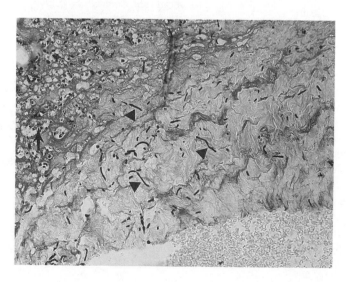

Figure 30.15. *Candida* sp. sepsis. Within and adjacent to an abscess (*arrow*) are numerous pseudohyphae (*arrowheads*), as highlighted by this periodic acid-Schiff stain.

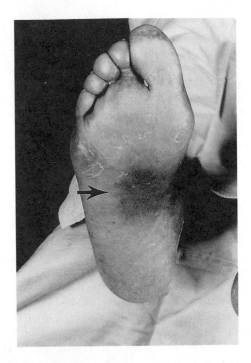

Figure 30.16. Septic embolus from *Aspergillus* sp. An ill-defined, hemorrhagic, necrotic patch (*arrow*) is present on the plantar surface of the foot.

tules over the chest, shoulders, and upper back (67). The eruption is generally pruritic. A skin biopsy specimen shows a dilated, keratin-filled follicle and large numbers of budding yeast measuring 2–4 microns. There is a surrounding inflammatory cell infiltrate of variable intensity. Mycelial elements are not seen.

OTHER FUNGI

Many other organisms are reported to cause invasive infections in patients treated with intensive chemotherapy. Cutaneous lesions may occur, but there are no distinguishing clinical characteristics to identify the various etiologies. Histologic characteristics, such as the broad nonseptate hyphae of *Mucor* (Fig. 30.17), or tissue culture results are required for identification of the pathogen. Other fungi involving the skin include *Fusarium* (68), *Torulopsis* (Fig. 30.18), *Alternaria*, *Scopulariopsis* (69), and *Henderson-*

ula. Adequate biopsy technique is essential for correct diagnosis, and specimens should include full thickness of the skin with some subcutaneous tissue. All biopsies should be sent for routine histologic evaluation and culture. Touching the base of the biopsy specimen firmly to a glass slide in several areas (touch preparation) may result in immediate identification of the infectious agent by gram stain and potassium hydroxide examination of the smear.

Viruses

Viruses are important pathogens after intensive chemotherapy. The herpesvirus group, including herpes simplex virus (HSV), varicella-zoster virus (VZV), and cytomegalovirus (CMV), commonly involve the skin. Prophylactic use of acyclovir and the use of CMV-seronegative blood products for seronegative patients have reduced the morbidity and mortality from these infections. A recent study of 81 allogeneic and autologous BMT patients, all of whom received acyclovir prophylaxis, documented 39 viral infections in 28 patients (70). Of these infections, 21 (53%) were due to CMV, VZV, or HSV. Other infections were caused by influenza viruses, rhinoviruses, adenoviruses, coxsackievirus, and papovavirus. Viral infections were similar in autologous and allogeneic recipients, with the exception of CMV, which did not occur in autologous BMT patients.

HERPES SIMPLEX VIRUS

HSV infections following BMT largely represent reactivation of virus in individuals who are seropositive before transplantation (71). Lesions may appear on the cutaneous or mucosal surfaces. There is often tingling or dysesthesia before appearance of the eruption. Lesions are usually grouped vesicles on an erythematous base and may become pustular. Lesions inside the oropharynx, especially those occurring early after conditioning and transplantation, may cause large areas of mucosal destruction, resem-

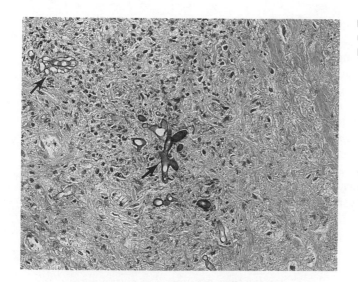

Figure 30.17. *Mucor* infection. Large nonseptate hyphae are seen (*arrow*) in this photomicrograph.

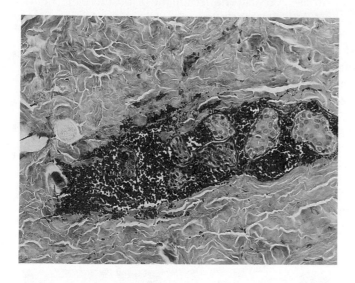

Figure 30.18. *Torulopsis glabrata* sepsis. This periodic acid-Schiff stain reveals numerous budding yeast in the dermis surrounding an eccrine coil. There is no significant inflammation.

bling primary herpetic infections rather than recurrent episodes (72). Disseminated lesions consist of erythematous papulovesicles.

VARICELLA-ZOSTER VIRUS

VZV infections are known to occur frequently in cancer patients, especially those with lymphoproliferative disorders. The incidence of varicella-zoster infections in BMT patients has decreased with the use of prophylactic acyclovir use (73). In a retrospec-

tive study of 153 patients undergoing autologous BMT, 43 (28%) developed VZV infections (74). Thirty-three had localized herpes zoster, and 10 had varicella. Infection became disseminated on the skin, and internal organ involvement was noted in some cases. No deaths occurred. The majority of cases occurred within 1 year of transplantation. In this study, the only significant risk factor for development of VZV infection was underlying illness, with most infections occurring in patients with lymphoma, as opposed to those with leukemia or solid tumors. Unlike HSV, VZV infections may occur in patients without preexisting antibody titers, indicating that a significant proportion of VZV infections represent primary infections and not reactivation of latent virus.

Varicella is characterized by successive crops of lesions that progress from macules to papules to vesicles to pustules to crusts (75). In immunosuppressed patients, the eruption is extensive, longer lasting, and may be accompanied by purpuric lesions. Lesions occur on the trunk but are also found on mucous membranes, including the oropharynx and vagina. The illness may be accompanied by high fever, constitutional signs, and visceral involvement.

Typical herpes zoster lesions begin as edematous erythematous macules. There is often a systemic prodrome of malaise, fever, and nausea and a cutaneous prodrome of burning, tingling, or pruritus. Grouped vesicles generally develop within 36 hours (75) and are on an erythematous base (Fig. 30.19). Vesicular fluid becomes turbid and purulent in 3–4 days. Lesions then become dry and crusted. The vesicles are generally located in a dermatomal distribution but may disseminate on the cutaneous surface or spread viscerally. Disseminated lesions are solitary erythematous papulovesicles. In immunosuppressed individuals, vesicles may last longer,

frank necrosis (Fig. 30.20) may develop, and healing may be delayed. Scarring may be severe. Postherpetic neuralgia, defined as persistent pain in the affected dermatome 2 months after the crusts have disappeared (75), occurs most frequently in older patients and those with herpes zoster ophthalmicus.

Local care of herpes zoster lesions include compressing with normal saline or astringent agents such as aluminum acetate, which allows gentle debridement. Topical antibiotics are helpful for preventing secondary infection. Pain control is essential. During the acute period, nonsteroidal antiinflammatory agents or narcotic medication is indicated. The role of oral corticosteroids in preventing postherpetic neuralgia is controversial. The treatment of postherpetic neuralgia includes tricyclic antidepressants, carbamazepine, biofeedback, sympathetic block, topical capsaicin, and acupuncture.

The diagnosis of herpesvirus infection can be made by Tzanck smear of the base of a vesicle or ulcer. It is essential to obtain epithelial cells, as the characteristic cytopathic changes of acantholysis, nuclear inclusions, and multinucleate giant cells are seen only in the epithelial cells (Fig. 30.21). Similar features may be seen in skin biopsy specimens. Both HSV and VZV may be isolated from skin biopsy specimens, but VZV is more difficult to isolate, and the Tzanck smear is more sen-

Figure 30.19.   Herpes zoster. Vesicles and bullae are arrayed in the dermatomal pattern typical of herpes zoster infection.

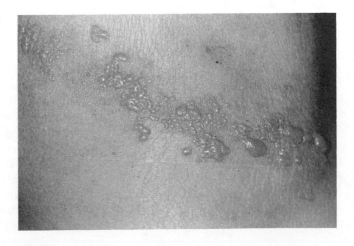

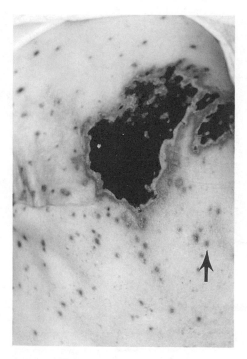

Figure 30.20. Necrotic ulcer due to herpes zoster. Large areas of necrosis covered by a thick, black eschar are typical of herpes zoster infection in severely immunocompromised patients. The surrounding papules (*arrow*) represent disseminated lesions of herpes zoster.

sitive for detection of infection (76). A direct immunofluorescence assay for VZV exists, which is more specific than the Tzanck smear (76).

CYTOMEGALOVIRUS

CMV is an important pathogen in this group of patients. No consistent specific cutaneous eruption is associated with CMV infection (77). Disseminated CMV infections have been reported to be associated with a morbilliform rash (78), with perianal ulcers (79), or with vesicular, indurated, or vasculitic lesions (80). One BMT patient had CMV present in a skin biopsy specimen from ill-defined erythematous macular lesions on the palms, soles, and ears (77). However, in one study (81) 60 skin biopsy specimens from patients with culture-proven (urine, blood, and/or bone marrow) CMV infection lacked CMV

by immunoperoxidase technique. CMV is reliably found, however, in the perianal ulcers of immunosuppressed patients (82). In summary, CMV infection should be strongly considered when a perianal ulcer is identified. Finding CMV in the skin is otherwise fortuitous.

CUTANEOUS GRAFT-VERSUS-HOST DISEASE

The cutaneous manifestations of GVHD occur in acute and chronic phases. Recognition of a cutaneous eruption as a GVHR is often the first clue to disease in other organs. Experience at the Johns Hopkins Medical Institutions indicates that an acute cutaneous GVHR is the only manifestation of acute GVHD in approximately 45% of patients. Establishing the diagnosis of a cutaneous GVHR requires observation of the eruption, histologic confirmation with a skin biopsy specimen, and consideration of other causes of rashes in BMT recipients. The clinical and histologic findings may vary markedly in degree in the same patient over time as well as between patients. For this reason, clinical-pathologic correlation is vital in determining the significance of a cutaneous eruption considered to be a GVHR.

Clinical Manifestations

The acute GVHR typically appears from 10–40 days after BMT (83). The patient may complain of tenderness or pruritus, or may be asymptomatic. The earliest sign of a cutaneous GVHR is faint erythematous macules, often located acrally. The macules progress in distribution and intensity over several days. The erythema remains blanchable unless, due to thrombocytopenia, there is sufficient erythrocyte extravasation to cause purpura. The macules may become papules over time as dermal edema gives the lesions palpable substance. Typical early cutaneous GVHR begins on the pinnae, palms, and soles, extending to involve the head, neck, and arms. This

Figure 30.21. Herpesvirus infection. HSV and VZV produce identical epidermal changes. An intraepidermal vesicle, filled with acantholytic (rounded and detached) keratinocytes, is present. An occasional multinucleated keratinocyte is seen (*arrow*). The dermis contains a polymorphous inflammatory cell infiltrate with numerous neutrophils.

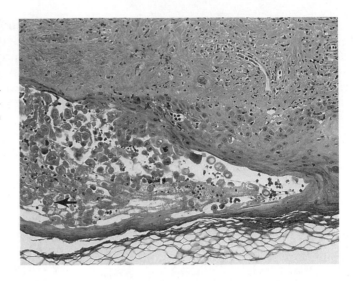

extension may progress to erythroderma. While such a sequence of progression is the usual scenario, other distributions may occur. Cutaneous GVHRs have been reported after autologous and syngeneic BMT (84). These eruptions tend to be more limited in extent and duration. As the eruptions resolve, desquamation and hyperpigmentation may occur. The dyschromia arises due to increased melanin and/or hemosiderin deposition and may be persistent.

Most patients developing a cutaneous GVHR after allogeneic BMT do not progress to erythroderma. Some patients develop vesicles and bullae within the erythematous macules, locally or widely distributed. Lateral pressure on the bullae may induce extension of the fluid in the plane of the skin (Nikolsky sign). This blistering form of cutaneous GVHD correlates with severe disease. Relying on the preceding descriptions a clinical grading system of acute cutaneous GVHD may be employed (Table 30.3).

The clinical differential diagnosis of erythematous macules and papules soon after BMT includes drug hypersensitivity and the cutaneous eruption of lymphocyte recovery. These entities are discussed below. Miliaria from sweat duct occlusion and bullae from hypoproteinemia and fluid deposition

Table 30.3. Clinical Grading of Acute Cutaneous Graft-Versus-Host Disease

Grade	Description
I	Erythematous macules and papules covering less than 25% of the skin
II	Eythematous macules and papules covering 25%–50% of the skin
III	Erythroderma
IV	Blisters

in the skin should not be confused with blistering due to a GVHR. Histologic examination of the skin aids in recognizing these conditions.

Chronic cutaneous GVHD generally develops 100 days or more after BMT (83). Lichenoid and sclerodermoid phases are identified based upon clinical and histologic findings. Lichenoid cutaneous GVHD is characterized by erythematous to violaceous papules and plaques distributed on the palms, soles, and occasionally more extensively (Fig. 30.22). The papules and plaques resemble lichen planus occurring in otherwise healthy individuals. Chronic cutaneous GVHD may appear after resolution of acute disease, may develop without a period of clearing, or may arise without identified antecedent acute GVHD. Resolution of the inflammatory phase

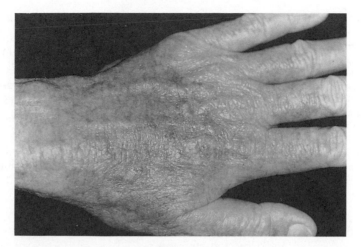

Figure 30.22. Lichenoid chronic GVHR. The acral location of this erythematous to violaceous plaque is typ- ical of a lichenoid chronic GVHR. (Reproduced with permission from Evan R. Farmer, M.D.)

of a lichenoid GVHR usually results in hyperpigmentation, often severe, due to increased melanin production and melanin deposition in the dermis.

Sclerodermoid GVHD resembles cutaneous scleroderma or morphea occurring in non-BMT patients. This form of chronic cutaneous GVHD tends to arise later than the lichenoid phase, which may or may not precede the sclerodermoid changes. The skin becomes indurated and thickened due to thickening and sclerosis of the dermal collagen. Pilosebaceous units and eccrine structures are lost over time. The epidermis becomes thinned, making cutaneous vessels prominent and imparting a shiny appearance. These changes may remain local or may generalize. In the latter setting, complications include joint contractures, infection, bullae, and difficulty with temperature regulation. Sclerodermoid GVHD may persist or may resolve spontaneously. While lichenoid and sclerodermoid GVHD have distinct clinical and histologic similarities with lichen planus and scleroderma, an etiologic link is not established.

Both acute and chronic GVHD may involve the oral mucosa and the conjuctivae. In the mouth, erythematous macules character- ize acute disease, while white macules and plaques, often reticulated, may develop with lichenoid chronic GVHD. In addition to the oral epithelium, the salivary glands may become involved, leading to sicca symptoms. The oral mucosa and salivary glands may be the primary or sole site of disease.

Histologic Changes

In the skin, the changes of an acute GVHR are those of an interface dermatitis with disruption of the dermal-epidermal junction and epidermal dysmaturation. The traditional framework for categorizing histologic changes in an acute cutaneous GVHR is shown in Table 30.4 (85). A superficial perivascular lymphocytic infiltrate is a common accompanying finding. Erythrocyte extravasation and endothelial cell swelling are variable findings. The normally sharp demarcation between epidermis and dermis is lost due to small vacuoles that form below the basilar epidermis (Fig. 30.23). These vacuoles fuse to form clefts in grade III changes (Fig. 30.24), and become confluent in grade IV disease. Lymphocytes migrate into the epidermis. A crucial element in the scheme above is the presence of dyskeratotic keratinocytes. These

Table 30.4. Histologic Grading of an Acute Cutaneous Graft-versus-Host Reaction

Grade	Description
0	Normal skin or changes unrelated to GVHD
I	Vacuolar alteration at the dermal-epidermal junction
II	Dyskeratotic keratinocytes in epidermis and/or follicular epithelium (Fig. 30.23 **A, B**)
III	Subepidermal cleft formation (Fig. 30.24)
IV	Separation of epidermis from dermis

cells are identified as brightly eosinophilic cells with pyknotic nuclei and retracted cytoplasm. An adjacent lymphocyte is variably identified (satellite cell necrosis) (Fig. 30.23B). As dyskeratotic cells may reside only in follicular epithelium, especially in early disease, careful examination of follicles is important. The presence of dyskeratotic cells (i.e., grade II change) is generally indicative of a GVHR.

The number of dyskeratotic cells in a given tissue section required to establish a grade II diagnosis is unclear. Dyskeratotic keratinocytes are occasionally found in skin specimens from patients receiving antineoplastic agents alone (85) and typically arise after ionizing radiation (86). Therefore, the scheme outlined above will not faultlessly identify GVHD to the exclusion of other processes. Interpretation of the tissue in conjunction with assessment of clinical status is a vital accompaniment. The histologic findings of a grade IV GVHR are indistinguishable from those of toxic epidermal necrolysis due to medications in otherwise healthy persons. Only in the setting of multiorgan disease and grade II changes elsewhere in the skin can this diagnosis be made.

Given the limitations noted above, histologic examination of the skin is extremely useful in patient management. The number of lymphocytes migrating into the epidermis (exocytosis) correlates with severity of disease and prognosis (87). The presence of dyskeratotic cells in the basilar epidermis suggests that the process is ongoing. Dysker-

atotic cells at higher epidermal levels in the absence of basilar involvement suggests that the acute insult has passed. Over time, these observations allow assessment of progression of disease and modification of therapy. Examination of frozen sections of skin is useful in rapidly establishing the presence of a grade II cutaneous GVHR.

In a lichenoid GVHR, the lymphocytic infiltrate becomes heavier and more readily identified as bandlike beneath the epidermis. The epidermal rete become pointed ("sawtoothed"), and the normally cuboidal basal keratinocytes become flattened ("squamotization"). The epidermis may be thickened, with a prominent stratum corneum and thickened granular cell layer. Beyond the earliest stages, melanin is usually found within dermal macrophages and free within the dermis. Such dermal deposition of pigment is typical of all inflammatory disorders affecting the dermal-epidermal junction. These findings are nearly identical to those of lichen planus, which generally displays a heavier inflammatory cell infiltrate. A sclerodermoid GVHR is characterized by homogenization and sclerosis of dermal collagen, which progresses from the papillary dermis downward (Fig. 30.25). This sequence is in distinction to scleroderma/morphea, in which the sclerosis progresses upward from a superficial panniculitis. In sclerodermoid GVHD, basal vacuolar change is noted. Adnexal structures are lost, pilosebaceous units first, then eccrine structures. Rarely, subepidermal bullae arise within the upper dermis due to edema.

Immunohistologic analysis of the epidermis during an acute cutaneous GVHR reveals induction of keratinocyte expression of HLA-DR (88) and intercellular adhesion molecule-1 (ICAM-1) antigens. Intraepidermal lymphocytes are largely CD8+, while dermal lymphocytes are mostly CD4+. The lymphocytes express lymphocyte function associated-1 antigen and are generally of the "memory" phenotype (i.e., CD45R+). The expression of these antigens is not specific as the induction of keratinocyte HLA-DR and

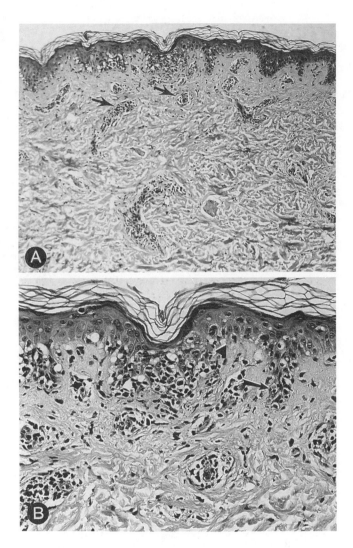

Figure 30.23. **A**, Photomicrograph of grade II acute GVHR. A superficial perivascular lymphocytic infiltrate (*arrow*) underlies epidermal changes. **B**, Photomicrograph of grade II acute GVHR. A closer view shows epidermal changes of basal vacuolization, dyskeratotic cells (*arrowhead*), and satellite cell necrosis (*arrow*).

ICAM-1 correlates with immunologic events affecting the epidermis in many cutaneous eruptions.

Laboratory Investigation Using the Skin

Models exist, utilizing the skin, to predict the development of GVHD after BMT in prospective donor-recipient pairs. An organ culture system coincubates various combinations of skin, trimmed of fat, with lymphocytes previously sensitized in bulk-mixed lymphocyte culture (89). A pattern of grade II GVHR in a sample of recipient skin incubated with sensitized donor lymphocytes is predictive of the subsequent development of GVHD. Epidermis derived from suction-blisters may be used to sensitize lymphocytes. The Langerhans cell is a potent antigen-presenting cell and is responsible for the allostimulatory activity of the epidermis. Prolifera-

Figure 30.24. Acute GVHR, grade III. There is significant necrosis of keratinocytes within the epidermis. Basal vacuolization has progressed to form the subepidermal clefts (*arrows*) characteristic of grade III changes. An accompanying bandlike lymphocytic infiltrate is present in the upper dermis.

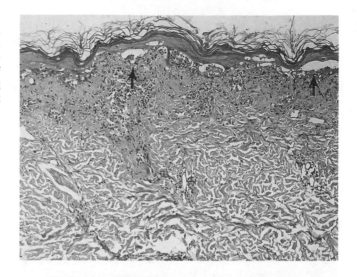

Figure 30.25. Chronic sclerodermoid cutaneous GVHR. The papillary and upper reticular dermis (*arrow*) display a subtle alteration in the tinctorial quality of the collagen. The individual collagen bundles are less distinct, giving a smudged or hyalinized appearance.

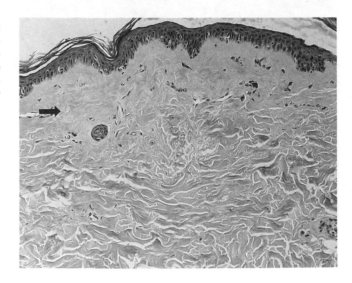

tion of donor lymphocytes in response to recipient epidermis may be a measure of future GVHD (90).

Why the skin should be commonly affected in GVHD is unclear. Severe cutaneous disease may develop in genotypic HLA-identical BMT. One possible explanation would be the existence of a skin-restricted alloantigen. In mice, Skn and Epa-1 are such skin-restricted antigens and most probably explain the phenomenon of "split tolerance" in chimeric animals (91). A similar antigen has not been identified in humans, however.

ORAL COMPLICATIONS

Oral GVHD, stomatitis, and infections involving the oral cavity are discussed above. Other oral complications include hemorrhage, tooth abnormalities, dental caries, and xerostomia. Osteoradionecrosis, taste abnormalities, and trismus are complications of radiotherapy of the head and neck and will not be discussed here.

Oral hemorrhage occurs frequently in patients treated with chemotherapeutic agents for hematologic malignancy. Thrombocytopenia is the most frequent cause (92), with hemorrhage frequently occurring when platelet counts are below 30,000 per cubic millimeter. Other etiologic factors include disseminated intravascular coagulation and combinations of thrombocytopenia and vitamin K deficiency or hypofibrinogenemia.

Hemorrhage is induced by trauma and can be seen anywhere in the oral cavity, with lips, tongue, and gingivae most commonly involved (92). Bleeding sites tend to ooze, with recurrent formation of soft clots. Treatment is with HLA-matched platelet transfusion or infusion of cryoprecipitates.

Dental abnormalities are reported in children receiving chemotherapy for cancer. Abnormalities include disturbed amelogenesis, bicuspid microdontia, and shortening, thinning, and blunting of roots (93). Dental caries are more common in treated children.

Xerostomia may occur as a result of chronic GVHD or following combination radio- and chemotherapy. The side effects include dental caries, infection (especially with *Candida* sp.) and difficulty in chewing, swallowing, or talking. Treatment includes saliva substitutes and sialogogues (94).

REFERENCES

1. Bronner AK, Hood AF. Cutaneous complications of chemotherapeutic agents. J Am Acad Dermatol 1983;9:645–663.
2. Dunagin WG. Dermatologic toxicity. In: Perry MC, Yarbro JW, eds. Toxicity of chemotherapy. New York: Grune & Stratton, 1984:125–154.
3. Robinson A, Jones W. Changes in scalp hair after cancer chemotherapy. Eur J Cancer Clin Oncol 1989; 25:155–156.
4. Dean JC, Salmon SE, Griffith KS. Prevention of doxorubicin induced hair loss with scalp hypothermia. N Engl J Med 1979;301:1427–1429.
5. Edelstyn GA, MacRae KD. Doxorubicin-induced hair loss and possible modification by scalp cooling. Lancet 1977;2:253–254.
6. Hussein AM, Jimenez JJ, McCall CA, Yunis AA. Protection from chemotherapy-induced alopecia in a rat model. Science 1990;249:1564–1566.
7. Peterson DE. Oral lesions. In: Perry MC, Yarbro JW, eds. Toxicity of chemotherapy. New York: Grune & Stratton, 1984:155–180.
8. Dose AM, Loprinzi CL, Cianflone S, et al. A controlled evaluation of an allopurinol mouthwash as prophylaxis against 5-fluorouracil (5-FU)-induced stomatitis: a North Central Cancer Treatment Group and Mayo Clinic study. Proc ASCO 1989;8:341.
9. Mills EED. The modifying effect of beta-carotene on radiation and chemotherapy induced oral mucositis. Br J Cancer 1988;57:416–417.
10. Loprinzi CL, Dose AM. Studies on the prevention of 5-fluorouracil-induced oral mucositis. NCI Monogr 1990;9:93–94.
11. Miaskowski C. Management of mucositis during therapy. NCI Monogr 1990;9:95–98.
12. Weiss RB, Bruno S. Hypersensitivity reactions to cancer chemotherapeutic agents. Ann Intern Med 1981;94:66–72.
13. Khan A, Hill JM, Grater W, et al. Atopic hyersensitivity to cis dichlorodiammineplatinum (II) and other platinum complexes. Cancer Res 1975;35:2766–2770.
14. Lakin JD, Cahill RA. Generalized urticaria to cyclophosphamide: type I hyersensitivity to an immunosupressive agent. J Allergy Clin Immunol 1976;58:160–171.
15. Kerker BJ, Hood AF. Chemotherapy-induced cutaneous reactions. Semin Dermatol 1989;8:173–181.
16. Braur MJ, McEvoy BF, Mitus WJ. Hypersensitivity to nitrogen mustards in the form of erythema multiforme. Arch Intern Med 1967;120:499–503.
17. Purpora D, Ahern MJ, Silverman N. Toxic epidermal necrolysis after mithramycin [Letter]. N Engl J Med 1978;299:1412.
18. Glovsky MM, Braunwald J, Opelz G, Alenty A. Hypersensitivity to procarbazine associated with angioedema, urticaria, and low serum complement activity. J Allergy Clin Immunol 1976;57:134–140.
19. Van Scott EJ, Kalmanson JD. Complete remissions of mycosis fungoides luymphoma induced by topical nitrogen mustard (HN$_2$): control of delayed hypersensitivity to HN$_2$ by desensitizaion and by induction of specific immunologic tolerance. Cancer 1973; 113:18–31.
20. Leshaw S, Simon RS, Baer RL. Failure to induce tolerance to mechlorethamine hydrochloride. Arch Dermatol 1977;113:1406–1498.
21. Hood AF. Cutaneous side effects of cancer chemotherapy. Med Clin North Am 1986;70:187–209.
22. D'Angio GJ. Potentiation of x-ray effects by actinomycin D. Radiology 1959;73:175–177.
23. Donaldson SS, Glick JM, Wilbur JR. Adriamycin activating a recall phenomenon after radiation therapy. Ann Intern Med 1974;81:407–408.

24. Yagoda A, Mukherji B, Young C, et al. Bleomycin, and antitumor antibiotic. Ann Intern Med 1972;77:861–870.

25. Frei E III. The clinical use of actinomycin. Cancer Chemother Rep 1974;58:49–54.

26. Kim YH, Aye MS, Fayos JV. Radiation necrosis of the scalp: a complication of cranial irradiation and chemotherapy. Radiology 197;124:813–814.

27. Solberg LA Jr, Wick MR, Bruckman JE. Doxorubicin-enhanced skin reaction after whole-body electron-beam irradiation for leukemia cutis. Mayo Clin Proc 1980;55:711–715.

28. Yung CW, Winston EM, Lorincz AL. Dacarbazine-induced photosensitivity. J Am Acad Dermatol 1981; 4:541–543.

29. Falkson G, Schulz EJ. Skin changes in patients treated with 5-fluorouracil. Br J Dermatol 1961;74:229–236.

30. Breza TS, Halprin KM. Taylor JR. Photosensitivity reaction to vinblastine. Arch Dermatol 1975;111:1168–1170.

31. Fuller B, Lind M, Bonomi P. Mitomycin C extravasation exacerbated by sunlight. Ann Intern Med 1981;94:542.

32. Korossy KS, Hood AF. Methotrexate reactivation of sunburn reaction. Arch Dermatol 1981;117:310–311.

33. Podoll LN, Winkler SS. Busulfan lung. Am J Roentgenol 1974;120:151–156.

34. Kyle RA, Schwartz RS, Oliner HL, et al. A syndrome resembling adrenal cortical insufficiency associated with long term busulfan (Myleran) therapy. Blood 1961;18:497–510.

35. Guillet G, Guillet M-H, De Meaux H, et al. Cutaneous pigmented stripes and bleomycin treatment. Arch Dermatol 1986;122:381–382.

36. Horn TD, Beveridge RA, Egorin MJ, Abeloff MD, Hood AF. Observations and proposed mechanism of N,N′,N″-triethylenethiophosphoramide (thiotepa)-induced hyperpigmentation. Arch Dermatol 1989;125:524–527.

37. Lotze MT, Matory YL, Rayner AA. Clinical effects and toxicity of interleukin-2 in patients with cancer. Cancer 1986;58:2764–2772.

38. Conlon KC, Urba WJ, Smith JW, Steis RG, Longo DL, Clark JW. Exacerbation of symptoms of autoimmune disease in patients receiving alpha-interferon therapy. Cancer 1990;65:2237–2242.

39. Tichelli A, Gratwohl A, Berger E, et al. Treatment of thrombocytosis in myeloproliferative disorders with interferon alpha-2a. Blut 1989;58:15–19.

40. Hirsh M, Lipton A, Harvey H, et al. Phase I study of interleukin-2 and interferon alpha-2a as outpatient therapy for patients with advanced malignancy. J Clin Oncol 1990;8:1657–1663.

41. Edwards L, Tucker SB, Perednia D, et al. The effect of an intralesional sustained release formulation of interferon alpha-2b on basal cell carcinomas. Arch Dermatol 1990;126:1029–1032.

42. Glaspy JA, Marcus SG, Ambersley J, Golde DW. Recombinant beta-serine-interferon in hairy cell leukemia compared prospectively with results with recombinant alpha-interferon. Cancer 1989;64:409–413.

43. Kinney P, Triozzi P, Young D, et al. Phase II trial of interferon-beta-serine in metastatic renal cell carcinoma. J Clin Oncol 1990;8:881–885.

44. Kaplan EH, Rosen ST, Norris DB, Roenigk HH, Saks SR, Bunn PA. Phase II study of recombinant human interferon gamma for treatment of cutaneous T cell lymphoma. J Natl Cancer Inst 1990;82:208–212.

45. Fierlbeck G, Rassner G, Muller C. Psoriasis induced at the injection site of recombinant interferon gamma. Results of immunologic investigations. Arch Dermatol 1990;126:351–355.

46. Horn TD, Burke PJ, Karp JE, Hood AF. Intravenous administration of recombinant human granulocyte-macrophage colony-stimulating factor causes a cutaneous eruption. Arch Dermatol 1991;127:49–52.

47. Crider MK, Jansen J, Norins AL, McHale MS. Chemotherapy-induced acral erythema in patients receiving bone marrow transplantation. Arch Dermatol 1986;122:1023–1027.

48. Kampmann KK, Graves TT, Rogers SD. Acral erythema secondary to high dose cytosine arabinoside with pain worsened by cyclosporine infusions. Cancer 1989;673:2482–2485.

49. Oksenhendler E, Landais P, Cordonnier C, et al. Acral erythema and systemic toxicity related to CHA induction therapy in acute myeloid leukemia. Eur J Cancer Clin Oncol 1989;25:1181–1185.

50. Harrist TJ, Fine J-D, Berman RS et al. Neutrophilic eccrine hidrandenitis. Arch Dermatol 1982;118:263–266.

51. Scallan PJ, Kettler AH, Levy ML, Tschen JA. Neutrophilic eccrine hidrandenitis. Evidence implicating bleomycin as a causative agent. Cancer 1988;62:2532–2536.

52. Epstein EH, Lutzner MH. Folliculitis induced by actinomycin D. N Engl J Med 1969;281:1094–1096.

53. Kyle RA, Dameshek W. Porphyria cutanea tarda associated with chronic granulocytic leukemia treated with busulfan. Blood 1964;23:776–785.

54. Guyotat D, Nicolas JF, Augey F, Fiere D, Thivolet J. Porphyria cutanea tarda after allogeneic bone marrow transplantation for chronic myelogenous leukemia. Am J Hematol 1990;34:69–70.

55. Peck GL, Herzig GP, Elias PM. Toxic epidermal necrolysis in a patient with graft-vs-host reaction. Arch Dermatol 1972;105:561–569.

56. Villada G, Roujeau J-C, Cordonnier C, et al. Toxic epidermal necrolysis after bone marrow transplantion: study of nine cases. J Am Acad Dermatol 1990;23:870–875.

57. Goldberg NS, Ahmed T, Robinson B, Ascensao J, Horowitz H. Staphylococcal scalded skin syndrome mimicking acute graft-vs-host disease in a bone marrow transplant recipient. Arch Dermatol 1989;125:85–87.

58. Horn TD, Groleau GE. Transient acantholytic dermatosis in immunocompromised febrile patients with cancer. Arch Dermatol 1987;123:238–240.

59. Horn TD, Redd JV, Karp JE, Beschorner WE, Burke PJ, Hood AF. Cutaneous eruptions of lymphocyte recovery. Arch Dermatol 1989;125:1512–1517.

60. Abel EA. Cutaneous manifestations of immunosuppression in organ transplant recipients. J Am Acad Dermatol 1989;21:167–179.

61. Lishner M, Patterson B, Kandel R, et al. Cutaneous and mucosal neoplasms in bone marrow transplant recipients. Cancer 1990;65:473–476.

62. Heimdahl A, Mattsson T, Dahllöf G, Lönnquist B, Ringden. The oral cavity as a port of entry for early infections in patients with bone marrow transplantation. Oral Surg Oral Med Oral Pathol 1989;68:711–716.

63. Winston DJ, Ho WG, Champlin RE. Current approaches to management of infections in bone marrow transplants. Eur J Cancer Clin Oncol 1989;25:S25–S35.

64. Wolf JE, Liu H, Rabinowitz LG. Ecthyma gangrenosum in the absence of *Pseudomonas* bacteremia in a bone marrow transplant recipient. Am J Med 1989;87:595–597.

65. Meyers JD. Fungal infections in bone marrow transplant patients. Semin Oncol 1990;17:10–13.

66. Kirk JL, Greenfield RA, Slease RB, Epstein RB. Analysis of early infectious complications after autologous bone marrow transplantation. Cancer 1988; 62:2445–2450.

67. Bufill JA, Lum LG, Caya JG. *Pityrosporum* folliculitis after bone marrow transplantation. Ann Intern Med 1988;108:560–563.

68. Merz WG, Karp JE, Hoagland M, Jett-Goheen M, Junkins JM, Hood AF. Diagnosis and successful treatment of fusariosis in the compromised host. J Infect Dis 198;158:1046–1055.

69. Neglia JP, Hurd DD, Ferrieri P, Snover DC. Invasive *Scopulariopsis* in the immunocompromised host. Am J Med 1987;83:1163–1166.

70. Taylor CE, Sviland L, Pearson ADJ, et al. Virus infections in bone marrow transplant recipients: a three year prospective study. J Clin Pathol 1990;43:633–637.

71. Saral R. Management of acute viral infections. NCI Monogr 1990;9:107–110.

72. Schubert MM, Peterson DE, Flournoy N, Meyers JD, Truelove EL. Oral and pharyngeal herpes simplex virus infection after allogeneic bone marrow transplantation: analysis of factors associated with infection. Oral Surg Oral Med Oral Pathol 1990;70:286–293.

73. Selby PJ, Powles RL, Easton D, et al. The prophylactic role of intravenous and long-term acyclovir after allogeneic bone marrow transplantation. Br J Cancer 1989;59:434–438.

74. Schuchter LM, Wingard JR, Piantadosi S, Burns WH, Santos GW, Saral R. Herpes zoster infection after autologous bone marrow transplantation. Blood 1989;74:1424–1427.

75. Liesegang TJ. The Varicella-zoster virus: systemic and ocular features. J Am Acad Dermatol 1984;11:165–191.

76. Sadick NS, Swenson PD, Kaufman RL, Kaplan MH. Comparison of detection of varicella-zoster virus by the Tzanck smear, direct immunofluorescence with a monoclonal antibody, and virus isolation. J Am Acad Dermatol 1987;17:64–69.

77. Horn TD, Hood AF. Clinically occult cytomegalovirus present in skin biopsy specimens in immunosuppressed hosts. J Am Acad Dermatol 1989;21:781–784.

78. Lin C-S, Penha P, Krishnan MN, Zak FG. Cytomegalic inclusion disease of the skin. Arch Dermatol 1981;117:282–284.

79. Nakoneczna I, Kay S. Fatal disseminated cytomegalic inclusion disease in an adult presenting with a lesion of the gastrointestinal tract. Am J Clin Pathol 1967;47:124–128.

80. Feldman PS, Walker AN, Baker R. Cutaneous lesions heralding disseminated cytomegalovirus infection. J Am Acad Dermatol 1982;7:545–548.

81. Horn TD, Farmer ER, Vogelsang GB, Wingard JR, Santos GW. Cutaneous graft-vs-host reaction lacks evidence of cutaneous cytomegalovirus by the immunoperoxidase technique. J Invest Dermatol 1989;93:92–95.

82. Horn TD, Hood AF. Cytomegalovirus is predictably present in perineal ulcers from immunosuppressed patients. Arch Dermatol 1990;126:642–644.

83. Farmer ER. Human cutaneous graft-versus-host disease. J Invest Dermatol 1985;85:124s–128s.

84. Hood AF, Vogelsang GB, Black LP, Farmer ER, Santos GW. Acute graft-vs-host disease. Development following autologous and syngeneic bone marrow transplantation. Arch Dermatol 1987;123:745–750.

85. Sale GE, Lerner KG, Barker EA, Shulman HM, Thomas ED. The skin biopsy in the diagnosis of acute graft-versus-host disease in man. Am J Pathol 1977;89:621–636.

86. LeBoit PE. Subacute radiation dermatitis: a histologic imitator of acute cutaneous graft-versus-host disease. J Am Acad Dermatol 1989;20:236–241.

87. Hymes SR, Farmer ER, Lewis PG, Tutschka PJ, Santos GW. Cutaneous graft-versus-host reaction: prognostic features seen by light microscopy. J Am Acad Dermatol 1985;12:468–474.

88. Breathnach SM, Katz SI. Immunopathology of cutaneous graft-versus-host disease. Am J Dermatopathol 1987;9:343–348.

89. Vogelsang GB, Hess AD, Berkman AW, et al. An in vitro predictive test for graft versus host disease in patients with genotypic HLA-identical bone marrow transplants. N Engl J Med 1985;313:645–650.

90. Bagot M, Cordonnier C, Vernant JP, Dubertret L, Rochant H, Levy JP. Mixed epidermal cell-lymphocyte reaction in prediction of acute graft-versus-host disease in bone marrow recipients. J Natl Cancer Inst 1986;76:1317–1319.

91. Tyler JD, Steinmuller D. Evidence of cell-mediated cytotoxicity to skin-specific alloantigens on mouse epidermal cells. Transplant Proc 1981;13:1082–1085.

92. Dreizen S. Description and incidence of oral complications. NCI Monogr 1990;9:11–15.

93. Rosenberg S. Chronic dental complications. NCI Monogr 1990;9:173–178.

94. Greenspan D. Management of salivary dysfunction. NCI Monogr 1990;9:159–161.

31

GENITOURINARY, GASTROINTESTINAL, AND OTHER COMPLICATIONS

Michael C. Perry

Higher doses of chemotherapeutic agents are used in an attempt to produce greater rates of response, higher complete response rates, and a greater proportion of long-term survivors or "cures." At conventional doses these same drugs have side effects that are usually predictable and reversible. (There are, of course, unanticipated allergic or idiosyncratic reactions). "Typical" toxicities include alopecia, mucositis, and myelosuppression (Table 31.1). At doses in excess of those usually given, however, some drugs display a new spectrum of toxicities. The use of "rescue" techniques, autologous bone marrow transplantation, and hematopoietic growth factors has considerably decreased myelosuppression as a significant cause of mortality and morbidity.

As an example, high doses of methotrexate, in the range of grams rather than milligrams per square meter, given with leucovorin rescue, do not produce the usual myelosuppression but may produce renal failure or CNS toxicity. Gastrointestinal toxicity, especially mucositis and diarrhea, remains a significant problem, however, and is often dose-limiting. This chapter will discuss by organ system some unique complications of high-dose therapy.

GENITOURINARY TOXICITY

Ifosfamide, an oxazaphosphorine analogue of cyclophosphamide, shares its potential for hemorrhagic cystitis, which may be dose limiting (1–3). Indeed, the incidence and severity may be greater than that associated with cyclophosphamide. This complication can be alleviated by fractionating the dose of ifosfamide, or more commonly, by the use of mesna (sodium-2-mercaptoethanesulfonate) and intravenous hydration. Mesna is an aliphatic carrier of two functional groups: the sulfo group leads to a rapid renal elimination, and the mercapto group binds acrolein and other toxic ifosfamide metabolites in the urinary tract (3). Oral mesna is rapidly oxidized to inert mesna disulfide during intestinal absorption or in the plasma (after intravenous administration), which is reduced to the pharmacologically active thiol form mesna in the renal tubular epithelium.

Most treatment programs using standard fractionated doses of ifosfamide include intravenous hydration and mesna at 20% of the ifosfamide dose prior to and every 4 hours after ifosfamide for a total of 3–5 doses. For continuous infusions a dose of mesna equal to 10% of the dose of ifosfamide should be given 15 minutes before ifosfamide, followed by a 24-hour infusion equal to 100% of the dose of ifosfamide. When mesna is given orally, the initial dose can be given intravenously, with subsequent oral doses at twice the intravenous dose at 4 and 8 hours after ifosfamide (2). This reduces the incidence of

Table 31.1. Complications Following Chemotherapy

Standard Dose	High Dose
Alopecia	Coagulation defects
Mucositis	Hepatic venoocclusive disease
Diarrhea	Hemorrhagic myocarditis
Myelosuppression	Encephalopathy
	Renal failure

gross hematuria to less than 5% and microscopic hematuria to 5–18% of courses.

It is also important to note that reactivation of the BK type of human polyomavirus is associated with hemorrhagic cystitis (4). The disease occurred in 50% of allogeneic marrow recipients and only 7% of syngeneic or autologous marrow recipients. Reactivation of BK virus may account for a substantial proportion of late-onset, long-lasting hemorrhagic cystitis.

Nephrotoxicity is both less common and less predictable than urotoxicity. At standard doses elevated levels of blood urea nitrogen (BUN) and creatinine are seen in a small percentage of patients, but acute tubular necrosis and even renal failure have been seen, especially in patients who are not adequately hydrated or who have preexisting renal impairment (5, 6).

High-dose ifosfamide by continuous infusion, on the other hand, has produced renal failure despite mesna use. Two of 42 patients treated with 8 g/m^2 of ifosfamide over 24 hours developed irreversible renal failure, and an additional 5 developed elevations in BUN or creatinine (7). Subclinical tubular nephrotoxicity despite mesna has also been documented (6, 8). It has been suggested that due to its concentration in the bladder bolus, mesna may be adequate to prevent hemorrhagic cystitis but may not be present in adequate levels in the kidney to prevent nephrotoxicity (9). Since ifosfamide and mesna are compatible in solution, they should be mixed and given continuously at equal dosage, and continued for 8–24 hours after the end of the ifosfamide infusion (9, 10).

In children, ifosfamide has induced both

renal tubular defects with the Fanconi syndrome and hypophosphatemic rickets (11–14).

High-dose cyclophosphamide therapy with autologous bone marrow transplantation has been implicated in the production of transient nephrogenic diabetes insipidus, usually at doses of >50 mg/kg (15). (See endocrine section, below).

Other novel toxicities associated with high-dose combination alkylating agents with autologous bone marrow support include hypertension, seen in 56% of patients and resistant to all classes of antihypertensives except nifedipine (16). By 60 days after transplantation, hypertension resolved and required no further therapy.

GASTROINTESTINAL TOXICITY

With the onset of autologous bone marrow support and hematopoietic growth factors, myelosuppression is no longer the dose-limiting toxicity for many chemotherapeutic drugs. In many patients stomatitis/mucositis has taken the place of myelosuppression as the dose-limiting toxicity (17–22). It may be severe enough to require the use of intravenous narcotics in addition to parenteral nutrition, and through ulceration it may predispose to infection.

Complete necrosis of the duodenal surface epithelium extending to involve the entire width of the mucosa has been seen following intensive chemotherapy followed by autologous marrow rescue (23). These dramatic changes reversed 18 days after the cessation of chemotherapy and prior to full bone marrow recovery. This intestinal toxicity may contribute to the morbidity of this form of therapy. Indeed, hyponatremia associated with fecal sodium loss has been seen following intensive chemotherapy and total body radiation (24).

Therapy of chemotherapy-induced mucositis consists of topical analgesics such as viscous lidocaine or a 50–50 mixture of benadryl and Maalox, and in many cases oral antifungal and/or antiviral therapy for complicating superinfections. To permit adequate nutrition patients may require either enteral supplementation through a feeding tube or total parenteral nutrition (TPN). TPN is not clearly superior to individualized enteral feeding, however, and it has been recommended that TPN be reserved for bone marrow transplant patients who are intolerant of enteral feeding (25). Intravenous narcotics, often given via patient-controlled analgesia (PCA), are necessary as well.

A shift of fluid from the intracellular to the extracellular fluid compartment during the first 4 weeks after bone marrow transplantation has been demonstrated (26). This was accompanied by a loss of body cell mass, perhaps due to inadequate nutrient intake. Thus over a short time period changes in body weight may not be sensitive enough to detect changes in body composition.

Infectious gastroenteritis is also a common problem in bone marrow transplant recipients, occurring in 40% in one series (27). Enteric pathogens that cause mild diarrhea in normal individuals may produce serious infections in marrow transplant recipients, and infectious etiologies should be sought in this setting.

Hemorrhagic colitis was encountered along with severe and even fatal hepatic necrosis as a complication of high-dose mitomycin therapy with autologous bone marrow transplantation (28). These severe nonhematologic toxicities were seen at three times the conventional dose of mitomycin, thus rendering it an unlikely agent for high-dose therapy.

ENDOCRINE TOXICITY

Since irradiation to the head and neck produces thyroid function abnormalities, it is not surprising that total body irradiation (TBI) in preparation for bone marrow transplantation produces similar problems (29). Asymptomatic uncompensated hypothyroidism with elevated thyroid-stimulating hormone and decreased thyroxine levels occurs

in 30%–60% of patients (Deeg). Single-dose (≥ 10 Gy) TBI appears to be most likely to cause thyroid dysfunction, and fractionated TBI least likely.

Gonadal function may also be adversely affected by the combination of TBI and cyclophosphamide (30). In 32 adults primary ovarian failure requiring hormone replacement therapy was produced in all females. In men, normal testosterone levels with increased levels of follicle-stimulating hormone suggestive of germinal aplasia were seen, confirmed by semen analysis in some patients. This is consistent with prior studies correlating impairment of ovarian function with both radiation dose and patient age.

High-dose cyclophosphamide (greater than 50 mg/kg) therapy may produce water intoxication as evidenced by hyponatremia, weight gain, and inappropriately concentrated urine (31). Since such patients receive extensive hydration to reduce the likelihood of uric acid nephropathy and hemorrhagic cystitis, this phenomenon should be anticipated.

There is also a single report of a pituitary abscess arising in a patient during recovery from autologous bone marrow transplantation.

NERVOUS SYSTEM TOXICITY

Several chemotherapeutic agents, especially ifosfamide, produce CNS toxicity at high doses. The spectrum of ifosfamide CNS toxicity includes mental status changes, cranial nerve defects, seizures, stupor, severe weakness, and ataxia. These symptoms are usually, but not always, reversible. The incidence of ifosfamide neurotoxicity has been reported at 0%–50%, without a clear-cut-dose-toxicity relationship, although high doses seem more likely to produce side effects (2, 33–35). Fatal CNS toxicity has been reported after single doses of 3–10 g/m^2 and a dose of 3.6 g/m^2 given over 2 days (36–38). Splitting the dose over 5 days seems to markedly reduce the likelihood of neurotoxicity. Oral administration, however, leads to an increased incidence of such toxicity, perhaps due to first-pass metabolism (39). Cerny et al. found the incidence of encephalopathy to be 43% with oral administration, 26% with intravenous administration, and only 7% with continuous intravenous infusion.

Other reported risk factors for encephalopathy include clinical or subclinical renal toxicity, especially following cisplatin therapy, hepatic disease, low serum albumin, and the presence of pelvic metastatic disease (40–44).

The etiology of ifosfamide encephalopathy is unclear. It has been suggested by Goren et al. that chloracetaldehyde, a metabolite of ifosfamide, was present in higher levels in the blood of patients who experienced neurotoxicity, compared to others without such toxicity (41). This explanation has not been universally accepted, however (39).

Therapy for established encephalopathy includes immediate cessation of ifosfamide and supportive care. During therapy every effort should be made to minimize other CNS-active drugs, such as antiemetics, sedatives, etc. (45).

Another alkylating agent, chlorambucil, has been implicated in the production of reversible CNS toxicity when used in high dose with autologous bone marrow transplantation for ovarian cancer (46). The spectrum of symptoms included generalized tremor, confusion, asterixis, hallucinations, and myoclonus. All three patients recovered spontaneously with residual deficits. The underlying mechanism behind chlorambucil neurotoxicity has not been determined, but the authors felt that the resolution of symptoms with discontinuation of the drug suggested toxicity rather than a structural lesion. They noted that a portion of the drug has lipophilic properties, raising the possibility that storage of the drug in fat may occur, explaining the prolonged toxic effects.

High-dose carmustine (BCNU) with autologous bone marrow transplantation used in the adjuvant treatment of high-grade gliomas produced CNS deterioration not due to tumor and characterized as diffuse encephalomyelopathy (47). This occurred in 2 of 18 patients, one a long-term survivor. The 22% incidence of fatal pulmonary toxicity led the investigators to abandon the protocol.

Mechlorethamine (nitrogen mustard) has been used as part of a preparative regimen for autologous bone marrow transplantation, but neurotoxicity proved to be dose limiting (48). Fourteen of 21 evaluable patients developed immediate toxicity a median of 4 days after treatment, which consisted of confusion, disorientation, headache, hallucinations, lethargy, tremors, paraplegia, seizures, and vertigo. Symptoms cleared in 11 of 14 recipients prior to death. Twelve patients survived more than 60 days; all 6 with previous acute changes developed new findings (personality change, confusion, seizure, diplopia, or dementia) a mean of 169 days after therapy.

Cerebrospinal fluid analysis in this group of patients was usually normal, but computed tomography (CT) scans showed ventricular enlargement and electroencephalograms diffuse slowing. Autopsy showed neuronal degenerative changes with increased vascularity, gliosis, and perivascular fibrosis. Neurotoxicity appeared to increase with age and dose and was more frequent in patients who also received procarbazine or cyclophosphamide.

Thiotepa was also implicated in the production of grade 3 somnolence in one patient and fatal brain injury (seizures and coma) in another when used with autologous bone marrow transplantation (19).

Six of eight glioma patients treated with high-dose etoposide and autologous bone marrow transplantation developed sudden neurologic deterioration (49). This occurred a median of 9 days after the initiation of therapy and consisted of confusion, papilledema, somnolence, exacerbation of motor deficits, and a sharp increase in seizure activity. No changes were seen in repeat CT scans. Abnormalities resolved within 12–48 hours after high-dose dexamethasone therapy. It was felt that even without CT evidence of increased intracranial pressure, this was the likely mechanism.

A "stroke like" syndrome of aphasia or hemiparesis occasionally with seizures has been described by Allen and Rosen in 8 of 31 patients receiving high-dose methotrexate (>200 mg/kg intravenously) for osteogenic sarcoma (50). The symptoms always occurred during the first three courses of therapy, resolved within 3 days, and did not recur with further therapy. CT scans were normal, but electroencephalogram abnormalities were noted. The authors postulated that the syndrome was due to necrosis of undetected pulmonary micrometastases that might have embolized to the brain.

Although CNS toxicity is a well-recognized complication of high-dose cytosine arabinoside therapy, peripheral neuropathy is rarely reported. Reversible ventilatory failure secondary to an acute, acquired Guillain-Barré-like polyneuropathy was seen in a patient undergoing bone marrow transplantation for chronic granulocytic leukemia (51). The onset of the neuropathy was temporally related to the use of high dose systemic cytosine arabinoside in the conditioning program.

Chemotherapeutic agents are not the only drugs to produce neurotoxicity in this setting. Acyclovir, the antiviral agent used to treat herpes simplex and varicella-zoster infections, has also been reported to produce neurologic symptoms of lethargy or agitation, tremor, disorientation, or transient hemiparesthesias (52). The only consistent laboratory finding was an abnormal electroencephalogram; five of six patients had an elevated myelin basic protein in cerebrospinal fluid. It was not clear what other factors, such as concomitant α-interferon or previous intrathecal methotrexate, contribute to this phenomenon.

There is also a report of the development of myasthenia gravis, thought to be of donor origin, following bone marrow transplantation (53). The possibility of other autoimmune diseases transmitted by this route must be considered.

HEMATOLOGIC TOXICITY

Temporary pancytopenia is an expected complication of bone marrow transplantation, but recovery is usual. Prolonged thrombocytopenia following transplantation may occur in up to 40% of patients, with a picture compatible with immune thrombocytopenic purpura (ITP) (54). The authors of this report suggested that this finding was more common than previously realized and emphasized its treatable nature. It has been suggested that these platelet-directed auto-antibodies are "due to transient immune-system imbalance common to both allografts and autografts in the early post-graft period" (55). Past cytomegalovirus infection was not predictive of the occurrence of prolonged thrombocytopenia (56).

Four patients who had received high-dose chemotherapy with autologous bone marrow transplantation developed posttreatment deficiencies of coagulation Factor XII and protein C (57). Three of the patients also had deficiencies of Factor VII, one deficiencies in Factors XII, X, IX, and VII and another deficiencies of both Factors XII and VII. Since three of these patients developed chemotherapy-related toxicity to lung, liver, or heart, the authors proposed that endothelial cell injury might be the underlying lesion responsible for these abnormalities. This, however, is still speculation. It is important to note that the Factor VII or Factor X deficiencies were severe enough to pose potential problems, either through hemorrhage or requiring factor replacement therapy prior to an invasive procedure.

In another study of the coagulation system 10 patients with breast cancer or melanoma who received high-dose chemotherapy with autologous bone marrow transplantation were studied to determine if such therapy was associated with an acquired platelet defect (58). Platelets underwent shape change and a primary wave of aggregation. High-dose chemotherapy was associated with the inhibition of secondary aggregation of platelets induced by adenosine diphosphate (ADP), arachidonic acid, prostaglandin H_2 analogue (U44619), and collagen.

Release of adenosine triphosphate (ATP) from dense granules was less than 20% of normal, although electron microscopy revealed normal morphology. This acquired platelet defect occurred before the onset of thrombocytopenia. The authors felt that this pattern of platelet inhibition was consistent with a platelet secretory defect and hypothesized that this defect could account for the complication of hemorrhagic myocarditis.

Functional asplenia as evidenced by five separate techniques was demonstrated in 6 of 15 allogeneic bone marrow transplant recipients (59). All the patients had evidence of chronic graft-versus-host disease, which presumably contributed to their four times greater incidence of bacterial infections.

MISCELLANEOUS

Three of 56 long-term survivors of bone marrow allografts developed second malignancies of the skin or oral mucosa, two squamous cell carcinomas and one melanoma (60). All had received a preparative regimen combining high-dose chemotherapy with total body irradiation and then immunosuppressive therapy for chronic graft-versus-host disease.

CONCLUSIONS

It is important to recall that there are individual variations in sensitivity to chemotherapeutic agents, and these variations may have profound implications. A genetic defect of pyrimidine-base degradation has been described, with resultant severe fluorouracil toxicity, even at reduced doses (61). Identification of similar deficiencies will be of utmost importance in dose modification.

In at least one situation it is possible to predict which individuals will experience toxicity. Fast acetylators of the investigational agent amonafide may have increased myelo-

suppression at standard doses. Ratain et al. have utilized caffeine to determine acetylator phenotype and predict amonafide toxicity (62). Using this assay, the standard amonafide dose appears to be too high for fast acetylators and too low for slow acetylators. If available for other drugs, this type of assay will permit accurate pretreatment prediction of toxicity.

REFERENCES

1. Van Dyck JJ, Falkson HC, van der Merwe AM, Falkson G. Unexpected toxicity in patients treated with iphosphamide. Cancer Res 1972;32:921–924.
2. Zalupski M, Baker LH. Ifosfamide. J Natl Cancer Inst 1988;80:556–566.
3. Scheulen ME, Niederle N, Bremer K, Schutte J, Seeber S. Efficacy of ifosfamide in refractory malignant diseases and uroprotection by mesna: results of a clinical phase II study with 151 patients. Cancer Treat Rev 1983;10(suppl A):93–101.
4. Arthur RR, Shah KV, Baust SJ, Santos GW, Saral R. Association of BK viruria with hemorrhagic cystitis in recipients of bone marrow transplants. N Engl J Med 1986;315:230–234.
5. Constanzi JJ, Morgan LH, Hokanson J. Ifosfamide in the treatment of extensive non-oat cell carcinoma of the lung. Semin Oncol 1982;9(suppl 1):61–65.
6. Patterson WP, Khojasteh A. Ifosfamide-induced renal tubular defects. Cancer 1989;63:649–651.
7. Stuart-Harris RC, Harper PG, Parsons CA, et al. High dose alkylation therapy using ifosfamide infusion with mesna in the treatment of adult advanced soft tissue sarcomas. Cancer Chemother Pharmacol 1985;11:69–72.
8. Goren MP, Wright RK, Horowitz ME, Pratt CB. Ifosfamide-induced subclinical tubular nephrotoxicity despite mesna. Cancer Treat Rep 1987;71:127–130.
9. Hilgard P, Burkert H. Sodium-2-mercaptoethane sulfonate(mesna) and ifosfamide nephrotoxicity. Eur J Cancer Clin Oncol 1984;20:1451–1452.
10. Klein HO, Dias Wickramanayake P, Coerper CL, et al. High dose ifosfamide and mesna as continuous infusion over 5 days—a phase I/II trial. Cancer Treat Rep 1983;10(suppl a):167–173.
11. Skinner R, Pearson ADJ, Price L, Coulthard MG, Craft AW. Nephrotoxicity after ifosfamide. Arch Dis Child 1990;65:732–738.
12. Burk CD, Restaino I, Kaplan BS, Meadows AT. Ifosfamide-induced renal tubular dysfunction and rickets in children with wilms tumor. J Pediatr 1990;117:331–335.
13. Pratt CB, Douglass EC, Etcubanas EL, et al. Ifosfamide in pediatric malignant tumors. Cancer Chemother Pharmacol 1989;24(suppl):S24–27.
14. Davies SM, Pearson ADJ, Craft AW. Toxicity of high-

dose ifosfamide in children. Cancer Chemother Pharmacol 1989;24(suppl):s8–s10.

15. Finn G, Denning D. Transient nephrogenic diabetes insipidus following high-dose cyclophosphamide chemotherapy and autologous bone marrow transplantation. Cancer Treat Rep 1987;71:220–221.

16. Peters WP, Eder J, Henner W, et al. Novel toxicities associated with high dose combination alkylating agents with autologous bone marrow support [Abstract]. Proc Am Soc Clin Oncol 1985;4:139.

17. Lu C, Braine HG, Kelzer H, Seral R, Tutschka PJ, Santos GW. Preliminary results of high-dose busulfan and cyclophosphamide with syngeneic or autologous bone marrow rescue. Cancer Treat Rep 1984;68:711–717.

18. Postmus PE, Mulder NH, Sleijfer DT, Meinecz AF, Vrissendorp R, de Vries EGE. High-dose etoposide for refractory malignancies: a phase I study. Cancer Treat Rep 1984;68:1471–1474.

19. Lazarus HM, Reed MD, Spitzer TR, Rabaa MS, Blumer JL. High-dose IV thiotepa and cryopreserved autologous bone marrow transplantation for therapy of refractory cancer. Bone Treat Rep 1987;71:689–695.

20. Elder JP, Antman K, Elias A, et al. Cyclophosphamide and thiotepa with autologous bone marrow transplantation in patients with solid tumors. J Natl Cancer Inst 1988;80:1221–1226.

21. Brown RA, Herzig RH, Wolff SN, et al. High-dose etoposide and cyclophosphamide without bone marrow transplantation for resistant hematologic malignancy. Blood 1990;76:473–479.

22. Viens P, Maraninchi D, Legros M, et al. High dose melphalan and autologous marrow rescue in advanced epithelial ovarian carcinomas: a retrospective analysis of 35 patients treated in France. Bone Marrow Transplant 1990;5:227–233.

23. Lubitz L, Ekert H. Reversible changes in duodenal mucosa associated with intensive chemotherapy followed by autologous marrow rescue [Letter]. Lancet 1979;2:532–533.

24. Taveroff A, McArdle AH, Alton-Mackay M, Rybka WB. Hyponatremia associated with fecal sodium loss following intensive cytotoxic therapy [Abstract]. Proc Am Soc Clin Oncol 1988;7:283.

25. Szeluga DJ, Stuart RK, Brookmeyer R, Utermohlen V, Santos GW. Nutritional support of bone marrow transplant recipients: a prospective, randomized clinical trial comparing total parenteral nutrition to an enteral feeding program. Cancer Res 1987;47:3309–3316.

26. Cheney CL, Gittere Abson K, Aker SN, et al. Body composition changes in marrow transplant recipients receiving total parenteral nutrition. Cancer 1987;59:1515–1519.

27. Yolken RH, Bishop CA, Townsend TR, et al. Infectious gastroenteritis in bone-marrow transplant recipients. N Engl J Med 1982;306:1009–1012.

28. Karanes C, Ratanatharathorn V, Schilcher RB, et al.

High-dose mitomycin-C with autologous bone marrow transplantation in patients with refractory malignancies. Influence of dose schedule on pharmacokinetics and nonhematopoietic toxicities. Am J Clin Oncol 1986;9:444–448.

29. Deeg HJ. Delayed complications and long-term effects after bone marrow transplantation. Hematol Oncol Clin North Am 1990;4:641–657.

30. Keilholz U, Korbling M, Fehrentz D, Bauer H, Hunstein W. Long-term endocrine toxicity of myeloablative treatment followed by autologous bone marrow/blood derived stem cell transplantation in patients with malignant lymphohematopoietic disorders. Cancer 1989;64:641–645.

31. DeFronzo RA, Braine H, Colvin OM, Davis PJ. Water intoxication in man after cyclophosphamide therapy. Ann Intern Med 1973;78:861–869.

32. Leff RS, Martino RL, Pollock WJ, Knight WA 3rd. Pituitary abscess after autologous bone marrow transplantation. Am J Hematol 1989;31:62–64.

33. Elias AD, Elder JP, Shea T, Begg CB, Frei E III, Antman KH. High-dose ifosfamide with mesna uroprotection: a phase I study. J Clin Oncol 1990;8:170–178.

34. Antman KH, Elias A. Dana-Farber Cancer Institute studies in advanced sarcoma. Semin Oncol 1990;17:7–15.

35. Pratt CB, Green AA, Horowitz ME, et al. Central nervous system toxicity following the treatment of pediatric patients with ifosfamide/mesna. J Clin Oncol 1986;4:1253–1261.

36. Meanwell CA, Mould JJ, Blackledge G, et al. Phase II study of ifosfamide in cervical cancer. Cancer Treat Rep 1986;70:727–730.

37. Wang JJ, Mittleman A, Twetrinon P, et al. Clinical trial of iphosphamide [Abstract]. Proc Am Assoc Cancer Res Soc Clin Oncol 1974;15:110.

38. Bremmer DN, McCormick J StC, Thomson JW. Clinical trial of isophosphamide (NSC-109724)—results and side effects. Cancer Chemother Rep 1974;58:889–893.

39. Cerny T, Castiglione M, Brunner K, Kupfer A, Martinelli G, Lind M. Ifosfamide by continuous infusion to prevent encephalopathy. Lancet 1990;335:175.

40. Salloum E, Flamant F, Ghosn M, et al. Irreversible encephalopathy with ifosfamide/mesna. J Clin Oncol 1987;5:1303–1304.

41. Goren MP, Wright RK, Pratt CB, Pell FE. Dechloroethylation of ifosfamide and neurotoxicity. Lancet 1986;2:1219–1220.

42. Lewis LD, Meanwell CA. Ifosfamide pharmokinetics and neurotoxicity. Lancet 1990;335:175–176.

43. Goren MP, Wright RK, Pratt CB, et al. Potentiation of ifosfamide neurotoxicity, hematotoxicity, and tubular nephrotoxicity by prior cis-diamminedichloroplatinum (II) therapy. Cancer Res 1987;47:1457–1460.

44. Meanwell CA, Blake AE, Kelly KA, Honigsberger L, Blackledge G. Prediction of ifosfamide/mesna as-

sociated encephalopathy. Eur J Cancer Clin Oncol 1986;22:815–819.

45. Watkin SW, Husband DJ, Green JA, Warenius HM. Ifosfamide encephalopathy: a reappraisal. Eur J Cancer Clin Oncol 1989;25:1303–1310.

46. Ciobanu N, Runowicz C, Gucalp R, et al. Reversible central nervous system toxicity associated with high-dose chlorambucil in autologous bone marrow transplantation for ovarian carcinoma. Cancer Treat Rep 1987;71:1324–1325.

47. Wolff SN, Phillips GL, Herzig GP. High-dose carmustine with autologous bone marrow transplantation for the adjuvant treatment of high-grade gliomas of the central nervous system. Cancer Treat Rep 1987; 71:183–185.

48. Sullivan KM, Storb R, Shulman HM, et al. Immediate and delayed neurotoxicity after mechlorethamine preparation for bone marrow transplantation. Ann Intern Med 1982;97:182–189.

49. Leff RS, Thompson JM, Daly MB, et al. Acute neurologic dysfunction after high-dose etoposide therapy for malignant glioma. Cancer 1988;62:32–35.

50. Allen JC, Rosen G. Transient cerebral dysfunction following chemotherapy for osteogenic sarcoma. Ann Neurol 1978;3:441–444.

51. Johnson NT, Crawford SW, Sargur M. Acute acquired demyelinating polyneuropathy with respiratory failure following high-dose systemic cytosine arabinoside and marrow transplantation. Bone Marrow Transplant 1987;21:203–207.

52. Wade JC, Meyers JD. Neurologic symptoms associated with parenteral acyclovir treatment after marrow transplantation. Ann Intern Med 1983;98:921–925.

53. Smith CI, Aarli JA, Biberfeld P, et al. Myasthenia gravis after bone-marrow transplantation. Evidence for a donor origin. New Engl J Med 1983;309:1565–1568.

54. Miller K, Braine R, Burns W, et al. Immune thrombocytopenic purpura (ITP) following autologous bone marrow transplantation (BMT) [Abstract]. Proc Am Soc Clin Oncol 1988;7:46.

55. Minchinton RM, Waters AH, Malfas JS, et al. Autoimmune thrombocytopenia after autologous bone-marrow transplantation [Letter] Lancet 1982;2:391.

56. Giannone L, Greer JP, Dessypris EN, Wolff SN. Prolonged thrombocytopenia (PT) following bone marrow transplantation (BMT): influence of cytomegalovirus (CMV) [Abstract]. Proc Am Soc Clin Oncol 1988;7:47.

57. Kaufman PA, Jones RB, Greenberg CS, Peters WP. Autologous bone marrow transplantation and factor XII, factor VII, and protein deficiencies: report of a new association and its possible relationship to endothelial cell injury. Cancer 1990;66:515–521.

58. Panella TJ, Peters W, White JG, Hannun YA, Greenberg CS. Platelets acquire a secretion defect after high dose chemotherapy. Cancer 1990;65:1711–1716.

59. Kalhs P, Panzer S, Kletter K, et al. Functional asplenia after bone marrow transplantation: a late complication related to extensive chronic graft-versus-host disease. Ann Intern Med 1988;109:461–464.

60. Lishner M, Patterson B, Kandel R, et al. Cutaneous and mucosal neoplasms in bone marrow transplant recipients. Cancer 1990;65:473–476.

61. Tuchman M, Stoeckeler JS, Kiang DT, O'Dea RF, Ramnaraine ML, Mirkin BL. Familial pyrimidinemia and pyrimidinuria associated with severe fluorouracil toxicity. New Engl J Med 1985;313:245–249.

62. Ratain MJ, Mick R, Berezin F, et al. Prospective correlation of acetylator phenotype with amonafide toxicity [Abstract]. Proc Am Soc Clin Oncol 1991;10:101.

32

GONADAL COMPLICATIONS

Catherine E. Klein and L. Michael Glode

It has long been recognized that both standard-dose chemotherapy and radiation therapy for the treatment of cancer produce reproductive system complications in patients who survive long enough to be evaluated. While radiation effects began to be studied as early as 1903 (1–4), the impact of chemotherapy on gonadal function was not appreciated until the initial trials of nitrogen mustard in the 1940s (5, 6). Since that time we have gained considerable insight into the mechanisms of cytotoxicity of these agents and have become increasingly aware of their potential detrimental effect on fertility. Much of what is observed might be predicted from these drugs' anticancer activity: Chemotherapeutic agents inflict damage on mitotic germ cells just as on neoplastic cells by interrupting DNA synthesis and cell division (7–11). As a consequence there is relative sparing of the less mitotically active stem spermatogonia and primordial ovarian follicles. The clinical correlate is that in general the prepubertal gonad is more resilient than the adult gonad.

Characteristically, women fare better than men, but for both sexes and all ages, the drug class, the administered dose, and the treatment duration all significantly influence the ultimate fertility of the patient. Other factors also affect the outcome: Radiation therapy even when given without chemotherapy, as for intracranial neoplasms, can result in secondary infertility (12). Theoretically, at least,

hypogonadism itself may potentiate the gonadal toxicity, particularly in the adult, because the compensatory increased gonadotropin release may actually recruit otherwise resting cells into the division cycle (13). While in rodents anthracyclines and procarbazine appear to be the most potentially toxic agents (7, 14), human studies implicate alkylating agents as particularly damaging. Antimetabolites do not appear to be associated with long-term damage.

Most of what is known regarding the reproductive-axis toxicity of cancer therapy is from a small number of patients treated with a variety of single agents and from larger series of patients treated with combinations of drugs with or without radiation therapy for such malignancies as Hodgkin's disease, breast cancer, acute leukemia, and testis cancer (15–20). Data are available on few of these drugs administered in high dose. These are generally reported in the setting of bone marrow transplantation, often with radiation therapy, and although exact incidence figures are difficult to obtain, it appears infertility and hypogonadism are common. In this chapter we will briefly review the well-documented effects of standard-dose chemotherapy and radiation and review the published data pertaining to high-intensity therapy.

THE HYPOTHALAMIC-PITUITARY-GONADAL AXIS

Regulation of the reproductive axis begins at the level of the hypothalamus (Figure

32.1). Here, neurosecretory cells synthesize and release gonadotropin-releasing hormone (GnRH) in a pulsatile fashion into the hypothalamo-hypophysial-portal circulation. Gonadotropes in the anterior pituitary respond by synthesizing and releasing the gonadotropins follicle-stimulating hormone (FSH) and luteinizing hormone (LH), which in turn control gonadal function. In women, ovarian follicles are stimulated to grow and mature by FSH, while LH stimulates ovulation and corpus luteum formation. In men, FSH initiates (and testosterone sustains) spermatogenesis, while LH controls androgen synthesis by the testicular Leydig cells (21). LH is increased in women with gonadal failure as the result of the loss of estrogen's negative feedback on the hypothalamus and pituitary, and in men from the loss of both androgen and estrogen feedback (22). In response to decreased levels of sex steroids and the loss of inhibition, FSH levels are also elevated following gonadal damage. Thus the hallmark of primary gonadal failure from any cause is elevation of gonadotropin levels, and this is the usual state in postpubertal patients receiving substantial doses of antineoplastic agents.

CHEMOTHERAPY EFFECTS IN CHILDREN

Histologic studies of testicular biopsies from boys receiving combination therapy for acute lymphoblastic leukemia or Hodgkin's disease commonly show seminiferous tubular damage, but clinically these patients generally progress normally through puberty without need for androgen replacement (23–25). Two major factors determine the degree

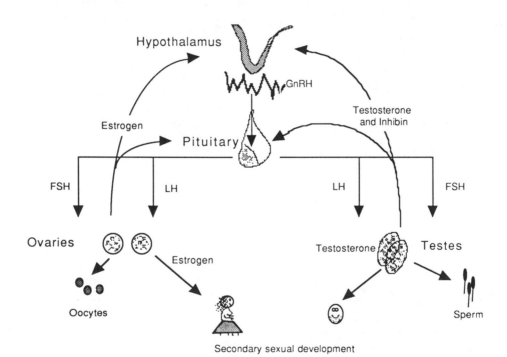

Figure 32.1. The hypothalmic-pituitary-gonadal axis. Pulsatile release of gonadotropin-releasing hormone from the hypothalamus results in pulsatile release of luteinizing hormone and follicle-stimulating-hormone from the pituitary gland. These gonadotropins result in production of gametes and sex steroid biosynthesis at the gonadal level. Feedback of sex steroids occurs at both the pituitary and hypothalamic level.

of testicular dysfunction among prepubertal boys. The first of these is the cumulative dose of chemotherapeutic drug, especially for the alkylating agents. In a recent metaanalysis of 30 studies evaluating gonadal function in 456 patients who received cyclophosphamide alone or in combination for renal disease, Hodgkin's disease, or leukemia, the cumulative dose of cyclophosphamide had a profound effect on the incidence of gonadal dysfunction. While less than 10% of prepubertal boys receiving under 400 mg/kg cyclophosphamide total dose demonstrated hypogonadism, this rose to 30% in those receiving over 400 mg/kg (26). This same study found a statistically significant relationship with pubertal stage. Overall, the reported incidence of dysfunction varies between 0% and 24% in prepubertal boys to as high as 68%–95% in sexually mature adults. Unfortunately, a confounding effect of nutritional status may also play an important role in determining the outcome of the spermatogenic epithelium in prepubertal boys who receive chemotherapy. Drug dose and patient developmental stage are therefore major determinants of the degree of damage to seminiferous epithelium (27). The nondividing Leydig cell population generally escapes severe damage when chemotherapy is administered at standard doses (24, 28, 29).

Overall, the ovarian effects of chemotherapy in prepubertal girls seem to be less than are seen in the reproductive axis of boys. Single-agent, standard-dose cyclophosphamide rarely delays puberty or produces infertility (30, 31). Procarbazine and nitrosoureas given for therapy of brain tumors may damage primary ovarian function, but most girls subsequently progress normally through puberty and achieve normal gonadotropin levels (32). Similarly, long-term survivors of standard-dose protocols including CNS radioprophylaxis for acute leukemia may have biochemical evidence of dysfunction but usually have normal menses, and some even have premature menarche (33).

CHEMOTHERAPY EFFECTS IN ADULT MEN AND WOMEN

In general, the effects of chemotherapeutic agents tend to be more profound on the adult than the prepubertal gonads. As in children, however, women tend to be less extensively damaged than men. Alkylating agents in particular have been widely recognized to produce permanent damage to the seminiferous epithelium and to oogonia. With the advent of curative and adjuvant combination chemotherapy, which often includes alkylators, multiple reports have appeared indicating permanent infertility among survivors of Hodgkin's disease, breast cancer, ovarian cancers, and the nonseminomatous testicular cancers.

Table 32.1 is a summary of the available studies on fertility effects of chemotherapy for these common neoplasms. As in children, there is relatively more infertility among male patients following chemotherapy than among their female counterparts. This comparison is particularly striking when the data relating to Hodgkin's disease are examined, since the two groups received comparable therapeutic regimens. Interestingly, however, recent reports from a randomized prospective study of MOPP versus ABVD provide convincing evidence that the latter combination produces less gonadal toxicity in men (34, 35). Since it is equally efficacious in bringing about long-term remissions, ABVD should be the treatment of choice in men who are concerned about preservation of reproductive potential. Although there are fewer data for treatment of non-Hodgkin's lymphomas, some evidence suggests that the CHOP regimen may have less gonadal toxicity (36).

The *precise* frequency of permanent amenorrhea and infertility in women depends not only on the drug given and total dose but also on concomitant radiation exposure and the age of the patient at the time therapy is administered. Among single agents studied, alkylating agents are the drugs most

Table 32.1.   Gonadal Dysfunction Following Standard-Dose Chemotherapy Regimens

Disease	Male			Female			References
	N	Permanent Azoospermia	(%)	N	Permanent Amenorrhea	(%)	
Hodgkin's disease	264	202	76	201	105	40	13, 28, 36, 94–97
Breast cancer				164	84	51	11, 48, 98
Ovarian cancer				57	4	7	46
Testis cancer	89	21	24				47, 99–102

commonly associated with premature ovarian failure as well as with mutagenesis and teratogenesis. Although nitrogen mustard may be the most toxic, cyclophosphamide is the agent best studied in this regard. Most series report amenorrhea within a month of starting therapy in 50%–75% of women treated with cyclophosphamide (15, 37, 38). There is, however, a striking age-related susceptibility. In one study the total dose of cyclophosphamide received before the onset of amenorrhea in women over 40 years was 5.2 g; in patients 30–39, the dose was 9.3 g, and for women 20–29, 20.4 g were administered before amenorrhea developed. Menses returned in 50% of those under 40 (11). Interestingly the ovarian function of prepubertal girls appears much more resilient. In this population, cyclophosphamide in doses used to treat nephrosis has been associated with no ovarian dysfunction (30, 31).

As in men, the largest data sets concerning standard-dose chemotherapy effects on gonadal function relate to combination chemotherapy. The reported incidence of amenorrhea in various series of women treated with MOPP, MVPP, or COPP for Hodgkin's disease ranges from 15%–80%, with a median of 50% (9, 10, 12–14, 34, 39–41) (Table 32.1). Two-thirds of those women develop amenorrhea during therapy, while the remainder develop it slowly over the next several years. The extent to which the cumulative dose administered alters the incidence of ovarian failure is unclear. In at least one study, there appeared to be no difference between women receiving three cycles

of MOPP and those receiving six (42). Age at the time of treatment, however, has repeatedly been shown to be an important variable affecting the incidence and time of onset of permanent amenorrhea. In general, patients over the age of 25 may expect a rate of amenorrhea between 60% and 100%. This typically begins during therapy, and menses do not reappear. In women under the age of 25 when therapy is initiated, ovarian failure is reported in 5%–30%, and menses gradually cease in these patients over the several months following treatment. Preliminary reports suggest that the alternative regimen, ABVD, for the treatment of Hodgkin's disease may have lower rates of prolonged amenorrhea (35).

Other forms of combination chemotherapy for ovarian germ cell tumors and some sarcomas have provided additional information on postchemotherapy reproductive potential. Women receiving cisplatin-containing therapy for germ cell tumors typically become amenorrheic during treatment, but over 90% restart menstruation within a few months after completing therapy (43–46). Among women with breast cancer, who may have age-related decreased reproductive potential to begin with (47), 80% receiving CMF become menopausal within 10 months of beginning therapy (48, 49). Those given Adriamycin and cyclophosphamide usually become anovulatory within 3 months, sooner if they are perimenopausal (50).

RADIATION THERAPY EFFECTS ON GONADAL FUNCTION

While direct radiation toxicity to the brain causes not only the well-documented impairment of intellectual function but also delay in sexual development, radiation exerts its most profound impact on gonadal function through its effects on the extremely radiosensitive spermatogenic epithelium. These effects on spermatogenesis have long been recognized in the mature gonad and have been extensively documented in both animals and human volunteers. More recently, the prolonged survival of boys with acute lymphoblastic leukemia who have suffered testicular relapse requiring gonadal radiation has led to substantial experience with radiation effects on the prepubertal testis. After demonstration that doses less than 1200 cGy were insufficient to control disease, most protocols now deliver 2400 rads to both testes. At these doses, permanent Leydig cell damage occurs and is manifested by delayed puberty, low or normal testosterone levels, and elevated FSH and LH levels in the majority of patients treated (42, 51, 52). These data are in contrast to those showing normal progression through puberty and normal Leydig cell function in boys receiving chemotherapy in childhood.

In adult men, single radiation doses in the range of 400–600 rads delivered to the testis may produce azoospermia lasting 2–5 years (4, 53). Fractionated radiation to the pelvis or lower extremities may result in substantial scatter to the testes as well. Shapiro documented oligo/azoospermia lasting up to 24 months after as little as 27 rads (54). These studies also showed Leydig cell dysfunction manifested by changes in LH values at gonadal doses greater than 200 cGy. FSH values increased even more markedly in a similar dose-dependent manner but, like LH values, tended to return to baseline during the 30-month follow-up period. Thus fractionated radiation appears to produce tubular damage similar to that seen with single doses. In children, Leydig cell dysfunction after 2400–3000 cGy can be significant enough to require hormonal replacement. Whether there are permanent effects to the surviving germ cells of male patients receiving radiation remains

controversial. Animal models suggest increased risk for common tumors following parental exposure to radiation and chemicals (55).

OVARIAN EFFECTS OF RADIATION THERAPY

Effects of radiation to the ovary depend not only on the dose delivered directly and indirectly by scatter but also, as with chemotherapy, upon the age of the patient at the time of treatment. Doses of 60 cGy or less produce essentially no change regardless of age. A dose of 150 cGy for women under age 40 is also unlikely to affect ovarian function but for women over 40 is associated with a moderate risk of menstrual problems. For women over 40, 600 cGy is virtually uniformly associated with menopausal symptoms. Women under 40 may tolerate up to 2000 cGy if delivered slowly over 5–6 weeks. Single doses of 800 cGy produce sterility in 100% of women (56). Radiation used therapeutically for Hodgkin's disease displays the same age-dependent toxicity. Women under age 20 receiving total lymphoid radiation generally regain menstrual function, but after age 20 there is a steady age-related decrease in return of function, reaching 0 at age 35 (57). One large review of survivors of childhood and adolescent cancer found no decrease in fertility when patients were compared to sibling controls for the group who had received alkylating therapy, but a 25% reduction in women who had received radiation therapy (56). From studies in patients receiving MOPP and total nodal radiation therapy, it appears that the combination induces significantly more persistent amenorrhea than does either therapy alone (57).

OUTCOME OF PREGNANCY

Chemotherapy

Several retrospective series have evaluated the outcome of pregnancy in women treated with chemotherapeutic agent as children or young adults, who completed therapy and then became pregnant (58). Somewhat fewer data are available for women who conceive during active cancer treatment or are pregnant at the time therapy is initiated. One of the largest studies of offspring of children treated for a variety of malignancies found that in a total of 286 subsequent pregnancies there was no increase in congenital anomalies, and chromosomal analysis was normal in 23 of 24 children tested (59). Women treated for trophoblastic tumors likewise appear to have no increased risk of congenital anomalies, spontaneous abortions or neonatal mortality (60, 61). Holmes and Holmes evaluated women treated for Hodgkin's disease and compared the 93 pregnancies in their chemotherapy-treated patients to 288 sibling-control pregnancies. Overall there was no difference between the groups, although when the subgroup who received both radiation and chemotherapy were analyzed separately, it appeared that combined treatment produced more spontaneous abortions in wives of male patients and that female patients were slightly more likely to produce abnormal offspring than control women (62). When large series are combined, nearly 1400 liveborn children have been reported to have a congenital defect incidence of about 4%, no different from the general population. Most of these anomalies represent common, nongenetic abnormalities.

Further follow-up to assess the longer-term morbidity in these children suggests that growth, development, and school performance are probably normal. A National Cancer Institute study to address the question of cancer in offspring of treated patients found a slight but statistically insignificant excess of cancers in these children when compared to offspring of sibling-matched controls (0.3% versus 0.23%), numbers not different from those expected in the general population. When analyzed by age and sex, however, it appeared that there was an excess of cancers diagnosed in male offspring under age 5. Five

cancers were detected in this group, with 1.7 expected (63). Some of these cancers potentially represented familial clustering of known hereditary cancers: retinoblastoma and Wilms' tumors.

Risk to the fetus exposed in utero to chemotherapy agents depends on gestational age as well as the drug and dose administered. Aminopterin has been consistently associated with teratogenic effects. It may be concentrated in the amniotic fluid and is associated with up to 100% fetal malformations, often in the CNS, when exposure is during the first trimester (64). Folate antagonists should not be administered during the first trimester. Other antimetabolities have rarely been associated with congenital abnormalities. First trimester exposure to 5-fluorouracil, cyclophosphamide, busulfan, and chlorambucil has been associated with low birth weight in infants and other abnormalities on rare occasion (64–66). Fetal myocardial necrosis has been reported following maternal administration of anthracyclines (67).

Whether the risk to the fetus is further increased with drug combinations is uncertain (68–72). Case reports and small series indicate that exposure in the second and third trimesters is associated with minimal risk to the fetus and that long-term development of these offspring is normal (68, 69, 71). One study of 16 children exposed to maternal antileukemic therapy could detect no difference in peripheral blood, bone marrow, cytogenetics, physical examination, neurologic assessment, school performance, or intelligence testing, when compared to sibling controls (73). Nonteratogenic effects including low birth weight, intrauterine growth retardation, and more subtle developmental abnormalities remain to be defined. In utero exposure to diethylstilbestrol has been linked to the development of clear cell carcinomas in the female offspring of these women, but other clear documentation of carcinogenesis from in utero exposure to chemotherapy is lacking. No information is available on the reproductive potential of these children.

Radiation Therapy

Most of what is known about the genetic effects of radiation therapy is inferred from data on survivors of atomic bomb exposure. While extensive data have been accumulated concerning the offspring, interpretation of these data is clouded by a variety of factors, particularly the calculation of gonadal dose. Nevertheless, it is apparent that the increase in "untoward pregnancy outcomes" (major congenital defects, stillbirth, death during the 1st week of life) is small, estimated at 0.00182 per gonadal rem (74). Small head size has been reported in these offspring (75) but has not been a consistent finding among offspring of women irradiated therapeutically during gestation. Among women treated with radiation therapy below the diaphragm, preterm delivery in up to 20% of pregnancies and an excess of low birth weight infants have been reported. That these adverse outcomes are often clustered in the first posttreatment year suggests they may result from local uterine or hormonal factors and may not be due to genetic defects (76). One large study of survivors of Wilms' tumor found an increase in perinatal death and low birth weight infants, findings that contributed to an overall 30% adverse outcome in these patients. These abnormalities were limited to women who had received pelvic radiation and were not seen among those who had been treated with chemotherapy alone (77).

In utero exposure produces the greatest risk of teratogenesis during the period of organogenesis from the 2nd to the 8th week, with growth retardation, eye problems, and microcephaly appearing as the predominant abnormalities. A "safe dose" has not yet been defined, but generally a therapeutic abortion is recommended for any uterine dose of 0.1 Gy during the first trimester. Supradiaphragmatic radiation is associated with considerable scatter to the fetus, much of which can probably be prevented with abdominal shielding. Local radiation to the neck and axilla may be safe during the first trimester (78).

Data on future fertility and carcinogenic potential in these offspring are unavailable.

EFFECTS OF INTENSIVE DOSE/ MARROW TRANSPLANTATION ON GONADAL FUNCTION

The long-term effects on gonadal function and fertility resulting from high-intensity (HI) chemotherapy have not been thoroughly described and in large measure are best reported in the bone marrow transplantation literature. Most of these patients have been treated as children or adolescents, so some conclusions can be drawn for these groups of patients, but relatively little is known about adults. Preparative regimens have for the most part been limited to HI cyclophosphamide with or without radiation therapy, which may confound interpretation of the outcomes. Little additional information is available for other drugs used in high intensity.

Follow-up studies of patients who received HI cyclophosphamide as their conditioning regimen suggest that both boys and girls, when treated in childhood, may experience delayed pubertal development, but ultimately most attain normal secondary sexual characteristics. The largest series of patients reported is from the Fred Hutchinson Cancer Research Center, where 155 consecutive children were followed after prepubertal transplantation. Of 16 girls progressing through puberty, 10 had significantly delayed pubertal development as measured by Tanner score. Six of the 16 achieved menarche (4 of whom received fractionated TBI as part of their conditioning regimen). Of 31 boys between the ages of 13 and 22 at the time of reporting, 21 demonstrated delayed development of secondary sexual characteristics (79). A small series of children treated with HI cyclophosphamide or HI melphalan from Austria similarly reported up to an 8-year delay in onset of puberty in girls. All who were postpubertal became permanently amenorrheic. Of 2 postpubertal boys treated, 1 became permanently azoospermic, the other recovered modest oligospermia with normal sperm motility (80). Other investigators have shown that testicular volume may be inappropriately small in up to 50% of men treated with HI cyclophosphamide regimens during puberty (81). Gynecomastia has not been reported.

In adults, the patterns of gonadal damage are similar to those described above for standard-dose chemotherapy: age-dependent toxicity in women and generally more damage to testes than ovaries. The short duration of preparative regimens may, however, be less toxic to testicular function than the use of intermittent long-term alkylating agent therapy. During and immediately following transplantation essentially 100% of postpubertal women develop amenorrhea (80, 82–86). From one study of 187 postpubertal, premenopausal transplants, 27 women conditioned with HI cyclophosphamide alone or with various additional drugs, including nitrogen mustard, procarbazine, and antithymocyte globulin, were between the ages of 13 and 25 at the time of transplantation. All 27 had the return of menses at a median of 6 months posttransplantation. All had normal gonadotropin levels. Sixteen women were between age 26 and 37 at the time of transplant. Nine had return of menstrual function at up to 18 months, and these women all had normal LH and FSH levels. Four women had return of irregular menses, but amenorrhea ultimately developed between 2 and 3 years later. Seven of these 16 never had return of menstrual function and maintained elevated gonadotropic hormone levels consistent with primary ovarian failure (83). Of 47 women treated at the Royal Marsden Hospital, 4 were treated with HI melphalan alone. All became amenorrheic, but 2 regained normal function within 1 year. The other 2 manifested ovarian failure over 2 years later (84).

Thirty-one men were treated with chemotherapy alone in similar fashion and were transplanted between the ages of 16 and 41. All had normal testosterone levels after trans-

plantation, and all but one had normal LH levels. Fifteen of these men had semen analyses: 5 remained azoospermic at up to 7 years, 10 had sperm counts between 5 and 245 million per milliliter (83). Fourteen of 14 men treated in West Germany with TBI and HI cyclophosphamide remained azoospermic at 2–28 months after transplant. All had normal testosterone and LH levels (86).

Small series and a number of case reports document fertility in both men and women treated with these HI cyclophosphamide regimens, and two successful pregnancies following conditioning with HI melphalan are documented (87). At least 51 pregnancies are reported in the literature (87–92). One was terminated by a spontaneous abortion, 5 by elective abortion, and the rest resulted in live births with only one reported congenital anomaly (a patent ductus arteriosus) (Table 32.2) (90).

Gonadal effects of HI methotrexate used to treat resected osteogenic sarcoma have been reported in 17 patients, 12 of whom also received vincristine (93). All women maintained normal menstrual function, both during and following therapy. Serum gonadotropins were normal. During therapy all men developed severe oligospermia, and half had gonadotropic hormone evidence of testicular failure. By 12 months spermatogenesis returned in all these men.

The effects of HI chemotherapy in the absence of total body or total lymphoid radiation are difficult to ascertain. Most reports relate 100% amenorrhea in women who receive single-fraction TBI, with menopausal symptoms of flushing and vaginal dryness within 6 months of therapy. Ovarian ultrasound examinations in these women show small ovaries and no demonstrable follicular activity (85). Similarly, among postpubertal men who receive TBI, azoospermia approaches 100% (83).

In summary relatively less information is available on the effect of high-dose chemotherapy on gonadal function and fertility. Most children who receive HI cyclophospha-

Table 32.2. Pregnancy Outcome after Bone Marrow Transplantation

Preparative Regimen	Patient Gender	Number	Number Pregnancies	Number Abortions	Number Live Births	Number Birth Defect	References
HI	Women	2	3	0	3	0	87
Melphalan	Men						
HI	Women	22	25	3	22	1[a]	88–92, 103
Cyclophosphamide	Men	14	16	0	16	0	103
HI	Women	3	4	3	0	0	103
Cyclophosphamide							
+ TBI	Men	1	3	0	3	0	103
Total	Women	27	32	6	25	1	
Total	Men	15	19	0	19	0	

[a]Patent ductus arteriosus.

mide (with or without other agents) as bone marrow transplantation conditioning regimens develop normal secondary sexual characteristics, but often after abnormal delay. Men may have slightly diminished testicular volume. Ovarian function in women is interrupted during therapy, but in most young women seems to recover normally. Women over the age of 26 appear to be at high risk for permanent, premature ovarian failure. Up to one-third of men become permanently azoospermic, although recovery of spermatogenesis is seen over time in the remainder. Addition of TBI greatly increases the incidence of gonadal failure. Fertility is reported both for treated men and women; offspring appear to be normal.

REFERENCES

1. Albers-Schonberg. Uber eine bisher unbekannte Wirkung der Rontgenstrahlen auf den Organismus der Tiere. Munch med Wochschr 1903;50:1859.
2. Clifton DK, Bremner WJ. The effect of testicular x-irradiation on spermatogenesis in man: a comparison with the mouse. J Androl 1983;4:387–392.
3. Oakberg EF. Sensitivity and time of degeneration of spermatogenic cells irradiated in various stages of maturation in the mouse. Radiat Res 1955;2:389.
4. Baker TG. Radiosensitivity of mammalian oocytes with particular reference to the human female. Am J Obstet Gynecol 1971;110(5):746–761.
5. Gilman A. The initial clinical trial of nitrogen mustard. Am J Surg 1963;105:574.
6. Spitz S. The histological effects of nitrogen mustards on human tumors and tissues. Cancer 1948; 1:383.
7. Gould SF, Powell D, Nett T, et al. A rat model for chemotherapy-induced male infertility. Arch Androl 1983;11:141–150.
8. Lee IP, Dixon RL. Antineoplastic drug effects on spermatogenesis studied by velocity sedimentation cell separation. Toxicol Appl Pharmacol 1972;23:20–41.
9. Meistrich ML. Critical components of testicular function and sensitivity to disruption. Biol Reprod 1986;34:17–28.
10. Goodpasture JC, Bergstrom K, Vickery BH. Potentiation of the gonadotoxicity of cytoxan in the dog by adjuvant treatment with a luteinizing hormone-releasing hormone agonist. Cancer Res 1988; 48:2174–2178.
11. Karashima T, Zalatnai A, Schally AV. Protective effects of analogs of luteinizing hormone-releasing hormone against chemotherapy-induced testicular damage in rats. Proc Natl Acad Sci USA 1988;85:2329–2333.
12. Qureshi MSA, Pennington, JH, Goldsmith HJ, et al. Cyclophosphamide therapy and sterility. Lancet 1972;2:1290–1291.
13. Ataya KM, McKanna JA, Weintraub AM, et al. A luteinizing hormone-releasing hormone agonist for the prevention of chemotherapy-induced ovarian follicular loss in rats. Cancer Res 1985;45:3651–3656.
14. Lu CC, Meistrich ML. Cytotoxic effects of chemotherapeutic drugs on mouse testis cells. Cancer Res 1979;39:3575–3582.
15. Andrieu JM, Ochoa-Molina ME. Menstrual cycle, pregnancies and offspring before and after MOPP therapy for Hodgkin's disease. Cancer 1983;52:435–438.
16. Horning SJ, Hoppe RT, Hancock SL, et al. Vinblastine, bleomycin, and methotrexate: an effective adjuvant in favorable Hodgkin's disease. J Clin Oncol 1988;6:1822–1831.
17. Koyama H, Wada T, Nishizawa Y, et al. Cyclophos-

phamide-induced ovarian failure and its therapeutic significance in patients with breast cancer. Cancer 1977;39:1403–1409.

18. Koziner B, Myers J, Cirrincione C, et al. Treatment of stages I and II Hodgkin's disease with three different therapeutic modalities. Am J Med 1986; 80:1067–1078.

19. Kreuser ED, Ziros N, Hetzel WD, et al. Reproductive and endocrine gonadal capacity in patients treated with COPP chemotherapy for Hodgkin's disease. J Cancer Res Clin Oncol 1987;113:260–266.

20. Whitehead E, Shalet SM, Blackledge G, et al. The effect of combination chemotherapy on ovarian function in women treated for Hodgkin's disease. Cancer 1983;52:988–993.

21. Hazum E, Conn PM. Molecular mechanism of gonadotropin-releasing hormone (GnRH) action. I. The GnRH receptor. Endocr Rev 1988;379–386.

22. Gooren K. Androgens and estrogens in their negative feedback action in the hypothalamo-pituitary-testis axis. Site of action and evidence of their interaction. J Steroid Biochem 1989;33(4B):757–761.

23. Lendon M, Palmer MK, Hann IM, et al. Testicular histology after combination chemotherapy in childhood for acute lymphoblastic leukemia. Lancet 1978;2:439–441.

24. Shalet SM, Hann IM, Lendon M, et al. Testicular function after combination chemotherapy in childhood for acute lymphoblastic leukemia. Arch Dis Child 1981;56:275–278.

25. Whitehead E, Shalet SM, Jones PH, et al. Gonadal function after combination chemotherapy for Hodgkin's disease in childhood. Arch Dis Child 1982;47:287–291.

26. Rivkees SA, Crawford JD. The relationship of gonadal activity and chemotherapy-induced gonadal damage. JAMA 1988;259(14):2123–2125.

27. Matus-Ridley M, Nicosia SV, Meadows AT. Gonadal effects of cancer therapy in boys. Cancer 1985; 55:2353–2363.

28. Sherins RJ, Olweny CLM, Ziegler JL. Gynecomastia and gonadal dysfunction in adolescent boys treated with combination chemotherapy for Hodgkin's disease. N Engl J Med 1978;299:12–16.

29. Whitehead E, Shalet SM, Blackledge G, et al. The effects of Hodgkin's disease and combination chemotherapy on gonadal function in the adult male. Cancer 1982;49:418–422.

30. Lentz RD, Bergstein J, Steffes MW. Postpubertal evaluation of gonadal function following cyclophosphamide therapy before and during puberty. J Pediatr 1977;91:385–394.

31. Pennisi AJ, Grushkin CM, Lieberman E. Gonadal function in children with nephrosis treated with cyclophosphamide. Am J Dis Child 1975;129:315–318.

32. Clayton PE, Shalet SM, Price DA, et al. Ovarian function following chemotherapy for childhood brain tumors. Med Pediatr Oncol 1989;17:92–96.

33. Quigley C, Cowell C, Jimenez M, et al. Normal or early development of puberty despite gonadal damage in children treated for acute lymphocytic leukemia. N Engl J Med 1989;321:143–151.

34. Santoro A, Bonadonna G, Valagussa P, et al. Long-term results of combined chemotherapy-radiotherapy approach in Hodgkin's disease: superiority of ABVD plus radiotherapy versus MOPP plus radiotherapy. J Clin Oncol 1987;5(1):27–37.

35. Viviani S, Santoro A, Ragni G, et al. Gonadal toxicity after combination chemotherapy for Hodgkin's disease. Comparative results of MOPP vs ABVD. Eur J Cancer Clin Oncol 1985;21(5):601–605.

36. Roeser HP, Stocks AE, Smith AJ. Testicular damage due to cytotoxic drugs and recovery after cessation of therapy. Aust NZJ Med 1978;8:250–254.

37. Schilsky RL, Lewis BJ, Sherins RJ. Gonadal dysfunction in patients receiving chemotherapy for cancer. Ann Intern Med 1980;93:109–114.

38. Uldall PR, Kerr DNS, Tacchi D. Amenorrhea and sterility. Lancet 1972;1:693–694.

39. King DJ, Ratcliffe MA, Dawson AA, et al. Fertility in young men and women after treatment for lymphoma: a population study. J Clin Pathol 1985; 38:1247–1251.

40. Lacher MJ, Toner K. Pregnancies and menstrual function before and after combined radiation and chemotherapy for Hodgkin's disease. Cancer Invest 1986;4:93–100.

41. Schilsky RL, Sherine RJ, Hubbard SM, et al. Long-term follow-up of ovarian function in women treated with MOPP chemotherapy for Hodgkin's disease. Am J Med 1981;71:552–556.

42. Blatt J, Sherins RJ, Niebrugge D, et al. Leydig cell function in boys following treatment for testicular relapse of acute lymphoblastic leukemia. J Clin Oncol 1985;3(9):1227–1231.

43. Davis TE, Loprinzi CL, Buchler DA. Combination chemotherapy with cisplatin, vinblastine, and bleomycin for endodermal sinus tumors of the ovary. Gynecol Oncol 1984;19:46–52.

44. Fossa SD, Aass N, Kaalhus O. et al. Long-term survival and morbidity in patients with metastatic germ cell tumors treated with cisplatin-based combination chemotherapy. Cancer 1986;58:2600–2605.

45. Gershenson DM. Menstrual and reproductive function after treatment with combination chemotherapy and malignant ovarian germ cell tumors. J Clin Oncol 1988;6:270–275.

46. Pektasides D, Rustin GJS, Mewlands ES, et al. Fertility after chemotherapy for ovarian germ cell tumours. Br J Obstet Gynaecol 1987;94:477–479.

47. Hansen PV, Trykker H, Helkjaer PE, et al. Testicular function in patients with testicular cancer treated with orchiectomy alone or orchiectomy plus cisplatin-based chemotherapy. J Natl Cancer Inst 1989;81:1246–1250.

48. Dnistrian AM, Schwartz MK, Frecchia AA. Endocrine consequences of CMF adjuvant therapy in premenopausal and postmenopausal breast cancer patients. Cancer 1983;51:803–807.

49. Samaan NA, DeAsis DN, Bugdar AO. Pituitary-ovarian function in breast cancer patients on adjuvant chemoimmunotherapy. Cancer 1978;41:2084–2087.

50. Schulz K, Schmidt-Rhode P, Weymar P, et al. The effect of combination chemotherapy on ovarian, hypothalamic and pituitary function in patients with breast cancer. Arch Gynaecol 1979;227:293–301.

51. Brauner R, Czernichow P, Cramer P. Leydig-cell function in children after direct testicular irradiation for acute lymphoblastic leukemia. N Engl J Med 1983;309:25–28.

52. Leiper AD, Grant DB, Chessells JM. The effect of testicular irradiation on Leydig cell function in prepubertal boys with acute lymphoblastic leukemia. Arch Dis Child 1983;58:906–910.

53. Rowley MJ, Leach DR, Warner GA. Effect of graded doses of ionizing radiation on the human testis. Radiat Res 1974;59:665–678.

54. Shapiro E, Kinsella TJ, Makuch RW, et al. Effects of fractionated irradiation on endocrine aspects of testicular function. J Clin Oncol 1985;3(9):1232–1239.

55. Nomura T. Of mice and men? Nature 1990;345:671.

56. Gabriel D, Bernard S, Lambert J, et al. Oopheropexy and the management of Hodgkin's disease. Arch Surg 1986;121:1083–1085.

57. Horning SJ, Hoppe RT, Kaplan HS, et al. Female reproductive potential after treatment for Hodgkin's disease. N Engl J Med 1981;304:1377–1381.

58. Byrne J, Mulvihill JJ, Myers MH, et al. Effects of cancer treatment on fertility in long-term survivors of childhood or adolescent cancer. N Engl J Med 1987;317:1315.

59. Li FP, Fine W, Jaffe N. Offspring of patients treated for cancer in childhood. J Natl Cancer Inst 1979;62:1193–1197.

60. Rustin GJS, Booth M, Dent J, et al. Pregnancy after cytotoxic chemotherapy for gestational trophoblastic tumours. Br Med J 1984;288:103–106.

61. Song HZ, Wu P, Wang Y, et al. Pregnancy outcomes after successful chemotherapy for choriocarcinoma and invasive mole: long term follow-up. Am J Obstet Gynecol 1988;158:538–545.

62. Holmes GE, Holmes FF. Pregnancy outcome of patients treated for Hodgkin's disease. Cancer 1978;41:1317–1322.

63. Mulvihill JJ, Connelly RR, Austin DF, et al. Cancer in offspring of long-term survivors of childhood and adolescent cancer. Lancet 1987;2:813–817.

64. Nicholson HO. Cytotoxic drugs in pregnancy. J Obstet Gynaecol 1968;75:307–312.

65. Jarrell J, YoungLai EV, McMahon A, et al. Effects of ionizing radiation and pretreatment of [D-Leu6,des-GlylO] luteinizing hormone-releasing hormone ethylamide on developing rat ovarian follicles. Cancer Res 1987;47:5005–5008.

66. Stephens JD, Globus MS, Miller TR. Multiple congenital anomalies in a fetus exposed to 5-FU during the first trimester. Am J Obstet Gynecol 1980;137:747–749.

67. Turchi JJ, Villasis C. Anthracyclines in the treatment of malignancy in pregnancy. Cancer 1988;61:435–440.

68. Blatt J, Mulvihill JJ, Ziegler JL, et al. Pregnancy outcome following cancer chemotherapy. Am J Med 1980;69:828–832.

69. Doll DC, Ringenberg S, Yarbro JW. Management of cancer during pregnancy. Arch Intern Med 1988;148:2058–2064.

70. Garrett MJ. Teratogenic effects of combination chemotherapy. Ann Intern Med 1974;80:667.

71. Reynoso EE, Shepherd FA, Messner HA, et al. Acute leukemia during pregnancy: the Toronto Leukemia Study Group experience with long-term follow-up of children exposed in utero to chemotherapeutic agents. J Clin Oncol 1987;5:1098–1106.

72. Schipira DS, Chudley AE. Successful pregnancy following continuous treatment with combination chemotherapy before conception and throughout pregnancy. Cancer 1984;54:800–803.

73. Aviles A, Niz J. Long-term follow-up of children born to mothers with acute leukemia during pregnancy. Med Pediatr Oncol 1988;16:3–6.

74. Schull WJ, Otake M, Neel JV. Genetic effects of the atomic bomb: a reappraisal. Science 1981;213:1220–1227.

75. Plummer G. Anomalies occurring in children exposed in utero to the atomic bomb at Hiroshima. Pediatrics 1952;10:687.

76. Mulvihill II, McKeen EA, Rosner F. Pregnancy outcome in cancer patients. Cancer 1987;60:1143–1150.

77. Li FP, Gimbrere K, Gelber RD, et al. Outcome of pregnancy in survivors of Wilms' tumor. JAMA 1987;257:216–219.

78. Jacobs C, Donaldson SC, Rosenberg SA. Management of the pregnant patient with Hodgkin's disease. Ann Intern Med 1981;95:669–675.

79. Sanders JE, Pritchard S, Mahoney P, et al. Growth and development following marrow transplantation for leukemia. Blood 1986;68:1129–1135.

80. Urban C, Schwingshandl I, Slavc A, et al. Endocrine function after bone marrow transplantation without the use of preparative total body irradiation. Bone Marrow Transplant 1988;3:291–296.

81. Sklar CA, Kim TH, Tamsey NCK. Testicular function following bone marrow transplantation performed during or after puberty. Cancer 1984;53:1498–1501.

82. Sanders JE, Buckner CD, Amos D, et al. Ovarian function following marrow transplantation for aplastic anemia or leukemia. J Clin Oncol 1988;6:813–818.

83. Sanders JE, Buckner CD, Leonard JM, et al. Late effects on gonadal function of cyclophosphamide, total-body irradiation, and marrow transplantation. Transplantation 1983;36:252–255.

84. Sklar CA, Kim TH, Williamson JF, et al. Ovarian function after successful bone marrow transplantation in postmenarcheal females. Med Pediatr Oncol 1983;11:361–364.

85. Nichols J, Maitland J, Nandi A, et al. Ovarian function following bone marrow transplantation. Bone Marrow Transplant 1986;1:221.

86. Schmeiser T, Kreuser ED, Heit W, et al. Endocrine and reproductive gonadal functions in male and female bone marrow transplant recipients. Bone Marrow Transplant 1987;2:256.

87. Milliken S, Powles R, Parikh P, et al. Successful pregnancy following bone marrow transplantation for leukemia. Bone Marrow Transplant 1990;5:135–137.

88. Schmidt H, Ehninger G, Dopfer R, et al. Pregnancy after bone marrow transplantation for severe aplastic anemia. Bone Marrow Transplant 1987;2:329–322.

89. Buskard N, Ballem T, Hill R, et al. Normal fertility after total body irradiation and chemotherapy in conjunction with a bone marrow transplant for acute leukemia. Clin Invest 1988;11:57.

90. Hinterberger-Fischer M, Hinterberger W, Kos M, et al. Three successful pregnancies after BMT for severe aplastic anemia. Bone Marrow Transplant 1987;2:259.

91. Jacobs P, Dubovsky DW. Bone marrow transplantation followed by normal pregnancy. Am J Hematol 1981;11:209–212.

92. Card RT, Holmes IH, Sugarman RG, et al. Successful pregnancy after high dose chemotherapy and marrow transplantation for treatment of aplastic anemia. Exp Hematol 1980;8:57–60.

93. Shamberger RC, Rosenberg SA, Seipp CA, et al. Effects of high-dose methotrexate and vincristine on ovarian and testicular functions in patients undergoing postoperative adjuvant treatment of osteosarcoma. Cancer Treat Rep 1981;65:739–746.

94. Chapman RM, Rees LH, Sutcliffe SB, et al. Cyclical combination chemotherapy and gonadal function. Lancet 1979;1:285–289.

95. Chapman RM, Sutcliff SB, Malpas JS. Male gonadal dysfunction in Hodgkin's disease. A prospective study. JAMA 1981;245:1323–1328.

96. Sherins RJ, DeVita VT. Effect of drug treatment for lymphoma on male reproductive capacity. Ann Intern Med 1973;79:216.

97. Waxman JHX, Terry YA, Wrigley PFM, et al. Gonadal function in Hodgkin's disease: long-term follow-up chemotherapy. Br Med J 1982;285:1612–1613.

98. Fisher B, Sherman B, Rockette H. L-phenylalanine mustard in the management of premenopausal patients with primary breast cancer. Cancer 1979;44:847–857.

99. Drasga RE, Einhorn LH, Williams SD, et al. Fertility after chemotherapy for testicular cancer. J Clin Oncol 1983;1(3):179–183.

100. Nijman JM, Schraffordt Koops H, Kremer H. Gonadal function after surgery and chemotherapy in men with stage II and III nonseminomatous testicular tumors. J Clin Oncol 1987;5(4):651–656.

101. Kreusar ED, Harsch V, Hetzel WD, et al. Chronic gonadal toxicity in patients with testicular cancer after chemotherapy. Eur J Cancer Clin Oncol 1986;22(3):289–293.

102. Johnson DH, Hainsworth JD, Linde RB, et al. Testicular function following combination chemotherapy with cis-platin, vinblastine, and bleomycin. Med Pediatr Oncol 1984;12:233–238.

103. Sanders J, Sullivan K, Witherspoon R, et al. Long term effects and quality of life in children and adults after marrow transplantation. Am J Hematol 1989;4:27–29.

Section IV

Clinical Applications of
High-Dose Therapy

33

HIGH-DOSE THERAPY FOR ACUTE MYELOCYTIC LEUKEMIA

N. C. Gorin

In the past 30 years, the treatment of acute myelocytic leukemias (AMLs) has evolved considerably (1). From the first already historical treatments with steroids, monochemotherapy, and exsanguino-transfusion, until the more complex strategies of today, the general evolution has invariably been in the direction of more aggressive therapy, culminating with the use of total body irradiation (TBI) or high-dose, "ablative" polychemotherapy regimens in conjunction with bone marrow transplantation (BMT).

Allogeneic BMT was first given in the seventies to patients with end stage overt AML (2, 3), with the initial, perhaps naive, idea of destroying the leukemic marrow and replacing it with a normal, HLA-identical, family-related marrow. Results were poor because of toxicity, including graft-versus-host disease (GVHD) (4–6) and also because of a very high rate of persisting and/or recurring leukemia. Moving allogeneic BMT to earlier in remission (7) to deliver the same high-dose therapy on a much lower residual tumor (i.e., in complete remission [CR]) has considerably improved the outcome. A very important finding, at least on theoretical grounds, has been that GVHD is associated with an antileukemic activity, the graft-versus-leukemia effect (GVL) (8, 9). However, while the occurrence of GVHD-GVL is associated with a lower incidence of leukemic recurrence, it has not yet brought a clear benefit to patients because of the increased toxic mortality resulting from GVHD per se.

Autologous bone marrow transplantation (ABMT), which developed later (3, 10–14), has been applied following the same principles previously used for allogeneic BMT: Marrow collected in remission has first been reinfused after high-dose therapy in patients in relapse (12, 15), producing high remission rates but no cure. Subsequently ABMT has been moved earlier in the disease to enable high-dose consolidation, again in CR. First essentially considered for patients with no HLA-identical available donor for an allograft, ABMT has recently been applied more widely in view of its reduced toxicity, in part linked to the absence of GVHD. However, a theoretical major impediment to ABMT has been the potential contamination of the marrow collected by residual leukemic cells and the risk of reinfusing them into the patient.

The introduction of techniques to purge the marrow of leukemic residual cells, using cyclophosphamide derivatives (4-hydroperoxycyclophosphamide) and mafosfamide (16–19), has led several teams, including ours, to systematically purge the marrow (20–23). In contrast, other teams relying on high-dose conventional chemotherapy consolidation courses given to the patient in remission prior to marrow collection, and referring to this as "in vivo purging," have advocated against unnecessary additional in vitro purging and obtained good results, raising controversy over whether purging indeed is necessary (24–27). However, in 1988, for the first time, analysis of the registry of the European cooperative Bone Marrow Transplantation Group (EBMTG) demonstrated that marrow purging with mafosfamide was associated with a lower relapse rate in patients with AML autografted in first CR (CR1) (28). This finding has been recently confirmed and the role of purging further defined in a subsequent EBMTG analysis of a population of 919 patients (29). Despite purging, ABMT, especially when done in second or third remission (CR2, CR3) may be associated with higher relapse rates than allogeneic BMT. This as well as the recent finding in the past 5 years that T cell depletion of the donor marrow for allografting, in an effort to reduce the incidence and severity of GVHD, is associated with an increased incidence of relapse (30), has further outlined the specific GVL potential of allografting, absent with ABMT.

Peripheral blood stem cell (PBSC) autografting has been introduced in the last 5 years, after the first observation that indeed a sufficient amount of stem cells could be collected by leukapheresis at time of recovery from aplasia after induction or consolidation courses and produce sustained engraftment (31, 32). While it has indeed produced more rapid engraftment than autologous marrow, with a clear benefit for the patient, the risk of reinfusing circulating leukemic cells with this unpurged material, supported by the observation of a possibly increased relapse rate over that observed with purged marrow, has at least for the moment reduced its use (33, 34).

While both allogeneic and autologous BMT was being developed, it must also be recognized that important progress was also being made in the field of conventional chemotherapy (35), for example, the promulgation of the concept of double induction (tandem chemotherapy), the demonstration that more than one consolidation course is needed, the development of the principles for early or late intensification, the introduction of new schedules for administration of existing drugs such as high-dose cytosine arabinoside (ARAC), and the introduction of new drugs for AML therapy such as idarubicin, mitoxantrone, and etoposide.

Therefore, the situation today is complex, and there is still controversy over which strategy should be applied for the treatment of AML. This situation is further clouded by the development of new research areas such as the administration of cytokines with chemotherapy (36) or post transplantation, the uses of interleukin-2 (37), and attempts to separate GVHD and GVL (9, 38) in allografting and to induce GVHD/GVL (39) in autografting. In this chapter, we will focus on allogeneic and autologous stem cell transplantation in AML. However, a brief review of the present status of chemotherapy is first necessary to understand the overall strategy.

FROM CHEMOTHERAPY TO STEM CELL TRANSPLANTATION

Chemotherapy of AML is divided in several successive steps. The induction regimen is given to reduce the tumor load to a level where no leukemic cells can be detected any longer on blood smears and marrow aspirates and a full recovery of normal hematopoiesis occurs. It has been calculated that the total tumor load at time of initial diagnosis is around 10^{12} leukemic cells and that CR as defined above corresponds to a persisting tumor load anywhere below 10^{10}. The more aggressive the induction regimen, the greater the tumor reduction and the lower the residual tumor burden. Therefore, CR is a very heterogeneous state in that the amount of residual tumor is variable. While a good indicator of the efficacy of an induction regimen is of course the rate of CR achieved, a probably even more important one (however, one quite difficult to assess) is the leukemic log cell kill obtained. Multiple chemotherapy combinations have been used to induce CR1; the generally accepted standard is the so-called 3 + 7, which combines daunorubicin 45 mg/ m^2 per day for 3 days and ARAC by continuous intravenous infusion of 200 mg/m^2 per day for 7 days, to achieve a CR rate around 60% when administered to previously untreated patients (Table 33.1). Reinforcement of this "standard" regimen, with the addition of etoposide (40) or the use of a more active analogue of daunorubicin, idarubicin (41), increases the rate up to 80%. A similarly high CR rate can also be obtained by the use of a double induction regimen in which different drugs are used sequentially, such as the TAD 9/HAM (42) combination of the BFM group, which follows the Goldie-Coldman hypothesis (43) predicting that the simultaneous use of all effective non-cross-resistant drugs prevents the emergence of resistant

clones. The TAD 9/HAM double induction consists of 6-thioguanine, conventional ARAC, and daunorubicin for the first cycle and high-dose ARAC and mitoxantrone for the second cycle.

Modern chemotherapy protocols use consolidation courses after CR is achieved to further reduce the amount of residual tumor. The optimal number of courses is unknown, but it is generally accepted that one consolidation course is not enough (44). The observations of the past 30 years (a) that cure of the disease is only observed in patients with long-lasting first (and not subsequent) CR and (b) that relapses, although occurring essentially in the first 2 years, nonetheless continue to occur steadily for up to 5 years (45) have raised the question of the length of therapy needed. Several protocols have administered chemotherapy for 3 years. A more recent approach has included intensification courses characterized by the administration

Table 33.1.   Treatment of Acute Myeloblastic Leukemia in Adults (<60 years) with Conventional Chemotherapy: Outcome in Relation to Intensity of Therapy[a]

Post initial diagnosis	Description	CR%	Long-term CR (cure rate %)	References
A: no treatment		0	0	160
B: lighter induction (no anthracycline)	ARAC-6 TG		<25	1
C: more aggressive induction (with anthracycline)	3 + 7	68		161
	3 + 10	Equivalent but CR rate after first course greater		162
	ADE	80		MRC 10 study (unpublished)
	Double induction TAD/HAM 77	77		42
No maintenance			0	163, 164
Maintenance/consolidation (≥2 courses)			<25	42, 161
Intensification	HD ARAC or AMSA Regular ARAC		47 in CR at 2 years	165
After First Relapse				
Aggressive salvage therapy + consolidation	Various	25–70	<10 (possibly 0) better results for late relapses	166, 167

[a]Abbreviations: ADE-ARAC, daunorubicin-etoposide; HAM, high-dose ARAC-mitoxantrone; HD ARAC, high-dose ARAC; TAD, 6-thioguanine-ARAC-daunorubicin; 6TG, 6-thioquanine.

of a combination of drugs different from the ones used at induction or in consolidation courses, and by its intensity, usually producing a phase of therapeutic aplasia comparable to the one after induction. Intensification is delivered early or late or both, with the same rationale already described above, i.e., to obtain the highest tumor reduction following the hypothesis of Goldie-Coldman. The principal interest of intensification courses is supposedly to shorten the duration of therapy to 1 year or less. Several studies have compared various protocols in relation to variations in the induction regimens, or in the number of consolidation courses, the use of intensification, and the total length of therapy with or without maintenance. The interested reader can refer to reviews of the subject (46–48); Table 33.1 gives a summary of the most-used induction regimens, with the remission rates reported, as well as (when available) the long-term disease-free survival.

A possible interim conclusion may be built on the three following observations:

1. In an analysis of 10 multicenter trials comprising 24 groups of patients, Büchner et al. (42) compared remission duration from maintenance strategies with postremission chemotherapy for longer periods (24–60 months) to those with shorter periods (0–16 months). They found (Fig. 33.1) a marked advantage of strategies using longer postremission chemotherapy, with median long-term remission rates after 4–6 years twice those of shorter therapies.
2. In contrast, in a large study of 760 patients of the Cancer and Leukemia Group B (45) addressing the issue of the usefulness of long-term maintenance (patients randomized either to receive chemotherapy for a total of 3 years or to discontinue all treatment after 8 months), despite a transient increase in the relapse rate in the latter group, the proportion of patients remaining in long-term remission was in the end identical in the two groups.
3. Recent protocols with high-dose intensi-

fication (with, however, an insufficient follow-up) show a rate of persisting remission at 2 years in the range of 40% (49, 50).

Thus, if relatively low dose chemotherapy is given, long administration is better than short, and in fact high-dose therapy is preferable. Within high-dose therapy, protocols combining consolidation and intensification achieve the best results. Table 33.2 summarizes some reasons for providing upfront aggressive therapy for the treatment of AML. Since, with some possible variations, the two most effective antileukemic regimens—cyclophosphamide + total body irradiation (TBI) at 10 Gy (2) and the combination of cyclophosphamide and busulfan (51), known to achieve a tumor cell kill of 6–9 logs—also are totally ablative, stem cell transplantation is required after their administration. High-dose therapy and stem cell transplantation, therefore, should be considered as a super-intensification that, if applied at time of minimal residual disease, can reduce the persisting tumor load to such a low level (probably lower than 10^5) that endogeneous mechanisms could control it and prevent new proliferation, thereby leading to cure. There is now considerable evidence that following high-dose therapy such as TBI, leukemic cells persist in the patient (52, 53). Animal models predict that a 1 log reduction (54) may result in an important difference in terms of disease-free survival in man. In this respect, it is interesting that mathematical calculations indicate that both GVL in the context of allografting and marrow purging in the context of autografting (55–57) produce antileukemic effectiveness of not more than this magnitude.

The techniques of allogeneic BMT and of autologous transplantation with marrow or peripheral blood stem cells, as well as the techniques of and problems raised by marrow purging, have been treated in previous

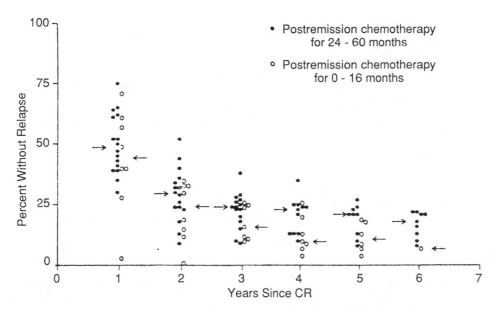

Figure 33.1. Probabilities of persisting remission in 10 multicenter studies comparing study arms with a longer (*closed circles*) and those with a shorter (*open circles*) postremission chemotherapy of any type. From Büchner T, Schellong G, Hiddemann W, Ritter J, eds. Acute leukemias II: prognostic factors and treatment strategies. Heidelberg: Springer-Verlag, 1990.

chapters and will not be detailed here. Table 33.3 compares the theoretical advantages and disadvantages of allogeneic and autologous BMT in AML. When dealing with transplantation, it is very clear that the quality of the transplanted stem cells not only is important for reingraftment of the patient in the early period, but also plays a role in preventing relapse, in that delayed hematopoiesis of donor origin allows a growth advantage for residual leukemic cells (58, 59). In this respect, the quality of cryopreservation (60), the dose of progenitors infused (17, 61), and purging (18, 62, 63) are variables of major importance for ABMT.

Finally, comparison of various therapeutic modalities for AML requires homogenization for prognostic factors. Table 33.4 lists some important recognized risk factors. Among them is age: results of conventional chemotherapy as well as allogeneic BMT are better in children. Comparison of allogeneic and autologous BMT must be matched for

population age. An important question, until now unanswered, is whether bone marrow transplantation suppresses the influence of risk factors previously defined during the chemotherapy era.

All considerations discussed above concern obtaining first CR (CR1) and the attempt, by any therapeutic means, to transform this CR1 into cure of the disease. After the first relapse, the prospect for cure with conventional chemotherapy is indeed dismal: Despite a CR2 rate that can reach up to 70% in the best-prognosis group (defined by a CR1 duration over 2 years [British Medical Research Council AML 9 trial]), the cure rate without BMT at this stage is <10% and possibly nil (Table 33.1). Therefore, while there is still some debate whether BMT should be used upfront in all patients at time of CR1, such a debate does not exist any longer after the first relapse, where the only therapeutic strategy with a potential for cure includes BMT.

Table 33.2.   Reasons for Providing Aggressive Therapy in AML Upfront

1. CR in AML cannot be obtained without a state of severe aplasia.
2. Attaining a first CR is an absolute prerequisite for long-term survival or cure.
3. The cure rate after relapse is low and possibly nil with conventional salvage chemotherapy (CT).
4. There is a steep dose-response curve for some drugs such as ARAC and etoposide. As an example, resistance to low-dose ARAC can be overcome with high-dose ARAC.
5. With conventional CT, the second major cause for not reaching CR (after death related to aplasia) is resistance of leukemic cells to drugs. In addition, 50%–70% of patients reaching CR will relapse, the majority in the first 2 years, which reflects an incomplete eradication of the original leukemic clone.
6. The CR and cure rates are lower in patients receiving less chemotherapy for whatever reason (older age, bad compliance, impaired tolerance, preceding hematologic disorders).
7. The Goldie-Coldman hypothesis predicts that the simultaneous use of all effective non-cross-resistant drugs will prevent the emergence of resistant clones.
8. In the past 20 years, introduction of new drugs (notably daunorubicin), increasing dosage, and multiple combinations in induction regimens have improved the CR rate, with the best results being presently achieved by double induction (also called tandem chemotherapy).
9. Comparison of the probabilities of persisting remission (cure) in 10 multicenter studies (see Figure 1 from Büchner et al. [42]) indicates better results in centers where postremission therapy is given for a longer period (>24 months).
10. In patients in first relapse, achievement of CR and median survival are better in those in whom the first CR lasted ≥18 months. This may be explained by the fact that late relapses occur from reactivated, quiescent drug-sensitive leukemic cells, while early relapses represent regrowth of uneradicated drug-resistant clones.
11. Total body irradiation (or equivalent "ablative" chemotherapy combinations) followed by infusion of stem cells (bone marrow transplantation [allogeneic or autologous] or peripheral autologous blood stem cells) combine the most aggressive tumor cytoreductive procedure with a highly potent supportive therapy, within an abbreviated time period, which allows for more tolerable toxicity.

ALLOGENEIC BONE MARROW TRANSPLANTATION

A considerable number of groups throughout the world have reported results of allogeneic BMT in AML. However, the biggest experience is probably that of the Fred Hutchinson Cancer Center in Seattle, and the biggest analysis comes from the European and international bone marrow transplantation registries. The Seattle group reported in 1977 the results of BMT using cyclophosphamide and TBI in 100 patients with end stage leukemia, of whom 54 had AML. The probability of cure at 10 years posttransplantation was 10%. This result, at first considered disappointing, established, however, that allogeneic BMT can cure some patients even at this stage (64). Later on, patients were transplanted in CR, first in CR3 and then in CR2, then as early as CR1, with considerably better results (65). This improvement, which was a direct consequence of the use of BMT earlier

in the disease, also resulted in part from other major advances in patient care, such as blood support; new antibacterial, antifungal, and antiviral agents; and, most of all, prevention of GVHD.

Present Results of Allogeneic Bone Marrow Transplantation in Acute Myelocytic Leukemia

The European registry as of October 1, 1990, contained information on 3966 allogeneic BMT procedures performed by 71 teams since January 1973; 1318 patients were transplanted for AML. Results presented confirmed previous reports from the EBMTG Leukemia Working Party (66, 67). With identical siblings for donors, the outcome depends essentially on the stage of the disease at transplant; the leukemia-free survival LFS at 5 years (Fig. 33.2) is roughly 50% in patients transplanted in CR1 but 25% in patients transplanted later, indicating that every effort

Table 33.3. Autologous and Allogeneic (Allo) BMT for Acute Leukemia: Advantages and Disadvantages

ABMT	ALLOBMT
Advantages	
Applicable to a large population	"Clean marrow"
	GVL effect
No rejection	
No GVHD	
Disadvantages	
Cryopreservation	Restricted to a minority
Contaminated marrow	Rejection
No GVL effect (?)	GVHD
	Severe immunosuppression

Common problems: Pretransplant regimens including TBI do not eradicate leukemia. Therefore, both the intensity of tumor load reduction pretransplant and immunosurveillance posttransplant play a major role in the final control of the disease (immunomodulators, growth factors).

should be made to perform the transplant as early as CR1, and also that beyond CR1 the only therapy with a potential for cure is BMT. Failure of therapy combines transplant-related mortality (TRM) and relapse or recurrence of leukemia. The relapse rate posttransplant is significantly correlated again to the stage of the disease at time of transplant (Fig. 33.3); patients transplanted in CR1 have a cumulated relapse rate below 25%, while patients transplanted in CR2 have a relapse incidence reaching 40%, and those trans-

planted later or in relapse have more than a 50% chance to have recurrent leukemia. In contrast, the TRM, although lower in patients transplanted earlier in CR1, is not strongly correlated with the stage at transplant and varies from 25%–45%, with a global incidence of 40% in the whole population of AML patients.

Factors Influencing Leukemia-Free Survival

Several factors are now known to influence the outcome.

AGE

The age of the recipient is of major importance. There is an increase of TRM decade by decade, with a marked increase above the age of 20–25. In an analysis of the first 75 patients transplanted in CR1, the Seattle team reported a LFS of 70% at 4 years in patients <20 years old compared to 50% in those aged 20–29 years and 30% for those older (68). This was later confirmed by many other groups, although not all (69), and apparently definitively established by both the EBMTG registry and the International Bone Marrow Transplant Registry (IBMTR) (Fig. 33.4). Interestingly, the age of the donor has also been

Table 33.4. Prognostic Factors to Consider When Selecting Treatment Strategy for AML

Factor	Association with Poor Prognosis	References
Age	>60 ⎫	
Performance status	Low ⎬ Reduces chemotherapy tolerance (incomplete treatment)	153
Previous hematologic disorder	Present ⎭	
Cytology FAB	M4, M5, M7[a]	154
Cytogenetics	t (9,22), trisomy 8	155, 156
	Abnormality chromosomes 5,7,11	
	Complex abnormalities (Inverted 16, t (8,21) and t (15,17) are good prognosis factors.)	
Auer rods	Absent	⎫
Peripheral blood count	High	⎬ 157–159
CNS leukemia	Present[a]	⎭
Number of induction courses or time to reach CR	Number >1 or longer time to CR	35

[a]These poor-risk factors are not universally accepted and may be influenced by the treatment used.

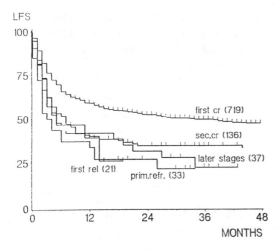

Figure 33.2. Leukemia-free survival following allogeneic BMT for AML, in relation to status of disease at transplant. (From Leukemia Working Party.)

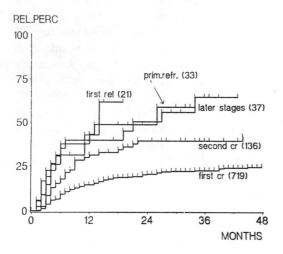

Figure 33.3. Probability of relapse after allogeneic BMT for AML, in relation to status of disease at transplant. (From European Cooperative Group for bone marrow transplantation, Leukemia Working Party.)

found to be associated with an increase in incidence and severity of GVHD (70).

SEX

When considering BMT in general, the sex match is an important prognostic factor. The risk of TRM is higher for male recipients of female marrow donors, and it is consid-

erably increased if the female donor has been previously pregnant and/or multitransfused. However, for some reason this general rule seems less important in AML (71, 72).

HEMATOLOGIC FACTORS

The outcome is worse for patients with an initial high white blood cell count (>75 × 10^9/liter) and the M4 or M5 FAB subtypes (73).

IMMUNOLOGIC FACTORS

The general problems raised by GVHD in BMT have been developed in other chapters and will not be detailed here. In brief, the general consensus is that GVHD is produced by the primary action of T lymphocytes of the donor marrow, essentially CD4+, CD8+, and natural killer (NK) cells that react against non-major HLA antigens if the donor recipient pair is totally HLA matched. The activation of these effector cells seems to be mediated by cytokines (74). Attempts to prevent GVHD, which occurs in almost 50% of patients and kills a quarter of them (71), have successively used the in vivo administration of methotrexate from day 1 to 100 posttransplant (referred to as "long methotrexate"); the administration of cyclosporine A (Cys A); the combination of Cys A and methotrexate, with methotrexate usually administered until day 11 only (referred to as "short methotrexate"); and more recently T cell depletion of the donor marrow. This last approach has resulted in a dramatic increase in both graft rejection and leukemic relapses, which in turn has reemphasized the prior observation that GVHD was at least in part associated with a GVL effect. While in rodents GVHD and GVL are produced by separate nonoverlapping cell populations (38), the situation is probably more complex in humans. Analyzing both the relapse rate and the disease-free survival versus the incidence and severity of GVHD and according to methods used for prevention has clearly demonstrated that the relapse incidence is lower in patients with GVHD and

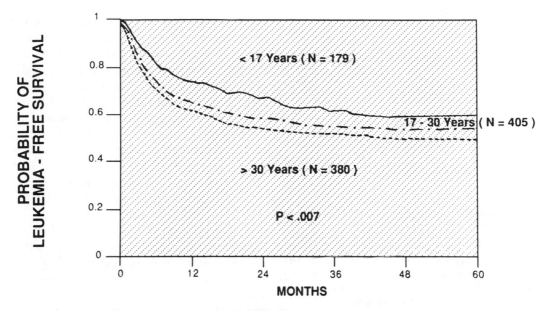

Figure 33.4. Probability of LFS after allogeneic BMT for AML, in relation to age at transplant. (From IBMTR, with permission.)

those with less GVHD prevention. (The maximum relapse was observed with T cell depletion, which is used now predominantly for transplanting marrow from unrelated donors). On the other hand, the TRM is increased by GVHD, so that the benefit of the antileukemic effect of GVHD is at the moment lost because of its adverse effect on survival. Figure 33.5 from the EBMTG indicates that in all patients transplanted for leukemia the highest LFS is observed with the combination of methotrexate + Cys A to prevent GVHD, while the worst corresponds to T cell depletion. Again, considering all leukemic patients, Figure 33.6 indicates that the probability of leukemia relapse is the highest with T cell depletion and the lowest for patients developing both acute and chronic GVHD. For AML patients autografted in CR1, the probability of relapse analyzed by the IBMTR was 24% in those with no GVHD, 27% in those with acute GVHD, 11% in those with chronic GVHD, and only 7% in those with acute and chronic GVHD (9). In Figure 33.7 the decrease in relapse rate observed with the in-

crease in the severity of GVHD is clearly neutralized by the increase in TRM. This finally led to the interesting observation that the best outcome is in patients developing grade I–II GVHD, which constitutes the rationale for trials to generate moderate GVHD in ABMT (see below).

THE ROLE OF THE TRANSPLANT REGIMEN

In the context of allogeneic BMT, the pretransplant regimen is usually termed the "conditioning regimen." This regimen, in addition to its optimal antileukemic activity (which is its major and possibly only role in the context of ABMT), must have other functions, such as immunosuppression to avoid graft rejection and making space to enable the homing of infused stem cells. This last property has been questioned but seems indeed credible when considering that better results are achieved when using a conditioning regimen in situations where it would be unnecessary on other theoretical grounds (BMT for

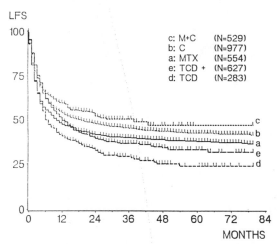

Figure 33.5. Leukemia-free survival in relation to GVHD prevention methods. (From Tura S, Bandini G, eds. Bone marrow transplantation for leukaemia in Europe in 1991. Bone Marrow Transplant 1991; 7(2): 161.)

immune deficiencies or BMT in aplastic anemia with identical twin marrow). Another very important property of any conditioning regimen is its lack of early and late toxicity. The ideal conditioning regimen for allografting AML (and for ABMT) was the optimal equilibrium of maximum antileukemic activity but minimum toxicities. For comparison between allogeneic and autologous BMT, we shall use the term "pretransplant regimen" for both.

Pretransplant regimens for AML can be divided between those using TBI and those using chemotherapy only.

Pretransplant Regimens with Total Body Irradiation

The standard pretransplant regimen was originally designed in Seattle. It combines cyclophosphamide at 60 mg/kg/day for 2 days (total 120 mg/kg) followed after a 2-day rest period by TBI at a dose of 10 Gy administered in a single fraction (STBI) (75). The two major toxicities of this regimen are interstitial pneumonitis (IP), developing early, and cataracts, occurring after several years. Analysis of risk factors for these complications has

led to modifications of the original TBI. A first modification has been a reduction in the dose rate of irradiation; Barrett et al. (76) showed that for delivery of a dose over 8 Gy to the lungs, the risk of developing fatal IP in the early posttransplant period correlated to the dose rate and was considerably increased for a rate >5 cGy/mn. It has, however, remained unclear whether the important variable was indeed the dose rate at the source or the mean dose rate received by the patient, taking into account the total duration of irradiation including intermediate rest periods.

A second way to reduce IP has been the introduction of lung shielding at 8 Gy when STBI is delivered. With lung shielding now routinely used, the incidence of IP has dramatically decreased, and reducing the dose rate may not be necessary any longer (77). Another important modification has been the introduction of fractionated (FTBI) or even hyperfractionated (HFTBI) TBI, in which the total dose administered is split in several fractions (two or three per day) over 2–6 days (75, 78, 79). For technical reasons, with this approach cyclophosphamide is usually given after rather than before irradiation, with no obvious difference. Lung shielding is begun at a level slightly higher than for STBI, usually 9 Gy. The rationale behind fractionated TBI is first to reduce toxicity, and this goal has been achieved not only when considering reduced IP rates but also rates for cataract formation. In a series of 181 TBI patients with a median follow-up of 47 months, 70 cataracts had developed. The Seattle group projected an estimated incidence of 80% with STBI opposed to only 19% in the group receiving FTBI (80).

However, while FTBI or HFTBI diminish toxicity, the question of the tumor cell kill achieved in comparison with the standard STBI remains. While it was initially believed that fractionation of doses would enable higher total doses for higher tumor cell kill, it now appears that part of the increase in the total dose over 10 Gy feasible with FTBI and HFTBI is in fact indispensable to achieve an effect

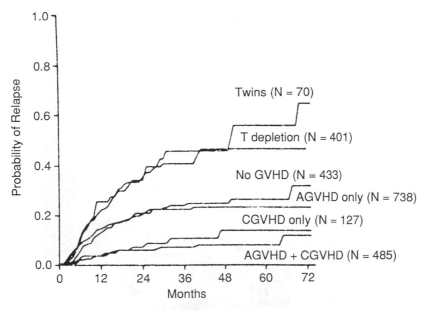

Figure 33.6. Actuarial probability of relapse after bone marrow transplantation for early leukemia according to type of graft and development of GVHD. (From Horowitz NM, Gale RP, Sondel PM. Graft versus leukemia reactions after bone marrow transplantation. Blood 1990;75:555–562.)

similar to STBI. While most teams using FTBI deliver a total dose of 12 Gy, the leukemic AML cell kill achieved may be inferior to the standard 10 Gy STBI (a situation possibly different in acute lymphoblastic leukemia (ALL). An increase in FTBI irradiation has therefore been attempted by several teams, and doses of 13.2 Gy and even 15.75 Gy have been delivered (69, 81–83). Results indicate that higher doses of TBI decrease the relapse incidence but unfortunately increase toxicity, with no global improvement in LFS. For instance, the Seattle group has conducted (83) a randomized trial in patients with AML in CR1 and chronic myelocytic leukemia in chronic phase, comparing 12 Gy to 15.75 Gy FTBI. The higher radiation dose was associated with a decrease in the probability of post-transplant relapse, an increase in the incidence of acute GVHD, an increase in TRM, and no global improvement in LFS. In patients with AML 50% of those receiving 12 Gy did receive 90%–100% of the prescribed posttransplant GVHD prophylaxis, while only 29% of those receiving 15.75 Gy did so. In those 50% and 29% of the patients

in each group who received "adequate GVHD prophylaxis," the incidence of acute GVHD was the same but the probability of relapse was 38% in the 12-Gy group versus 0% in the 15.75-Gy group. The reduction in relapse rate was due to the increase in irradiation but this benefit in a minority of patients was counterbalanced by the inability to deliver sufficient doses of methotrexate and Cys A in the remaining majority. Similarly, in a recent study of 175 transplanted patients in Genoa, the dose effect of TBI on relapse rate appeared evident after stratifying for chronic GVHD and TBI doses (84). This last study demonstrated elegantly that both the radiobiologic and the immunologic effects (TBI + GVH/GVL) are active and indeed combine to eradicate leukemia (84).

Other attempts to increase the antileukemic activity of the pretransplant regimens with TBI or FTBI have used other chemotherapeutic agents in place of or in addition to cyclophosphamide (64). For obvious ethical reasons, these regimens have been first tested in poor-prognosis patients with ad-

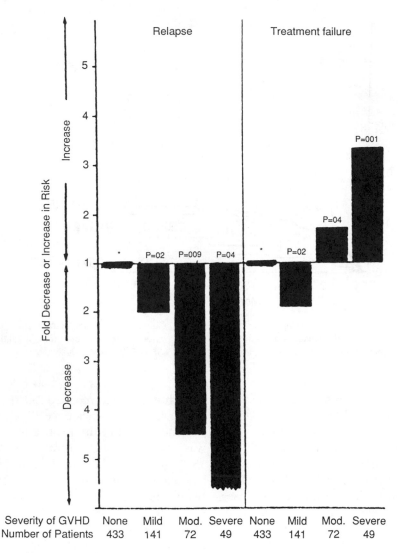

Figure 33.7. Fold increase and decrease in risk of relapse and treatment failure after BMT for early leukemia among patients with both acute and chronic GVHD as compared with patients without GVHD. (From Horowitz NM, Gale RP, Sondel PM. Graft versus leukemia reactions after bone marrow transplantation. Blood 1990;75:555–562.)

vanced disease. One of the most interesting studies has introduced etoposide (VP-16) at 60 mg/kg given in a single infusion as a substitute for CY in combination with FTBI at 13.2 Gy. As of June 1990, of a total of 69 patients with acute leukemia with a median age of 28 years and a median posttransplant follow-up of 17 months, 48 were alive in CR, with an actual disease-free survival of 65% at 3 years.

Three of 28 patients with AML had relapsed (82, 85). Other regimens have included high-dose ARAC (3 g/m^2 every 12 hours for 12 doses) (86) or piperazinedione (87), but they have been used for ALL. In our institution we usually replace the second dose of CY 60 mg/kg by high-dose melphalan (140 mg/m^2) whenever there is a previous history or an increased risk of CNS involvement. In fact the most important challenge to TBI is the chemotherapy-only combination of busulfan and CY, detailed below.

Pretransplant Regimens without Total Body Irradiation: The Combination of Busulfan and Cyclophosphamide

In 1983 the Baltimore group described initial results in patients with AML who received a combination of busulfan and CY (BU-CY) in preparation for allogeneic BMT. The schedule of administration consisted of busulfan 4 mg/kg/day orally for 4 consecutive days, followed by CY 50 mg/kg/day for 4 additional days (51). In an updated report on 99 AML patients with this original regimen, the probability of remaining in CR at 3 years was 87% and the LFS 45% in patients transplanted in CR1. The probabilities were 68% and 31%, respectively, in those transplanted in later stages (CR2, CR3, early relapse). The use of Cys A for GVHD prophylaxis further improved results in patients in CR1, with an increase of LFS to 64% as opposed to those treated previously without Cys A who had an LFS of only 30%. Interestingly (see above problems raised by GVHD prevention and GVL in AML), the probability of relapse was higher with Cys A, and therefore in patients transplanted in later stages, the overall LFS was not improved despite a reduction in incidence and severity of GVHD (88) (Figs. 33.8, 33.9). Early complications observed with this regimen by the Baltimore group, including IP and liver venoocclusive disease (VOD), appeared similar in frequency and severity to those observed with TBI, but this has been questioned. The Columbus transplant team, in an attempt to reduce toxicity while maintaining similar antileukemic activity, modified the original Baltimore regimen by reducing CY administration to 60 mg/kg/day for 2 days only and reported similar efficacy (89). However, a recent trial comparing this modified BU-CY2 (as opposed to the original BU-CY4) regimen to standard TBI, conducted in France by the Groupe D'Etude sur la Greffe de Moelle Osseuse (GEGMO) group, has just been interrupted because of an increased incidence of leukemic relapse in the BU-CY2 arm. Therefore, the consensus at the present time is that BU-CY4 is very likely to be at least equivalent to TBI, while BU-CY2 needs further evaluation. Because BU-CY4 is more flexible than TBI and can be administered in institutions where facilities for TBI do not exist, its use is spreading rapidly.

OTHER FACTORS INFLUENCING THE OUTCOME POSTTRANSPLANTATION

There are several other recognized factors that may influence overall survival, among them complications such as IP, liver VOD, infections (including cytomegalovirus), all of which are grouped under the term TRM. These also occur (although their incidence may be different) with ABMT and will be detailed below. Other factors may well be still unrecognized. For instance, the Leukemia Working Party of the EBMTG, in an analysis of 1904 allogeneic HLA-identical sibling donor bone marrow transplants performed in 52 European centers between 1979 and 1986, grouped patients into six distinct geographical locations. They observed a significant difference in relapse incidence from region to region with no effect on LFS and TRM. There is no logical explanation for this other than that pretransplant factors probably affect outcome more than was previously realized (90).

AUTOLOGOUS BONE MARROW TRANSPLANTATION

In the past 15 years, as an alternative to allogeneic BMT, which was felt to have improved the prognosis of acute leukemia in patients with HLA-identical siblings, several teams, including ours, have developed ABMT to allow patients with no available donor a chance to receive high-dose consolidation therapy. Results of ABMT from various institutions and the European registry now indicate that this goal has been achieved and fur-

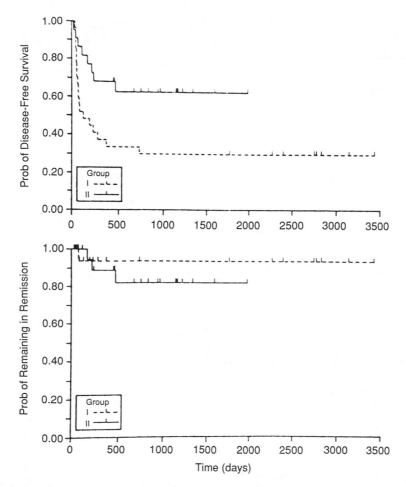

Figure 33.8. Allogeneic BMT in patients with AML in first remission. Actuarial probability of disease-free survival and of remaining in remission for 49 patients who received allogeneic transplants in first CR. Comparison of 27 patients in group 1 and 22 in group II. Tick marks represent censored patients. Group I: no cyclosporine A. Group II: cyclosporine A administration. (From Geller RB, Saral R, Piantadosis, et al. Allogeneic bone marrow transplantation after high dose busulfan and cyclophosphamide in patients with acute nonlymphocytic leukemia. Blood 1989;73:2207–2218.)

ther, it is now possibly advisable to extend ABMT even to AML patients who have donors for allogeneic BMT. However, a potential major impediment to ABMT in leukemias is that the bone marrow extracted during CR may include residual malignant cells that can only rarely be detected by techniques whose power of resolution is higher than that of cytology (e.g., chromosome studies, immunofluorescence, cell sorting, blast colony cultures, and more recently polymerase chain reaction [PCR]). Therefore, the reinfusion of such a bone marrow, in the absence of an effective in vitro method to purge leukemic cells, bears the potential risk of inducing recurrence of leukemia.

Several in vitro treatment methods have been developed in the past decade. With the exception of a few attempts with monoclonal antibodies (91), most teams have concentrated on CY derivatives, mainly 4-hydroxy-cyclophosphamide (4HC) in the United States (21) and mafosfamide (supposedly more stable for in vitro use) in Europe (20, 22, 92).

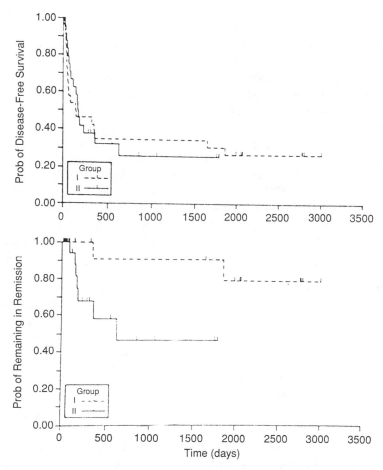

Figure 33.9. Allogeneic BMT in patients with AML in second and third remissions and early relapse. Actuarial probability of disease-free survival and of remaining in remission for 50 patients who received allogeneic transplants in second and third CRs and early relapse. Comparison of 26 patients in group I and 24 patients in group II. Tick marks represent censored patients. Group I: no cyclosporine A. Group II: cyclosporine A administration. (From Geller RB, Saral R, Piantadosis, et al. Allogeneic bone marrow transplantation after high dose busulfan and cyclophosphamide in patients with acute nonlymphocytic leukemia. Blood 1989;73:2209–2218.)

In vitro treatment with CY derivatives has been performed either using a constant dose per milliliter of marrow or with attempts to adjust the level of the drug to the individual sensitivity of normal hematopoietic stem cells, in an effort to induce maximum antileukemic activity yet spare sufficient amounts of normal counterparts to ensure successful engraftment. This has been our own approach (17, 93, 94). In numerous animal models (and in particular the BNML rat leukemia model of human AML) (16) marrow purging, reducing leukemic cell contamination in marrow collected in CR or in artificial marrow tumor cell mixtures, results in cure of leukemia by ABMT. The important question of the efficacy of marrow purging in the human situation has remained unanswered for several years. Indeed, up to now, a majority of teams have performed ABMT with unpurged marrow, relying on optimal in vivo purging by aggressive consolidation chemotherapy courses given prior to marrow collection, which may render unnecessary further in vitro purging. As indicated in the introduction of this chapter, in 1988 the first analysis of the European registry demonstrated the value of marrow purging with mafosfamide in AML autografted in CR1 (28). This demonstration was later confirmed by the 1989 (95) and further extended by the 1990 EBMTG analysis (29). We will first review historical data on ABMT for acute leukemia in relapse. We will successively summarize results of ABMT for AML in CR in some institutions where purging is not used, review data using purged marrow, especially our own results with levels of mafosfamide individually adjusted, and finally present the last European survey that confirmed the efficacy of marrow purging in AML in CR1.

Autologous Bone Marrow Transplantation for Acute Myelocytic Leukemia in Relapse: A Brief History

Retrospective analysis (96–98) clearly indicates that high-dose therapy at time of leukemic relapse, followed by reinfusion of marrow collected earlier in CR, results in a very small percentage with long-term survival (<10%), although it produces a high rate of CR. Pooled data from our institution, Houston, TX, and Besançon, France, showed remission rates of 55% following TBI and of 78% following high-dose chemotherapy with thioguanine (100 mg/m^2 every 12 hours for seven doses), ARAC (200 mg/m^2 by continuous infusion every 12 hours for seven doses), CY (45 mg/kg/day for four doses), and lomustine (250 mg/m^2 for a single dose) (TACC). The best results (CR rates of 71%–90%) were obtained when ABMT was performed to treat the first relapse, with marrow collected at the beginning of CR1. From the first French survey in 1981 (97), we established that CR obtained with ABMT developed parallel to the kinetics of recovery of

hematopoiesis typical of autologous engraftment, suggesting a link between the two events. Complete disappearance of blast cells was documented in 30 of 33 evaluable patients. Unfortunately, all patients in these studies have relapsed, and none has been cured. The first survey for the EBMTG in 1983 (98) showed similar results. Of the 135 patients with acute leukemia who were treated with ABMT, 37 with AML had autografting at relapse. Survival was 0% at 68 months. An international survey in July 1983 (Dicke K, unpublished data) identified 95 patients with end stage acute leukemia treated with ABMT. The CR rate was 60%, and the median duration of CR was 6 months; only 4 patients were disease-free after 2 years.

These early trials, although disappointing, did demonstrate the feasibility of ABMT in patients with leukemia, as well as the sensitivity of blast cells to high-dose cytotoxic therapy and the possibility of achieving a much higher remission rate than that obtained with conventional chemotherapy. Most patients did not receive maintenance chemotherapy post-ABMT. The duration of remission obtained with TACC plus ABMT appeared very similar to that of the previous remission during which the marrow was collected. The results suggested, though, that in patients with acute leukemia in relapse, a cure can only rarely be achieved. One of our patients with an AML (FAB classification 2) diagnosed in May 1976, who was treated with conventional chemotherapy for a CR1 of 19 months, achieved a CR2 lasting 4 years with TACC plus ABMT. In May 1982 he developed a meningeal infiltration, which was treated with local therapy and a second ABMT. He died in December 1983, 7.5 years post initial diagnosis and 6 years post systemic relapse and first treatment with ABMT, from CNS leukemic infiltration, having been in persisting systemic CR and under maintenance chemotherapy for the whole course of his disease.

Although one does conclude from these early trials that high-dose therapy plus ABMT brings few if any benefits to patients with AML in relapse, there are also some other lessons. For example, high-dose therapy plus ABMT can be used occasionally to induce a new CR in end stage leukemia with a probably higher rate than any other conventional salvage regimen.

Autologous Bone Marrow Transplantation in Complete Remission

PRETRANSPLANT REGIMENS

Pretransplant regimens used for ABMT are for the major part those used for allogeneic BMT, first of all TBI with all possibly variations (STBI, FTBI, HFTBI) and second the BU-CY combination. These regimens indeed can be considered standard, and their use enables easier comparisons between allogeneic and autologous BMT. However, in the context of ABMT where antileukemic activity is a priority while immunosuppression (which is indispensable for allogeneic BMT) is not needed, other interesting polychemotherapy regimens have been designed with good results in terms of relapse rate and LFS. These are essentially the University College Hospital (UCH) (London) and the BAVC regimen established in Rome. Details of these high-dose regimens appear in Table 33.5. Results presently available, in particular from the

Table 33.5. High-Dose Polychemotherapy Regimens Used for Autografting Patients with AML

Regimen (Origin)	Description
BAVC (Rome)	BCNU 800 mg/m² × 1
	AMSA 150 mg/m² × 3
	VP-16 150 mg/m² × 3
	ARAC 300 mg/m² × 3
UCH (University College Hospital, London)	CY 1.5 g/m² × 3
	BCNU 300 mg/m² × 1
	ARAC 200 mg/m² × 4
	6-TG 200 mg/m² × 4
	ADR 50 mg/m² × 1
BU + CY4 (Johns Hopkins, Baltimore)	Busulfan 4 mg/kg × 4
	+ CY 50 mg/kg × 4
BU + CY2 (Columbus)	Busulfan 4 mg/kg × 4
	+ CY 60 mg/kg × 2

EBMTG registry, indicate that all these regimens can at least for the moment be considered effective, although not necessarily equivalent.

AUTOLOGOUS BONE MARROW TRANSPLANTATION WITH NONPURGED MARROW IN INDIVIDUAL CENTERS

The overall LFS for AML patients autografted in CR1 is around 50%. Analysis of results from individual centers is of interest in several respects but is unfortunately hampered by the small number of patients in most series: In 25 patients autografted in CR1 between 1984 and 1988 at Genoa, using CY + STBI, Carella et al. reported six toxic deaths, six relapses, an LFS of 56% at 5 years, and a 32% relapse incidence (27). In 20 patients autografted in CR1 with the BU-CY2 combination, the 3-year LFS was 55% and the probability of leukemic recurrence 38%. It was felt, however, that this regimen had significant, albeit manageable, nonhematologic toxicity (99). Thirty-nine pts with AML in CR1 have been autografted in Rome either using the BAVC regimen (n = 25) or CY + STBI (n = 14) (100). All patients had received the same induction and consolidation regimens in the pretransplant period. There were six toxic deaths, five with TBI and one with BAVC. At the time of analysis 12 of 25 BAVC patients and one of nine TBI patients had relapsed. With a median follow-up of 4 years, the LFS rates were 48% and 57% for BAVC and TBI, respectively. This comparison suggests that TBI may have better antileukemic activity, while BAVC is less toxic. The same group has obtained impressive results with BAVC in CR2, which again seems essentially linked to a very low TRM (101). The London UCH team reported on 72 patients autografted in CR1 (25); the design of the study was special in that a double autograft was initially planned. Marrow for the second ABMT was to be reharvested after the first, to take advantage of the in vivo purge (see above) produced. Unfortunately only 26 patients received the second ABMT and completed the protocol. The TRM was 7% in those 66 patients with no preceding myelodysplastic syndrome, and the LFS 66% in those (however selected) that received the double transplant. Individual series are too small to give valuable information on ABMT in CR2.

AUTOLOGOUS BONE MARROW TRANSPLANTATION WITH PURGED MARROW IN INDIVIDUAL CENTERS

We developed in our own institution (St. Antoine, Paris) a technique for adjusting the dose of mafosfamide to individual patients, the rationale being to treat each individual marrow at the highest possible level in an effort to obtain a maximum tumor kill and yet spare a sufficient population of stem cells to ensure proper engraftment. This dose was defined as the colony-forming units of granulocyte-macrophages (CFU-GM) LD95 (sparing 5% CFU-GM) (20). Pretesting in each patient 15 days prior to marrow harvesting indicated a wide range of sensitivity from patient to patient ($20-170$ μg per 2×10^7 cells). With this approach, from January 1983 to January 1990 100 patients with acute leukemia (63) (AML, 55 patients, and ALL, 45 patients) have been consolidated while in CR with CY 60 mg/kg/day $\times$ 2 and TBI followed by the reinfusion of their purged marrow. The median interval from remission to transplant was 5 months. Figure 33.10 describes the protocol we followed. Patients with AML autografted in CR1 had at 6 years a probability of persisting remission and an LFS of 69 $\pm$ 7% and 56 $\pm$ 7%. The figures for patients autografted in CR2 were 20 $\pm$ 17% and 17 $\pm$ 14% (Fig. 33.11). The toxic death rate was 18%. Patients with AML had significantly delayed engraftment compared to ALL: recovery of reticulocytes to 0.1% on day 20 versus 18, of leukocytes to 10^9/liter on day 28 versus 20, platelets to 50 $\times$ 10^9/liter on day 80 versus 39 ($p <$ .0001 for each parameter).

Further, 21 patients received marrow totally depleted of CFU-GM post in vitro

treatment. While of all evaluable patients with ALL engrafted within normal range, 50% of those with AML did not recover a platelet count $>50 \times 10^9$/liter. We found that the CFU-GM LD95 was lower in AML than in ALL, supporting a specific defect of the AML stem cell pool. The best results in terms of LFS and relapse rates were observed in patients receiving the richest marrows evaluated at time of collection (Fig. 33.12) and possibly the lowest residual CFU-GM percentage recoveries after purging. In particular, patients receiving marrow containing less than 0.71% residual CFU-GM post in vitro treatment had a significantly lower relapse rate (28 $\pm$ 8% versus 52 $\pm$ 7%, $p <$ .02). We concluded that ABMT with marrow treated in vitro by mafosfamide is an effective therapy for patients with acute leukemia, with an LFS and a probable cure rate considerably higher than the rates previously obtained in our institution with conventional chemotherapy. We also observed that high initial richness in collected marrow possibly followed by heavy treatment with mafosfamide reduced the relapse rate, but that total depletion of CFU-GM resulted in unacceptable toxicity in AML. We therefore felt that this experience supports an individual adjustment of the dose of mafosfamide for in vitro treatment of the marrow.

The Parma team in Italy designed a specific study to determine the efficacy of marrow purging in patients with AML in CR1 treated with either CY + STBI or BU-CY followed by ABMT. They compared 52 patients grafted with untreated marrow to 49 patients receiving marrow purged with mafosfamide. In 36 of these patients, the mafosfamide was used at a standard dose, while in 13, they adjusted the dose to the individual sensitivity of normal blast colonies according to the technique of Gordon et al. (102) with the same rationale we had. They found an LFS of 37% in patients transplanted with unpurged marrow, 48% in those receiving marrow purged with a standard dose and 75% in those grafted with the adjusted dose methodology. To explain part of the efficacy of purging, they re-

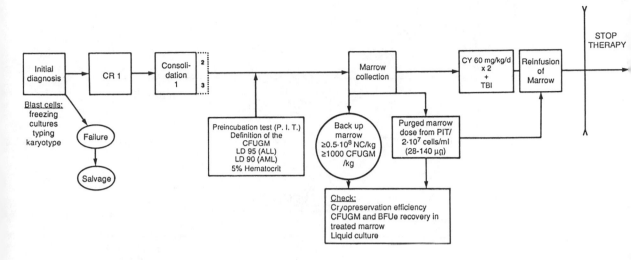

Figure 33.10. ABMT with marrow purged by mafosfamide for adult acute leukemia in CR1. Adjustment of the dosage of mafosfamide and clinical protocol.

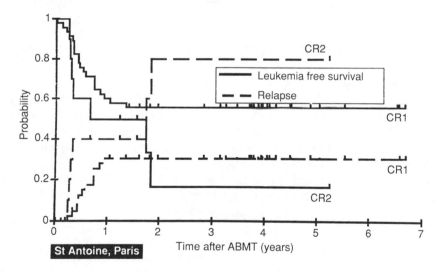

Figure 33.11. LFS and relapse rate in AML patients autografted with mafosfamide-purged marrow.

ported an enhancement of NK-mediated cytotoxicity post-ABMT in patients receiving marrow treated with mafosfamide (23).

The Hopkins group has investigated in depth marrow purging with 4HC both in animal models and in humans for AML in CR2 or beyond. Twenty-five patients with AML, including 20 in CR2 and 5 in CR3, were treated by BU-CY4 followed by infusion of marrow purged with 4HC. Five died of toxicity, 9 re-

lapsed before 1 year posttransplant, and 11 remained in CR for an LFS of 40% (21). Recently the same team (54) using the IPC 81 AML subline, which can be grown in clonogenic assays and maintained in suspension culture, reevaluated the BNML rat model that has initially been used to demonstate the value of 4HC to purge marrow and cure leukemia. They showed a relationship between the effects of 4HC on the growth of leukemic cells

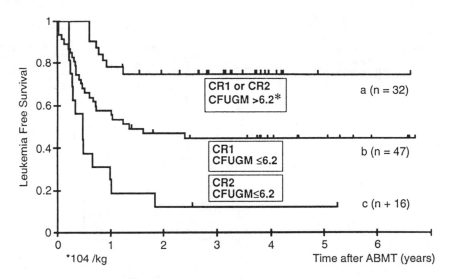

Figure 33.12.   LFS in 100 leukemic patients autografted with mafosfamide-purged marrow. Model 1 for prognosis (without CFU-GM recovery post purging).

in vitro, the dose of leukemic cells infused, and survival. In particular, a decrement of 1 log in the dose of AML cells infused resulted in a 5- to 7-day increase in median survival time. In their work the doses of 4HC used to eradicate leukemia and yet enable engraftment were within narrow limits. After incubation of the marrow—AML cell mixtures with 24 µg/ml of 4HC, no CFU-GM were recovered and yet animals engrafted, while doses of 30 µg/ml were constantly associated with engraftment failure. They indicated that a CFU-GM content of at least 1% of control values in treated bone marrow suspensions was adequate for engraftment, and they further suggested as a reasonable strategy in human trials a selection of drug concentrations similar to the one we and the Parma team use.

Overall there are several indications that marrow purging may indeed improve the outcome after ABMT in AML. However, none of the studies presented above, including ours, has been designed in such a way as to definitively demonstrate its value. Even retrospective analysis is impossible because all series are small. This last obstacle, however, has been

circumvented by the analysis of the European registry.

EUROPEAN SURVEYS: OVERALL RESULTS AND EVIDENCE IN FAVOR OF MARROW PURGING FOR ACUTE MYELOCYTIC LEUKEMIA IN FIRST REMISSION

Fifty-nine European teams have reported 919 autografts for consolidation of AML as of December 31, 1989 (29). The distribution for marrow transplant (ABMT) was as follows: (*a*) CR1, 671; CR2, 196; (*b*) pretransplant regimens—TBI, 456; BU-CY, 174; (*c*) marrow purging with mafosfamide: 269, corresponding to 26% in CR1 and 41% in CR2. The overall results were as follows: For patients autografted in CR1 with no high-risk factor (standard risk), the LFS and relapse rate at 7 years were 48% and 41%, respectively. For patients autografted in CR2, the LFS and relapse rate were 34% and 54%, respectively (Fig. 33.13). Age, sex, and FAB classification were not prognostic factors despite a trend in favor of better results for children autografted in CR2. With the restriction of a shorter follow-up, results achieved with the BU-CY

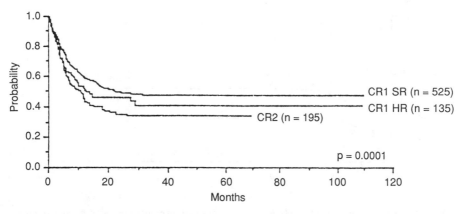

Figure 33.13. LFS following ABMT for AML. (From Gorin NC, Labopin M, Meloni G, et al. Autologous bone marrow transplantation for acute myeloblastic leukemia in Europe: further evidence of the role of marrow purging by mafosfamide. Leukemia 1991;5:896–904.)

combination did not differ from those with TBI or other chemotherapy combinations. LFS and relapse rates were correlated with several pretransplant intervals: In CR1, patients reaching CR more rapidly (≤40 days) had a better LFS (53% versus 42%, p = .03) and a lower relapse rate (46% versus 57%, p = .03). In patients autografted at less than 3 months, 3–6 months, and more than 6 months post induction of CR, the LFS was respectively 26%, 49%, and 55%, and the relapse rates 63%, 38%, and 36% (p < .0001 for both). In CR2, patients autografted more than 18 months post initial diagnosis had a better LFS (42% versus 24%, p < .001) and a lower relapse rate (45% versus 65%, p < .001). For those autografted less than 3 months, 3–6 months, and more than 6 months post initiation of CR, LFS was respectively 30%, 30%, and 50% (p = .06), and the relapse rates 63%, 50%, and 36% (p = .01).

Multivariate analysis of relapse rates in several subpopulations showed the efficacy of marrow purging in AML in CR1. In patients transplanted prior to January 1988 (minimum follow-up, 2 years), the relapse rate with purged marrow was 35 ± 5% versus 47% ± 3% (p = .006). In patients autografted after TBI only it was 29% ± 5% versus 50% ± 4% (p < .0001) (Fig. 33.14), and 16% ± 6% ver-

sus 60% ± 6% (p < .0001) in those autografted within 6 months from induction of CR. In patients autografted after TBI who reached CR1 with a delay from diagnosis to CR1 > 40 days, the figures were 20% ± 8% versus 61% ± 6% (p = .001) in favor of purging, while relapse rates with and without purging were similar in those who initially reached CR1 within 40 days. Results were also significant in multivariate analyses, though at lower levels, when considering all patients autografted until December 1989.

Finally, patients with AML in CR1 autografted post TBI and nonrelapsing at 1 year had a 91% probability of cure with purged marrow versus 80% with nonpurged marrow. This difference was not significant (p = .1) (Fig. 33.15). Relapse patterns were different in that the plateau for persisting remission started at 23 months with purged marrow versus 32 months with unpurged marrow. These results on 671 AML in CR1 patients confirmed the initial finding on a smaller series of patients transplanted before January 1987 and analyzed in 1988 (28). Marrow purging was effective in situations when residual tumor is more likely to persist (initial diagnosis to CR1 > 40 days, CR1 to ABMT ≤ 6 months). In CR2, marrow purging also was associated with a better LFS in patients re-

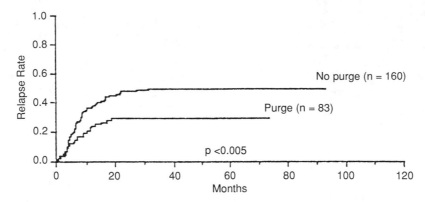

Figure 33.14. Relapse rates in patients with AML in CR1 autografted after TBI with purged or unpurged marrow; patients transplanted before January 1988. (From Gorin NC, Labopin M, Meloni G, et al. Autologous bone marrow transplantation for acute myeloblastic leukemia in Europe: further evidence of the role of marrow purging by mafosfamide. Leukemia 1991;5:896–904.)

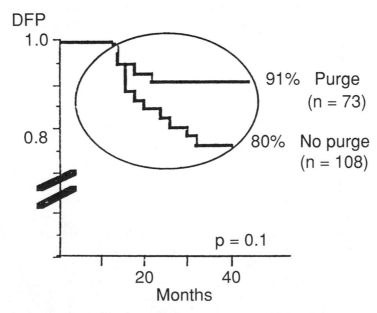

Figure 33.15. Probability of persisting remission in patients with AML in CR1, autografted with TBI, still in persisting CR1 year post-ABMT, according to whether they received purged or unpurged marrow. (From Gorin NC, Labopin M, Meloni G, et al. Autologous bone marrow transplantation for acute myeloblastic leukemia in Europe: further evidence of the role of marrow purging by mafosfamide. Leukemia 1991;5:896–904.)

ceiving TBI (32% ± 8% versus 16% ± 7%, p = .03 in univariate analysis), but the relapse rate was not significantly different (57% ± 9% versus 68% ± 9%, p = .07). Overall, patients with AML who have not relapsed at 1 year post-ABMT performed in CR1 or CR2 with purged or unpurged marrow have a probability of being cured greater than 80%. Interestingly, the EBMT analysis of purging in ALL did not detect any influence of purging (be it with CY derivatives as for AML or with monoclonal antibodies) on outcome.

PRESENT SITUATION AND FUTURE PROSPECTS CONCERNING PURGING

There are presently several arguments in favor of purging with CY derivatives in ABMT for AML, in contrast to ALL. The strongest argument is probably the favorable results obtained with purged marrow in AML in CR2 and the EBMTG surveys indicating fewer relapses with purged marrow in AML in CR1. However, results in AML in CR2 such as those obtained by the Baltimore team (21) are criticized in that the influence of purging is unknown since all patients received purged marrow, and results from the EBMTG in CR1 are questioned since they were obtained from a registry and therefore rely on nonrandomized comparisons of less than optimally controlled information (a general comment pertinent to all registries). Indeed, in Europe 70% of the teams still perform ABMT without purging. In such a situation they rely essentially on in vivo purging procured by consolidation courses given prior to marrow collection. Of interest are the poor results obtained when ABMT is done very early after achieving CR, usually only after one consolidation course. The conclusion of the EBMTG surveys that the influence of marrow purging is important and its efficacy more pronounced when the interval from CR to ABMT is shorter and the number of consolidation courses smaller is credible if in vivo purging has been insufficient or the amount of residual tumor is more likely to be great. The

finding in the field of chemotherapy that only one course of consolidation is not enough strengthens this interpretation (44).

While many teams do not purge marrow in CR1, some still have a bias in favor of purging (as reflected by the EBMTG analysis of the distribution of marrow purging by status of the disease (29): CR1 standard risk 25.1%, high risk 30.3%; CR2 standard risk 39.7%, high risk 55.2%). If indeed some teams would select purging for higher risk patients, this would further support rather than argue against a favorable role of purging in AML. Finally, recent comparisons of relapse rates in patients autografted with peripheral blood stem cells versus marrow, which indicate that the relapse rate is lower with purged marrow and similar with unpurged marrow or PBSCs, further support purging (see below). Unfortunately, these last studies are also retrospective (33, 34).

The consensus is that all information available at the present time should set the stage for randomized trials comparing infusion of purged marrow versus unpurged marrow. Two such trials exist, one in the United States, presently ongoing, and one in Europe, presently planned. Figure 33.16 represents a typical scheme. To avoid any bias, in vitro manipulation of the marrow should be done in both arms, one with the drug verum and the other with a placebo. Because of the potential importance of both in vivo and in vitro purging, ABMT should not, as least in our view, be compared to allogeneic BMT. The need to reduce residual disease may be more important prior to ABMT than prior to allogeneic BMT in CR1, especially in CR2, where results of allogeneic BMT have been similar for patients transplanted in CR2 or in early relapse where ABMT is impossible (65).

AUTOGRAFTING IN ACUTE MYELOCYTIC LEUKEMIA WITH PERIPHERAL BLOOD STEM CELLS

After some early concern about the possibility of obtaining sustained engraft-

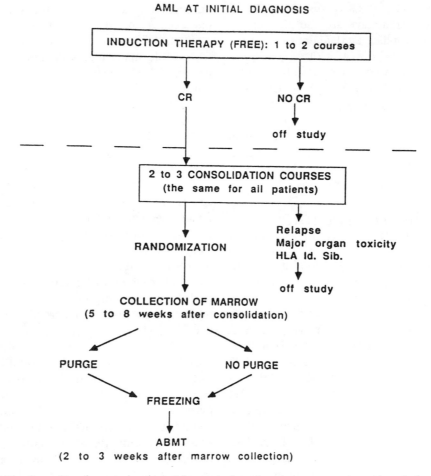

Figure 33.16.   Proposition for a randomized trial to study the value of marrow purging with mafosfamide in AML in CR1.

ment with PBSCs, this technique has become routinely used since 1985 (30, 103–107). At the present time PBSCs are usually collected after chemotherapy, sometimes followed by administration of hematopoietic growth factors, and are used for autografting in the case of solid tumors and lymphomas.

In the context of AML the initial rationale was appealing, for two reasons. First, the contamination of peripheral blood by leukemic clones at time of CR was likely to be less important than the estimated contamination of marrow, or even nil; therefore, the risk of reinfusing tumor would be less or

nonexistent, and purging would no longer be necessary. The second reason was related to the long duration of aplasia observed with ABMT, which has a median duration of thrombocytopenia around 100 days necessitating platelet support sometimes for as long as a year; preliminary results of PBSC autografting had indicated very rapid kinetics of recovery of hematopoiesis. Therefore, several teams started collecting PBSCs at time of recovery from aplasia, after either induction or consolidation courses. The yields of CFU-GM collected were better after induction and decreased after each additional consolidation course. Since the minimum dose for safe engraftment was considered to be $>10^5$ CFU-GM per kilogram, 3–6 leukaphereses were usually needed requiring considerable effort in terms of harvesting, freezing, storage facilities, and hence finances.

The initial experience of our own team was disastrous (108). In a 1-year period, six patients with AML (four in CR1 and two in CR2) and four patients with acute lymphocytic leukemia (two in first, one in second, and one in third remission) underwent 49 leukaphereses done after induction of remission and after one course of consolidation. The median dose of progenitor cells (in CFU-GM $\times$ 10^4/kg) collected per patient was 4.6 (range 0.02–26.9). The yields were better in CR1 than in CR2 or CR3 (145.2 versus 0.7). The four patients with AML in CR1 were given PBSC autografts 3–5 months after the initial diagnosis (Table 33.6). The pretransplant regimen consisted of CY 60 mg/kg daily $\times$ 2 plus TBI (10 Gy, lung shielding after 8 Gy). Engraftment was rapid in three patients (white cell count above 10^9/liter by day 13, reticulocytes above 0.1% by day 13, and platelet count above 50 $\times$ 10^9/liter by day 14). However, three patients relapsed rapidly, at 4, 4, and 5 months posttransplant. The fourth one is probably cured—still in unmaintained CR 4 years later.

We postulated, when the six patients with AML relapsed, that in opposition to the starting hypothesis of an absence of or reduction in contamination of peripheral blood by leukemic cells, that in fact leukemic clonogenic cells might circulate in peripheral blood precisely at time of marrow regeneration, especially after induction. We considered that the large volume of blood processed (15 or so liters per patient) may have increased the probability of collecting tumor cells. Finally, we suggested that leukapheresis should be done after additional courses of consolidation, to take advantage of in vivo purging. In a recent review, Reiffers et al. (34) identified 28 patients (mean age 38 years, range 18–50) with AML in CR1 who were transplanted with PBSCs collected after induction and/or consolidation therapy. They were prepared with either busulfan (4 mg/day $\times$ 4) associated with CY (120–200 mg/kg) or melphalan (n = 9) or with CY associated with FTBI (n = 19). The main characteristics for these patients (age or sex, FAB morphology, interval from diagnosis to CR, or from CR to BMT or PBSC autograft, conditioning regimen) did not differ significantly from those of 683 patients who received ABMT for AML in CR1. After PBSC autograft, the median time to recover 500 polymorphonuclear leukocytes per cubic millimeter was 15.5 days (9–60), which was shorter than that observed after ABMT (27 days). Platelet engraftment was similar after either PBSC autograft (58.5 days) or ABMT. After PBSC autograft, the estimated chance of surviving at 2 years was 39 $\pm$ 10% without disease, and the actuarial risk of relapse was 50 $\pm$ 10%. These results did not differ significantly from those observed after ABMT with unpurged marrow but were possibly inferior to those of purged ABMT (DFS = 47 $\pm$ 0.04%).

Table 33.6. Four Cases of PBSC Autotransplantation in AML in First Remission[a]

Case	PBSC dose[b]	PMN >0.5 10^9/liter[c]	WBC >10^9/liter	Retic. >10^9/liter	Plat. >50 10^9	Outcome
1 (20,M)	27.6	18	17	16	100	CR (4 years +)
2 (39,F)	47.9	14	13	13	15	R (4 mos)
3 (45,M)	142	13	11	11	13	R (5 mos)
4 (35,M)	56	14	13	13	13	R (4 mos)

[a]Abbreviations: Plat., platelets; PMN, polymorphonuclear cells; R, relapse; Retic., reticulocytes; WBC, white blood cells.
[b]In 10^4 CFU-GM/kg.
[c]Days.

This indeed appeared more clearly in a comparative study conducted by M. Körbling, where patients with AML in CR1 received either infusion of PBSCs (n = 20) or ABMT with marrow purged with mafosfamide (n = 23) (33). In both cases the pretransplant regimen combined CY and FTBI at a higher dosage than usual (14.4 Gy). The major differences in the two approaches were the following:

1. The blood stem cell autograft contained 17-fold more mononuclear cells.
2. White blood cell reconstitution was initiated earlier with PBSCs. The median time to reach 10^9/liter was 10 days with PBSCs versus 28 days with purged ABMT.
3. Platelet reconstitution occurred faster following PBSC infusion compared with purged ABMT, although the significance was borderline.
4. The patients' hospital stay was significantly shorter following PBSC autografting: 45 days versus 73 days for purged ABMT.
5. However, more relapses occurred following PBSC autografting, and the LFS at 2 years was higher in the group receiving purged marrow: 51% compared to 35%.

Thus the only advantage of PBSC infusion over ABMT seems to be to shorten the duration of granulocytopenia, certainly not to decrease the risk of relapse. This suggests that the leukemic contamination of peripheral blood stem cells is not different from that of bone marrow, and the question arises again as to the origin of leukemic relapse. At present time, PBSC autografting plays a minor role in the general management of AML. In an effort to take advantage of PBSCs to speed up the recovery of hematopoiesis and yet avoid the risk of reinfusing leukemic cells in our own institution, where all marrows are purged with mafosfamide, we recently designed a pilot study and transplanted a few consecutive patients with both purged marrow and the product of a single leukapheresis done in steady state 15 days prior to marrow collec-

tion, so that in vivo purging would be equal for marrow and peripheral blood and stimulation and recirculation of blast cells after aplasia and regeneration would be avoided. While the study is far from completion, we still have the same feeling that infusion of PBSCs, for whatever reason, may in fact increase the relapse rate.

ALLOGENEIC BONE MARROW TRANSPLANTATION WITH MISMATCHED RELATED OR MATCHED UNRELATED DONORS

It is usually estimated that allogeneic BMT if performed in all AML patients with a related HLA-identical donor would involve not more than 15% of the patients (considering, in addition to the existence of a donor, the age limitation linked essentially to GVHD). Another alternative has been considered, namely, allogeneic BMT using HLA-mismatched family donors, or the use of HLA-identical unrelated donors identified through large computerized registries of volunteers who have agreed to be marrow donors. In Europe, the worldwide bone marrow dictionary now includes 500,000 donors with HL A and B types for all, and for Dr in an increasing proportion (109). For HLA-mismatched related donors, the Seattle team has attempted to analyze the influence of HLA compatibility on the outcome of 280 such transplants, which included patients with AML (110, 111): 10% of the recipients were phenotypically but not genotypically identical to their donors, 42% were mismatched for one antigen, 37% were mismatched for two antigens, and 10% were mismatched for three antigens. With a follow-up of at least 2 years, it is clear that for both phenotypically matched and one-antigen-mismatched patients, the probability of survival was indistinguishable from that of patients who received HLA genotypically identical marrow. However, one-antigen-mismatched patients had an increased probability of rejection and of developing GVHD. The lack of impact of this increased GVHD upon survival did not appear to be due to a beneficial influence of GVHD on posttransplant leukemia relapse. Patients transplanted from two- or three-antigen-mismatched donors had a much worse probability of survival than patients with the same disease status transplanted from HLA-identical donors. Since most such transplants were in critical clinical settings, there is clearly a role for transplants from HLA-mismatched donors, particularly in younger patients, in which GVHD seems to be less severe. The incidence of both graft rejection and GVHD increases with the degree of antigenic disparity.

The conclusion of this study is that a phenotypically matched or a one-antigen-mismatched family donor can be considered as favorably as a totally matched family donor for an allogeneic BMT in AML.

In contrast, results of allogeneic BMT with unrelated HLA-identical donors are presently poor. In a recent analysis of about 200 such BMTs performed in France, the disease-free survival at 1 year was only 28%. This led to the conclusion that marrow-unrelated donor (MUD) BMT should be done only with fully matched donors with a negative mixed lymphocyte reaction. Very clearly, in the management of AML, BMT or aggressive chemotherapy is to be considered first before a MUD transplant.

COMPLICATIONS OF HIGH-DOSE THERAPY IN ACUTE MYELOCYTIC LEUKEMIA AND RECENT IMPROVEMENTS IN MANAGEMENT

It is far beyond the scope of this chapter to review all complications that can occur following chemotherapy, TBI, or allo- or autografting, since for the most part they are not specific for AML. In addition they have been reviewed in other chapters. However, high-dose therapy in AML bears certain spe-cific risks that we would like to emphasize. GVHD will not be addressed here.

High-dose chemotherapy or any pre-transplant regimen results in a *4- to 6-week period of aplasia* with usually some degree of organ damage, essentially mucositis, which may be improved by prophylactic administration of pentoxifylline (112). Approximately 50% of transplanted patients develop *bacterial or fungal infection* during this period. This risk is considerably reduced by the use of laminar airflow rooms and the administration of nonabsorbable broad-spectrum antibiotics (113, 114).

Death from sepsis may occur but is a rare event with the present aggressive use of several antibiotics very quickly in the absence of fever resolution or persistence of fibrinogen elevation. Our present approach to treating fever in transplanted patients is to introduce as first line a combination of ticarcillin-clavulanic acid (a penicillin active against Pseudomonas and an inhibitor of the β-lactamases produced by most gram-positive bacteria, including *Staphylococcus*) and amikacin (an aminoglycoside). With persisting fever, in the absence of an apparent source we introduce vancomycin and finally amphotericin B. With this approach, we obtain resolution of the fever in over 90% of cases. Indeed, death from sepsis is usually combined with other serious complications such as liver VOD, viral infection, or GVHD. *Hematopoietic growth factors such as granulocyte-macrophage colony-stimulating factor (GMCSF) or granulocyte colony-stimulating factor (GCSF)* reduce the duration of neutropenia by 7–10 days (115–118) and may be useful to reduce mucositis. One of our patients allografted following the BU-CY4 regimen developed a drug (non-GVHD) related toxic epidermal necrolysis (Lyell's syndrome) as early as day 4 and recovered successfully under GMCSF therapy (unpublished). In addition, GMCSF is now the first-line therapy for delayed engraftment or engraftment failure, to be considered prior to a second transplant (120). In our experience GMCSF partly prevents myelosuppression from ganciclovir when administered for cytomegalovirus (CMV) infection (121). Finally, we have been able in a few highly selected cases of progressing non-Hodgkin's lymphomas with marrow involvement precluding ABMT to administer a high-dose chemotherapy pretransplant regimen (BEAM) followed by GMCSF in place of ABMT (122, 123).

Overall, GMCSF in our experience as well as GCSF in the experience of others (124–126) have considerably increased the safety in the transplant ward. In the context of AML the use of hematopoietic growth factors has been first cautioned against and even considered unethical since about 50% of leukemic blast cells bear receptors for these cytokines (127–128), and it was feared that their administration might induce leukemic proliferation. While this has been indeed observed in occasional cases of myelodysplastic syndromes, hematopoietic growth factors have been introduced successfully in the early management of AML in elderly patients, with two aims: when given prior to induction chemotherapy, to recruit leukemic clones in S phase and increase tumor killing, and when given post chemotherapy to reduce the duration of the neutropenic period (129, 130). Here again this has not induced any detectable enhancement of leukemic clone proliferation and has in fact resulted in an improvement in terms of shortening of the aplasia duration post chemotherapy, while the outcome in terms of long-term LFS remains unknown. Currently, it seems reasonable to consider that hematopoietic growth factors are very likely to be used soon in AML patients receiving high-dose therapy, for chemotherapy or allogeneic or ABMT, when no leukemic cells are detected, especially when a marrow transplant is performed in remission. Similarly, hematopoietic growth factors may be used for engraftment failure, also in the context of AML. In summary, the increased safety contributed by hematopoietic growth factors in the transplant setting, now

only benefiting patients with nonmyeloid hematologic malignancies, is very likely to eventually benefit AML patients.

The most important viral infections associated with high-dose therapy in AML are infections with herpesvirus (HSV), which can produce encephalitis, and CMV, which can produce *interstitial pneumonitis* (IP), often leading to death. HSV infection has been almost totally prevented by the introduction of prophylactic acyclovir (131), and further, the use of high-dose prophylactic acyclovir has somewhat unexpectedly reduced the CMV infection rate posttransplant (132). The incidence (especially for IP) and mortality from CMV infection are significantly lower in patients who receive ABMT than allogeneic BMT (133). CMV infection usually develops from reactivation of latent viruses but also can be transmitted by blood products used for transfusion support. Pretransplant, approximately 50% of patients are CMV seronegative. If submitted to allogeneic BMT (and not ABMT), about half of them will receive marrow from a CMV-seronegative donor. Therefore, about 25% of allogeneic BMT and 50% of ABMT patients will be CMV seronegative immediately posttransplant. These patients may be totally protected against CMV by the use of blood products exclusively from seronegative donors (134). One of the major risks of CMV infection in the early posttransplant period is myelosuppression or delayed engraftment or graft rejection. The only antiviral agent effective against active CMV infection, ganciclovir (DHPG), also carries a serious risk of secondary myelosuppression, usually developing after the administration of the initial 14-day course. Therefore, the decision to introduce DHPG in a patient with CMV in blood or urine in the absence of any other sign of infection is difficult. Our current policy in this situation is the administration of specific hyperimmune anti-CMV immunoglobulins (0.25 g/kg/day bolus followed by a half dose every week until day 100) without DHPG, while patients with active infection receive the combination of both. In a recent study of this combination for the treatment of CMV IP, confirmed by CMV detection after bronchoalveolar lavage, of 25 recipients of allogeneic BMT 14 patients survived, indicating improved survival in comparison to historical controls. As indicated above, the most serious side effect was myelodepression (135). Trials are now in progress to evaluate the role of DHPG given as maintenance for several weeks after curative administration in patients with documented CMV infection and the role of preventive DHPG in transplanted patients (136).

Another major complication of high-dose therapy in AML is *liver VOD,* which has a death rate of approximately 50%. The incidence of VOD has varied from as high as 21% after allogeneic BMT to only 6% after ABMT (95, 137–145). In these series, identified predisposing factors have included age over 15 years, female sex, previous history of liver disease (non-A, non-B (C) and B hepatitis), abnormal alanine aminotransferase levels before ABMT, and underlying malignancy other than ALL, acute leukemia in other situations than CR1, and allogeneic rather than autologous BMT (25% versus 4.8%) (137). (In particular, in a recent European survey [95], the incidence of VOD was higher in AML [4.3%] as compared to ALL [1.6%]). The incidence of VOD is also reportedly higher after preparative regimens using unfractionated rather than fractionated TBI and ARAC or thioguanine. Of interest in this respect is that preparative regimens with CY and busulfan are not associated with an increased incidence of VOD when compared to CY and TBI. Finally, in allogeneic BMT, for GVHD prophylaxis, methotrexate and/or Cys A has been incriminated, although GVHD per se cannot be excluded.

Until now there has not been any effective curative measure for clinical VOD. Several trials have been conducted with heparin. In our institution (145), we studied the potential role of continuous intravenous administration of low-dose heparin for VOD prevention in 234 consecutive patients who underwent ABMT. The population consisted of 98 patients autografted before October 1984 who did not receive heparin and a series of 136 patients autografted from October 1984 to March 1989, containing 98 patients included in a randomized trial comparing heparin administration (n = 52) and no heparin (n = 46), and an additional group of 38 patients who received nonrandomized heparin in view of their high risk of developing VOD (n = 31) or other reasons unrelated to VOD (n = 7). Overall, 90 patients (38%) received heparin, and 144 (62%) did not. The global incidence of VOD was 13 of 234 (5.5%). Heparin did not reduce the risk of VOD in all subgroups studied. In particular, in the randomized trial, the incidence of VOD was 2.2% in the group without heparin versus 7.7% in the group receiving heparin. We analyzed in depth the 13 patients who developed VOD, and we compared them to a control group of 13 patients pair-matched for age, sex, diagnosis, and preparative regimen, who did not develop VOD. We found that abnormal liver function tests before ABMT predisposed patients to VOD; refractoriness to platelet transfusion was observed in 85% of the patients in the VOD group versus 15% in the control group ($p < .05$). VOD patients had an increased requirement for red cell and platelet transfusions, a lower recovery (R < 25%) after the second and third platelet transfusion, and shorter intervals separating the first four platelet transfusions. Further, the platelet reconstitution after ABMT in the VOD group was slower in comparison to the control group ($p < .01$). Again, in this pair-matched analysis, continuous infusion of low-dose heparin did not prevent VOD. Therefore, the best way to avoid liver VOD is still prevention: Patients with an increased risk of developing VOD as described above either receive high-dose CT or pretransplant regimens selected for less hepatic damage, or usually have their liver shielded when receiving TBI to receive less radiation (6 Gy for STBI, 8 Gy for FTBI). Whether this protocol indeed does reduce the incidence or severity of VOD remains unknown. In the context of AML one must remember that any shielding (for lungs, skull, or liver with an unavoidable parallel shielding of ribs) would diminish by 2–3 logs the leukemic burden reduction. Present trials in progress evaluate the therapeutic, curative, and preventive role of prostaglandin and prostacyclin derivatives, with apparently favorable preliminary observations (146, 147).

Late side effects seen after transplants involving TBI include growth retardation in children, early menopause, sterility, cataract formation, and an increased incidence of secondary malignancies. Although each of these side effects is serious, treatment (i.e., hormone substitution and cataract surgery) or a low incidence (secondary malignancies) result in most posttransplant patients having an excellent performance status.

CHEMOTHERAPY VERSUS ALLOGENEIC BONE MARROW TRANSPLANTATION VERSUS AUTOLOGOUS BONE MARROW TRANSPLANTATION: WHAT IS THE CHOICE?

While after a first relapse BMT (allogeneic or autologous) seems to be superior to chemotherapy, which is associated with a minimal and possibly nil cure rate, the situation is more complex in CR1. Advocates of modern aggressive but still conventional chemotherapy argue that a 40% disease-free survival can be achieved in good-prognosis categories, especially in children. Even with a disease-free survival around 20% in adults, which corresponds to the experience of a majority of teams, it can be argued that this poor result does not differ from the apparently better 40%–50% disease-free survival achieved with BMT, when one considers that the disease-free survival curves of chemotherapy start at diagnosis while in transplanted patients they start later, at time of BMT. This induces a selection bias in that all poor-risk patients that relapse early are excluded from the BMT group. A simple correction would consist of comparing the outcome of transplanted patients to the outcome of those selected patients treated by chemotherapy that are still in CR at the time when BMT would be performed (median 3–6 months). Even so it is our own judgment that results of both allogeneic and autologous BMT are still superior chemotherapy in CR1, notwithstanding that patients transplanted, especially those submitted to ABMT, have a much shorter overall treatment duration, which in spite of the considerable psychologic stress of BMT may be counted as a benefit. Comparisons of the three therapeutic approaches and also comparisons between allogeneic and autologous BMT are of importance. Considering ABMT, because of the risk of reinfusing tumor cells, we believe that comparisons should only consider reinfusion of "clean" marrow, as achieved with purged marrow, or if the marrow infused is unpurged, with marrow collected in CR and not in partial remission, following several consolidation courses for in vivo purge. Obviously, ABMT carries more technical risks for failure than the other techniques. Unfortunately this has not been always considered in numerous studies.

In a combined European Bone Marrow Transplant Group and European Organization for Research on the Treatment of Cancer (EBMTG-EORTC) retrospective analysis (148), patients with AML, treated in CR1 with chemotherapy or with allogeneic or autologous BMT were compared with respect to their LFS from CR. Two hundred and thirty-six patients treated with chemotherapy according to the EORTC AML 5 and AML 6 trials were included. The data of the transplanted patients were taken from two EBMTG registries, 453 with an allogeneic and 182 with an autologous BMT. In this study several precautions were taken in an effort to avoid a selection bias. First of all, since the study concentrated on LFS from CR, patients not reaching CR were not included in the evaluation of the chemotherapy cohort. Second, since BMT patients must have remained in remission from time of CR to time of BMT (while no such requirement held for the chemotherapy group), a time-dependent covariate was introduced in the proportional hazards analysis. Finally, to reach a better comparability of the groups, age at diagnosis was restricted to between 15 and 45 years. The result of the overall log rank test showed significant differences in LFS between the three groups. More than 6 months after transplant, patients allografted had a statistically significant higher LFS than those receiving chemotherapy. Patients autografted tended also to have a better LFS over CT, but the p value was not significant. In a recent analysis of their own experience on a total of 140 transplanted patients with AML in CR1, the Genoa team observed a similar LFS at 7 years (47% and 48%) for both ABMT with unpurged marrow and allogeneic BMT (Fig. 33.17). In the allogeneic BMT group, the relapse rate was higher in patients receiving doses of TBI < 10 Gy (50% versus 18%) and in those with no chronic GVHD (35% versus 10%). When comparing autologous to allogeneic BMT, the relapse rate in ABMT (39%) was identical to the relapse rate in allogeneic BMT in the absence of

chronic GVHD (37%) but higher than in allogeneic BMT with chronic GVHD (30%). The beneficial reduction in relapse rate brought by chronic GVHD was balanced by a higher toxic death rate.

Obviously adequate comparison of autologous and allogeneic BMT requires randomized studies. Such a study has been conducted by several Dutch centers (149). The comparative value of ABMT with unpurged marrow and allogeneic BMT was assessed in 117 patients with AML included from initial diagnosis. Of 90 patients achieving CR, 37 were not transplanted for various reasons, 32 were autografted, and 21 were allografted. The LFS was higher in allogeneic transplant recipients (51% versus 35% at 3 years, p = NS), and the relapse rate higher in the ABMT group (60% versus 34%, p = .03). Preliminary analysis of other trials in progress with a similar design and unpurged marrow appear confirmatory (150, 151). An Eastern Cooperative Oncology Group (ECOG) trial is currently evaluating ABMT with marrow purged with 4HC; in this trial, patients with de novo AML ages 15–55 receive one or two induction course(s) with daunorubicin, ARAC, and thioguanine. One to 3 months post-CR, they then either receive ABMT or undergo allogeneic BMT if they are less than 41 years of age and have a histocompatible sibling. In an interim analysis recently presented, the CR rate was 74%. Thirty-five patients underwent ABMT and 16 allogeneic BMT. The Kaplan-Meier estimate of event-free survival at 2 years was 52% ± 29% versus 46% ± 26% for ABMT and allogeneic BMT, respectively (152). Taken with the results of the trials using nonpurged marrow, this might indeed indicate that using purged marrow improves the outcome. This question, however, needs a separate trial. There is at least one such trial in progress at the moment comparing purged and unpurged marrow for AMBT in AML in CR1.

It is actually difficult to draw a valuable conclusion since the field is evolving quickly. However we propose our own approach as a possible strategy for the management of AML:

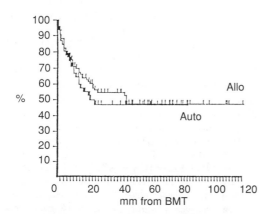

Figure 33.17. LFS after autologous or allogeneic BMT for patients with AML in CR1. The Genoa experience on 148 patients. (From AM Carella, F Frassoni, Van Lint MT, et al. Autologous and allogeneic bone marrow transplantation in acute myeloid leukemia in first complete remission: an update of the Genoa experience on 159 patients [Abstract]. Paper presented at 5th International Symposium on Therapy of Acute Leukemias, Rome, Nov 1991).

We consolidate in CR1 all adult patients with AML and all children with poor-risk features by CY 60 mg/kg/day × 2 and single-dose TBI at 10 Gy with lung shielding at 8 Gy, followed by ABMT with marrow purged by mafosfamide. We believe that marrow should be collected after a minimum of two consolidation courses to take advantage of in vivo purging. We even recommend this procedure in CR1 for a patient having an HLA-indentical related sibling since the transplant-related mortality is lower with ABMT. We use exactly the same approach in CR2. We would recommend allografting for patients with an available HLA-identical sibling only in CR3 or in early relapse after CR2. We never consider allografting with an HLA-identical unrelated donor for AML.

Acknowledgments
The author wishes to express his gratitude to Mrs. V. Skalli for typing this manuscript.

REFERENCES

1. Clarkson BD, Gee T, Mertelsmann K, et al. Current status of treatment of acute leukemia in adults. an overview of the Memorial experience and review of literature CRC. Crit Rev Oncol Hermatol 1986; 4:221.
2. Thomas ED, Storb R, Clift RA, et al. Bone marrow transplantation. New Engl J Med 1975;292:832–843, 895–902.
3. Santos G. History of bone marrow transplantation. Clin Haematol 1983;12:611–638.
4. Mathe G, Bernard J, De Vries MJ. Nouveaux essais de greffe de moëlle osseuse homologués après irradiation totale chez des enfants atteints de leucémie aiguë en rémission. Le problème du syndrome secondaire chez l'homme. Rev Fr et Clin Biol 1960;15:115.
5. Atkinson K, Horowitz MM, Biggs JC, et al. The clinical diagnosis of acute graft versus host disease: a diversity of views amongst marrow transplant centers. Bone Marrow Transplant 1988;3:5–10.
6. Atkinson K, Horowitz MM, Gale RP, et al. Consensus among bone marrow transplanters for diagnosis grading and treatment of chronic graft versus host disease. Bone Marrow Transplant 1989;4:247–254.
7. Thomas ED, Büchner CD, Clift RA, et al. Marrow transplantation for acute non lymphoblastic leukemia in first remission. New Engl J Med 1979;301:597–599.
8. Weiden PL, Flournoy N, Thomas ED, et al. Antileukemia effect of graft versus host disease in human recipients of allogeneic marrow grafts. N Engl J Med 1979;300:1068.
9. Horowitz NM, Gale RP, Sondel PM. Graft versus leukemia reactions after bone marrow transplantation. Blood 1990;75:555–562.
10. Gorin NC, Najman A, Duhamel G. Autologous bone marrow transplantation in acute myelocytic leukemia. Lancet 1977;14:1050.
11. Gorin NC, Herzig G, Bull MI, et al. Long term preservation of bone marrow and stem cell pool in dogs. Blood 1978;51:257–265.
12. Dicke KA, Zander A, Spitzer G, et al. Autologous bone marrow transplantation in relapsed adult acute leukemia. Lancet 1979;1:514–517.
13. Goldstone AH ed. Autologous bone marrow transplantation. Clin Haematol 1986;1:15.
14. Masson L'autograffe, ed. de moëlle osseuse. Paris: Barcelone, 1987.
15. Gorin NC, David R, Stachowiak J, et al. High dose chemotherapy and autologous bone marrow transplantation in acute leukemias, malignant lymphomas and solid tumors: a study of 23 patients. Eur J Cancer 1981;17:557–568.
16. Sharkis SJ, Santos GW, Colvin OM. Elimination of acute myelogenous leukemia cells from marrow and tumor suspensions in the rat with 4 hydroperoxycyclophosphamide. Blood 1980;55:521–523.
17. Douay L, Mary JY, Giarratana MC, et al. Establishment of a reliable experimental procedure for bone marrow purging with mafosfamide (Asta Z 7557). Exp Hematol 1989;17:429–432.
18. Jones RJ, Zuehldorf M, Rowley SD et al. Variability in 4 hydroperoxycyclophosphamide activity during clinical purging for autologous bone marrow transplantation. Blood 1987;70:1490–1494.
19. Carlostella C, Mangoni L, Almici C, et al. Differential sensitivity of adherent CFU-blast, CFU-mix, BFUE and CFU-GM to mafosfamide: implications for adjusted dose purging in autologus bone marrow transplantation. Exp Hematol 1992, in press.
20. Gorin NC, Douay L, Laporte JP, et al. Autologous bone marrow transplantation using marrow incubated with Asta Z 7557 in adult acute leukemia. Blood 1986;67:1367–1376.
21. Yeager AM, Kaizer H, Santos GW, et al. Autologous bone marrow transplantation in patients with acute non lymphoblastic leukemia using ex vivo marrow treatment with 4 hydroperoxycyclophosphamide. New Engl J Med 1986;315:141–147.
22. Körbling M, Hunstein W, Fliedner JM, et al. Disease free survival after autologous bone marrow transplantation in patients with acute myelocytic leukemia. Blood 1989;74:1898–1904.
23. Rizzoli V, Mangoni L, Carlo Stella C, et al. Autologous bone marrow transplantation in first remission acute myeloid leukemia using marrow purging with mafosfamide: 17th annual meeting of the

EBMT. Cortina d'Ampezzo Italy, January 27–31 1991, 47, 87a.

24. Burnett AK, Tansey P, Watkins R, et al. Transplantation of unpurged autologous bone marrow in acute myeloid leukemia in first remission: Lancet 1984;2:1068–1070.

25. McMillan AK, Goldstone AH, Linch DC, et al. High dose chemotherapy and autologous bone marrow transplantation in acute myeloid leukemia. Blood 1990;76:480–488.

26. Meloni G, Fabritiis DC, Carella AM. Autologous bone marrow transplantation in patients with AML in first complete remission. Results of two different conditioning regimens after the same induction and consolidation therapy. Bone Marrow Transplant 1990;5:29–32.

27. Carella AM, Gaozza E, Santini G, et al. Autologous unpurged bone marrow transplantation for acute non-lymphoblastic leukemia in first complete remission. Bone Marrow Transplant 1988;3:537–541.

28. Gorin NC, Aegerter P, Auvert B, et al. Autologous bone marrow transplantation for acute myelocytic leukemia in first remission: a European survey of the role of marrow purging. Blood 1990;75:1606–1614.

29. Gorin NC, Labopin M, Meloni G, et al. for the European Cooperative Group of Bone Marrow Transplantation. Autologous bone marrow transplantation for acute myeloblastic leukemia in Europe: further evidence of the role of marrow purging by mafosfamide. Leukemia 1991;5:896–904.

30. Goldman JM, Gale RP, Horowitz MM, et al. Bone marrow transplantation for chronic myelogenous leukemia in chronic phase. Increased risk of relapse associated with T cell depletion. Ann Intern Med 1988;108:806–814.

31. Juttner CA, To LB, Haylock DN, et al. Circulating autologous stem cells collected in very early remission from acute non lymphoblastic leukemia produce prompt but incomplete haematopoietic reconstitution after high dose melphalan or supralethal chemoradiotherapy. Br J Haematol 1985;61:739–745.

32. Kessinger A, Armitage JO, Landmark JD, et al. Autologous peripheral hematopoiesis stem cell transplantation restores hematopoietic function following marrow ablative therapy. Blood 1988;71:723–727.

33. Körbling M, Fliedner TM, Holle R, et al. Autologous blood stem cell (ABSCT) versus purged bone marrow transplantation (p ABMT) in standard risk AML: influence of source and cell composition of the autograft on hemopoietic reconstitution and disease free survival. Bone Marrow Transplant 1991;7:343–349.

34. Reiffers J, Körblung M, Labopin M, Gorin NC, on behalf of the EBMT Working party on Autologous Bone Marrow Transplantation. Bone Marrow Transplant 1991;7(suppl 2):144.

35. Büchner T, Schellong G, Hiddemann W, Ritter F, eds. Acute leukemias II: prognostic factors and treatment strategies. Heidelberg: Springer-Verlag, 1990.

36. Büchner T, Hiddemann W, Koenigsmann M, et al. Recombinant human GMCSF following chemotherapy versus chemotherapy alone in patients with high risk AML. Blood 1990;76(suppl 1):529a.

37. Foa R, Meloni G, Tosti S, et al. Treatment of acute myeloid leukemia with recombinant IL2: clinical and biological findings. Blood 1990;76(suppl 1):1071a.

38. Slavin S, Naparstek E, Or E, Weiss L. Prevention of GVHD and induction of graft versus leukemia effects: will it ever be possible? Bone Marrow Transplant 1988;3(suppl 1):208.

39. Jones RJ, Vogelsang GB, Hess AD, et al. Induction of graft versus host disease after autologous bone marrow transplantation. Lancet 1989;1:754–757.

40. Bishop JF, Lowenthal RM, Jochua D, et al. Etoposide in acute non lymphocytic leukemia. Blood 1990;75:27–32.

41. Carella AM, Berman E, Maraone MP, Ganzina T. Idarubicin in the treatment of acute leukemias: an overview of preclinical and clinical studies. Haematologica 1990;75:1–11.

42. Büchner T, Hiddemann W, Blasius S, et al. Adult AML: the role of chemotherapy intensity and duration. Two studies of the AML cooperative group. Haematol Blood Transfusion 1990;33:261–266.

43. Goldie JH, Coldman AJ, Gudauskas GA. Rationale for the use of alternating non cross-resistant chemotherapy. Cancer Treat Rep 1982;66:439.

44. Büchner T, Urbanitz D, Hiddemann W, et al. Intensified induction and consolidation with or without maintenance therapy for acute myeloid leukemia: two multicenter studies of the German AML Cooperative Group. J Clin Oncol 1985;3:1583.

45. Preisler H, Davis KB, Kirshner J, et al. Comparison of three remission induction regimens and two postinduction strategies for the treatment of acute nonlymphocytic leukemia: a Cancer and Leukemia Group B study. Blood 1987;69:1441.

46. Rees JKH. Chemotherapy of the leukemias. In: Freireich EJ, ed. New approaches to the treatment of leukemia. ESO monograph. Berlin: Springer Verlag, 1990.

47. Tricot GJK. Treatment of acute non lymphocytic leukemia. In: Hoffman R, Benz EJ, Shattil SJ, Furie B, Cohen HJ, eds. Hematology, basic principles and practice. New York: Churchill Livingstone, 1991:732–748.

48. Gale RP, Foon KA. Therapy of acute myelogenous leukemia. Semin Hematol 1987;24:40.

49. Grier HE, Gelber RD, Camitta BM, et al. Prognostic factors in childhood acute myelogenous leukemia. J Clin Oncol 1987;5:1026.

50. Wolff SN, Herzig RH, Philips GL, et al. High dose

cytosine-arabinoside and daunorubicin as consolidation therapy for acute non lymphocytic leukemia in first remission: an update. Semin Oncol 1987; 14(suppl 1):12–17.

51. Santos GW, Tutschka PJ, Brookmeyer R, et al. Marrow transplantation for acute non lymphocytic leukemia after treatment with busulfan and cyclophosphamide. N Engl J Med 1983;309:1347–1353.

52. Marmont AM, Gale RP, Butturini A, et al. T cell depletion in allogeneic bone marrow transplantation, progress and problems. Haematology 1989;74:235–248.

53. Kamani N, Lange B, August CS, Nowell P. Leukemic relapse in host cells almost 7 years after bone marrow transplantation for acute promyelocytic leukemia in first complete remission. Bone Marrow Transplant 1989;4:455–456.

54. Wiley JM, Yeager AM. Predictive value of colony forming unit assays for engraftment and leukemia free survival after transplantation of chemopurged syngeneic bone marrow in rats. Int J Cell Cloning Exp Hematol 1991;19:179–186.

55. Schultz FW, Vriesendorp HM, Hagenbeck A. On the quantitative role of graft versus host disease in decreasing the leukemia relapse rate after allogeneic bone marrow transplantation submitted for publication.

56. Schultz FW, Martens ACM, Hagenbeek A. The contribution of residual leukemic cells in the graft to leukemia relapse after autologous bone marrow transplantation: mathematical considerations. Leukemia 1989;3:530–534.

57. Martens ACM, Van Bekkum DW, Hagenbeek A. Minimal residual disease in leukemia: studies in an animal model for acute myelocytic leukemia (BNML). Int J Cell Cloning 1990;8:27–38.

58. Hale G, Cobbold S, Waldmann H. T Cell depletion with campath 1 in allogeneic bone marrow transplantation. Transplantation 1988;45:753–759.

59. Frassoni F, Sessarego M, Bacigalupo A. Competition between recipient and donor cells after bone marrow transplantation for chronic myeloid leukemia. Br J Haematol 1988;69:471–475.

60. Gorin NC. Collection, manipulation and freezing of hemopoietic stem cells. Clin Haematol 1986;15:19–48.

61. Douay L, Gorin NC, Mary JY, et al. Recovery of CFUGM from cryopreserved marrow and in vivo evaluation after autologous bone marrow transplantation are predictive of engraftment. Exp Hematol 1986;14:358–365.

62. Rowley SD, Zuehlsdorf M, Braine HG, et al. CFUGM content of bone marrow graft correlates with time to hematologic reconstitution following autologous bone marrow transplantation with 4 hydroperoxycyclophosphamide = purged bone marrow. Blood 1987;70:271–275.

63. Laporte JP, Gorin NC, Douay L, et al. Autologous bone marrow transplantation in acute leukemia using marrow incubated with mafosfamide at levels individually adjusted: correlations of engraftment, leukemia free survival and relapse rate to characteristics of marrow transplanted. Paper submitted for presentation at the 18th Annual Meeting of the European Cooperative Group for Bone Marrow Transplantation, Stockholm 1992.

64. Thomas ED, Buckner CD, Banaji M, et al. One hundred patients with acute leukemia treated by chemotherapy, total body irradiation and allogeneic bone marrow transplantation. Blood 1977; 49:511.

65. Clift RA, Buckner CD, Thomas ED, et al. The treatment of acute non lymphoblastic leukemia by allogeneic bone marrow transplantation. Bone Marrow Transplant 1987;2:243.

66. Working Party on Leukemia—European Group for Bone Marrow Transplantation. Allogeneic bone marrow transplantation for leukemia in Europe. Lancet 1988;1:1379–1382.

67. Gratwohl A, Hermans J, Zwaan F. Bone marrow transplantation for AML in Europe. In: Acute Myelogenous Leukemia II: progress and controversies. New York: Wiley-Liss, 1990:381–390.

68. Thomas ED, Appelbaum FR, Buckner CD et al. Marrow transplantation for acute non lymphocytic leukemia. In: Gale RP, ed. Recent advances in bone marrow transplantation. Proceedings of the UCLA symposia. New York: Alan R. Liss, 1983:61.

69. McGlave PB, Haake RJ, Bostrom BC, et al. Allogeneic bone marrow transplantation for acute non lymphocytic leukemia in first remission. Blood 1988;72:1512–1517.

70. Gratwohl A, for The Leukemia Working Party, unpublished paper, 1990.

71. Gale RP, Bortin MM, Van Bekkum DW, et al. Risk factors for acute graft versus host disease. Br J Haematol 1987;67:397–406.

72. Zwaan FE, Hermans J, Gratwhol A. The influence of donor recipient sex mismatching on the outcome of allogeneic BMT in leukemia. Bone Marrow Transplant 1989;3(suppl 2):8.

73. International Bone Marrow Transplant Registry. Transplant or chemotherapy in acute myelogenous leukemia ? Lancet 1989;1:1119–1121.

74. Barret AJ. Graft versus host disease: clinical features and biology. Bone Marrow Transplant 1990; 4(suppl 4):18–21.

75. Thomas ED, Clift RA, Hersman J, et al. Marrow transplantation for acute non lymphoblastic leukemia in first remission using fractionated or single dose irradiation. Int J Radiat Oncol Biol Phys 1981;7:1695–1701.

76. Barret A. Total body irradiation (TBI) before bone marrow transplantation in leukemia. A cooperative

study from the European Group. Br J Radiol 1982;55:562–567.

77. Oszahin M, Pene F, Touboul E. Total body irradiation prior to bone marrow transplantation: comparison of two instantaneous dose rates (157 patients). Cancer, 1992, in press.

78. Shank B, Hoplan S, Kim JH, et al. Hyperfractionated total body irradiation for bone marrow transplantation: I early results in leukemia patients. Int J Radiat Oncol Biol Phys 1981;7:1109–1115.

79. Vitale V, Bacigalupo A, Van Lint MT et al. Fractionated total body irradiation in marrow transplantation for leukemia. Br J Haematol 1983;55:547–554.

80. Deeg HJ, Flournoy N, Sullivan KM et al. Cataracts after total body irradiation and marrow transplantation: a sparing effect of dose fractionation. Int J Radiat Oncol Biol Phys 1984;10:957–996.

81. Brochstein JA, Kernan NA, Groshen S, et al. Allogeneic bone marrow transplantation after hyperfractionated total body irradiation and cyclophosphamide in children with acute leukemia. New Engl J Med 1987;317:1618–1624.

82. Blume KG, Forman SJ, O'Donnell MR, et al. Total body irradiation and high dose etoposide: a new preparative regimen for bone marrow transplantation in patients with advanced hematologic malignancies. Blood 1987;69:1015–1020.

83. Buckner CD, Clift RA, Appelbaum FR et al. An increased dose of total body irradiation decreased relapses in marrow allograft recipients with acute and chronic myeloid leukemia. Paper read at 17th annual meeting of the EBMT, Cortina d'Ampezzo, Italy, January 27–31, 1991.

84. Frassoni F, Bacigalupo A, Vitale V et al. The effect of total body irradiation dose and chronic graft versus host disease on leukemic relapse after allogeneic bone marrow transplantation. Br J Haematol 1989;73:211–216.

85. Forman SJ, Blume KG. Allogeneic bone marrow transplantation for acute leukemia. Bone Marrow Transplant 1990;4:517–533.

86. Herzig RH, Bortin MM, Barett AJ et al. Bone marrow transplantation in high risk acute lymphoblastic leukaemia in first and second remission. Lancet 1987;1:786.

87. Horwitz LJ, Kantarjian HM, Jagannath S, et al. Piperasinedione plus total body irradiation: an alternative separative regimen for allogeneic bone marrow transplantation in advanced phases of chronic myelogenous leukemia. Bone Marrow Transplant 1989;4:101–105.

88. Geller RB, Saral R, Piantadosi S, et al. Allogeneic bone marrow transplantation after high dose busulfan and cyclophosphamide in patients with acute non lymphocytic leukemia. Blood 1989;73:2209–2218.

89. Tutschka PJ, Copelan EA, Klein JP. Bone marrow transplantation for leukemia following a new busulfan and cyclophosphamide regimen. Blood 1987;70:1382–1388.

90. Gratwohl A, Hermans J, Barret AJ et al. Allogeneic bone marrow transplantation for leukemia in Europe: regional differences. Report from the Leukemia Working Party of the EBMT. Bone Marrow Transplant 1990;5:159–165.

91. Ball ED. In vitro purging of bone marrow for autologous marrow transplantation in acute myelogenous leukemia using myeloid specific monoclonal antibodies. Bone Marrow Transplant 1988;3:387–392.

92. Rizzoli V, Mangoni L. Pharmacological-mediated purging with mafosfamide in acute and chronic myeloid leukemias. In: Gross SR, Gee AP, Worthington-White DA, eds. Bone marrow purging and processing. New York: Alan R. Liss, 1990:21–38.

93. Douay L, Gorin NC, Laporte JP et al. Asta Z 7557 (INN mafosfamide) for the in vitro treatment of human leukemic bone marrow. Invest New Drugs 1984, 2, 187–190.

94. Lopez M, Dupuy-Montbrun MC, Douay L et al. Standardization and characterization of the procedure for in vitro treatment of human bone marrow with cyclophosphamide derivatives. Clin Lab Haematol 1985;7:327–334.

95. Gorin NC, Aegerter P, Auvert B. Autologous bone marrow transplantation for acute leukemia in remission: an analysis of 1322 cases. Haematol Blood Transfusion 1990;33:660–666.

96. Gorin NC. Autologous bone marrow transplantation in hematological malignancies. Eur J Cancer 1983;20:1–9.

97. Gorin NC, Herve P, Philip T. High dose therapy and autologous bone marrow transplantation in France. In: Touraine JL, ed. Bone marrow transplantation in Europe–Symposia II. Fondation Mérieux 6. Amsterdam: Excerpta Medica, 1981:42–50.

98. Gorin NC. Autologous bone marrow transplantation for acute leukemia in Europe. Exp Hematol 1984;12(suppl 15):123–125.

99. Beelen DW, Quabeck K, Gralven U, et al. Acute toxicity and first clinical results of intensive post induction therapy using a modified busulfan and cyclophosphamide regimen with autologous bone marrow rescue in first remission of acute myeloid leukemia. Blood 1989;74:1507–1516.

100. Meloni G, De Fabritiis P, Carella AM, Petti MC, et al. Autologous bone marrow transplantation in patients with AML in first complete remission. Results of two different conditioning regimens after the same induction and consolidation therapy. Bone Marrow Transplant 1990;5:29–32.

101. Meloni G, De Fabritiis P, Petti MC, et al. BAVC regimen and autologous bone marrow transplantation in patients with acute myelogenous leukemia in second remission. Blood 1990;12:2282–2285.

102. Gordon MY, Hibbin JA, Kearny LU, et al. Colony formation by primitive haemopoietic progenitors in cultures of bone marrow cells and stromal cells. Br J Haematol 1985;60:129.

103. Bell AJ, Hamblin TJ, Oscier DG. Circulating stem cell autograft. Bone Marrow Transplant 1986;1:103–110.

104. Castaigne S, Calvo F, Douay L, et al. Successful haematopoietic reconstitution using autologous peripheral blood mononucleated cells in a patient with acute prolymphocytic leukaemia. Br J Haematol 1986;63:209–211.

105. Körbling M, Dorken B, Ho AB, et al. Autologous transplantation of blood derived hemopoietic stem cells after myeloablative therapy in a patient with Burkitt's lymphoma. Blood 1986;67:529–532.

106. Reiffers J, Bernard P, David B, et al. Successful autologous transplantation with peripheral blood haematopoietic cells in a patient with acute leukaemia. Exp Hematol 1986;14:312–315.

107. To LB, Juttner CA. Peripheral blood stem cell autografting: a new therapeutic option for AML ? Br J Haematol 1987;66:285–288.

108. Laporte JP, Gorin NC, Feuchtenbaum J, et al. Relapse after autografting with peripheral blood stem cells [Letter]. Lancet 1987;2:1393.

109. Van Rood JJ, De Planque M, Van Leen, Wen A, et al. Unrelated bone marrow donor files. Bone Marrow Transplant 1989;4(suppl 2):6a.

110. Beatty PG, Clift RA, Mickelson EM, et al. Marrow transplantation from related donors other than HLA identical siblings. New Engl J Med 1985;313:765–771.

111. Beatty PG, Anasetti C, Thomas ED et al. Marrow transplantation from donors other than HLA identical siblings. Hematol Oncol Clin North Am 1990;3:677–686.

112. Bianco J, Nemunaitis J, Brown P, et al. Pentoxifylline and GMCSF decrease tumor necrosis factor alpha levels in patients undergoing allogeneic bone marrow transplantation. Blood 1990;76(suppl 1):522a.

113. Petersen FB, Thornquist M, Buckner CD, et al. The effects of infection prevention regimens on early infectious complications in marrow transplant patients: a four arm randomized study. Infection 1988;16:199–208.

114. Meyers JD, Thomas ED. Infection complicating bone marrow transplantation. In: Rubin RH, Young LD, eds. Clinical approach to infection in the immunocompromised host. New York: Plenum Press, 1988:525–566.

115. Link H, Boogaerts M, Carella AM, et al. Recombinant human granulocyte-macrophage colony-stimulating factor after autologous bone marrow transplantation for acute lymphoblastic leukemia or malignant lymphoma: an international double-blind placebo-controlled trial 1991. Blood, submitted, 1992.

116. Brandt SJ, Peters WP, Atwater SK, et al. Effect of recombinant human granulocyte-macrophage colony-stimulating factor on hematopoietic reconstitution after high dose chemotherapy and autologous bone marrow transplantation. N Engl J Med 1988;318:869–876.

117. Nemunaitis J, Singer JW, Buckner CD, et al. Use of recombinant human granulocyte-macrophage colony-stimulating factor in autologous marrow transplantation for lymphoid malignancies. Blood 1988;72:834–836.

118. Nemunaitis F, Rabinowe S, Singer JW, et al. Recombinant granulocyte-macrophage colony stimulating factor after autologous bone marrow transplantation for lymphoid cancer. New Engl J Med 1991;324:1773–1778.

119. Gorin NC, Coiffier B, Hayab M, et al. Recombinant human granulocyte-macrophage colony stimulating factor after autologous bone marrow transplantation with unpurged and purged marrow in non-Hodgkin's lymphoma: a double blind placebo controlled trial. Blood 1992, in press.

120. Nemunaitis J, Singer JW, Buckner CD, et al. Use of recombinant human granulocyte-macrophage colony-stimulating factor in graft failure after bone marrow transplantation. Blood 1990;76:245–253.

121. Fouillard L, Gorin NC, Laporte JP, et al. GMCSF and ganciclovir for cytomegalovirus infection after autologous bone marrow transplantation. Lancet 1989;2:1273.

122. Fouillard L, Gorin NC, Laporte JP, et al. Recombinant human granulocyte-macrophage colony-stimulating factor plus the BEAM regimen instead of autologous bone marrow transplantation. Lancet 1989;1:1460.

123. Laporte JP, Fouillard L, Douay L, et al. RHU GMCSF instead of autologous bone marrow transplantation after the BEAM pretransplant regimen in resistant non Hodgkin's lymphoma. Lancet 1991;338:601–602.

124. Morstyn G, Souza LM, Keech, J, et al. Effect of granulocyte colony stimulating factor on neutropenia induced by cytotoxic chemotherapy. Lancet 1988;1:667–672.

125. Gabrilove JL, Jakubowski A, Scher H, et al. Effect of granulocyte colony-stimulating factor on neutropenia and associated morbidity due to chemotherapy for transitional cell carcinoma of the urothelium. New Engl J Med 1988;318:1414–1422.

126. Teshima H, Ishikawa J, Kitayama H, et al. Clinical effects of recombinant human granulocyte colony-stimulating factor in leukemia patients: a phase I/II study. Exp Hematol 1989;17:853–858.

127. Vellenga E, Young DC, Wagner K, et al. The effects of GMCSF and G CSF in promoting growth of clonogenic cells in acute myeloblastic leukemia. Blc 1987;69:1771–1776.

128. Miyauchi J, Kelleher CA, Yang YC, et al. The effects

of three recombinant growth factors, IL3, GMCSF and G CSF on the blast cells of acute myeloblastic leukemia maintained in short term suspension culture. Blood 1987;70:657–663.

129. Büchner T, Hiddemann W, Koenigsmann M, et al. Recombinant human granulocyte-macrophage colony-stimulating factor after chemotherapy for acute leukemias at higher age or after relapse. Haematol Blood Transf. In: Büchner T, Schellong G, Hiddemann W, Ritter T, eds. Acute leukemia II. Berlin: Springer-Verlag, 1990;33:724–731.

130. Estey EH, Kantarjian HM, Beran M, et al. Treatment of poor prognosis, newly diagnosed acute myelogenous leukemia with high dose cytosine arabinoside (Ara-C) and rHUGM-CSF. In: Büchner T, Schellong G, Hiddemann W, Ritter T, eds. Acute leukemia II. Berlin: Springer-Verlag, 1990;33:732–735.

131. Hann IM, Prentice HG, Blaclock HA, et al. Acyclovir prophylaxis against herpes virus infections in severely immunocompromised patients: randomized double blind trial. Br Med J 1983;287:384–388.

132. Meyers JD, Reed EC, Shepp DH, et al. Acyclovir for prevention of cytomegalovirus infection and disease after allogeneic marrow transplantation. N Engl J Med 1988;318:70–75.

133. Pecego R, Hill R, Appelbaum FR, et al. Interstitial pneumonitis following autologous bone marrow transplantation. Transplantation 1986;42:515–517.

134. Bowden RA, Sayers M, Flournoy M, et al. Cytomegalovirus immune globulin and seronegative blood products to prevent primary cytomegalovirus infection after marrow transplant. N Engl J Med 1986;314:1006–1010.

135. Schmidt GM, Horak DA, Zaia JA, et al. Ganciclovir (GCV) and immunoglobulin (IG) treatment of human cytomegalovirus pneumonia (HCMV-IP) after allogeneic bone marrow transplantation (BMT): an update. Bone Marrow Transplant 1989;4(suppl 2):66a.

136. Schmidt GM, Horak DA, Niland JC, et al. Prophylactic ganciclovir for pulmonary cytomegalo-virus infection in allogeneic bone marrow transplant recipients: a randomized controlled trial. Blood 1990;76(suppl 1):564a.

137. Dulley FL, Kanfer EJ, Appelbaum FR, et al. Venocclusive disease of the liver after chemotherapy and autologous bone marrow transplantation. Transplantation 1987;43:870–873.

138. Berk PD, Popper H, Krueger GRF, et al. Venocclusive disease of the liver after allogeneic bone marrow transplantation. Possible association with graft versus host disease. Ann Intern Med 1979;90:158–164.

139. Lazarus HM, Gottfried MR, Herzig RH, et al. Venocclusive disease of the liver after high dose mitomycin C therapy and autologous bone marrow transplantation. Cancer 1982;42:1789–1795.

140. Rio B, Zittoun R, Ifrah N, et al. Fréquence et gravité des maladies veino-occlusives du foie après greffe de moëlle osseuse. Presse Méd 1984;13:2648.

141. McDonald GB, Sharma P, Matthews DE, et al. The clinical course of 53 patients with venocclusive disease of the liver after bone marrow transplantation. Transplantation 1985;39:603–608.

142. Baume D, Cosset JM, Pico JL, et al. Maladie veinoocclusive du foie après greffe de moëlle osseuse. Intérêt du fractionnement de l'irradiation totale. Presse Med 1987;16:1759.

143. Jones RJ, Lee KSK, Beschorner WE, et al. Venoclusive disease of the liver following bone marrow transplantation. Transplantation 1987;44:778–783.

144. Brugieres L, Hartmann O, Benhamou E, et al. Complications hépatiques après chimiothérapie lourde et autogreffe de moëlle dans les tumeurs solides de l'enfant. Presse Med 1988;17:1305–1308.

145. Marsa-Vila L, Gorin NC, Laporte JP, et al. Prophylactic heparin does not prevent liver veno-occlusive disease following autologous bone marrow transplantation. Eur J Hematol 1991;67:346–354.

146. Ibrahim A, Pico JL, Maraninchi D, et al. Hepatic venocclusive disease (VOD) following bone marrow transplantation (BMT), treated by prostaglandin E1 (PGE 1). Paper read at 17th annual meeting of the EBMT. Cortina d'Ampezzo, Italy, January 27–31, 1991.

147. Klier F, Weiss M, Bunjes D. Use of prostaglandin E1 for the prevention and therapy of venocclusive disease of the liver after allogeneic bone marrow transplantation. Paper read at 7th annual meeting of the EBMT. Cortina d'Ampezzo, Italy, January 27–31, 1991.

148. Hermans J, Suciu S, Stynen TH. Treatment of acute myelogeneous leukemia: an EBMT-EORTC retrospective analysis of chemotherapy versus allogeneic or autologous bone marrow transplantation. Eur J Cancer Clin Oncol 1989;25:545–550.

149. Löwenberg B, Verdonck LJ, Dekker AW, et al. Autologous bone marrow transplantation in acute myeloid leukemia in first remission: results of a Dutch propsective study. J Clin Oncol 1990;8:287–294.

150. Mitus AJ, Miller KB, Schenkein DP, et al. Multicenter trial of allogeneic versus autologous bone marrow transplantation for the treatment of ANLL in first remission. A preliminary report. Blood 1990;76(suppl 1):554a.

151. Ferrant A, Martiat PH, Doyen C, et al. Allogeneic or autologous bone marrow transplantation for acute non lymphocytic leukemia in first remission. Blood 1990;76(suppl 1):538a.

152. Casileth PA, Anderson J, Lazarus HM. An ECOG trial of autologous bone marrow transplantation in first remission of acute myeloid leukemia. Blood 1990;76(suppl 1):532a.

153. Curtis JE, Messner HA, Hasselback R, et al. Contri-

butions of host and disease-related attributes to the outcome of patients with acute myelogenous leukaemia. J Clin Oncol 1984;2:253–259.

154. Amaki I, Hattoni K, Bennett JM, et al. FAB classification of acute leukaemias correlates with response to chemotherapy. Acta Haematol Jpn 1984;47:206–238.

155. Fourth international workshop on chromosomes in leukemia: a prospective study of acute non lymphocytic leukemia. Cancer Genet Cytogenet 1984;11:249.

156. Schiffer CA, Lee EJ, Tomiyasu T, et al. Prognostic impact of cytogenetic abnormalities in patients with de novo acute non lymphocytic leukemia. Blood 1989;73:263.

157. Rai KR, Holland JF, Glidewell OJ, et al. Treatment of acute myelocytic leukemia: a study by the cancer and leukemia group B. Blood 1981;58:1203.

158. Schwartz RS, Mackintosh FR, Halpern J, et al. Multivariate analysis of factors associated with outcome of treatment for adults with acute myelogenous leukemia. Cancer 1984;54:1672.

159. Keating MJ, McCredie KB, Bodey GP, et al. Improved prospects for long term survival in adults with acute myelogenous leukemia. JAMA 1982;248:2481.

160. Tivey H. The natural history of untreated acute leukemia. Ann NY Acad Sci 1955;60:322.

161. Petti MC, Broccia G, Carona F, et al. Therapy of acute myelogenous leukaemia in adults. Haematol Blood Transfusion 1990;33:249–253.

162. Preisler HD, Priore R, Azarnia N, et al. Prediction of response of patients with acute non lymphocytic leukaemia to remission induction therapy: use of clinical measurements. Br J Haematol 1986;63:625.

163. Cassileth PA, Harrington DP, Hines JD, et al. Maintenance chemotherapy prolongs remission duration in adult acute nonlymphocytic leukemia. J Clin Oncol 1988;6:583.

164. Cassileth PA, Harrington DP, Hines JD. Comparison of post remission therapies in adult acute myeloid leukaemia: preliminary analysis of an ECOG study. Haematol Blood Transfusion 1990;33:267–270.

165. Preisler HD, Raza A, Early A, et al. Intensive remission consolidation therapy in the treatment of acute non lymphocytic leukemia. J Clin Oncol 1987;5:722.

166. Kantarjian HM, Keating MJ, Walters RS, et al. The characteristics and outcome of patients with late relapse acute myelogenous leukemia. J Clin Oncol 1988;6:232.

167. Davis CL, Rohatiner AZS, Amess J, et al. Treatment of recurrent acute myelogenous leukemia at a single centre over a 10 year period. Haematol Blood Transfusion 1990;33:339–341.

34

HIGH-DOSE THERAPY IN ACUTE LYMPHOBLASTIC LEUKEMIA

Amy L. Billett

Approximately 2000 children in the United States are diagnosed with acute lymphoblastic leukemia (ALL) each year. Marrow transplantation is usually not recommended for children with ALL in first remission because with current chemotherapy regimens more than 70% of these patients are expected to remain in long-term continuous remission (1). Even children with high-risk ALL have at least a 50% chance of cure with chemotherapy.

However, several prognostic factors predict a very poor outcome for children with ALL (2). The most important of these is relapse. Most children with ALL after relapse might benefit from marrow transplantation since chemotherapy after relapse cures very few children. Marrow relapse accounts for the majority of recurrences in childhood ALL, and only 5%–25% of such patients can be cured by further chemotherapy (3). Marrow transplantation can thus play an important role in the treatment of children after a medullary relapse.

Isolated extramedullary relapses, either CNS or testicular, are less common, but such children may also benefit from marrow transplantation. For example, children with ALL in first marrow remission who experience an isolated CNS relapse usually cannot be successfully treated. Retreatment with intensive systemic chemotherapy and another course of CNS irradiation results in only a 30% likelihood of long-term leukemia-free survival (4). The most frequent site of subsequent relapse after an aggressive retreatment approach is in the marrow. Results from a study of ALL carried out by the Children's Cancer Study Group suggest that children who had inadequate primary CNS prophylaxis, such as intrathecal methotrexate alone, may have a somewhat better prognosis than those children whose initial CNS prophylaxis included cranial irradiation (5).

Based on the poor outcome with conventional therapy, some investigators have recommended marrow transplantation for children with an isolated CNS relapse. However, transplantation has also been associated with a high risk of relapse in several studies (6, 7). Many of these patients had combined CNS and marrow relapse before transplant and therefore are not totally comparable to others transplanted in first marrow remission. Since the risk of CNS relapse following transplant is highest in patients with prior CNS leukemia, the Seattle group has recommended giving intrathecal chemotherapy after marrow transplant (8). Giving intrathecal methotrexate following marrow transplantation may reduce the incidence of CNS relapse, but it has occasionally been associated with severe leukoencephalopathy. At present, the data are insufficient to decide whether marrow transplantation or intensive chemotherapy together with repeat irradiation of the CNS is better for the child with an isolated CNS relapse of ALL.

Another example is provided by boys with ALL who develop an isolated testicular relapse while on chemotherapy. These children have a very poor rate of long-term survival after treatment with additional chemotherapy and testicular irradiation (9). The majority of such patients experience marrow relapse within 1 year of testicular relapse and eventually die from their disease. Marrow transplantation should be considered for these patients, although there are insufficient data to indicate whether this approach would be beneficial.

Marrow transplantation is currently being investigated for patients with ALL in first remission who are at extremely high risk for relapse (e.g., Philadelphia-chromosome-positive ALL, or adults with ALL). These include the B cell type of ALL, the presence of the Ph chromosome, or other specific chromosomal translocations, such as t(4, 11), and age less than 12 months at the time of diagnosis. Marrow transplantation has been recommended by some investigators for treatment of these very high risk patients. Although the European experience regarding transplantation in patients with the B cell type of ALL in first remission is promising (10), there is little published documentation of the posttransplant survival rate for these groups of patients.

TREATMENT OPTIONS FOR RELAPSED ACUTE LYMPHOBLASTIC LEUKEMIA

Conventional-Dose Chemotherapy

Early relapse on therapy or within 2 years of diagnosis is associated with survival rates of less than 20% in most series (11–20). Butturini and colleagues reviewed 36 published reports of children with relapsed ALL; 18% of 600 children treated with chemo-

therapy survived (21). Survival was 1% for children who relapsed within 18 months of diagnosis, as compared to 25% for those with a later relapse. Since 1980 newer multidrug chemotherapy regimens have been used in treating children with relapsed ALL. Results from one of these studies showed that for patients whose initial remission was less than 24 months, the 6-year probability of maintaining remission was 18%. But for patients whose initial remission lasted more than 24 months, the probability of survival at 5.5 years was 31% (22).

Although late relapse has a somewhat better prognosis, only two studies have shown event-free survival rates significantly greater than 50% (18, 23). In both studies, patients had an initial remission of at least 36 months, and follow-up was reported at a median of 36 months.

Allogeneic Marrow Transplantation

Numerous studies from various centers have clearly demonstrated that high-dose chemotherapy plus total body irradiation in conjunction with allogeneic marrow transplantation represents an effective and curative therapy for some patients with hematologic malignancies (24–26). The earliest candidates for marrow transplantation were patients with advanced leukemia resistant to conventional therapy. Even though leukemic cells were refractory to standard chemotherapy, ablative chemotherapy and total body irradiation could achieve significant tumor cell eradication and a small percentage of long-term cures if marrow toxicity could be circumvented by infusion of normal marrow cells from an identical twin (syngeneic marrow transplant) (24, 27). Thomas and colleagues in Seattle in 1977 reported long-term disease-free survival in 11 of 110 patients with end stage acute leukemia who underwent marrow transplantation from a histocompatible (allogeneic) donor (28). The major cause of treatment failure was relapse (in more than 60% of patients). Overwhelming infection early after marrow transplantation, graft ver-sus-host disease, and interstitial pneumonia also caused a significant number of deaths. These results, however, were superior to those obtained with existing alternative therapies.

Since a few patients with refractory ALL were cured by marrow transplantation, trans-plantation earlier in the course of the disease at a time when patients were not debilitated from progressive leukemia, infections, or toxicity from intensive chemotherapy seemed logical for patients whose prognosis was known to be poor, such as those in second or subsequent remission. The results of transplanting such remission patients were compared to those obtained with concurrent patients with ALL who were transplanted in relapse. Results from Seattle showed a sur-vival rate of 27% for the patients transplanted in remission, compared to a rate of 15% for patients transplanted in relapse (29).

Disease-free survival after allogeneic marrow transplantation from matched sibling donors ranges from 30% to 75% for children with ALL in second or subsequent remission (16, 30–36). The one group reporting the highest disease-free survival in a group of 31 children in second complete remission uti-lized a conditioning regimen of fractionated total body irradiation followed by high-dose cyclophosphamide (30). Graft-versus-host disease causes significant toxicity, and the in-cidence of fatal complications ranges from 20% to 30% in most series.

The major obstacle to success in mar-row grafting for treatment of ALL in second or subsequent remission remains relapse, which occurs in 30%–50% of patients (31, 37). Therefore, recent efforts have focused on im-proving the antileukemic efficacy of the pre-transplant chemoradiotherapy regimen. Hy-perfractionated total body irradiation followed by cyclophosphamide, used at the Memorial Sloan-Kettering Cancer Center (30), and high-dose cytosine arabinoside (32) combined with fractionated total body irradiation, used in Cleveland, appear to have resulted in an im-provement in leukemia-free survival for chil-dren with ALL transplanted in second remis-sion. It remains to be seen if these results will be confirmed by studies carried out by other groups, especially as the prior therapy of patients has become increasingly intensive over the past decade.

The survival rate of patients who re-lapse after marrow transplantation is ex-tremely low. However, some patients with ALL who relapsed after transplantation have been successfully reinduced into complete remis-sion using a chemotherapy regimen consist-ing of vincristine, prednisone, L-asparaginase, and daunorubicin (38). The median length of survival was 4 months, with a range from 3–22 months. Interestingly, there was a positive correlation between the disease-free interval from marrow transplantation and the overall duration of survival following relapse.

COMPARISONS OF CONVENTIONAL CHEMOTHERAPY WITH MARROW TRANSPLANT IN ACUTE LYMPHOBLASTIC LEUKEMIA

Comparisons with chemotherapy are difficult because the lack of sibling donors prevents truly randomized comparisons and because patients who undergo transplanta-tion include only those who achieve remis-sion and then stay in remission for several months until transplantation can be per-formed. Patients with the worst prognosis are thus excluded from transplant series. Several groups have reported disease-free survivals after allogeneic marrow transplantation for patients who had a matched donor compared to chemotherapy for those who did not.

Two studies of patients treated between 1976 and 1980 compared the use of combi-nation chemotherapy to marrow transplan-tation in children with a marrow relapse of ALL while receiving maintenance chemother-apy. In a Seattle study, children in a second or subsequent remission were given a mar-row transplant if a matched sibling donor was available (16). After a minimum follow-up of 3 years, 8 of 24 transplant recipients compared to 0 of 21 treated with chemotherapy were leukemia-free survivors (39). However, possible risk factors in these two groups of patients were not entirely comparable. The chemotherapy group had a higher frequency of high-risk features at diagnosis and shorter initial remissions compared to the transplant group. The marrow transplant recipients who survived all had initial complete remissions of more than 20 months (and 4 were longer than 3 years). Leukemic relapse was the most frequent cause of failure in this study after either chemotherapy or marrow transplantation.

The University of Minnesota study also showed that transplanted patients had a significantly increased likelihood of leukemia-free survival compared to a conventionally treated group of patients (7). Significant risk factors for predicting relapse after marrow transplantation included an initial leukocyte count of over 50,000 per microliter and presence of extramedullary leukemia. The authors of the Seattle and Minnesota marrow transplantation studies both concluded that marrow transplantation offered the best chance of long-term remission and cure for a patient with relapse of ALL in the marrow while still receiving chemotherapy.

Chessells reported a study comparing marrow transplantation with chemotherapy in 53 children with marrow relapse of ALL in second marrow remission (13). Five of 13 (39%) with HLA-compatible donors who were eligible for marrow transplantation survive, compared with 16 of 40 (40%) who received further chemotherapy. The lengths of first and second remissions in both groups were similar. In a subsequent update, the same author reported improved outcome in the marrow transplantation group due to a higher rate of late relapses in the chemotherapy arm (40). Similar results were observed in a study from Italy in which 46% of patients who underwent marrow transplantation survived, compared to 22% of those who received chemotherapy only (41).

Controlled trials are needed to com-

pare the results of chemotherapy with marrow transplantation in patients who are stratified for various prognostic variables. Such trials are needed to clarify the relative efficacy of chemotherapy and marrow transplantation in children with ALL in second remission (Table 34.1).

In one review of 36 reports of 871 children with relapsed ALL, including data from the International Bone Marrow Transplant Registry, 18% of children treated with chemotherapy survived as compared to 36% of 200 children who underwent matched allogeneic marrow transplantation. However, the outcome after treatment with either marrow transplantation or chemotherapy correlated with risk factors present at diagnosis and with length of the first remission. Marrow transplantation seemed superior only in patients who relapsed within 18 months of first remission (21).

Historically, patients with ALL who had very late relapse (>3 years from diagnosis) represented a group with a relatively favorable prognosis after retreatment with chemotherapy. Whether chemotherapy will be adequate for this previously favorable group relapsing on current programs after intensive chemotherapy remains to be determined.

We currently favor marrow transplantation over chemotherapy for children with ALL in second or subsequent remission.

Table 34.1. Comparison of Survival Rates for Chemotherapy and Allogeneic Marrow Transplantation in Children with Acute Lymphoblastic Leukemia[a,b]

Disease Status: Second Remission	Chemotherapy (Survival Rate)	Marrow Transplantation (Survival Rate)
Total group	10%–30%	30%–60%
If first remission lasted		
less than 18 months	0%–10%	20%
more than 18 months	10%–55%	30%–60%

[a]Adapted with permission from Weinstein HJ. Use of bone marrow transplantation in leukemias. In: Johnson FL, Pochehedly C, eds. Bone marrow transplantation in children. New York: Raven Press, 1990;207.
[b]Approximate range of leukemia-free survival determined from literature review.

However, the choice of therapy for the patient in second remission after a long initial remission (>3 years) must be made on an individual basis.

LIMITATIONS OF ALLOGENEIC MARROW TRANSPLANTATION

The major limitation of allogeneic marrow transplant is the requirement for histocompatibility between donor and recipient. Since transplantation across histocompatibility barriers usually results in severe morbidity and mortality from graft-versus-host disease (GVHD), allogeneic marrow transplant cannot generally be offered to the 60%–80% of patients without histocompatible donors. Only 15% of pediatric patients have had matched donors in more recent national trials (42). Unfortunately even when the donor and recipient are histocompatible, GVHD often subsequently develops. The incidence and severity of GVHD increase with age. Thus in patients more than 10 years of age, significant morbidity and mortality result with some frequency from both acute and chronic GVHD despite identity of all major histocompatibility antigens (HLA-A, B, C, and D/DR) (43–45). This complication occurs because of an attack by donor immune cells present in the marrow infusate against the cells of the recipient's skin, liver, and gastrointestinal tract. The elimination or reduction of the incidence and severity of the GVHD reaction was therefore thought likely to improve the survival of marrow transplant recipients as well as to reduce their morbidity.

Programs that have successfully decreased the incidence of severe acute GVHD by intensive immunoprophylaxis post-transplantation or by T lymphocyte depletion of the marrow inoculum have by and large not influenced the overall disease-free survival (46–48). This appears due to increased regimen-related toxicity, relapse (46–49), failure of engraftment (50–52), and lymphoproliferative disease (53, 54). No studies confined to ALL have been published, however.

Because over 60% of patients do not have histocompatible sibling donors, various experimental methods have been developed to circumvent the lack of a matched related donor. Attempts to expand the applicability of allogeneic marrow transplant, including the use of marrow from mismatched related donors and matched unrelated donors, have met with mixed success (55–57). Potential unrelated donors are identified through either national or local registries with computer search for individuals with similar HLA type. Several centers are exploring different techniques to overcome the problems of graft failure and significant GVHD with T cell depletion. Even if these techniques meet with success, the donor pool remains limited. Only 15% of patients who seek donors through the National Bone Marrow Donor Registry eventually undergo marrow transplantation.

Autologous Marrow Transplantation

Extending therapy of comparable intensity to larger numbers of patients could also be approached by using autologous marrow harvested in remission to rescue patients from the hematologic toxicity of high-dose preparative regimens. Although this technique could be applicable to more patients and have decreased toxicity because of the lack of GVHD and less severe immunosuppression, several theoretical disadvantages exist. The lack of graft-versus-leukemia effect, the potential inability of heavily pretreated patient marrow to sustain adequate hematologic reconstitution, and the high probability that the reinfused remission marrow would contain residual leukemic cells remain potential obstacles.

Only one controlled study has compared autologous marrow transplant to allogeneic transplant in ALL. Kersey and colleagues transplanted 91 patients with high-risk or refractory leukemia: 45 patients without a matched donor received autologous purged marrow and 46 patients with a donor received an allogeneic marrow (33). All patients were treated with cyclophosphamide 60 mg/kg × 2 and fractionated total body irradiation 1320 cGy. Overall survival at 4 years did not differ significantly between the two groups, although the cause of failure did. In the autologous group, 31 patients died of relapse and 3 of toxicity. In contrast, the 30 deaths in the allogeneic group were divided evenly between relapse and toxicity. Relapse rates were similar in patients in the autologous group (79%) and in patients in the allogeneic group who did not develop GVHD (75%).

Many centers have utilized autologous marrow transplantation with or without in vitro purging of the marrow to treat patients with ALL (Table 34.2). Transplantation in first remission has been used primarily for children with very high risk features and adults. Disease-free survival for transplantation after relapse ranges from 11%–57% with variable follow-up. The European Cooperative Group for Bone Marrow Transplantation has recently reported the results of autologous marrow transplantation in 560 patients with ALL. The disease-free survival for patients with standard risk (N = 173) and high-risk (N = 41) features autografted in second complete remission was 31% ± 4 at 5 years and 23% ± 8 at 30 months, respectively. For children grafted in second remission, survival was 42% ± 6 at 52 months. There were trends in favor of increased disease-free survival in patients receiving purged versus unpurged marrow and in patients receiving fractionated versus single-dose total body irradiation.

DANA-FARBER CANCER INSTITUTE EXPERIENCE

From 1980–1990 we have treated 66 children with ALL with autologous marrow transplantation with high-dose chemotherapy and radiotherapy and marrow purged with two cycles of two monoclonal antibodies, anti-J5 and anti-J2 (directed against CD10 [CALLA] and CD9 [GP26]), and complement. The conditioning regimen included VM-26, cytara-

bine, cyclophosphamide, and total body irradiation. Cytarabine was administered as a continuous infusion in the first 28 patients and at 3 gm/m^2 every 12 hours for a total of six doses subsequently. After the first 12 patients, the total body irradiation dose was changed from 850 cGy single-dose to fractionated total body irradiation with a total dose of 1200–1400 cGy. Of the 66 patients, the first 30 patients will be described as the early group. The latter 36 received both high-dose cytarabine and 1400 cGy fractionated total body irradiation and will be described as the current group.

All patients except 1 who did not achieve first remission until day 104 were transplanted in second (N = 42) or subsequent (N = 23) remission. Seven had an isolated extramedullary relapse; all others had at least one marrow relapse. Forty-seven were male and 19 female. The median age was 8 years (range 3–18). Median duration of first remission was 32 months.

A median of 9.7 × 10^7 (range 2.76–4,300 × 10^6) mononuclear cells per kilogram was infused. All patients demonstrated hematopoietic engraftment. Median time to an absolute neutrophil count >500 per microliter was 26 days (range 10–68), to reticulocyte count >0.4% was 28 days (range 3–69), and to platelet count >20,000 per microliter was 33 days (range 12–100). The median time to platelet count >20,000 per microliter was 28 days for current patients as compared to 41 days for patients treated previously.

Twelve patients died from complications, including disseminated aspergillosis, hemorrhage, idiopathic interstitial pneumonitis, venoocclusive disease, *Candida* sepsis, and cardiovascular collapse. Toxicity was decreased significantly from 30% in the early group to 8% currently ($p < .05$). This decrease in toxicity may have occurred because of improvements in supportive care, the shorter duration of conditioning (8 versus 10–12 days), or changes in the patient population.

Relapse after marrow transplantation

Table 34.2. Characteristics and Results of ABMT for ALL[a]

Team	Median N	Median Age	Status 1	Status 2	Status ≥3[b]	Purging MoAb	Purging Drug	Purging None	Conditioning TBI	Conditioning HiDAC	Conditioning CTX	Conditioning Other	DFS 1st CR	DFS >2nd CR
Boston	66	8	1	42	23	+	−	−	F1400 mixed	Y	Y	VM-26		30%
GDR (58)	15	7	6	7	2	1	−	14	2 none	−	Y	−		13 ± 20%
Besançon (59)	44	12	14	26	4	+	+	−		−		−	57%	
Pittsburgh/ Montefiore (60)	10	33	1	6	3	−	+	−	F1200	−	Y	−	1/1	2/9
Hopkins (59)	29	22	10	19	0	−	+	−	NA	NA	NA	NA	20%	11%
Minnesota	28	9	0	10	18	+	−	−	F1365	N	Y	N		22%
Minnesota	23	10	2	18	3	+	−	−	S850	Y	N	N		15%
Minnesota	18	8	1	12	5	+	+	−	S850	Y	N	N		42%
Total Minnesota (59)	69	9	3	40	26	+	+	−	All	Some	Some	N		22%
EBMTG children (61)	438	15	233	205	0	+	+	+	N/A	N/A	N/A	N/A	SR 42% ± 5% / HR 41 ± 7%	SR 31 ± 4% / HR 23 ± 8% / 42 ± 6%
Seattle (59)	41	15	3	40	26	+	−	−	N/A	N/A	N/A	N/A	53%	28%/0%[c]
Genoa (62)	13	24	7	4	2	−	+	+	Some	−	Some	BCNU	0/7	1/6
Italian Study Group (63)	82	21	37	42	0	−	+	+	S1000 / F1200	N	Y	N	38%	27%
Uppsala (64)	54	3–55	21	29	3	+	−	−	Mixed	Some	Most	Various	65%	31%
Westminster (59)	18	18	7	10	1	+	−	−	N/A	N/A	N/A	N/A	28%	45%

[a]Abbreviations: CR, complete remission; DFS, disease-free survival; HR, high-risk: MoAB, monoclonal autibodies; N/A, not applicable; SR, standard-risk.
[b]Includes patients in relapse.
[c]Patients in 3rd CR.

occurred in 26 patients at a median of 6 months (range 2–80). The five extramedullary relapses tended to occur later (8, 12, 14, 24, and 25 months) than isolated marrow relapses. Only three marrow relapses occurred after 1 year. Overall event-free survival was 32% ± 8 with a median follow-up of 27 months. Thirteen patients maintained a remission after transplantation longer than their first remission. Three of these subsequently relapsed.

The single most important predictor of outcome after autologous marrow transplantation was duration of initial remission. Patients with a first remission of less than 24 months had a significantly increased risk of both toxic death and relapse. Predicted event-free survival in this group was 0%, as compared to 47% for patients with a longer first remission.

Since duration of initial remission was a prognostic factor in multiple chemotherapy and transplant studies, we thought our findings could reflect a higher residual leukemic burden in the early relapse group. We thus developed a new protocol designed to treat these patients more intensively. This high-risk protocol combined elements from a number of other successful marrow transplantation programs, including starting conditioning with fractionated total body irradiation and adding high-dose etoposide (65). When we started this protocol there were few data about the use of high-dose etoposide in children, and we thus designed a phase I dose escalation study. Because we did not want to increase the total duration of the conditioning regimen, we elected to give the high-dose cytarabine in conjunction with asparaginase as a cycle of chemotherapy prior to marrow harvest. Four patients have been entered on this protocol. None experienced unexpected toxicity, and all remain in remission at 1+, 7+, 12+, and 19+ months.

PURGING

The majority of studies utilized in vitro purging of the marrow, and combined re-sults suggest a trend to better disease-free survival when purging is used. However, purging has never been evaluated in a randomized comparative trial. A variety of techniques to purge the marrow of residual leukemia cells have been developed, including pharmacologic manipulations with techniques that utilize mafosfamide or 4-hydroperoxycyclophosphamide (4-HC) (66, 67), photolysis, and photoradiation (68) and immunologic approaches with monoclonal antibodies directed against leukemia cell antigens to target the residual leukemia cells. Removal or destruction of these cells can then be accomplished by the addition of complement (69), linking the antibodies to magnetic beads (70), or linking the antibodies to a toxin such as ricin (71).

Preclinical in vitro studies have shown that purging can reduce leukemic cell contamination of marrow by 3–4 logs (69). Using very sensitive techniques to measure minimal residual disease, however, Uckun and colleagues have found that marked variability in the efficacy of ex vivo purging in marrows treated with monoclonal antibodies, complement, and 4-HC (72). The efficacy of purging in the clinical setting has never been conclusively demonstrated but is strongly suggested from recent results with adult lymphoma patients (73).

Leukemia cells from 80%–85% of ALL patients originate from B-lineage cells. The majority of B-lineage ALL cells express one or more of the following antigens: Ia, CD 19 (B4), CD10 (CALLA), CD9 (GP26), and CD24 (74, 75). CD19 is an antigen expressed on normal B cells from the earliest pre–B cell until differentiation into a plasma cell. CD19 expression is detected on 96% of non-T ALL Cells (76). Within the hematopoietic system, CD19 is not expressed on normal or neoplastic T or myeloid cells. In addition, an anti-CD19 monoclonal antibody and complement did not decrease numbers of stem cells in long-term Dexter cultures (77). There was also no evidence of depletion of erythroid or myeloid precursors.

An anti-CD19 monoclonal antibody, designated B4, was developed at Dana-Farber Cancer Institute in 1981 (78, 79). This monoclonal antibody was capable of detecting most ALL cells with very high specificity and thus could be a potentially ideal antibody for in vitro marrow purging. Most in vitro immunologic purging methods rely on complement to lyse the targeted cells. Unfortunately, the B4 antibody could not activate complement and was incapable of cytotoxicity against target cells.

Current complement-mediated autologous marrow purging can only be performed in a highly specialized laboratory where immunologic and clonogenic evaluation methods have been mastered. Simplification of the treatment process would decrease risks of the current procedure and increase availability of this treatment modality to other centers. In addition, since cells from 20% of patients with B-lineage ALL do not express CD10 or CD9, a significant number of patients cannot benefit from current procedures. Since CD19+ ALL cells include both CD10+ and CD10-cells, current purging procedures may not be optimal.

The toxic lectin ricin has been extensively studied as a component of antibody-toxic conjugates (78–82). Ricin consists of two subunits, the A and B chains. The A chain is an enzyme that inactivates the 60S subunit of eukaryotic ribosomes, and the B chain binds to oligosaccharides that are ubiquitous on eukaryotic cell surfaces. The intact molecule is a potent cytotoxin because it binds to all cells through the B chain. Purified A chain conjugated to an antibody has markedly diminished cytotoxicity because the B chain participates in the transport of the A chain into the cytoplasm. Toxins linked to monoclonal antibodies may be ideal reagents for in vitro elimination of residual leukemia lymphoblasts prior to autologous marrow transplantation.

In summary, results of most studies of autologous marrow transplantation have demonstrated that high-dose chemotherapy with marrow support is feasible and effective for many children with ALL who experience relapse. Many centers report results that compare favorably with chemotherapy and are not significantly different from many studies of allogeneic marrow transplantation in patients with matched sibling donors.

REFERENCES

1. Clavell LA, Gelber RD, Cohen HJ, et al. Four-agent induction and intensive asparaginase therapy for treatment of childhood acute lymphoblastic leukemia. N Engl J Med 1986;315:657–626.
2. Chessels JM. Acute leukemia in children. Clin Haematol 1986;15:727–753.
3. Buchanan GR. Diagnosis and management of relapse in acute lymphoblastic leukemia. Hematol Oncol Clin North Am 1990;4(5):971–995.
4. Kun LE, Camitta BM, Mulhern RH, et al. Treatment of meningeal relapse in childhood acute lymphoblastic leukemia. Results of craniospinal irradiation. J Clin Oncol 1984;2:359–364.
5. Nesbit ME, D'Angio GJ, Sather HN, et al. Effect of isolated central nervous system leukemia on bone marrow remission and survival in childhood acute lymphoblastic leukemia. Lancet 1981;1:1386–1391.
6. Spruce WE, Forman SJ, Krance RA, et al. Outcome of bone marrow transplantation in patients with extramedullary involvement of acute leukemia. Blut 1983;48:75–79.
7. Woods WG, Nesbit ME, Ramsay NKC, et al. Intensive therapy followed by bone marrow transplantation for patients with acute lymphocytic leukemia in second or subsequent remission. Determination of prognostic factors. Blood 1983;61:1182–1189.
8. Thompson CB, Sanders JE, Flournoy N, et al. The risks of central nervous system relapse and leukoencephalopathy in patients receiving marrow transplants for acute leukemia. Blood 1986;67:195–199.
9. Bowman WP, Aur RJA, Hustu HO, et al. Isolated testicular relapse in acute lymphocytic leukemia of childhood. Categories and influence in survival. J Clin Oncol 1984;2:924–929.
10. Zwann FE, Hermans J. Factors associated with relapse following allogeneic bone marrow transplantation for acute leukemia in remission. In: Hagenbeck A, Lowenberg B, ed. Minimal residual disease in acute leukemia. Dordrecht, Netherlands: Martinus Nihjoff Publishers, 1984:293–310.
11. Amato KR, Sallan SE, Lipton JM. Combination chemotherapy in relapsed childhood acute lymphoblastic leukemia. Cancer Treat Rep 1984;68:411–412.
12. Baum E, Nachman J, Ramsay N, et al. Prolonged second remissions in childhood acute lymphocytic leukemia: a report from the Children's Cancer Study Group. Med Pediatr Oncol 1983;11:1–7.

13. Chessells JM, Rogers DW, Leiper AD, et al. Bone marrow transplantation has a limited role in prolonging second remission in childhood lymphoblastic leukemia. Lancet 1986;1:1239–1241.

14. Dini G, Bernardi B, Comelli A, et al. First isolated bone marrow relapse in children receiving chemotherapy for ALL. Haematologica 1983;68:202–213.

15. Gustafsson G, Kreuger A. Prognosis after relapse in acute lymphoblastic leukemia in childhood. Pediatr Hematol Oncol 1986;3:119–126.

16. Johnson FL, Thomas ED, Clark BS, Chard RL, Harrmann JR, Storb R. A comparison of marrow transplantation with chemotherapy for children with acute lymphoblastic leukemia in second or subsequent remission. N Engl J Med 1981;305:845–851.

17. Rivera GK, Buchanan G, Boyett JM, et al. Intensive retreatment of childhood acute lymphoblastic leukemia in first bone marrow relapse. N Engl J Med 1986;315:273–278.

18. Rossi MR, Masera G, Zurlo MG, et al. Randomized multicentric Italian study on two treatment regimens for marrow relapse in childhood acute lymphoblastic leukemia. Pediatr Hematol Oncol 1986;3:1–9.

19. Wagner B, Baumgartner C, Beck D, et al. Treatment of relapsing acute lymphoblastic leukemia in childhood. I: Experiences with 82 first bone marrow and 17 isolated central nervous system relapses observed 1968–80. Helv Paediatr Acta 1987;42:349–361.

20. Von Der Weid N, Wagner B, Baumgartner C, et al. Treatment of relapsing acute lymphoblastic leukemia in childhood. II: Experiences with 45 first bone marrow and 24 isolated central nervous system relapses observed 1981–84. Helv Paediatr Acta 1987; 42:363–370.

21. Butturini A, Rivera GK, Bortin MM, Gale RP. Which treatment for childhood acute lymphoblastic leukaemia in second remission? Lancet 1987;1:429–432.

22. Henze G, Fengler R, Hartmann R, et al. Six-year experience with a comprehensive approach to the treatment of recurrent childhood acute lymphoblastic leukemia (ALL-REZ BFM 85) A relapse study of the BFM Group. Blood 1991;78(5):1166–1172.

23. Bleyer WA, Sather H, Hammond GD. Prognosis and treatment after relapse of acute lymphoblastic leukemia and non-Hodgkin's lymphoma: 1985. A report from the Children's Cancer Study Group. Cancer 1986;58:590–594.

24. Fefer F, Buckner CD, Thomas ED, et al. Cure of hematologic neoplasia with transplantation of marrow from identical twins. N Engl J Med 1977;297:146–148.

25. Thomas ED, Buckner CD, Banaji M, et al. One hundred patients with acute leukemia treated by chemotherapy, total body irradiation and allogeneic marrow transplantation. Blood 1977;49:511–533.

26. Blume KB. Bone marrow ablation and allogeneic marrow transplantation in acute leukemia. N Engl J Med 1980;302:1041–1046.

27. Fefer A, Cheever MA, Thomas ED, et al. Bone marrow transplantation for refractory acute leukemia in 34 patients with identical twins. Blood 1981;57:421–429.

28. Thomas ED. Marrow transplantation for malignant disease. J Clin Oncol 1983;1:517–531.

29. Thomas ED, Sanders JE, Flournoy N, et al. Marrow transplantation for patients with acute lymphoblastic leukemia: a long-term follow-up. Blood 1983;62:1139–1141.

30. Brochstein J, Kernan N, Groshen S, et al. Allogeneic bone marrow transplantation after hyperfractionated total body irradiation and cyclophosphamide in children with acute leukemia. N Engl J Med 1987;317:1618.

31. Barrett AJ, Joshi R, Kendra JR, et al. Prediction and prevention of relapse of acute lymphoblastic leukaemia after bone marrow transplantation. Br J Haematol 1986;64:179–186.

32. Coccia P, Strandjord S, Warkentin P, et al. High-dose cytosine arabinoside and fractionated total body irradiation: an improved preparative regimen for bone marrow transplantation of children with acute lymphoblastic leukemia in remission. Blood 1988;71:888–893.

33. Kersey JH, Weisdorf D, Nesbit ME, et al. Comparison of autologous and allogeneic bone marrow transplantation for treatment of high-risk refractory acute lymphoblastic leukemia. N Engl J Med 1987;317:461–467.

34. Niethammer D, Klingebiel T, Dopfer R, et al. Allogeneic bone marrow transplantation in childhood leukemia: results and strategies in the Federal Republic of Germany. Hamatol Bluttransfus 1990;33:638–648.

35. Wingard JR, Piantadose S, Santos GW, et al. Allogeneic bone marrow transplantation for patients with high-risk acute lymphoblastic leukemia. J Clin Oncol 1990;8:820–830.

36. Sanders JE, Thomas ED, Buckner CD, et al. Marrow transplantation for children with acute lymphoblastic leukemia in second remission. Blood 1987;70:324–326.

37. Sanders JE, Flournoy N, Thomas ED, et al. Marrow transplantation experience in children with acute lymphoblastic leukemia: an analysis of factors associated with survival, relapse and graft-vs.-host disease. Med Ped Oncol 1985;13:165–172.

38. Barrett AJ, Joshi R, Tew C. How should acute lymphoblastic leukemia relapsing after bone marrow transplantation be treated? Lancet 1985;1:1188–1190.

39. Johnson FL, Thomas ED, Clark BS, et al. Treatment of relapsed acute lymphoblastic leukemia in childhood. N Engl J Med 1984;310:263–264.

40. Chessells JM. A reply to D. Pinkel. Allogeneic bone marrow transplantation in childhood leukemia: another form of intensive treatment. Leukemia 1989; 3:543–544.

41. Bacigalupo A, Lint MTV, Frassoni F, et al. Allogeneic bone marrow transplantation versus chemotherapy for childhood acute lymphoblastic leukaemia in second remission: an update. Bone Marrow Transplant 1990;6:353–354.

42. Graham-Pole J. Treating acute lymphoblastic leukaemia after relapse: bone marrow transplantation or not? Lancet 1989;2:1517–1518.

43. Ramsey NKC, Kersey JH, Robison LL, et al. A randomized study of the prevention of acute graft-versus-host disease. N Engl J Med 1982;307:392–397.

44. Storb H, Deeg HJ, Fisher L, et al. Cyclosporine vs methotrexate for graft-vs-host disease prevention in patients given marrow grafts for leukemia: long-term follow-up of three controlled trials. Blood 1988; 71:293–298.

45. Bross DS, Tutschka PJ, Farmer ER, et al. Predictive factors for acute graft versus-host disease in patients transplanted with HLA-identical bone marrow. Blood 1987;63:1265–1270.

46. Hale G, Cobbold S, Waldmann H, et al. T cell depletion with Campath-1 in allogeneic bone marrow transplantation. Transplantation 1988;45:753.

47. Maranichi D, Gluckman E, Blaise, et al. Impact of T cell depletion on outcome of allogeneic bone-marrow transplantation for standard-risk leukaemias. Lancet 1987;2:175.

48. Mitsuyasu R, Champlin Gale R, et al. Treatment of donor bone marrow with monoclonal anti T-cell antibody and complement for the prevention of graft-versus-host disease. Ann Intern Med 1986;105:20.

49. Bacigalupo A, Van Lint M, Occhini D, et al. Increased risk of leukemia relapse with high-dose cyclosporine A after allogeneic marrow transplantation for acute leukemia. Blood 1991;77:1423.

50. Ash R, Casper J, Chitambar C, et al. Successful allogeneic transplantation of T-cell depleted bone marrow from closely HLA-matched unrelated donors. N Engl J Med 1990;322:485.

51. Bacigalupo A, Hows J, Gordon-Smith E. Bone marrow transplantation for severe aplastic anemia from donors other than HLA identical siblings. Bone Marrow Transplant 1988;3:531.

52. Hows J, Yin Y, Marsh J, et al. Histocompatible unrelated volunteer donors compared with HLA non-identical family donors in marrow transplantation for aplastic anemia and leukemia. Blood 1986;68:1322.

53. Kapoor N, Jung L, Engelhard D, et al. Lymphoma in a patient with severe combined immunodeficiency with adenosine deaminase deficiency following unsustained engraftment of histoincompatible T cell depleted bone marrow. J Pediatr 1986;108:435.

54. Shapiro R, McClain, Frizzera, et al. Epstein-Barr virus associated B cell lymphoproliferative disorders following bone marrow transplantation. Blood 1988; 71:1234.

55. Gingrich RD, Ginder GD, Goeken NE, et al. Allo-geneic marrow grafting with partially mismatched, unrelated marrow donors. Blood 1988;71:1375.

56. Beatty PG, Clift RA, Mickelson EM, et al. Marrow transplantation from related donors other than HLA-identical siblings. N Engl J Med 1985;313:765.

57. Powles RL, Clink HEM, et al. Mismatched family donors for bone marrow transplantation as treatment for acute leukemia. Lancet 1983;1:612–615.

58. Zintl F, Hermann J, Fuchs D, et al. Comparison of allogeneic and autologous bone marrow transplantation for treatment of acute lymphocytic leukemia in childhood. Haematol Blood Transfusion 1990; 33:692–698.

59. Ramsay N, LeBien T, Weisdorf D, et al. Autologous BMT for patients with acute lymphoblastic leukemia: In: Bone marrow transplantation: current controversies. New York: Alan R Liss, 1989;57–66.

60. Gonzales-Chambers R, Przepiorka D, Shadduck RK, et al. Autologous bone marrow transplantation with 4-hydroperoxycyclophosphamide-purged marrow for acute lymphoblastic leukemia. Med Pediatr Oncol 1991;19:160–164.

61. Gorin NC, Aegerter P, Auvert B. Autologous bone marrow transplantation for acute leukemia in remission: an analysis of 1322 cases. Haematol Blood Transfusion 1990;33:660–666.

62. Carella AM, Martinengo M, Santini G, et al. Autologous bone marrow transplantation for acute leukemia in remission, the Genoa experience. Haematologica 1988;73:119–124.

63. Rizzoli V, Mangoni L, Carella AM, et al. Drug-mediated marrow purging: mafosfamide in adult care leukemia in remission. The experience of the Italian study. Bone Marrow Transplant 1989;4(suppl 1):190–194.

64. Simonsson B, Burnett AK, Prentice HG, et al. Autologous bone marrow transplantation with monoclonal antibody purged marrow for high risk acute lymphoblastic leukemia. Leukemia 1989;3(9):631–636.

65. Blume K, Forman S, O'Donnell S, et al. Total body irradiation and high-dose etoposide: a new preparatory regimen for bone marrow transplantation in patients with advanced hematologic malignancies. Blood 1987;69:1015–1020.

66. Kaizer H, Stuart RK, Brookmeyer R, et al. A phase I study of in vitro treatment of marrow with 4-hydroperoxycyclophosphamide to purge tumor cells. Blood 1985;65(6):1504–1510.

67. Douay L, Mary JY, Giarratana MC, et al. Establishment of a reliable experimental procedure for bone marrow purging with mafosfamide. Exp Hematol 1989;17:429.

68. Gulliya KS, Pervaiz S. Elimination of clonogenic tumor cells from HL-60, Daudi, and U-937 cell lines by laser photoradiation therapy: implications for autologous bone marrow purging. Blood 1989;73:1059.

69. Blast JRC. Elimination of malignant clonogenic cells

from human marrow using multiple monoclonal antibodies and complement. Cancer Res 1984;45:499–503.

70. Kvalheim G, Sorenson O, Fodstad O, et al. Immunomagnetic removal of G-lymphoma cells from human bone marrow: a procedure for clinical use. Bone Marrow Transplant 1988;3:31.

71. Strong RC, Uckun F, Youle RJ, et al. Use of multiple T cell-directed intact ricin immunotoxins for autologous bone marrow transplantation. Blood 1985; 66:627–635.

72. Uckun FM, Kersey JH, Waddick KG, Ramsay NKC. Residual acute lymphoblastic leukemia blasts in autologous remission marrow grafts. J Cell Biochem 1988;12C(suppl):124.

73. Gribben JG, Freidman AS, Neuberg D, et al. Immunologic purging of marrow assessed by PCR before autologous bone marrow transplantation for B-cell lymphoma. N Engl J Med 1991;325:1525–1533.

74. Abramson C, Kersey JH, LeBien TW. A monoclonal antibody (BA-1) primarily reactive with cells of human B lymphocyte lineage. J Immunol 1981;126:83.

75. Kersey JH, Lebien TW, Abramson CS, et al. A human hemopoietic progenitor and acute lymphoblastic leukemia-associated cell surface structure identified with a monoclonal antibody. J Exp Med 1981;153:726.

76. Freedman AS, Nadler LM. Cell surface markers in hematologic malignancies. Semin Oncol 1987;14:193.

77. Kiesel S, Dorken B, Messner H. Personal communication.

78. Nadler LM. C cell/leukemia panel workshop: summary and comments. In: Reinherz EL, Haynes FB, Nadler L, Bernstein ID, eds. Leukocyte typing II. Vol. 2. New York: Springer-Verlag, 1986.

79. Nadler LM, Anderson KC, Mariti G, et al. B4 a human B lymphocyte-associated antigen expressed on normal mitogen-activated and malignant B lymphocytes. J Immunol 1983;131:244.

80. Vitetta ES, Fulton RJ, May RD, et al. Redesigning nature's poisons to create anti-tumor reagents. Science 1987;238:1098.

81. Dillman RO, Johnson DE, Shawler DL. Comparisons of drug and toxin immunoconjugates. Antibody Immunol Radiopharmacol 1988;1:65–77.

82. Blakely DC, Thorpe PE. An overview of therapy with immunotoxins containing ricin or its A chain. Antibody Immunol Radiopharmacol 1988;1:1–16.

35

INTENSIVE THERAPY OF CHRONIC MYELOGENOUS LEUKEMIA

Robert Peter Gale and Anna Butturini

We review results of intensive therapy of chronic myelogenous leukemia (CML). Two approaches are considered: high-dose chemotherapy alone and high-dose chemotherapy, with or without radiation, followed by a bone marrow transplant.

Results of high-dose chemotherapy alone are comparable to those of conventional treatment, with no evidence of increased survival or cures. In contrast, results of intensive therapy followed by a transplant are markedly superior to conventional treatment; relapses are uncommon, and many subjects are cured.

Two variables may account for these diverse results: The more intensive therapy used pretransplant or an immune-mediated antileukemia effect of the graft. Analysis of data following transplants from different donors (e.g., HLA-identical siblings, twins, autotransplants) suggests that most of the increased efficacy of transplants is immune mediated. However, there may be a small direct antileukemia effect of intensive treatment.

Cytogenetic and molecular biologic studies of transplant recipients without leukemia relapse indicate prolonged persistence of at least some cells related to the leukemia clone in most instances. These data suggest that it may not be necessary to eradicate all leukemia cells to cure CML.

These observations suggest it may be reasonable to reexamine the possible role of very intensive therapy in chronic-phase CML.

INTRODUCTION

CML is a common leukemia with an age-adjusted incidence of about 1.4 per 100,000. CML accounts for about 20% of all leukemias and about one-third of those in adults (1, 2). CML is caused by a consistent acquired genetic rearrangement between the ABL and BCR genes in a pluripotent hematopoietic stem cell. This rearrangement creates a chimeric BCR/ABL gene that is expressed as a novel tyrosine kinase (3). Introduction of this chimeric gene into mice results in a disease resembling CML (4). The BCR/ABL rearrangement is most easily recognized by the t(9;22) translocation and resulting Philadelphia or Ph1-chromosome found in over 95% of cases of CML.

CML has two phases, chronic and acute. The chronic phase is characterized by an accumulation of mature myeloid cells, whereas the acute phase resembles acute leukemia. About one-third of persons have an intermediate accelerated phase. Because the accelerated phase is difficult to precisely define and its biologic import is unknown, our discussion focuses predominantly on therapy of the chronic and acute phases of CML.

CONVENTIONAL THERAPY

Chronic Phase

The overproduction of mature myeloid cells that characterizes the chronic phase is relatively easily controlled with myleran or hydroxyurea. However, there is no evidence that this treatment results in recovery of normal hematopoiesis or that duration of the chronic phase is increased. Because there is no effective therapy of the acute phase, this treatment has no effect on survival and results in no cures (5).

Interferon is also used to treat chronic-phase CML. Interferon controls myeloid proliferation but, unlike myleran and hydroxyurea, sometimes results in partial or complete restoration of normal hematopoiesis. This is manifest as a reduced proportion of bone marrow cells with the t(9;22) translocation and/or Ph1-chromosome. About one-quarter of persons treated with interferon over several months have a substantial reduction in the proportion of CML cells. Usually this is both incomplete and transient. However, 5% to 20% of subjects seem to have complete disappearance of CML cells for several months or even years (6). There are not yet convincing data that interferon treatment prolongs duration of the chronic phase, increases survival, or cures persons with CML—even those who become Ph1-chromosome negative.

In summary, although it is relatively easy to control the chronic phase, treatment is without effect on its duration. Because this is the major determinant of survival, therapy of the chronic phase is only of modest benefit, and cures are not achieved.

Acute Phase

In acute-phase CML the leukemia cells fail to mature. The two predominant forms of the acute phase are myeloid and lymphoid. However, detailed studies indicate that both lineages are often involved, reflecting leukemia progression in a pluripotent stem cell (7).

Conventional therapy of the acute phase is unsatisfactory. The myeloid acute phase is typically treated with cytarabine and an anthracycline or anthracinedione used singly and combined (reviewed in 1, 2, 5). Plicamycin and hydroxyurea are sometimes used (8). Although the chronic phase is reestablished in about 25% of cases, duration is typically brief, without cures.

The lymphoid acute phase is typically treated with vincristine and corticosteroids, sometimes with other drugs. Although the chronic phase is reestablished in about 50% of cases, duration is again brief, without cures.

INTENSIVE CHEMOTHERAPY OF CHRONIC PHASE

There are several studies of intensive chemotherapy of chronic-phase CML (9–13). Most regimens, patterned after therapy of acute myelogenous leukemia (AML), used conventional-dose cytarabine and an anthracycline, sometimes with other drugs like vincristine, prednisone, 6-mercaptopurine, or thioguanine, methotrexate, amsacrine, and 5-azacytidine. More recent studies use new anthracyclines, like idarubicin and mitoxantrone. Results of these studies are disappointing. Many subjects had no or only a slight reduction in the proportion of bone marrow cells with the Ph1-chromosome. Although others had more substantial reductions, few became completely Ph1-chromosome negative. Furthermore, most responses were brief, with rapid reappearance of cells with the Ph1-chromosome along with clinical features of CML. Most discouraging was lack of convincing data of increased duration of the chronic phase, improved survival, or cures, even in responders.

The sole encouraging data from intensive treatment are from persons accidentally receiving overdoses of myleran. Several survived for many years without evidence of the

Ph1-chromosome or with mixed, stable chimerism (14–16).

BONE MARROW TRANSPLANTS

Human-Leukocyte-Antigen-Identical Transplants

CHRONIC PHASE

Bone marrow transplants are commonly used to treat chronic phase CML. Most transplants are from HLA-identical sibling donors; smaller numbers are from HLA-matched alternative related and unrelated donors (17).

Results of transplants in CML are summarized in Figures 35.1 and 35.2. Transplants in chronic-phase CML are remarkably effective in eradicating leukemia: 5-year actuarial probability of relapse after HLA-identical sibling transplants is about 10% (for example, 18–20). Graft-versus-host disease (GVHD) is the major determinant of relapse, which is about 15% in persons with little or no GVHD versus 5% in those with GVHD (21). T cell depletion of the graft is also associated with increased relapse, an effect persisting even

after adjustment for GVHD (22). Variables without detectable effect on relapse include hematologic parameters at diagnosis and pretransplant, like white blood cells and percent immature cells, splenomegaly or splenectomy, duration of the chronic phase pretransplant, conditioning regimen, and posttransplant immune suppression (after adjusting for GVHD).

Five-year leukemia-free survival after chronic phase transplants is about 50% (Fig. 35.1) and is highest in younger persons. Use of cyclosporine and methotrexate posttransplant is also associated with improved leukemia-free survival (20). Other variables are of little influence. Persons transplanted within 1 year of diagnosis have a modestly better outcome than those transplanted later but while still in chronic phase (18–20). This is not the result of fewer relapses, however.

ACCELERATED/ACUTE PHASE

Transplants in accelerated and acute-phase CML are associated with more relapses and lower leukemia-free survival (Figs. 35.1, 35.2). Relapse rates after transplants in accel-

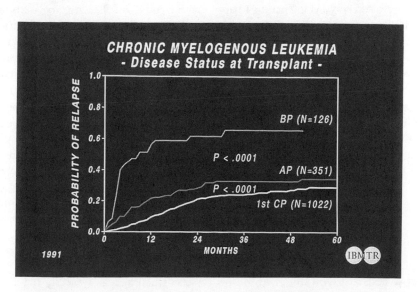

Figure 35.1.   Relapse following HLA-identical sibling bone marrow transplants for CML. (Data courtesy of the International Bone Marrow Transplant Registry.)

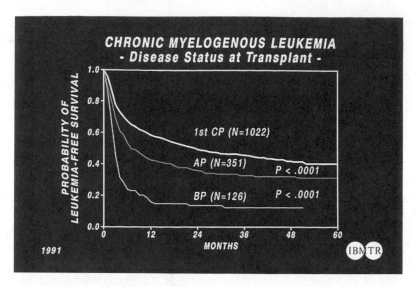

Figure 35.2.   Leukemia-free survival after HLA-identical sibling bone marrow transplants for CML. (Data courtesy of the International Bone Marrow Transplant Registry.)

erated and acute phase are about 20% and about 40%, respectively. Leukemia-free survival rates are similar, about 30% (23).

Twin Transplants

Transplants from genetically identical twin donors are also reported in chronic-phase CML (24). Relapses, about 60%, are considerably greater than after comparable transplants from HLA-identical siblings even after adjusting for GVHD. Five-year leukemia-free survival is about 40%. Although some data suggest fewer relapses when dimethylmyleran is added to standard pretransplant conditioning, this is uncertain. There are insufficient data to comment on results of twin transplants in more advanced CML.

Autotransplants

There are considerable data regarding results of autotransplants in CML in chronic or acute phase (reviewed in 25). Although bone marrow cells are typically used, blood stem cells are sometimes substituted for or added to the graft. In an attempt to avoid in-

fusing CML cells, bone marrow or blood cells used for autotransplants are often obtained following intensive chemotherapy or interferon treatment when all or a proportion of these cells are Ph1-chromosome negative. In other studies, attempts were made to remove CML cells from the graft by in vitro treatment with drugs or following in vitro culture.

Most persons receiving autotransplants in the chronic phase become partially or completely Ph1-chromosome negative posttransplant. Responses are often incomplete and transient. Three-year leukemia-free survival is less than 5%. Most relapses are probably from residual CML cells in the subject. Whether leukemia contamination of the graft is important in causing relapse is unknown. There is little evidence that any pretransplant therapy, conditioning regimen, in vitro treatment of the graft, or posttransplant manipulation is superior. Furthermore, there is little proof that any is effective.

Autotransplants in acute phase reestablish the chronic phase in about 80% of subjects. This effect is typically brief, with a median duration of less than 6 months before the acute phase recurs. Most data suggest that acute-phase recurrence is from persisting acute-phase cells in the subject rather than evolution from chronic phase cells (26).

LEUKEMIA ERADICATION

Analyses of transplant data provide important insights into how CML is cured. One issue is the role of immune-mediated antileukemia effects. Considerable data from allograft recipients with and without GVHD indicate a potent associated antileukemia effect, a notion supported by the high relapse rate after twin transplants (24). The very high relapse rate after T-cell-depleted transplants suggests an additional T-cell-mediated antileukemia effect independent of GVHD. Additional support for this notion comes from treatment of relapse after T-cell-depleted transplants. Here, discontinuing cyclosporine or infusing of donor T cells sometimes results in remission (27, 28). In summary, transplants for CML are associated with two potent immune-mediated antileukemia effects: GVHD and an independent T cell effect.

One important issue is whether intensive pretransplant treatment plays a role in leukemia eradication after transplants. The answer is uncertain. It is very likely that intensive treatment is needed to reduce the leukemia mass sufficiently for immune-mediated mechanisms to operate. Whether intensive therapy alone can cure CML is less certain. The about 40% freedom-from-relapse after twin and T-cell-depleted transplants, where immune-mediated effects are likely small, suggests that intensive treatment alone may be effective. There are caveats to this conclusion, however. One is that without data from T-cell-depleted twin transplants, it is impossible to exclude that immune-mediated effects cure leukemia even in twins. A second disturbing consideration is that diverse pretransplant therapies result in similar relapse risks. This means either that all regimens are similarly effective or that none are effective. A possible exception is a report of fewer relapses after very high dose radiation

(29). However, interpretation of these data is complicated by confounding effects of GVHD on relapse. Another issue is whether the intensity of treatment required to cure CML might not cause unacceptable damage to normal stem cells. Were this so, cure of CML by intensive pretransplant treatment might not be achievable without a transplant.

Detailed cytogenetic and molecular studies after bone marrow transplants also provide clues as to how CML is cured (30–33). These observations indicate that some CML cells remain following intensive pretransplant therapy even in persons with no clinical evidence of relapse for 5 or more years posttransplant. Unknown is whether immune mechanisms control or eradicate these residual CML cells or other mechanisms prevent relapse.

STRATEGIES TO CURE CHRONIC MYELOGENOUS LEUKEMIA

Several conclusions emerge from these data. First, conventional therapy neither prolongs survival nor cures CML. Second, some persons with CML are cured by transplants. This effect is predominantly the result of immune-mediated antileukemia mechanisms. However, the very intensive treatment given pretransplant is likely important in reducing the leukemia mass so that immune-mediated effects can operate. Whether some persons are cured by intensive treatment alone is unknown but may be possible based on results of twin and T-cell-depleted transplants.

Is it time to reconsider intensive chemotherapy for CML? For this approach to succeed there should be an exploitable therapeutic margin between normal and CML stem cells. It is not possible to know if this is so from transplant data since subjects are "rescued" with normal bone marrow containing both hematopoietic stem cells and immune cells. Also unknown is what dose of intensive chemotherapy is needed to cure CML. Although we know what doses are used for transplants, it is unknown if treatment intensity is necessary. However, most data suggest that therapy will need to be reasonably intensive. For example, few if any persons with Ph1-chromosome-positive acute lymphoblastic leukemia, some with an identical BCR/ABL rearrangement as CML (34), are cured with current intensive chemotherapy (reviewed in 35, 36).

The doses needed to cure CML are likely to be associated with substantial morbidity and mortality. This risk is, however, unlikely to exceed the current 30% mortality associated with transplants from imperfectly HLA-matched related or unrelated donors. Perhaps these risks can be decreased by prophylactic antibiotics, protected environments, and hematopoietic growth factors. Caution is needed since CML cells may also respond to these factors.

Although intensive chemotherapy alone may not cure CML, it may when combined with immune-mediated antileukemia effects. How to achieve these without a transplant is uncertain. Perhaps immune modulators, like interleukin-2 or tumor necrosis factor, might be effective. Recall however, that the transplant-related immune-mediated effects we discuss appear to operate only in the context of genetic disparity between the immune system (donor) and leukemia cells (recipient). Whether they would operate in a genetically identical setting is unknown.

Another approach to cure CML might be to use antiproliferative agents like interferon after intensive chemotherapy. This strategy appears to work in multiple myeloma (37); it is untested in CML. A final strategy might involve use of factors that regulate myelopoiesis after intensive therapy.

Acknowledgments

Supported in part by a grant from the Center for Advanced Studies in Leukemia. Robert Peter Gale is the Wald Foundation Scholar in Biomedical Communications. Becky Beckham prepared the typescript.

REFERENCES

1. Clarkson B. The chronic leukemias. In: Wyngaarden JB, Smith LH Jr, eds. Cecil textbook of medicine. 18th ed. Philadelphia: WB Saunders, 1988:988–1001.
2. Cannellos GP, ed. Chronic leukemias. Hematol Oncol Clin North Am 1990;4:319–506.
3. Kurzrock R, Gutterman JU, Talpaz M. The molecular genetics of Philadelphia chromosome positive leukemias. N Engl J Med 1988;319:990–998.
4. Daley CQ, van Etten RA, Baltimore D. Induction of chronic myelogenous leukemia in mice by the P210 BCR-ABL gene of the Philadelphia chromosome. Science 1990;247:824–830.
5. Spiers ASD. The management of chronic myelogenous leukemia. In: Henderson ES, Lister TA, eds. Leukemia. 5th ed. Philadelphia: WB Saunders, 1990:515–564.
6. Talpaz M, Kantarjian H, Kurzrock R, Trujillo JM, Gutterman JU. Interferon alpha produces sustained cytogenetic responses in chronic myelogenous leukemia. Ann Intern Med 1991;114:532–538.
7. Sato Y, Kitano K, Tsunoda S, et al. Karyotype evolution and multi-lineage involvement of Philadelphia chromosome positive clones in blastic transformation of two patients with chronic myelocytic leukemia. Blood 1988;71:1561–1567.
8. Keller CA, Miller DM. Preliminary observation on the therapy of the myeloid blast phase of chronic granulocytic leukemia with Plicamicyn and hydroxyurea. N Engl J Med 1986;315:1433–1438.
9. Smalley RV, Vogel J, Huguley CM, Miller D. Chronic myelogenous leukemia: cytogenetic conversion of the bone marrow with cycle specific chemotherapy. Blood 1977;50:107–113.
10. Cunningham I, Gee T, Dowling M, et al. Results of treatment of Ph'+ chronic myelogenous leukemia with an intensive treatment regimen (L-5 Protocol). Blood 1979;53:375–394.
11. Goto T, Gee T, Dowling M, et al. Growth characteristic of leukemia and normal hematopoietic cells in Ph' positive chronic myelogenous leukemia and effects of intensive treatment. Blood 1982;59:793–803.
12. Sharp JC, Joyner MV, Wayne AW, et al. Karyotypic conversion in Ph1 positive chronic myeloid leukemia with combination chemotherapy. Lancet 1979;1:1370–1372.
13. Kantarjian HM, Vellekoop L, McCredie KB, et al. Intensive combination chemotherapy (ROAP 10) and splenectomy in the management of chronic myelogenous leukemia. J Clin Oncol 1985;3:192–200.
14. Finney R, McDonald GA, Baikie AG, Douglas AS. Chronic granulocytic leukemia with Ph1 negative cells in bone marrow and a ten year remission after busulfan hypoplasia. Br J Haematol 1972;23:283–288.
15. Benjamin D, Djaldetti M, Mammom Z, et al. Prolonged busulfan-induced remissions in chronic myeloid leukemia. Acta Haematol 1979;62:119–120.
16. Bennett M, Lewis D, Walker H. Prolonged survival in chronic granulocytic leukemia after busulfan induced hypoplasia and karyotype conversion. Br J Haematol 1985;59:738–740.

17. Champlin RE, Bortin MM, Horowitz MM, for the International Bone Marrow Transplant Registry. Trends in bone marrow transplantation for leukemia. Exp Hematol 1991;19:569.

18. Thomas ED, Cliff RA, Fefer A, et al. Marrow transplantation for the treatment of chronic myelogenous leukemia. Ann Intern Med 1986;104:155–153.

19. McGlave P, Arthur D, Haoke R, et al. Therapy of chronic myelogenous leukemia with allogeneic bone marrow transplantation. J Clin Oncol 1987;5:1033.

20. Goldman JM, Gale RP, Horowitz MM, et al. Bone marrow transplantation for chronic myelogenous leukemia in chronic phase: increased risk of relapse associated with T-cell depletion. Ann Intern Med 1988;108:806–814.

21. Horowitz MM, Gale RP, Sondel PM, et al. Graft-versus-leukemia reactions after bone marrow transplantations. Blood 1990;75:555–562.

22. Marmont AM, Horowitz MM, Gale RP, et al. T cell depletion of HLA identical transplants in leukemia. Blood 1991;78:2120–2130.

23. Martin PJ, Clift RA, Fisher LD, et al. HLA identical bone marrow transplantation during accelerate phase chronic myelogenous leukemia: analysis of survival and remission duration. Blood 1988;72:1978–1991.

24. Gale RP, Goldman JM, Horowitz MM, for the International Bone Marrow Transplant Registry. Identical twin transplants in chronic myelogenous leukemia in chronic phase. Exp Hematol 1991;19:573.

25. Butturini A, Keating A, Goldman JM, Gale RP. Autotransplants in chronic myelogenous leukemia: strategies and results. Lancet 1990;1:1255–1257.

26. Reiffers J, Bernard P, David B, Broustet A. Autografting for chronic myelogenous leukemia in transformation. Am J Hematol 1985;18:105–106.

27. Frassoni F, Sessarego M, Bacigalupo A, et al. Competition between recipient and donor cells after bone marrow transplantation for chronic myelogenous leukemia. Br J Haematol 1988;69:471–475.

28. Kolb HJ, Mittermuller J, Clemm CH, et al. Donor leukocyte transfusions for treatment of recurrent chronic myelogenous leukemia in marrow transplant patients. Blood 1990;76:2462–2465.

29. Clift RA, Buckner CD, Appelbaum FR, et al. Allogeneic bone marrow transplantation for patients with chronic myeloid leukemia in chronic phase: a randomized trial of two irradiation regimens. Blood 1991;77:1660–1665.

30. Arthur CK, Apperley JF, Guo AP, et al. Cytogenetic events after bone marrow transplantation for chronic myelogenous leukemia in chronic phase. Blood 1988;71:1179.

31. Zaccaria A, Rosti G, Sessarego M, et al. Relapse after allogeneic bone marrow transplantation for Philadelphia chromosome positive chronic myeloid leukemia: cytogenetic analysis of 24 patients. Bone Marrow Transplant 1988;3:413–423.

32. Gabert J, Thuret I, Lafage M, Carcassonne Y, Maraninchi D, Mannoni P. Detection of residual BCR-ABL translocation by polymerase chain reaction in chronic myeloid leukemia patients after bone marrow transplantation. Lancet 1989;2:1125–1128.

33. Hughes TP, Morgan GJ, Martiat P, Goldman JM. Detection of residual leukemia after bone marrow transplant for chronic myeloid leukemia: role of polymerase chain reaction. Blood 1991;77:874–878.

34. Maurer J, Janssen JWG, Thiel E, et al. Detection of chimeric BCR-ABL genes in acute lymphoblastic leukemia by the polymerase chain reaction. Lancet 1991;337:1055–1061.

35. Champlin RE, Gale RP. Acute lymphoblastic leukemia: recent advances in biology and therapy. Blood 1989;73:2051–2066.

36. Gale RP, Hoelzer D. Acute lymphoblastic leukemia: current controversies, future directions. Leukemia 1989;3:681–686.

37. Mandelli F, Avissati G, Amadori S, et al. Maintenance treatment with recombinant interferon alpha-2b in patients with multiple myeloma responding to conventional induction chemotherapy. N Engl J Med 1990;322:1430–1434.

36

High-Dose Therapy and Allogeneic Bone Marrow Transplantation in Chronic Lymphocytic Leukemia

Giuseppe Bandini and Mauricette Michallet

Chronic lymphocytic leukemia (CLL) is a hematologic neoplasm characterized by proliferation and accumulation of small, relatively mature appearing, immunologically incompetent lymphocytes, usually of B-lineage. In nearly 5% of cases the malignant transformation involves T lymphocytes; T-CLL's morphologic, clinical, and hematologic expression differs strikingly from that of the commoner B-CLL to which this chapter is primarily devoted. Clonality of CLL is confirmed by the expression of a single immunoglobulin light chain, either κ or λ on the cell surface membrane (1); unique immunoglobulin idiotype specificities (2); a single pattern of glucose 6-phosphate dehydrogenase activity (3); clonal chromosomal abnormalities (4); and, finally, clonal immunoglobulin gene rearrangements (5). Also, patients with T-CLL demonstrate unique clonal rearrangements of one chain of the T cell receptor (6).

CLL belongs to the category of low-grade malignant lymphomas and is, in many cases, of an indolent nature. A typical survival curve of an unselected population of patients, such as those observed by us between 1966 and 1978, shows that annual mortality is about 8%, median survival is nearly 6 years, and 20% of patients survive more than 10 years (7). Treatment has not been aimed, with good reasons, at curing the disease but instead at prolonging survival and improving the quality of life. These goals have been achieved satisfactorily, but we are left with the dilemma of whether this disease is curable or not. The widely held assumption that CLL is incurable could just be a consequence of the fact that effective treatments have not been used.

If CLL were curable, the next step would be to explore the feasibility and practicality of a therapeutic approach aimed at this goal; treatment would be based on the administration of an aggressive, high-dose therapy, since increasing doses are increasingly effective in chemosensitive tumors (8). The whole procedure of bone marrow transplantation (BMT) represents the best example of very high dose therapy administered over a short period of time; it has been shown able to cure thousands of patients with acute myeloid and lymphoid leukemias, chronic myelogenous leukemia, and other hematologic malignancies, and therefore could be applied to CLL. However, few transplants—slightly over two dozen, including two syngeneic and one mismatched case, worldwide—have been performed for CLL (9); considering that this neoplasm is the commonest form of adult leukemia in the Western world, it appears that

CLL can still be considered at the moment an orphan disease with regard to BMT. To try to understand why, in the first part of this chapter we examine the conceptual basis for performing BMT—or not—in CLL; in the second part we examine the results of a series of 21 patients who received allogeneic BMT at different European centers and had a close follow-up after transplant. There are few points to be discussed, and we shall do it separately, although they overlap to a considerable extent.

AGE

The median age of onset of CLL is 60 years, clearly beyond the upper limit not only of BMT but also of other highly aggressive chemotherapy regimens now commonly used for hematologic malignancies. However, a proportion of patients are <50 years at diagnosis, and their number increases as routine hematochemical screening is being undertaken more and more frequently in our health-conscious society. The proportion of patients <50 years was 12% in an Eastern Cancer Oncology Group (ECOG) study including 182 patients (10) and 9% in a study from the MD Anderson Hospital on 325 patients (11). The prognosis of these younger patients is much better than that of the general population with CLL; in fact, the median survival was not reached at 60+ months in the ECOG study (versus 50 months for the remaining population) and was 9 years in the MD Anderson study (versus 6.2 years for those between 51 and 60 years, 5.2 years for those aged 61–70 years, and 3.3 years for those >70 years). This presents one dilemma of CLL. Younger patients may tolerate aggressive therapies better than older ones, but in the case of BMT results are progressively worse with age, and the 40- to 50-year range represents nowadays the upper limit of BMT (12, 13). The passage of time may be an advantage for these younger patients who are diagnosed today, simply because new, effective drugs could come into use, just to mention

one reason, but may also be a disadvantage because transplantation cannot be applied later, when the risk of toxic death becomes unacceptably high.

PROGNOSTIC FACTORS

The clinical course of CLL is so highly variable that the search of potential prognostic factors, in order to design optimal therapeutic strategies, has been very thorough. There are two well-known staging systems. The five-stage Rai classification (14) basically divides patients into low-risk (0), intermediate-risk (I, II), and high-risk (III, IV) groups, on the basis of presence or absence of adenopathy, hepatomegaly, splenomegaly, anemia, and thrombocytopenia. These groups constitute approximately 25%, 50%, and 25% of patients, respectively. Other investigators prefer the three-stage Binet system (15), which identifies patients at low (A), intermediate (B), and high (C) risk on the basis of the number of lymphoid sites involved and a slightly different definition of anemia and thrombocytopenia compared to the Rai system. The main limitation of these staging systems is that the intermediate group is heterogeneous with respect to prognosis, some patients having a survival similar to that of the low-risk and other patients having a survival comparable to that of the high-risk patients.

These staging systems can be supplemented with other documented prognostic factors such as sex (16), lymphocyte count at diagnosis (7), chromosomal findings (17), and pattern of marrow infiltration (18); as a result, it is possible to identify patients with a survival comparable to that of their age and sex-matched population (19) or a median survival of less than 2 years (18). If a patient is considered a potential candidate for BMT, on the basis of age, for example, as much prognostic information as possible should be obtained; this would make the final decision, and the timing of BMT, a logically constructed process. Clearly, patients with the worst risk factors would be candidates for early BMT.

EVALUATION OF RESPONSE

The concept of complete response in CLL is not as straightforward as it might appear at first glance. A major problem is the lack of uniform response criteria; without them it is difficult, if not impossible, to compare and evaluate individual therapeutic studies. For many years the concept of complete response was based on the normalization of blood counts, marrow aspirate and biopsy, resolution of organomegaly, and absence of constitutional symptoms. However, looking at the definition of complete response used by different institutions or study groups, it appears that the required levels of lymphocytes in the peripheral blood or bone marrow differ considerably. For example, peripheral blood lymphocytes may vary between $<2.5 \times 10^9$ (MD Anderson Hospital) to $<15 \times 10^9$ per liter (Cancer and Acute Leukemia Group B). The bone marrow lymphocytes should be $<20\%$ (MD Anderson Hospital, Mayo Clinic), $<25\%$ (European Organization for Research and Treatment of Cancer), or $<30\%$ (ECOG, South Western Oncology Group, Memorial Sloan-Kettering Cancer Center). There are also differences, although to a lesser extent, in the physical examination requirements, usually centered around disappearance of adenopathies or their reduction to <1 cm and, sometimes, disappearance of disease-related symptoms. A good table of complete response criteria is found in reference 20. The definition of partial response is more variable and can be summarized as 50%–75% decrease in peripheral blood lymphocytes, a 50% decrease in palpable disease, hemoglobin >11 g/dl, and platelet count $>100 \times 10^9$ per liter (21). These definitions, however, are clinical ones and only apply to a setting of conventional treatment, where the aim is to control the disease and its symptoms.

It must be repeated, however, that the absence of standardized and rigorous criteria of response makes it difficult to appreciate if, for example, achievement of complete remission gives a better survival than partial remission. But if the aim of treating CLL is the elimination of the neoplastic clone, more stringent criteria of response than the previously mentioned ones are needed. Indirect evidence of the disappearance of the disease includes normalization of T and B cells and the κ/λ light chain ratio and occurrence of very low numbers of cells phenotypically characteristic of B-CLL (for example, CD5– CD20) by dual marker analysis. Finally, direct evidence is provided only by resolution of markers of the neoplastic clone. Cytogenetic analysis has more conceptual than practical value, because of the low mitotic yield commonly observed in CLL, but it nonetheless should be applied when possible; immunoglobulin gene rearrangements occur very frequently in CLL (22), and their study can detect very low proportions (1%–2%) of malignant cells, if the pattern of each individual patient was known before transplant. By use of the polymerase chain reaction it is possible to amplify the rearrangements and thus to detect residual tumor at a much lower threshold level; this has already been done in the acute lymphoid malignancies (23) and can theoretically be applied to CLL also. Obviously, all these studies should be performed in transplant patients before and after the procedure, in order to gain knowledge of the nature of remission in CLL and its relationship to the long-term cure of the disease.

THERAPY OF CHRONIC LYMPHOCYTIC LEUKEMIA

There are two main modalities of treatment in CLL: chemotherapy and radiation therapy. (BMT will be discussed later.)

Chemotherapy

A large number of antineoplastic agents are active in CLL: chlorambucil, cyclophosphamide, busulfan, corticosteroids, vincristine, melphalan, anthracycline antibiotics (reviewed in 21). Chlorambucil, introduced in 1952, has remained the most popular drug; an aromatic derivative of nitrogen mustard absorbed orally, it can be used daily until the disease is controlled or in short courses (4–7 days) every 4 weeks. Lymphocyte count is reduced in 70% of patients, while lymphoadenopathy is reduced in 50% and splenomegaly is reduced in 25%. Cyclophosphamide is probably as effective as chlorambucil and has a lesser tendency to produce thrombocytopenia or anemia than the former drug. Busulfan also has activity in CLL, but at a lower degree than the two previously mentioned agents. Corticosteroids have the unique capacity of causing lysis of lymphoid cells and reduction of tumor masses without bone marrow depression. They are particularly useful when immune-mediated anemia and thrombocytopenia accompany CLL but should not be used alone because they aggravate, in the long term, the immunosuppression of these patients, rendering them more susceptible to infections caused by defective antibody production.

In the past few years two new drugs, used as single agents, have given very promising results. Fludarabine-monophosphate (9-β-D-arabinofuranosyl-2-fluoroadenine monophosphate), a fluorinated analogue of adenine that is resistant to deamination by adenosine deaminase, has given response rates of over 50% even in previously treated patients in Rai stages III and IV (24). The drug has recently been approved with orphan drug status for therapy of CLL. Treatment is well tolerated, and the only major toxicity is associated with infections, which, in turn, are associated with neutropenia. A recent case of concurrent cytomegalovirus and *Pneumocystis carinii* pneumonia after therapy with this agent has been reported in a patient with CLL (25), probably because of a selective depletion of CD4 cells caused by fludarabine (26), and this event points to a new possible kind of complication—infections with opportun-

istic agents—in the modern therapy of this neoplasm. 2-Chlordeoxyadenosine (27), a lymphocyte-selective drug, is an adenosine-deaminase-resistant purine analogue that selectively accumulates in cells rich in deoxycytidine kinase; its cytotoxic activity is independent of cell division. Its first reported use in CLL was in 18 patients with advanced refractory disease, and there was an overall 55% response (complete responses, partial responses, and clinical improvement). The drug exerts a minor degree of marrow toxicity, and its general toxicity has been shown to be low, also in patients with non-Hodgkin's lymphomas and hairy cell leukemia (28). These two new drugs are very likely to have a major role to play in the management of CLL, and this will be assessed by ongoing treatment phase II and phase III trials, but at the moment they remain investigational.

More intensive combination therapies have been used in CLL. Cyclophosphamide, vincristine, and prednisone (COP) have been moderately effective in ameliorating advanced CLL (29, 30), but one controlled study of untreated patients with advanced CLL failed to show superiority of COP over conventional regimens (31). Controlled studies of the M 2 protocol, an aggressive five-drug combination (vincristine, carmustine [BCNU], cyclophosphamide, melphalan, and prednisone) in stage C CLL have shown that "complete responses" can be induced in 17% of patients and "partial responses" in 44%. Median survival of patients achieving complete response, partial response, or no response were 73, 40, and 14 months, respectively (32). Although survival was certainly better for patients responding more completely, there was no advantage in that study when survival was compared to stage at the beginning of therapy with respect to what was initially described by Rai et al. (14). The M 2 protocol, although effective in controlling the disease, did not result in significant improvement of survival (20). Promising results of therapy with an intensive regimen containing the anthracycline antibiotic adriamycin and cytosine arabinoside combined with COP (POACH) were reported several years ago (33), but a recent paper shows survivals similar to those commonly observed in CLL (34).

In summary, there are many agents that are active in CLL, but the key question with regard to the use of high-dose therapy and BMT is whether a dose-response effect, an ideal prerequisite for applying high-dose therapy, has been demonstrated in this disease. The more intensive regimens employed in CLL, such as those including moderately high doses of cyclophosphamide, vincristine, cytosine-arabinoside, and anthracycline antibiotics, have not shown a survival advantage over conventional treatment in the majority of published studies; however, there is an exception, represented by a prospective, randomized study of the French group on CLL, where the cyclophosphamide, adriamycin, vincristine, and prednisone (CHOP) regimen was clearly superior in inducing a response to the COP regimen (which does not contain the anthracycline) in advanced CLL patients, with a statistically better survival of $52 \pm 9\%$ SD for CHOP versus $14 \pm 7\%$ SD ($p = .0005$) for COP at 5 years (35). Thus the answer to the question of the existence of a dose-response effect can be at least a cautiously affirmative one.

Radiotherapy

Lymphocytes of CLL are as radiosensitive as, or more so than, their normal counterparts, and the lytic effect of radiation is independent of the cell cycle. Since the introduction of the very practical and effective combination of prednisone and chlorambucil, radiotherapy has played only a secondary role in the management of CLL, being used with palliative intent for massive and painful splenomegaly, large nodal masses, or masses producing obstructive symptoms. Radiotherapy has been used in several innovative forms in the treatment of CLL. Total body irradiation (TBI) (which, remarkably, was started in the early decades of this century

(36)), mediastinal irradiation (37), low-dose splenic irradiation (38), thymic irradiation (39), hemibody irradiation (40), radioisotopic irradiation (41), and extracorporeal blood irradiation (42) all have been claimed to produce good, albeit temporary, results. The considerable interest in TBI was revived in the late 1960s (43), but two controlled studies have shown no superiority of TBI over cyclophosphamide and prednisone (20) or chlorambucil and prednisone (44). An interesting observation associated with the use of TBI is that one study (45) reported a return of the immunoglobulins to the normal range in 80% of patients who had depressed levels before therapy. Although usually not regarded as a criterion of complete response, such an immunologic improvement has rarely been seen after chemotherapy. All these data do suggest that a conditioning regimen incorporating TBI should be used before transplant; the severe myelotoxicity commonly observed after radiation therapy, due to a poor marrow reserve, would not be a problem in this case, since a complete marrow aplasia is precisely the object of the conditioning treatment.

Results of chemotherapy and radiotherapy trials give us a rational basis for applying aggressive therapy, followed by BMT, in selected patients with CLL, with the aim of cure.

BONE MARROW TRANSPLANTATION AS THERAPY FOR CHRONIC LYMPHOCYTIC LEUKEMIA

Twenty-one patients, 16 males and 5 females, with a mean age of 41 years (range 32–58) underwent allogeneic BMT for CLL: 19 were B, one T, and one unclassified. Hematologic and immunologic characteristics and the Rai classification at diagnosis and just prior to the conditioning regimen are shown in Table 36.1. Eighteen patients were resistant to previous therapy, including chlorambucil, COP, CHOP, and local irradiation.

Table 36.1. Hematologic and Immunologic Classification and Rai Classification of Patients[a]

Patient	Age/Sex	Immunological Photype	Stage at Diagnosis	Conventional Chemotherapy	Splenectomy Yes/No	Stage Pre-Graft	Interval from Diagnosis to BMT (Months)
1	37/F	B, IgML	II	Chlorambucil, TNI	Y	IV	64
2	46/M	B, IgMK	II	Chlorambucil, TNI	Y	IV	46
3	39/M	B, IgMDK	II	Chlorambucil	N	IV	44
4	40/M	B, IgML	I	Chlorambucil, TNI	Y	I	25
5	35/M	B, IgML	IV	CHOP	N	IV	28
6	43/F	B, IgMK	III	No treatment	N	III	5
7	43/M	B, IgMDL	II	Chlorambucil	Y	I	39
8	36/M	B, IgMK	II	Chlorambucil, COP	N	III	48
9	43/M	B, L	IV	CHOP, Chlorambucil	N	II	29
10	36/F	Unknown	I	CHOP, Chlorambucil, COP	N	IV	87
11	41/F	T	III	Chlorambucil	Y	III	51
12	48/F	B, IgGK	0	No treatment	N	0	25
13	36/M	B	III	CHOP, COP	N	III	24
14	32/M	B, IgMK	III	Chlorambucil, COP	Y	IV	41
15	49/M	B, IgML	III	Chlorambucil, CHOP	N	IV	41
16	32/M	B	II	Chlorambucil	N	II	96
17	49/M	B	Unknown	Chlorambucil, Cyclo	N	IV	51
18	33/M	B	I	No treatment	N	I	38
19	43/M	B, IgML	IV	Chlorambucil	N	IV	15
20	44/M	B	III	CHOP	N	III	20
21	58/M	B	I	CHOP, Local Irradiation	N	IV	21

[a]Abbreviations: Cyclo, cyclophosphamide; TNI, total nodal irradiation.

Among these 18 patients, 6 were splenectomized, and 3 had received previous total nodal irradiation. All of these patients were grafted in active phase. Three patients, one stage I, one stage III, and one stage 0, were grafted without any previous therapy at 5, 25 and 38 months, respectively, after diagnosis. At the time of BMT all 21 patients were classified according to the Rai classification as follows: 10 in stage IV, 5 in stage III, 2 in stage II, 3 in stage I, and 1 in stage 0. The interval between diagnosis and BMT was 45 months (range 5–120). All patients received fully matched allogeneic BMT from identical sibling donors; the donors were 15 males and 6 females with a mean age of 39 years (range 29–52).

In all patients except one, the conditioning regimen included TBI (8–14 Gy) with lung shielding. Chemotherapy was standard (16), using cyclophosphamide in 14 patients, with reinforcement in 6 patients using chlorambucil (1 patient), etoposide (4 patients),

or melphalan (1 patient). One patient received cyclophosphamide with busulfan.

Graft-versus-host disease (GVHD) prophylaxis was long methotrexate in 1 case, cyclosporine alone in 2 cases, cyclosporine and short methotrexate in 15 cases, and cyclosporine and physical removal of T cells in 3 cases. Eleven patients were evaluable for chimerism: 3 by red blood cell markers, 5 by sex markers, and 3 by restriction fragment length polymorphism.

For one patient (patient 11), a variable number of tandem repeats probe was used to detect polymorphism on chromosome 2 at locus D2S44 (46). DNA from donor and host peripheral blood before and after BMT was prepared by standard techniques. DNA was digested by the restriction enzyme HaeIII under manufacturer's conditions. DNA fragments were separated by electrophoresis on 1% agarose gel and transferred by the Southern method to Hybond N+ nylon membrane. Hybridization was carried out with a dCTPP32-radiolabeled probe p YNH24.

One study for immunoglobulin gene rearrangements (patient 8) was performed in one patient. High molecular weight DNA was extracted from cryopreserved leukemic cells and peripheral lymphoid cells after transplantation. DNA was prepared using standard procedures. DNA was digested with Bam HI, electrophoresed on 0.8% agarose gels, transferred to nitrocellulose filters, and hybridized with nick-translated JH and Cβ probes, which were provided by Dr. Rabbitts and Dr. T.W. Mak.

Results

Eighteen patients had evidence of successful engraftment. Three patients were nonevaluable: one experienced early death at day 15, one developed graft failure at day 34, and one patient with refractory lymphocytosis died from venoocclusive disease (VOD) at day 67. The mean day to achieve a granulocyte count of 0.5×10^9 per liter was day 26 (range 12–41). The platelet count was 50×10^9 per liter by day 67 (range 30–395). Lymph nodes, splenomegaly, and/or hepatomegaly disappeared between the 3rd–20th day post-BMT except in one patient presenting persistent adenopathies. Lymphocytosis decreased slowly and disappeared from the 13th–28th day after BMT, except in one patient who died from CLL and VOD at day 67 with a white blood cell count of 40×10^9 per liter, 80% of which were lymphocytes.

Three patients developed temporary polyclonal lymphocytosis post-BMT. One patient could be studied (B cell Ig M λ); lymphocytosis was related to cytomegalovirus hepatitis with development of a monoclonal immunoglobulin Ig G1 λ that disappeared completely by the 300th day post-BMT. A study of allotypic immunoglobulin markers revealed that this monoclonal immunoglobulin was of donor origin. Of the 19 evaluable patients, 16 had acute GVHD: 5 grade I, 6 grade II, 3 grade III that resolved, and 2 grade IV who died. One case of grade I, 1 grade II, and 3 grade III evolved toward chronic GVHD.

Of the 21 patients, 1 patient died early at day 15, leaving 20 patients who were evaluable for response to BMT. Two patients were refractory, and died, 1 from CLL at day 66 and 1 from CLL and VOD at day 67. Eighteen patients were in CR, of whom 7 died, 1 from graft failure at day 34, 1 from intracerebral hemorrhage at day 31, 2 from acute GVHD at days 71 and 82, 1 in CR from sepsis at day 107, and 2 from relapse. Eleven patients are alive and well in CR with a median follow-up of 32.3 months (8–60) (Table 36.2, Fig. 36.1).

Complete chimerism was obtained in 9 evaluable patients (3 donor red blood cells, 3 donor sex, 3 restriction fragment polymorphism). Two patients had no marker, and 2 patients had autologous reconstitution, 1 complete at 7 months post-BMT (host RBC) and 1 partial at 12 months post-BMT (host sex). These last 2 patients had received T-cell-depleted marrow. Finally, for 2 patients with follow-up in CR of 31 and 60 months, molecular biology studies were performed. One patient (patient 8) was studied before and after BMT using JH region rearrangement and the B probe. In leukemic cells, the JH probe detected a rearranged fragment (Fig. 36.2), while the Cβ2 probe showed the germ line configuration. In the peripheral lymphoid cells studied after BMT, both immunoglobulin and TCR genes were in the germ line configuration, demonstrating the absence of residual disease. For the other patient (patient 11), the results are shown in Figure 36.3: Donor DNA (lane 7) and host DNA before BMT (lane 5) showed very different genotypes, providing respectively 2 donor and 2 host genetic markers in cell populations. In post-BMT host DNA (lane 6), the donor genotype was present exclusively. As we were able to detect as little as 100 ng of pre-BMT host DNA (lane 2) that could not be seen in 10 μg of post-BMT host DNA, we concluded that chimerism was complete, with a 1% sensitivity level.

Two patients relapsed. One patient relapsed 7 months after BMT and died at 8 months. The other relapsed 54 months after BMT and died at 60 months after a second

Table 36.2. Results of Trial[a]

Patient	Donor Age/Sex	Chemotherapy	TBI Dose	Number of Fractions	Year of BMT	GVHD Prevention	GVHD Acute	Chronic	Evolution After BMT
			Conditioning Regimen						
1	44/F	Cyclo	8	5	84	MTX	II	No	Relapse, dead 60 months
2	44/M	Cyclo	9.5	5	86	CSA	II	Nonevaluable	Intercerebral hemorrhage, dead day 31
3	39/M	Cyclo	14	5	86	CSA	IV	Nonevaluable	AGVHD, dead day 71
4	40/M	Cyclo	12	5	86	CSA + MTX	IV	Nonevaluable	AGVHD, dead day 82
5	33/F	Cyclo-Etoposide	12	6	86	CSA + Tdepletion[b]	I	No	Cr 52 months alive
6	36/F	Cyclo-Etoposide	12	6	87	CSA + Tdepletion	I	No	CR 41 months alive
7	43/M	Cyclo	14	6	87	MTX + CSA	III	Limited	CR 51 months alive
8	39/M	Cyclo Chlorambucil	10	1	86	MTX + CSA	I	No	Cr 60 months alive
9	38/M	Cyclo	12	6	87	CSA + MTX	III	Limited	Cr 43 months alive
10	22/M	Cyclo	12	6	88	CSA + MTX	II	No	Relapse, dead 8 months
11	14/M	Cyclo	12	5	88	CSA + MTX	I	Extensive	CR 31 months alive
12	50/M	Cyclo-Etoposide	12	3	89	CSA + Tdepletion	I	No	CR 26 months alive
13	38/M	Cyclo	12	6	89	CSA + MTX	II	Limited	CR 16 months alive
14	43/M	Cyclo	12	6	88	CSA + MTX	II	Nonevaluable	Infection refractory, dead day 66
15	41/M	Cyclo-Etoposide	12	6	88	CSA + MTX	Nonevaluable		Graft failure, dead day 34
16	37/M	Cyclo	10	1	89	CSA + MTX	III	Limited	CR 19 months alive
17	44/F	Cyclo-Melphalan	12	6	89	CSA + MTX	Nonevaluable		Hepatic and renal failure, dead day 15
18	31/M	Cyclo	12	3	90	CSA + MTX	0	No	CR 11 months alive
19	39/F	Cyclo	12	5	90	CSA + MTX	II	No	CR, dead day 107 (sepsis)
20	40/M	Cyclo	10	6	90	CSA + MTX	0	Limited	CR 6 months alive
21	52/M	Busulfan + Cyclo			90	CSA + MTX	0	Nonevaluable	Refractory VOD Dead day 67

[a]Abbreviations: CSA, cyclosporine A; Cyclo, cyclophosphamide; MTX, methotrexate; TBI, total body irradiation.
[b]Splenic irradiation.

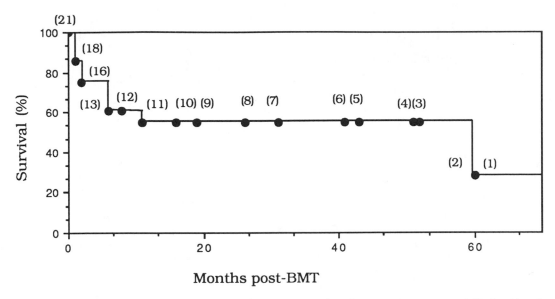

Figure 36.1.   Survival of chronic lymphocytic leukemia patients after allogeneic BMT (21 cases) (Kaplan-Meyer).

BMT was performed with the same donor. In the case of early relapse after BMT we observed a progression of lymphadenopathy and secondarily an increased leukocytosis and lymphocytosis with CD19, CD20, CD24, and HLA-DR cells in blood and bone marrow.

Summary and Conclusions

BMT was performed in 21 patients with CLL: 18 had resistant disease and 3 were untreated. Sixteen were males and 5 females, with a mean age of 41 years (range 32–58). The conditioning regimens and GVHD prophylaxis used varied. Successful engraftment was obtained in 18 evaluable cases. Lymphocytosis decreased slowly and disappeared in all but 1 case. Clinical symptoms subsided in all but 1 case. Of 19 evaluable patients, 16 developed acute GVHD. Of the 21 grafted, one early death occurred at day 15 after BMT, and 2 patients with refractory disease died at 66 and 67 days after BMT. Of the remaining 18 patients in CR, 5 died of GVHD, hemorrhage, sepsis, and graft failure, and 2 relapsed at 7 and 54 months and then died. Eleven patients are alive in CR with a mean follow-up

of 32 months (range 8–60). Chimerism was complete in 9 evaluable patients and partial in the two T-depleted cases. In one patient, alive in CR at 60 months after BMT, immunoglobulin gene rearrangement studies showed no residual disease.

This series of patients is of course too small to allow many speculations and also cannot be compared to series of refractory CLL patients treated with "conventional" chemotherapy regimens or phase I–II new drugs. However, these 21 patients receiving a fully matched allogeneic BMT represent the largest, most homogeneous group of patients with CLL treated in this way. A few observations can be made. First, BMT can be successfully performed in CLL; the main causes of death have been transplant-related mortality occurring early after BMT, a finding similar to that observed after BMT for multiple myeloma (47). It can be expected that improved modalities of transplantation will enable us to reduce transplant-related mortality also in this disease. Second, overall results were better, although not at a level of statistical significance, in patients with a shorter history of the disease, and this finding is perhaps self-ex-

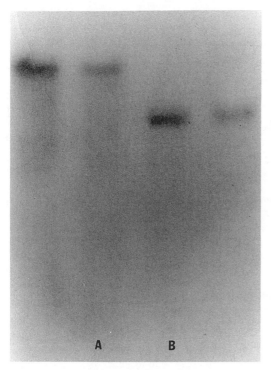

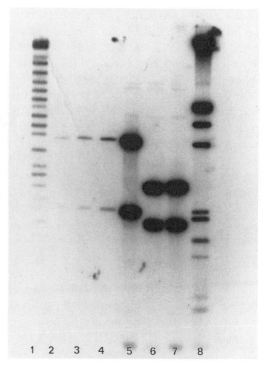

Figure 36.2. Southern blot hybridization of JH probe to normal lymphoid and leukemic cell DNA. Lane A: Germ line. JH probe. Normal lymphoid cells post-BMT. Lane B: Rearranged band JH probe (leukemic cells).

Figure 36.3. Southern blot showing DNA polymorphism detected by probe pYNH24 on donor and host peripheral blood DNAs. Lane 1: "Binning" molecular weight DNA marker (from PROMEGA), a mixture of Pvu II- and Pst II-digested DNA and various digests of O X 174 DNA. Lanes 2, 3, 4, 5: 100 ng, 250 ng, 500 ng, and 10 µg of Hae III-digested pre-BMT host DNA. Lane 6: 10 µg of Hae III-digested post-BMT host DNA. Lane 7: 10 µg of Hae III-digested donor DNA. Lane 8: Hind III/Eco R1-digested DNA.

planatory since patients with long-standing CLL will have probably received more antineoplastic agents, will have a higher degree of immunosuppression, and will have a poorer performance status at transplant than patients with CLL of relatively shorter duration. As a consequence, it would probably be advantageous to perform BMT earlier in the course of the disease.

The choice of the conditioning regimen is an important issue in BMT in general and of course in CLL. Whether a basic regimen based on cyclophosphamide and TBI is better than a reinforced one cannot be answered from this series; of 14 patients receiving standard regimens, 7 are alive in CR, while 4 of 6 of those who received a reinforced regimen are alive in CR. It is interesting to note that etoposide was used in 4 pa-

tients with good results: this drug is usually not employed in the treatment of CLL. One patient only received a regimen without TBI and died at day 67 of VOD, with refractory disease, but no conclusions can be drawn from this single case. The incidence of acute GVHD was high, with 5 patients having grade III–IV disease, and this finding could perhaps be anticipated in view of the high median age, which carries an increased risk of GVHD (48). Finally, these data indicate that BMT is effective in the treatment of refractory CLL.

A complete disappearance of the neoplastic clone could be documented with the most sensitive techniques of molecular biology in 1 patient; this unprecedented finding meets, in our view, the criteria for complete remission as discussed earlier in this chapter. Other patients have no signs of disease, with follow-up times ranging from 11–52 months; in particular, 4 patients have follow-up times between 41 and 50 months. One of them received BMT as the initial treatment of CLL, but the others had very advanced disease, and it is unlikely, in view of the well-known poor results of conventional treatments in this kind of patient, that their long periods of CR would be compatible with a condition of hidden or minimal disease. Similar results have not been reported with any kind of chemotherapy and show that the neoplastic clone of CLL can be eliminated. We think that further studies of the use of BMT in selected patients with CLL are justified and should be encouraged.

References

1. Aisemberg AC, Bloch KJ. Immunoglobulins on the surface of neoplastic lymphocytes. N Engl J Med 1976;287:272–276.
2. Giardina SL, Kipps TS, Schroff RW, et al. The generation of monoclonal anti-idiotype antibody to human B-cell derived leukemias and lymphomas. J Immunol 1985;135:653–658.
3. Fialkow PJ, Najfeld V, Redd A, Singer J, Steinmann L. Chronic lymphocytic leukemia: clonal origin in a committed B-lymphocyte progenitor. Lancet 1978; 2:444–446.
4. Gahrton, Robert K-H, Friberg K, Zech L, Bird AG. Non random chromosomal aberrations in chronic lymphocytic leukemia revealed by polyclonal B-cell-mitogen stimulation. Blood 1980;56:640–647.
5. Waldmann TA, Korsmeyer SJ, Bakhshi A, Arnold A, Kirsch IR. Molecular genetic analysis of human lymphoid neoplasms. Immunoglobulin genes and the c-myc oncogene. NIH Conference. Ann Intern Med 1985;102:497–510.
6. Foa R, Pellicci PG, Migone M, et al. Analysis of T-cell receptor beta chain (T) gene rearrangements demonstrate the monoclonal nature of T-cell chronic lymphoproliferative disorders. Blood 1986;67:247–250.
7. Baccarani M, Cavo M, Gobbi M, Lauria F, Tura S. Staging of chronic lymphocytic leukemia. Blood 1982;59:1191–1196.
8. Frei E III, Canellos GP. Dose: a critical factor in cancer chemotherapy. Am J Med 1980;69:585–594.
9. Bandini G, Michallet M, Rosti G, Tura S. Bone marrow transplantation for chronic lymphocytic leukemia. Bone Marrow Transplant 1991;7:101–103.
10. Bennett JM, Raphael B, Oken MM, Rubin PH, Silber R. The prognosis and therapy of chronic lymphocytic leukemia under age 50 years. Nouv Rev Fr Hematol 1988;30:411–412.
11. Lee JS, Dixon DO, Kantarjian HM, Keating MJ, Talpaz M. Prognosis of chronic lymphocytic leukemia: a multivariate regression analysis of 325 untreated patients. Blood 1987;63:929–936.
12. Klingemann HG, Storb R, Fefer A, et al. Bone marrow transplantation in patients aged 45 years and older. Blood 1986;7:770–776.
13. International Bone Marrow Transplant Registry. Transplant or chemotherapy in acute myelogenous leukaemia. Lancet 1989;1:1119–1122.
14. Rai KR, Sawitsky A, Cronkite EP, Chanana A, Levy RN, Pasternack BS. Clinical staging of chronic lymphocytic leukemia. Blood 1975;46:219–234.
15. Binet J, Auquier A, Dighiero G, et al. A new prognostic classification of chronic lymphocytic leukemia derived from multivariate survival analysis. Cancer 1981;48:198–206.
16. Catovsky D, Fooks J, Richards S for the MRC Working Part on Leukaemia in adults. Prognostic factors in chronic lymphocytic leukemia: the importance of age, sex, and response to treatment in survival. A report from the MRC CLL 1 trial. Br J Haematol 1989;72:141–149.
17. Juliusson G, Robert KH, Gaharton G. Cytogenetic abnormalities in chronic lymphocytic leukemia. N Engl J Med 1984;311:123.
18. Rozman C, Montserrat E. Bone marrow biopsy in chronic lymphocytic leukemia. Nouv Rev Fr Hematol 1988;30:369–371.
19. Montserrat E, Vinolas N. Reverter JC, Rozman C. Natural history of chronic lymphocytic leukemia: on the progression and prognosis of early clinical stages. Nouv Rev Fr Hematol 1988;30:359–361.
20. Kempin SJ. Treatment strategy in chronic lymphocytic leukemia. In: Polliak A, Catovsky D, eds. Chronic lymphocytic leukemia. London: Harwood Academic, 1988:159–172.
21. Gale RP, Foon KA. Chronic lymphocytic leukemia. Recent advances in biology and treatment. Ann Intern Med 1985;103:101–120.
22. Rechavi G, Mandel M, Katzir N, et al. Immunoglobulin heavy chain gene rearrangements in chronic lymphocytic leukaemia: correlation with clinical stage. Br J Haematol 1989;72:524–529.
23. Campana D, Yokota S, Coustan-Smith E, Hansen-Hagge TE, Janossy G, Bartram CR. The detection of residual acute lymphoblastic leukemia cells with immunologic methods and polymerase chain reaction: a comparative study. Leukemia 1990;9:609–614.
24. Keating MJ, Kantarjian H, Talpaz M, et al. Fludarabine: a new agent with major activity against chronic lymphocytic leukemia. Blood 1989;74:19–25.

25. Schilling PJ, Vadhan-Raj Saroj. Concurrent cytomegalovirus and pneumocystis pneumonia after fludarabine therapy for chronic lymphocytic leukemia. N Engl J Med 1990;323:833–834.

26. Boldt DH, Von Hoff DD, Kuhn JG, Hersh M. Effects on human peripheral lymphocytes of in vivo administration of 9-B-D-arabinofuranosyl-2-fluoroadenine-5'-monophosphate (NSC 312887), a new purine antimetabolite. Cancer Res 1984;44:4661–4666.

27. Piro LD, Carrera CJ, Beutler E, Carson DA. 2-Chlorodeoxyadenosine: an effective new agent for the treatment of chronic lymphocytic leukemia. Blood 1988;72:1069–1073.

28. Piro L, Carrera CJ, Carson D, Beutler E. Lasting remissions in hairy-cell leukemia induced by a single infusion of 2-chlorodeoxyadenosine. N Engl J Med 1990;322:1117–1121.

29. Liepman N, Votaw ML. The treatment of chronic lymphocytic leukemia with COP chemotherapy. Cancer 1978;41:1664–1669.

30. Oken MM, Kaplan ME. Combination chemotherapy with cyclophosphamide, vincristine and prednisone in the treatment of refractory chronic lymphocytic leukemia. Cancer Treat Rep 1979;63:441–447.

31. Montserrat E, Alcala A, Parody R, et al. Treatment of chronic lymphocytic leukemia in advanced stages: a randomized trial comparing chlorambucil plus prednisone vs cyclophosphamide, vincristine and prednisone. Cancer 1985;56:2369–2375.

32. Kempin S, Lee BJ III, Koziner B, et al. Combination chemotherapy of advanced chronic lymphocytic leukemia: the M-2 protocol (vincristine, BCNU, cyclophosphamide, melphalan and prednisone). Blood 1982;60:1110–1121.

33. Scouros M, Murphy S, Hester J. Complete remission (CR) in chronic lymphocytic leukemia (CLL) treated with combination chemotherapy [Abstract]. Proc Am Soc Clin Oncol 1980;21:441.

34. Keating MJ, Scouros M, Murphy S, et al. Multiple agent chemotherapy (POACH) in previously treated and untreated patients with chronic lymphocytic leukemia. Leukemia 1988;2:157–164.

35. French Cooperative Group on Chronic Lymphocytic Leukaemia. Long-term results of the CHOP regimen in stage C chronic lymphocytic leukaemia. Br J Haematol 1989;73:334–340.

36. Heublein AC. Preliminary report on continuous irradiation of entire body. Radiology 1932;18:1051–1060.

37. Sawitsky A, Ray KR, Aral I, et al. Mediastinal irradiation for chronic lymphocytic leukemia. Am J Med 1976;61:892–896.

38. Byhardt RW, Brace CK, Wiernik PM. Role of splenic irradiation in chronic lymphocytic leukemia. Cancer 1975;35:1621–1625.

39. Richards F II, Spurr CL, Pajak TF, Blake DD, Rabeu M. Thymic irradiation. An approach to chronic lymphocytic leukemia. Am J Med 1974;57:862–869.

40. Duchesne GM, Harmer CL. Hemibody irradiation in lymphomas and related malignancies. Int J Radiat Oncol Biol Phys 1985;11:2003–2006.

41. Osgood EE. Relative dosage required of total body x-ray versus intravenous p32 for equal effectiveness against leukemic cells of lymphocytic and granulocytic series in chronic leukemia. Nucl Med 1961;6:421–432.

42. Chanana AD, Cronkite EP, Rai KR. The role of extracorporeal irradiation of blood in the treatment of leukemia. Int J Radiat Oncol Biol Phys 1976;1:539–548.

43. Radiotherapy for chronic lymphatic leukaemia [Editorial]. Lancet 1979;1:82–83.

44. Rubin P, Bennett JM, Begg C, Bozdech MJ, Silber R. The comparison of total body irradiation versus chlorambucil and prednisone for remission induction in active chronic lymphocytic leukemia. An ECOG study: Part I: total body irradiation-response and toxicity. Int J Radiat Oncol Biol Phys 1981;7:1623–1632.

45. Johnson RE. Treatment of chronic lymphocytic leukemia by total body irradiation alone and combined with chemotherapy. Int J Radiat Oncol Biol Phys 1978;5:159–164.

46. Nakamura Y, Gillilan S, O'Connel P, Lathrop GM, Lalouel JM, White R. Isolation and mapping of a polymorphic DNA sequence pYNH244 on chromosome 2 (D2S44). Nucleic Acids Res 1987;15:10073–10077.

47. Tura S, Cavo M, Gobbi M, et al. High-dose chemoradiotherapy and allogeneic bone marrow transplantation in multiple myeloma. Eur J Haematol 1990;43(suppl 51):191–195.

48. Gale R, Bortin MM, Van Bekkum DW, et al. Risk factors for acute graft-versus-host disease. Br J Haematol 1987;67:397–406.

High-Dose Therapy, Autologous Stem Cells, and Hematopoietic Growth Factors for the Management of Multiple Myeloma

Sundar Jagannath, David Vesole, and Bart Barlogie

Until recently, patients with multiple myeloma were not considered for intensive-dose regimens because of their usually advanced age and frequently incapacitated clinical condition. Oral melphalan and prednisone had been the mainstay of treatment, effecting remissions in approximately 40% of patients and a median survival duration not exceeding 3 years (1). Complete remissions occurred in no more than 10% of patients; about 5% survived 10 years, typically when tumor burden at diagnosis was low and initial tumor cytoreduction profound (2, 3).

Past clinical trials had evaluated whether additional alkylating agents and anthracyclines could improve disease control and extend survival. Although individual drug doses were relatively low and thus myelosuppression usually mild, such combination regimens were not superior to melphalan and prednisone (4).

DOSE-RESPONSE EFFECTS IN MULTIPLE MYELOMA

Dose-response questions had not been addressed in myeloma until the development of the VAD regimen and trials with high-dose melphalan administered intravenously. The VAD regimen, combining continuous infusions of standard doses of vincristine and adriamycin together with frequent pulses of high doses of dexamethasone, represented the first attempt to overcome drug resistance by increasing markedly the dose intensity of glucocorticoids (5). The result was impressive in that about 50% of patients with alkylating-agent-resistant myeloma achieved marked and speedy tumor cytoreduction, typically by 75%–90%. Dexamethasone alone was equally effective in patients with primary refractory disease, although VAD induced more frequent remissions in relapsing patients (6). VAD as initial therapy for untreated myeloma induced responses in 60%–70% of patients and in up to 80% among those presenting with low tumor mass (7, 8).

McElwain et al. were the first to evaluate efficacy and toxicity of a single high dose of intravenously administered melphalan (140 mg/m^2) without hematopoietic stem cell support (9). The marked antitumor activity also in refractory myeloma prompted additional high-dose therapy studies (10–13). Remission rates (≥75% reduction in myeloma protein production and disappearance of Bence

Jones proteinuria) increased with melphalan dose intensity and especially with added total body irradiation (TBI), from 34% to 72%; the corresponding complete remission rates were 4% and 11%, respectively (Table 37.1). Relapse-free survival duration was extended from a median of 3 months after melphalan at 70 mg/m^2 to 12 months following chemoradiotherapy with melphalan and TBI; the overall median survival was prolonged from 4 to 12 months. Despite a marked increase in cytotoxic dose intensity, autologous bone marrow support prevented a further increase in treatment-related mortality, which was in fact eliminated in a recent trial with melphalan at 200 mg/m^2 and combined marrow and blood stem cell grafts as well as hematopoietic growth factor support (Table 37.1).

HIGH-DOSE PREPARATIVE REGIMENS

Considering the potentially lethal toxicity associated with intensive therapy, cytotoxic regimens should be maximally effective. Among the alkylating agents investigated extensively in refractory myeloma, melphalan was superior to cyclophosphamide at maximum tolerated doses and equally effective as the CBV regimen with added carmustine and etoposide, requiring hematopoietic stem cell support (Table 37.2). Because of its hematopoietic stem cell-sparing properties, cyclophosphamide can be administered at maximum tolerated doses of 6–7 gm/m^2 and

can even be combined with etoposide at 1.8 gm/m^2 with profound but not protracted myelosuppression and in fact predictably rapid hematologic recovery. The associated hematopoietic stem cell mobilization can be further augmented by granulocyte-macrophage colony-stimulating factor (GM-CSF) and has hence been used successfully for blood stem cell apheresis.

Among TBI-containing trials, melphalan was superior to thiotepa, producing more complete and durable remissions, especially among patients receiving consolidation therapy in remission from prior standard dose therapy (Table 37.3, Fig. 37.1).

ROLE OF TOTAL BODY IRRADIATION

TBI in combination with alkylating agents (cyclophosphamide, melphalan, thiotepa) can effect cure in several hematologic malignancies (14). In myeloma, strictly defined complete remissions (by immunofixation) were obtained more frequently with melphalan (140 mg/m^2) and TBI (850 cGy) than with a single course of melphalan alone at a higher dose of 200 mg/m^2, although remission durations and survival times were comparable (Table 37.4). The Royal Marsden group reported a 50% complete response rate when melphalan 200 mg/m^2 was applied after induction therapy with VAMP (vincristine, adriamycin, methylprednisolone) (15). Trials are currently underway to determine whether

Table 37.1. Melphalan Dose Escalation in Refractory Myeloma[a]

Melphalan Dose (mg/m^2)	Graft	N	%ED	%R	%CR	Median Months RFS	Median Months SURV
70	—	23	26	34	4	3	4
90–100	—	45	20	38	7	5	8
140	ABMT	8	13	63	0	4	8
200	ABMT + PSCT + GM-CSF	14	0	50	0	7	12
140 + TBI	ABMT	18	28	72	11	12	12

[a]Abbreviations: %ED, percent early death within 2 months from treatment; %R, percent response, ≥75% tumor cytoreduction; %CR, percent complete response, no monoclonal protein by immunofixation; RFS, relapse-free survival; SURV, overall survival; ABMT, autologous bone marrow transplant; PSCT, autologous peripheral blood stem cell transplant.

Table 37.2. Efficacy of Different Alkylating Agents in Refractory Myeloma[a]

Regimen	N	Graft	%ED	%R	%CR
Cyclophosphamide					
6 gm/m²	23	—	4	17	0
CBV[b]	11	PSCT	18	36	0
Melphalan ≤ 100 mg/m²	68	—	22	37	6

[a]See Table 37.1 for abbreviations.
[b]CBV = cyclophosphamide 6 gm/m², carmustine (BCNU) 300 mg/m², etoposide (VP16) 750 mg/m².

Table 37.3. Melphalan or Thiotepa with TBI in Responsive Myeloma[a]

TBI Regimen with	N	%ED	%R	%CR	RFS	p	SURV	p
Melphalan								
140 mg/m²	19	5	58	37	NR		NR	
						.002		.08
Thiotepa								
750 mg/m²	15	0	47	13	8		23	

Median Months header spans RFS, p, SURV, p.

[a]See Table 37.1 for abbreviations; NR, median not reached.

"tandem transplants" with melphalan alone at 200 mg/m² may provide superior antitumor effect to TBI-containing regimens at markedly reduced toxicity. Busulfan-cyclophosphamide combinations have been used successfully with allogeneic marrow transplantation in myeloma, but autografting experience is limited (16).

TIMING OF BONE MARROW TRANSPLANTATION

Timing of high-dose therapy has proven critical for the long-term prognosis of patients with lymphoma and acute leukemia (17–19). In multiple myeloma, melphalan and TBI effected longer remissions and survival times when applied for response consolidation rather than as salvage therapy (Fig. 37.2) (20).

BONE MARROW PURGING

With autologous transplantation for hematologic malignancies, disease relapse may originate from tumor cells present in auto-

grafts or from expansion of residual tumor cells remaining in the patient despite high-dose therapy. The nature of relapse after autografting can only be determined with the help of genetic marker studies. In myeloma, most tumor cells are terminally differentiated B cells with low proliferative potential (1). Using autografts with up to 30% plasma cells, remission and survival times were not affected adversely by increasing proportions of tumor cells in the harvested bone marrow, regardless whether transplants were performed for sensitive or resistant myeloma (20). In vitro purging with B cell monoclonal antibodies with rabbit complement (21), immunotoxin conjugates (22), or 4-hydroperoxycyclophosphamide (23) did not compromise hematopoietic engraftment among small groups of patients studied to date. However, relapses have occurred within 6 months of bone marrow transplantation applied in remission, with or without purging, suggesting that the removal of tumor cells from autografts may not be critical in preventing relapse.

PROGNOSTIC FACTORS WITH HIGH-DOSE THERAPY FOR MULTIPLE MYELOMA

Considering the potential for marked toxicity from intensive therapy, assessment of favorable and adverse prognostic factors is important. Hence, clinical and laboratory variables were examined pertaining to host features (age, performance status), disease variables (time from diagnosis, β-2-microglobulin, lactic dehydrogenase (LDH), immunoglobulin isotype, responsiveness or resistance to standard doses of therapy), and treatment regimen (lower versus higher intensity regimens with TBI or high-dose melphalan at 200 mg/m²) (Table 37.5). Early mortality was highest among patients exhibiting unfavorable parameters such as poor performance (Zubrod >1), age >50 years, and high tumor mass (Tables 37.5, and 37.6). Complete remission was highest when high-

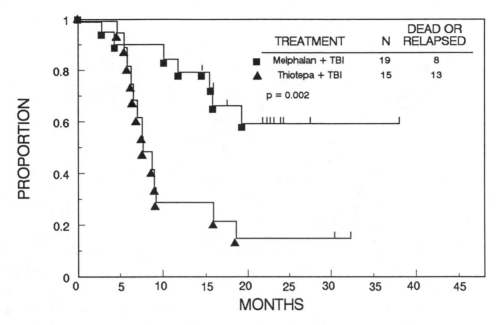

Figure 37.1. Response consolidation with chemoradiotherapy and marrow autografts was more effective when TBI was combined with melphalan rather than with thiotepa (p = .002).

Table 37.4. Role of TBI in Multiple Myeloma[a]

Disease Status	Regimen	N	%ED	%R	%CR	Median Months RFS	SURV
Sensitive	Melphalan 140 mg/m² +TBI 850 cGy	19	5	58	37	NR	NR
	Melphalan 200 mg/m²	11	0	55	0	NR	NR
Resistant	Melphalan 140 mg/m² +TBI 850 cGy	18	28	72	11	12	12
	Melphalan 200 mg/m²	14	0	50	0	7	12

[a]See Table 37.1 for abbreviations; NR, median not reached.

intensity regimens were applied for responsive rather than resistant disease. Relapse-free and overall survival shortened progressively as the number of adverse parameters present prior to intensive therapy increased (Table 37.6). Among 45 patients receiving high-intensity therapy for responsive myeloma, the degree of further cytoreduction (especially attainment of complete remission) did not influence relapse-free and overall survival durations. Whether the persistence of monoclonal gammopathy noted posttransplantation reflects residual myeloma or the reestablishment of a preceding benign disorder such as monoclonal gammopathy of undetermined significance (MGUS) awaits further follow-up (1). A multivariate analysis was carried out to define the parameters most significantly associated with early mortality, attainment of complete remission, as well as relapse-free and overall survival durations (Table 37.7). Mortality within the first 2 months after transplantation was highest among patients with poor performance. A low β-2-microglobulin level was the single most favorable parameter for achieving complete remission as well as for extended relapse-free and overall survival. A low level of LDH was

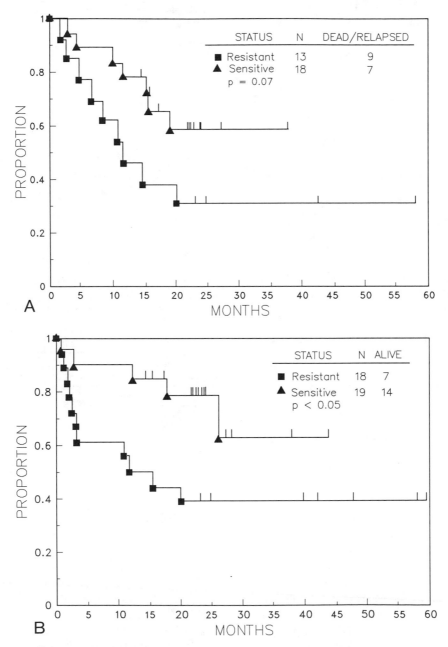

Figure 37.2. Relapse-free survival (**A**) and overall survival (**B**) was significantly longer among patients receiving melphalan 140 mg/m² and TBI 850 cGy for remission consolidation treatment ("sensitive") than for salvage of refractory disease ("resistant").

Table 37.5. Prognostic Factors with High-Dose Therapy[a]

Parameter	N	%ED	%R	(%CR)	Median Months			
					RFS	p	SURV	p
Age (years)								
<50	69	7	56	(10)	16	.001	28	.01
50–60	62	18	42	(11)	9		11	
>60	39	21	54	(3)	5		9	
Performance status								
≤1	128	9	51	(12)	10	.0001	24	.0001
>1	42	31	50	(0)	3		3	
β-2 microglobulin								
≤3.0 mg/liter	93	7	54	(12)	15	.0001	33	.0001
>3.0 mg/liter	77	22	47	(5)	4		6	
LDH								
≤250 U/liter	119	11	53	(7)	9	.04	23	.0001
>250 U/liter	51	22	45	(14)	5		6	
Light chain								
κ	104	12	53	(11)	9	.04	23	.009
λ	53	19	48	(6)	6		9	
Status at treatment								
Responsive	45	2	53	(20)	16	.0001	26	.0001
Resistant	125	18	50	(5)	6		1	
Intensity of therapy[b]								
High	80	8	59	(14)	15	.0001	25	.0001
Low	90	20	43	(4)	4		7	

[a]See Table 37.1 for abbreviations.
[b]High intensity: TBI with melphalan or thiotepa; melphalan 200 mg/m^2; low intensity: other regimens.

an additional independent feature associated with longer durations of relapse-free and overall survival. Using only these readily assessable laboratory parameters, three risk groups with good, intermediate, and poor prognosis could be defined according to whether none, one, or both variables were elevated (Fig. 37.3).

PERIPHERAL BLOOD STEM CELL PROCUREMENT IN MYELOMA

Gianni et al. reported on the usefulness of high doses of cyclophosphamide (7 gm/m^2) followed by GM-CSF administration to increase markedly the concentration of hematopoietic stem cells in peripheral blood of untreated patients with lymphoma (24, 25). Stem cell mobilization was accompanied by an increase in the proportion of CD34+ cells in the blood, which correlated closely with the concentration of hematopoietic progeni-

tor cells in the colony-forming units, granulocyte-macrophage (CFU-GM) assay (Fig. 37.4) (25). Sixty patients were treated with cyclophosphamide at 6 gm/m^2 initially without and in later stages with GM-CSF support (24 patients). Twenty-two patients had been diagnosed within 12 months, while the remainder had longer prior chemotherapy exposure. Peripheral blood stem cell mobilization was greatest among the 11 patients with limited prior drug exposure who also received GM-CSF; with longer time intervals from diagnosis or without GM-CSF, the stem cell yield after cyclophosphamide priming declined, reaching its lowest levels in the 25 patients who had been treated for more than 12 months and who did not receive GM-CSF (Table 37.8) Impairment in blood stem cell mobilization was also reflected in progressive delays in platelet recovery. Thus among the 37 patients recovering at least 50,000 platelets per microliter within 17 days, more

Table 37.6. Risk Factors for Outcome after High-Dose Therapy[a]

Number of Adverse Variables[b]	N	%ED	p	%R	%CR	p	Median Months			
							RFS	p	SURV	p
0 or 1	43	2	.07	56	21	.004	19	.0001	44+	.0001
2 or 3	77	13		53	6		7		20	
4 or 5	50	26		42	2		3		5	

[a]See Table 37.1 for abbreviations.
[b]β-2-microglobulin >3.0 mg/liter, age >50, resistant disease, lower intensity therapy (not TBI or melphalan 200 mg/m²), λ light chain.

Table 37.7. Prognostic Parameters with High-Dose Therapy, Multivariate Analysis

End point	Variable	p
Early death	Performance status >1	<.001
Complete response	β-2-Microglobulin ≤3.0 mg/liter	.002
	LDH ≤250 U/liter	.03
Relapse-free survival	β-2-Microglobulin ≤3.0 mg/liter	<.0001
	Age ≤50 years	<.0001
		<.0001
	Higher intensity of therapy	.04
	LDH ≤250 U/liter	
Survival	β-2-Microglobulin ≤3.0 mg/liter	<.0001
		<.0001
	Performance status <1	<.0001
	LDH ≤250 U/liter	.001
	Age ≤50 years	

than 80% had adequate stem cell mobilization as opposed to fewer than 20% among the 23 with delayed platelet recovery (*p* < .001).

PERIPHERAL BLOOD STEM CELLS IN SUPPORT OF HIGH-DOSE THERAPY

Peripheral blood stem cells have been used successfully as autografts in support of marrow-ablative therapy with or without TBI. Peripheral blood has been advocated as a preferred source of hematopoietic stem cells for malignancies arising in or having metastasized to the bone marrow. In the case of myeloma, circulating tumor cells have been detected in the blood even in early disease stages (1), although comparisons between marrow and blood concentrations of clonogenic tumor stem cells have not been performed. Reiffers and coworkers treated 24 recently diagnosed patients mainly with melphalan 140 mg/m² and added TBI (1050 cGy), of whom 17 received only blood and 7 both blood and marrow autografts (because of poor blood stem yield) (26). Thirteen patients achieved complete and 10 attained partial remission. Eighteen patients continue in complete or partial remission with a median follow-up of 17.5 months, regardless of disease stage prior to transplantation and the use of blood alone or blood combined with marrow stem cells.

Fermand et al. have treated 42 patients with limited prior therapy and sensitive disease; 22 patients received lomustine (CCNU) 120 mg/m², etoposide 75 mg/m², melphalan 140 mg/m², and TBI 1200 cGy, and 20 were treated, in addition, with cyclophosphamide (27). Blood stem cell autografts had been obtained during recovery from a brief drug-induced marrow aplasia using an intensive CHOP regimen with cyclophosphamide, doxorubicin, vincristine, and prednisone. Rapid recovery within 3 weeks was assured when more than 7.5 × 10⁴ CFU-GM per kilogram body weight had been transplanted. Twenty percent of patients attained complete remission. After a median follow-up of 26 months, 31 patients remained either in remission or with stable residual disease. The CBV regimen (as initially reported for Hodgkin's disease; 18) was evaluated with blood stem cell support in 11 patients with advanced and refractory myeloma. Four pa-

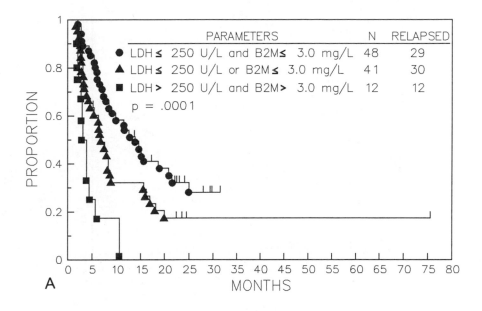

A

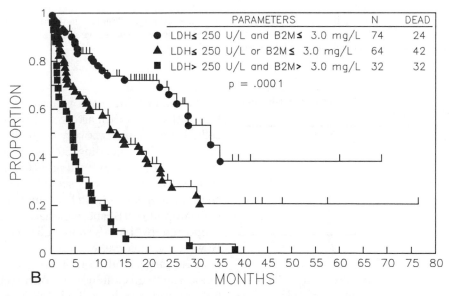

B

Figure 37.3. Pretreatment serum LDH and β-2-microglobulin levels distinguish risk groups for both relapse-free survival (**A**) and overall survival (**B**). The best clinical outcome was observed among patients with low levels for both parameters, and the highest risk pertained to patients with elevated levels of both LDH and β-2-microglobulin.

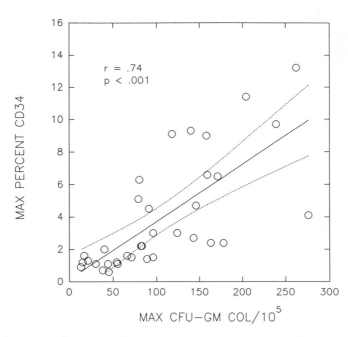

Figure 37.4. Correlation exists between in vitro CFU-GM colony growth and CD34 antigen expression by mononuclear blood cells after high-dose cyclophospha-mide and GM-CSF administration. Only the maximum values noted upon successive apheresis are indicated.

Table 37.8. Blood Stem Cell Mobilization with High-Dose Cyclophosphamide

Months from Diagnosis	GM-CSF		N	Percent of Patients	
				MAX CFU-GM $>50 \times 10^5$	MAX CD34+ $>2.0\%$
≤12	and	+	11	100	91
>12	or	−	24	61	56
>12	and	−	25	36	13
p				<.002	<.002

tients achieved partial remission (>75% cytoreduction) with a median relapse-free survival of 3 months and a median overall survival of all treated patients of 9 months.

Hematopoietic engraftment has been reported to proceed faster with blood than with bone marrow stem cells. A comparison was made between three groups of patients mainly with refractory myeloma who received either bone marrow autografts, blood stem cells, or both marrow and blood stem cells. Hematologic recovery to median granulocyte levels exceeding 500 per microliter and platelet levels exceeding 50,000 per microliter was about 4 weeks and hence similar among patients receiving bone marrow grafts with support of TBI and melphalan and those supported by blood stem cells after CBV. However, granulocyte recovery occurred about 1 week earlier with combined marrow and blood stem cells, often with concurrent GM-CSF support, which resulted in elimination of treatment-related mortality (see Table 37.1). When applied as first remission consolidation, the latter approach afforded engraftment within 14 days of transplantation (Fig. 37.5).

While the quality of blood stem cell procurement was largely determined by he-

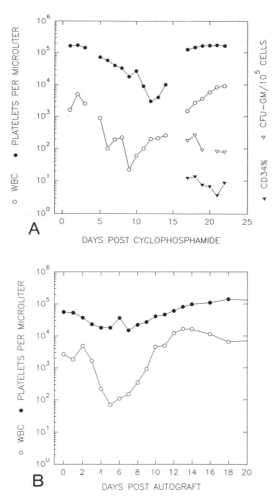

Figure 37.5. Blood stem cell mobilization (CD34, CFU-GM) after cyclophosphamide and GM-CSF (**A**). Rapid engraftment after melphalan 200 mg/m² and combined marrow and blood autograft plus GM-CSF (**B**).

matopoietic stem cell reserve, concurrent GM-CSF administration could partially offset the stem cell compromise in patients with more than 1 year of prior alkylating agent therapy (see Table 37.8). However, these two variables (duration of prior therapy and GM-CSF after cyclophosphamide) also influenced the recovery kinetics after melphalan at 200 mg/m² among 25 patients receiving both bone marrow and blood stem cells. The speed of platelet recovery after cyclophosphamide, which also correlated with the extent of blood stem cell mobilization, was another pretreat-

ment variable that predicted for platelet recovery after melphalan (Table 37.9). Thus when platelet levels of at least 50,000 per microliter were reached in less than 18 days after cyclophosphamide, engraftment proceeded within slightly more that 2 weeks; otherwise, platelet recovery was delayed to a median of over 2 months.

INTERFERON-α

Interferon-α has demonstrated antitumor activity in newly diagnosed patients pre-

Table 37.9. Post-Cyclophosphamide Platelet Recovery Reflects Hematopoietic Stem Cell Reserve

Post-Cyclophosphamide Platelet Recovery to >50,000/µl	N	Melphalan 200 mg/m² and Marrow Plus Blood Stem Cells, Median Days to	
		Granulocytes >500/µl	Platelets >50,000/µl
≤17 days	15	16	16
>17 days	10	21	75
p		.3	.006

senting with low-tumor-mass myeloma (29, 30). Beneficial effects have also been reported from interferon-α as maintenance therapy (31) and, together with combination alkylating agent therapy, for remission induction (32). These observations have prompted trials with interferon-α after transplantation. In a randomized trial of 48 patients induced with VAMP (methylprednisolone instead of dexamethasone in VAD), the Royal Marsden group reported only two relapses among 24 patients receiving interferon-α compared to nine among 20 patients followed on no treatment after high-dose melphalan at 200 mg/m² and autologous bone marrow transplantation (D Cunningham, unpublished observation).

REPEATED HIGH-DOSE THERAPY FOR RELAPSE

Twenty patients with advanced and refractory myeloma received a second course of high-dose therapy upon disease progression (33). The median time interval between the two treatments was 10 months, (range, 3–51 months). At least one cycle was supported by hematopoietic stem cells. Eight patients received autografts with both courses, 3 only with the first, and 9 with the second cycle. Eighty percent achieved >75% tumor cytoreduction with the first cycle (complete remission, 15%), and the median progression-free survival was 6 months; 75% responded to the second cycle with a median progression-free survival of 3.5 months. The overall median survival from the first high-dose therapy was 22 months.

PLANNED DOUBLE HIGH-DOSE THERAPY

Harousseau et al. had attempted administration of two cycles of high-dose melphalan (140 mg/m²) to increase the frequency of complete remission and extend relapse-free survival (34). In order to achieve in vivo purging, marrow stem cells were obtained after the first course of melphalan without autografting to be available in support of the second cycle of melphalan. Ninety-one patients from nine French centers received a first course of melphalan, including 50 receiving front-line therapy for stage III disease and 41 with relapsed or refractory myeloma in earlier disease stages. Of 67 responders, 31 received a second course with autologous bone marrow (24 patients) or with blood stem cells (7 patients). The preparative regimen consisted of melphalan at 140 mg/m² in 14 patients and was marrow-ablative in 17 patients (16 received TBI). Among all 91 patients, the median survival was 23 months with a projected 5-year survival rate of 38%, while the expected 5-year survival among the subset of newly diagnosed patients was 50%. Among the 31 transplanted patients, a 5-year survival rate of 44% was projected (median, 31 months) with a significantly superior outcome among newly diagnosed compared to previously treated and refractory patients (77% versus 11%, p = .02).

CONCLUSIONS

High-dose therapy induced marked tumor cytoreduction including some complete remissions even in advanced and refractory multiple myeloma. There was a steep dose-response effect for melphalan, which, as a single agent, appears superior to cyclophosphamide and thiotepa. Addition of TBI to melphalan increased the frequency of complete remission and the durations of relapse-free and overall survival. As in other malignancies, greater benefit was seen when high-dose therapy was applied in remission when tumor burden was low and resistance had not yet developed.

The median age of onset of myeloma is 65 years. If high-dose therapy is to play a significant role in the management of myeloma, patients up to the age of 70 should be eligible for such therapy. The use of growth factors in conjunction with autologous bone marrow and blood stem cell transplantation has made high-dose therapy safer and thus an option even for elderly patients. High-dose cyclophosphamide proved to be a useful in vivo tolerance test to determine hematopoietic stem cell reserve. Fast platelet recovery post cyclophosphamide was associated with efficient stem cell procurement and predicted for fast and complete hematologic reconstitution after transplantation. In the absence of treatment-associated mortality, high-dose cyclophosphamide may therefore help identify patients with poor stem cell reserve due to prior therapy, who should not be subjected to potentially fatal toxicities from marrow-ablative treatment. Once a preparative regimen with superior tumor cytoreduction has been identified (using single or double transplantation) and the tolerance of such therapy further improved (e.g., by marrow and blood stem cells with growth factor support), comparative trials will be required to determine whether high-dose therapy early in the disease course is justified by marked prolongation of disease-free and overall survival. Advances in the understanding of cellular and humoral factors involved in myeloma growth control (e.g., immunoglobulin binding factor and various cytokines) will provide exciting new opportunities for posttransplant immune modulation to achieve cure for multiple myeloma.

Acknowledgments

The authors grafefully acknowledge the excellent technical assistance of Kimberly Pruitt and the dedicated secretarial assistance of Emma Searcy and Rosemary Linder. Supported in part by CA37161-01 and CA23077 from the National Institutes of Health, Bethesda, Maryland.

REFERENCES

1. Barlogie B, Epstein J, Selvanayagam P, Alexanian R. Plasma cell myeloma: new biological insights and advances in therapy. Blood 1989;73:865–879.
2. Kyle RA. Long-term survival in multiple myeloma. N Engl J Med 1983;308:314–316.
3. Alexanian R. Ten year survival in multiple myeloma. Arch Intern Med 1985;145:2073–2074.
4. Boccadoro M, Marmont F, Tribalto M, et al. Multiple myeloma: VMCP/VBAP alternating combination chemotherapy is not superior to melphalan and prednisone even in high-risk patients. J Clin Oncol 1991;9:444–448.
5. Barlogie B, Smith L, Alexanian R. Effective treatment of advanced multiple myeloma refractory to alkylating agents. New Engl J Med 1984;310:1353–1356.
6. Alexanian R, Barlogie B, Dixon D. High dose glucocorticoid treatment for resistant multiple myeloma. Ann Intern Med 1986;105:8–11.
7. Samson D, Newland A, Kerney J, et al. Infusion of vincristine and doxorubicin with oral dexamethasone as first-line therapy for multiple myeloma. Lancet 1989;2:882–885.
8. Alexanian R, Barlogie B, Tucker S. VAD-based regimens as primary treatment for multiple myeloma. Am J Hematol 1990;33:86–89.
9. McElwain TJ, Powles RL. High-dose intravenous melphalan for plasma-cell leukemia and myeloma. Lancet 1983;1:822–823.
10. Selby P, McElwain TJ, Nandi AC, et al. Multiple myeloma treated with high dose intravenous melphalan. Br J Haematol 1987;66:55–62.
11. Barlogie B, Alexanian R, Smallwood L, et al. Prognostic factors with high dose melphalan for refractory multiple myeloma. Blood 1988;72:2015–2019.
12. Barlogie B, Jagannath S, Dixon D, et al. High dose melphalan and GM-CSF for refractory multiple myeloma. Blood 1990;76:677–680.
13. Barlogie B, Hall R, Zander A, Dicke A, Alexanian R. High dose melphalan with autologous bone marrow transplantation for multiple myeloma. Blood 1986;67:1298–1301.
14. Buckner CD, Fefer A, Bensinger WI, et al. Marrow transplantation for malignant plasma cell disorders: summary of the Seattle experience. Eur J Haematol 1989;43:(suppl 51):186–190.
15. Gore ME, Selby PJ, Viner C, et al. Intensive treatment of multiple myeloma and criteria for complete remission. Lancet 1989;2:879–885.
16. Bensinger WI, Buckner CD, Cliff R. Allogeneic marrow transplantation for multiple myeloma using busulfan and cyclophosphamide. Blood 1990;76(suppl 1):527a.
17. Philip T, Armitage JO, Spitzer G, et al. High dose therapy and autologous bone marrow transplantation after failure of conventional chemotherapy in

adults with intermediate grade or high-grade non-Hodgkin's lymphoma. N Engl J Med 1987;316:1493–1498.

18. Jagannath S, Armitage JO, Velasquez WS, Hagemeister FB. The role of bone marrow transplantation in management of Hodgkin's disease and non-Hodgkin's lymphomas. In Fuller LM, Hagemeister FB, Sullivan MP, Velasquez WS, eds. Hodgkin's disease and non-Hodgkin's lymphomas in adults and children. New York: Raven Press, 1988;440–450.

19. Gorin NC, Aegerter P, Auvert B, et al. Autologous bone marrow transplantation for acute myelocytic leukemia in first remission: a European survey of the role of marrow purging. Blood 1990;75:1606–1614.

20. Jagannath S, Barlogie B, Dicke KA, et al. Autologous bone marrow transplantation in multiple myeloma: identification of prognostic factors. Blood 1990; 76:1860–1866.

21. Anderson K, Barut B, Ritz J, et al. Monoclonal antibody purged autologous bone marrow transplantation for multiple myeloma. Blood 1991;77:712–720.

22. Gobbi M, Cavo M, Tazzari PL, et al. Autologous bone marrow transplantation with immunotoxin-purged marrow for advanced multiple myeloma. Eur J Haematol 1989;43(suppl 51):176–181.

23. Reece DE, Barnett MJ, Connors JM, et al. Intensive therapy with busulfan, cyclophosphamide and melphalan (bucy + mel) and 4-hydroperoxycyclophosphamide (4HC) purged autologous bone marrow transplantation (AUTOBMT) for multiple myeloma (MM) [Abstract]. Blood 1989;74:754a.

24. Gianni AM, Siena S, Bregni M, et al. Granulocyte-macrophage colony-stimulating factor to harvest circulating haemopoietic stem cells for autotransplantation. Lancet 1989;2:580–584.

25. Siena S, Bregni M, Brando B, Ravagnani F, Bonadonna G, Gianni AM. Circulation of CD34(+) hematopoietic stem cells in the peripheral blood of

high-dose cyclophosphamide-treated patients: enhancement by intravenous recombinant human granulocyte-macrophage colony-stimulating factor. Blood 1989;74:1905–1914.

26. Reiffers J, Marit G, Boiron JM, Autologous blood stem cell transplantation in high-risk multiple myeloma. Br J Haematol 1989;72:296–297.

27. Fermand JP, Levy Y, Gerota J, et al. Treatment of aggressive multiple myeloma by high-dose chemotherapy and total body irradiation followed by blood stem cell autologous graft. Blood 1989;73:20–23.

28. Ventura GJ, Barlogie B, Hester JP, et al. High dose cyclophosphamide, BCNU and VP-16 with autologous blood stem cell support for refractory multiple myeloma. Bone Marrow Transplant 1990;5:265–268.

29. Mellstedt, Bjorkholm M, Johansson B, Ahre A, Holm G, Strander H. Interferon therapy in myelomatosis. Lancet 1979;1:245.

30. Quesada JR, Alexanian R, Hawkins M, et al. Treatment of multiple myeloma with recombinant α-interferon. Blood 1986;67:275–278.

31. Mandelli F, Avvisati G, Amadori S, et al. Maintenance treatment with recombinant interferon α-2b in patients with multiple myeloma responding to conventional induction chemotherapy. New Engl J Med 1990;322:1430–1434.

32. Oken MM, Kyle RA, Greipp PR, Kay NE, Tsiatis A, O'Connell MJ. Alternating cycles of VBMCP with interferon (rIFN-α 2) in the treatment of multiple myeloma [Abstract]. Proc Am Soc Clin Oncol 1988;7:868a.

33. Jagannath S, Barlogie B. Repeated high dose therapy in refractory myelomatosis. In: Dicke K, Armitage J, Dicke-Evinger MJ, eds. Autologous bone marrow transplantation. Vol. 5. Omaha, NE: University of Nebraska Medical Center, 1990:571–580.

34. Harousseau JL, Milpied N, Garand R, Bourhis JH. High dose melphalan and autologous bone marrow transplantation in high risk myeloma. Br J Haematol 1987;67:493.

38

AUTOLOGOUS BONE MARROW TRANSPLANTATION FOR HODGKIN'S DISEASE

Julie M. Vose, Gordon L. Phillips, and James O. Armitage

With the use of MOPP (mechlorethamine, vincristine, procarbazine, and prednisone) (1), MOPP alternatives such as MVPP (mechlorethamine, vinblastine, procarbazine, and prednisone) (2) and ChlVPP (chlorambucil, vinblastine, procarbazine, and prednisone) (3), ABVD (doxorubicin, bleomycin, vinblastine, and decarbazine) (4), or hybrid regimens such as MOPP/ABV (5), the majority of patients with advanced Hodgkin's disease can now be cured of their disease. However, Hodgkin's disease can be primarily refractory or alternatively can relapse in a percentage of these patients. For those patients who were initially treated with MOPP alone who develop MOPP-resistant disease, the use of ABVD or similar combinations has resulted in a 20% 3-year disease-free survival (4). Patients with disease resistant to both MOPP and ABVD occasionally respond to third-line regimens; however, long-term disease-free survival is very uncommon with the administration of other conventional chemotherapeutic agents (6, 7). Approximately 7400 patients per year are diagnosed in the United States with Hodgkin's disease. Of these patients, 30% will ultimately fail therapy, and 80% of these patients will be under age 60 and eligible for transplant. With these estimates, approximately 1660 patients could poten-tially receive high-dose therapy with transplantation for relapsed Hodgkin's disease.

The success of high-dose therapy with bone marrow transplantation in other malignancies such as the non-Hodgkin's lymphomas, testicular carcinoma, and some acute leukemias has led to the use of this technique in patients with relapsed Hodgkin's disease who were thought to be incurable with conventional therapy. Experience utilizing this technique has greatly expanded over the last several years. The early studies have now allowed physicians to evaluate prognostic factors and to build on this knowledge in an attempt to improve clinical outcomes. This article will outline the clinical studies of bone marrow transplantation for Hodgkin's disease and discuss ongoing transplant studies as well as possibilities for future improvements in this area of transplantation.

AUTOLOGOUS BONE MARROW TRANSPLANTATION IN HODGKIN'S DISEASE: BACKGROUND

Many of the first transplant protocols for Hodgkin's disease utilized the CBV regimen (cyclophosphamide, carmustine [BCNU], and etoposide). These drugs are attractive due to the relatively low nonhematologic toxicity profile associated with their administration and because most Hodgkin's patients have not previously received these agents. The original CBV regimen developed by physicians at MD Anderson included cyclophosphamide 6 gm/m^2, carmustine 300 mg/m^2, and etoposide 750 mg/m^2 (8). Jagannath et al. (8) treated 30 heavily pretreated patients with the CBV protocol followed by autologous bone marrow transplantation. They reported a 50% complete response rate in this original patient population, with 1 patient in a remission of more than 44 months. In this heavily pretreated patient population there was a 7% toxic death rate.

A larger follow-up to this trial included patients treated with this protocol at the University of Nebraska Medical Center and the MD Anderson Cancer Center (9). In this series Bierman et al. evaluated 128 patients with relapsed Hodgkin's disease who were treated with the CBV regimen plus autologous bone marrow transplantation (ABMT) (9). Ten of the patients were in second or subsequent complete remission and received CBV and ABMT as consolidation therapy. Of the total 128 patients, 65 (51%) were in complete remission and 32 (27%) achieved partial remission after transplantation. An additional 7 patients received post-ABMT localized radiotherapy, with a complete response being obtained following the radiation. At the time of publication with a median follow-up of 21 months, 41 (32%) of the patients were alive in continuous complete remission following high-dose CBV and ABMT (9).

An augmented CBV regimen has been evaluated by investigators in Vancouver. In this regimen the cyclophosphamide dose has been increased by 20% to 7.2 gm/m^2, the carmustine increased 100% to 600 mg/m^2, and the etoposide increased by 300% to 2.4 gm/m^2 (10). This evaluation reported that 44 of the 56 patients (80%) achieved a complete remission, with 12 of 56 (21%) patients suffering a toxic death due to sepsis or interstitial pneumonia. With a median follow-up of 3.5 years (range 2.5–5.0 years), the event-free survival 5 years posttransplant is 47% (10). Although this augmented CBV regimen did have a higher complete remission rate (80%), compared with the lower-dose CBV regimen (51%) there was a higher toxic death rate (21% versus 7%). It is also difficult to compare the two studies due to differences in the patient population. In the University of Nebraska/MD Anderson study, the patients were for the most part heavily pretreated; however, in the Vancouver study most patients were in first relapse after having failed the MOPP/ABV hybrid regimen.

Many other regimens have subsequently been utilized for the treatment of relapsed Hodgkin's disease. Several studies have utilized high-dose melphalan in the preparative regimen. A study by Gribben et al. (11) evaluated 44 patients treated with the BEAM protocol (BCNU, etoposide, cytarabine, and melphalan). The complete response rate in this trial was 50%. With a median follow-up of 22 months, 20 of the 44 patients were alive without evidence of disease (11). Both the complete remission (CR) rate and the disease-free survival in this trial of the BEAM regimen are similar to those of the original CBV trials published. Another melphalan-containing regimen has been evaluated by Zulian et al. (12). The regimen of high-dose melphalan, BCNU, and etoposide with ABMT was utilized in this study for 38 patients with relapsed Hodgkin's disease. This regimen had a similar CR rate at 46%; however, there was a higher incidence of respiratory failure in this trial, with seven toxic deaths due to pulmonary toxicity (12). The disease-free survival in this trial was 31%, with a 12-month median follow-up. Several other transplantation conditioning regimens are outlined in Table 38.1.

Total body irradiation (TBI) has been utilized only in a few studies due to the fact that many Hodgkin's patients have already received thoracic radiation by the time they have reached the transplantation stage. Comparisons are difficult between the various studies

Table 38.1. ABMT for Hodgkin's Disease: Regimens and Results[a]

Ref.	Patients	Regimen	CR Rate	DFS (F/U)
8	30	CBV	50%	11 of 30 (3–44 mo.)
9	128	CBV	51%	32% (median 21 mo.)
10	54	CBV (augment)	80%	56% (median 15 mo.)
13	26	Cy/TBI	69%	27% (3.5–6.5 years)
14	14	Cy/ARA-C/TBI or Cy/ARA-C/VP	57%	7% (median 40 mo.)
11	44	BEAM	50%	20 of 44 (median 22 mo.)
12	38	MBE	46%	31% (median 12 mo.)
33	17	Cy/BCNU/ARA-C/6TG	53%	3 of 17 (25–66 mo.)
34	50	CBV	48%	45% (median 24 mo.)

[a]Abbreviations: CBV = cyclophosphamide, carmustine (BCNU), etaposide (VP-16); Cy/TBI = cyclophosphamide, total body irradiation; ARA-C = cytarabine; BEAM = BCNU, VP-16, cytarabine, melphalan; MBE = melphalan, BCNU, VP-16; 6TG = 6-thioguanine; CR, complete remission; DFS, disease-free survival; F/U, follow-up.

as the patient populations are very diversified. A report by Phillips et al. (13) evaluated 26 patients with progressive Hodgkin's disease after conventional chemotherapy who received high-dose chemoradiotherapy consisting of cyclophosphamide and TBI followed by ABMT. Eighteen of the 26 patients (69%) obtained a CR with this protocol. Seven of these patients were continuously disease-free with a median follow-up of 4.5 years (range 3.5–7 years). Three of the patients died of idiopathic interstitial pneumonitis—all had received previous localized mediastinal irradiation. Another study by Broun et al. (14) evaluated either (a) cyclophosphamide, cytarabine, and TBI or (b) cyclophosphamide, cytarabine, and Etoposide as the conditioning regimen in refractory lymphoma patients. In this study, the patients received the TBI-containing protocol if they had not had previous radiation therapy that precluded the use of TBI. If they had previously received the maximum radiation tolerated by vital organs, the patients received the chemotherapy-only regimen. Once again the CR rate was similar in this trial at 57%; however, the overall relapse-free survival was only 7% (14). Also very significantly, among patients receiving TBI, there were no survivors, and 4 of 5 early deaths were secondary to pulmonary complications.

It is difficult to compare these trials as the patient populations were very different, as well were the supportive care methods. Truly comparative studies are needed to evaluate different transplantation preparative regimens utilized for the treatment of relapsed Hodgkin's disease in order to choose the most effective method of preparation for transplantation.

PROGNOSTIC CHARACTERISTICS

Following the initial evaluation of high-dose chemotherapy with ABMT for the treatment of relapsed Hodgkin's disease, subsequent studies have focused on ways to improve on these initial results. In addition to the evaluation of different transplantation preparative regimens, the identification of patients for whom this procedure is likely to be beneficial has also been very important.

Jagannath et al. described the risk factors that influenced the overall response and survival when treated with CBV and ABMT for relapsed Hodgkin's disease (15). In this analysis, performance status, number of prior chemotherapies failed, and sensitivity to the last therapy all had a significant impact on the prognosis of the patients in this evaluation. The fact that extensive prior chemotherapy was an adverse determinant is probably related to the selective growth of drug-resistant tumor cells. Although high-dose chemotherapy can overcome some of this resistance, certainly the use of this method earlier in a patient's clinical course, before resistance becomes a problem, seems warranted.

A more recent evaluation of 70 patients treated at the University of Nebraska Medical Center treated for relapsed Hodgkin's disease using CBV followed by ABMT evaluated the optimal timing for transplantation. Thirty-six patients were transplanted "early" after only one or two previous chemotherapy regimens and with no site of bulky disease >10 cm. Thirty-four patients were transplanted "late" after three or more treatment regimens and/or had bulky disease >10 cm. Chemotherapy sensitivity was not able to be evaluated in all of the patients. The patients who were transplanted early had a CR rate of 69% (25 of 36) and an early death rate of 6% (2 of 36). With a median follow-up of 3 years, the 19 patients continuing in CR have a disease-free survival of 51% and the 3-year survival was 76%. In contrast, the patients transplanted late had a CR rate of 44% (15 of 34) and an early death rate of 18% (6 of 34), and the proportion of patients in CR at 3 years was 22%, with a 3-year overall survival of 38% (Fig. 38.1). This trial also confirmed that heavily pretreated patients did not benefit from transplantation to the same extent as patients who were transplanted at an earlier time in their disease course.

Several other studies have also evaluated the importance of prognostic factors for patients undergoing high-dose therapy and transplantation. The study by Gribben et al. (11) performed univariate and multivariate analysis on their population treated with the BEAM regimen. They found that the only important factor when the others were controlled for was the size of the tumor mass at ABMT. In the study by Phillips et al. (13) utilizing cyclophosphamide and TBI, a multivariate analysis showed that the Karnofsky score and the duration of disease were independent predicators of survival.

One very interesting study from Vancouver evaluated the risk factors of patients who were treated by several different methods including high-dose therapy and ABMT at the time of first relapse from their Hodgkin's disease (17). In this analysis, the presence or absence of any one of three risk factors had a strong negative impact on outcome: stage IV disease at primary diagnosis, B symptoms at relapse, or a time from primary treatment to relapse of less than 1 year. These risk factors were predictive of the outcome with conventional salvage therapy as well as high-dose chemotherapy with ABMT (17). The prognostic factors found important in the various studies are outlined in Table 38.2.

STRATEGIES TO IMPROVE AUTOLOGOUS BONE MARROW TRANSPLANTATION RESULTS FOR HODGKIN'S DISEASE

With the recognition that certain patient populations obtained a higher benefit with transplantation for Hodgkin's disease in the early trials, several concepts have been developed to try to improve the results in the good- and poor-prognosis groups. These include different chemotherapeutic agents included in the transplant preparative regimen, the use of sequential or "double" transplants, the addition of radiolabeled antibodies to standard transplant regimens, the utilization of allogeneic transplantation instead of autologous transplantation, or the use of he-

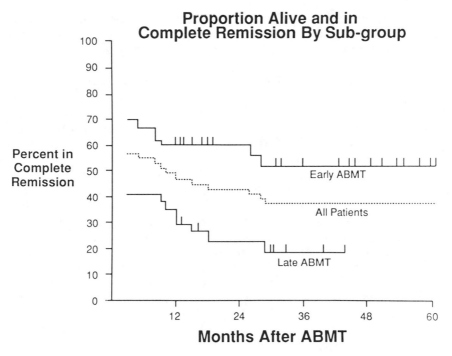

Figure 38.1. The three curves represent the patients continuing in CR for the early subgroup, late subgroup, and all treated patients. Tic marks on the curves represent patients continuing in CR to that interval. (Adapted from Vose JM, Bierman PJ, Armitage JO, et al. The importance of early autologous bone marrow transplantation (ABMT) in the management of patients (Pts) with Hodgkin's disease (HD). Proc ASCO 1990;9:256a.)

Table 38.2. Prognostic Factors for Transplantation in Hodgkin's Disease[a]

Reference	Regimen	Prognostic Factors
Jagannath (15)	CBV	Performance status
		Failed prior therapies ≥2
		Chemotherapy sensitivity
Vose (16)	CBV	Failed prior therapies ≥2
		Bulky disease ≥10 cm
Gribben (11)	BEAM	Tumor mass at ABMT
Phillips (13)	Cy/TBI	Performance status
		Disease duration

[a]See Table 38.1 for abbreviations.

Table 38.3. Strategies for Improvement of ABMT for Hodgkin's Disease

1. Changes in the preparative regimen:
   A. Chemotherapy only versus TBI containing
   B. Dose augmentation
   C. Newer chemotherapeutic agents added
2. Sequential transplantations
3. Radioimmunoconjugate added to the preparative regimen
4. Allogeneic versus autologous transplantation
5. Hematopoietic growth factor utilization
6. Peripheral stem cell transplantation

matopoietic growth factors to allow the escalation of drug doses safely (Table 38.3).

Alternate Chemotherapeutic Preparative Regimens

Several alternate chemotherapy programs have been utilized in an attempt to improve on the initial results of high-dose therapy and ABMT in this patient population. A few studies have utilized TBI-containing regimens. One such study by Phillips et al. (13) (discussed above) treated 26 patients with relapsed Hodgkin's disease utilizing a regimen of cyclophosphamide 60 mg/kg × 2 and TBI ranging from 1000 to 1400 cGy. The results with this regimen included six early transplant-related toxic deaths, with three of these from idiopathic interstitial pneumonitis on days +21, +34, and +132 (13). Overall at the time of the analysis, 10 of the 26 patients were alive and disease-free, with 7 of the 10 continuously disease-free. Another study that utilized TBI in some patients undergoing high-dose therapy and transplantation for Hodgkin's disease was reported by Broun et al. (14). In this analysis, patients who were eligible for a TBI-containing regimen received the TBI as part of their conditioning regimen. Alternatively, if the patients' prior radiation therapy prohibited the use of TBI, they received etoposide as a substitution in their transplant regimen. The overall survival at the time of the report was 21%, with only 7% of the patients surviving disease-free. There were no survivors among the patients receiving the TBI-containing regimen, with a majority of the patients treated with TBI dying of pulmonary complications (14).

There have also been several other studies of chemotherapy-only regimens. The BEAM regimen (BCNU 300 mg/m^2 day -6, etoposide 200 mg/m^2, and cytarabine 400 mg/m^2 on days -5 to -2, melphalan 140 mg/m^2 on day -1) has been utilized extensively in Europe. As discussed above, one analysis of 44 patients treated with this regimen was reported by Gribben et al. (11). Twenty-two patients (50%) entered CR within 6 months of the transplant, with only 2 patients having a subsequent relapse from CR at the time of the analysis. Only 2 patients died of sepsis during the aplastic phase of the transplant (4.5%). This regimen also utilized localized involved field irradiation following the transplant to sites of prior bulk disease. This allows the use of radiation therapy without the added toxicity of the TBI-containing regimens. Other chemotherapy-only protocols have been utilized with some success as well. Several of these are outlined in Table 38.1.

Sequential Transplantation

One approach to the high-risk Hodgkin's patient has been the use of double or sequential transplants. The strategy behind this concept consists of utilizing non-cross-resistant regimens in an attempt to overcome chemotherapeutic resistance to a greater extent. These studies have been carried out and reported by Ahmed et al. (18). In this group of studies, patients with sensitive relapses who were in CR after the first ABMT received no further treatment. However, patients who had evidence of residual disease by computerized tomography (CT) scan or biopsy following the first transplant, or who alternatively had poor prognostic features such as disease that was not sensitive to salvage therapy, failing > two prior regimens, or bone marrow involvement, were eligible to participate in a second sequential marrow transplant trial. The patients were transplanted with one of two potentially non-cross-resistant regimens that included thiotepa, cytarabine, and vinblastine (TAVe) or thiotepa, mitoxantrone, and carboplatin (TMJ).

In a recent analysis, 25 high-risk patients had undergone two sequential transplants as described (18). Twelve of the 25 had received the TAVe regimen, and 13 were treated with the TMJ regimen for the second transplant. Twelve of these 25 patients were alive in continuous CR with a follow-up of 40+ months. Ahmed then compared this group to a historical control group of poor-prognosis Hodgkin's patients who had undergone a single transplant and found that the sequential transplant group seemed to have a superior survival (18). There were 5 of 12 early transplant-related deaths with the TAVe regimen and 2 of 13 early deaths with the TMJ regimen as the second transplant regimen.

A sequential transplant may be beneficial in certain subsets of patients with Hodgkin's disease. Further analysis of the appropriate patient population to utilize this technique as well as analysis of the long-term follow-up data will be needed.

Radiolabeled Antibody Studies

A technique that has recently been developed for the treatment of Hodgkin's disease is the use of ratiolabeled antibodies. A trial at Johns Hopkins utilized yttrium-90-labeled antiferritin for the treatment of multiply relapsed Hodgkin's disease. They reported a 60% response rate with a mean response duration of 6 months (19). The dose-limiting side effect was hematologic toxicity. With this is mind, a program was developed to combine this radiolabeled immunoconjugate with high-dose therapy and bone marrow transplantation. In a pilot study, 11 poor-prognosis Hodgkin patients were treated with 20–30 mCi of yttrium-90-labeled antiferritin antibody, which was followed several days later with conventional high-dose CVB chemotherapy and bone marrow transplantation. This initial small study had promising results, with 5 of 8 evaluable patients achieving response to the treatment (20). The toxicity was not out of the expected range for this poor patient population. Further studies utilizing a dose escalation of the antibody and new linker methods as well as new antibody conjugates are ongoing.

Allogeneic versus Autologous Transplantation

Studies utilizing high-dose therapy with an allogeneic bone marrow transplant for acute leukemias and chronic myelogenous leukemia show evidence for an antitumor effect that is independent from that of the pretransplant cytotoxic therapy (21). The mechanisms responsible for this graft-versus-leukemia effect are not completely understood. A similar graft-versus-lymphoma effect may also exist; however, prospective randomized trials comparing the two are not available. One study by Phillips et al. (22) evaluated eight patients with refractory Hodgkin's disease who were treated with an allogeneic transplant. One of the eight patients was alive and free of progression 29 months after transplantation.

There have been a few nonrandomized trials comparing autologous and allogeneic transplantation for Hodgkin's disease. An early

nonrandomized study by Appelbaum et al. (23) did not demonstrate a survival advantage for lymphoma patients treated with allogeneic bone marrow transplant compared with autologous transplant. There was a trend toward a decreased relapse rate in the allogeneic patients; however, this was not statistically significant (23). In that study only a total of 18 Hodgkin's disease patients were treated (syngeneic = 2, autologous = 5, and allogeneic = 11). With these small numbers it is difficult to evaluate the role of allogeneic transplantation effectively in Hodgkin's disease. In a more recent study by Jones et al. (24), 118 consecutive patients with relapsed Hodgkin's disease or non-Hodgkin's lymphoma undergoing an autologous or an allogeneic transplant were evaluated. The overall results show a significant difference in the relapse rate between the allogeneic patients—actuarial probability of relapse 18%, compared to a 46% actuarial probability of relapse in the autologous group (24). However, this did not translate into a survival advantage as the allogeneic patients had a 47% actuarial event-free survival compared to a 41% actuarial event-free survival for the autologous transplant group (Fig. 38.2). Again in this trial there was a relatively small population of Hodgkin's patients (autologous = 20, allogeneic = 9).

Although both of these trials showed at least a hint of an advantage to the allogeneic transplant patients as far as decreasing the relapse rate, neither trial could show a difference in the event-free survival, probably due to increased transplant and graft-versus-host-disease related deaths in the allogeneic group. More cases of allogeneic transplantation for relapsed Hodgkin's disease have now been reported to the International Bone Marrow Transplant Registry and are under evaluation.

Because bone marrow contamination with Hodgkin's disease is a poor prognostic indicator in many trials, selection bias may be present in trials comparing transplantation methods utilized in patients with bone marrow contamination (i.e., allogeneic trans-

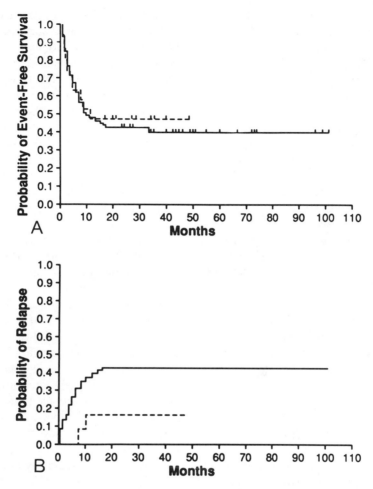

Figure 38.2. Actuarial probability of event-free survival (**A**) and relapse (**B**) in patients who underwent autologous bone marrow transplantation (*solid line*) and patients who underwent allogeneic bone marrow transplantation (dashed line) for lymphomas in sensitive relapse. (Reprinted with permission from Jones JR, Ambincler RF, Piantadouis, Santos S. Evidence of a graft-versus-lymphoma effect associated with allogeneic bone marrow transplantation. Blood 1991;77:649–653.)

plants or peripheral stem cell transplants) to the standard autologous transplantation techniques. A careful analysis of patient characteristics is necessary for a full evaluation of such studies.

Hematopoietic Growth Factor Utilization

With the utilization of hematopoietic growth factors, the dosages and types of drugs that can be utilized for high-dose therapy and transplantation may change. For example, the initial randomized trial utilizing GM-CSF with autologous transplantation demonstrated a 7-day decrease in hospitalization time as well as a significant decrease in infectious complications (25). With decreases in the transplant-related complications, myelosuppressive drugs may be dose escalated even higher. This dose escalation may translate into improved results as the drug resistance seen in rclapsed lymphoma is overcome. One study from MD Anderson specifically addressed the use of granulocyte colony-stimulating factor (G-CSF) to accelerate recovery after ABMT for Hodgkin's disease (26). In this study 18 patients who were undergoing high-dose CBV chemotherapy and ABMT were treated with G-CSF for a maximum of 28 days beginning on day 1 posttransplant. The G-CSF significantly accelerated the absolute granulocyte count (AGC) compared with historical controls, with recovery to 500 AGC per microliter at a median of 13 days compared to 22 days in historical controls (26). The platelet recovery was not significantly altered by the G-CSF administration. As with most other hematopoietic growth factor trials, few side effects were noted other than mild bone pain and myalgias.

Another possibility would be to utilize higher doses of therapy with growth factor support without the use of bone marrow for reconstitution. This has been tried in a few circumstances with some early success (27, 28). One study by Neidhart et al. (28) evaluated 24 patients who received chemotherapy regimens at doses that would normally need bone marrow transplantation support. Ten of the patients received G-CSF in a dose escalation study, while the other patients served as controls. The patients not receiving G-CSF had a median of 8.5 days of severe granulocytopenia. Those patients receiving 40 μg/kg of G-CSF had a median of 7.0 days of neutropenia, while the patients receiving 60 μg/kg of G-CSF had a median of 5.5 days of neutropenia ($p < .007$) (30). Recovery to a granulocyte count of at least 500 per cubic millimeter took a median of 12 days in the control group and 8 days in the patients receiving G-CSF at 60 mg/kg. In order to assess the most efficacious use of hematopoietic growth factors during transplantation, more studies will need to be undertaken in this new, exciting area of oncology.

Peripheral Stem Cell Transplantation

In patients who have bone marrow involvement with Hodgkin's disease, or who alternatively have had extensive pelvic irradiation, an autologous bone marrow harvest may not be possible. In these instances, autologous peripheral blood stem cell transplantation has been utilized to facilitate recovery following high-dose therapy. Several studies have now utilized this technique in the Hodgkin's disease population undergoing transplantation (29–31). Korbling et al. (29) evaluated 12 patients with relapsed Hodgkin's disease who were treated with CVB plus autologous peripheral stem cell transplantation. Of the 11 evaluable patients in this series, 7 are in unmaintained CR at a median disease-free follow-up of 318 days (29). These results compare favorably with published reports of Hodgkin's patients who were transplanted utilizing autologous bone marrow.

There may also be some additional benefits from utilizing autologous peripheral stem cells, as the natural killer (NK) cell activity in this product is at a high level (32). One study by Kessinger et al. (30) evaluated 56 Hodgkin's patients treated with CVB plus peripheral stem cell transplantation. In this study the patients were divided into two groups, those receiving a peripheral stem cell transplant due to bone marrow involvement with Hodgkin's disease (N = 26) and those with prior pelvic irradiation (N = 30). Of the subgroup with no marrow involvement, the actuarial event-free survival was 47% at 3 years (27). This compares favorably to published reports of Hodgkin's patients undergoing bone marrow transplantation with similar prognostic factors. Although this study does not directly address the role of NK cell activity in peripheral stem cell transplantation, this early analysis may hint at an advantage for peripheral stem cell transplantation in Hodgkin's patients. A prospective randomized trial will be needed to validate this information.

CONCLUSIONS

Despite the advances made in the primary therapy of Hodgkin's disease in the last 2 decades, a percentage of patients will fail to be cured. The strategy of high-dose therapy with autologous marrow rescue has now been evaluated in this clinical situation over the past decade. With the background evaluation completed in heavily pretreated patients, newer studies are now utilizing this promising therapy in patients more likely to benefit, such as those less heavily pretreated, those with less bulky disease, and in high-risk patients as part of their primary therapy. Over the next decade many of these will be evaluated, including the utilization of different preparative regimens, labeled antibody adjunctive therapy, sequential transplants, and peripheral stem cell techniques. It is hoped that the utilization of these newer techniques will increase the long-term disease-free survival among patients transplanted for Hodgkin's disease.

REFERENCES

1. DeVita VT, Serpick A, Carbone PO, et al. Combination chemotherapy in the treatment of advanced Hodgkin's disease. Ann Intern Med 1970;73:881–893.
2. Sutcliffe SB, Wrigley PF, Peto J, et al. MVPP chemotherapy regimen for advanced Hodgkin's disease. Br Med J 1978;1:679–685.
3. Vose JM, Bierman PJ, Anderson JR, et al. CHLVPP plus involved field irradiation for Hodgkin's disease: comparable results with less toxicity. Proc ASCO 1991;10:272a.
4. Bonadonna G, Zucali R, Monfardini S, et al. Combination chemotherapy of Hodgkin's disease with adriamycin, bleomycin, vinblastine, and imidazole carboxamide versus MOPP. Cancer 1975;36:252–259.
5. Klimo P, Connors JM. MOPP/ABV hybrid program: Combination chemotherapy based on early introduction of seven effective drugs for advanced Hodgkin's disease. J Clin Oncol 1985;3:1174–1182.
6. Tseng A, Jacobs C, Coleman CN, et al. Third-line chemotherapy for resistant Hodgkin's disease with lomustine, etoposide and methotrexate. Cancer Treat Rep 1987;71:475–478.
7. Hagemeister FB, Tannir N, McLaughlin P, et al. MIME chemotherapy (methyl-GAG, ifosfamide, methotrexate, etoposide) as treatment for recurrent Hodgkin's disease. J Clin Oncol 1987;5:556–561.
8. Jagannath S, Dicke DA, Armitage JO, et al. High-dose cyclophosphamide, carmustine, and etoposide and autologous bone marrow transplantation for relapsed Hodgkin's disease. Ann Intern Med 1986; 104:163–168.
9. Bierman PJ, Jagannath S, Dicke KA, et al. High dose cyclophosphamide, carmustine and etoposide (CBV) in 128 patients with Hodgkin's disease. Blood 1988; 72:239a.
10. Reece D, Barnett M, Connors J, et al. Intensive chemotherapy with cyclophosphamide, BCNU, and etoposide followed by autologous bone marrow transplantation for relapsed Hodgkin's disease. J Clin Oncol 1991;9:1871–1879.
11. Gribben JG, Linch DC, Singer DRJ, et al. Successful treatment of refractory Hodgkin's disease by high-dose combination chemotherapy and autologous bone marrow transplantation. Blood 1989;73:340–344.
12. Zulian GB, Selby P, Milan S, et al. High dose melphalan, BCNU and etoposide with autologous bone marrow transplantation for Hodgkin's disease. Br J Cancer 1989;59:631–635.
13. Phillips GL, Wolff SN, Lazarus HM, et al. Treatment of progressive Hodgkin's disease with intensive chemoradiotherapy and autologous bone marrow transplantation. Blood 1989;73:2086–2092.
14. Broun ER, Tricot G, Akard L, et al. Treatment of refractory lymphoma with high dose cytarabine, cyclophosphamide and either TBI or VP-16 followed by autologous bone marrow transplantation. Bone Marrow Transplant 1990;5:431–344.
15. Jagannath S, Armitage JO, Dicke KA, et al. Prognostic factors for response and survival after high-dose cyclophosphamide, carmustine and etoposide with autologous bone marrow transplantation for relapsed Hodgkin's disease. J Clin Oncol 1989;7:179–185.
16. Vose JM, Bierman PJ, Armitage JO, et al. The importance of early autologous bone marrow transplantation (ABMT) in the management of patients (Pts) with Hodgkin's disease (HD). Proc ASCO 1990;9:256a.
17. Lohri A, Barnett M, Fairey RN, et al. Outcome of treatment of first relapse of Hodgkin's disease after primary chemotherapy: identification of risk factors from the British Columbia Experience 1970 to 1988. Blood 1991;77:2292–2298.
18. Ahmed T, Ascensao JL, Feldman EJ, et al. Marrow transplantation for Hodgkin's disease: studies with sequential transplantation. Proc Fifth Int ABMT Sym 1991;5:487–499.
19. Vriesendorp HM, Herpst JM, Leichner PK, et al. Polyclonal yttrium-90 labeled antiferritin for refractory Hodgkin's disease. J Radiat Oncol Biol Phys 1989;17:815–819.
20. Bierman PJ, Vriesendorp HM, Vose JM, et al. High-dose chemotherapy and polyclonal yttrium-90 labeled antiferritin (Y-90) followed by autologous bone marrow transplantation (ABMT) for Hodgkin's disease (HD). Blood 1990;76:258a.
21. Butturini A, Bortin MM, Gale RP. Graft-versus-leukemia following bone marrow transplantation. Bone Marrow Transplant 1987;2:233–242.
22. Phillips GL, Reece DE, Barnett MJ, et al. Allogeneic marrow transplantation for refractory Hodgkin's disease. J Clin Oncol 1989;7:1039–1045.

23. Appelbaum FR, Sullivan KM, Buckner CD, et al. Treatment of malignant lymphoma in 100 patients with chemotherapy, total body irradiation, and marrow transplantation. J Clin Oncol 1987;5:1340–1347.

24. Jones RJ, Ambinder RF, Piantadosi S, Santos GW. Evidence of a graft-versus-lymphoma effect associated with allogeneic bone marrow transplantation. Blood 1991;77:649–653.

25. Nemunaitis J, Rabinowe SN, Singer JW, et al. Recombinant granulocyte-macrophage colony stimulating factor after autologous bone marrow transplantation for lymphoid malignancy: results of a multicenter randomized, double-blind, placebo controlled trial. N Engl J Med 1991;324:1773–1778.

26. Taylor KM, Jagannath S, Spitzer G, et al. Recombinant human granulocyte colony-stimulating factor hastens granulocyte recovery after high-dose chemotherapy and autologous bone marrow transplantation in Hodgkin's disease. J Clin Oncol 1989;7:1791–1799.

27. Fouillard L, Gorin NC, Paporte J, et al. Recombinant granulocyte-macrophage colony stimulating factor plus the BEAM regimen instead of autologous bone marrow transplantation. Lancet 1989;1:1460.

28. Neidhart J, Mangalik A, Kohler W, et al. Granulocyte colony-stimulating factor stimulates recovery of granulocytes in patients receiving dose-intensive chemotherapy without bone marrow transplantation. J Clin Oncol 1989;7:1685–1692.

29. Korbling M, Holle R, Haas R, et al. Autologous blood stem-cell transplantation in patients with advanced Hodgkin's disease and prior radiation to the pelvic site. J Clin Oncol 1990;8:978–985.

30. Kessinger A, Bierman PJ, Vose JM, Armitage JO. High-dose cyclophosphamide, carmustine and etoposide followed by autologous peripheral stem cell transplantation for patients with relapsed Hodgkin's disease. Blood 1991;77:2322–2325.

31. Lasky LC, Hurd DD, Smith JA, Haake R. Peripheral blood stem cell collection and use in Hodgkin's disease: comparison with marrow in autologous transplantation. Transfusion 1989;29:323–327.

32. Talpaz M, Spitzer G. Low natural killer cell activity in the bone marrow of healthy donors with normal natural killer cell activity in the peripheral blood. Exp Hematol 1984;12:629–632.

33. Philip T, Dumont J, Teillet F, et al. High dose chemotherapy and autologous bone marrow transplantation in refractory Hodgkin's disease. Br J Cancer 1986;53:737–742.

34. Carella AM, Congiu AM, Gaozza E, et al. High-dose chemotherapy with autologous bone marrow transplantation in 50 advanced resistant Hodgkin's disease patients: an Italian group report. J Clin Oncol 1988;6:1411–1416.

HIGH-DOSE THERAPY FOR THE TREATMENT OF NON-HODGKIN'S LYMPHOMA

A. H. Goldstone, A. K. McMillan, and R. Chopra

High-dose chemotherapy, with the use of stored autologous bone marrow to rescue the patient from otherwise lethal hematologic toxicity, began to be used in significant numbers of patients with non-Hodgkin's lymphoma (NHL) in the late 1970s (1, 2). The procedure was initially performed in apparently hopeless patients, for whom it offered the only prospect of cure, and there was therefore an inevitably high procedure-related toxicity. In the early 1980s the results of larger studies from collaborating, pioneering centers in cooperative groups began to suggest that remissions, if not cures, were possible (3). The end of this first stage of the development of the technique was signaled by the realization that the response to previous salvage chemotherapy was critical in determining outcome of autologous bone marrow transplantation (ABMT) (4). The second phase of evaluation of ABMT has been the presentation of the results from large single centers (5–8) and from the collection of data on over 900 patients by the European Bone Marrow Transplant Group registry of ABMT in lymphoma. The third and most recent stage is now underway with the Parma international randomized prospective study, which was commenced following the successful pilot study (9).

In the future, if ABMT does become a valuable part of the treatment of this disease, then its utilization earlier in the disease will have to be examined. For this to be successful more will have to be known about the identification of poor-prognosis patients at an early stage in the disease, and the procedure-related mortality will have to be reduced. The inevitable mortality rate for patients beyond first remission is around 10%, and we are not aware of any convincing data *yet* that this can be reduced by the use of recombinant hematopoietic growth factors.

CONVENTIONAL SALVAGE THERAPY FOR HIGH- AND INTERMEDIATE-GRADE LYMPHOMAS

The evidence of the success of regimens such as CHOP and its very many would-be replacements is that long-term survival is seen in a proportion of patients. This proportion in most studies with long follow-up is described as between 30% and 40%, with the initial stage, age, performance status, and histology of the patients being important in determining the outcome (10). The next generation of regimens, exemplified by MACOP-B (11), has not been reliably shown to be superior to CHOP when like cases are compared, and the results of several prospective trials of CHOP versus MACOP-B type regimens are eagerly awaited. Hence 60%–70%

of patients will either fail to remit or will relapse after first-line therapy. The outcome of conventional salvage therapy is best assessed by examining the three studies from the MD Anderson Hospital during the 1980s, which detail the results of the IMVP16, MIME, and DHAP regimens (12–14). The projected overall disease-free survivals were approximately 15% (at 12 months), <10% (at 2 years), and <10% (at 2 years) for the three trials, respectively. Even for the most recent regimen, DHAP, the disease-free survival (in the patients achieving complete remission [CR]) was still only about 25% at 2 years, with no sign of a plateau on the life table plot. Thus the long-term prognosis of conventional salvage therapy is grim.

THEORETICAL BASIS AND CHOICE OF HIGH-DOSE THERAPY CONDITIONING REGIMEN

The basic principles on which the practice of dose escalation is based were first proposed by Skipper et al. (15) from their experiments on the transplantable mouse leukemia L1210. They proposed that for a given tumor a particular dose of a chemotherapeutic drug will yield a certain number of logs reduction in the tumor cell burden; thus the tumor cell burden of the animal, or in the case of their experiments the initial inoculum, will determine whether the animal is "cured" by a certain dose. For example, if a 4-log reduction results in the residual number of tumor cells being 10^2, then no animals would be cured, but if there were 2 logs fewer cells to begin with then some animals would be expected to have all tumor cells eradicated. In addition, they suggested that dose escalation will result in a greater log kill and therefore may render some animals curable even with a greater initial inoculum. In a second paper (16) they discuss the importance of the mechanism of action of drugs; for example, single-dose escalation of a cell cycle–specific agent such as cytosine arabinoside does not result in greater cell kill because

the cells out of cycle will not be killed even at the higher dose level, whereas alkylating agents, radiation, and the nitrosoureas, which are non-cycle-specific, are most effective at the single highest tolerated dose. These experiments are based on a transplantable laboratory leukemia with a high growth fraction, and consideration of the different kinetics of human leukemias is necessary, but the fundamental principles remain as valid as when they were proposed over 20 years ago.

The choice of the drugs or radiation used in the conditioning regimen must be based on the mechanisms of action of the drugs rather than on their efficacy in the conventional dose treatment of a tumor. For example, the intercalating agents, which are probably the single most valuable component of primary lymphoma therapy, are of little value in the context of ABMT because of their dose-limiting cardiac toxicity. Similarly, for the reasons outlined above the cell-cycle-specific agents such as the vinca alkaloids are of limited value because they "miss" cells that are out of cycle. This leaves the non-cycle-specific drugs such as the alkylating agents and nitrosoureas, as well as total body irradiation, as the cornerstones of high-dose therapy. They are especially suitable since at conventional dose levels their dosage is limited by hematologic toxicity, so that with ABMT the doses can be escalated until other vital organ toxicity (e.g., to the gastrointestinal tract and lungs) become dose limiting.

These then are the theoretical considerations in the choice of drugs for the conditioning regimens. Unfortunately there are no good comparative data on the efficacy of differing regimens in practice. Unlike Hodgkin's disease, relatively few patients have received radiation as part of their first-line treatment, so total body irradiation is available as an option. The impression from the published literature and the EBMTG register is that regimens that are "more intensive" within the context of the high doses used in ABMT procedures may increase the remission rate but that this is often offset by a higher early death rate caused by nonhematologic toxicity, especially from interstitial pneumonitis. There is current interest as to whether myelopoietic growth factors may exert a protective effect on the host, enabling further dose escalation without concomitant toxicity.

REPORTED RESULTS OF HIGH-DOSE THERAPY AND AUTOLOGOUS BONE MARROW TRANSPLANTATION IN NON-HODGKIN'S LYMPHOMA

An effective assessment of the outcome of ABMT from a review of the literature is made difficult by the number of variables that can alter the expected outcome. Most important of these is the selection of patients to be included in any given study; for example, with the increasing acceptance of the value of treating patients with responding disease, it has become the policy of some institutions to exclude more resistant or refractory patients from ABMT. The results reported by these centers therefore are apparently superior to those reporting unselected series; for example, Colombat et al. (17) and Freedman et al. (18) report projected disease-free survivals at 3 years of 60% and 50%, respectively, for chemosensitive patients. Other variables of possible significance include histology, stage at ABMT, and conditioning regimen.

Another confounding feature of reported series is the decision to report together series that include both patients with NHL and those with Hodgkin's disease, especially as it is not always possible from results sections to establish the separate outcome of patients in these different groups. In particular, our own experience has been that the prognostic significance for outcome of disease status at ABMT in NHL cannot always be extrapolated to Hodgkin's disease and so joint series must now be regarded as inappropriate. Table 39.1 shows the results of various unselected series that have been published in the major journals.

For the reasons discussed above, there is little more to conclude from these studies other than the general conclusion that long-term remissions can be achieved in apparently otherwise "incurable" patients, and that apparently the chance of such a remission is closely related to chemoresponsiveness at the time of referral for ABMT. Thus there is a need to proceed with randomized prospective trials to confirm these views.

DATA FROM THE EUROPEAN BONE MARROW TRANSPLANT GROUP REGISTRY FOR AUTOLOGOUS BONE MARROW TRANSPLANTATION IN LYMPHOMA (1991)

The results of ABMT in patients that have been reported to the European Bone Marrow Transplant Group's (EBMTG) registry for ABMT in lymphoma give further corroboration to these views. To January 1991, 938 patients with NHL had been reported to the registry. Two hundred and fifty patients underwent ABMT in first remission and 688 were beyond first remission at the time of ABMT. The overall survival for the latter group at 6 years is 37% (Fig. 39.1). The response to ABMT again shows that patients with disease that is chemoresponsive (partial responders or responding relapse) at the time of ABMT have a satisfactory outcome (42% overall survival), but patients with chemoresistant disease have only a 20% chance of long-term survival (Fig. 39.2). Nevertheless, this still means that further dose escalation may nonetheless benefit 1 of 5 patients with chemoresistant disease. This is, however, contrary to our own, single-center experience with 50 patients undergoing BEAM and ABMT in which we have seen no long-term survivors in patients who were truly chemoresistant to salvage therapy prior to ABMT (19).

Table 39.1. Single-Center Reports of Unselected Series Published in Peer-Reviewed Journals[a]

Center	High-dose Therapy	No. of Patients	Early Deaths	Outcome
Seattle (52) DFS (Includes 20 Hodgkin's patients)	Various	101	21%	11% at 5 years
UCH, London (5)	BEAM BEAC UCH 1	50	20%	OS 26% at 4 years
Omaha (7)	Various	41	19.5%	T cell: 28% B cell:17% DFS at 2 years 28%
Boston (8)	CBV	28	10%	13 of 28 alive at 9 months DFS 41%
Iowa (53)	BVAC	21	50%	2.5 years
New York (54)	Cyclo/TBI	17	29%	DFS 22% at 3 years

[a]Abbreviations: DFS, disease-free survival; OS, overall survival.

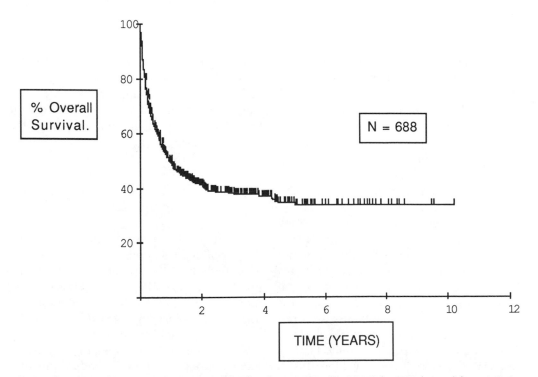

Figure 39.1. Overall survival of patients reported to the EBMTG after ABMT for NHL beyond first remission.

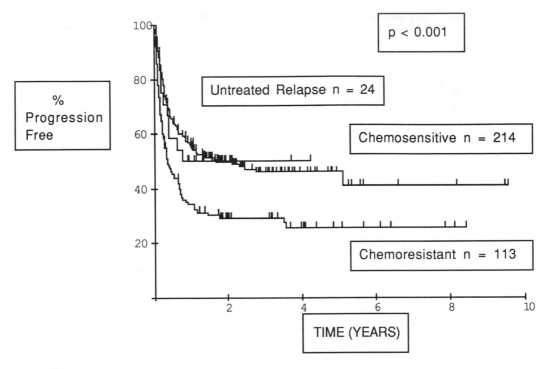

Figure 39.2. Progression-free survival after ABMT for NHL by status at ABMT.

Indeed, when the registry data are examined closely, it appears that the patients with primary refractory disease have a better prognosis than those with relapsed and resistant disease (Fig. 39.2). We suspect that this may indicate misclassification of some patients on the registry. The most likely explanation of this is that some patients with residual masses are labeled as primary refractory when there is no active disease present. This phenomenon is well recognized in lymphoma therapy (20, 21). Analysis of the recent LNH 84 trial of 737 patients receiving front-line chemotherapy shows that 150 of 533 (27%) patients achieving a CR had computerized tomography (CT) scan abnormalities (22). The status of such patients could only be assessed retrospectively. Retrospective reappraisal of the status at ABMT of the patients on the EBMTG registry is therefore necessary (and this is being currently undertaken), before final conclusions about the chemoresistant group

can be drawn. The EBMTG data confirm the conclusions from other centers that the procedure-related mortality from high-dose chemotherapy and ABMT varies according to the patient status at the time of transplantation (see Table 39.2).

AUTOLOGOUS VERSUS ALLOGENEIC BONE MARROW TRANSPLANTATION

The relative roles of ABMT and allogeneic bone marrow transplantation (alloBMT) after high-dose therapy are not clearly defined. There have been few reports of significant numbers of patients undergoing allogeneic transplantation in NHL (6, 23, 24). One of these studies in particular has suggested a graft-versus-leukemia (GVL)-like effect (23), but this study looked at a mixture of histologies and included patients with Hodgkin's disease as well as NHL. In addition

Table 39.2. Procedure-Related Mortality in NHL by Status at ABMT (n = 938) (EBMTG 1991)

Status at ABMT	Procedure-Related Mortality
First remission	7%
Chemo-responsive (2 CR, partial response, responding relapse)	14%
Chemo-resistant (primary refractory or resistant relapse)	23%

they gave no information about the distribution of histologies in the patients with NHL between the allogeneic and autologous groups, and in any case the number of patients in each histologic subgroup must have been small and may not therefore have afforded a meaningful conclusion.

Our group has carried out a direct comparison between the patients reported to the EBMTG allogeneic and autologous bone marrow transplant registries (Chopra et al., in preparation). A major problem in making a comparison between ABMT and AlloBMT in lymphoma is that the distribution of status and histology in the patients undergoing alloBMT or ABMT is not comparable. For example, the EBMTG allogeneic registry has a preponderance of children and patients with lymphoblastic lymphoma in first remission. Furthermore, a greater proportion of patients undergoing alloBMT have received total body irradiation as their conditioning therapy. The autologous registry, on the other hand, is based mainly on adult patients with intermediate- and high-grade lymphoma treated in relapse. With the increasing numbers of patients being reported to the two registries, it is now possible to carry out a case-controlled study by comparing the 101 NHL allografted patients on the EBMTG allogeneic registry with the closest matched 101 patients of the 938 autografted patients on the EBMTG autologous registry, taking account of those factors deemed to be most prognostically important by multivariate analysis for outcome after autologous or allogeneic transplantation. By carrying out this matching process

using the main prognostic factors, namely, status at transplant, stage at transplant, histology, and conditioning therapy, we were also able to match for age, sex, and length of time between diagnosis and transplantation. The results show that there is no difference in the progression-free survival in this closely matched group of patients between ABMT and alloBMT, for all histologic categories of NHL. The number of patients evaluated with Burkitt's lymphoma and low-grade NHL makes any meaningful conclusion in this small group very difficult. In the group of patients with intermediate- and high-grade NHL, although the procedure-related mortality is significantly higher for the alloBMT group, the relapse and progression rates are similar. In the lymphoblastic lymphoma patients, the relapse and progression rates are greater for the ABMT patients (48% ABMT versus 24% alloBMT, $p = .0035$). The progression-free survival is, however, not significantly different. The higher relapse/progression rate in the ABMT group is offset by the high procedure-related mortality in the alloBMT group. The difference in the relapse/progression rates between ABMT and alloBMT for all the lymphoblastic lymphoma patients is due either to reinfusion of viable lymphoma cells with autologous grafts or to a graft-versus-lymphoma effect analogous to the graft-versus-leukemia effect that is postulated to occur after allogeneic bone marrow transplantation for leukemia (25). The similar progression-free survival rate combined with the greater long-term morbidity seen after alloBMT would suggest that the use of alloBMT should probably be reserved for situations when ABMT is impossible, due to, for example, persistent bone marrow involvement.

DOSE ESCALATION IN FIRST REMISSION

High- and Intermediate-Grade Lymphoma

The advent of dose intensification with marrow transplantation has sharpened the debate about dose escalation in high- and intermediate-grade lymphoma that has been raging for some years. Standard CHOP therapy in high- and intermediate-grade lymphoma has resulted in overall complete response rates for stage II–IV disease of around 60%, with long-term disease-free survival in two-thirds of this 60% of patients (26). It has been suggested that dose intensification of conventional therapy has improved the results from some centers with second- and third-generation first-line regimens, but there is in fact little evidence that such regimens are superior to CHOP, and the results of several large randomized studies by cooperative groups are eagerly awaited. For those patients who do not go into remission on first-line therapy or who relapse from complete remission, the prognosis with conventional therapy is very poor, and the role of ABMT and high-dose therapy has up till now been concentrated on these patients, as discussed earlier. The achievement of at least some durable complete responses with high-dose therapy and ABMT in these patients has turned attention to whether a group of patients can be identified whose prognosis on current conventional therapy is sufficiently poor to justify the use of dose intensification in first remission. The search for reliable prognostic factors on which to base such a selection has attracted much attention and debate (27, 28), and there is a consensus that the performance status of patients, the lactate dehydrogenase level (LDH) at presentation, and the tumor extent and bulk may provide independent prognostic information about the risk of relapse from complete remission, in addition to the probability of patients' achieving remission in the first place.

It must be emphasized that prediction of overall survival at time of diagnosis is mainly dependent on the achievement of remission and that therefore when considering patients who have already achieved CR, any prognostic index must be able to predict for relapse from remission in patients achieving CR. In addition, patients having advanced peripheral T cell lymphoma also represent a poor prognostic category even if they achieve remission (29, 30). The largest analysis of prognostic factors has been the French/Belgian LNH 84 trial (22), and in this trial patients who were considered to be in the poor-prognosis group at presentation had only a 40% survival at 3 years, with, as suggested above, the major problem being failure to achieve CR in the first place. The authors found that the same factors at presentation also predict for relapse, and in the worst prognostic group the relapse rate was 45%. The problem, however, of selecting this group of patients for ABMT is that in order to improve the survival of this 45% one has to treat at least some of the 55% of patients who are already cured, who thereby incur the risk of a procedure-related death even if for these patients it might be possible that this risk could be kept to around 5%. In terms of cost-to-benefit analysis, the comparison between two alternative strategies can be considered. In the first case patients achieving remission can be observed, with ABMT reserved for patients remaining chemoresponsive at relapse. This strategy will minimize the number of ABMT procedures and only treat patients who are unlikely to be cured by any other means. In the second case all patients in first remission (CR1) are treated with ABMT as consolidation. This strategy will increase the number of ABMT procedures and the number of "already cured" patients treated, but some additional patients may be cured. The margin of this improvement can be expressed as

(Increase in no. of patients free from relapse) = (No. of patients free from relapse after ABMT in CR1)

− (no. of patients in continuous CR after first-line therapy or free from relapse after salvage ABMT) − (increased number of procedure-related deaths due to increased no. of ABMTs)

The reader can insert into this equation his or her own hypothetical figures, but from published results one might estimate that in a group of 100 patients in CR, the following might obtain:

(Increase in no. of = (80% of 100
patients free from   patients free from
relapse)   relapse after ABMT
                               in CR1)

− 55% in continuous   − 5% of 100 ABMT
   CR after first-line   in CR1 − 10% of
   therapy +30% of   30 ABMT in
   30 patients   chemo-sensitive
   salvaged in chemo-   relapse
   sensitive relapse

(Increase in no. of = 80   − 65 − 2
patients free from   = 13/100
relapse)

Thus in the extreme scenario, where all first-remission patients are treated with ABMT, this hypothetical model predicts that only 13 more patients in every 100 achieve long-term survival, at a cost of an additional 70 ABMT procedures. This shows that an aggressive transplant policy would make a relatively modest impact on survival at a large cost, not only in terms of resources used but also in terms of "already cured" patients treated. Identification of the poor-risk patients would reduce the number of ABMT procedures performed from this extreme but would also decrease the improvement, as it is not likely that all patients who will relapse can be identified in advance. The size of these hypothesized differences also underlines the need for large randomized studies to be performed to justify definite conclusions on the relative outcomes of differing treatment strategies. A further alternative to be considered is dose escalation after the start of conventional therapy but before its completion, for example after 6 weeks of a MACOP-B type regimen. This strategy would enable early selection of poorly responding patients and reduce the

total amount of treatment received in the dose escalation group.

Special Histologies: Lymphoblastic and Small Non-Cleaved Cell Lymphoma

These tumors require more intensive therapy than the large cell lymphomas and need CNS-directed therapy at an early stage of treatment. Patients with stage IV lymphoblastic lymphoma (LBL) and bone marrow involvement, CNS disease, or a significantly raised LDH level at presentation do particularly badly, with less than 20% long-term survival. These patients must be differentiated from the remainder who do remarkably well, with over 80% disease-free survival on standard multiagent acute lymphoblastic leukemia-type therapy (31). Two European cooperative groups in France (32) and Italy (33) have shown that the outcome of poor-risk patients may be improved to around 60% by dose intensification with autologous or allogeneic bone marrow rescue, but prospective studies are needed so that all patients are included from diagnosis (as distinct from following patients from bone marrow transplantation) and so that the study is confined to patients with precisely the poor-risk criteria that were defined by Coleman. Though these pilot studies justify the organization of such prospective studies, these have, however, proved difficult to recruit to, for two main reasons. Firstly, patients are treated on a variety of protocols before they are referred to a transplant center, and, second, with the pilot studies reported showing good results, there is a reluctance to enter a randomized trial in which there is a 50% chance of randomization to the nontransplant arm.

In the case of small non-cleaved cell (SNCC) lymphomas the data are less clear than for LBL. It is certainly true that following any form of relapse, these patients are difficult if not impossible to treat by conventional therapy. Also, adults who present with CNS disease certainly have a poor long-term survival, and it seems appropriate that with this histology in adult patients those presenting with advanced disease should be considered for ABMT in first remission.

DOSE ESCALATION IN CHILDHOOD NON-HODGKIN'S LYMPHOMA

Childhood NHL is represented virtually always by SNCC lymphoma, LBL, or large cell lymphoma. Chemotherapy has improved so much in the last 2 decades that even advanced stage III and IV disease (if bone marrow is negative) does excellently on conventional therapy, with good long-term survival. Recent reports from the Societé Française d'Oncologie Pédiatrique (SFOP) (34) suggest that even patients with CNS or marrow involvement can achieve excellent results with modern chemotherapy, and it is now very difficult to define a patient group, in children, who should have dose escalation in first remission. Probably dose escalation with marrow rescue should be confined only to those patients obtaining a partial remission to first-line therapy (35) or with chemosensitive relapse in whom a long-term survival of around 25% might be anticipated (36).

DOSE ESCALATION FOR LOW-GRADE LYMPHOMA

It has traditionally been accepted that virtually no patients with advanced-stage low-grade lymphoma are curable by conventional therapy. These stage III and IV patients may often achieve a CR with standard conventional therapy, but the median duration of this CR is often only 1–3 years, with frequent relapse leading, to a disease-free survival of less than 25% at 5 years. The value of aggressive chemotherapy has been debatable, for although it achieves a higher CR rate, this does not translate into prolonged overall survival. Patients with low-grade lymphoma are still responsive to conventional chemotherapy following first relapse of the disease, but many

series show an inexorable decline in the duration of later remissions. In addition, between 50% and 70% of patients with low-grade lymphoma will undergo histologic transformation to a higher-grade histology at some stage, and this is normally associated with profound resistance to treatment.

Although it is now accepted that ABMT or alloBMT can cure some patients with relapsed high- or intermediate-grade lymphoma, the use of this approach in low-grade lymphoma has only been investigated more recently. This is possibly because it is known that many patients out of first remission, even with active disease, can live for many years with a good performance status. Investigators have been reluctant to subject such patients to the risks of dose intensification procedures in the same way that, in the early days of alloBMT for chronic granulocytic leukemia, there was anxiety because of the risk of early death when quality of life in early chronic phase was good. A further reason for the reluctance to investigate dose intensification of treatment in low-grade lymphoma is the long time span needed for any study to compare outcome to that of conventional management; this must be on the order of 5–8 years even for patients in first relapse or second CR. Therefore, single-arm trials are very difficult to assess, and randomized studies would need to be very large to have the statistical power to identify differences within a reasonable time duration.

Nonetheless, since low-grade lymphoma is inevitably fatal, some transplant centers have now advocated dose intensification in young patients after first relapse or in second remission (17, 37–39). These studies have reported the outcome of patients treated with minimal residual disease, with selection based on careful restaging. It is possible that they may therefore represent a group of patients with an excellent prognosis anyway had they been treated with conventional therapy, and this must be remembered when the outcomes are compared with historical "control groups." The frequency of bone marrow involvement with tumor (e.g., 61% at harvest and 47% at ABMT for the Boston series) is consistent with the pattern seen in low-grade lymphoma. The outcome of the patients whose disease transforms to a more aggressive histology is not clear as there are conflicting outcomes in these series. Suffice it to say that where a difference is detectable, this transformation is an adverse prognostic indicator. The procedure-related mortality overall seems to be around 10%. The disease-free survival with short follow-up seems to be between 50% and 60%. The results of these studies will be followed with great interest, and if the outcome is positive they should be used as the basis of a prospective randomized trial to confirm any value of this approach. These single-center nonrandomized studies cannot answer this question because of the problem of the bias introduced by patient selection for transplant, not only in transplant centers but probably also in referring centers as well.

If an early answer to the question of the value of dose escalation in low-grade lymphoma is to be found, it may be in the analysis of patients with more advanced disease, which have been reported in modest numbers to the EBMTG registry. The analogy that can be drawn here is with the early trials of alloBMT in relapsed AML, for we are looking for a small number of cured patients in an otherwise "hopeless" group as evidence of efficacy of the procedure. There do appear to be some such patients with advanced disease who remain disease-free after ABMT in low-grade lymphoma in a situation where this would not be expected with conventional therapy, and the data on them are currently being examined in more detail.

GROWTH FACTORS AND HIGH-DOSE THERAPY IN NON-HODGKIN'S LYMPHOMA

The human hematopoietic growth factors (HGFs) are glycoproteins implicated in the control of proliferation and differentia-tion of the cells of the hematopoietic system. Their role in the regulation of hematopoiesis has recently been reviewed (40). As well as the effects on primitive cells, the HGFs have a range of effects on the function of mature myeloid cells. Granulocyte-macrophage colony-stimulating factor (GM-CSF) has been shown to enhance phagocytosis and augment neutrophil superoxide production in response to physiologic chemoattractants such as f-met-leu-phe, the bacterial peptide, and to significantly impair neutrophil migration in vivo (41). In patients with malignant lymphoma, GM-CSF has been shown to cause not only an expansion in the absolute granulocyte count but also an increase in absolute lymphocyte counts (42). Accompanying this increase, there was a marked rise in sIL-2 receptor and a moderate rise in sCD8 concentrations, with changes in surface membrane antigens on peripheral mononuclear cells indicating that GM-CSF may activate lymphocytes, particularly T cell lymphocytes, bearing interleukin-2 (IL-2) receptors in vivo. The significance of this activation on the rate and duration of remissions in malignant lymphoma patients is not known but may become clearer once the survival data from these patients are published. The *potential* uses of HGFs in the context of high-dose therapy in NHL may include the following:

1. reduction of the period of bone marrow aplasia following ABMT or alloBMT
2. enablement of dose intensification in patients receiving multiple cycles of salvage chemotherapy by reducing myelotoxic and other side effects
3. enhancement of the collection of peripheral blood stem cells for use with high-dose therapy (see below)
4. augmentation of phagocyte response against infection
5. enhancement of host antitumor response

Although an increasing number of studies are now being reported of the use of HGFs in bone marrow transplantation in lymphoid malignancies and solid tumors, very few of these studies include randomized controls. Both granulocyte- (G-) and GM-CSF have been shown to decrease the duration of neutropenia in ABMT (43–46). There is no impact on platelet engraftment. There may be documented decrease in the rate of infections, but there appears to be no proven impact on mortality. Macrophage colony-stimulating factor (M-CSF) has also been used in patients undergoing ABMT for lymphoma (Khwaja et al., submitted). While overall there was no significant effect of M-CSF on hematologic recovery, there was a marked correlation between the number of nucleated marrow cells reinfused and platelet recovery in the M-CSF group. In patients receiving M-CSF, who were reinfused with greater than 2×10^8 nucleated cells, the time to achieve a platelet count of greater than 50×10^9 was shortened to 20 days from 40 days in 20 matched controls ($p < .05$), with a shortening of inpatient stay by 9 days. The time to attain 0.5×10^9 neutrophils was not significantly different when compared to the control group. These data suggest that M-CSF maybe acting on reinfused accessory cells (monocytes/macrophages) to produce cytokines that stimulate marrow (especially platelet) recovery, but that large infusions of cells are required to see this effect. IL-3 has recently been used in a phase-I setting with a suggestion of some enhancement of platelet recovery (47).

Overall, although there is undoubtedly earlier recovery of neutrophil counts in patients receiving HGFs after ABMT, there is no proven benefit in terms of mortality or morbidity. In our experience most procedure-related mortality occurs before day 14–15 after ABMT, when it may be too early, in heavily pretreated patients, to see hematopoietic recovery even with HGFs (Chopra et al., in preparation). The interpretation of trials measuring the number of days spent in hospital is complicated by the tendency for the discharge date to be governed by absolute neutrophil counts (ANCs), so that if control patients show slow rises in ANCs between 0.5

and 1.0×10^9 per liter, they may be kept in hospital for an unusually long time to meet the set criteria. Final justification of the use of these expensive new therapies is still awaited.

ALTERNATIVES TO CONVENTIONAL MARROW RESCUE

The advent of the recombinant growth factors and a greater understanding of the use of peripheral stem cells have in the last few years combined to increase the options available to the physician for hematopoietic reconstitution after myeloablative therapy. These two approaches can be used separately, but increasingly they are used in combination.

It has been apparent for some years that long-term hematologic reconstitution can be achieved using stem cells harvested from the peripheral circulation. These are genuine stem cells by virtue of their ability to self-renew and differentiate into all the mature cells of the hematopoietic system. The number of stem cells harvested can be increased, as measured by the granulocyte-macrophage colony-forming unit assay (GMCFC), by either the use of hematopoietic growth factors such as GM-CSF or by harvesting cells in the recovery phase after intermediate-dose chemotherapy, such as single-agent cyclophosphamide. These strategies can increase the yield of GM-CFCs by as much as 100-fold.

The enthusiasm for peripheral stem cells has been based on two possible advantages: First, hematopoietic reconstitution, including platelet recovery, may be accelerated by up to 1–2 weeks, and, second, patients excluded from conventional bone marrow harvesting may be included. In this second category, patients who have received previous wide-field pelvic irradiation can clearly be helped. However, it is also argued that cells can be harvested from peripheral circulation of patients with bone marrow involvement, with a decreased risk of tumor contamination. It is the opinion of our group that there is a lack of convincing data to substantiate this proposition, especially as in most cases 10 times the number of nucleated cells are reinfused with a peripheral stem cell harvest. In addition, patients with marrow involvement may be poor candidates for high-dose therapy independently of the risk of reinfusing tumor cells, as the persistent marrow involvement may reflect disease resistance to salvage therapy. For this reason at our institution we have adopted a strategy of treating such patients with an intermediate-dose salvage regimen in an attempt to achieve marrow remission before proceeding to ABMT (Chopra et al., submitted for publication). However, equally there are reports of the successful use of peripheral stem cells for use with high-dose therapy in patients with bone marrow involvement (48).

The significant shortening of the time from marrow hypoplasia to recovery is a much more important clinical finding in terms of the numbers of patients who might benefit. The advantages of shorter inpatient stay not only would accrue to the individual patient but also would increase the potential numbers of patients that could be treated and reduce the financial cost of their treatment.

In the case of chemotherapy-induced mobilization of stem cells, however, there has been a problem in choosing the time of the stem cell collection, for the peak of maximum yield may only last a short period of time. This could not be predicted in advance, and the yield of GMCFC from cultures takes up to 2 weeks to determine. The choice of the leukapheresis days is therefore informed guesswork. However, in a recent important paper, the Milan group have suggested that this problem can be overcome by flow cytometric analysis of the patient's blood, collected to determine whether a satisfactory yield of CD34+ cells has been obtained (49).

The use of chemotherapy to induce mobilization of stem cells is not without morbidity or indeed mortality from the complications of the neutropenia even before the high-dose procedure, so that increasingly GM-CSF is being used to mobilize the stem cells, either alone or in combination with chemotherapy, as the two approaches show a synergy that can lead to collection of greater numbers of progenitors than is possible with either technique alone.

A further advance may be the work of Gianni and coworkers (50), who have used a combination of bone marrow and peripheral blood-derived stem cells and thereby have apparently achieved the advantages of early reconstitution without the anxiety of late graft failure, which it has been suggested might occur with peripheral stem cells due to the collection of committed stem cells with a limited capacity for self-renewal. Their results have been very encouraging, with regeneration times for both granulocytes and platelets of under 12 days from the time of stem cell reinfusion. However, it should be remembered that it is unlikely that regeneration times as quick as these will be possible with advanced patients who have received multiple courses of alkylating agents, as these initial results have mainly been in patients with solid tumors or lymphomas treated at a relatively early stage of their disease. Second, the total period of hospitalization when the single agent cyclophosphamide is included may actually exceed that seen with conventional ABMT in comparable patients, and it is debatable how much antitumor effect is achieved by the use as a single agent of a drug to which most of the patients have already been exposed in their primary chemotherapy.

The ultimate goal of some investigators seems to be to deliver myeloablative doses of high-dose chemotherapy without the need for stem cell rescue. A preliminary report of the use of a standard BEAM regimen with GM-CSF infusion without stem cell rescue in patients with persistent bone marrow involvement in NHL has just been published (51). Of the five patients treated, full hematologic regeneration was achieved in three, but the other two died in aplasia on days 40 and 50, respectively. This report indicates that high-dose therapy without stem cell support can be given, but it unlikely that patients or doctors would be able to accept a 40% procedure-related mortality if these small numbers were representative of the outcome that could be expected if larger numbers of patients were treated in this way.

The real question is not simply the time for hematopoietic recovery to occur following stem cell reinfusion but whether the whole process of, on the one hand, ABMT versus, on the other hand, growth factor mobilization with or without chemotherapy, multiple peripheral stem cell collections, and then rescue, with or without bone marrow, in the end produces a safer result with lesser morbidity and more economic use of resources. In our own group we find that the collection and reinfusion of bone marrow is a modest procedure of little morbidity or expense. Some investigators are not convinced that leukopheresis is a procedure that should supplant marrow harvest too easily.

CONCLUSIONS

In the context of a variety of tumors retaining sensitivity to salvage therapy, the non-Hodgkin's lymphomas appear to be the major candidates for the use of dose escalation. Unfortunately many of the earlier series have documented the poor outcome of patients treated in advanced chemoresistant relapse when they were irretrievable even to high-dose therapy, and this has tended to obscure the success of dose escalation in the group of less advanced patients who can definitely be helped. However, the last 10 years have seen advances in conventional salvage therapy that make prospective trials important to define the place of high-dose therapy. There is circumstantial evidence for the use of dose escalation for some poor-risk patients in first remission, but the application of high-dose therapy in this context will inevitably require the treatment of a significant number of cured but unidentified patients.

Whether high-dose therapy can be given without stem cell rescue by the use of the hematologic growth factors remains to be determined. Unless or until this is reliably demonstrated to be an acceptable alternative, the use of bone marrow or peripheral stem cells will continue to be necessary if the limits of dose escalation are to be tested in this disease.

REFERENCES

1. Appelbaum FR, Herzig GP, Ziegler JL, et al. Successful engraftment of cryopreserved autologous bone marrow in patients with malignant lymphoma. Blood 1978;52:85–92.
2. Kaizer H, Levanthal B, Wharam ND. Cryopreserved autologous bone marrow transplantation in the treatment of selected paediatric malignancies. A preliminary report. Transplant Proc. 1979;1:208–211.
3. Philip T, Biron P, Maraninchi D, et al. Massive chemotherapy with autologous bone marrow transplantation in 50 cases of bad prognosis non-Hodgkin lymphoma. Br J Haematol 1985;60:599–609.
4. Philip T, Armitage JO, Spitzer G, et al. High dose therapy and ABMT after failure of conventional therapy in adults with intermediate grade or high grade non-Hodgkin's lymphoma. N Engl J Med 1987; 316:1493–1498.
5. Gribben JG, Goldstone AH, Linch DC, et al. Effectiveness of high dose combination chemotherapy and autologous bone marrow transplantation for patients with non-Hodgkin's lymphoma who are still responsive to conventional dose chemotherapy. J Clin Oncol 1989;7:1621–1629.
6. Appelbaum FR, Sullivan KM, Buckner CD, et al. Treatment of malignant lymphoma in 100 patients with chemotherapy, total body irradiation and marrow transplantation. J Clin Oncol 1987;5:1340.
7. Vose JM, Peterson C, Bierman PJ, et al. Comparison of high dose therapy and autologous bone marrow transplantation for T-cell and B-cell non Hodgkin's lymphomas. Blood 1990;76:424–431.
8. Wheeler C, Antin JH, Churchill W, et al. Cyclophosphamide, carmustine, and etoposide with autologous bone marrow transplantation in refractory Hodgkin's disease and non Hodgkin's lymphoma: a dose finding study. J Clin Oncol 1990;8:648.
9. Philip T, Chauvin F, Bron D, et al. PARMA International Protocol Pilot study on 50 patients and preliminary analysis on the ongoing randomized study (62 patients). Ann Oncol 1990, in press.
10. Coltman CA, Dahlberg S, Jones SE, et al. CHOP is curative in thirty percent of patients with large cell lymphoma: a twelve year Southwest Oncology Group followup. In: Skarin AT, ed. Advances in cancer chemotherapy. New York: Park Row, 1986.
11. Klimo P, Connors JM. MACOP-B chemotherapy for

the treatment of diffuse large cell lymphoma. Ann Intern Med 1985;102:596–602.

12. Cabanillas F, Hagemeister FB, Bodey GP, Freireich EJ. IMVP 16: an effective regimen for patients with lymphoma who have relapsed after initial combination chemotherapy. Blood 1982;60:693–697.

13. Cabanillas F, Hagemeister FB, McLaughlin P, et al. Results of MIME salvage regimen for recurrent or refractory lymphoma. J Clin Oncol 1987;5:407–412.

14. Velasquez WS, Cabanillas F, Salvador P, et al. Effective salvage therapy for lymphoma with cisplatin in combination with high dose Ara C and dexamethasone (DHAP). Blood 1988;71:117–122.

15. Skipper HE, Schabel FM Jr, Wilcox WS. Experimental evaluation of potential anticancer agents XII. On the criteria and kinetics associated with "curability" of experimental leukaemia. Cancer Chemother Rep 1964;35:1–111.

16. Skipper HE, Schabel FM Jr, Mellet LB, et al. Implications of biochemical, cytokinetic, pharmacologic, and toxicologic relationships in the design of optimal therapeutic schedules. Cancer Chemother Rep 1970;54:431–450.

17. Colombat P, Gorin NC, Lemonnier MP, et al. The role of autologous bone marrow transplantation in 46 adult patients with non-Hodgkin's lymphomas. J Clin Oncol 1990;8:630–637.

18. Freedman AS, Takvorian T, Anderson KA, et al. Autologous bone marrow transplantation in B cell non-Hodgkin's lymphoma: very low treatment-related mortality in 100 patients in sensitive relapse. J Clin Oncol 1990;8:784–791.

19. McMillan A, Chopra R, Linch DC, Goldstone AH. Update on results of ABMT in NHL. In: Powles R, Gordon-Smith E, eds. Critical papers in bone marrow transplantation. London Royal Marsden Hospital, in press.

20. Canellos GP. Residual of mass in lymphoma may not be residual disease [Editorial]. 1988;6:931–932.

21. Surbonne A, Longo DL, DeVita V, et al. Residual abdominal masses in aggressive non-Hodgkin's lymphoma after combination chemotherapy: significance and management. 1988;6:1832–1837.

22. Coiffier B, Gisselbrecht C, Herbrecht R, et al. LNH-84 regimen, a multicentre study of intensive chemotherapy in 737 patients with aggressive malignant lymphoma. 1989;7:1018–1026.

23. Jones R, Ambinder R, Piantodosi S, Santos G. Evidence of a graft versus lymphoma effect associated with allogeneic bone marrow transplantation. 1991;77:649–653.

24. Copelan EA, Kapoor N, Gibbins B, Tutschka PJ. Allogenic marrow transplantation in non-Hodgkin's lymphoma. Bone Marrow Transplant 1990;5:47–50.

25. Horowitz M. Evidence for a graft versus leukaemia effect in clinical bone marrow transplantation. Exp Haematol 1988;16:547a.

26. Linch D, Vaughan-Hudson B. The management of Hodgkin's disease and the non Hodgkin's lymphomas. In: Hoffbrand AV, ed. Recent advances in haematology. Edinburgh: Churchill Livingstone, 1988.

27. Shipp MA, Harrington DP, Klatt MM, et al. Identification of major prognostic subgroups of patients with large cell lymphoma treated with m-BACOD or M-BACOD. Ann Intern Med 1986;104:757–765.

28. Coiffier B, Gisselbrecht C, Vose JM. Prognostic factors in aggressive malignant lymphomas: description and validation of a prognostic index that could identify patients requiring a more intensive therapy. J Clin Oncol 1991;9:211–219.

29. Armitage JO, Vose JM, Linder J, et al. Clinical significance of immunophenotype in diffuse aggressive non-Hodgkin lymphomas. J Clin Oncol 1989;7:1783–1790.

30. Coiffier B, Brousse N, Peuchmaur M, et al. Peripheral T cell lymphomas have a worse prognosis than B cell lymphomas: a prospective study of 361 immunophenotyped patients treated with the LNH 84 regime. Ann Oncol 1991, in press.

31. Coleman CN, Picozzi VJ, Cox RS, et al. Treatment of lymphoblastic lymphoma in adults. J Clin Oncol 1987;4:1628–1637.

32. Milpied N, Ifrah N, Kuentz M, et al. Bone marrow transplantation for adult poor prognosis lymphoblastic lymphoma in first complete remission. Br J Haematol 1989;73:82–87.

33. Santini G, Coser P, Chisesi T, et al. Autologous bone marrow transplantation for advanced stage adult lymphoblastic lymphoma in first complete remission. A pilot study of the Non Hodgkin Lymphoma Co-Operative Study Group (NHLCSG). Bone Marrow Transplant 1989;4:399–404.

34. Gentet JT, Patte C, Quintana E, et al. Phase II study of cytarabine and etoposide in children with refractory or relapsed non Hodgkin's lymphoma: study of SFOP. J Clin Oncol 1990;8:661–5.

35. Philip T, Hartmann O, Biron P, et al. High dose therapy and autologous bone marrow transplantation in partial remission after first line induction therapy for diffuse non-Hodgkin's lymphoma. J Clin Oncol 1988;6:1118–1124.

36. Blay JY, Louis D, Buffet E, et al. Management of paediatric non Hodgkin lymphoma. Blood Rev 1991, in press.

37. Freedman AS, Ritz J, Neuburg K, et al. Autologous bone marrow transplantation in 69 patients with a history of low grade B cell non Hodgkin lymphoma. Blood 1991;77:2524–2529.

38. Schouten HC, Bierman PH, Vaughan WP, et al. Autologous bone marrow transplantation in follicular non-Hodgkin's lymphoma before and after histological transformation. Blood 1989;74:2579–2584.

39. Rohatiner AZ, Price CG, Dorey E, et al. Therapy with ABMT as consolidation therapy for follicular lymphoma. In: Fifth International Symposium on Au-

tologous Bone Marrow Transplantation. Omaha, NE: University of Nebraska, 1991, in press.

40. Devalia V, Linch DC. Haemopoietic regulation by growth factors. In: Newland A, ed. Cambridge medical reviews: haematological oncology. Cambridge: Cambridge University Press, 1991.

41. Addison I, Johnson B, Devereux S, et al. GM-CSF inhibits neutrophil migration in vivo. Clin Exp Immunol 1989;76:149.

42. Ho AD, Haas R, Wulf G, et al. Activation of lymphocytes induced by recombinant human granulocyte-macrophage colony-stimulating factor in patients with malignant lymphoma. Blood 1990;75:203–212.

43. Brandt SJ, Peters WP, Atwater S, et al. Effect of recombinant human granulocyte-macrophage colony-stimulating factor on haematopoietic reconstitution after high dose chemotherapy and autologous bone marrow transplantation. N Engl J Med 1988;318:869–875.

44. Devereux S, Linch DC, Gribben JG, et al. GM-CSF accelerates neutrophil recovery after autologous bone marrow transplantation. Bone Marrow Transplant 1989;4:49–54.

45. Nemunaitis J, Rabinowe SN, Singer JW, et al. Recombinant granulocyte-macrophage colony-stimulating factor after autologous bone marrow transplantation for lymphoid cancer. New Engl J Med 1991;324:1773–1778.

46. Taylor K, Spitzer G, Jagganath S, et al. Phase II study of recombinant human granulocyte colony-stimulating factor in Hodgkin's disease after high dose chemotherapy with ABMT. Blood 1988;72:452.

47. Ganser A, Lindemann A, Ottomann OG, et al. Effect of recombinant human interleukin-3 in vivo — a phase 1 trial. Exp Haematol 1989;17:40.

48. Kessinger A, Armitage JO, Smith DM, et al. High dose therapy and autologous peripheral blood stem cell transplantation for patients with lymphoma. Blood 1989;74:1260.

49. Siena S, Bregni M, Brando B, et al. Flow cytometry for clinical estimation of circulating hematopoietic progenitors for autologous transplantation in cancer patients. Blood 1991;77:400–409.

50. Gianni AM, Bregni M, Siena S, et al. Rapid and complete haemapoietic recovery following combined transplantation of autologous blood and bone marrow cells: a changing role for high dose chemo-radiotherapy. Haematol Oncol 1989;7:139.

51. Laporte JP, Fouillard L, Douay L, et al. GM-CSF instead of autologous bone marrow transplantation after the BEAM regimen. Lancet 1991;338:601–602.

52. Petersen FB, Appelbaum FR, Hill R, et al. Autologous bone marrow transplantation for malignant lymphoma: a report of 101 cases from Seattle. J. Clin Oncol 1990;8:638–647.

53. Gingrich RD, Ginder GR, Burns LJ, Chen-Wen B, Fyfe MA. BVAC ablative therapy followed by autologous bone marrow transplantation for patients with advanced lymphoma. Blood 1990;75:2276–2281.

54. Gulati SC, Shank B, Black P, et al. Autologous bone marrow transplantation for patients with poor-prognosis lymphoma. J Clin Oncol 1988;6:1303–1313.

40

HIGH-DOSE THERAPY IN BURKITT'S LYMPHOMA

Jean-Yves Blay and Thierry O. Philip

Burkitt's lymphoma (BL) is the most frequent (45%) non-Hodgkin's lymphoma (NHL) of children in Europe (1). Although its frequency in the whole adult NHL population is much lower (4%–7%), 20% of NHL in adults before 40 years demonstrates the characteristic diffuse, small, noncleaved cellular morphology and behaves in a similar fashion with regard to clinical presentation and treatment (2). Until 1980 less than 40% of patients with BL were cured by conventional chemotherapy regimens (2). Most of the relapses occured in the first 8 months. After this date, a patient alive in remission was likely to be cured (2).

The first trials of massive therapy and bone marrow transplantation (BMT) in BL were reported 15 years ago (3, 4). At this time, the cure rate of patients with relapsing or refractory BL was considered to be very low (5). The rationale for massive therapy in cancer came from the observation of a steep dose-response curve for both radiotherapy and cytotoxic drugs in several models of human tumor in vivo and in vitro (6, 7). The clinical efficacy of such an approach had been demonstrated by reports of higher survival rates in patients with acute leukemia treated with massive therapy and allogeneic BMT.

The results of massive therapy in acute leukemia have driven investigators to explore the concept of dose-effect in chemo-therapy in Burkitt's lymphoma. Considering the acute sensitivity of this lymphoma to both cytotoxic drugs and radiotherapy, BL was an obvious candidate for the assessment of the efficacy of high-dose chemotherapy and bone marrow transplantation.

The first reports of Appelbaum et al. clearly demonstrated a dose-response relationship for chemotherapy in NHL and especially in BL (3, 4). Several other groups have since confirmed the efficacy of high-dose therapy for NHL with different chemotherapeutic regimens, sometimes including total body irradiation (TBI) (8–17). Interestingly, high response rates were observed in patients with relapsing lymphomas resistant to second-line regimens at conventional doses, but response in these cases was never associated with cure (8–18). The observations of long-term survival and probable cure in patients treated with high-dose therapy and autologous BMT when still chemosensitive to conventional rescue protocols at relapse or in first partial remission demonstrated the potential for cure via massive chemotherapy in BL (18).

In 1992 massive chemotherapy and BMT are still, from our point of view, the optimal treatment for 15%–20% of patients with BL. However, the place of BMT in the treatment of BL remains controversial in several clinical situations. Furthermore, the nature of massive therapy as well as the efficacy of the purging of bone marrow are still matters of debate.

In this chapter we will focus on three major points: the optimum massive regimen for BMT in BL, indications for high-dose therapy in patients with BL, and the value of bone marrow purging.

WHICH MASSIVE THERAPY REGIMEN SHOULD BE USED IN BURKITT'S LYMPHOMA?

Multiple conditioning regimens have been tested, including high doses of a single agent or combinations of drugs with or without TBI (Table 40.1). New chemotherapeutic agents are usually introduced into treatment after the completion of phase I and phase II studies at normal dose ranges demonstrating significant effectiveness in relapsed or resistant disease. New combinations of conventional chemotherapeutic agents, with the exception of those based upon kinetic or in vitro synergism, are often constructed rather empirically on the assumption that the cumulative antitumor effect will outweigh any enhanced toxicity. Such an approach, using a combination of conventional high doses, has produced impressive results in the treatment of NHL of children (19). Few trials have evaluated the toxicity and efficacy of very high doses of a single agent, such as carmustine (BCNU) (20), melphalan (21), cyclophosphamide (22), or etoposide (23), in phase I/II studies. Most of these trials involved a limited number of patients and seemed to offer very few chances of long-term survival.

Hence most of the massive regimens for NHL combine multiple drugs, with limited or tolerable extrahematopoietic toxicity, in order to increase the probability of durable response. Table 40.1 indicates the regimes used for massive therapy of BL. The BACT regimen reported by Appelbaum combines carmustine, cytarabine, cyclophosphamide, and thioguanine (3, 4). This regimen has next been further intensified with a threefold increase in carmustine with no major enhancement of antitumor effect but with an apparent increase in morbidity (8, 15). The BACT-derived TACC regimen, in which lomustine replaced carmustine, tested by a French group, was withdrawn because of cardiac toxicity (24).

The BEAM regimen incorporated two agents, etoposide and melphalan, that were effective at high doses in phase I/II studies and were introduced in an attempt to reduce the toxicity of the BACT combination (25–28). Other conditioning regimens, such as BAVM (similar to BEAM but with no etoposide and with the addition of vindesine), CBV or ABV (a combination of cyclophosphamide, carmustine, etoposide, or cytarabine) and BAC (carmustine, cytarabine, cyclophosphamide) have also been used (17, 26). Review of the arguments for these different regimens favors BEAM, from our point of view.

Several studies have assessed the effect of massive therapy regimens containing TBI

Table 40.1   High-Dose Chemotherapy Regimens with or without TBI used in Burkitt's Lymphoma[a]

Regimen	References
Without TBI	
BACT	Appelbaum et al. (4)
BACT/incr. dose BCNU	Hartmann et al. (15)
	Philip et al. (8)
BEAM	Philip et al. (18, 26)
CPM	Philip (34)
CPM/DXR/VBL/CTA/MTX	Eckert et al. (14)
CPM/BCNU	Barbasch et al. (16)
With additional TBI	
CPM/TBI	Phillips et al. (31)
	Appelbaum et al. (3)
	Takvorian et al. (30)
	Fenaux et al. (38)
	Jones et al. (60)
CPM/CTA/BCNU/TBI	O'Leary et al. (37)
CPM/VBL/DXR/TBI	Philip et al. (34)
CPM/DXR/TBI	Kaiser et al. (9)
CPM/VBL/TBI	Gale et al. (10)
	Douer et al. (12)
BACT/TBI	Philip. (34)

[a]Abbreviations: BACT: carmustine, cytosine arabinoside, cyclophosphamide, thiotepa; BEAM: carmustine, etoposide, cytosine arabinoside, melphalan; BCNU: carmustine; CTA: cytosine arabinoside; CPM: cyclophosphamide; DXR: doxorubicine; MTX: methotrexate, VBL: vinblastine, incr.: increased.

for BL and other NHL with various fractionations and doses (6, 29–33). In 1991 the use of TBI in conditioning regimens before BMT in BL remains controversial. TBI-containing regimens have not demonstrated their superiority to massive chemotherapy alone for BL or NHL in terms of response rate or longterm survival (33, 34). Furthermore, TBI enhances the rate of severe nonhematologic toxicities such as interstitial pneumonitis and encephalopathies (6, 26). Review of studies of TBI in combination with chemotherapy does not favor TBI-containing regimens to prepare patients with BL for ABMT. Moreover, in young children, the long-term sequelae must be taken in consideration (35). Table 40.2 depicts the massive chemotherapy regimens used for BL in Lyon.

There are few indications for localized irradiation before or after BMT in BL. However, in the case of BL with CNS involvement either at diagnosis or relapse, cranial irradiation is still considered necessary in conjunction with BMT. In rare cases of atypical sites of involvement, such as bone localization, boost x-rays can also be performed.

The use of a double autograft has been proposed for lymphoma in relapse (36, 37). However, in BL only one graft is possible in most cases because of the rapid turnover of BL cells. Two patients with resistant relapse have been treated at the Centre Leon Berard with a double high-dose regimen and two consecutive autologous BMTs. Both relapsed in the 1st month following the second autologous BMT (unpublished results).

Table 40.2. Massive Chemotherapy Regimens Used for Patients with Burkitt's Lymphoma in Lyon between 1980 and 1989 (n = 65)[a]

Drugs		Days							Number of Courses
		1	2	3	4	5	7	8	
Appelbaum BACT									
BCNU	200 mg/m²	*							
Cytosine arabinoside	200 mg/m²		*	*	*	*			
Cyclophosphamide	50 mg/kg		*	*	*	*			3
6-Thioguanine	200 mg/m²		*	*	*	*			
ABMT							*		
Increased dose BACT									
BCNU	200 mg/m²	*	*	*					
Cytosine arabinoside	200 mg/m²		*	*	*	*			
Cyclophosphamide	50 mg/kg		*	*	*	*			16
6-Thioguanine	200 mg/m²		*	*	*	*			
ABMT							*		
BEAM protocol									
BCNU	300 mg/m²	*							
Cytosine arabinoside	200 mg/m²		*	*	*	*			
Melphalan	140 mg/kg						*		24
VP16	200 mg/m²		*	*	*	*			
ABMT							*		
BEAC protocol									
BCNU	300 mg/m²	*							
Cytosine arabinoside	200 mg/m²		*	*	*	*			
Cyclophosphamide	35 mg/kg		*	*	*	*			5
VP16	200 mg/m²		*	*	*	*			
Mesna	50 mg/kg		*	*	*	*			
ABMT							*		

[a]One patient received high-dose cyclophosphamide alone; three patients received busulphan and cyclophosphamide; three patients received various cyclophosphamide-containing regimens.

Our conclusion is that BEAM is the regimen of choice in BL treatment.

SELECTION OF PATIENTS WHO WILL BENEFIT FROM AUTOLOGOUS BONE MARROW TRANSPLANTATION

Patients included in the early clinical studies of BMT in BL were refractory to conventional therapy, i.e., in relapse or uncontrolled by first-line therapy (4, 8, 29). In these series, almost 33% (range 0%–50%) of these patients with very poor prognosis are long-term survivors after high-dose therapy and BMT (Table 40.3). Massive therapy regimens were effective in terms of achieving response in 75% or more of patients with NHL in relapse or uncontrolled by first- or second-line treatment (26–32). However, the response was very short-lived in most of the patients. Subsequent trials have included patients with BL at an early phase of their disease, such as first complete remission, with features of poor prognosis or patients in first partial remission (18, 26, 28, 38, 39). The clinical experience gained with studies including a larger number of patients has allowed the characterization of subgroups with very different prognoses in the population of "refractory lymphomas" (26, 27, 30). We will review first the role of high-dose therapy in the first-line

Table 40.3. Early Studies of High-Dose Therapy for Poor-Prognosis Burkitt's Lymphoma

Study	Reference	Number of Cases	Number of Patients Alive
Appelbaum et al.	4	18	4
Mascret et al.	11	19	7
Barbasch et al.	16	1	1
Douer et al.	12	1	0
Eckert et al.	14	3	1
Philip et al.	8	8	4
Kaiser et al.	9	1	1
Phillips et al.	29	8	2
Total		59	20 (33%)

treatment of BL and then its place in the treatment of relapses.

Bone Marrow Transplantation as Consolidation of First-Line Treatment

Patients with BL or non-BL refractory to primary treatment experience response, sometimes complete, after massive therapy but invariably relapse in most studies (18, 30, 31). None of the 15 patients with BL grafted for refractory disease survived more than 8 months after BMT, in the Lyon experience (40, 41). A single report mentions long-term survivors in patients with "primary refractory" lymphoma (32). However, since the precise nature of the "histologic" response to therapy is not indicated in this study, these patients could have been partial or even complete responders with residual fibrotic masses, as previously reported (42). It is generally believed by most transplant teams that patients refractory to primary treatment as previously defined (26), i.e., with progressive disease, are not good candidates for BMT and also are incurable with current approaches.

Patients who achieve partial response at the end of induction treatment for BL are good candidates for massive therapy. This population of patients is known to have a poor prognosis, with less than 25% long-term survivors with conventional regimens (43, 44). Although these patients have been considered as having "refractory" lymphoma, this terminology is inaccurate since they are undoubtedly sensitive to chemotherapy and continue to respond after each course. A French study of ABMT of lymphoma in first partial remission, including 10 cases of BL, has demonstrated a 75% overall survival at 24 months and 70% for BL (45). Results of this study are presented in Figure 40.1. These patients represent a limited fraction of the whole BL population treated with modern intensive treatment (46, 47). However, they must be individualized since they un-

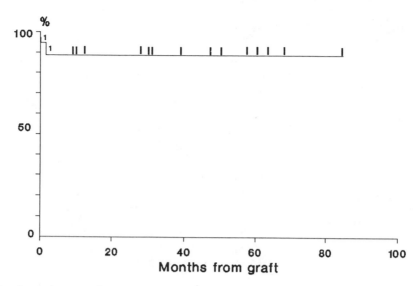

Figure 40.1. Survival curve of 17 patients who received high-dose therapy and autologous BMT in Lyon as consolidation in first partial remission on induction chemotherapy.

doubtedly benefit from massive therapy and ABMT.

Several groups have evaluated the efficacy of high-dose therapy with BMT for patients in first complete remission with poor prognosis due to a delay in obtaining complete remission, the presence of a massive infiltration of bone marrow (infiltration by type 3 lymphoblasts (L3 blasts) > 25% defines B-acute lymphocytic leukemia (B-ALL), and/or initial CNS involvement. Eighteen patients were grafted in Lyon because of CNS involvement at diagnosis, long delay (>3 months) to complete remission, or BL leukemia. Fifty-five percent are alive. Two additional patients who were grafted in first partial remission with initial CNS involvement are also long-term survivors. Figure 40.2 presents the survival rates of the 18 patients grafted in first complete remission in Lyon.

Another French group has reported seven long-term survivors among nine patients with CNS+ Burkitt leukemia treated with cyclophosphamide, TBI, and allogeneic BMT (39). Although none of these studies included a control group, these results demonstrate the efficacy of high-dose therapy in the treatment of BL with initial CNS involvement or isolated CNS relapse and compare favorably with previous published results (47). However, a French group has recently reported comparable results with five courses of intensive polychemotherapy induction followed by cranial irradiation and maintenance therapy with or without consolidation with high-dose chemotherapy and ABMT (48). In conclusion, the role of massive therapy in the first-line treatment of B-ALL and BL with bone marrow and CNS involvement is not established at the present time, and autologous BMT should be compared to the LMB86 protocol in a randomized trial.

We thus do not recommend use of massive therapy and autologous BMT as consolidation for BL in first complete remission, outside of a controlled study.

Bone Marrow Transplantation for the Treatment of Burkitt's Lymphoma in Relapse

The prognosis of BL in relapse was very poor until 1980, with a cure rate close to 0% (2, 5). The first cases of long-term disease-

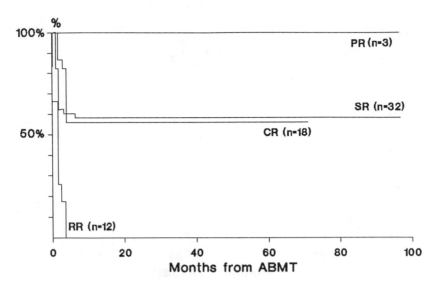

Figure 40.2. Survival of 65 patients with BL treated in Lyon with massive therapy and autologous BMT according to clinical status at BMT. PR, partial remission after first-line chemotherapy; CR, complete remission after first-line chemotherapy; SR, sensitive relapse (i.e., partial or complete remission after salvage chemotherapy for relapse); RR, resistant relapse (i.e., progressive after salvage chemotherapy for relapse).

free survival for BL in relapse were reported after autologous BMT (8–17). Long-term disease-free survival rates were close to 25% (range 0%–50%) in most of these studies. Figure 40.3 presents the survival curves of 16 patients with relapsing BL treated with or without BMT between 1978 and 1980 at the Centre Leon Berard. Pooling of the results of the early studies of BMT in BL (8–17) indicates a mean of 33% of long-term survival (Table 40.3).

These results clearly demonstrated the capacity of massive therapy and BMT to cure NHL after relapse. Analysis of large studies of high-dose therapy and BMT for BL and other NHLs has demonstrated that response in reinduction cytotoxic treatment is a major prognostic criterion (26, 30–32). In all these studies, patients with BL (and other NHL) in relapse who achieve partial or complete response to reinduction treatment (i.e., sensitive relapse) have a very significantly improved outcome compared to patients with NHLs refractory to reinduction (i.e., resistant relapse) (Table 40.4).

We have reported 62% survival for sensitive relapse versus 14% for resistant relapse in a series of 100 patients with relapsing NHL of various histologies (26). Other studies confirm these observations, with 44%–62% of long-term survivors for patients in sensitive relapse and 0%–10% for patients in resistant relapse (Table 40.4).

Forty-four patients with BL in relapse were treated with a high-dose polychemotherapy regimen and autologous BMT in Lyon from 1980–1989. All 12 patients with resistant relapse who progressed at the time of autologous BMT died of progressive disease in the 3 months following transplantation. Fifty-six percent of the 32 patients grafted in sensitive relapse are alive with nonevolving disease (Fig. 40.2). The type of response to second-line treatment (partial or complete remission) at the time of transplant did not influence survival. It is of interest to consider all patients treated in Lyon during this period who were potential candidates for BMT. Six additional patients were not included in the BMT program because of early deaths (2 pa-

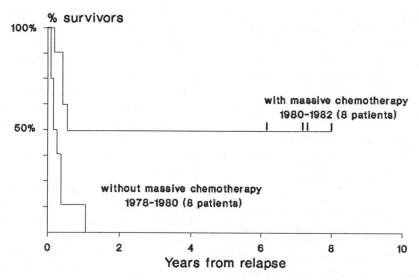

Figure 40.3. Survival curve at Centre Leon Berard of 16 patients with BL in relapse between 1978 and 1982. Eight received second-line chemotherapy without mas-sive therapy between 1978 and 1980. Eight received massive therapy as their second-line treatment (1980–1982).

Table 40.4   Survival after BMT According to Response to Second-Line Regimen

Study (Reference)	Number of patients (% of RFS[a])	
	SR	RR
Philip et al. (26)	44 (38%)	22 (14%)
Gribben et al. (27)	20 (60%)	29 (10%)
Colombat et al. (28)	21 (62%)	8 (0%)
Freedman et al. (61)	100 (61%)	—
Jones et al (60)	80 (44%)	38 (0%)

[a]RFS, relapse-free survival.

tients), resistant relapse during rescue protocol treatment (3 patients), or bone marrow involvement at relapse (1 patient).

Considering this total experience of BMT for BL in Lyon, the overall survival between 1980 and 1990 in Lyon for patients with indications for BMT in BL was 48%. A selection process in favor of autologous BMT is then obvious. The only way to examine the role of selection in the outcome of BL after relapse is to isolate the evolution of all relapses in a prospective group of patients. Twenty-six of the 216 children (13%) included in the So-

ciété Française Oncologie Pediatrique (SFOP) LMB84 protocol (46, 49) have relapsed. Fifteen have received massive therapy as consolidation after two or three courses of a conventional second-line regimen. Four of these 15 patients are alive (27%). In contrast, none of the 11 patients treated without massive therapy are alive. This indicates that patients with BL in relapse after a highly efficient first-line chemotherapy regimen (46) can be cured with a second-line protocol including high-dose chemotherapy. Such a second-line protocol appears to be the best available treatment for these patients.

Taken together, these data led us to separate patients with BL in relapse in two different subgroups with a completely different treatment and prognosis:

1. Patients with BL in relapse who are sensitive to second-line conventional chemotherapy regimens must receive a massive chemotherapy regimen followed by autologous BMT as consolidation after the second remission. The BEAM protocol is the optimal regimen and must be given as

soon as possible after two courses of second-line conventional chemotherapy.

2. Patients with BL in relapse who are resistant to conventional second-line chemotherapy regimens do not achieve cure with high-dose therapy regimens and should be offered for phase I or II trials.

TOXICITY OF MASSIVE CHEMOTHERAPY FOR BURKITT'S LYMPHOMA

Toxic deaths and complications observed in the first 35 patients treated with the BACT or BEAM regimen with or without TBI at the Centre Leon Berard are listed in Table 40.5. As expected, there has been a steady decline over the years in the morbidity of ABMT as both the supportive therapy and the general condition of patients entering the program have improved. Under current conditions, the treatment-related mortality is around 10%, which is only moderately higher than that of most modern intensive conventional chemotherapy regimens.

BONE MARROW PURGING

The theoretical risk of autologous BMT for malignant tumor is reinfusing clonogenic malignant cells with the bone marrow. In the case of BL, this potential risk is increased considering the observations of the presence

Table 40.5. Complications of Massive Therapy in the 35 First Cases of Burkitt's Lymphoma Treated at the Centre Leon Berard, Lyon[a]

Toxic deaths	3
Interstitial pneumonitis	5
Myocardiopathy	2
Hemorrhagic cystitis	2
Delayed hematologic recovery	2
Leukoencephalitis	2
Hepatitis	1
Venoocclusive disease	1
Postradiation encephalopathy	1
Subarachnoid hemorrhage	1

[a]Some patients had more than one complication.

of BL cells in long-term liquid cultures of histologically "normal" marrows (50, 51). In 7 of 37 patients in whom conventional techniques failed to show any disease, there was clear evidence, using morphologic, immunologic, and cytogenetic criteria, of significant BL cell growth in culture (52). Whether such a level of contamination is capable of causing disease relapse is a separate question, but evidence in animal studies suggests that it can (53).

The potential risk of BL cell reinfusion was also suggested by observations of "exploding" bone marrow and leukemic relapse of BL after BMT (34). However, we have also observed such BM and leukemic relapse in two patients treated with massive therapy followed by allogeneic BMT (unpublished data). These latter observations suggest that such relapses are rather due either to the inefficacy of cytotoxic regimens to treat BL or to a possible contribution of immunodepression associated with aplasia.

A variety of purging procedures have been devised, including physical separation, cytotoxic agents, and monoclonal antibodies.

Cytotoxic agents such as mafosfamide, 4-hydroperoxycyclophosphamide, etoposide, and ricin have been used for bone marrow purging (54, 55). Treatment of BM with these drugs generally results in an inhibition of in vitro colony formation but generally allows hematopoietic reconstitution (54). Bone marrow purging can also be performed with monoclonal antibodies and complement-mediated lysis or with antibody-coated magnetic microspheres. In Lyon we have evaluated three purging procedures: (a) asta-Z, (b) complement-mediated lysis, and (c) magnetic microsphere removal. The details of these techniques are summarized in Table 40.6. Complement and monoclonal antibody-mediated lysis is the most effective and reliable technique in our hands (34). Bone marrow purging techniques are clearly efficient in a wide number of patients in terms of reducing bone marrow infiltration to an undetectable level. However, we had some evidence

Table 40.6. Bone Marrow Purging Procedures Studied at the Centre Leon Nerard, Lyon

Asta-Z	Concentration	100 µg/mL
	Incubation time	30 mn at 37°C
	Procedure duration	1 hour
	Quality of purging (log)	2–4
Microsphere	Monoclonal cocktail	B1, Y29/55, AL2
	Incubation time with beads (followed each time by magnetic separation)	30 mn × 2 at 4°C
	Procedure duration	5–6 hours
	Quality of purging (log)	4
Complement lysis	Monoclonal cocktail	B1, Y29/55, AL2
	Incubation time with monoclonals	30 mm at 24°C
	Incubation time with complement	60 mn at 24°C × 2
	Procedure duration	4 hours
	Quality of purging (log)	4

of failure of such procedures to purge cytologically clear bone marrow effectively (41), possibly due to heterogeneity of BL cell immunophenotype.

A major problem has been how to assess the efficacy of bone marrow purging in terms of reduction of BMT indication, especially with minimal bone marrow infiltration (34). Liquid culture assay appears to be the most sensitive method, with which up to $1/10^6$ cells are detectable in vitro (34). It is obvious that the sensitivity of the method is a major parameter for defining the efficiency of purging. Hence a randomized study is not possible unless standardization of purging and detection procedures is obtained.

Takvorian et al. have reported a 62% relapse-free survival in a series of NHL patients in sensitive remission treated with massive therapy followed by CD20-purged autologous BMT (30). We have not observed any differences in survival or relapse in a nonrandomized study of 24 patients receiving

purged or unpurged marrow (Fig. 40.4) (41). However, due to the inefficiency of the purging procedure for several patients, no conclusions can be drawn. Studies of bone marrow purging with cytotoxic agents for NHL do not permit one to conclude for or against the efficacy of these procedures. However, none of these clinical studies of bone marrow purging in lymphoma have demonstrated the efficiency of this technique to prevent relapse or to increase survival.

In conclusion, the capacity of available BM purging techniques to completely eliminate malignant cells from the bone marrow has not been demonstrated, nor has it been demonstrated that this achievement was effective in reducing relapse or increasing survival, since an important proportion of patients grafted for relapse with unpurged bone marrow do not relapse. The observation that 81% of relapses occur at sites of previous disease rather suggests that relapse after BMT is due to failure of the conditioning regimen to eradicate the disease (56). Bone marrow purging cannot be considered a routine procedure, and it requires further investigation in order to make conclusions as to its efficacy. We do not recommend using purging procedures for autologous BMT to treat BL in 1992 when marrow is cytologically and histologically normal.

ALLOGENEIC BONE MARROW TRANSPLANTATION

A limited number of studies of allogeneic BMT for BL and NHL are available (Table 40.7). Appelbaum et al. (57) have reported a series of 100 patients, including 36 patients with high-grade lymphoma, who received allogeneic BMT (60%), autologous BMT (27%), and syngeneic BMT (13%). This study does not show any difference in survival or relapse between the groups. O'Leary et al. (37) have reported a series of 10 patients, including 6 with BL, who received an allogeneic transplant, with 3 long-term survivors in the BL subgroup. Three other groups have re-

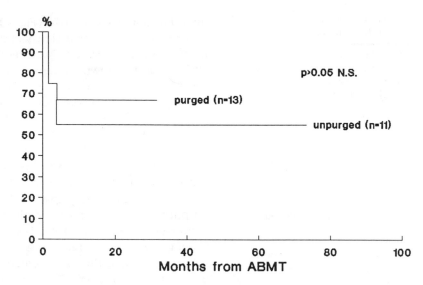

Figure 40.4. Survival of patients with BL in sensitive relapse treated with high-dose therapy followed by purged (n = 13) or unpurged (n = 11) autologous BMT in Lyon.

Table 40.7. Allogeneic BMT for Non-Hodgkin's Lymphoma and Burkitt's Lymphoma

Study (Ref.)	No. of Patients Allogeneic (BL)	Probability of Relapse	Probability of DFS[a]
Mascret (11)	11 (1)	.28	.14
O'Leary (37)	10 (6)	.20	.50
Phillips (58)	14 (4)	.28	.14
Appelbaum (57)	49 (NI)	.50	.27
Ernst (59)	25 (NI)	.28	.52
Troussard (39)	9 (9)	.0	.77
Jones (60)	10 (NI)	.16	.47

[a]DFS, disease-free survival.

ported their experience in the treatment of BL and other NHL with poor prognosis (11, 58, 59). The survival rates are comparable to those obtained with autologous BMT, but toxicity appears to be higher in these series. All these studies included various types of lymphoma treated with various chemotherapy and TBI-containing regimens and showed no evidence for the superiority of allogeneic BMT compared to autologous BMT in term of survival or relapse in BL or any other NHL.

However, two recent studies have re- newed interest in allogeneic BMT for NHL. A French group has reported seven long-term survivors in nine patients with L3 ALL and CNS involvement treated with massive therapy and allogeneic BMT in consolidation after re- sponse to a conventional regimen (39). Such patients have a poor prognosis with the same induction treatment and no consolidation. However, this protocol must be evaluated in a larger series of patients since similar sur- vival rates have been recently reported with an intensive regimen that does not include BMT (48).

The second study reported by Jones et al. (60), which did not include BL, has com- pared relapse and survival in a series of pa- tients treated with the same massive therapy regimen followed by autologous or alloge- neic BMT. A significant superiority of allo- geneic BMT in term of relapse-free survival is observed in this study but without survival advantages. This report suggests the exis- tence of a graft-versus-lymphoma effect of al- logeneic BMT and should stimulate addi- tional work on this field, in BL and other NHL. Low toxicity of the cyclophosphamide/TBI conditioning regimen has been reported (61).

PERSPECTIVES

The indications for high-dose therapy in BL are currently restricted to patients in sensitive relapse or in partial response to first-line regimens. At least 50% of these patients will be cured with the procedure. Patients with primary or secondary "refractory" tumors cannot be cured with the high-dose therapy programs available in 1991. The current goal for clinical research and evaluation is thus the treatment of this limited subgroup of patients with BL. Although considerable progress was achieved in the past 10 years for the understanding of the gene dysregulation operating in BL, no obvious perspective of "gene therapy" applicable to humans is currently in view. Intensification of cytotoxic treatment with the use of hematopoietic growth factors must now be evaluated in this disease. Immunotherapy using antiproliferative or immunomodulatory cytokines or allogeneic BMT may also have an important role for the treatment of these patients.

CONCLUSIONS

Major progress has been made in the treatment of BL since 1980. More than 80% of the patients are definitely cured at the end of first-line treatment with today's regimens. The improvement of conventional chemotherapy has led to a reduction in the indications for high-dose therapy and BMT in BL. However, in 1992 some patients are still candidates for these treatments, of whom 40%–50% will be cured. The optimal high-dose chemotherapy regimen is the BEAM regimen.

Two major indications are clearly characterized: partial remission to first-line treatment and sensitive first or second relapse.

REFERENCES

1. Philip T, Lenoir GM, Bryon PA, et al. Burkitt's type malignant lymphoma in France: individualisation among Caucasian childhood non Hodgkin's lymphoma. Br J Cancer 1982;45:670–678.
2. Philip T. Burkitt's lymphoma in Europe. In: Lenoir GM, O'Connor GT, Olweny CLM, eds. Burkitt's lymphoma: a human cancer model. Lyon: IARC, 1985:303–326.
3. Appelbaum FR, Herzig GP, Ziegler JL, et al. Successful engraftment of cryopreserved autologous bone marrow in patients with malignant lymphoma. Blood 1978;52:85–95.
4. Appelbaum FR, Deisseroth AB, Graw RG, et al. Prolonged complete remission following high dose chemotherapy of Burkitt's lymphoma in relapse. Cancer 1987;41:1059–1063.
5. Murphy SB. Classification, staging and end results of treatment of childhood non Hodgkin's lymphoma: dissimilarities from lymphomas in adults. Semin Oncol 1980;7:332–339.
6. Appelbaum FR, Thomas ED. Review of the use of marrow transplantation in the treatment of non Hodgkin's lymphoma. J Clin Oncol 1983;1:440–447.
7. Goldie JH, Coldman AJ. Quantitative model for multiple levels of drug resistance in clinical tumors. Cancer Treat Rep 1983;67:923–931.
8. Philip T., Biron P., Herve P., et al. Massive BACT therapy with autologous bone marrow transplantation in 17 cases of non Hodgkin's lymphoma with very bad prognosis. Eur J Cancer Clin Oncol 1983;19:1371–1379.
9. Kaiser H, Warham MD, Munoz RJ. Autologous bone marrow transplantation in the treatment of selected human malignancies: the John Hopkins Oncology Cancer Program. Exp Haematol 1979;7(suppl 5):309–320.
10. Gale RP, Graze PR, Wells J. Autologous bone marrow transplantation in patients with cancer. Exp Haematol 1979;7(suppl 5):351–359.
11. Mascret, B, Maraninchi D, Gastaut JA, et al. Treatment of malignant lymphoma with high doses of chemo or chemoradiotherapy and bone marrow transplantation. Eur J Cancer Clin Oncol 1980;22:461–471.
12. Douer D, Champlin RE, Ho WG, et al. High dose combined modality therapy and autologous bone marrow transplantation in resistant cancer. Am J Med 1981;71:973–976.
13. Phillips G, Herzig G, Lazarus H, et al. Cyclophosphamide, total body irradiation and autologous bone marrow transplantation for refractory malignant lymphoma. Blood 1981;58:175a.
14. Eckert H, Ellis WM, Waters KD, Tauro GP. Autologous bone marrow rescue in the treatment of advanced tumor of childhood. Cancer 1982;49:603–609.
15. Hartmann O, Pein F, Philip T, Lemerle J. The effect of high dose poly chemotherapy with autologous bone marrow transplantation in 18 children with relapsed lymphoma. Eur J Cancer Clin Oncol 1982;18:1044–1045.
16. Barbasch A, Higby DJ, Brass C. High dose cytoreductive therapy and autologous bone marrow transplantation in advanced malignancies. Cancer Treat Rep 1983;67:143–148.

17. Tannir NM, Spitzer G, Zander AR, et al. High dose chemoradiotherapy and bone marrow transplantation in patients with refractory lymphoma. Eur J Cancer Clin Oncol 1983;19:1091–1096.

18. Philip T, Biron P, Philip I, et al. Massive therapy and ABMT in Burkitt lymphoma (30 courses on 28 patients: a 5 years experience). Eur J Cancer Clin Oncol 1986;22:1015–1027.

19. Patte C, Philip T, Rodary C, et al. Improved survival rate in children with stage III and IV B cell non Hodgkin lymphoma and leukemia using multi-agent chemotherapy: results of a study of 114 children from the French pediatric oncology society. J Clin Oncol 1984;4:1219–1226.

20. Spitzer G, Dicke K, Verma DS, et al. High dose BCNU therapy with autologous bone marrow infusions: preliminary observations. Cancer Treat Rep 1979; 63:1257–1264.

21. Mac Elwain TH, Hedley DW, Cordon MY, et al. High dose melphalan and non cryopreserved autologous bone marrow treatment of melanoma and neuroblastoma. Exp Haematol 1979;7(suppl 5):360–371.

22. Souhami RL, Harper PG, Linch DC, et al. High dose cyclophosphamide with autologous bone marrow transplantation for small cell carcinoma of the bronchus. Cancer Chemother. Pharmacol 1983;10:205–207.

23. Wolff SN, Fer MF, McKay CM, et al. High dose VP16-213 and ABMT for refractory malignancies: a phase I study. J Clin Oncol 1983;1:701–705.

24. Cazin B, Gorin NC, Laporte JP, et al. Cardiac complications after bone marrow transplantation; a report of 63 consecutive transplantations. Cancer 1986;57:2061–2069.

25. Biron P, Goldstone A, Colombat P, et al. A phase II study of a new cytoreductive conditioning regimen with autologous bone marrow transplantation for lymphomas: the BEAM protocol. In: Dicke K, Spitzer G, Jaganath S, eds. Autologous bone marrow transplantation. Houston: 1987:593–600.

26. Philip T, Armitage O, Spitzer G, et al. High dose therapy and autologous bone marrow transplantation after failure of conventional chemotherapy in adults with intermediate-grade or high grade non Hodgkin's lymphoma. N Engl J Med 1987;316:1493–1498.

27. Gribben JG, Goldstone AH, Linch DC, et al. Effectiveness of high dose combination chemotherapy and autologous bone marrow transplantation for patients with non Hodgkin's lymphoma who are still responsive to conventional dose therapy. J Clin Oncol 1989;11:1621–1629.

28. Colombat P, Gorin NC, Lemonnier MP, et al. The role of autologous bone marrow transplantation in 46 adult patients with non Hodgkin's lymphomas. J Clin Oncol 1990;8:630–637.

29. Phillips GL, Herzig RH, Lazarus HM, et al. Treatment of resistant malignant lymphoma with cyclophosphamide, total body irradiation, and transplantation of cryopreserved autologous marrow. N Engl J Med 1983;310:1557–1561.

30. Takvorian T, Canellos GP, Ritz J, et al. Prolonged disease free survival after autologous bone marrow transplantation in patients with non Hodgkin's lymphoma with a poor prognosis. N Engl J Med 1987;316:1499–1505.

31. Phillips GL, Fay JW, Herzig RH, et al. The treatment of progressive non Hodgkin's lymphoma with intensive chemoradiotherapy and autologous bone marrow transplantation. Blood 1990;75:831–838.

32. Petersen FB, Appelbaum FR, Hill R, et al. Autologous marrow transplantation for malignant lymphoma: a report of 101 cases from Seattle. J Clin Oncol 1990;8:638–647.

33. Phillips GL, Wolff SN, Herzig RH, et al. The role of total body irradiation in the treatment of lymphoma. In: Dicke KA, Spitzer G, Zander AR, et al., eds. Autologous bone marrow transplantation. Proceedings of the first international symposium. Houston: University of Texas, 1986:117–123.

34. Philip T, Pinkerton R, Hartmann O, et al. The role of massive therapy with autologous bone marrow transplantation in Burkitt's lymphoma. Clin Hematol 1986;15:205–218.

35. Deeg HJ. Bone marrow transplantation: a review of delayed complications. Br J Haematol 1984;57:185–208.

36. Goldstone AH, Souhami RL, Linch DC, et al. Intensive chemotherapy and ABMT for relapsed lymphoma. Exp Haematol 1984;12(suppl 15):137.

37. O'Leary M, Ramsay NKC, Nesbit ME. Bone marrow transplantation for non Hodgkin's lymphoma in children and young adults. Am J Med 1983;74:497–501.

38. Fenaux P, Lai JL, Zandecki M, et al. Burkitt acute leukemia in adults: a report of 18 cases. Br J Haematol 1989;71:371–376.

39. Troussard X, Leblond M, Kuentz N, et al. Allogeneic bone marrow transplantation in adults with Burkitt's lymphoma or acute lymphoblastic leukemia in first complete remission. J Clin Oncol 1990;8:809–812.

40. Philip T, Bouffet E, Biron P, et al. Review of the 73 bone marrow transplantations in B lymphoma and T lymphoma. Bone Marrow Transplant 1989;4:55.

41. Philip T, Biron P, Maraninchi D, et al. Massive therapy with ABMT in 50 cases of bad prognosis non Hodgkin's lymphoma. Br J Haematol 1985;60:599–610.

42. Surbone A, Longo D, De Vita C Jr, et al. Residual masses in aggressive non Hodgkin's lymphoma after combination chemotherapy: signification and management. J Clin Oncol 1988;6:1832–1837.

43. Fischer RI, DeVita VT, Hubbard SM, et al. Diffuse aggressive lymphomas: increased survival after alternating flexible sequences of ProMACE and MOPP chemotherapy. Ann Intern Med 1983;93:304–309.

44. Coiffier B, Bryon PA, Berger F, et al. Intensive and

sequential combination chemotherapy for aggressive malignant lymphoma (protocol LNH 80). J Clin Oncol 1986;4:147–153.

45. Philip T, Hartmann O, Biron P, et al. High dose therapy and autologous bone marrow transplantation in partial remission after first line induction therapy for diffuse non Hodgkin's lymphoma. J Clin Oncol 1988;6:1118–1124.

46. Patte C, Philip T, Rodary C, et al. High survival rate in advanced stage B cell lymphoma and leukemias without CNS involvement with a short intensive polychemotherapy: results from the French Pediatric Oncology Society of a randomized trial of 216 children. J Clin Oncol 1991;9:123–132.

47. Patte C, Rodary C, Sarrazin D, et al. Resultats du traitement de 178 lymphomes malins non Hodgkiniens de l'enfant de 1973 à 1978. Arch Fr de Pediatr 1978;38:321–330.

48. Patte C, Perel Y, Leverger G, et al. High survival rate of B-cell non Hodgkin's lymphoma with CNS involvement and B-ALL. Results of the protocol LMB86 of the French Pediatric Oncology Society [Abstract]. In: Cavalli F, ed. Fourth International Conference on Malignant Lymphoma. 1990:39.

49. Gentet JC, Patte C, Quintana E, et al. Phase II of study of cytarabine and etoposide in children with refractory or relapsed non-Hodgkin's lymphoma: a study of the SFOP. J Clin Oncol 1990;8:661–665.

50. Benjamin D, Magrath I, Douglas EC, et al. Derivation of lymphoma cell lines from microscopically normal bone marrow in patients with undifferentiated lymphoma: evidence of occult bone marrow involvement. Blood 1983;61:1017–1019.

51. Philip I, Philip T, Favrot M, et al. Establishment of lymphomatous cell lines from bone marrow samples from patients with Burkitt's lymphoma. J Natl Cancer Inst 1984;73:835–841.

52. Philip I, Favrot MC, Combaret V, et al. Use of a liquid cell culture assay to measure the in vitro Burkitt cell elimination from the BM in preclinical and clinical procedure. In: Dicke K, Spitzer G, Zander AR, eds. Proceedings of the Second International Symposium on ABMT. Houston: 1986:341–347.

53. Bast RC, Ritz J, Lipton JM, et al. Elimination of leukemic cells from human bone marrow using monoclonal antibodies and complement. Cancer Res 1983;43:1389–1392.

54. Santos GW, Kaiser H. In vitro chemotherapy as a prelude to autologous bone marrow transplantation in haematological malignancy. In: Lowenberg B, Hagenbeek A, eds. Minimal residual disease in acute leukemia. Boston: Nijhoff, 1984:165–181.

55. Williams J. The role of bone marrow transplantation in non Hodgkin's lymphomas. Semin Oncol 1990; 17:88–95.

56. Goldstone AH. EBMT experience of autologous bone marrow transplantation in non Hodgkin's lymphoma and Hodgkin's disease. In: Autologous bone marrow transplantation. London: Churchill-Livingstone, 1989: 289–292.

57. Appelbaum FR, Sullivan KM, Buckner CD, et al. Treatment of malignant lymphoma in 100 patients with chemotherapy, total body irradiation and marrow transplantation. J Clin Oncol 1987;5:1340–1347.

58. Phillips GL, Herzig RH, Lazarus HM, et al. High dose chemotherapy, fractionated total body irradiation, and allogeneic marrow transplantation for malignant lymphoma. J Clin Oncol 1986;4:480–488.

59. Ernst, P, Maraninchi D, Jacobsen N, et al. Marrow transplantation for non Hodgkin's lymphoma: a multicenter study from the European Cooperative Bone Marrow Transplant Group. Bone Marrow Transplant 1986;1:81–86.

60. Jones RJ, Ambinder RF, Piantadosi S, Santos GW. Evidence of a graft versus lymphoma effect associated with allogeneic bone marrow transplantation. Blood 1991;77:649–653.

61. Freedman AS, Takvorian T, Anderson KC, et al. Autologous bone marrow transplantation in B cell non Hodgkin's lymphoma: very low treatment related mortality in 100 patients in sensitive relapse. J Clin Oncol 1990;8:784–791.

41

HIGH-DOSE CHEMOTHERAPY IN THE MANAGEMENT OF MALIGNANT GERM CELL TUMORS

E. Randolph Broun and Craig R. Nichols

Germ cell neoplasms serve as model of a curative neoplasm (1). Overall, 80% of patients with disseminated germ cell cancer will be cured with cisplatin-based chemotherapy coupled, when necessary, with postchemotherapy surgery. In those few patients with disease not responsive to primary chemotherapy or the 10% of patients who recur after chemotherapy-induced complete remission, the outlook is less hopeful. Standard salvage chemotherapy in this setting with cisplatin and ifosfamide-based regimens may cure 25%–30% of patients, but those patients not cured with salvage therapy or those patients with cisplatin-resistant disease are destined to die of their illness (2).

Preliminary studies using high-dose chemotherapy in patients with refractory germ cell cancer had mixed results. In early studies using high-dose cyclophosphamide, etoposide, or thiotepa, high rates of response were obtained, but these responses were uniformly brief (3). Subsequent studies in Europe and the United States using principles and chemotherapy combinations more specific to germ cell cancer had more favorable results. We will review the recent and current studies using high-dose chemotherapy in germ cell cancer using supportive autologous bone marrow transplantation, he-matopoietic growth factors, and high-dose therapy without specific efforts to modulate myelosuppression.

HIGH-DOSE CHEMOTHERAPY IN GERM CELL NEOPLASMS

The rationale for very high dose chemotherapy in testis cancer comes in part from laboratory evidence that suggests a steep dose-response curve for cisplatin and other agents commonly used in the treatment of germ cell neoplasms (4). As well, several clinical trials (5, 6) have suggested improved outcome for patients with germ cell cancer who receive more dose-intensive regimens. Unfortunately, there are only a handful of randomized prospective trials adequately testing this hypothesis.

One of the most important trials in this regard is the trial conducted jointly by the Southeastern Cancer Study Group (SECSG) and the Southwest Oncology Group (SWOG) (7). This trial was a straightforward comparison of cisplatin dose intensity in patients with germ cell cancer. This trial enrolled only patients with poor-risk (Table 41.1) disease, a group of patients that had previously been shown to have a relatively poor outcome with conventional therapies (8). It was hoped that

Table 41.1.   Indiana Classification System

Advanced Disease
7. Advanced pulmonary metastases—Mediastinal mass >50% of the intrathoracic diameter or >10 nodules per lung field or multiple pulmonary metastases >3 cm (± nonpalpable abdominal disease)
   Mediastinal nonseminomatous germ cell tumor
8. Palpable abdominal disease + pulmonary metastases
9. Hepatic, osseous, or CNS metastases

Table 41.2.   Therapeutic Outcome

	Standard Dose (n = 77)	High Dose (n = 76)
Complete remission	36(47%)	35(46%)
NED-teratoma[a]	15(19%)	15(20%)
NED-cancer	5(6%)	1(1%)
Partial remission	14(18%)	20(26%)
Stable/progression	7(9%)	4(5%)
Continuously NED	48(62%)	48(62%)
Presently NED	52(68%)	53(70%)
Dead	20(26%)	20(26%)

Table 41.3.   Hematologic Toxicity

	Standard Dose (n = 77)	High Dose (n = 76)
White blood cell count <1.0 × 10⁹/liter	12(16%)	27(36%)
Platelet count <20 × 10⁹/liter	2(3%)	16(21%)
Red blood cell transfusions, number of patients	19(25%)	48(63%)
Platelet transfusions, number of patients	2(3%)	21(28%)
Granulocytopenic fever, number of episodes	13	47
Episodes of sepsis	2	7

Table 41.4.   Toxic Manifestations, Grade 3 or 4

	Standard Dose (n = 77)	High Dose (n = 76)
Ototoxicity	0	24(32%)
Neurotoxicity	1(1%)	20(26%)
Renal toxicity	2(3%)	2(3%)
Gastrointestinal toxicity	3(4%)	20(26%)

dose-escalation of cisplatin would result in higher cure rates in this poor-risk subgroup to a degree sufficient to justify the expected increase in therapy-related morbidity.

Of the 159 patients entered on this trial, 153 were fully eligible and evaluable for toxicity and response. The results are outlined in Table 41.2. There was no improvement of outcome using the higher-dose cisplatin regimen. Overall, 61% of patients receiving standard-dose therapy are continuously free of disease, and 63% of patients receiving high-dose therapy are continuously free of disease. The median duration of follow-up is 24 months, with 87% of patients having greater than 1 year of follow-up and 55% having greater than 2 years. There was no significant difference between the two treatment groups ($p = .9$).

Granulocytopenia and thrombocytopenia were significantly more common in patients receiving high-dose cisplatin therapy (Table 41.3). Biologic consequences of this myelosuppression were seen more frequently in the high-dose arm. Granulocytopenic fever and sepsis were three times more common on the high-dose arm. Red blood cell transfusions were required on 142 separate occasions in 48 patients receiving the high-dose cisplatin compared to 34 occasions in 19 patients receiving standard-dose therapy. Likewise, platelet transfusions were required on 44 occasions by 21 patients on high-dose therapy compared to 3 occasions in 2 patients receiving standard-dose therapy.

As shown in Table 41.4, patients receiving high-dose therapy had significantly more ototoxicity, neurotoxicity, and gastrointestinal toxicity ($p < .001$). Severe hearing loss or disabling tinnitus was confined to the high-dose arm, with 24 patients (32%) experiencing this toxicity. In general, tinnitus resolved slowly over a period of months. Disabling peripheral neuropathy manifest as numbness, pain, and small motor dysfunction was seen in 20 patients (26%) receiving high-dose therapy compared to 1 patient on the standard-dose arm. Severe nausea and vomiting necessitating hospitalization or weight loss of greater than 30 pounds over the course of treatment occurred significantly more often in patients receiving high-dose therapy.

Dose intensity analysis was performed for each drug in the treatment regimen (Table 41.5). Treatment courses in 72 patients receiving high-dose therapy could be analyzed for dose intensity. Overall dose intensity was calculated for each arm and comparisons made for the most important single agent, cisplatin, the two most important agents, cisplatin and etoposide, and the overall dose intensity of all three agents (Table 41.6). In all these analyses, the agents were given equal weight in consideration of dose intensity. The three univariate logistic regression analyses investigating the relationship between dose intensity and treatment were unable to conclude that dose intensity had an effect on response; cisplatin ($p = .42$); cisplatin and eto-

Table 41.5. Median Dose Delivered

	High Dose (n = 72)	Standard Dose (n = 76)
Cisplatin	60 mg/m^2/week	33 mg/m^2/week
>90%	47%	91%
>80%	79%	95%
Etoposide	152 mg/m^2/week	166 mg/m^2/week
>90%	49%	91%
>80%	79%	95%
Bleomycin	14 units/m^2/week	14 units/m^2/week
>90%	44%	48%
>80%	75%	75%

Table 41.6. Relative Dose Intensity

	Standard Dose (n = 76)	High Dose (n = 72)
Cisplatin	1.00	1.80
Cisplatin + etoposide	1.00	1.35
Cisplatin + etoposide + bleomycin	0.97	1.21

Median dose delivered relative to
cisplatin 33 mg/m^2/week
etoposide 167 mg/m^2/week
bleomycin 16 units/m^2/week

poside ($p = .33$); cisplatin, etoposide, and bleomycin ($p = .15$).

This trial provides one of the best examples of a prospective analysis of dose intensity. The straightforward comparison of one variable (cisplatin dose intensity) simplifies the analysis. The randomized format ensured that poor prognostic features (and inherent inability to tolerate aggressive treatment) were distributed equally between the two treatment arms. There was a full accounting of dose actually delivered. The young age of the patients and the experience of the investigators allowed for maintenance of dose intensity in both treatment groups. Indeed, the median dose intensity for the entire combination in the standard arm was 0.97. The difference in dose intensity between the two arms (0.97–1.21) was substantially greater than the usual comparisons of dose intensity, which cluster in the range of 0.6–0.8 relative dose intensity. This difference is even more striking when one considers the most important component in the BEP combination, cisplatin, for which the relative dose intensity was 1.82 and 1.00 in the high-dose and standard arms, respectively, or even when the comparison is made with the two most important drugs, cisplatin and etoposide, for which the difference in relative dose intensity was 1.35–1.00.

The impact of achieving high cisplatin dose intensity in this study was clear. There was a marked increase in ototoxicity, neurotoxicity, gastrointestinal complications, and severe myelosuppression. Therapy-related deaths, while rare, occurred more commonly in the high-dose arm. This increase in therapy-induced toxicity was not compensated by an increase in complete remission rate or survival. With identical therapeutic results achieved with much less toxicity, cisplatin (100–120 mg/m^2 per course), etoposide, and bleomycin remains the standard regimen for poor-risk germ cell cancer. Higher doses of cisplatin should not be used outside the context of a controlled clinical trial.

The results of this trial must be reconciled with those of other trials exploring the role of cisplatin dose intensity in germ cell cancer. One trial frequently cited as validation of the concept of dose intensity in cancer therapy is the study of the SWOG (6). Patients with disseminated germ cell cancer were randomly assigned to receive vinblastine, bleomycin, and either cisplatin 120 mg/m^2 every 4 weeks (30 mg/m^2/week) or cisplatin 75 mg/m^2 every 4 weeks (19 mg/m^2/week). There was a statistically significant increase in the complete remission (CR) rate and survival for patients receiving the higher-dose therapy. This advantage was most apparent when the group of patients with maximal disease was considered (57% CR compared to 34% CR, $p = .02$). While this trial addresses a different question than the more recent SECSG/SWOG trial mentioned above, it clearly demonstrates that halving the standard cisplatin dose intensity does not maintain therapeutic outcome. As a point of reference, the low-dose cisplatin arm of this trial has a relative cisplatin dose intensity of 0.58 compared to standard BEP.

The second important and frequently cited trial in this regard is the trial conducted at the National Cancer Institute (5). This trial was designed in a manner similar to the SECSG/SWOG trial and asked whether maximum escalation of chemotherapy doses resulted in superior outcome relative to standard therapy. Fifty-two patients with poor-risk germ cell cancer were randomized to receive high-dose therapy with high-dose cisplatin (40 mg/m^2 daily $\times$ 5), etoposide (100 mg/m^2 daily $\times$ 5), vinblastine (0.2 mg/kg day 1), and bleomycin (30 units days 1, 8, and 15), or standard therapy with cisplatin (20 mg/m^2 daily $\times$ 5), vinblastine (0.3 mg/kg day 1), and bleomycin (30 units days 1, 8, and 15). Patients were randomized in a 2:1 fashion. Of 34 patients randomized to the high-dose therapy, 30 (88%) obtained disease-free status compared to 12 of the 18 patients (67%) who randomized to the standard-dose therapy ($p = .14$). Sixty-eight percent of patients (23 of 34) randomized to the high-dose therapy arm remained alive and continuously free

of disease compared to 33% (6 of 18) of patients randomized to the standard dose therapy ($p = .02$). This small study with this particular design illustrates some of the difficulty in dose intensity analysis of regimens containing different drugs. In this study, it is difficult to ascribe the apparent improvement in outcome to the high-dose cisplatin component of the regimen since full-dose etoposide was the other addition to the high-dose regimen. In particular, since the randomized comparison of cisplatin, bleomycin, and either etoposide or vinblastine in advanced germ cell cancer performed by the SECSG showed an advantage for the etoposide-containing arm, one might argue that the seeming improvement in outcome is due to the inclusion of etoposide rather than to the doubling of the cisplatin dose (9). Of note, this trial of the SECSG demonstrated a complete remission rate of 63% in advanced disease patients with standard-dose BEP, and our current trial had a 73% CR rate, with 62% of patients being continuously disease-free with standard-dose BEP. We and other investigators have noted continued improvements in remission rate and survival rates using identical doses of chemotherapy.

Other trials of cisplatin dose intense regimens conducted at single institutions, demonstrate mixed results. Modern large trials of cisplatin, etoposide, and bleomycin-based therapy in untreated poor-risk germ cell tumor (5, 9–13) are plotted in Figure 41.1 comparing percent disease-free to relative *planned* dose intensity, using standard-dose BEP as a reference. As can be seen from this figure, the dose-response relationship over the span of relative dose intensity of 1.00–1.8 is shallow and, with the exception of two small studies, would be flat or negative.

The trials in patients with poor-risk germ cell cancer highlight two important points in reference to high-dose chemotherapy in this disease. First, with modern standard-dose chemotherapy, 75% of patients obtain disease-free status. We at Indiana University have been unable to define a subgroup that had

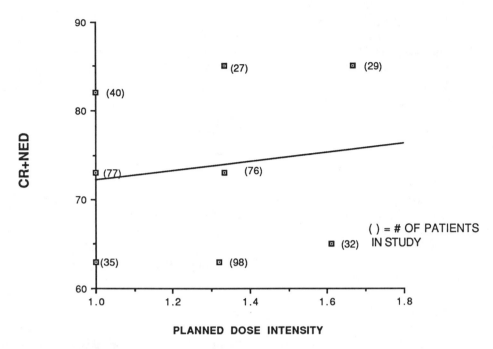

Figure 41.1.   Impact of dose intensity in poor-risk germ cell cancer.

less than a 50% likelihood of successful outcome. Thus it is extremely unlikely that very high dose chemotherapy with its atendant risk and expense will influence the primary care of patients with germ cell cancer. Second, the results of this recent study and analysis of dose intensity in therapy of testis cancer suggest that the dose-response relationship is relatively shallow and that minor modifications of doses of existing therapy (20%–50% increase in delivered dose intensity) are unlikely to improve therapeutic outcome. More likely, improved results will come with either new drug combinations or major increases in dose intensity of existing agents (300%–400%).

HEMATOPOIETIC GROWTH FACTORS AS AN ADJUNCT TO THERAPY IN GERM CELL CANCER

The use of hematopoietic growth factors to ameliorate myelosuppressive consequences of chemotherapy in germ cell cancer has been limited. Primary treatment programs are highly successful at current conventional doses. This curative therapy, while quite myelosuppressive, only rarely results in biologic consequences of myelosuppression. For example, in a recent large chemotherapy trial in patients with good-risk features, only 1 patient of the 188 entered died due to neutropenic sepsis (14). In the recent poor-risk trial of the SEGSG and SWOG, only one patient of the 159 entered died due to sepsis while granulocytopenic. In these trials, approximately 15% of patients treated with standard-dose BEP had a febrile neutropenic event (7).

In the setting of recurrent disease or prior radiotherapy, however, subsequent chemotherapy is associated with a much higher incidence of febrile neutropenic events. Using vinblastine, ifosfamide, and cisplatin as salvage treatment, about 40% of patients will experience myelosuppressive complications (2). Thus it is in this setting that the use of hematopoietic growth factors could be expected to be beneficial.

The use of recombinant human granulocyte-macrophage colony-stimulating factor (rhGM-CSF) has been tested recently in this setting (15). Investigators entered patients with recurrent testicular cancer who received standard doses of ifosfamide, cisplatin, and either etoposide or vinblastine (VIP or VeIP). Patients were allocated at random to receive rhGM-CSF with either the first and second cycles or the third and fourth cycles. Preliminary review of this trial suggests a decrease in the number of major infections and antibiotic use, and an increase in the number of patients receiving chemotherapy on schedule associated with the administration of rhGM-CSF. Further analysis of this trial is pending, but in the setting of recurrent disease where conventional-dose treatment still has the potential for cure, the hematopoietic growth factors may be useful in diminishing myelosuppressive consequences of therapy and maintaining treatment intensity.

HIGH-DOSE CHEMOTHERAPY WITH AUTOLOGOUS BONE MARROW TRANSPLANTATION IN TESTICULAR CANCER

Indiana University Studies

Investigations into the use of high-dose carboplatin and etoposide with autologous bone marrow support began at Indiana University in 1986. Initial investigations were in patients who were heavily pretreated and for whom no other curative therapeutic options existed. Subsequent studies have explored modification of the initial regimen in refractory patients and the efficacy of this regimen in patients in first relapse after conventional therapy. Important insights into the need for patient selection, the particular problem of primary nonseminomatous mediastinal germ cell tumors, and the value of intervention early in the course of the disease for these toxic, expensive, yet potentially curative modes of therapy have been gained.

The initial phase I/II dose escalation study was done in collaboration with Vanderbilt University (16). This trial examined the use of two courses of high-dose carboplatin and etoposide in patients with germ cell tumors refractory to cisplatin (defined as progression within 4 weeks of the last cisplatin dose) or recurrent after a minimum of two prior regimens containing cisplatin. Thirty-three patients were entered on this trial. The initial 13 patients were treated with varying doses of carboplatin (Table 41.7) to establish the maximum tolerated dose in combination with etoposide at a fixed dose of 1200 mg/m^2. The subsequent 20 patients were treated with etoposide 1200 mg/m^2 and the phase II dose of carboplatin of 1500 mg/m^2 given in three divided doses on days -7, -5, and -3. Toxicities seen in the protocol were the expected severe myelosuppression, moderate enterocolitis, and stomatitis. Grade 3 hepatic toxicity (more than five-fold increase in liver enzymes), usually in association with massive infections, was observed in 8 of 33 (24%) patients. Of interest, significant ototoxicity, neurotoxicity, or nephrotoxicity was not seen despite extensive prior exposure to cisplatin in this patient population. Overall, 7 of 33 (21%) of patients died as a consequence of treatment, 2 on the phase II portion of the study. Deaths were primarily due to infection; however, 1 patient died of venoocclusive disease of the liver (Table 41.8). Of note, this was a very heavily pretreated patient population, with over half of the patients having received three or more prior chemotherapy regimens, and 67% of patients were cisplatin refractory. There were 8 patients who obtained a CR and 6 a

Table 41.7.   Phase I Trial of High-Dose Carboplatin/Etoposide

| | Dose (mg/m^2) | | No. of Patients |
	Carboplatin	Etoposide	
Phase I	900	1200	3
	1350	1200	4
	1800	1200	5
	2000	1200	1
Phase II	1500	1200	20

Table 41.8.   Causes of Death: Phase I/II Study

Carboplatin (mg/m^2)	Day No.	Cause
1500	+13	Streptococcal sepsis
1500	+19	Venoocclusive disease
1500	+5	Streptococcal sepsis
1500	+5	*Candida* sepsis, hemorrhage
1500	+11	Pulmonary infection
1800	+15	*Candida* sepsis
2000	+20	*Candida* sepsis

partial remission (PR), for an overall response rate of 44% (95% confidence intervals, 27%–63%). Of the 8 patients obtaining CR, 3 are long-term disease-free survivors, and a fourth patient died at 22 months free of germ cell cancer from a therapy-related acute non-lymphocytic leukemia. Review of responding patients reveals that CR was achieved despite advanced stage or disease refractory to cisplatin.

The conclusions that can be drawn from these data are that the use of high-dose carboplatin and etoposide can result in long-term disease-free survival in a small percentage of patients for whom high-dose therapy represents third- or fourth-line therapy and that overt cisplatin resistance can sometimes be overcome with high doses of carboplatin and etoposide. The results in this group of very heavily pretreated, unfavorable-prognosis patients are reminiscent of the reports by the bone marrow transplant group in Seattle, who carried out initial studies into the use of allogeneic bone marrow transplantation (BMT) in the treatment of acute nonlymphocytic leukemia. In each study, a small number of very poor prognosis patients doing well led to further investigations in more favorable patients.

Following the phase I/II study, a larger multiinstitutional phase II trial was carried out through the Eastern Cooperative Oncology Group (ECOG), utilizing the same dose and schedule of agents as in the phase II portion of the initial study (17). Again, patients had to have failed at least two prior cisplatin-based

regimens, at least one of which contained ifosfamide, or be cisplatin refractory. Forty patients were entered on this multiinstitution cooperative group effort between July 1988 and September 1989. Two patients were ineligible due to insufficient prior therapy (1) and incorrect histologic diagnosis (1). Twenty-two of 38 (58%) evaluable patients proceeded to a second course of high-dose therapy. Toxicity was similar to that seen in the phase I trial, with 5 of 38 (13%) patients dying of treatment-related causes. Infection (1), hemorrhage (2), and hepatic toxicity (2) accounted for the deaths. All treatment-related deaths occurred in the first course of therapy. Other extramyeloid toxicities were comparable to those seen in the initial study. Nine patients (24%) achieved a CR, including 2 patients rendered disease-free with post-BMT surgical resection, and 8 achieved a PR, for an overall response rate of 45%. Of note, three of the CRs occured on BMT no. 1, and 4 patients converted to CR on BMT no. 2. Five of 9 are alive and free of disease with a minimum follow-up of 18 months. All PRs recurred, with a median duration of remission of 2.5 months. Achievement of a CR was associated with testicular rather than extragonadal primary, absence of liver metastases, and embryonal cell type.

A striking finding in these studies was the poor outcome in patients with nonseminomatous primary mediastinal germ cell tumors. Eleven patients with this diagnosis were enrolled in the Phase II study, and none obtained durable remission. This parallels the institutional experience at Indiana University with patients with nonseminomatous mediastinal germ cell tumors treated in second or greater relapse with high-dose chemotherapy and autologous BMT (18). Since 1987 12 such patients were treated on serial protocols of high-dose carboplatin and estoposide with or without ifosfamide. Seven of the 12 failed to receive the planned second course of therapy due to tumor progression or therapy-related toxicity. No patient achieved a CR, and the median survival post high-dose chemotherapy was 3.5 months. This subgroup has been identified as having poor outcome with other conventional salvage therapies, and such patients should be the focus of investigation of new approaches in treatment (19). At Indiana University, patients with primary mediastinal germ cell tumor who fail primary therapy are treated with two rounds of high-dose carboplatin and etoposide with high-dose ifosfamide as initial salvage therapy.

The results with high-dose carboplatin/ etoposide/autologous BMT in patients with recurrent and refractory germ cell cancer indicated that a fraction of patients could be rendered permanently disease-free. In view of the known activity of ifosfamide in recurrent and refractory germ cell tumors and its favorable side effect profile for dose escalation in the setting of BMT, investigators at Indiana University added high-dose ifosfamide to the CBDCA/VP-16 treatment template. Ifosfamide, as a single agent, has been shown to produce responses in patients with recurrent and cisplatin-resistant germ cell cancer (20). Seven patients were entered on a phase II trial of carboplatin and etoposide in the previously described doses and schedule with the addition of ifosfamide beginning at 2 gm/ m^2 daily $\times$ 5 with mesna (21). The patients were treated with one or two courses of high-dose therapy. Due to excessive renal toxicity at the first dose level, escalation of the ifosfamide dose was impossible. Of the seven patients treated, four had a marked decline in their renal function, with three of the four requiring hemofiltration or hemodialysis. Six of the seven patients had decline of serum biomarkers, indicating a response to treatment, but all responses have been brief, perhaps due to the truncated treatment course necessitated by the toxicity encountered.

A second attempt at dose escalation was made in patients with less prior therapy. To date, 27 patients have been entered in a careful dose escalation trial of carboplatin and etoposide without reaching dose-limiting extramedullary toxicity. The current dose achieved in this trial is carboplatin 700 mg/

m^2 and etoposide 650 mg/m^2 for three doses on days -6, -5, -4. Further studies will focus on improvement of therapeutic results by the addition of new agents, alkylating agents, newer cisplatin analogues, and the development of a second non-cross-resistant regimen for use in the double autologous BMT setting. Additionally, we will explore the use of newer cytokines to improve supportive care.

In the treatment of acute leukemia, bone marrow transplants were initially used in end stage, heavily pretreated patients with refractory disease. In this setting, responses were observed but there were only 13% long-term survivors. When this treatment was used in more favorable patients, the response rate improved and about 50% were cured. In like fashion, the use of high-dose therapy with autologous BMT in the treatment of multiply relapsed and refractory germ cell tumors has resulted in an overall response rate of about 50%, with a fraction of patients cured of their disease. A logical progression of this therapy is to move it earlier in the sequence of treatment for germ cell tumors.

Since the overall cure rate for patients with recurrent testis cancer treated with ifosfamide and cisplatin-based salvage chemotherapy is in the range of 25%–30%, the inclusion of high-dose chemotherapy as a portion of initial salvage therapy seemed a logical next step to improve outcome in this group of poor-risk patients. Based on preliminary pilot data at Indiana University and principles from high-dose studies in other disease sites, ECOG is opening a trial of conventional-dose salvage therapy for two cycles (VIP $\times$ 2) followed by a single round of high-dose chemotherapy with carboplatin in the doses and schedule employed in the previous double autologous transplant protocol.

A number of conclusions can be drawn from the series of studies performed at Indiana University. First, a small percentage of patients with multiply relapsed or cisplatin-resistant germ cell cancer can be cured with high-dose chemotherapy. The initial attempt to increase the therapeutic ratio of the regimen with the addition of ifosfamide was unsuccessful in this patient population. Analysis of prognostic factors from these and other studies suggests that patients with primary mediastinal nonseminomatous germ cell cancer have a particularly poor prognosis, and such patients should be entered into clinical trials of more intense therapy or combinations with newer agents. Finally, previous experience in other disease sites and some preliminary studies would suggest that the use of high-dose chemotherapy earlier in the course of recurrent disease may result in a better outcome.

INSTITUT GUSTAVE-ROUSSY

Similar studies from other institutions provide further substantiation of the curative potential of high-dose chemotherapy in refractory germ cell cancer. Serial studies at the Institut Gustave-Roussy have demonstrated activity in recurrent germ cell cancer. These investigators developed a regimen using cisplatin 40 mg/m^2 days 1–5, etoposide 350 mg/m^2 days 1–5, and cyclophosphamide 1600 mg/m^2 days 2–5 (PEC). Sixteen patients with recurrent germ cell cancer were enrolled (22). All had received prior therapy with cisplatin-based treatments. Five of the 15 evaluable for response were long-term disease survivors. The succeeding study enrolled untreated patients felt to be at high risk of treatment failure with conventional therapy (12). Brief conventional induction therapy was followed by a single round of high-dose chemotherapy with PEC. Of 32 poor-risk patients entered, 15 remain free of disease at a median follow-up of 18 months. Based on what the investigators felt were promising results, this group has embarked on a phase III trial in patients with untreated poor-risk germ cell cancer. All patients receive induction therapy with high-dose cisplatin, etoposide, vinblastine, and bleomycin and are subsequently randomized to receive consolidation with the PEC regimen or observation.

OTHER EUROPEAN STUDIES

Two other trials have incorporated principles of the French studies and the studies from Indiana University and ECOG. A large study by Rosti and colleagues expanded the basic carboplatin and etoposide protocol skeleton with the addition of ifosfamide (23). In this study 21 patients were entered after failing primary and usually secondary therapy for germ cell tumors. Therapy consisted of a similar dose and schedule of carboplatin and etoposide as used in our trial, but, recently, has added ifosfamide at a dose of 12 gm/m^2 over 3 days. Again, the primary toxicity was myelosuppression, and no significant renal toxicity, ototoxicity, or neurotoxicity was encountered. Overall, 13 patients received one course, 7 received two courses, and 1 received three courses. There was one therapy-related death due to venoocclusive disease. There were eight CRs including 3 patients who had unresectable PRs with prior therapy. The durations of CRs were 2, 4, 4, 1+, 2+, 4+, 5+, 5+, and 33+ months.

A preliminary report from Linkesch and colleagues in Austria combines features of the PEC protocol and the protocols from Indiana University along with rh GM-CSF (24). In this study, high-dose chemotherapy with carboplatin (2000 mg/m^2), etoposide (1500 mg/m^2), and cyclophosphamide (60 mg/kg × 2) was given to patients with recurrent and refractory germ cell cancer. Twelve patients received the high-dose chemotherapy with autologous marrow rescue and an additional 4 patients received the same treatment with rhGM-CSF along with autologous marrow rescue. The hematologic toxicity appeared successfully modulated by the use of rhGM-CSF. Of the 12 patients receiving therapy without the hematopoietic growth factor, the median time to an absolute granulocyte count > 500 was 20 days compared to 12 days for the 4 patients receiving identical therapy plus GM-CSF. The median time to hospital discharge was 24 days in the group of patients not receiving GM-CSF compared to 15 days in the group receiving GM-CSF. Nonhematologic toxicity included grade 3 and 4 diarrhea in 4 patients, renal toxicity in 2 patients, and ototoxicity in 2 patients. There was no significant neurotoxicity, hepatotoxicity, or cardiac toxicity, and there were no therapy-related deaths. Overall, 8 patients achieved a PR and 3 achieved durable CRs lasting 7+, 9+, and 14+ months.

FUTURE DIRECTIONS

There is now ample evidence that high-dose chemotherapy (PEC, high-dose carboplatin/etoposide) can cure patients who are incurable with conventional salvage regimens. However, in this heavily pretreated population the impact of such therapy has been small (15%–20% long-term disease-free survivors), and the toxicity has been substantial. The next logical step in the development of better therapy for patients with germ cell cancer is to consider use of such high-dose treatments earlier in the course of recurrent disease, prior to the development of bulky drug-resistant disease and at a time when performance status and organ function are maintained.

One of the first reports of such an approach is from Barnett, Coppin, and colleagues at the Cancer Control Agency of British Columbia (25). These investigators report the results of using high-dose chemotherapy as part of initial salvage chemotherapy. In this trial, 18 patients with recurrent or persistent germ cell cancer after cisplatin-based primary therapy were given conventional induction chemotherapy with cisplatin, etoposide, vincristine, and bleomycin given on a weekly schedule or vinblastine, ifosfamide, and cisplatin combinations. At the completion of conventional salvage chemotherapy, consolidation with high-dose chemotherapy was given with autologous marrow support. Patients received high-dose carboplatin, etoposide, and either high-dose cyclophosphamide or ifosfamide. There were two toxic deaths, 2 patients were too early to evaluate, and 8 of 14

remained free of progression from germ cell cancer.

ECOG has begun a similar trial in which patients with recurrent germ cell cancer (non-cisplatin-resistant) receive two courses of conventional salvage chemotherapy (with VIP or PVB). Responding patients will then receive a single round of high-dose etoposide and carboplatin as described earlier. Relative to the preceding ECOG trial, this trial will enter a group of patients who have had much less prior therapy, have better performance status, and have responding smaller-volume disease.

Memorial Sloan Kettering has begun to use high-dose chemotherapy as a portion of initial treatment in selected patients. Patients are given conventional chemotherapy (VAB-6), and those patients in whom there is a suboptimal decline in serum human chorionic gonadotropin or α-fetoprotein after two to three cycles of treatment are given high-dose carboplatin and etoposide with autologous marrow support. To date, the majority of patients entered on the protocol have required transplantation, and there is early evidence of improved outcome relative to a comparable group of patients from earlier trials.

Acknowledgments
    The authors wish to thank Dr. Guido Tricot, Dr. Ron Hoffman, and Dr. Lawrence Einhorn for continued guidance and support of autologous bone marrow transplantation at Indiana University and the nurses, social workers, and data managers on 5N and the Bone Marrow Transplantation Unit at Indiana University for superb care of our patients.

REFERENCES

1. Einhorn LH. Testicular cancer as a model for a curable neoplasm: the Richard and Hinda Rosenthal Foundation Award lecture. Cancer Res 1981;41:3275–3280.
2. Munshi N, Loehrer P, Roth B, et al. Vinblastine, ifosfamide and cisplatin (VeIP) as second line chemotherapy in metastatic germ cell tumors (GCT). Proc Am Soc Clin Oncol 1990;9:134.
3. Cheson B, Lacerna L, Leyland-Jones B, Sarosy G, Wittes R. Autologous bone marrow transplantation: current status and future directions. Ann Intern Med 1989; 110:51–65.

4. Frei III E, Teicher BA, Holden SA, et al. Preclinical studies and clinical correlation of the effect of alkylating dose. Cancer Res 1988;48:6417–6423.

5. Ozols RF, Ihde DC, Linehan M, Jacob J, Ostchega Y, Young RC. A randomized trial of standard chemotherapy v a high-dose chemotherapy regimen in the treatment of poor prognosis nonseminomatous germcell tumors. J Clin Oncol 1988;6(6):1031–1040.

6. Sampson MK, Rivkin SE, Jones SE, et al. Dose-response and dose-survival advantage for high versus low-dose cisplatin combined with vinblastine and bleomycin in disseminated testicular cancer A Southwest Oncology Group study. Cancer 1984; 53:1029–1035.

7. Nichols C, Williams S, Loehrer P, et al. Randomized study of cisplatin dose intensity in advanced germ cell tumors: a Southeastern Cancer Study Group and Southwest Oncology Group protocol. J Clin Oncol 1991;9:1163–1172.

8. Birch R, Williams S, Cone A, et al. Prognostic factors for favorable outcome in disseminated germ cell tumors. J Clin Oncol 1984;4:400–407.

9. Williams SD, Birch R, Einhorn LH, Irwin L, Greco FA, Loehrer PJ. Treatment of disseminated germ-cell tumors with cisplatin, bleomycin and either vinblastine or etoposide. N Engl J Med 1987;316:1435–1440.

10. Pizzocaro G, Piva L, Salvoioni R, Zanoni F, Milani A. Cisplatin, etoposide, bleomycin first-line therapy and early resection of residual tumor in far-advanced germinal testis cancer. Cancer 1985;56:2411–2415.

11. Daugaard G, Rorth M. High-dose cisplatin and VP-16 with bleomycin, in the management of advanced metastatic germ cell tumors. Eur J Cancer Clin Oncol 1986;22:477–485.

12. Droz J, Pico J, Ghosn M, et al. High complete remission (CR) and survival rates in poor prognosis (PP) non seminomatous germ cell tumors (NSGCT) with high dose chemotherapy (HDCT) and autologous bone marrow transplantation (ABMT). Proc Am Soc Clin Oncol 1989;8:130.

13. Schmoll HJ, Schubert I, Arnold H, et al. Disseminated testicular cancer with bulky disease: results of a phase II study with cisplatin ultra high dose/VP-16/bleomycin. Int J Androl 1987;10:311–317.

14. Einhorn LH, Williams SD, Loehrer PJ, et al. Evaluation of optimal duration of chemotherapy in favorable-prognosis disseminated germ cell tumors: a Southeastern Cancer Study Group protocol. J Clin Oncol 1989;7(3):387–391.

15. Nichols C, Bajorin D, Schmoll H, Pizzocaro G, Bosl G, Einhorn L. VIP chemotherapy with/without GM-CSF for poor risk, relapsed, or refractory germ cell tumors (GCT): preliminary analysis of a random controlled trial. Proc Am Soc Clin Oncol 1991;10:167.

16. Nichols CR, Tricot G, Williams SD, et al. Dose-intensive chemotherapy in refractory germ cell cancer—a phase I/II trial of high dose carboplatin and etoposide with autologous bone marrow transplantation. J Clin Oncol 1989;7:932–939.

17. Nichols C, Anderson J, Lazarus H, et al. High dose carboplatin and VP-16 with autologous bone marrow transplantation in patients with recurrent and refractory germ cell cancer: an Eastern Cooperative Oncology Group study. J Clin Oncol, 1991, in press.

18. Broun E, Nichols C, Einhorn L, Tricot G. Salvage therapy with high dose chemotherapy and autologous bone marrow support in the treatment of primary nonseminomatous mediastinal germ cell tumors (EGGCT). Cancer 1991;68:1513–1515.

19. Munshi N, Loehrer P, Williams S, et al. Ifosfamide combination salvage chemotherapy in extragonadal germ cell tumors (EGGCT). Proc Am Soc Clin Oncol 1991;10:182.

20. Wheeler B, Loehrer P, Williams S, Einhorn L. Ifosfamide in refractory male germ cell tumors. J Clin Oncol 1986;4:28–34.

21. Broun E, Nichols C, Tricot G, Loehrer P, Williams S, Einhorn L. High dose carboplatin/VP-16 plus ifosfamide with autologous bone marrow support in the treatment of refractory germ cell tumors. Bone Marrow Transplantation 1991;7:53–56.

22. Pico J, Droz J, Gouyette A, et al. 25 high dose chemotherapy regimens (HDCT) followed by autologous bone marrow transplantation for treatment of relapsed or refractory germ cell tumors. Proc Am Soc Clin Oncol 1986;5:111.

23. Rosti G, Salvioni R, Pizzocaro G, Valzania F, Marangolo M. High dose chemotherapy (HDC) with carboplatin (CBP) and VP-16 in germ cell tumors: the Italian experience. In: Dicke K, Armitage JO, Dicke-Euinger MJ, eds. Autologous bone marrow transplantation: proceedings of the fifth international symposium. Omaha, NE 1990:186.

24. Linkesch W, Kuhrer I, Wagner A. rhu-GM-CSF after ultra-high dose carboplatin, VP-16, cyclophosphamide with ABMT in refractory germ cell cancer. Proc Am Soc Clin Oncol 1990;9:141.

25. Barnett M, Coppin C, Murray N, et al. Intensive therapy and autologous bone marrow transplantation (BMT) for patients with poor prognosis nonseminomatous germ cell tumors. Proc Am Soc Clin Oncol 1991;10:165.

42

DOSE-INTENSIVE THERAPY
IN BREAST CANCER

Karen H. Antman

Breast cancer currently develops in one of nine American women. While less common in Japan, the incidence there is increasing, as well. Rates for Europeans fall between those for Americans and Japanese women. The TMN classification is used for staging breast cancer and is shown in Table 42.1.

Relapse rates at 10 years increase proportionally to the number of axillary lymph nodes, from approximately 20% for patients with no positive lymph nodes to 60% for one to three involved lymph nodes to more than 85% for four or more axillary lymph nodes. Women with stage II disease with more than 10 positive lymph nodes and locally advanced or inflammatory breast cancer have a very poor prognosis with standard therapy. Relapse tends to occur earlier for patients with higher numbers of lymph nodes involved, and some risk of relapse remains for at least 20 years after mastectomy. Prognosis is worse for patients with poorly differentiated tumors and those with high nuclear grade, greater than a diploid number of chromosomes, high fraction of cells synthesizing DNA (S-phase fraction), and extra copies of Her 2/neu oncogene.

Women with metastatic breast cancer are essentially incurable with standard therapy, with a median survival of about 2 years after documentation of metastases (1, 2). The median survival of women with metastatic disease has not changed in the 5 decades for which statistics are available. While generally sensitive to initial chemotherapy regimens, metastatic breast cancer virtually always progresses with shorter and less complete remissions with subsequent regimens. Women with estrogen-receptor-positive tumors (median 2.3 years) and those who achieve a complete response with standard-dose therapy (median 2.5 years) or who have only small amounts of local disease (median >4 years) have a somewhat better survival (2). Metastatic breast cancer therefore represents a major public health problem, as well as a frightening personal dilemma for women afflicted with the disease.

From the late 1960s through the mid-1970s, chemotherapy regimens were developed for metastatic breast cancer utilizing agents with nonoverlapping toxicities based on the superiority of combinations over single agents in the laboratory to decrease the emergence of drug resistance (3–6). Generally administered in an outpatient setting, regimens were designed to achieve maximal objective clinical response rates with acceptable toxicity (i.e., infrequent admissions for fever and neutropenia and rare need for platelet transfusions).

Conventional-dose chemotherapy regimens tend to be either doxorubicin (e.g., FAC) or methotrexate (e.g., CMF or CMFVP) based.

Table 42.1. Staging of Primary Breast Cancer

Tumor (T)

T_0 No evidence of tumor

T_{is} Carcinoma in situ or Paget's disease of nipple with no tumor

T_1 ≤2 cm
- T_{1a} < 0.5 cm
- T_{1b} > 0.5–1 cm
- T_{1c} > 1–2 cm

T_2 >2–5 cm

T_3 >5 cm

T_4 Any size; direct extension to chest wall (excluding pectoral muscle); skin infiltration; *peau d'orange;* satellite nodules

T_{4a} Extension to chest wall

T_{4b} Edema or ulceration of skin or presence of satellite nodules

T_{4c} Both T_{4a} and T_{4b}

T_{4d} Inflammatory carcinoma

Nodes (N)

N_0 No regional lymph node metastasis

N_1 Metastasis to movable ipsilateral axillary lymph node or nodes

N_2 Metsatasis to ipsilateral axillary node or nodes fixed to one another or to other structures

N_2 Metastasis to ipsilateral internal mammary node or nodes

Metastasis (M)

M_0 No distant metastases

M_1 Distant metastasis, including metastasis or ipsilaterial supraclavicular lymph node or nodes

	T	N	M
Stage 0	T_{is}	N_0	M_0
Stage I	T_1	N_0	M_0
	T_0	N_1	
	T_1	N_1	
Stage IIA	T_2	N_0	M_0
	T_2	N_1	
	T_3	N_0	
	T_0	N_2	
Stage IIB	T_1	N_2	M_0
	T_2	N_2	
Stage IIIA	T_3	N_1, N_2	
	T_4	Any N	
Stage IIIB	Any T	N_3	M_0
Stage IV	Any T	Any N	M_1

In previously untreated patients, these regimens produce 40%–75% objective response rates (complete remission and partial remission), with median durations of 6–12 months. Doxorubicin-based regimens generally have somewhat higher overall response rate than methotrexate-based regimens, though at greater cost in toxicity (7).

These results should be considered in context. The majority of trials excluded patients with coexisting medical and psychologic illness, poor performance status, organ system dysfunction, or older age. Furthermore, reported results for standard regimens were largely derived in populations with no prior adjuvant chemotherapy. Thus the current prognosis for metastatic breast cancer is even more dismal than statistics reported from clinical trials.

RATIONALE FOR DOSE-INTENSIVE THERAPY IN BREAST CANCER

In laboratory models of breast cancer and other malignancies, the delivery of the highest possible doses of chemotherapy is essential to achieving curative therapy. Theory, and experimental and clinical data suggest that breast cancer recurs despite an initial response to chemotherapy because of resistance to the chemotherapy drugs. In the laboratory, resistance to alkylating agents can often be overcome by using a 5- to 10-fold higher dose. Laboratory models have been recently reviewed (8).

Clinically, some correlation between chemotherapy dose and response has long been recognized (9). Systematic analysis of dose-response relationships in the clinic has proven problematic, and until recent years few attempts had been made to quantify dose-response relationships in patients with metastatic breast cancer.

In 1984 Hryniuk and Bush introduced the concept of dose intensity for the purpose of quantifying dose-response effects, using metastatic breast cancer as a model (10). They argued that quantitation of dose-response effects required that dose be viewed as a function of the time (i.e., dose intensity) expressed in drug dose administered per square meter per week. Assumptions included (*a*) that all drugs in a given regimen are therapeutically equivalent, (*b*) that synergy and cross-resistance between drugs and scheduling play no role; (*c*) that area under the curve (AUC) is more important than peak drug concentrations; and (*d*) that scheduling has no importance other than as relates to total dose intensity. Their analysis of both methotrexate- and doxorubicin-based regimens in metastatic breast cancer suggested that dose intensity correlated with response, and that response correlated significantly with survival. They concluded that chemotherapy regimens should be designed to maximize dose intensity, the overall dose administered over time, rather than peak dose (in contrast to the philosophy underlying high-dose chemotherapy and autologous marrow transplantation).

The dose intensity hypothesis and methodology have been extensively debated based on both practical and theoretical concerns (11, 12). Given these concerns, a review of randomized clinical trials in which dose intensity is the sole or most important variable seems appropriate (Table 42.2). These trials are difficult to interpret because the increased doses planned varied from 10% to two- to threefold over the low-dose arms. Because serum levels for a given dose of drug commonly vary fivefold, serum levels of drug achieved on these trials must overlap considerably. In addition the actually delivered dose (which is often not included in the manuscript) is frequently not significantly different from that delivered on the lower-dose arm. While some of these trials have shown an increased response rate for regimens with greater dose intensity, few trials demonstrate a significantly increased overall survival. In the trial by Tannock et al., randomization resulted in an excess of patients with brief durations between initial diagnosis and relapse on the low-dose-intensity arm, causing the authors to advise caution in the interpretation of their observations (13). Carmo-Pereira et al. demonstrated a statistically significant difference in median survival (8 months versus 20 months) for patients receiving two different doses of doxorubicin (14). The overall lack of evidence for an improvement in survival for the higher-dose-intensity arms may reflect the relatively minor differences in dose administered, or the lack of any major effect of standard chemotherapy regimens on median survival in metastatic breast cancer. These randomized trials suggest that modest increments in dose intensity produce, at best, only modest effects on survival. However, the trial by Tannock et al. suggests also that increased response rates are associated with an improved quality of life (13).

DOSE-INTENSIVE TREATMENT WITH HEMATOPOIETIC GROWTH FACTOR SUPPORT

The introduction of hematopoietic growth factors may facilitate the clinical evaluation of the importance of dose intensity in a nontransplant setting (Table 42.3). In a small pilot trial, Bronchud et al. reported that use of granulocyte colony-stimulating factor (G-CSF) allows the administration of outpatient

Table 42.2. Randomized Studies of Dose in Breast Cancer[a]

	Prior Chemotherapy	No.	Drugs	Relative Dose	% RR Low	% RR High	S (Months) Low	S (Months) High	Reference
Tannock	None	133	CMF	2	**11**	**30**	**13**	**16**	13
Hoogstraten	None	283	CMFVPr	3	**40**	**59**	14	14	15
Tormey	None	165	CMF ± Pr	1.13	57	63	**14**	**16**	16
Malik	None	60	FAC × 3	1–3	39	70	22	19	17, 18
Focan	None	160	ECF	1–2	**43**	**67**			19
Becher		125	CE	1.5	40	40			20
Beretta	Limited	103	CMF	1.3	32	50			21
Ebbs	Limited	53	E	2	34	37	**10**	**21**	22
Habeshaw	Limited	202	E, Pr	2	**23**	**41**	10	11	23
Carmo-Pereira		48	A	2	25	58	**20**	**8**	14
O'Bryan	Limited	103	A	1.9	32	25			24
O'Bryan	Extensive	68	A	2	6	24			24
Forastiere	Extensive	37	P	2	0	21			25
Samal	Extensive	23	P	1.6	0	0			26

[a]Significant differences in boldface.
[b]Abbreviation: A, doxorubicin (adriamycin); C, cyclophosphamide; F, 5-fluorouracil; M, methotrexate; E, epirubicin; P, cisplatin; Pr, prednisone; RR, objective response rate; S, survival (in months); V, vincristine.

Table 42.3. High-Dose-Intensity Chemotherapy Regimens

Doxorubicin and G-CSF repeated every 12–14 days (27)

	mg/m^2	
Doxorubicin	75–150	day 1
G-CSF	10, 5 μg/kg/day	continuous intravenous infusion day 1–12

Dana-Farber high-dose CAF and G-CSF. Cycles repeated every 28 days (28)

	mg/m^2	
Doxorubicin	60–120	Dose split over day 1 and 2 intravenously
Cyclophosphamide	1000–4000	day 1 intravenously
5-Fluorouracil	600	day 1 intravenously
G-CSF	10 μg/kg/day	Subcutaneously day 3 until recovery

Duke AFM regimen: Cycles repeated every 21 days (29)

	mg/m^2	
5-Fluorouracil	750	continuous intravenous infusion for 5 days
Doxorubicin	25	per day, day 3–5 intravenously
Methotrexate	250	day 15 intravenously
Folinic acid	12.5	Orally every 6 hours × 6 doses day 16

Hopkins Regimen: Cycles repeated every 14 days (30)

Cyclophosphamide	100	Orally every day for 7 days
Doxorubicin	40	day 1 intravenously
Vincristine	1	day 1 intravenously
Methotrexate	100	day 1 intravenously
5-Fluorouracil	600	Day 2
Leucovorin rescue		
5-Fluorouracil	300	Continuous infusion days 8 and 9

doxorubicin at high doses of up to 150 mg/m^2 on an every 12–14 day schedule, with a high complete and overall response rate in patients with metastatic breast cancer (27).

DOSE-INTENSIVE TREATMENT WITH HEMATOPOIETIC STEM CELL SUPPORT

Rationale for Stem Cell Support

Because the limiting toxicity of higher chemotherapy doses is myelosuppression, many authors have used autotransplants to ensure prompt marrow recovery after high doses of chemotherapy. Breast cancer is an optimal tumor for studies of the role of high-dose therapy, based on its sensitivity at conventional chemotherapy doses.

Principles in the Design of a High-Dose Regimen for Breast Cancer

The principles of *dose-response* and *combination chemotherapy* were basic to the design of the initial curative treatment regimens for malignancies that are now curable with chemotherapy (e.g., leukemias, lymphomas, testis cancer, and breast cancer in the adjuvant setting) (31–34). Skipper estimated the spontaneous rate of mutation to resistance to a single drug as $1/10^6$ to 10^7 cancer cells (3–6). The likelihood of spontaneous mutations conferring resistance is high in patients with visually apparent tumor. Thus combinations of active non-cross-resistant agents are essential to decrease the emergence of drug resistance. Agents were selected with *different dose-limiting toxicities,* resulting in subadditive toxicity in combination. A fourth principle in the design of curative regimens is to combine agents with *different mechanisms of action* to avoid cross-resistance.

Alkylating agents exhibit a steep linear-log dose-response curve, and nonhematologic toxicity varies among the different agents. Combinations of alkylating agents produce significant therapeutic synergy and subadditive toxicity in a variety of experimental tumor systems. Full utilization of the dose-response curve for many alkylating agents is limited by myelosuppression. Thus marrow autografting permits dose escalation of agents with dose-limiting myelosuppression. While many antimetabolites and other cycle-specific agents are schedule dependent in experimental and clinical trials, alkylating agents are non-cycle-specific and less schedule dependent.

Significant resistance to alkylating agents is not believed to result from either gene amplification or pleiotropic drug resistance (documented mechanisms of resistance against antimetabolites, antibiotics, and vinca alkaloids) (35). Goldenberg and coworkers (36), Vistica and colleagues (37), and Redwood and Colvin (38) have documented decreased active transport of alkylating agents into resistant tumor cells. Colvin has observed enhanced cyclophosphamide degradation (39). Other mechanisms of tumor resistance include increased intracellular glutathione with binding of melphalan and cisplatin and enhanced excision of adducts for nitrosoureas.

Although most alkylating agents at conventional doses share a common dose-limiting toxicity (myelosuppression), marrow autografting permits dose escalation to the level of dose-limiting nonhematologic toxicity. The dose-limiting organ toxicity of the various alkylating agents used at high dose differs substantially (pulmonary fibrosis and hepatic toxicity for carmustine [BCNU], cardiotoxicity for cyclophosphamide, nephrotoxicity for cisplatin, and stomatitis and enterocolitis for melphalan). Thus nonoverlapping toxicity may allow a combination of alkylating agents at full or nearly full transplant doses.

Bone Marrow Involvement

More than 40% of patients with metastatic breast cancer and about 55% of those with a positive bone scan or metastases evident on bone x-rays have bone marrow involvement detected by conventional studies of bone marrow biopsies, aspirations, or clot sections (40, 41). Investigational techniques to evaluate marrow involvement by tumor include monoclonal antibodies to keratin or other cytoskeletal elements (42, 43). Approximately 30% of patients without bone marrow metastases by standard criteria were determined to have bone marrow involvement at the time of diagnosis using more sensitive, but possibly less specific, techniques (44). Tumor cells have been grown in vitro from a histologically normal bone marrow sample of a patient with breast cancer (45).

The importance of either overt or occult bone marrow involvement in the setting of autologous bone marrow transplantation is unknown. Chemotherapy given prior to bone marrow procurement may reduce or eliminate tumor cells in vivo and permit autotransplantation.

CLINICAL TRIALS OF DOSE-INTENSIVE THERAPY WITH AUTOLOGOUS STEM CELL SUPPORT

Failed or Refractory Breast Cancer

SINGLE AGENTS

There are 12 studies of high doses of alkylating agents and 5 of nonalkylating agents followed by autotransplantation in women with advanced breast cancer (Table 42.4). All complete responses were obtained with alkylating agents (melphalan or thiotepa), although partial responses were observed with all drugs evaluated. The response rate for alkylating agents was 39% compared to 16% for nonalkylating agents.

COMBINATIONS OF DRUGS WITH OR WITHOUT TOTAL BODY RADIATION

Multiple combinations of high-dose chemotherapy with or without total body irradiation (TBI) have been reported in 238 patients with failed or refractory breast can-

cer (Table 42.5). Regimens of two or more alkylating agents seemed to produce the highest response rates. The response rate for radiation-containing regimens (12 of 19, 63%) was not significantly different from that of regimens without radiation (152 of 219, 69%).

Autologous Bone Marrow Transplantation for Previously Untreated or Responding Metastatic Breast Cancer

Theoretically the use of an induction regimen reduces tumor bulk, may decrease the number of cells resistant to the high-dose regimen, and allows the selection of patients with sensitive tumors for high-dose therapy. Alternatively, several cycles of conventional dose therapy could induce multidrug or specific resistance or allow the growth of partially resistant clones. A number of investigators have chosen either strategy.

NO PRIOR CHEMOTHERAPY FOR METASTATIC BREAST CANCER

There are four studies of combination chemotherapy in 53 previously untreated patients with inflammatory or metastatic breast cancer (Table 42.6). (Some patients had received prior adjuvant therapy.) One patient was treated by Peters at Dana-Farber Cancer Institute (DFCI) and is included in reports from both Duke and DFCI. She is shown here with the DFCI data.

BREAST CANCER RESPONDING TO STANDARD-DOSE CHEMOTHERAPY

Multiple regimens have been used in patients responding to induction therapy. A total of 58% of these patients have achieved complete responses, and 28% were in continuous complete response at the time of data analysis (Table 42.7).

Results in the Dana-Farber Cancer Institute Study

In the phase II study, CTCb was demonstrated to be an intensification regimen with

Table 42.4. Failed or Refractory Breast Cancer[a]

Author	Institution	Drug	No. Pts. Treated	No. in CR	RR %	RR No.	% Dur.	Median Months Resp.	mg/m²	Reference
Nonalkylating agents										
Mulder	Groningen	Etoposide	3	0	0	1	33	1.5	1000–1500	46
Wolf	Vanderbilt	Etoposide	3	0	0	0	0	—	1500–2700	47
Fraschini	MDAH	Etoposide	15	0	0	1	7	NA	900–1350	48
Total		**Etoposide**	**21**	**0**	**0**	**2**	**10**			
Tannir	MDAH	AMSA	16	0	0	2	13	7, 11	600–750	49
Ariel	NY Med Col	Hydroxyurea	8	0	0	3	38	NA	40,000	50
Total			**45**	**0**	**0**	**7**	**16**			
Alkylating agents										
Corringham	R Free, London	Melphalan	4	3	75	3	75	9–23+	120–140	51
Maraninchi	Marseilles	Melphalan	4	1	25	1	25	24	140	52, 53
Knight	San Antonio	Melphalan	6	1	17	3	50	(1–4)	180	54, 55
Lazarus	NATG	Melphalan	6	0	0	4	67	(2–14)	120–225	56, 57
Tannir	MDAH	Mitomycin C	15	0	0	1	7	<3	30–50	58
Schilcher	Wayne State	Mitomycin C	2	0	0	0	0	—	60	59, 60
LeMaistre	NATG	Thiotepa	18	1	6	8	44	4 (2–7)	180–1575	61, 62
Lazarus	Case Western	Thiotepa	2	0	0	1	50	4	270–810	63
Slease	Oklahoma	Cyclophosphamide	6	0	0	3	50	3, 4, 8	7800	64
Collins	Seattle	Cyclophosphamide	2	0	0	1	50	NA	5000[b]	
Peters	Duke	Dibromodulcitol	7	0	0	0	14	1	1500–4800	
Shea	DFCI	Carboplatin	2	0	0	1	50	NA	500–2400	65
Total			**74**	**6**	**8**	**27**	**36**			

[a]Abbreviations: CR, complete response; DFCI, Dana-Farber Cancer Institute; MDAH, MD Anderson Hospital; NATG, North American Transplant Group; NA, data not available; RR, objective response rate.
[b]P. Collins, personal communication.

Table 42.5. Combinations of Drugs with or without Total Body Radiation[a]

Author	Institution	Drug	No.	CR No.	CR %	RR No.	RR %	Med. Mos Dur. Resp.	Reference
			TBI Regimens						
Stewart	Seattle	C	5	2	40	2	40	(5–6)	66
Kessinger	Nebraska	CP	5	0	0	3	60	(3–9)	
Niederwieser	Innsbruck	C[b]	4	4	100	4	100	(3–34)	67
Bearman	Seattle	C	2	0	0	2	100	3	
Douer	UCLA	CA/Vb	2	1	50	1	50	5	68
Vaughan	Nebraska	CT	1	0	0	0	0	—	
Total			**19**	**7**	**37**	**12**	**63**		
			Combination Chemotherapy						
Eder	DFCI	CBP	14	3	21	10	71	5	69
Slease	Oklahoma	CB	10	2	20	8	80	(2–7)	70
Eder	DFCI	CT	7	0	0	5	71	2(1–3)	71
Mukaiyama	Tokyo (JFCR)	CT	4	1	25	2	50	3	72
Fay	NATG	CT	9	1	11	9	100	4(3–11)	73
Peters	Duke	CTP	6	1	17	3	50	2	74
Kaizer	Rush	CTP	9	1	11	6	67	(1–9)	75
Eder	DFCI	CTCb	4	0	0	4	100	1–3+	76
Vaughan	Nebraska	CT ± H	7	0	0	4	57	(1–6)	
Eder	DFCI	CTL	1	0	0	1	100	3	71
Kaminer	Chicago	CT/LorB	19	2	11	14	74	3(1–12)	77–79
Lazarus	ECOG	LE	4	2	50	4	100	1–4+	
Peters	Duke	CLP	8	3	38	7	88	(2–6)	
Maraninchi	Marseilles	CL	5	3	60	3	60	(3–8)	52
Maraninchi	Marseilles	CL/Mitox	2	1	50	2	100	(3–25+)	52
Langleben	McGill	CLP/Mitox	4	2	50	3	75	6–11+	80
Dunphy	MDAH	TE/Mitox	28	7	25	22	79	(3–10+)	81
Spitzer	MDAH	T/Mitox	24	3	13	16	67	6+	
Mulder	Groningen	Mitox/CorL	2	2	100	2	100	11+–25+	82
Spitzer	MDAH	T/Mitox	24	3	13	16	67	6+	
Tajima	Tokai	ACU/EP	16	1	6	7	44	4(2–42)	
Tobias	DFCI	CA	3	0	0	1	33	NA	83
Lazarus	Case W Res	BP	3	0	0	0	0	—	
Robinson	Denver	FMV/HN/Ad	1	0	0	1	100	NA	84
Slease	Oklahoma	CPEB	3	0	0	1	33	2	
Jacobs	Pittsburg	CPE	4	0	0	2	50	NA	85
Kessinger	Nebraska	CPE	3	0	0	3	100	4	
Bearman	Seattle	BU/C	4	1	25	1	25	10	
Total			**228**	**39**	**17**	**157**	**69**		

[a] Abbreviations: see Table 42.2. B, carmustine; Cb, carboplatin; CorL, designates patients who received either cyclophosphamide or melphalan; CR, complete response; H, hydroxyurea; L, melphalan (L-PAM); LorB, designates patients who received either melphalan (L-PAM) or BCNU; mitox, mitoxantrone; HN, nitrogen mustard; NA, data not available; T, thiotepa; U, uracil mustard; Vb, vinblastine.
[b] Three in CR prior to bone marrow transplantation (two liver treatment, one lobectomy).

Table 42.6.   High-Dose Chemotherapy with Marrow Support in Untreated Stage IV Breast Cancer

Author	Institution	Agents	No.	CR No.	CR %	RR No.	RR %	No.	CCR %	CCR Mos.	Deaths	References
Peters[b]	Duke	CBP	21	11	52	14	67	2	10	42, 58	5	86
Eder	DFCI	CBP	4	3	75	4	100	1	25	72	0	69
Tajima	Tokai	CAU	23	7	30	17	74	4	17	17–82	0	87–89
Kaizer	Rush	CTP	5	4	80	5	100	2	40	(13, 37+)	0	75
Total			**53**	**25**	**47**	**40**	**75**	**9**	**17**		**5**	

[a]Abbreviations: see Tables 42.2 and 42.5.
[b]One patient reported in both Duke and DFCI data shown here with DFCI.

a low mortality that achieves the goal of delivery of significantly increased doses of agents known to be active at conventional doses in breast cancer. While profound myelosuppression and some mucositis were considered acceptable, agents with organ toxicity such as doxorubicin or BCNU were avoided in the construction of this transplant regimen (78). Nevertheless, a 21%–28% incidence was observed of transient, moderate renal, cardiac, and hepatic toxicity. The use of continuous infusions of the three drugs may decrease peak drug levels associated with toxicity. For example, a divided dose schedule of cyclophosphamide is less cardiotoxic in primates than the same dose given as a single bolus infusion (90). The cytotoxicity of cyclophosphamide, unlike most alkylating agents, is enhanced in actively proliferating cancer cells (91). Cyclophosphamide also differs from other alkylating agents in that cytotoxicity is enhanced when a given total dose is divided and administered in multiple doses in vivo, but not in tissue culture (92). Because cyclophosphamide induces its own metabolism, the half-life is shortened and the total alkylating capacity (AUC) is significantly increased when administered as multiple daily doses, particularly at high total doses (93). This may explain the lack of schedule effect in vitro using the "activated" 4-hydroxycyclophosphamide (4HC). A multiple dose (i.e., continuous infusion) schedule may thus exploit these unique properties of cyclophosphamide.

As predicted by modeling experiments and also observed in studies of marrow transplant in patients with leukemia and lymphoma, the duration of partial responses was short. The impact of less than 2 logs of tumor cytotoxicity (i.e., a partial response) is small if tumor growth kinetics are assumed to be Gompertzian (94). Complete responses (whether achieved after induction or after intensification) appeared to be relatively durable, as did responses in patients with only residual positive bone scans and sclerosis on x-ray.

There are too few patients to draw any conclusions regarding prognostic variables (Table 42.8). Nevertheless, none of the eight patients without progression after transplant had received prior adjuvant doxorubicin (and five had no adjuvant chemotherapy). Visceral versus soft tissue disease did not seem to predict for durability of remission; the predominant sites of disease were different in each of these eight patients. While patients with large bulky tumors or many sites of disease responded to both standard and high-dose therapy, they seemed less likely to achieve complete or durable responses. These currently available published trials have now documented that dose-intensive chemotherapy with hematopoietic autotransplantation is an effective treatment for metastatic breast cancer. Several high-dose regimens tested in patients with no prior chemotherapy for stage 4 disease or responding to standard-dose treatment have resulted in a complete response rate higher than generally reported with standard-dose treatment. While partial

Table 42.7. Dose-intensive Therapy with Autologous Marrow Support in Metastatic or Recurrent Breast Cancer Responding to Conventional-Dose Chemotherapy

Author	Institution	Agents	No.	After induction CR No.	CR %	RR No.	RR %	After ABMT No. CR	No. RR	No progression No.	%	Dur. (Mo.)	Toxic Deaths	References
Gisselbrecht	Paris	C/TBI	5	1	20	5	100	5	100	1	20	30	0	95, 96
Livingston	Seattle	C/TBI	7	2	29	7	100	3	43	1	14	42+	0	97
Vaughan	Nebraska	CP/TBI	2	2	100	2	100	2	100	1	50	40	0	
Vaughan	Nebraska	CT/TBI	5	1	20	3	60	2	40	0	0	—	3	
Vincent	R Marsden	L	15	7	47	14	93	12	80	1	7	18	3	98
Russell	Calgary	L	1	1	100	1	100	1	100	0	0	—	0	
Maraninchi	Marseille	CL	1	1	100	1	100	1	100	0	0	—	0	
Maraninchi	Marseille	CL/Mitox	4	0	0	1	25	4	100	3	75	(4–18)	0	
Gisselbrecht	Fr Autol Gp	CL Mitox	18	6	33	14	78	11	61	9	50	(1–18)	2	
Kotasek	Adelaid	CLCb	5					1	20	1	20	3	0	
Spitzer	MDAH	CPE	58	20	34	49	84	31	53	13	22	40	2	81, 99–101
Jones	Duke	CPB	39	17	44	35	90	25	64	10	26	20 (9–34)	8	102–104
Williams	U. Chicago	CT	27	4	15	19	70	12	44	5	19	19 (12–36)	4	105, 106
Kennedy	J Hopkins	CT	24	8	33	24	100	13	54	4	17	(1–28)	0	30, 107, 108
Vaughan	Nebraska	CTH	12	3	25	12	100	3	25	3	25	(2–10)	2	
Antman	DFCI	CTCb	53		0	29	55	28	53	19	36	(1–45)	2	
Rosti	Ravenna	C/MC/Vb	9	4	44	7	78	6	67	5	56	1–9+	0	109–111
Willemse	Groningen	CE/tam	10	10	100	10	100	10	100	3	30	21	1	112, 113
Slease	Oklahoma	CB	11	5	45	11	100	7	64	6	55	10 (2–21)	2	115
Total			**306**	**92**	**30**	**244**	**80**	**177**	**58**	**85**	**28**		**29**	

[a] Abbreviations: See Tables 42.2 and 42.5. Fr Autol Gp, French Autologous Group; MDAH, MD Anderson Hospital; tam, tamoxifen.

Table 42.8. Summary of Patient Outcome of Women Treated with High-Dose Cyclophosphamide, Thiotepa, and Carboplatin (CTCB) at the Dana-Farber Cancer Institute[a]

Number of women transplanted	53	
Toxic deaths	2	4%
Evaluable for response	51	
CR or PR*[b]	29	57+
Without progression	20	39%
Transplanted prior to 9/1/90		
(i.e., 2–4 year follow-up)	30	
Without progression	8	27%

[a]Abbreviations: CR, complete remission.
[b]PR* is defined as complete response save for residual abnormal bone scan; once abnormal, bone scans do not again become normal, even if disease responds, for extended periods of time.

responses have been brief, complete responses have proven relatively durable. A quarter to a half of those achieving complete response have no evidence of progression with follow-up intervals in the range of 2–4 years in trials at multiple institutions. Because of the toxicity (and costs) associated with this treatment, patients should be selected carefully. It appears clear at present that those with refractory or bulky disease are unlikely to achieve a complete response.

Autotransplants in Patients with Inflammatory or Stage III Breast Cancer

Five regimens have been used in 56 women with breast cancer responding to conventional-dose (induction) therapy at the time of transplant (Table 42.9). A total of 79% of these patients were in complete remission after standard dose-therapy prior to the transplant (Pre), and 89% were in complete response after high-dose therapy. Of the total, 54% were in continuous complete response at the time of data analysis with relatively short follow-up times of 1–37 months.

Adjuvant Dose-Intensive Treatment

Four institutions are studying adjuvant high-dose therapy in patients with 10 or more involved lymph nodes at the time of primary treatment (Table 49.10). A total 88% were in continuous complete response at the time of data analysis, although with the exception of the Japanese study, the follow-up on these studies is too short to draw any conclusions.

SUMMARY OF CURRENT RESULTS IN BREAST CANCER

From the experience gained so far, several regimens designed for breast cancer yield both a high complete response rate and durable remissions in patients responding to standard-dose chemotherapy. While response rates of 30%–50% in refractory breast cancer (with complete responses in 10%–20% of patients) do provide evidence of a dose-response relationship, long-term disease-free survival of patients treated for refractory disease is rare (as in high-dose therapy for leukemia and lymphoma). Patients with advanced refractory disease (which more easily justifies a higher risk therapy for some physicians) are least likely to benefit from the treatment. Transplant early in the course of the illness, after a good response to standard-dose therapy, yields a complete response rate higher than the 10%–20% reported with standard-dose therapy. With follow-up intervals of 18–40 months from the time of transplant (24–44 months from the beginning of 2–4 cycles of induction therapy), these unmaintained responses appear to be relatively durable (28% in continuous complete response). While any treatment-related mortality is to be avoided, metastatic breast cancer is invariably fatal, with a median duration of remission of 8 months and a median survival of 1.6 years. Mortality of conventional-dose chemotherapy for metastatic disease is in the range of 2%–4%. Mortality for dose-intensive therapy in breast cancer has ranged from 3 to 24%. Mortalities of 50% are acceptable in the setting of allogeneic marrow transplant for second remission acute myelocytic leukemia with a cure rate of approximately 20%–30%.

Table 42.9. Dose-Intensive Therapy in Inflammatory Breast Cancer Stage III[a]

Author	Institution	Agents	No.	CR Pre	CR Post	No.	%	Mos.	Deaths	References
Gisselbrecht	Paris	C/TBI	9	9	9	3	33	37	0	95, 96
Mulder	Groningen	CE/tam	18	18	17	12	67	27	1	112, 113
Maraninchi	Marseille	CL ± mitox	11	4	8	4	36	(5–25)	0	
Gisselbrecht	Fr Autol Gp	CL/Mitox	13	12	11	6	46	(5–12)	1	
Gianni	Milan	L ± TBI	5	1	5	5	100	24 (2–32)	0	115
Total			**56**	**44**	**50**	**30**	**54**		**2**	

[a]Abbreviations: See Tables 42.2, 42.5, and 52.7.

Table 42.10. Autotransplant in Women with Stage II Breast Cancer with 10 or Greater Positive Lymph Nodes[a]

Author	Institution	Agents	No.	Continuous, CR No.	%	Mos.	Deaths	References
Gianni	Milan	L	14	14	100	6 (1–17)	0	
Fay	NATG	CT	5	5	100	(4–24)	0	73
Peters	Duke	CBP	52	47	90	(1–36)	4	116
Tajima	Tokai	CAU	18	12	67	(6–102)	NA	87–89, 117
Total			**89**	**78**	**88**		**4**	

[a]Abbreviations: See Tables 42.2 and 42.5. NA, data not available.

Concurrent studies of prophylactic antibiotics, colony-stimulating factors, and peripheral blood stem cell support may substantially decrease the morbidity and the length of admissions for these patients, significantly decreasing the cost of this mode of therapy. A preliminary analysis of costs based on 3-year data from the Duke program compared to standard-dose therapy on Cancer and Leukemia Group B studies estimates that the current cost of dose-intensive therapy per year of life saved is $85,000. (The cost of conventional-dose therapy and dose-intensive therapy were estimated at $31,500 and $73,300 respectively.) Thus current costs are "very high and greater than most but not all acceptable therapies." If the complete remissions prove to be durable and growth factors and peripheral blood progenitor cell support significantly lower the costs, dose-intensive therapy may prove both effective and cost-effective (118).

FUTURE DIRECTIONS

For patients with metastatic disease, attempts to further improve the therapeutic index of high-dose chemotherapy utilizing other active agents, modulation of chemotherapeutic agents to address mechanisms of resistance, or two or more high-dose treatments are currently under study.

From the experience gained so far, several regimens designed for breast cancer yield both a high complete response rate and durable remissions in patients responding to standard-dose chemotherapy. Certainly the study of a high-dose regimen with documented activity in metastatic disease as primary or adjuvant therapy for patients with inflammatory or stage III disease or stage II disease with multiple positive lymph node involvement is now totally appropriate. Stage II and III patients with no macroscopic metastatic disease, whose primary lesions can be adequately treated with local therapy, provide an optimal group in which to test the efficacy of dose or dose rate in a prospective randomized trial. Unlike most patients with metastatic disease, such patients have not received prior adjuvant chemotherapy and have only microscopic metastatic disease, and their performance status is generally excellent.

Table 42.11.   Randomized Trials of Dose-Intensive Therapy with Stem Cell Support Planned or Underway

Stage	Group	Standard Dose Induction	Responding Patients Randomized To:
II > 10 positive LNs[a]	CALGB	CAF × 4	High-dose CBP vs. standard dose CBP
	ECOG	CAF × 4	High-dose CT vs. no further therapy
III	CALGB	G-CSF × 4	Very high dose CTCb vs. high-dose CTC × 4
IV	Duke	AFM × 4	CRs only to CBP vs. observation
	Philadelphia Group	CAF × 6	CTCb vs. no further treatment
	SWOG	CAF × 6	CTCb vs. no further treatment

[a]Abbreviations: See Tables 42.2 and 42.5. LNs, lymh nodes.

Randomized trials in stage II (with 10 or more positive nodes), III, and IV breast cancer are currently planned or under way. The Cancer and Leukemia Group B (CALBG) trial in women with stage II disease with 10 or more positive nodes, chaired by Dr. Peters, is accruing patients to a regimen that includes cyclophosphamide, doxorubicin, and 5-fluorouracil followed in responders by high-dose cyclophosphamide, cisplatin, and BCNU. The Eastern Cooperative Oncology Group (ECOG) trial planned includes a similar induction followed by cyclophosphamide and thiotepa. A pilot study in stage III is currently under way at DFCI, applying high-dose doxorubicin and G-CSF for four cycles followed in responders by high-dose cyclophosphamide, thiotepa, and carboplatin. The control arm for this proposed randomized trial within CALGB is currently under discussion. In metastatic disease, randomized trials are currently under way by the Philadelphia group and planned by the Southwest Oncology Group (SWOG). These trials are designed to address the impact of dose or dose rate, as well as to delineate optimal timing for dose-intensive therapy (Table 42.11).

Other critical issues that also need to be addressed in single-institution trials include the design of more effective regimens. Since the majority of women with metastatic breast cancer continue to relapse despite dose-intensive therapy, reasonable strategies include the incorporation of new drugs and repetitive high-dose cycles.

Major advances in supportive care in the last 2 years have significantly decreased the time to reengraftment, morbidity, and cost associated with transplant. In multiple randomized trials, hematopoietic growth factors have been found to decrease the time to reengraftment. Even more effective in achieving these aims has been the addition of peripheral stem blood cells (addressed in Chapter 11). Indeed, for the first time, the strategies of increased dose can be efficiently and relatively safely tested in breast cancer. The use of regimens with 5- to 10-fold increments in dose can be compared to conventional-dose chemotherapy regimens, while in the past, even a 1.5- to 2-fold escalation in dose resulted in substantial myelosuppression.

REFERENCES

1. Clark G, Sledge GW, Osborne CK, McGuire WL. Survival from first recurrence: relative importance of prognostic factors in 1,015 breast cancer patients. J Clin Oncol 1987;5:55–61.
2. Mick R, Begg CB, Antman K, Korzun AH, Frei III E. Diverse prognosis in metastatic breast cancer: who should be offered alternative initial therapies? Breast Cancer Res Treat 1989;13:33–38.
3. Skipper HE, Schabel FM, Jary R, Wilcox WS. Experimental evaluation of potential anticancer agents. Cancer Chemother Rep 1964;35:1–111.
4. Skipper HE. Criteria associated with destruction of leukemia and solid tumor cells in animals. Cancer Res 1967;27:2636–2645.
5. Skipper HE. Combination therapy: some concepts and results. Cancer Chemother Rep 1974;4:137–145.
6. Skipper HE. Stepwise progress in the treatment of disseminated cancers. Cancer 1983;51:1773–1776.
7. Hayes DF, Henderson IC. CAF in metastatic breast

cancer: standard therapy or another effective regimen? J Clin Oncol 1987;5:1497–1499.

8. Frei III E, Antman K, Teicher B, Eder P, Schnipper L. Bone marrow autotransplantation for solid tumors—prospects. J Clin Oncol 1989;7:515–526.

9. Frei III E, Canellos GP. Dose, a critical factor in cancer chemotherapy. Am J Med 1980;69:585–594.

10. Hryniuk WM, Bush H. The importance of dose intensity in chemotherapy of metastatic breast cancer. J Clin Oncol 1984;2:1281–1287.

11. Cohen M, Rajendra R, Ahuja N, Nguyen D. Chemotherapy dose intensity (CT-DI) and median survival (MS) in advanced breast cancer: no apparent relationship. Proc Am Soc Clin Oncol 1990;9:34.

12. Henderson IC, Hayes DF, Gelman R. Dose-response in the treatment of breast cancer: a critical review. J Clin Oncol 1988;6:1501–1510.

13. Tannock IF, Boyd NF, Deboer G, et al. A randomized trials of two dose levels of cyclophosphamide, methotrexate, and fluorouracil chemotherapy for patients with metastatic breast cancer. J Clin Oncol 1988;6:1377–1387.

14. Carmo-Pereira J, Costa FO, Henriqiues E, et al. A comparison of two doses of Adriamycin in the primary chemotherapy of disseminated breast carcinoma. Br J Cancer 1987;56:471–473.

15. Hoogstraten B, George SL, Samal B, et al. Combination chemotherapy and Adriamycin in patients with advanced breast cancer. Cancer 1976;38:13–20.

16. Tormey DC, Gelman R, Band PR, et al. Comparison of induction chemotherapies for metastatic breast cancer: an Eastern-Cooperative Oncology Group trial. Cancer 1982;50:1235–1244.

17. Malik R, Blumenschein GR, Legha SS, et al. A randomized trial of high dose 5-fluorouracil (F), doxorubicin (A) and cyclophosphamide (C) vs conventional FAC regimen in metastatic breast cancer [Abstract 303]. Proc Am Soc Clin Oncol 1982;1:79.

18. Hortobagyi GN, Bodey SP, Buzdar AU, et al. Evaluation of high-dose versus standard FAC chemotherapy for advanced breast cancer in protected environment units: a prospective randomized study. J Clin Oncol 1987;5:354–364.

19. Focan C, Closon MT, Andrien JM, et al. Dose response relationship with epirubicin (E) as first line chemotherapy for advanced breast cancer (BC). A randomized trial. Ann Oncol 1990;1(suppl):S18.

20. Becher R, Wandl U, Kloke O, et al. Randomized study of different doses of epirubicin and identical doses of cyclophosphamide in advanced breast cancer. Proc Am Soc Clin Oncol 1990;9:47.

21. Beretta G, Gambrosier P, Tabiodon D, Luporini G. Therapeutic response after two dose levels of intravenous CMF in metastatic breast carcinoma [Abstract]. Proc Am Soc Clin Oncol 1986;5:77.

22. Ebbs SR, Saunders JA, Graham H, A'Hern RPA, Bates T, Baum M. Advanced breast cancer. A randomised trial of epidoxorubicin at two different dosages and two administration systems. Acta Oncol 1989;28:887–892.

23. Habeshaw T, Jones R, Stallard S, et al. Epirubicin (Epi) at 2 dose levels with prednisolone (P) as treatment for advanced breast cancer (ABC): results of a randomised trial. Proc Am Soc Clin Oncol 1990;9:43.

24. O'Bryan RM, Baker LH, Gottlieb JE, et al. Dose response evaluation of Adriamycin in human neoplasia. Cancer 1977;39:1940–1948.

25. Forastiere AA, Hakes TB, Wittes JT, et al. Cisplatin in the treatment of metastatic breast carcinoma: a prospective randomized trial of two dosage schedules. Am J Clin Oncol 1982;5:243–247.

26. Samal B, Vaitevicius V, Singhakowinta A, et al. CIS-diamiminedichloroplatinum (CDDP) in advanced breast and colorectal carcinomas [Abstract]. Proc Am Soc Clin Oncol 1978;19:347.

27. Bronchud MH, Howell A, Crowther D, Hopwood P, Souza L, Dexter TM. The use of granulocyte colony-stimulating factor to increase the intensity of treatment with doxorubicin in patients with advanced breast and ovarian cancer. Br J Cancer 1989;60:121–125.

28. Demetri GD, Younger J, McGuire BW, et al. Recombinant methionyl granulocyte-CSF (r-metG-CSF) allows an increase in the dose intensity of cyclophosphamide/doxorubicin/5-fluorouracil (CAF) in patients with advanced breast cancer [Abstract 153]. Proc Am Soc Clin Oncol 1991;70.

29. Jones RB, Shpall EJ, Shogan J, et al. The Duke AFM program: intensive induction chemotherapy for metastatic breast cancer. Cancer 1990;66:431–436.

30. Beveridge RA, Abeloff MD, Donehower RC, Damron DJ, Fetting JH, Waterfield, W. Sixteen week dose intense chemotherapy for breast cancer [Abstract 47]. Proc Am Soc Clin Oncol 1988;7:13.

31. Pinkel D. Ninth annual David Karnofsky lecture: treatment of acute lymphocytic leukemia. Cancer 1979;43:1128–1137.

32. Frei III E, Freireich EJ. Progress and perspectives in the chemotherapy of acute leukemia. Adv Chemother 1965;2:269–289.

33. Frei III E, Karon M, Levin RH, et al. The effectiveness of combinations of antileukemic agents in inducing and maintaining remission in children with acute leukemia. Blood 1965;26:642–656.

34. Feireich EJ, Henderson ES, Karon M, Frei III E. The treatment of acute leukemia with respect to cell population kinetics. In: The proliferation and spread of neoplastic cells; 21st Annual Symposium on Fundamental Cancer Research. Houston: University of Texas Press, 1968:441–452.

35. Teicher B, Cucchi C, Lee J, et al. Alkylating agents. In vitro studies of cross-resistance patterns in human tumor cell lines. Cancer Res 1986;46:4379–4383.

36. Goldenberg GJ, Vanstone CL, Israels LG, et al. Evidence for a transport carrier of nitrogen mustard in nitrogen mustard sensitive and resistant L51784 lymphoblasts. Cancer Res 1970;30:2285–2291.

37. Vistica DT, Rabinowitz M. Amino acid-conferred protection against melphalan—characterization of melphalan transport and correlation of uptake with cytotoxicity in cultured L1210 murine leukemia cells. Biochem Pharmacol 1978;27:2865–2870.

38. Redwood WR, Colvin M. Transport of melphalan by sensitive and resistant L1210 cells. Cancer Res 1980;40:1144–1149.

39. Colvin M. The alkylating agents. In: Chabner B, ed. Pharmacologic principles of cancer treatment. Philadelphia: WB Saunders, 1982:276–308.

40. Ingle JN, Tormey DC, Tan KH. The bone marrow examination in breast cancer: diagnostic considerations and clinical usefulness. Cancer 1978;41:670–674.

41. Ellis G, Ferguson M, Yamanaka E, Livingston RB, Gown AM. Monoclonal antibodies for detection of occult carcinoma cells in bone marrow of breast cancer patients. Cancer 1989;63:2509–2514.

42. Kufe D, Inghirami G, Hayes AM, Wheeler J, Schlom J. Differential reactivity of a novel monoclonal antibody (DF3) with human malignant versus benign breast tumors. Hybridoma 1984;3:223–232.

43. Hilkens J, Buijs F, Hilgers J, et al. Monoclonal antibodies against human milk-fat globule membranes detecting differentiation antigens of the mammary gland and its tumors. Int J Cancer 1983;34:197–206.

44. Redding WH, Monoghan P, Imrie SF, et al. Detection of micrometastases in patients with primary breast cancer. Lancet 1983;2:1271–1274.

45. Mann SL, Joshi SS, Weisenburger DD, et al. Detection of tumor cells in histologically normal bone marrow of autologous transplant patients using culture techniques [Abstract 771]. Exp Hematol 1986;14:54.

46. Mulder NH, Meinesz AP, Sleijfer DT, et al. High-dose etoposide with or without cyclophosphamide and autologous bone marrow transplantation in solid tumors. In: McVie JG, Dalesio O, Smith EI, eds. Autologous bone marrow transplantation and solid tumors. Vol. 14. New York: Raven Press, 1984:125–130.

47. Wolff S, Fer M, McKay C. High-dose VP-16-213 and autologous bone marrow transplantation for refractory malignancies: a phase I study. J Clin Oncol 1983;1:701–705.

48. Fraschini G, Esparza L, Holmes F, Tashima C, Theirault R, Hortobagyi G. High-dose etoposide in metastatic breast cancer [Abstract 39]. Breast Cancer Res Treat 1989;14:142.

49. Tannir N, Spitzer G, Schell F, Legha S, Zander A, Blumenschein GC. Phase II study of high-dose amsacrine and autologous bone marrow transplantation in patients with refractory metastatic breast cancer. Cancer Treat Rep 1983;67:599–600.

50. Ariel I. Treatment of disseminated cancer by intravenous hydroxyurea and autogenous bone-marrow transplants: experiences with 35 patients. J Surg Oncol 1975;7:331–335.

51. Corringham R, Gilmore M, Prentice H, Boesen E. High-dose melphalan with autologous bone marrow translant: treatment of poor prognosis tumors. Cancer 1983;52:1783–1787.

52. Maraninchi D, Piana L, Blaise D, et al. Phase I and II studies of high dose alkylating agents in poor risk patients with breast cancer with autologous bone marrow transplantation. In: Dicke K, Spitzer TR, Jaggannath S, eds. Autologous bone marrow transplantation: proceedings of the third international symposium. Houston: University of Texas MD Anderson Hospital Press, 1987:475–480.

53. Maraninchi D, Gastuat JA, Herve P, et al. High-dose melphalan and autologous marrow transplantation in adult solid tumors: clinical responses and preliminary evaluation of different strategies. In: McVie JG, Dalesio O, Smith IE, ed. Autologous bone marrow transplantation and solid tumors. Vol. 14. New York: Raven Press, 1984:145–150.

54. Knight WA, Page CP, Kuhn JG, et al. High dose L-PAM with autologous bone marrow infusion for advanced, steroid hormone receptor negative breast cancer [Abstract]. Breast Cancer Res Treat 1984;4:336.

55. Knight W, Page CP, Kuhn JG, et al. High dose L-PAM and autologous marrow infusion for refractory solid tumors [Abstract]. Proc Am Soc Clin Oncol 1984;3:150.

56. Lazarus J, Herzig R, Graham-Pole J, et al. Intensive melphalan chemotherapy and cryopreserved autologous bone marrow transplantation for the treatment of refractory cancer. J Clin Oncol 1983;2:359–367.

57. Herzig R, Phillips G, Lazarus H, et al. Intensive chemotherapy and autologous bone marrow transplantation for the treatment of refractory malignancies. In: Dicke K, Spitzer G, Zander A, ed. Autologous bone marrow transplantation; proceedings of the first international symposium. Houston: University of Texas MD Anderson Cancer Center Press, 1985:197–202.

58. Tannir N, Spitzer G, Dicke K, Schell F, Distefano A, Blumenschein G. Phase I-II study of high-dose mitomycin with autologous bone marrow transplantation in refractory metastatic breast cancer. Cancer Treat Rep 1983;68:805–806.

59. Schilcher RB, Young JD, Ratanatharathorn V, Karanes C, Baker LH. Clinical pharmacokinetics of high dose mitomycin C. Cancer Chemother Pharmacol 1984;13:186–190.

60. Schilcher RB, Young JD, Ratanathorathorn V, Baker

LH. High dose mitomycin C and autologous bone marrow transplantation: clinical results and pharmacokinetics. Blut 1982;45:183.

61. Le Maistre CF, Herzig GP, Herzig RH, et al. High dose thiotepa and autologous bone marrow rescue for the treatment of refractory breast cancer [Abstract]. Breast Cancer Res Treat 1987;10:89.

62. Brown R, Herzig R, Fay J, et al. A phase I-II study of high-dose N, N1, N2 triethylenethiophosphoramide (thio-tepa) and autologous marrow transplantation for refractory malignancies [Abstract 494]. Proc Am Soc Clin Oncol 1986;5:127.

63. Lazarus HM, Reed MD, Spitzer TR, Rabaa MS, Blumer JL. High-dose IV thiotepa and cryopreserved autologous bone marrow transplantation for therapy of refractory cancer. Cancer Treat Rep 1987; 71:689–695.

64. Slease RB, Reitz CL, Hughes WL, et al. Autologous bone marrow transplantation for metastatic breast carcinoma; autotransplantation for breast carcinoma. In: Dicke K, Spitzer G, Jagannath S, eds. Autologous bone marrow transplantation: proceedings of the third international symposium. Houston: University of Texas MD Anderson Hospital Press, 1987.

65. Shea TC, Flaherty M, Elias A, et al. A phase I clinical and pharmacological study of high-dose carboplatin and autologous bone marrow support. J Clin Oncol 1989;7:651–661.

66. Stewart P. Autologous bone marrow transplantation in metastatic breast cancer. Breast Cancer Res Treat 1982;2:85–92.

67. Neiderwieser D, Aulitzky FH, et al. Bone marrow transplantation in the treatment of haematological malignancies and solid tumors. Wien Klin Wochenschr 1987;99:49–53.

68. Douer YD, Champlin R, Ho W, et al. High-dose combined-modality therapy and autologous bone marrow rescue or refractory solid tumors. Am J Med 1981;71:973–976.

69. Eder JP, Antman K, Peters W, et al. High dose combination alkylating agent chemotherapy with autologous bone marrow support for metastatic breast cancer. J Clin Oncol 1986;4:1592–1597.

70. Slease RB, Benear JB, Selby GB, et al. High-dose combination alkylating agent therapy with autologous bone marrow rescue for refractory solid tumors. J Clin Oncol 1988;6:1314–1320.

71. Eder JP, Antman K, Elias A, et al. Cyclohosphamide and thiotepa with autologous bone marrow transplantation with solid tumors. J Natl Cancer Inst 1988;80:1221–1226.

72. Mukaiyama T, Ogawa M, Horikoshi N, et al. A study to overcome drug resistance using high-dose chemotherapy with autologous bone marrow transplantation. Gan To Kagaku Ryoho (Jpn J Cancer Chemother) 1989;16:2013–2018.

73. Fay JW. Personal communications.

74. Peters W, Jones R, Shpall E, Shogan J. Dose intensification using high-dose combination alkylating agents and autologous bone marrow support for the treatment of breast cancer. In: Dicke K, Spitzer G, Jagannath S, Evinger-Hodges M, eds. Autologous bone marrow transplantation; proceedings of the fourth international symposium. Houston: University of Texas MD Anderson Cancer Center Press, 1989:389–399.

75. Kaizer H, Ghalle R, Adler SS, Korenblit AD, Richman CM. High dose chemotherapy and bone marrow transplantation in the treatment of metastatic breast cancer. J Cell Biochem 1990;14A:321.

76. Eder JP, Elias A, Shea TC, et al. A phase I/II study of cyclophosphamide, thiotepa and carboplatin with autologous bone marrow transplantation in solid tumor patients. J Clin Oncol 1990;8:1239–1245.

77. Kaminer L, Williams S, Beschorner J, O'Brien S, Golick J, Bitran J. High dose chemotherapy with autologous hematopoietic stem cell support in the treatment of stage IV breast carcinoma [Abstract 174]. Proc Am Soc Clin Oncol 1989;8:45.

78. Kaminer L, Williams S, Beschorner J, Golick J, O'Brian S, Bitran J. High dose chemotherapy with autologous hematopoietic stem cell support in the treatment of refractory stage IV breast carcinoma [Abstract 62]. Breast Cancer Res Treat 1988;12:122.

79. Bitran J, Kaminer L, Williams S. High dose chemotherapy with autologous hematopoietic stem cell rescue in stage IV breast cancer: the University of Chicago experience. In: Dicke K, Spitzer G, Jagannath S, Evinger-Hodges, M. eds. Autologous bone marrow transplantation; proceedings of the fourth international symposium. Houston: University of Texas MD Anderson Cancer Center Press, 1989:367–371.

80. Langleben A, Ahlgren P, Shustik C, Fauser A. Autologous bone marrow transplantation for metastatic breast cancer—a phase I study [Abstract 149]. Proc Am Soc Clin Oncol 1988;7:38.

81. Dunphy F, Spitzer G, Buzdar A, et al. High-dose therapy with ABMT in metastatic breast cancer; clinical features of prolonged progression-free survival [Abstract 91]. Proc Am Soc Clin Oncol 1989;8:25.

82. Mulder POM, Sleijfer, DT, Willemse PH, de Vries EG, Uges DRA, Mulder NH. High dose cyclophosphamide or melphalan with escalating doses of mitoxantrone and autologous bone marrow transplantation for refractory solid tumors. Cancer Res 1989;49:4654–4658.

83. Tobias J, Weiner F, Griffiths C. Cryopreserved autologous marrow infusion following high-dose cancer chemotherapy. Eur J Cancer 1977;13:269–277.

84. Robinson W, Hartmann D, Mangalik A, et al. Autologous non frozen bone marrow transplantation after intensive chemotherapy: a pilot study. Acta Haematol 1981;66:145–153.

85. Jacobs S, Earle M, Shadduck R, Stoller R. A phase I-II trial of ablative chemotherapy with cyclophosphamide, etoposide, cis-platinum and autologous bone marrow rescue in advanced solid tumors [Abstract 53]. Proc Am Soc Clin Oncol 1989;8:15.

86. Peters WP, Shpall EJ, Jones RB, et al. High-dose combination alkylating agents with bone marrow support as initial treatment for metastatic breast cancer. J Clin Oncol 1988;6:1368–1376.

87. Tajima T, Sonoda H, Kubnota M, et al. High-dose combination chemotherapy with autologous bone marrow transplantation in breast carcinoma. Gan To Kagaku Ryoho (Jpn J Cancer Chemother) 1983; 10:840–847.

88. Tajima T, Sonoda K, Tokuda Y, et al. High-dose chemotherapy supported by autologous bone marrow transplantation in solid tumors. Tokai J Exp Clin Med 1988;8:41–51.

89. Tajima T, Tokuda Y, Ohta M, et al. Role of autologous bone marrow transplantation in cancer chemotherapy. Low Temp Med 1989;15:44–50.

90. Storb R, Buckner C, Dillingham L, Thomas ED. Cyclophosphamide regimens in Rhesus monkeys with and without marrow infusions. Cancer Res 1970;30:2195–2203.

91. Bruce WR, Meeker BE, Valeriote FA. Comparison of the sensitivity of normal hematopoietic and transplanted lymphoma colony forming cells to chemotherapeutic agents administered in vivo. J Natl Cancer Inst. 1966;37:233–245.

92. Teicher BA, Holden SA, Eder JP, Brann TW, Jones SM, E Frei III. Influence of schedule on alkylating agent cytotoxicity in vitro and in vivo. Cancer Res 1989;49:6994–6998.

93. Wagner T, Ehninger G. Self-induction of cyclophosphamide and ifosfamide metabolism by repeated high-dose treatment. 1987;26:69–75.

94. Norton L, Day R. Potential innovations in scheduling of cancer chemotherapy. In: DeVita Jr VT, Hellman S, Rosenberg SA, eds. Important advances in Oncology 1991. Philadelphia: JB Lippincott, 1991:57–72.

95. Gisselbrecht C, Lepage E, Espie M, et al. Cyclophosphamide, total body irradiation with autologous bone marrow support for metastatic breast cancer [Abstract 255]. Proc Am Soc Clin Oncol 1987;6:65.

96. Gisselbrecht C, LePage E, Extra J, et al. Inflammatory and metastatic breast cancer: cyclophosphamide and total body irradiation (TBI) with autologous bone marrow transplantation (ABMT). In: Dicke K, Spitzer G, Jagannath S, Evinger-Hodges M, eds. Autologous bone marrow transplantation; proceedings of the fourth international symposium. Houston: University of Texas MD Anderson Cancer Center Press, 1989:363–367.

97. Livingston R, Schulman S, Griffin B, et al. Combination chemotherapy & systemic irradiation consolidation for poor prognosis breast cancer. Cancer 1987;9:1249–1254.

98. Vincent MD, Trevor J, Powles R, Coombes R, McElwain T. Late intensification with high-dose melphalan and autologous bone marrow support in breast cancer patients responding to conventional chemotherapy. Cancer Chemother Pharmacol 1988;21:255–260.

99. Spitzer G, Buzdar A, Auber M, et al. High dose cyclophosphamide/VP-16/platinum intensification for metastatic breast cancer. Breast Cancer Res Treat 1987;10:89.

100. Spitzer G, Dunphy F II, Ellis J, et al. High-dose intensification for stage IV hormonally-refractory breast cancer. In: Dicke K, Spitzer G, Jagannath S, Evinger-Hodges M, eds. Autologous bone marrow transplantation; proceedings of the fourth international symposium. Houston: University of Texas MD Anderson Cancer Center Press, 1989:399–405.

101. Dunphy FR, Spitzer G, Dicke K, Buzdar A, Hortobagyi G. Tandem high-dose chemotherapy as intensification in stage IV breast cancer. In: Bone marrow transplantation: current controversies. New York: Alan R Liss, 1989:245–251.

102. Jones RB, Shpall EJ, Peters WP. AFM—intensive induction chemotherapy for advanced breast cancer [Abstract]. Breast Cancer Res Treat 1987;10:90.

103. Jones RB, Shpall EJ, Shogan J, Gockerman J, Peters WP. AFM Induction chemotherapy followed by intensive consolidation with autologous bone marrow support for advanced breast cancer [Abstract 29]. Proc Am Soc Clin Oncol 1988;7:8.

104. Jones RB, Shpall EJ, Ross M, Bass R, Affronti M, Peters WP. AFM induction chemotherapy, followed by intensive alkylating agent consolidation with autologous bone marrow support (ABMS) for advanced breast cancer, current results [Abstract 30]. Proc Am Soc Clin Oncol 1990;9:9.

105. Williams S, Mick R, Dresser R, Golick J, Beschorner J, Bitran J. High dose consolidation therapy with autologous stem cell rescue in stage IV breast cancer. J Clin Oncol 1989;7:1824–1830.

106. Bitran JD, Williams SF. A phase II study of induction chemotherapy followed by intensification with high dose chemotherapy with autologous bone marrow rescue (ABMR) in stage IV breast cancer [Abstract]. Breast Cancer Res Treat 1987;10:88.

107. Kennedy M, Beveridge R, Rowley S, Abeloff M, Davidson N. Dose-intense cytoreduction followed by high dose consolidation chemotherapy and rescue with purged autologous bone marrow for metastatic breast cancer [Abstract 3]. Breast Cancer Res Treat 1989;14:133.

108. Kennedy MJ, Beveridge R, Rowley S, et al. High dose consolidation chemotheraphy and rescue with purged autologous bone marrow following dose-

intense induction for metastatic breast cancer [Abstract 69]. Proc Am Soc Clin Oncol 1989;8:19.

109. Rosti G, Galligioni E, Argnani M, et al. Autologous bone marrow transplantation as intensification therapy in breast cancer: an Italian cooperative experience. In: Dicke K, Spitzer G, Jagannath S, Evinger-Hodges M, eds. Autologous bone marrow transplantation; proceedings of the fourth international symposium. Houston: University of Texas MD Anderson Cancer Center Press, 1989;357–363.

110. Rosti G, Tumolo S, Figoli F, et al. High dose chemotherapy and autologous bone marrow transplantation in advanced breast cancer [Abstract]. Breast Cancer Res Treat 1987;10:110.

111. Leoni M, Rosti G, Flamini E, et al. High-dose chemotherapy and ABMT in advanced breast cancer: a pilot study [Abstract]. Bone Marrow Transplant 1988;3:299.

112. Mulder NH, Sleijfer DT, de Vries EG, Willemse PH. Intensive induction chemotherapy and intensification with autologous bone marrow reinfusion in patients with stage IIIB and IV breast cancer [Abstract 26]. Proc Am Soc Clin Oncol 1988;7:8.

113. Willemse PHB, de Vries EGE, Sleijfer DT, Mulder POM, Sibinga CTS, Mulder NH. Intensive induction chemotherapy and intensification with autologous bone marrow reinfusion in patients with stage IIIB and IV breast cancer [Abstract 163]. Breast Cancer Res Treat 1988;12:147.

114. Slease R, Selby G, Saez R, Keller A, Benear J, Epstein R. Autologous bone marrow transplantation for metastatic breast carcinoma in complete on partial remission [Abstract 58]. Breast Cancer Res Treat 1989;14:147.

115. Bonadonna G. Karnofsky Memorial Lecture. J Clin Oncol 1989;10:1380–1397.

116. Peters WP, Davis R, Shpall EJ, et al. Adjuvant chemotherapy involving high dose combination cyclophosphamide, cisplatin, and carmustin (CPA/CDDP/BCNU) and autologous bone marrow support (ABMS) or stage II/III breast cancer involving ten or more lymph nodes (CALGB): a preliminary report. Proc Am Soc Clin Oncol 1990;9:23.

117. Tajima T, Tokuda Y, Kubota M, Mitomi T. Adjuvant chemotherapy supported by autologous bone marrow transplantation in breast cancer [Abstract 116]. Proc Am Soc Clin Oncol 1990;9:31.

118. Hilner BE, Smith TJ, Desch CE. Estimating the cost-effectiveness of autologous bone marrow transplantation for metastatic breast cancer [Abstract 60]. Proc Am Soc Clin Oncol 1991;10:46.

High-Dose Chemotherapy with Autologous Bone Marrow Support for Lung Cancer

Gary Spitzer, Verneeda Spencer, and Frank R. Dunphy

Improvements in lung cancer therapy utilizing conventional doses of drugs or irradiation have been modest (1–4). Some minor enthusiasm has been recently initiated as a consequence of a potential increase in the survival of patients with limited disease (small-cell carcinoma) who were treated with concurrent radiation and chemotherapy (4). Much research revolves around the concept of optimizing dosage and timing of irradiation in relation to chemotherapy (4). In non-small-cell lung cancer, combination chemotherapy incorporating cisplatin reproducibly induces response rates of more than 20% in extensive disease and even higher in limited disease. Recent studies suggest that adjuvant therapy increases the proportion of survivors with inoperable limited disease (5–8). Overall there appears to be a new attitude to our approach to lung cancer. Subgroups of patients with less volume of disease appear to have a modest improvement in survival with chemotherapy. This may be improved even further by more intensive therapy incorporating early irradiation. The thinking that therapy other than surgery was worthwhile in non-small-cell lung cancer and that more aggressive approaches to both non-small-cell and small-cell lung cancer were associated with increased survival evolved slowly. Many patients and years of clinical research were needed to determine advances or subgroups of patients able to benefit from new therapy. An overriding principle was that patients with early disease and better performance status were optimal. The probability of extensive clonal evolution in more advanced disease, with its associated drug resistance, makes this group of patients less likely to have durable responses.

This chapter will attempt to place in perspective the studies of high-dose therapy in small-cell bronchogenic cancer (SCBC), the deficiencies in design of a number of these studies, the differences from other solid tumor types, the difficulties of studying patients who receive high-dose therapy, and the potential patient groups worthy of study, given our advances in drug selection for high-dose therapy and methods of toxicity modification since the early trials. Some emphasis will be placed on our strategy of high-dose intensification. We can only hint at a place for high-dose therapy in non-small-cell lung cancer, given the infancy of studies incorporating multidisciplinary aggressive therapies.

TANDEM (DOUBLE) HIGH-DOSE THERAPY IN SOLID TUMORS

Some of the difficulty in clearly demonstrating potential improvements with high-dose therapy is caused by the shallow dose-response curve with a number of non-hematologic tumors. Almost a decade ago, we began developing the technique of tandem (double) high-dose chemotherapy (9–12). This strategy was developed in part because of an early skepticism that the dose-response curve of most human solid tumors was not steep enough to warrant expectations that a single cycle of high-dose therapy would achieve results significantly different from those of standard chemotherapy in advanced stage disease. Newer strategies were needed to approach drug resistance that is not overcome by one cycle of high-dose therapy. Dose intensity over time may be important for reasons not generally considered in transplant approaches. Tandem high-dose therapy offers a potential means of circumventing kinetic resistance related to the presence of a proportion of G_0 cells in a tumor population. Theoretically, the first course of therapy may initiate the cycling of some of these cells to coincide with the second cycle of therapy. Furthermore, drug delivery to the center of tumor masses might be problematic, and tumor reduction by the first cycle of chemotherapy might enhance the effects of subsequent cycles.

Our first efforts were focused on testing whether identical high doses of chemotherapeutic agents could be administered in tandem within a short period of time and on determining the maximum tolerated doses (MTDs) feasible using such an approach. Simultaneously, we anticipated modifications of our chemotherapy that would include a different, but hopefully non-cross-resistant, combination of agents in the second cycle. Drug resistance might be overcome in a proportion of patients by alternative drugs.

A second aspect of our approach to high-dose escalations in this and our other successful high-dose therapy programs (13–15) has been a more cautious and conservative philosophy than that of most investigators in this field. In our initial studies we were searching for the MTD for high-dose chemotherapy that would equal that dose unassociated with life-threatening extramedullary toxicity, i.e., below the critical level at which a consistent percentage of patients experience extramedullary toxic effects. The unacceptable dose is the dose escalation point we term the "ceiling dose," which is regularly associated with a clinically worrisome frequency of extramedullary toxic effects such as cardiovascular, pulmonary, hepatic, and neurologic vasculitis. These effects would be unacceptable in the treatment of early disease such as stage II breast cancer, where the patient's median survival is lengthened significantly by conservative therapy. Unlike cases of acute leukemia, relapse of solid tumors such as breast cancer is not necessarily associated with early death. Median disease-free intervals are longer in patients with solid tumors than in those with acute leukemia. In a patient group with lung cancer, an obvious alternative strategy other than the classical methods of high-dose intensity must be available. Mortality rates of 10% in patients with good respiratory reserve would translate into unacceptable rates in this patient population. Drugs for dose escalation would be limited to those not associated with pulmonary toxicity because of the associated reduction in pulmonary reserve in patients with lung cancer.

The practice of defining the MTD for high-dose chemotherapy at a level unassociated with life-threatening extramedullary toxicity is supported by the lack of clinical evidence that long-term disease-free survival is improved by the super-high doses associated with high mortality rates. In leukemia, for instance, no clear evidence exists that any particular cytoreductive program is superior to the founding program of cyclophosphamide and total body irradiation (TBI), despite obvious increases in such programs' intensity when extra drugs are added or replace the TBI. This is exemplified by the therapy's new and increasingly toxic effects (16–18). The combination of busulfan and cyclophosphamide employing a cyclophosphamide dose approximately 50% of that used in initial studies has an equivalent antileukemic effect (19). Ongoing studies are examining therapies that use higher doses of cyclophosphamide, carmustine (BCNU), and etoposide (VP-16) (CBV) in patients with relapsed Hodgkin's disease than those used in our original description of CBV (13–15). When we evaluate outcome in identical subgroups (equivalent number of relapses, prior therapies, and tumor bulk), we find no convincing evidence that super-CBVs are associated with a higher proportion of long-term disease-free survivors than is lower-dose therapy, but they are certainly associated with a higher rate of early mortality (20, 21).

This lack of evidence that escalation to the level of serious extramedullary toxicity increases the therapeutic ratio within a single cycle further strengthened our conviction to develop and build programs based on the principle of what we now call tandem high-dose chemotherapy (i.e., below ceiling dose, with acceptable toxicity).

INITIAL STUDIES OF TANDEM HIGH-DOSE THERAPY IN SMALL-CELL BRONCHOGENIC CANCER

The initial combination chemotherapy we evaluated was cyclophosphamide and etoposide, drugs with reversible myeloid toxic effects and, if administered below certain doses, free of serious extramedullary toxicity. This combination was initially tested in small-cell lung cancer and formed our founding studies of high-dose intensification response in solid tumor patients (22).

We published some years ago on the use of high-dose cyclophosphamide, etoposide, and vincristine in 32 patients with limited SCBC following induction therapy with Adriamycin and alkylator agent therapy (Fig. 43.1) (23). The complete remission (CR) rate to induction was 41%. Classical of high-dose intensification studies, the CR rate was increased to approximately 70% and the overall response rate to 100% before subsequent

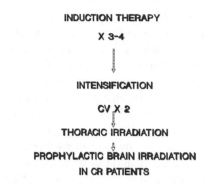

Figure 43.1.   Schema of our initial high-dose intensification with subsequent thoracic and brain irradiation in patients with small-cell bronchogenic carcinoma.

radiation therapy. Six of the 32 limited-disease patients have been off therapy for more than 4 years. These are unmaintained responses of approximately 7–8 years. With therapy at this level of intensity, in patients with minimal residual disease (the CR patients to induction therapy) 5 of 13 subsequently remained in CR following intensification. Only 1 of the 9 partial responders to induction therapy who converted to CR by intensification is still a long-term disease-free survivor. Not one patient died during this therapy, and a number were nursed without isolation.

Several points are worthy of emphasis. First, the intensity of therapy is less than that employed today for high-dose intensification. With more intense therapy, patients with less than CR to induction therapy may also potentially benefit, not just the patients in CR at the time of intensification. Furthermore, patients specifically excluded from this study were those eligible for surgery after two to three courses of induction therapy or those who had no evaluable disease (NED) from surgery before therapy. This excluded the most restricted of the limited-disease patients, the patients with the best prognosis, who in our experience have a disease-free survival of 50%–60% (24–26). Of the 13 patients intensified in CR, only 8 received the maximum therapeutic intensity intended by the protocol: two cycles of intensification and radiation within a short period after completion of intensification. Five of these 8 patients (over 50%) are surviving. The 5 patients not receiving the maximum dose have all relapsed. Reasons for not receiving the full therapy intensity include the following: (a) first-cycle toxicity and our extreme degree of conservatism at this early developmental stage with regard to repeating the cycle and (b) patient refusal and our hesistancy to encourage the second cycle. This analysis of the dose intensity received by the long-term survivors suggests that for optimal results therapy intensity should approach that received by the first 8 patients.

During the period of these investigations, other patients (nonparticipants) did not enter the program who matched study patients in most aspects, e.g., limited disease, less than 65 years of age, with a performance status of 2 or less. The CR rate of the first three cycles of therapy in nonparticipants was higher. The reason for this unfavorable selection factor was that patients achieving only partial remission (PR), and not CR, were encouraged more than were patients who achieved CR to undergo the unknown consequences of high-dose therapy. In nonparticipants, the CR median survival was equivalent, the median response duration was a little shorter, and there was only one patient with long-term progression-free survival. Although these patients had undergone conservative therapy and were in a more favorable group (achieving a higher CR rate to conventional therapy), there were fewer long-term disease-free survivors than in our study of modestly intense therapy.

To understand further directions, we examined relapse sites in patients who achieved CR. Relapses were systemic and occurred in the brain despite prophylactic brain irradiation, suggesting that the intensity of systemic therapy remained a problem. Further improvements in outcome with this approach will require the ability to administer even more intense therapy with acceptable toxicity (Table 43.1).

OTHER STUDIES OF HIGH-DOSE THERAPY IN SMALL-CELL BRONCHOGENIC CANCER

The effectiveness of dose intensity in SCBC has been the subject of many reviews with negative conclusions. In this review, we would like to address some questions of clinical design regarding most of these studies. Radiotherapy trials are not considered adequate unless the methodology has been correct. Trials with inadequate dose-intense methodology cannot be used to refute the principle. Most studies that attempt to address the question of high-dose therapy in SCBC do not approach the intensity of therapy that is administered for hematologic malignancy with either autologous or allogeneic marrow transplants. Many studies addressing this question have used cyclophosphamide doses of 2.0 g/m^2 rather than 5.0 g/m^2, single intensification agents, or relatively minor dose escalations (27–36). Studies incorporating these doses must be looked at quite critically because only when dose is adequate can the effectiveness of dose intensity be proven or disproved.

A major technical problem is inherent in addressing this question in this patient population. A greater propensity to toxicity and mortality from associated pulmonary and cardiovascular disease renders these patients more susceptible to serious pneumonia and fatal outcomes. Methods must be defined to determine the effectiveness of dose intensity in these individuals. These important clinical realities limit our ability to aggressively escalate therapy.

Some of these studies also incorporated a number of patients with extensive disease and only a small proportion of patients in complete remission. A durable response from high-dose therapy would be most anticipated in patients with minimal residual

Table 43.1.   Autologous Bone Marrow Transplantation in Small-Cell Bronchogenic Carcinoma, Sites of Relapse in Complete Remission Patients

	CR Induction CR Intensification		PR[a] Induction CR Intensification	
	Number of Patients		Number of Patients	
Single Sites				
Lung	1[b,c]	—	0	—
Brain	1[d]	—	3[d]	—
Liver	1	—	1	—
		Site		Site
Multiple Sites	3[c]	Lung/soft tissue	3	Brain/soft tissue
		Lung/liver		Brain/liver/lung
				Marrow/adrenal/renal
		Cause		Cause
Died in CR	1[c]	Hepatitis	2	Radiation pneumonitis
				Pericarditis
Total number of patients	13		9	

[a]PR, partial remission.
[b]Patient did not receive thoracic irradiation.
[c]Patient received only one course of intensification.
[d]All patients had received prophylactic brain irradiation.

Table 43.2.   High-Dose Late Intensification Therapy and Autologous Bone Marrow Transplantation in SCBC[a]

	Conditioning Regimen	Conclusions
Smith (34)	CTX	Negative: low dose
Postmus (31)	CTX-VP-16	Negative: low dose, wrong patients
Ihde (30)	CTX-VP-16 Local irradiation	Negative: low dose, extensive disease
Stewart (38)	CTX-TBI ± hydroxyurea	Predominantely extensive disease
Klastersky (27)	CDDP-VP-16 Adriamycin	Negative: low dose, mainly extensive disease

[a]Abbreviation: ABMT, autologous bone marrow transplantation; CTX, cyclophosphamide; CDDP, cisplatin; VP-16, etoposide.

Table 43.3.   Example of Doses Used for High-Dose Therapy in SCBC

Smith (34)	Cyclophosphamide 7 g/m^2 × 1 CDDP 120–180 mg/m^2
Klastersky (27)	Doxorubicin 90–135 mg/m^2 Etoposide 240–360 mg/m^2
Idhe (30)	Cyclophosphamide 60 mg/kg days 1–2 Etoposide 200 mg/m^2 days 1–3 XRT[a] to primary site, 200 rad/5 fractions

[a]XRT, Radiation.

disease at the time of intensification and known marked sensitivity to induction therapy. Criticisms of several of these studies are listed in Table 43.2. Representative doses in some of these studies are provided in Table 43.3.

Souhami (28, 29) reports the results of several trials of high-dose therapy in SCBC that are informative for several reasons. Most of these studies incorporated modestly high doses of cyclophosphamide at 4.5–5 g/m^2 as initial treatment or intensification after a small number of cycles of conventional therapy. The overall response is not increased, but CR is increased by either a second cycle of high-dose therapy or intensification. Arguments are proposed that this strategy only decreases the sensitive component of the tumor and not the resistant component. Therefore, long-term survival is not different. These studies raise many questions about how to best approach high-dose therapy; the role, selection, and number of courses of induction therapy; the choice of drugs; single agent versus drug combination; the dose intensity needed to ensure the elimination of sensitive tumors; and the methods to eliminate resistant tumors.

There has been only one randomized study of high-dose therapy versus conventional therapy in SCBC (37). Patients received induction therapy, three courses of doxorubicin (Adriamycin), cyclophosphamide, and vincristine followed by two courses of cisplatin and etoposide. They were then randomized to one additional course of conventional therapy or intensification with cyclophosphamide at 6 g/m², BCNU at 300 mg/m², and etoposide at 900 mg/m² (Fig. 43.2). Although the therapy was with multiple drugs at intensive doses, the patient characteristics were not ideal, because only a small number of patients had limited disease in CR. A significant proportion of the patients had extensive disease or had achieved only partial remission at the time of intensification (38). As is usual with high-dose therapy, there was a significant conversion of patients from PR to CR. Progression-free survival with limited disease in the high-dose arm was superior. Survival favored the high-dose therapy arm but did not reach statistical significance.

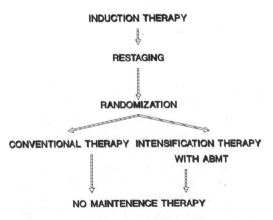

Figure 43.2. Design of high-dose intensification radomization for small-cell brochogenic carcinoma. Patients received five induction cycles (see text), followed by radomization to high-dose therapy with cyclophosphamide, carmustine, and etoposide versus another cycle of conventional-dose therapy.

An overview of multiple studies of high-dose therapy in SCBC shows that patients intensified in CR after induction therapy, despite inadequate clinical designs such as single drugs for intensification or minimal dose escalation, realize an approximate 39% disease-free survival, potentially higher than the proportion of long-term disease-free survival in CR patients with limited disease with SCBC (Table 43.4). Patients with PR or less at intensification achieve only a 6% disease-free survival. Patients with extensive disease and CR have a small proportion with long-term disease-free survival (37).

Patients with limited disease would be an appropriate group to evaluate when advances in the modification of toxicity have been made so that early mortality could be reduced and greater dose intensity administered.

OUR PRESENT DIRECTIONS

More recent data suggest that cisplatin provides significant extra cytoreduction when added to high-dose cyclophosphamide and etoposide in treating extensive SCBC (39). We subsequently incorporated cisplatin because of its theoretical synergism with the other two drugs and its activity across a broad range of tumor types. We have evaluated this combination, termed CVP, in 199 patients at four dosage levels with tumors of various types (Table 43.5). Table 43.6 compares the doses of one course at the highest dose of CVP to the classic single dose, initial STAMP therapy, and other commonly used intensification

Table 43.4. Autologous Marrow Transplantation for Responding SCBC, Limited Disease in CR at Time of Transplantation

1. 39% disease-free survival, most with greater than 2-year follow-up despite variable dose intensity.
2. 20%–40% expected with standard chemoradiotherapy.
3. This would be the upper limit of expectations with conventional therapy.

Table 43.5. Double CVP, 199 Patients, December 1990[a]

First relapse (breast)	103
Second or subsequent relapse (breast)	24
ER+ metastatic breast cancer	16
SCBC	18
Adenocarcinoma (unknown primary)	6
Others (gastric, other gastrointestinal, sarcoma, adenocarcinoma, lung lymphoma)	32

[a]Abbreviations: CVP, cyclophosphamide, etoposide, cisplatin; ER, estragon receptor positive.

Table 43.6. Dose-Intensity Comparison of CVP[a]

	Protocol		
CVP	CYT 6 g/m^2	CDDP 165 mg/m^2	VP-16 1500 mg/m^2
STAMP 1	CYT 5.6 g/m^2	CDDP 165 mg/m^2	BCNU 600 mg/m^2
STAMP V	CYT 6 g/m^2	Carboplatin 800 mg/m^2	Thiotepa 500 mg/m^2
CT	CYT 5.25 g/m^2		Thiotepa 675 mg/m^2

[a]Abbreviations: Cyt, cyclophosphamide; CDDP, cisplatin; VP-16, etoposide.

protocols in solid tumors (40). Compared to STAMP 1 the cyclophosphamide doses we employed are slightly higher and the cisplatin doses are equivalent; any differences in effect, therefore, are almost totally attributed to the third drug. A carefully chosen third drug can bring the therapeutic effects of a single cycle of our regimen to an equivalent or near equivalent intensity to that of other high-dose single-administration chemotherapy for human solid tumors.

A further question one could ask of our strategy is, did we choose the appropriate cytoreductive therapy? Alternatives to CVP include similar combinations such as ifosfamide, carboplatin, and etoposide (STAMP 2), STAMP 5 variants that replace the nitrosourea with thiotepa and use carboplatin instead of cisplatin, and busulfan plus cyclophosphamide and TBI in combination with many drugs. We chose etoposide rather than a nitrosourea such as BCNU because of BCNU's life-threatening pulmonary toxicity, particu-

larly in patients who have undergone prior radiotherapy, as the dose is escalated above 450 mg/m^2, and because of BCNU's propensity to produce other extramedullary toxic effects such as venoocclusive disease and vasculitis. Tandem CVP appears at least therapeutically equivalent to alternatives in other tumor types (10). The choice of high-dose chemotherapy approaches may ultimately be decided on the basis of which therapy can be administered with the fewest toxic effects and, therefore, can be used in the greatest variety of patients because of the lower risk of death. This would be of particular importance in patients with lung cancer.

DETECTION OF TUMOR CELLS IN BONE MARROW AND THEIR REMOVAL

Some of the reasons for treatment failure in SCBC may be the propensity for this tumor to involve bone marrow. The maximum sensitivity for the morphologic detection of tumor cells is 0.1% or less. If we were to collect 10^{10} marrow cells for transplantation, there could be as many as 10^7 tumor cells in the marrow inoculum, hence the continuing research emphasis in detection of marrow tumor cells and their removal. Favrot's group (41) studying neuroblastoma, another tumor type that frequently involves marrow, could detect marrow involvement in approximately 50% of patients by more extensive marrow sampling (four aspirates and biopsies). Biopsy was found to be more sensitive than was aspirate. The frequency of this marrow involvement is even more impressive and surprising since the evaluation was performed following response. A recent manuscript confirms these data (42). Nine of 12 neuroblastoma patients had circulating tumor cells at diagnosis, detected by examination of the mononuclear cells with immunoperoxidase staining using a panel of antibodies reactive to neuroblastoma cells. Eight of 23 peripheral blood specimens (35%) were still positive during therapy. A significant proportion of patients following therapy also had either histologically or immunocytologically positive marrow. All had positive marrow biopsies. Circulating tumor cells were detected even when there was scant or no detectable marrow disease. The level of marrow disease quantitated by aspirate examination from both these studies gives a poor estimate of the potential for reinfusion of tumor cells.

Despite prejudice about reasons for relapse following a CR after autologous bone marrow transplantation (ABMT), the frequency of marrow or blood involvement is a concern. This problem is not unique to neuroblastoma. A recent report evaluated a cocktail of seven monoclonal antibodies to detect small cell carcinoma cells in mononuclear preparations of marrow cells from patients with limited disease in CR (43). Most surprising was the detection of tumor cells in the majority of patients despite the examination following therapy and achievement of maximal response. The few patients with negative findings had a tendency for local relapse. Those with positive marrow had a tendency for systemic relapse. We postulated that failure in marrow transplantation is related to reinfusion of tumor cells.

Other antibodies have been used to detect tumor cells, and immunomagnetic beads and monoclonal antibodies can eliminate detectable disease as evaluated by two-parameter flow cytometry (44–47). Since the sensitivity of this method is 1 in less than 10^5, there could be up to 10^5 tumor cells reinfused. Other alternative strategies for purging include drugs, monoclonals, combinations thereof, and light-activated merocyanine 540 phototreatment in combination with antithiols. These studies generally incorporate malignant cell line and marrow hematopoietic progenitor survival as end points to document efficiency. These artificial in vitro systems are probably less representative than is documentation of the removal of tumor cells from clinical specimens. Nevertheless, the true proportion of cells with self-renewal poten-

tial among these contaminating tumor cells, the efficiency of any method in removing this subpopulation, and the necessary numbers to reproduce the disease in vivo remain undetermined.

Because of this obvious potential for tumor contamination and the unknown efficiency of purging techniques of marrow in patients with solid tumors, this aspect is worthy of significant investigation in SCBC.

CONCLUSIONS

Few adequate studies testing the hypothesis of dose intensity in SCBC exist. Only one was randomized. The impact shown has been minimal, but valuable insights into future research directions and better clinical design are now apparent. More tolerable yet active drugs, such as cisplatin and carboplatin, are now available for escalation. The use of recombinant growth factors and peripheral blood cells has modestly reduced the toxicity of high-dose therapy. This may be more important in reducing complications in this group than in other, more robust patient populations. The aggressive approach to limited but inoperable non-small-cell carcinoma with chemotherapy, irradiation, and surgery would suggest that patients who have tumor shrinkage with this approach but still experience systemic relapse should be considered as new patient groups for high-dose intensification approaches. Prognostic factors identifying those patients with limited disease, non-small-cell and small-cell lung cancer with high probability of relapse despite multimodal therapy should be available soon. The challenge will be to devise dose-intensive therapy adequate to eradicate residual disease and methods to modify the toxicity of this therapy.

REFERENCES

1. Goodman GE, Miller TP, Manning MM, Davis SL, McMahon IJ. Treatment of small cell lung cancer with VP-16, vincristine, doxorubicin (Adriamycin), cyclophosphamide (EVAC), and high-dose chest radiotherapy. J Clin Oncol 1983;1:483–488.

2. Niiranen A. Long-term survival in small cell carcinoma of the lung. Eur J Cancer Clin Oncol 1988; 24:749–752.

3. Seifter EJ, Ihde DC. Therapy of small cell lung cancer: a perspective on two decades of clinical research. Semin Oncol 1988;15:278–299.

4. Vokes EE, Weichselbaum RR. Concomitant chemoradiotherapy: rationale and clinical experience in patients with solid tumors. J Clin Oncol 1990;8:911–934.

5. Bonomi P, Rowland K, Taylor SG IV, et al. Phase II trial of etoposide, cisplatin, continuous infusion 5-fluorouracil, and simultaneous split-course radiation therapy in stage III non-small-cell bronchogenic carcinoma. Semin Oncol 1986;13(suppl 3):115–120.

6. Martini N, Kris MG, Gralla RJ, et al. The effects of preoperative chemotherapy on the resectability of non-small cell lung carcinoma with mediastinal lymph node metastases (N2 MO). Ann Thorac Surg 1988; 45:370–379.

7. Taylor SG IV, Trybula M, Bonomi PD, et al. Simultaneous cisplatin fluorouracil infusion and radiation followed by surgical resection in regionally localized stage III, non-small cell lung cancer. Ann Thorac Surg 1987;43:87–91.

8. Weiden PL, Piantadosi S. Preoperative chemotherapy (cisplatin and fluorouracil) and radiation therapy in stage III non-small-cell lung cancer: a phase II study of the lung cancer study group. J Natl Cancer Inst 1991;83:266–272.

9. Dunphy FR, Spitzer G, Buzdar AU, et al. Treatment of estrogen receptor-negative or hormonally refractory breast cancer with double high-dose chemotherapy intensification and bone marrow support. J Clin Oncol 1990;8:1207–1216.

10. Dunphy FR, Spitzer G, Dicke KA, Buzdar AU, Hortobagyi GN. Tandem high-dose chemotherapy as intensification in stage IV breast cancer. In: Gale RP, Champlin R, eds. Bone marrow transplantation: current controversies. UCLA Symposia on Molecular and Cellular Biology, New Series. New York: Wiley-Liss, 1988;87:245–51.

11. Spitzer G, Dunphy FR, Ellis JK, et al. High-dose intensification for stage IV hormonally-refractory breast cancer. In: Dicke KA, Spitzer G, Jagannath S, eds. Autologous bone marrow transplantation: proceedings of the Fourth International Symposium. Houston: University of Texas MD Anderson Cancer Center, 1989:399–403.

12. Spitzer G, Huan S, Dunphy F, et al. Double high-dose therapy in human solid tumors: an emphasis on breast cancer. In: Champlin RE, Gale RP, eds. New strategies in bone marrow transplantation. New York: Alan R. Liss, 1990:437–446.

13. Spitzer G, Dicke KA, Litam J, et al. High-dose combination chemotherapy with autologous bone marrow transplantation in adult solid tumors. Cancer 1980;45:3075–3085.

14. Jagannath S, Dicke KA, Armitage JO, et al. High-dose cyclophosphamide, carmustine, etoposide, and autologous bone marrow transplantation for relapsed Hodgkin's disease. Ann Intern Med 1986;104:163–168.

15. Jagannath S, Armitage JO, Dicke KA, et al. Updated results of CBV and autologous bone marrow transplantation for Hodgkin's disease. In: Dicke KA, Spitzer G, Jagannath S, eds. Proceedings of the Third International Symposium on Autologous Bone Marrow Transplantation. Houston: The University of Texas Press, 1987:217–221.

16. Thomas ED, Buckner CD, Clift RA, et al. Marrow transplantation for acute non-lymphocytic leukemia in first remission. N Engl J Med 1979;301:597–599.

17. Santos GW, Tutschka PJ, Brookmeyer R, et al. Marrow transplantation for acute non-lymphocytic leukemia after treatment with busulfan and cytoxan. N Engl J Med 1983;309:1347–1353.

18. Maranchi DI, Blaise DI, Guyotat D, et al. Prospective study randomizing CY-TBI vs little BUS-CY prior to allogeneic bone marrow transplantation (BMT) for acute myeloid leukemia (AML) in first complete remission (CR). Exp Hematol 1990;18:706.

19. Tutschka PJ, Copeland EA, Klein JP. Bone marrow transplantation for leukemia following a new busulfan and cyclophosphamide regimen. Blood 1987; 70:1382–1388.

20. Phillips G, Barnett M, Buskard M, et al. Augmented cyclophosphamide, BCNU and etoposide and autologous bone marrow transplantation for progressive Hodgkin's disease. J Cell Biochem 1988;12c:K418.

21. Wheeler C, Antin JH, Churchill WH, et al. Cyclophosphamide, carmustine, and etoposide with autologous bone marrow transplantation in refractory Hodgkin's disease and non-Hodgkin's lymphoma: a dose finding study. J Clin Oncol 1990;8:648–656.

22. Farha P, Spitzer G, Valdivieso M, et al. High-dose chemotherapy and autologous bone marrow transplantation for the treatment of small-cell lung carcinoma. Cancer 1983;52:1351–1355.

23. Spitzer G, Farha P, Valdivieso M, et al. High-dose intensification therapy with autologous bone marrow support for limited small-cell bronchogenic carcinoma. J Clin Oncol 1986;4:4–13.

24. Davis S, Wright PW, Schulman SF, Scholes D, Thorning D, Hammar S. Long-term survival in small-cell carcinoma of the lung: a population experience. J Clin Oncol 1985;3:80–91.

25. Baker RR, Ettinger DS, Ruckdeschel JD, et al. The role of surgery in the management of selected patients with small-cell carcinoma of the lung. J Clin Oncol 1987;5:697–702.

26. Comis RL. The role of surgery in small-cell lung cancer: a reappraisal. Clin Oncol 1985;4:141–151.

27. Klastersky J, Nicaise C, Longeval E, Stryckmans P. The EORTC Lung Cancer Working Party. Cisplatin, Adriamycin, and etoposide (CAV) for remission induction

of small-cell bronchogenic carcinoma: evaluation of efficacy and toxicity and pilot study of a "late intensification" with autologous bone marrow rescue. Cancer 1982;50:652–658.

28. Souhami RL, Harper PG, Linch D, et al. High-dose cyclophosphamide with autologous marrow transplantation as initial treatment of small-cell carcinoma of the bronchus. Cancer Chemother Pharmacol 1982;275:1–4.

29. Souhami RL, Finn G, Gregory WM, et al. High-dose cyclophosphamide in small-cell carcinoma of the lung. J Clin Oncol 1985;3:958–963.

30. Ihde DC, Deisseroth AB, Lichter AS, et al. Late intensive combined modality therapy followed by autologous bone marrow infusion in extensive-stage small cell lung cancer. J Clin Oncol 1986;4:1443–1454.

31. Postmus PE, Mulder NH, De Vries-Hospers HG, et al. High-dose cyclophosphamide and high-dose VP 16-213 for recurrent or refractory small-cell lung cancer: a phase II study. Eur J Cancer Clin Oncol 1985;21:1467–1470.

32. Glode LM, Robinson WA, Hartmann DW, Klein JJ, Thomas MR, Morton N. Autologous bone marrow transplantation in the therapy of small-cell carcinoma of the lung. Cancer Res 1982;42:4270–4275.

33. Marangolo M, Rosti G, Amadori D, et al. High-dose etoposide and autologous bone marrow transplantation as intensification treatment in small-cell lung cancer: a pilot study. Bone Marrow Transplant 1989;4:405–408.

34. Smith IE, Evans BD, Harland SJ. High-dose cyclophosphamide ($7g/m^2$) with or without autologous bone marrow rescue after conventional chemotherapy in the treatment of patients with small-cell lung cancer. Cancer Treat Rev 1983;10:79–81.

35. Postmus PE, De Vries EGE, De Vries-Hospers HG, et al. Cyclophosphamide and VP 16-213 with autologous bone marrow transplantation: a dose escalation study. 1984;20(6):777–782.

36. Spitzer G, Valdivieso M, Farha P, Dicke KA, Zander AR. High-dose chemotherapy with and without autologous bone marrow support for small-cell bronchogenic lung cancer: a review. Ann Clin Conf Cancer 1986;28:301–315.

37. Humblet Y, Symann M, Bosly A, et al. Late intensification chemotherapy with autologous bone marrow transplantation in selected small-cell carcinoma of the lung: a randomized study. J Clin Oncol 1987;5:1864–1873.

38. Stewart P, Buckner CD, Thomas ED, et al. Intensive chemoradiotherapy with autologous marrow transplantation for small-cell carcinoma of the lung. Cancer Treat Rep 1983;67:1055–1059.

39. Johnson DH, DeLeo MJ, Hande KR, Wolff SN, Hainsworth JD, Greco FA. High-dose induction chemotherapy with cyclophosphamide, etoposide, and cisplatin for extensive-stage small-cell lung cancer. J Clin Oncol 1987;5:703–709.

40. Peters WP, Eder JP, Henner WD, et al. High-dose combination alkylating agent chemotherapy with autologous bone marrow support for metastatic breast cancer. J Clin Oncol 1986;4:646–654.

41. Combaret V, Favrot MC, Kremens B, et al. Immunological detection of neuroblastoma cells in bone marrow harvested for autologous transplantation. Br J Cancer 1989;59(6):844–847.

42. Moss TJ, Sanders DG, Lasky LC, Bostrom B. Contamination of peripheral blood stem cell harvests by circulating neuroblastoma cells. Blood 1990;76:1879–1883.

43. Leonard RCF, Duncan LW, Hay FG. Immunocytochemical detection of residual marrow disease at clinical remission predicts metastatic disease in small-cell lung cancer. Cancer Res 1990;50:6545–6548.

44. Bernal SD, Speak J, Mabry MM, Stahel RA, Cualing HM, Elias AD. Small-cell carcinoma antigens. In: Biology of lung cancer. Vol. 37. New York: Marcel Dekker, 1988;213–236.

45. Combaret V, Kremens B, Favrot MC, Laurent JC, Philip T. S-L 11.14: a monoclonoal antibody recognizing neuroectodermal tumors with possible value for bone marrow purging before autograft. Bone Marrow Transplant 1988:3:221–227.

46. Meagher RC, Rothman SA, Paul P, Koberna P, Willmer C, Baucco PA. Purging of small-cell lung cancer from human bone marrow using ethiofos (wr-2721) and light-activated merocyanine 540 phototreatment. Cancer Res 1989;49:3637–3641.

47. Vredenburgh JJ, Ball Ed. Elimination of small-cell carcinoma of the lung from human bone marrow by monoclonal antibodies and immunomagnetic beads. Cancer Res 1990;50:7216–7220.

HIGH-DOSE CHEMOTHERAPY AND AUTOLOGOUS MARROW TRANSPLANTATION FOR COMMON EPITHELIAL OVARIAN CARCINOMA

Patrice Viens and Dominique Maraninchi

Common epithelial ovarian carcinoma is the most frequent of ovarian neoplasms. The first-line treatment of advanced stages (FIGO III and IV) is now well established and must include initial debulking surgery followed by cisplatin-based combination chemotherapy. After this first-line therapy, 30%–50% of patients will achieve a complete remission, and of these patients, about 50% appear to be cured. For patients with residual disease after first-line therapy, prognosis is worse. Chemotherapy (intraperitoneal or intravenous) leads to a median survival of 29 months (1) and abdominopelvic radiotherapy to a 3-year disease-free survival of 30% (2). Finally, there is no available treatment for relapsing and primary refractory disease.

However, ovarian carcinoma is a chemosensitive tumor, and various drugs have a good effect (Table 44.1). Among them, alkylating agents have been extensively used at a conventional dosage and have produced an objective response rate ranging from 33% to 63% (3, 4). Cisplatin and more recently carboplatin have also shown high efficiency in ovarian cancer (6, 11). A dose-response relationship is a general property of alkylating agents (12, 13), and their main toxicity, which

is hematologic, can be overcome by autologous marrow rescue. Such a relationship has been shown for cisplatin in ovarian carcinoma, but nonhematologic toxicities limit the use of high-dose cisplatin (7). Utilization of high-dose carboplatin may be an alternative to high-dose cisplatin (11).

The efficiency of chemotherapy in ovarian cancer has been shown with high-dose alkylating agents, and more recently high-dose carboplatin with marrow support has been used in ovarian cancer by several groups, including ours, with the aim of improving the cure rate of chemosensitive disease, or of salvaging refractory disease.

THE MARSEILLE EXPERIENCE

Patients

Twenty-six patients with common epithelial ovarian carcinoma received high-dose chemotherapy and autologous bone marrow transplantation. Their median age at time of high-dose chemotherapy was 45 years (range 24–57). The first-line treatment included, for all patients, debulking surgery and cisplatin-based combination chemotherapy (4–8 cycles). Twelve patients, with an initial FIGO

Table 44.1. Single Drugs Active in Ovarian Carcinoma

Drugs	Percent Response (%CR)[a]	Reference
Melphalan	47 (20)	3
Thiotepa	65	3
Cyclophosphamide	49	3
Ifosfamide	20 (7)	4
Etoposide	32	5
Cisplatin	27	6
Cisplatin (high dose)	32 (11)	7
Carboplatin	50 (17)	8–10
Carboplatin[b] (high dose)	27 (13)	11

[a]CR, complete response.
[b]Patients previously treated with cisplatin.

stage III or IV, responded to first-line therapy (complete remission [CR]: 4; partial remission [PR]: 8) and received high-dose chemotherapy as consolidation or for minimal residual disease. Seven patients with primary refractory disease and seven patients with resistant relapse received high-dose chemotherapy as a salvage therapy.

High-Dose Chemotherapy

Nine patients received melphalan alone (140 mg/m^2 in 8, 200 mg/m^2 in 1). Fifteen patients received cyclophosphamide (60 mg/kg/day × 2 days) followed by melphalan (140 mg/m^2). Two patients received etoposide (350 mg/m^2/day × 5 days), carboplatin (400 mg/m^2/day × 4 days), and cyclophosphamide (1600 mg/m^2/day × 4 days) (Table 44.2). All patients were well hydrated with continuous intravenous fluid, and patients who received cyclophosphamide received mesna. All patients had a central venous line. Melphalan was given as an intravenous bolus, etoposide and cyclophosphamide as a 1-hour infusion, and carboplatin as a continuous infusion over 22 hours.

Bone Marrow Procedure and Supportive Care

In patients who received melphalan alone, marrow was collected immediately before high-dose chemotherapy and was stored 24 hours at room temperature before infusion (14). In the other patients, marrow cells were cryopreserved with dimethylsulphoxide (15) prior to infusion. In all cases, marrow was morphologically normal. Patients were managed in single rooms with reverse isolation. All blood products, except marrow, were irradiated to 15 Gy. Packed red blood cells and platelets were administered to maintain hemoglobin level >8 g/dl and platelet count >20 × 10^9/liter. If patients became febrile, they were promptly treated with intravenous broad-spectrum antibiotics; amphotericin B was added if they remained so for more than 48 hours. Parenteral nutrition was given if oral intake was inadequate.

Results

TOXICITY

All patients experienced profound aplasia. One patient had a slow neutrophil recovery (45 days) and one a very slow platelet recovery (10 months) (Table 44.3).

All patients had nausea and vomiting after high-dose chemotherapy. Ten patients experienced moderate or severe mucositis and 9 diarrhea. Bacteremia occured in 10 patients. One patient treated with etoposide-carboplatin-cyplophosphamide had a supraventricular arrhythmia and did not receive the last day of cyclophosphamide.

Three patients (12%) died directly from the treatment: 2 from disseminated aspergillosis (day +52 and day +68) and one from hepatitis (day +60).

RESPONSE

Thirteen patients were not evaluated for response: 3 died from treatment toxicity, 10 had no radiologically evaluable tumor at time of high-dose chemotherapy. Thirteen were evaluable: 7 responded to high-dose chemotherapy (CR: 4, PR: 3, response rate: 55%). Median duration of response was 10 months (range 3–53).

Table 44.2. Conditioning Regimens Used in Marseille for Ovarian Carcinomas[a]

Days	−7	−6	−5	−4	−3	−2	−1	0
Conditioning regimen 1							Mel 140 mg/m²	ABMT
Conditioning regimen 2				Cy 60 mg/kg	Cy 60 mg/kg	Mel 140 mg/m²		ABMT
Conditioning regimen 3	VP16 350 mg/m²	VP16 350 mg/m² Cy 1600 mg/m² CP 400 mg/m²	VP16 350 mg/m² Cy 1600 mg/m² CP 400 mg/m²	VP16 350 mg/m² Cy 1600 mg/m² CP 400 mg/m²	VP16 350 mg/m² Cy 1600 mg/m² CP 400 mg/m²			ABMT

[a]Abbreviations: ABMT, autologous bone marrow transplantation; CP, carboplatin; Cy, cyclophosphamide; Mel, melphalan.

Table 44.3. Toxicity after Autologous Bone Marrow Transplantation for Ovarian Carcinoma (Marseille)

Days with granulocytes < 0.5 × 10⁹/liter	13 (6–45)
Days with platelets < 50 × 10⁹/liter	26 (13–300)
Mucositis, moderate or severe	35%
Diarrhea, moderate or severe	30%
Bacteremia	32%
Cardiac toxicity	4% (1 patient)
Toxic death	12% (3 patients)
Median of hospitalization (days)	35 (21–70)

Five of 12 patients with chemosensitive disease at time of high-dose chemotherapy are alive without progression from 12 to 30 months after high-dose chemotherapy. In this group of patients, a very late relapse was seen: 53 months after high-dose chemotherapy. The 3-year progression-free survival of this group is 50% (Kaplan-Meier method) (Fig. 44.1).

In the group of 14 patients with primary refractory disease or resistant relapse at time of high-dose chemotherapy, 3 patients are alive without progression at 1 month, 2 months, and 18 months after high-dose chemotherapy. Other patients progressed very soon after high-dose chemotherapy.

OVERVIEW AND DISCUSSION

Autologous bone marrow transplantation offers the opportunity of using the dose-effect relationship in the therapy of cancer.

The main limitations to this approach are (*a*) the necessity for using drugs known to have a dose-dependent antitumor effect (i.e., mainly alkylating agents) and (*b*) the risk of infusion of tumor cells with the marrow transplant, which could be involved in advanced neoplasms.

Ovarian carcinoma is a tumor where bone marrow involvement is rare and where chemosensitivity to alkylating agents and/or platinin derivatives has been extensively demonstrated. Such a disease, in advanced stages, is a good candidate for dose intensification with autologous marrow transplant support. Table 44.4 presents data from 116 patients reported in the literature who received various high-dose chemotherapy regimens with autologous marrow support. Despite several of the patients' being treated aggressively at an advanced stage of the disease, the procedure-related mortality (4%) is relatively low and similar to transplant-related mortality in the treatment of several other tumors.

In a review of the literature, including our experience, 49 patients were clearly evaluable for response (Table 44.5); most of them had refractory disease at time of high-dose chemotherapy. With a 53% response rate (37% CR rate), such dose escalations of chemotherapy clearly represent an efficient salvage therapy for some chemoresistant ovarian carcinomas. It is, however, not possible at the present time to evaluate the comparative ef-

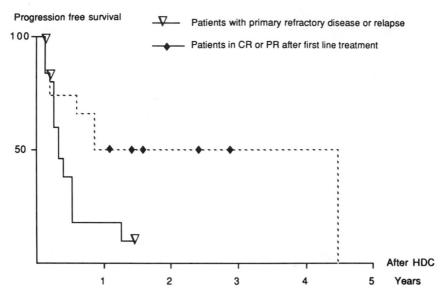

Figure 44.1.   Progression-free survival after high-dose chemotherapy.

fects on response of the various chemotherapies used.

In patients with refractory disease at the time of high-dose chemotherapy, despite antitumor activity, duration of response is short, median 3 months in our group and ranging from 3 to 75 months in the literature, with few patients remaining free of progression 1 year after autologous marrow transplant. In patients who received high-dose chemotherapy in advanced but still chemosensitive disease, median duration of response is clearly longer, with progression-free survival at 3 years after high-dose chemotherapy ranging from 30% to 50%. These rates of progression-free survival are superior to those observed with conventional therapy (1, 2, 26, 27) in similar situations. Thus several combinations of high-dose chemotherapy have been studied in ovarian carcinomas. Current promising approaches of intensive chemotherapy in ovarian cancer include combinations of high-dose alkylating agents with carboplatin, with or without etoposide (Tables 44.2, 44.4; 28).

The 5% mortality seen in patients extensively treated is low, and morbidity of high-dose chemotherapy should decrease with the extensive use of hematopoietic growth factors. This low mortality and the results obtained in patients with chemosensitive disease allow the introduction of high-dose chemotherapy for patients with an initial FIGO stage III or IV and with a very low probability of being cured. This poor-prognosis population could include patients with chemosensitive disease but with residual tumor after first-line therapy and some patients with initial bulky disease, residual tumor after initial debulking surgery, and high histologic grade in CR after first-line therapy. In this population, randomized studies versus conventional therapy are needed to evaluate the impact of high-dose chemotherapy and autologous marrow transplant in common epithelial ovarian carcinoma.

SUMMARY AND CONCLUSIONS

Common epithelial ovarian carcinoma is often diagnosed at an advanced stage (FIGO III or IV). Cure of advanced stages is uncommon, particularly for patients with residual disease after adequate first-line therapy (in-

Table 44.4.   High-Dose Chemotherapy in Ovarian Carcinoma[a]

Author (Reference)	n	Status at time of HDC	Conditioning regimen	Response/ Evaluable (CR)	Duration of Response
Extra (16)	21	Res	Cy-AI (16) Cy-AI-Mel (3) Cy-AI-CP (1) Cy-Mel-CP (1)	NA	Progression-free survival: 30% 3 years after HDC
Mulder (17)	11	Ref	Cy-VP16	6/11 (6)	Median duration of CR: 15 months (8, 75+)
Mulder (18)	6	Ref	Cy-Mx	4/5 (2)	3, 3, 13, 5+, 9+ (months)
Dauplat (19)	14	Res 12 Ref 2	Mel	NA	Progression-free survival: 33% 3 years after HDC
Ellis (20)	3	Ref	Cy-T-Mx	1/3 (1)	—
Lazarus (21)	2	Ref	Mel	0/0	5, 6.5 (months)
Corringham (22)	2	Ref	Mel	1/2 (1)	8, 35 (months)
Barnett (23)	5	Ref 4 Res 1	CP-VP16-Mel	0/0	3+, 9+, 10+, 29+ (months)
Shea (24)	12	Ref	CP	6/11 (1)	Median time to tumor progression: 3 months
Oberling (25)	9	Res	Mel	0/0	3−, 4−, 9+, 10−, 10+, 23+, 23+, 32+, 32+ (months)
Herve (25)	2	Ref	Mel	0/2	2−, 3− (months)
Philip (25)	3	Ref 2 Res 1	Mel	1/2	2−, 10−, 32+ (months)
Maraninchi (present study)	26	Ref 14 Res 12	Mel Cy-Mel Cy-VP16-CP	7/13 (4)	Progression-free survival: 50% 3 years after HDC for responders at time of HDC
Total	116	Res 56 Ref 60		26/49 (15)	

[a]Abbreviations: n, number of patients; HDC, high-dose chemotherapy; Res, responder; Ref, refractory; Cy, cyclophosphamide; AI, abdominal irradiation; Mel, melphalan; CP, carboplatin; Mx, mitoxantrone; T, thiotepa; NA, not available.

Table 44.5.   Response and Toxic Death

Total Number of Patients	Toxic Death (%)	Patients Evaluable for Response	CR (%)	PR (%)	Objective Response (%)
116	5 (4)	49	15 (31)	111 (22)	26 (53)

should be tested prospectively in patients with residual tumor after first-line therapy and in some patients with complete response but with poor-prognosis disease at presentation.

REFERENCES

1. Louie KG, Ozols RF, Myers CE, et al. Long-term results of a cisplatin containing combination chemotherapy regimen for the treatment of advanced ovarian carcinoma. J Clin Oncol 1986;4:1579–1585.
2. Schray MF, Martinez A, Howes AE, et al. Advanced epithelial ovarian cancer: salvage whole abdominal irradiation for patients with recurrent or persistent disease after combination chemotherapy. J Clin Oncol 1988;6:1433–1439.
3. Young RC, Hubbard SP, De Vita VT. The chemotherapy of ovarian carcinoma. Cancer Treat Rev 1974;1:99–110.
4. Sutton GP, Blessing JA, Homesley HD, Berman ML, Malfetano J. Phase II trial of ifosfamide and mesna in advanced ovarian carcinoma. A Gynecologic Oncology Group study. J Clin Oncol 1989;7:1672–1676.

cluding debulking surgery and cisplatin-based combination chemotherapy). High-dose chemotherapy and autologous marrow transplant lead to a high response rate (53%) in patients with refractory disease and allows progression-free survival from 30% to 50% at 3 years after high-dose chemotherapy in patients with chemosensitive disease. The impact of high-dose chemotherapy, including at least an alkylating agent and carboplatin, followed by autologous marrow transplant,

5. Hillcoat BL, Campbell JJ, Pepperell R, Quinn MA, Bishop JF, Day A. Phase II trial of VP-16-213 in advanced ovarian carcinoma. Gynecol Oncol 1985; 22:162–166.

6. Ozols RF, Young RC. Chemotherapy of ovarian cancer. Semin Oncol 1984;11:251–263.

7. Ozols RF, Ostchega Y, Myers CE, Young RC. High dose cisplatin in hypertonic saline in refractory ovarian cancer. J Clin Oncol 1985;3:1246–1250.

8. Wiltshaw E, Evans BD, Jones AC, Baker JW, Calvert AH. JM8, successor to cisplatin in advanced ovarian carcinoma? Lancet 1983;1:587.

9. Canetta RM, Carter SK. Developing new drugs for ovarian cancer: a challenging task in a changing reality. Cancer Res Clin Oncol 1984;107:111–124.

10. Thigpen JT, Vance RB, Balducci L, Khansur T. New drugs and experimental approaches in ovarian cancer treatment. Semin Oncol 1984;11:314–326.

11. Ozols RF, Ostchega Y, Curt G, Young RC. High dose carboplatin in refractory ovarian cancer patients. J Clin Oncol 1987;5:197–201.

12. Frei E, Canellos GP. Dose a critical factor in cancer chemotherapy. Am J Med 1980;69:585–594.

13. Griswold DP Jr, Trader MW, Frei E III, et al. Response of drug sensitive and resistant L 1210 leukemias to high dose chemotherapy. Cancer Res 1987;47:2323–2327.

14. Maraninchi D, Abecassis M, Gastaut JA, et al. High dose melphalan with autologous bone marrow rescue for the treatment of advanced adult solid tumors. Cancer Treat Rep 1984;68:471–474.

15. Herve P, Coffe C, Tamayo E, et al. Collection and cryopreservation of bone marrow and clinical applications in therapy of acute leukemia. In: Proceedings of the 2nd International Symposium. Rome: 1977:592–597.

16. Extra JM, Dieras V, Espie M, et al. Intensification therapeutique avec autogreffe médullaire au cours des adénocarcinomes ovariens: étude de phase I–II de 21 sujets. Cahiers Cancer 1989;1:81–84.

17. Mulder POM, Willemse PHB, Aalders JG, et al. High dose chemotherapy with autologous bone marrow transplantation in patients with refractory ovarian cancer. Eur J Cancer Clin Oncol 1989;25:645–649.

18. Mulder POM, Sleijfer DT, Willemse PHB, De Vries EGE, Uges DRA, Mulder NH. High dose cyclophosphamide or melphalan with escalating doses of mitoxantrone and autologous bone marrow transplantation for refractory solid tumors. Cancer Res 1989;49:4654–4658.

19. Dauplat J, Legros M, Condat P, Ferriere JP, Ben Ahmed S, Plagne R. High dose melphalan and autologous bone marrow support for treatment of ovarian carcinoma with positive second-look operation. Gynecol Oncol 1989;34:294–298.

20. Ellis ED, Williams SF, Moormeier JA, Kaminer LS, Bitran JD. A phase I–II study of high dose cyclophosphamide, thiotepa and escalating doses of mitoxantrone with autologous stem cell rescue in patients with refractory malignancies. Bone Marrow Transplant 1990;6:439–442.

21. Lazarus HM, Herzig RH, Graham-Pole J, et al. Intensive melphalan chemotherapy and cryopreserved autologous bone marrow transplantation for the treatment of refractory cancer. J Clin Oncol 1983; 1:359–367.

22. Corringham R, Gilmore M, Prentice HG, Boesen E. High dose melphalan with autologous bone marrow transplant. Treatment of poor prognosis tumors. Cancer 1983;52:1783–1787.

23. Barnett MJ, Swenerton KD, Hoskins PJ, et al. Intensive therapy with carboplatin, etoposide and melphalan (CEM) and autologous stem cell transplantation (SCT) for epithelial ovarian carcinoma (EOA). Proc ASCO 1990;9:168.

24. Shea TC, Flaherty M, Elias A, et al. A phase I clinical and pharmacokinetic study of carboplatin and autologous bone marrow support. J Clin Oncol 1989;7:651–661.

25. Viens P, Maraninchi D, Legros M, et al. High dose melphalan and autologous marrow rescue in advanced epithelial ovarian carcinomas: a retrospective analysis of 35 patients treated in France. Bone Marrow Transplant 1990;5:227–233.

26. Wils J, Blijham G, Naus A, et al. Primary or delayed debulking surgery and chemotherapy consisting of cisplatin, doxorubicin and cyclophosphamide in stage III–IV epithelial ovarian carcinoma. J Clin Oncol 1986;4:1068–1073.

27. Conte PF, Bruzzone M, Chara S, et al. A randomized trial comparing cisplatin plus cyclophosphamide versus cisplatin, doxorubicin and cyclophosphamide in advanced ovarian cancer. J Clin Oncol 1986;4:965–971.

28. Elias A, Ayash LJ, Eder JP, et al. A phase I study of high dose ifosfamide and escalating doses of carboplatin with autologous bone marrow support. J Clin Oncol 1991;9:320–327.

45

MYELOABLATIVE TREATMENT SUPPORTED BY MARROW INFUSIONS FOR CHILDREN WITH NEUROBLASTOMA

John R. Graham-Pole

Neuroblastoma (NBL) is the commonest extracranial cancer of the childhood years, affecting about 10 per million children per year in the United States. Its biologic behavior continues to fascinate the laboratory researcher and frustrate the clinical therapist. While it has the highest spontaneous remission rate of any cancer, two-thirds of children present with widespread disease that often progresses quickly despite treatment.

We have learned a lot about the biology of NBL in the past 10 years. We now recognize the clinical significance of molecular markers, several national screening programs for its early detection have been developed, and many multicenter clinical trials have been completed that have improved the results for children at all clinical stages.

Because these clinical trials have mostly resulted in more responses but only temporary remissions in those with unfavorable forms of NBL, there has been interest for more than a decade in the use of dose-intense marrow-ablative chemoradiotherapy supported by autologous or allogeneic marrow infusions.

This chapter will review the relevant biology of this disease and the rationale and current results of this form of treatment for patients with NBL. Some conclusisons about its current use and what studies are needed for its further evaluation are presented.

BIOLOGY

The outcome for children with NBL depends mostly on age and the distribution of the disease at diagnosis. The definition of prognostic factors is an essential guide to de termining treatment. This is particularly important because most affected children are less than 5 years old at diagnosis (1), and their rapidly growing tissues are especially vulnerable to high-dose cytotoxic treatment.

Several clinicopathologic staging criteria have been used to help define prognosis and guide clinical management. The recently described International NBL Staging System (2), developed by consensus of all major pediatric oncology groups, promises to make it easier to compare clinical and laboratory studies between different centers and cooperative groups throughout the world. It should also form a sound basis for refining staging systems that will increasingly use molecular biology markers of tumor activity. Table 45.1 shows the system adopted for clinicopathologic staging at diagnosis. Relevant to dose-intense treatment for patients with NBL with unfavorable prognosis is the description of stage 4 (metastatic) and stage 3 disease. Stage 3 disease has not been further subclassified because different patterns of spread within

Table 45.1.   International Neuroblastoma Staging System[a]

Stage 1: Localized tumor confined to the area of origin; complete gross excision, with or without microscopic residual disease; identifiable ipsilateral and contralateral lymph nodes negative microscopically.

Stage 2A: Unilateral tumor with incomplete gross excision; identifiable ipsilateral and contralateral lymph nodes negative microscopically.

Stage 2B: Unilateral tumor with complete or incomplete gross excision; with positive ipsilateral regional lymph nodes; identifiable contralateral lymph nodes negative microscopically.

Stage 3: Tumor infiltrating across the midline with or without regional lymph node involvement; or, unilateral tumor with contralateral regional lymph node involvement; or, midline tumor with bilateral regional lymph node involvement.

Stage 4: Dissemination of tumor to distant lymph nodes, bone, bone marrow, liver, and/or other organs (except as defined in stage 4S).

Stage 4S: Localized primary tumor as defined for stage 1 or 2 with dissemination limited to liver, skin, and/or bone marrow.

[a]From Brodeur G, Seeger RC, Barrett A, et al. International criteria for diagnosis, staging, and response to treatment in patients with neuroblastoma. J Clin Oncol 1988;6:1874.

this category were not thought to have prognostic significance. So far dose-intense chemoradiotherapy supported by marrow infusion has been mostly reserved for patients with stage 4 disease. A recent publication from the Children's Cancer Study Group (3) using the same criteria as above for defining stage 3 disease showed such patients had a 5-year survival of 44%, so marrow-ablative chemotherapy may be appropriate for stage 3 patients. Those with disease confined to one side of the midline, which in earlier classifications would have been called stage 3 disease, had a much better prognosis than those with bilateral disease, so it is probably only indicated for the latter.

Brodeur et al. also reached a consensus on defining response to treatment (Table 45.2) (2), which had not been included in previous staging systems. They recommended adhering closely to tests used previously for defining clinicopathologic stage at diagnosis. They emphasized the need for thoroughly assessing both primary and metastatic sites to give an overall evaluation and unifying the timing of evaluations across studies (e.g., before induction, before and after surgery, before and after myeloablative therapy). The knotty problem of quantitating the extent of marrow involvement was also recognized, as well as the increasing value of serial measurement of tumor markers in body tissues, including urinary catecholamine metabolites, serum ferritin, ganglioside GD_2, and nonspecific enolase (NSE) (4–7).

These clinicopathologic criteria should allow us to evaluate new diagnostic and prognostic tools that will refine staging in the future. New markers measurable within NBL cells are already helping define the best treatment for these children, including immunophenotyping, N-myc gene expression and copy number, and DNA index (8–10). For example, N-myc copy number in NBL cells seems to be a prognostic factor independent of clinicopathologic stage (11). Patients with multiple N-myc copies have a poor prognosis and probably need more dose-intense treatment to have a chance of being cured. The amount of tumor cell DNA also predicts outcome in infants, who as a group do much better than older children (12, 13). A recent multivariate analysis of clinical and biologic predictors of outcome in a group of 59 unselected patients showed that only N-myc amplification and DNA index were independent predictors of relapse (Table 45.3) (14).

The presence of high RNA levels of the MDR1 gene, which encodes a multidrug transporter responsible for drug efflux from the cells, has also been reported recently to be associated with poorer responses to treatment (15). The level of MDR1 gene expression in RNA did not correlate closely with N-myc expression in these patients, so these two may be independent factors. MDR1 gene expression sometimes increases soon after induction treatment (16), suggesting rapid acquisition of drug resistance by NBL cells. These molecular markers therefore seem to

Table 45.2.   Definition of Response to Treatment[a,b,c]

Response	Primary	Metastases	Markers
1. CR	No tumor	No tumor (chest, abdomen, liver, bone, bone marrow, nodes, etc)	HVA/VMA normal
2. VGPR	Reduction >90% but <100%	No tumor (as above except bone); no new bone lesions, all preexisting lesions improved	HVA/VMA decreased >90%
3. PR	Reduction 50%–90%	No new lesions; 50%–90% reduction in measurable sites; 0 to 1 bone marrow samples with tumor; bone lesions same as VGPR	HVA/VMA decreased 50% to 90%
4. MR	No new lesions; >50% reduction of any measurable lesion (primary or metastases) with <50% reduction in any other; <25% increase in any existing lesion[d]		
5. NR	No new lesions; <50% reduction but <25% increase in any existing lesion[d]		
6. PD	Any new lesion; increase of any measurable lesion by >25%; previous negative marrow positive for tumor		

[a]From Brodeur G, Seeger RC, Barrett A, et al. International criteria for diagnosis, staging, and response to treatment in patients with neuroblastoma. J Clin Oncol 1988;6:1874.
[b]Note: Evaluations of primary and metastatic disease as outlined.
[c]Abbreviations: HVA, homovanillic acid; MR, mixed response; PD, progressive disease; VGPR, very good partial response; VMA, vanillylmandelic acid.
[d]Quantitative assessment does not apply to marrow disease.

have significance independent of the clinicopathologic stage and patient age. The study of N-myc amplification, MDR1 gene expression, and DNA index is therefore relevant to selecting treatment for children with NBL.

REVIEW OF RECENT TREATMENT

Treatment of children with widespread NBL remains a distressing experience for patients and pediatric oncologists alike. Relapse after initial response is still the rule despite the availability of many treatment options.

Early clinical trials of chemotherapy regimens including vincristine, doxorubicin, and cyclophosphamide produced responses in children with stage 4 disease but almost no survivors beyond 2 years (17, 18). The sequential use of cyclophosphamide and doxorubicin based on kinetic studies indicating recruitment of resting cells into cycle (18) produced a higher number of clinical responses, and some were maintained longer than previously achieved without changing survival. The introduction of teniposide and cisplatin (19, 20) and recent use of high initial doses of cisplatin (21), etoposide (22), carboplatin (23), and ifosfamide (24) have

resulted in complete or partial responses in about three-quarters of the children over 1 year of age with newly diagnosed stage 4 NBL. We do not yet know if current clinical trials in North America and Europe will show that these more frequent and complete responses will translate into indefinite remissions.

Dose-dependent effects have been shown for several drugs in patients with NBL (21, 25). These dose escalations may be facilitated by the availability of hematopoietic growth factors that enhance recovery from marrow suppression. This may allow more rapid drug delivery and minimize intervals between courses (26, 27) and may decrease the likelihood of drug-resistant cancer cell clones emerging. Whether such drug resistance can be overcome by using agents that block MDR expression is the subject of current studies (28).

In addition to the development of new chemotherapy regimens, there has been a focus on the best way to manage the primary tumor. Relapses are often in sites of initial disease, suggesting failure to eradicate bulk tumor masses. Most clinical trials include an attempt at postinduction surgery to try to resect residual disease, but a controlled study

Table 45.3. Relationship between Clinical and Biologic Factors and Relative Risk of Relapse[a]

	No.	RR1[b]	RR2
Age (yr)			
<1	23	1[c]	
≥1	36	6.3 (.01)[d]	(NS)
Stage (Evans)			
I, II, IV-S	17	1[c]	
III	10	5.3 (.14)	
IV	32	10.4 (.02)	(NS)
N-myc (copy number)			
<3	50	1[c]	1[c]
≥3	9	7.7 (<.001)	3.1 (.02)
Ploidy index			
Near-triploid	28	1[c]	1[c]
Diploid or			
near-diploid[e]	31	9.09 (<.001)	9.1 (.01)

[a]From Bourhis J, DeVathaire F, Wilson GD, et al. Combined analysis of DNA ploidy index and N-myc genomic content in neuroblastoma. Cancer Res 1991;51:33–36.
[b]RR1, relative risk of relapse in univariate analysis; RR2, relative risk of relapse taking into account for the factors of the table previously selected by a stepwise procedure (with enter and remove limits of $P = .1$ and .15, respectively); NS, not significant.
[c]Reference category.
[d]Numbers in parentheses, probability.
[e]This group also included 1 hypotetraploid neuroblastoma.

of this approach has not been possible (29). NBL is a very radiosensitive cancer, suggesting the value of using radiation therapy to residual disease sites (30, 31), but this treatment has also not been subject to prospective controlled trials. There has been much interest in the use of targeted radioisotope therapy, notably iodine-131 monoiodobenzylguanidine (^{131}I-mIBG), based on the specific uptake of mIBG by neuroectodermal cells (32). Though designed as tumor specific, this treatment produces generalized effects, particularly myelosuppression, as well as being labor intensive and needing special facilities.

A fourth treatment modality being used to treat children with metastatic NBL is that of biologic response modifiers and other nonchemotherapeutic agents. These include interleukin-2 (33), *cis*-retinoic acid (34), desferoxamine (35), and immunotoxins (36, 37). The latter consists of NBL-directed monoclonal antibodies convalently linked to a toxin able to kill cancer cells.

This wide variety of treatment reflects tremendous ingenuity in the clinical application of our better understanding of the biology of NBL. Given the rarity of this cancer, it also raises the major problem of comparing these different approaches with each other. With this background the current status of myeloablative chemoradiotherapy supported by autologous or allogeneic bone marrow infusions will be reviewed, with an assessment of its current place as an alternative or adjuvant to other forms of treatment.

DOSE-INTENSE TREATMENT WITH MARROW INFUSIONS

Rationale

Because of the low cure rate achieved with the conventional treatments described above, several centers have explored over more than a decade the use of dose-intense chemoradiotherapy supported by either autologous or allogeneic marrow infusions (38–45). This cancer meets generally accepted criteria for considering autotransplant. First, it is sensitive to both radiation and classes of chemotherapy that have as their dose-limiting toxicity myelosuppression. Second, a dose-response effect has been shown between NBL and several drugs and radiation. Third, clinical remissions can usually be achieved with induction regimens during which marrow, overtly free or rendered free in vitro of cancer cells, can be harvested and frozen for later reinfusion.

NBL shows a steep dose-response curve to chemotherapy, particularly alkylating agents, both in experimental systems and clinically (25, 46, 47). It is also highly radiosensitive, making the use of both local and systemic irradiation (total body irradiation, TBI) a rational approach (30, 31, 38). A dose-response effect has been shown for TBI in an experimental myeloid leukemia model, in which a further log of cancer cells can be killed by increasing the TBI dose 37% (49). A similar dose-effect of TBI has been suggested though not conclusively proved in clinical studies of children with NBL (50). In vitro studies using NBL cell lines have shown the efficacy of escalating doses of radiation therapy (51). Escalation is limited primarily by myelosuppression.

Children differ from adults as candidates for myeloablative therapy. Severity of acute toxicity tends to correlate with age; early death from complications affects about 10% of children but about twice the percentage of adults. Long-term toxicity, on the other hand, is potentially worse in children, particulary after TBI, which severely limits growth and development. Suppression of pituitary, thyroid, and gonadal function is common and often requires long-term hormone replacement, which is not always effective. Dental development is also commonly arrested in young children, and another concern is carcinogenesis. A secondary cancer was seen in 35 (1.6%) of 2246 marrow transplant recipients followed at the Fred Hutchinson Cancer Center, occurring 1.5 months–14 years after treatment (52). In planning high-dose regimens the extent of damage to young and rapidly developing normal tissues must be carefully weighed. Finally, childhood cancers are rare compared with adult cancers, and the use of many different therapeutic approaches makes carefully planned multicenter clinical trials a necessity.

History

The first report of high-dose chemotherapy with autologous marrow infusions for children with advanced NBL used melphalan (L-phenylalanine mustard) alone (38). A more rapid hematologic recovery had previously been achieved when melphalan was given to adults with myeloma in a dose of 180 mg/m^2 supported by marrow infusions, compared with those given 140 mg/m^2 without marrow (54). Melphalan was chosen for NBL because of its efficacy in adult cancers, its steep dose-response curve, the possibility that its chemical structure would cause it to block ty-

rosine metabolism within NBL cells, and its dose-limiting toxicity, which is myelosuppression. The use of melphalan in a dose of 180 mg/m^2 seemed tolerable as consolidation treatment in these children. Their median survival was about 2 years, but most then relapsed in sites of previous disease.

A French pilot study published soon after used the same single-drug regimen and reported longer remissions in several patients (41). Alternative and additional drugs were then tested in dose-intense regimens, including peptichemio, bulsulfan, cyclophosphamide, cisplatin, teniposide (VM26), etoposide (VP16), and doxorubicin. A more aggressive approach to residual cancer was also adopted, including extensive surgery and local irradiation as well as TBI.

Figure 45.1 shows the worldwide escalation in the number of autotransplants for NBL over the past decade, which now number about 750. Several multicenter clinical trials have been conducted. The French group based in Lyon treated 56 unselected children with advanced NBL with a new induction regimen followed by dose-intense consolidation for the 37 who achieved clinical remission (44). They used melphalan as a 180 mg/m^2 bolus and vincristine as a 4 mg/m^2 infusion, to which they added fractionated TBI in a total dose of 12 Gy . The latter had been previously piloted mostly in children with recurrent NBL at the Children's Hospital of Philadelphia, with promising results (39). In vitro marrow purging was also adopted, using monoclonal antibodies specific for NBL cells linked with paramagnetic microspheres. This was based on preliminary work with this immunomagnetic purging technique reported from London and Oslo (54), which had seemed to be efficacious in vitro and safe in vivo.

The French group in Lyon reported a significantly better relapse-free survival probability than in their previously treated patients not given such dose-intense treatment. They also found that patients in more complete remission when they received this

Figure 45.1. Escalating use of high-dose therapy and marrow infusions in children with advanced NBL. (From Graham-Pole J. Autologous marrow transplants in pediatric tumors. In: Champlin RE, Gale RP, eds. New strategies in bone marrow transplantation. New York: Wiley-Liss, Inc., 1991:413–422. Copyright © Wiley-Liss, 1991.)

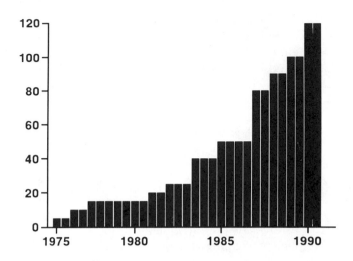

treatment remained well longer. They noted that the immunomagnetic purging technique did not seem to slow hematologic recovery, though seven (19%) of the 37 died of toxicity (44). Late follow-up by the French group has shown that their patients have continued to relapse up to 7 years after completing treatment, with a current plateau at about 20% relapse-free survival (55).

Recent and Current Studies

There have been recent reports of this treatment from the North American Children's Cancer Study Group (CCSG; 56) and Pediatric Oncology Group (POG; 50), and also from France, Italy, Britain, and Japan (21, 42, 45, 55, 57, 60–63). Almost all have been single-arm pilot studies and have explored high-dose consolidation regimens based mostly on melphalan or another alkylating agent together with TBI and sometimes additional drugs. Most have included in vitro immunomagnetic marrow purging (54, 58). Not all these investigators have seen late relapses beyond 2 years after completing treatment.

The CCSG has recently reported results of myeloablation with autologous marrow infusions in 101 children, using first teniposide, doxorubicin, melphalan, and cisplatin

and later etoposide, melphalan, and cisplatin, both with TBI (56). Close to 50% have relapsed. The projected survival is 40% at 39 months median for the first group and 51% at 10 months median for the latter group. No individual prognostic factor for outcome was identified, but relapse was noted to be commonest at sites involved at diagnosis, supporting other evidence of inadequate eradication of bulk disease.

In the POG study (50) 56 of the 100 subjects have relapsed, 14 have died of complications, and 30 remain in remission, all more than 2 years since completing treatment. With a median follow-up for the survivors of 42 (range 29–80) months, there has so far been no relapse beyond 2 years. This study confirmed that patients receiving high-dose treatment in first remission have a significantly better outcome than those treated after a relapse (Fig. 45.2). The relapse-free survival probability by Kaplan-Meier analysis for the 65 in first remission is currently 37% compared with 13% for the 35 who had had prior relapses ($p < .001$). There was also a suggestion that the timing of high-dose chemoradiotherapy was important, those treated after a longer prior remission having a significantly better outcome. Half the children receiving myeloablation more than 9 months

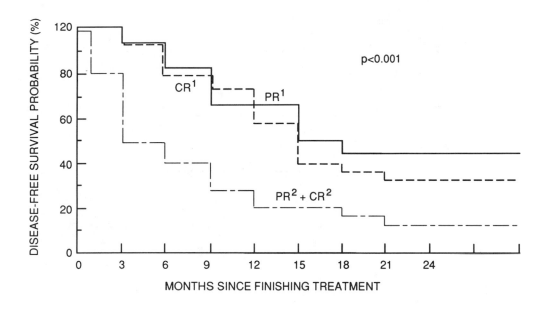

CR¹   =1st complete remission
PR¹   =1st partial remission
CR² or PR² =2nd complete or partial remission

100 patients receiving myeloablative chemoradiotherapy plus marrow infusions for metastatic
neuroblastoma (minimum follow-up 28 months; updated to 5/1/91)

Figure 45.2.   Probability of disease free survival according to remission status at time of autotransplant in 100 children with NBL (update of POG 8340).

after diagnosis remain alive and well, compared with only a quarter of those treated less than 9 months after diagnosis. This could be due to selection, in that those who received this treatment later may as a group have had a slower disease pace or remained chemoresponsive for longer. It is also possible that prolonging the premyeloablative induction achieved a lower tumor burden, thus improving the efficacy of the end-intensification.

The POG study also suggested that the radiosensitivity of NBL can be exploited in high-dose regimens. By univariate analysis, significantly more patients receiving a higher TBI dose (12 Gy) remain relapse-free (34%) than those receiving a lower dose (9 Gy; 17% relapse-free). Also, those patients who received extra irradiation to residual disease sites

had a better relapse-free survival probability than those not given such irradiation boosts. Figure 45.3 shows an updated analysis of the effect of using local irradiation boosts in patients entered on POG 8340 in first remission who received local irradiation before myeloablative treatment. This is of particular interest because those chosen to receive such boosts were mostly in partial rather than complete remission after induction. These observations are supported by other reports of the value of local irradiation in improving primary disease control and outcome in stage 3 (59) and stage 4 (48) NBL.

Another recent pilot study in Japan in which 21 children were given high-dose chemotherapy with or without TBI in first remission has resulted in a 78% 2-year survival. This promising result was attributed to the

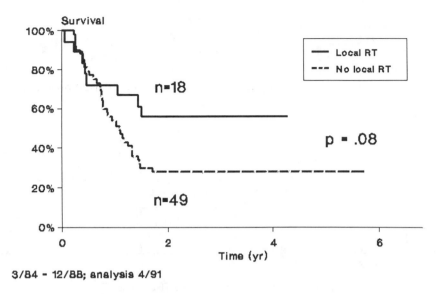

3/84 - 12/88; analysis 4/91

Figure 45.3.   Effect of including local irradiation boosts in children receiving high-dose treatment for NBL (up-date of POG 8340). (Data and figure courtesy of Robert Marcus, Jr., M.D.)

intensive induction that preceded the mye-loablation (57). Thus there appears to be a trend for recent studies using better induction regimens to show improvement over earlier trials of myeloablative consolidation.

The use of dose-intense treatment seems generally tolerable by children, at least in the short term, but relapses are still frequent. This had led to recent trials of repeated courses of myeloablative therapy. Hartmann et al. treated 33 children with metastatic NBL after prolonged induction (6–10 courses of chemotherapy) with a consolidation of either one (n = 33) or two (n = 16) courses of melphalan (180 mg/m^2) together with tenipo-side 1 gm/m^2 and carmustine (BCNU) 300 mg/m^2 (42). After a median follow-up of 28 months, 16 patients are alive and free of relapse. Although the second course seems to have been tolerated as well as the first, there is no evidence yet of an advantage to two courses. A French group is conducting a randomized study of double versus single courses of myeloablative treatment, but there is as yet no advantage of one over the other in terms of disease-free survival (60).

The European Neuroblastoma Study Group has recently completed the only randomized trial so far of myeloablative chemotherapy and marrow infusions versus conventional treatment in chilren with stage 3 and 4 NBL (61). One hundred and forty children aged at least 6 months received a common induction and surgical debulking. Ninety-five (68%) achieved clinical remissions, of whom 65 were randomized to receive either melphalan 140 mg/m^2 and autologous unpurged marrow or no further treatment. On initial analysis, significantly more children treated with melphalan remained relapse-free than those treated conventionally ($p = .03$, log rank analysis). On longer follow-up this difference has been maintained, but it is no longer significant (62).

Table 45.4 summarizes recent results of myeloablative treatment with marrow infusions in over 400 children with advanced NBL in first remission using different regimens, most including melphalan and TBI. About a third of these children are clinically free of disease 3–4 years after autograft, but late relapses are being reported. Only one of these

Table 45.4. Recent Results of Myeloablative Treatment With Marrow Infusions in Children with NBL in First Remission

Group/Series	Patients	Disease-Free (Actual or Estimated)	Comments (Regimen, Use of Purging)
CCSG (56)	46	40% at 4 years	VM26-Doxo-Mel-CPDD(VAMP)-TBI; purged
European (ENSG) (62)	32	34% at 6 years	Melphalan, no TBI; unpurged
Italian (AIEOP) (45)	53	29% at 5 years	VAMP-TBI; unpurged; similar result to maintenance
Japanese (57)	21	63% at 4 years	Various regimens, stage 3 and 4 patients; ? purged
LMCE (44)	62	39% at 2 years	VCR-Mel-TBI; purged
		20% at 5 years	
LMCE (60)	17	50% at 2 years	2 courses of myeloablation; purged
French multicenter (42)	33	40% at 2 years	Mel-VM26-BCNU, no TBI; 18 received 2 courses; purged
Philadelphia (40)	41	27% at 4 years	VAM or VAMP, TBI; unpurged
POG (50)	54	37% at 3 years	Mel-TBI; purged
Worldwide (66)	125	30% at 3 years	Allogeneic; various regimens

studies was a randomized comparison with nonmyeloablative treatment.

Several comparative clinical trials are underway or planned in North America. The POG has been conducting a prospective study for the past 2 years. It compares the use of high-dose melphalan and TBI supported by purged marrow infusions with less intensive maintenance treatment in children with stage 4 NBL over 1 year old. All patients receive the same induction. Those who achieve a clinical remission and are treated at an institution with a marrow transplant facility are assigned to the high-dose arm, whether or not they actually receive high-dose therapy. They are being compared statistically for relapse-free survival with patients achieving a remission with induction therapy at institutions not using marrow infusions. The latter are automatically assigned to continue on maintenance and cannot by design of the trial be referred elsewhere for autotransplant.

The CCSG has just opened a more ambitious randomized clinical trial for all children with NBL at high risk of relapse (63). This includes patients with stage 4 disease over 1 year of age, infants and older children with stage 3 disease whose tumors have multiple copies of N-myc or unfavorable histology, and children with high serum ferritin at diagnosis. They receive a common multidrug in-

duction treatment, followed by randomization to either continue maintenance treatment or to receive autotransplant with a combination of melphalan, etoposide, carboplatin, and TBI supported by purged autologous marrow infusions. All patients are being transferred to one facility for marrow harvest and immunomagnetic purging, and then receive their myeloablation at designated CCSG centers.

The next POG group-wide phase 3 trial will examine the question raised by the earlier pilot study about the timing of myeloablative treatment. All children with metastatic NBL will receive a common induction using the best induction arm of the current study. Those achieving complete or partial remissions will be randomized to an intensive consolidation regimen including ifosfamide, etoposide, and high-dose cisplatin for either a short or a long course. They will then receive myeloablative chemoradiotherapy with purged autologous marrow infusions either at about 24 weeks (early) or about 40 weeks (late). All patients will therefore be receiving autotransplants. The question addressed is whether a longer period of consolidation and delay of dose-intense treatment, potentially reducing the tumor burden, offers an advantage over shorter consolidation, with earlier intensive therapy, potentially preventing the early acquisition of multiple-drug resistance in residual NBL cells.

Controversies and Questions

There are several unresolved questions about the place of dose-intense myeloablative treatment supported by marrow infusions in the treatment of children with advanced NBL.

DOES IT CURE MORE PATIENTS THAN CONVENTIONAL-DOSE TREATMENT?

This question remains unresolved. Almost all therapeutic trials so far have been uncontrolled, although several studies contained enough patients to indicate an impact of this treatment on survival duration. Some studies have suggested that remaining well for 2–3 years off treatment is equated with an indefinite survival, while others have reported a continuing albeit lower risk of relapse as late as 10 years after treatment. This issue should be resolved in the next several years both by prospective trials and by retrospective analysis of patients reported to the bone marrow transplant registries. Recent expansion of the International Bone Marrow Transplant Registry to include patients receiving autologous as well as allogeneic marrow infusions should allow enough patients with NBL to be studied to resolve these questions.

WHO SHOULD RECEIVE THIS TREATMENT?

In the absence of proof of superior efficacy, it is possible to select patients at higher risk of disease progression who might benefit most from high-dose treatment. These include children with metastatic NBL (excluding infants, who have a significantly better outcome with less dose-intense chemotherapy). Those who have unfavorable prognostic indicators on the basis of molecular biology studies (multiple N-myc copies, high RNA MDR1 gene expression, unfavorable histol-

ogy) may also be good candidates regardless of stage and age. Patients who have relapsed, particularly early or during first-line treatment, have rarely done well even with subsequent myeloablative treatment. They might still be candidates for phase 1 and 2 studies of new drug/radiation combination.

IS AUTOLOGOUS OR ALLOGENEIC MARROW MORE SUITABLE FOR ACHIEVING HEMATOLOGIC RECOVERY?

There are theoretical advantages for using allogeneic rather than autologous marrow to support patients given dose-intense treatment. Studies in leukemia have shown a clear-cut graft-versus-leukemia effect that may augment chemoradiotherapy in improving disease control (64). There have also been reports of prolonged delays in hematologic recovery after autologous marrow infusions (65). Figure 45.4 shows the hematologic recovery time of 123 children undergoing high-dose therapy and autologous marrow reinfusions. Recovery, particularly of platelets, was delayed in almost 20%. Delayed reengraftment was significantly related to the amount of chemotherapy received before marrow harvest and the sex of the patient, although there was no apparent adverse effect of the purging procedure.

The problem is that histocompatible sibling donors can be found for only about 20% of these young children. The percentage may be decreasing with the trend to smaller family size. Also, no clear benefit has emerged from the use of allogeneic rather than autologous marrow for support. A retrospective survey of the use of allogeneic marrow infusions in children with NBL collected data on 125 such patients (66). There was no apparent advantage when compared with data from all patients with NBL reported to the Autologous Bone Marrow Transplant Registry who received autologous marrow. Relapses occurred with equal frequency, and fatal toxicity was commoner in the allografted patients.

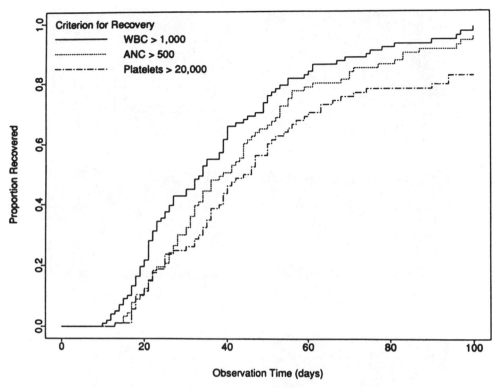

Figure 45.4. Analysis of hematologic recovery (white blood cell count >1000, absolute neutrophil count >500, platelets >20,000/mm³) in 123 patients with metastatic neuroblastoma undergoing high-dose treatment and autologous marrow reinfusions. (From Graham-Pole J, et al. Myeloablative chemoradiotherapy and autologous bone marrow infusions for treatment of neuroblastoma: factors influencing engraftment. Blood 1991;78:1607–1614.)

IS MARROW PURGING NEEDED?

Although in vitro purging is widely used, there is no proof it is beneficial. Relapses following autologous marrow infusions in children with NBL are mostly thought to be due to failure to eradicate persisting disease in vivo. Marrow-purging methods, of which the immunomagnetic technology has been most widely adopted, seem to be highly effective in vitro and safe clinically. A recent report shows that cells removed from the marrow at the time of purging almost always contain enough clonogenic cells to establish new NBL cell lines, even though the marrow was in most cases morphologically free of tumor (67). Figure 45.5 shows several such cell lines, which have been characterized as NBL by oncogene and cytogenetic analysis. A preliminary study of the purged material collected after in vitro immunomagnetic purging in 17 children with NBL revealed clonogenic cells (median number 12.5 × 10⁶ NBL cells) in all 17 cases. Because relapses are still common in children with NBL and we still need to establish whether dose is an important variable in the treatment of NBL, there is a case for optimizing conditions by including in vitro purging. If and when we can reduce relapse frequency, a prospective trial comparing purging with no purging may be appropriate. Alternatively, retrospective analysis of registry data from centers who either do or do not use purging may resolve this issue.

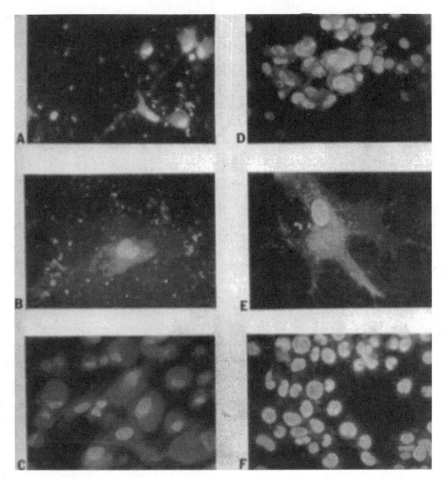

Figure 45.5. Cell lines established from the purged material obtained from marrow harvests of six children with metastatic NBL. All have been characterized as being NBL cell lines. (Figure courtesy of Yair Gazitt, Ph.D.)

CONCLUSIONS

Approximately 750 children with advanced NBL have received myeloablative chemoradiotherapy over the past 12 years. About a quarter of them are apparently living happy and healthy lives 2–10 years later. This figure has probably improved in recent years with better patient selection and better specific and supportive treatment. Despite the lack of randomized clinical trials, these results seem better than those achieved with other available forms of treatment.

It is helpful to remember that dose-intensive treatment is not given in isolation. That the drug-dose tumor response relationships seen in vitro in NBL are relevant clinically has generally been upheld. However, improved results from high-dose treatment will probably come not from even more dose-intense myeloablative regimens but from improvements in other aspects of treatment. Examples include more extensive knowledge of this cancer's biology, allowing us to develop more selective treatment; improved initial induction regimens, allowing a higher percentage of more complete initial remissions; refining our use of surgery and radiation therapy to eradicate bulky disease sites that may receive inadequate doses of chemotherapy; and the use of biologic response modifiers as adjuvants to other forms of treatment.

REFERENCES

1. Gross RE, Farber S, Martin LW. American Academy of Pediatrics Proceedings Neuroblastoma Sympatheticum: a study and report of 217 cases. Pediatrics 1959;23:1179–1191.
2. Brodeur GM, Seeger RC, Barrett A, et al. International criteria for diagnosis, staging, and response to treatment in patients with neuroblastoma. J Clin Oncol 1988;6:1874–1881.
3. Evans AE, D'Angio GJ, Sather HN, et al. A comparison of four staging systems for localized and regional neuroblastoma: a report from the Children's Cancer Study Group. J Clin Oncol 1990;8:678–688.
4. Hann HWL, Evans AE, Cohen IJ, et al. Biologic differences between neuroblastoma stage IVS and IV, measurement of serum ferritin and E-rosette inhibition in 30 children. N Engl J Med 1981;305:425–429.
5. Evans AE, D'Angio GJ, Propert K, Anderson J, Hann H-WL. Prognostic factors in neuroblastoma. Cancer 1987;59:1853–1859.
6. Moss TJ, Seeger RC, Kindler-Rohrborn A, et al. Immunohistologic detection and phenotyping of neuroblastoma cells in bone marrow using cytoplasmic neuron-specific enolase and cell surface antigens. Prog Clin Biol Res 1985;175:367–378.
7. Philip T, Helson L, Bernard J-L, et al. Definition of response and remission in children over 1 year of age with advanced neuroblastoma: proposition for a scoring system. Pediatr Hematol Oncol 1987;4:25–31.
8. Shimada H, Chatten J, Newton WA Jr, et al. Histopathologic prognostic factors in neuroblastic tumors: definition of subtypes of ganglioneuroblastoma and an age-linked classification of neuroblastomas. J Natl Cancer Inst 1984;73:405–416.
9. Donner K, Triche TJ, Israel MA, et al. A panel of monoclonal antibodies which discriminate neuroblastoma from Ewings' sarcoma, rhabdomyosarcoma, neuroepithelioma, and hematopoietic malignancies. Prog Clin Biol Res 1985;175:367–378.
10. Brodeur GM, Seeger RC, Schwab M, et al. Amplification of N-myc in untreated human neuroblastomas correlates with advanced disease stage. Science 1984;224:1121–1124.
11. Seeger RC, Brodeur GM, Sather H, et al. Association of multiple copies of the N-myc oncogene with rapid progression of neuroblastomas. N Engl J Med 1985;312:1111–1116.
12. Look AT, Hayes FA, Nitschke R, et al. Cellular DNA content as a predictor of response to chemotherapy in infants with unresectable neuroblastoma. N Engl J Med 1984;311:231–235.
13. Oppedal B, Strom-Mathisen I, Lie S, Brandtzaeg P. Prognostic factors in neuroblastoma. Cancer 1988; 62:772–780.
14. Bourhis J, DeVathaire F, Wilson GD, et al. Combined analysis of DNA ploidy index and N-myc genomic content in neuroblastoma. Cancer Res 1991;51:33–36.
15. Goldstein LJ, Fojo AT, Ueda K, et al. Expression of the multidrug resistance, MDR1, gene in neuroblastomas. J Clin Oncol 1990;8:128–136.
16. Bourhis J, Benard J, Hartmann O, et al. Expression of a human multidrug resistance gene, MDR1, correlates with chemotherapy in neuroblastoma. J Natl Cancer Inst 1989;81:1401–1405.
17. Finkelstein J, Klemperer M, Evans A, et al. Multiagent chemotherapy for children with metastatic neuroblastoma; a report from Children's Cancer Study Group. Med Pediatr Oncol 1979;6:179–188.
18. Green AA, Hayes FA, Hustu HO. Sequential cyclophosphamide and doxorubicin for induction of complete remissions in children with disseminated neuroblastoma. Cancer 1981;48:2310–2317.
19. Hayes FA, Green AA, Casper J, et al. Clinical evaluation of sequentially scheduled cisplatin and VM26 in neuroblastoma; response and toxicity. Cancer 1981;48:1715–1718.
20. Shafford EA, Rogers DW, Pritchard J. Advanced neuroblastoma: improved response rate using a multiagent regimen (OPEC) including sequential cisplatin and VM-26. J Clin Oncol 1984;2:742–747.
21. Pinkerton CR. Where next with therapy in advanced neuroblastoma? Br J Cancer 1990;61:351–353.
22. Philip T, Ghalie R, Pinkerton R, et al. A phase II study of high-dose cisplatin and VP-16 in neuroblastoma: a report from the Societe Francaise d'Oncologie Pediatrique. J Clin Oncol 1987;5:941–950.
23. Pinkerton CR, Lewis IJ, Pearson ADJ, Stevens MC, Barnes J. Carboplatin or cisplatin? Lancet 1989;2:161.
24. Kellie SJ, DeKraker J, Lilleyman JS, Bowman A, Pritchard J. Ifosfamide in previously untreated neuroblastoma. Eur J Cancer Clin Oncol 1988;24:903–908.
25. Kushner BH, Helson L. Coordinated use of sequentially escalated cyclophosphamide and cell-cycle-specific chemotherapy (N4SE protocol) for advanced neuroblastoma: experience with 100 patients. J Clin Oncol 1987;5:1746–1751.
26. Pearson ADJ, Craft AW. Ultra high dose induction regime for disseminated neuroblastoma—'Napoleon'. Med Pediatr Oncol 1988;16:414.
27. Pinkerton CR, Zucker JM, Hartmann O, et al. Short duration, high dose, alternating chemotherapy in metastatic neuroblastoma (ENSG 3C induction regimen). Br J Cancer 1990;62:319–323.
28. Hartmann O, Boccon-Gibod L, Lemerle J, et al. High levels of human MDR1 gene transcripts are related

to previous chemotherapy in neuroblastoma. Proc ASCO 1989;8:298.

29. LeTourneau JN, Bernard JL, Hendren WH, Carcassone M. Evaluation of the role of surgery in 130 patients with neuroblastoma. J Pediatr Surg 1985;20:244–249.

30. Rosen EM, Cassady JR, Frantz CN, et al. Neuroblastoma: the Joint Center for Radiation Therapy/Dana-Farber Cancer Institute/Children's Hospital experience. J Clin Oncol 1984;2:719–732.

31. Jacobson HM, Marcus RB, Thar TR, et al. Pediatric neuroblastoma: postoperative radiation therapy using less than 2,000 rad. Int J Radiat Oncol 1983;9:501–505.

32. Mastrangelo R, Troncone L, Lasorella A, Riccardi R, Montemaggi P, Ruffini V. ^{131}I-metaiodobenzylguanidine in the treatment of neuroblastoma at diagnosis. Am J Pediatr Hematol Oncol 1989;11:28–31.

33. Favrot MC, Floret D, Negrier S, et al. Systemic interleukin-2 therapy in children with progressive neuroblastoma after high dose chemotherapy and bone marrow transplantation. Bone Marrow Transplant 1989;4:499–503.

34. Thiele CJ, Reynolds CP, Israel MA. Decreased expression of N-myc precedes retinoic acid-induced morphological differentiation of human neuroblastoma. Nature 1985;313:404–406.

35. Donfrancesco A, Deb G, Dominici C, Pileggi D, Castello MA, Helson L. Effects of a single course of deferoxamine in neuroblastoma patients. Cancer Res 1990;50:4929–4930.

36. Kemshead JT, Coakham HB, Lashford LS. Clinical experience of iodine-131 monoclonal antibodies in treating neural tumours. Front Radiat Ther Oncol 1990;24:166–181.

37. Cassano WF, Zaytoun AM. Specific killing of neuroblastoma cells *in vitro* by immunotoxins. In: Gross S, ed. Bone marrow purging and processing. New York: Alan R. Liss, 1990:217–223.

38. Pritchard J, McElwain TJ, Graham-Pole J. High-dose melphalan with autologous marrow for treatment of advanced neuroblastoma. Br J Cancer 1982;45:86–94.

39. August CS, Serota FT, Koch PA, et al. Treatment of advanced neuroblastoma with supralethal chemotherapy, radiation, and allogeneic or autologous marrow reconsititution. J Clin Oncol 1984;2:609–616.

40. Graham-Pole J, Lazarus HM, Herzig RH, et al. High-dose melphalan therapy for the treatment of children with refractory neuroblastoma and Ewing's sarcoma. Am J Ped Hematol Oncol 1984;6:17–26.

41. Hartmann O, Kalifa C, Benhamou E, et al. Treatment of advanced neuroblastoma with high-dose melphalan and autologous bone marrow transplantation. Cancer Chemother Pharmacol 1986;16:165–169.

42. Hartmann O, Benhamou E, Beaujean F, et al. Repeated high-dose chemotherapy followed by purged autologous bone marrow transplantation as consolidation therapy in metastatic neuroblastoma. J Clin Oncol 1987;5:1205–1211.

43. Seeger RC, Moss TJ, Feig SA, et al. Bone marrow transplantation for poor prognosis neuroblastoma. In: Evans AE, D'Angio GJ, Knudsen AG, et al, eds. Advances in neuroblastoma research. New York: Alan R. Liss, 1988:203–213.

44. Philip T, Bernard JL, Zucker JM, et al. High-dose chemoradiotherapy with bone marrow transplantation as consolidation treatment in neuroblastoma: an unselected group of stage IV patients over 1 year of age. J Clin Oncol 1987;5:266–271.

45. Dini G, Lanino E, Garaventa A, et al. Unpurged ABMT for neuroblastoma: the AIEOP-BMT experience. Bone Marrow Transplant 1991;7(suppl 3):109–111.

46. Worthington-White DA, Graham-Pole JR, Stout SA, Riley CM. In vitro studies with melphalan and pediatric neoplastic and normal bone marrow cells. Int J Cancer 1986;37:819–823.

47. Frei E, Antman K, Teicher B, et al. Bone marrow autotransplantation for solid tumors—prospects. J Clin Oncol 1989;7:515–526.

48. Kushner BH, O'Reilly RJ, Mandell LR, Gulati SC, LaQuaglia M, Cheung N-KV. Myeloablative combination chemotherapy without total body irradiation for neuroblastoma. J Clin Oncol 1991;9:274–279.

49. Hagenbeck J, Martens A, Schulz FW. How to prevent a leukemia relapse after bone marrow transplantation in acute leukemia: preclinical and clinical model studies. In: Baum SJ, Dicke KA, Lotzoua E, et al., eds. Experimental hematology today. New York: Springer-Verlag, 1988:147–151.

50. Graham-Pole J, Casper J, Elfenbein G, et al. High-dose chemoradiotherapy supported by marrow infusions for advanced neuroblastoma: a Pediatric Oncology Group Study. J Clin Oncol 1991;9:152–158.

51. Deacon JM, Wilson PA, Peckham MJ. The radiobiology of human neuroblastoma. Radiother Oncol 1985;3:201–209.

52. Sanders J, Sullivan K, Witherspoon R, et al. Long term effects and quality of life in children and adults after marrow transplantation. Bone Marrow Transplant 1989;4(suppl 4):27–29.

53. McElwain TJ, Hedley DW, Burton G, et al. Marrow autotranplantation accelerates haematological recovery in patients with malignant melanoma treated with high-dose melphalan. Br J Cancer 1979;40:72–80.

54. Treleaven JG, Gibson FM, Ugelstad J, et al. Monoclonal antibodies and magnetic microspheres for the removal of tumor cells from bone marrow. Lancet 1984;1:70–73.

55. Philip T, Zucker JM, Bernard JL, Gentet JC, Michon J, Bouffet E for the LMCE group. High dose chemotherapy with BMT as consolidation in neuroblastoma—the LMCE 1 unselected group of patients revisited with a median follow up of 55 months after BMT. Bone Marrow Transplant 1990;5(suppl 2):38.

56. Seeger RC, Matthay KK, Villablanca JG, et al. Intensive chemoradiotherapy and autologous bone marrow transplantation (ABMT) for high risk neuroblastoma. Proc ASCO 1991;10:310.

57. Sawaguchi S, Kaneko M, Uchino J-i, et al. Treatment of advanced neuroblastoma with emphasis on intensive induction chemotherapy. Cancer 1990;66:1879–1887.

58. Seeger RC, Reynolds CP, Vo DD, et al. Depletion of neuroblastoma cells from bone marrow with monoclonal antibodies and magnetic immunobeads. Prog Clin Biol Res 1985;175:443–458.

59. Castleberry RP, Kun LE, Shuster JJ, et al. Radiotherapy improves the outlook for patients older than 1 year with Pediatric Oncology Group stage C neuroblastoma. J Clin Oncol 1991;9:789–795.

60. Zucker JM, Philip T, Bernard JL, et al. Single or double consolidation treatment according to remission status after initial therapy in metastatic neuroblastoma. Bone Marrow Transplant 1991;7(suppl 2):91.

61. Pinkerton CR, Pritchard J, DeKraker J, et al. ENSG 1—randomized study of high doses melphalan in neuroblastoma. In: Dicke KA, Spitzer G, Jagannath S, eds. Autologous bone marrow transplantation. Houston: University of Texas Press, 1987:401.

62. Pinkerton CR. ENSG1—randomized study of high-dose melphalan in neuroblastoma. Bone Marrow Transplant 1991;7(suppl 3):112–113.

63. Matthay K. Personal communication. 1991.

64. Gale RP, Armitage JO, Dicke KA. Autotransplants: now and in the future. Bone Marrow Transplant 1991;7:153–157.

65. Graham-Pole J, Gee A, Janssen W, Lee C, Gross S. Immunomagnetic purging of bone marrow: a model for negative cell selection. Am J Pediatr Hematol Oncol 1990;12:257–261.

66. Graham-Pole J. Autologous marrow transplants in pediatric tumors. In: Gale RP, Champlin RE, eds. New strategies in bone marrow transplantation. New York: Wiley-Liss, 1991:413–422.

67. Gazitt Y, Chang L, He Y-J, Kedar A, Gross S. Coexpression of C-myc and N-myc oncoproteins in newly established neuroblastoma (NB) cell lines: a study by two color immunofluorescence and flow cytometry. Fed Assoc Soc Exp Biol J 1991;5:A1442.

46

DOSE-INTENSIVE THERAPY FOR ADVANCED MELANOMA

Roger H. Herzig

Standard treatment for metastatic malignant melanoma has been disappointing. A wide variety of agents have been tried, with dacarbazine (DTIC) most extensively evaluated. The response rate (complete and partial) in patients receiving DTIC, alone or in combination, is about 20% (1–3). One approach to improve cytotoxic therapy is intensification of therapy (4). This effect can be accomplished by decreasing the interval between dose administration (frequency intensification) or by increasing the dose administered (dose intensification). Cytotoxic agents that are predominantly myelosuppressive can be dose intensified with marrow support to ensure hematopoietic recovery (5). Alkylating agents have been used most frequently not only because they are limited by myelosuppression but also because they exhibit steep, log-linear dose-response curves (in animal and tissue culture systems), resistance is difficult to induce, and generally they lack cross-resistance (4, 6). Over the past 30 years, many investigators have explored dose-intensive therapy with alkylating agents with the hope of improving the response and survival in patients with metastatic malignant melanoma. This chapter will summarize the phase I–II trials with dose-intensive regimens.

CLINICAL TRIALS

Single-Agent Phase I–II Trials

The treatment of patients with advanced melanoma was one of the first applications of intensive therapy and autologous marrow support (7). A number of alkylating agents have been used in single-agent studies, including cyclophosphamide, amsacrine (AMSA), carmustine (BCNU), melphalan, and triethylene thiophosphoramide (thiotepa), with both cryopreserved and fresh autologous marrow (7–20). The results of these studies are shown in Table 46.1. Most of the patients in these studies had far advanced disease, yet there was substantial antitumor activity demonstrated for BCNU, melphalan, and thiotepa. However, the duration of the responses was brief, generally 3 months. In Table 46.2, the responses reported with standard-dose therapy are compared with the results obtained in the collaborative trials of the North American Marrow Transplant Group (NAMTG) (13, 19, 20, and summarized in 21). Compared to conventional-dose therapy, the responses are statistically better ($p < .05$ by confidence interval). In the NAMTG studies, the responses with melphalan and thiotepa were higher than with BCNU. The difference can be accounted for by a significantly poorer response of patients who had received prior therapy before high-dose BCNU (Table 46.3). There were also better responses observed in patients who had more limited disease (soft tissue involvement, i.e., confined to skin and/or lymph node) compared to patients with visceral metastatic disease. Overall, 10 of 15 (67%) with skin and/or lymph node disease

Table 46.1. Advanced Melanoma: High-dose Single-Agent Therapy with Autologous Marrow Transplantation

Ref	Drugs[b]	Dose[c]	Number of Patients	CR	PR	RR (%)
8	CY	4200	2	0	0	0
9	AMSA	600–1000	4	0	0	0
10	Mustard	33	4	1	1	50
11	BCNU	600–750	5	0	1	20
12	BCNU	1200	6	0	1	17
13	BCNU	1200	31	4	10	45
14	BCNU	800	9	1	3	44
7	L-PAM	100 mg	31	0	11	35
15	L-PAM	140–260	27	2	10	44
16	L-PAM	120–200	3	0	0	0
17	L-PAM	140	2	0	2	100
18	L-PAM	180	3	0	2	100
19	L-PAM	180–225	26	6	12	69
20	Thiotepa	180–1575	55	4	25	53
	Total		208	18	79	47

Response[a]

[a]CR is complete response; PR is partial response; RR, response rate, determined by dividing the total number of patients responding by the total number evaluable and multiplying the fraction by 100 to yield percent. 95% CI is the 95% confidence interval.
[b]CY, cyclophosphamide; AMSA, amsacrine; mustard, nitrogen mustard; BCNU, carmustine; L-PAM, melphalan.
[c]In mg/m^2 except reference 7; the same dose was given to all patients.

Table 46.2. Advanced Melanoma: Comparison of Responses to Conventional-Dose and High-Dose Therapy with Autologous Marrow Transplantation

Drug[a]	Number of Patients	Rate (%)	95% C.I.
BCNU	110	15	10–23
BCNU/ABMT	31	45	29–62
Melphalan	24	17	7–36
Melphalan/ABMT	26	69	56–90
Thiotepa	55	16	9–28
Thiotepa/ABMT	55	53	40–65

Response

[a]Conventional dose is presented on the top line; high dose with autologous bone marrow transplantation (ABMT) is presented below.

Table 46.3. Advanced Melanoma: Effect of Prior Therapy and Extent of Disease on the Response to High-Dose Therapy with Autologous Marrow Transplantation

	BCNU	Melphalan	Thiotepa
Prior therapy[b]	2/15 (13)	10/16 (63)	16/31 (52)
No prior therapy	12/16 (75)	8/10 (80)	13/24 (54)
Skin ± lymph[c]	3/5 (60)	1/2 (50)	6/8 (75)
Visceral disease	11/26 (42)	17/24 (71)	23/47 (49)

Response Rate (%)[a]

[a]Number of patients responding/number patients evaluable; percent in brackets.
[b]Patients who received previous chemotherapy.
[c]Skin and/or lymph node involvement only; visceral disease refers to visceral organ metastases.

responded, while 51 of 97 (53%) with visceral metastases responded. The median duration of unmaintained response was similar for all three agents: BCNU, 6 months (range 2–46+ mos.); melphalan, 4 months (range 2–14 mos); thiotepa, 4 months (range 2–31+ mos). Of note, l0%–15% of the patients had responses that lasted more than 1 year.

Multi-Agent Phase I–II Trials

The dose-limiting toxicities from the phase I portion of these studies were hepatic (acute yellow atrophy) and pulmonary (interstitial fibrosis) with BCNU, mucositis with melphalan, and CNS dysfunction (organic brain syndrome) with thiotepa. Since there were no overlapping nonmyeloid toxicities, a series of phase I–II combination alkylator studies was started. A summary of the clinical trials using high-dose combinations can be found in Table 46.4. The results are not significantly better than those obtained with single agents, except that there seems to be a trend for improved duration of response. The NAMTG trials illustrate the progression and common problems of these studies. The first, CARMEL, involved combining melphalan and BCNU (25, 26). The initial dose selected was 50% of the maximally tolerated doses from the phase I single-agent studies (melphalan 90 mg/m^2, BCNU 600 mg/m^2). Each agent was escalated individually. While it was hoped to escalate each drug to the full single-dose level, this expectation was unrealistic if the phase I trial had truly identified the single-agent maximum tolerated dose. The pattern of marrow recovery was similar to that observed with each agent alone. The pulmonary

Table 46.4. Advanced Melanoma: High-Dose Combination Regimens with Autologous Marrow Transplantation

Ref	Drugs[b]	Number of Patients	Response[a] CR	PR	RR (%)
22	CY, CDDP, BCNU ± L-PAM	19	1	10	65
23	CY, BCNU	5	0	2	40
24	BCNU, L-PAM	17	2	5	41
25, 26	BCNU, L-PAM	58	6	28	59
27	CY, Thiotepa	2	1	0	50
28	CY, Thiotepa	6	3	2	83
29	Thiotepa, L-PAM	7	0	4	57
30	CY, Thiotepa, L-PAM	1	1	0	100
31	CY, CDDP, L-PAM	10	1	5	60
31	CY, CDDP, Thiotepa	4	0	2	50
	Total	129	15	58	57

[a]CR is complete response; PR is partial response; RR, response rate, determined by dividing the total number of patients responding by the total number of evaluable and multiplying the fraction by 100 to yield percent. 95% CI is the 95% confidence interval.
[b]CY, cyclophosphamide; CDDP, cisplatin; BCNU, carmustine; L-PAM, melphalan.

(noninfectious diffuse interstitial pneumonitis and respiratory distress syndrome) and gastrointestinal (diarrhea) toxicities were increased in frequency at the highest level (100% melphalan and BCNU) compared to the lower combination levels or the single-agent frequencies. Overall, there were 58 patients entered, with 6 complete responses and 28 partial responses, for a response rate of 59%. The response rate showed a trend for improved responses with increasing doses (44% at the lowest, 59% at the highest levels), but too few patients were entered at each level to be statistically significant. The response rate resembled that for melphalan alone and was marginally better than that for BCNU alone, but the duration of response resembled that for BCNU with a median duration of unmaintained response of 5 months (range: 2–30+ months), with 15% of patients responding for more than 1 year.

The significant dose escalation possible and the dose response seen with thiotepa prompted the second NAMTG study using

melphalan and thiotepa, MELT (29). With the recognition of an inability to reach full maximally tolerated doses when used in combination, we started at 50% melphalan (90 mg/m^2) and 80% thiotepa (900 mg/m^2). Seven patients were treated, but no escalations were accomplished because of significant liver and lung toxicity not previously encountered with these drugs.

When the availability of intravenous melphalan was diminished because of formulation problems, the NAMTG substituted cyclophosphamide (150–180 mg/kg) in combination with thiotepa (28). The regimen consists of thiotepa 300 mg/m^2 and cyclophosphamide 50–60 mg/kg daily for 3 days with marrow rescue after 3 days' rest. As part of a broad phase II study, six patients with melanoma have been treated. Marrow recovery occurred within 4 weeks, and none of these patients had severe grade 3 or 4 toxicity. Five of the six (83%) responded, with three with complete remission and two with partial remission. Three patients had skin and/or lymph node involvement. All three responded (two with complete remission), and the responses were of 8+, 15, and 24+ months. The responses of patients with visceral metastases were all less than 6 months in duration.

Combined Modality Trials

In an effort to improve the results, the investigators at Washington University have added interleukin-2 (IL-2) to the approach (32). The treatment scheme included the administration if IL-2 for two cycles, followed by high-dose thiotepa (900 mg/m^2) with marrow support and then two more cycle of IL-2. Eight patients have been entered since December 1988. Six had visceral disease, two had prior chemotherapy, and one had previously received a biologic response modifier. All eight patients received the first two cycles of IL-2. None of the eight responded. Two patients did not go on to receive the high-dose thiotepa, one because of severe toxicity from IL-2 and one because of progressive disease on IL-2. Six patients underwent the high-dose portion of the protocol; five are evaluable; one had a partial response. Only one patient has received the last two cycles of IL-2 and has had stable disease. Four patients did not get the second IL-2 cycle due to toxicity from the high-dose chemotherapy, previous IL-2 toxicity, progressive disease, or patient refusal. Thus while it is an interesting concept to combine different therapeutic approaches, there are many problems that will have to be addressed to permit wider application of this approach.

FUTURE DIRECTIONS

Since patients with limited disease appear to have the best results with the dose-intensive approach, it would seem more practical to extend this type of therapy to patients with less extensive disease but with a poor prognosis for cure. One such group would include patients who achieve a complete response to initial therapy (surgery, radiotherapy, and/or chemotherapy) for recurrent disease. Another suitable situation might be the use of high-dose therapy in the adjuvant setting for high-risk stage II patients. Such a trial has been recently closed at Duke University. The results are now being analyzed (32).

CONCLUSIONS

Dose escalation is possible with marrow support. There is a dose-response effect observed for patients with advanced melanoma treated with high doses of alkylating agents, singly or in combination. Unfortunately, the duration of unmaintained response is short, regardless of chemotherapy regimen; about 10% of patients have responses of more than 1 year. Initial efforts to improve the results with the addition of the biologic response modifier IL-2 have not yet been successful, but the trial is still ongoing. Another approach, multiple courses of dose-

intensive therapy, has been tried in a few patients. No conclusions can be drawn from these preliminary studies. Melanoma patients with minimal disease or at high risk for recurrence are likely to be the beneficiaries of the approach of dose intensity.

REFERENCES

1. Comis RL. DTIC (NSC 45388) in malignant melanoma: a perspective. Cancer Treat Rep 1976;60:165–176.
2. Wittes RE, Wittes JT, Golbey RB. Combination chemotherapy in metastatic melanoma. A randomized study of three DTIC-containing combinations. Cancer 1978;41:415–421.
3. Amer MN, Serraf M, Vaitkevicius VK. Metastatic sites and survival in patients with advanced metastatic melanoma. Surg Gynecol Obstet 1979;149:687–692.
4. Frei E III, Canellos GP. Dose: a critical factor in cancer chemotherapy. Am J Med 1980;69:585–594.
5. Thomas ED. Marrow transplantation for malignant disease. J Clin Oncol 1983;1:517–531.
6. Schabel FN Jr, Trader NW, Laster WR, et al. Patterns of resistance and therapeutic synergism among alkylating agents. Antibiot Chemother 1978;23:200–215.
7. Ariel IM, Pack GT. Treatment of disseminated melanoma with phenylalanine mustard (melphalan) and autogenous bone marrow transplants. Surgery 1962;51:582–591.
8. Buchner CD, Rudolph RH, Fefer A, et al. High-dose cyclophosphamide therapy for malignant disease: toxicity, tumor response, and the effects of stored autologous marrow. Cancer 1972;29:357–365.
9. Zander A, Spitzer G, Legha S, et al. High dose AMSA and autologous bone marrow transplantation (ABMT) in leukemia (L) and solid tumors (ST) [Abstract]. Proc AACR/ASCO 1980;21:366.
10. Thomas MR, Robinson WA, Glode LM, et al. Treatment of advanced malignant melanoma with high-dose chemotherapy and autologous bone marrow transplantation. Am J Clin Oncol 1982;5:611–622.
11. Spitzer G, Dicke KA, Verma DS, et al. High-dose BCNU therapy with autologous bone marrow infusion: preliminary observations. Cancer Treat Rep 1979;63:1257–1264.
12. Barbasch A, Higby DJ, Brass C, et al. High-dose cytoreductive therapy with autologous bone marrow transplantation in advanced malignancies. Cancer Treat Rep 1983;67:143–148.
13. Phillips GL, Fay JW, Herzig GP, et al. A phase I–II study; intensive BCNU (1, 3-bis (2-chloroethyl)-1-nitrosourea, NSC 409962) and autologous bone marrow transplantation for refractory cancer. Cancer 1983;52:1792–1802.
14. Lakhani S, Selby P, Bliss JM, et al. Chemotherapy for

malignant melanoma: combinations and high doses produce more responses without survival benefit. Br J Cancer 1990;61:330–334.

15. Cornbleet MA, McElwain TJ, Kumar PJ, et al. Treatment of advanced malignant melanoma with high-dose melphalan and autologous bone marrow transplantation. Br J Cancer 1983;48:329–334.

16. Corringham R, Gilmore M, Prentice HG, et al. High-dose melphalan with autologous bone marrow transplant: treatment of poor prognosis tumors. Cancer 1983;52:1783–1787.

17. Maraninchi D, Gastaut JA, Herve P, et al. High dose melphalan and autologous marrow transplantation in adult solid tumors: clinical response and preliminary evaluation of different strategies. In: McVie JG, Dalesio O, Smith IE, eds. Autologous bone marrow transplantation and solid tumors. New York: Raven Press, 1984:145–150.

18. Knight WA III, Page CP, Kuhn JG, et al. High dose L-PAM and autologous marrow infusion for refractory solid tumors [Abstract]. Proc ASCO 1984;3:150.

19. Lazarus HM, Herzig RH, Wolff SN, et al. Treatment of metastatic malignant melanoma using intensive melphalan (NSC #8806) and autologous bone marrow transplantation. Cancer Treat Rep 1985;69:473–477.

20. Wolff SN, Herzig RH, Fay JW, et al. High-dose thiotepa with autologous bone marrow transplantation for metastatic malignant melanoma: results of phase I and II studies of the North American Bone Marrow Transplantation Group. J Clin Oncol 1989;7:245–249.

21. Herzig RH, Brown RA, Wolff SN, et al. Dose intensive therapy for advanced melanoma. In: Dicke KA, Armitage JO, Dicke-Evinger MJ, eds. Autologous bone marrow transplantation. Omaha, NE: University of Nebraska Medical Center, 1990:661–667.

22. Shea TC, Antman KH, Eder JP, et al. Malignant melanoma: treatment with high-dose combination alkylating agent chemotherapy and autologous bone marrow support. Arch Dermatol 1988;124:878–884.

23. Slease RB, Benear JB, Selby GB, et al. High-dose combination alkylating agent therapy with autologous bone marrow rescue for refractory solid tumors. J Clin Oncol 1988;6:1314–1320.

24. Thomas MR, Robinson WA, Glode LM, et al. Treatment of advanced malignant melanoma with high dose BCNU and melphalan and autologous bone marrow transplantation—preliminary results phase I [Abstract]. Clin Res 1983;31:69A.

25. Herzig R, Phillips G, Wolff S, et al. Treatment of metastatic melanoma with intensive melphalan-BCNU combination, combination chemotherapy and cryopreserved autologous bone marrow transplantation [Abstract]. Proc ASCO 1984;3:264.

26. Herzig RH, Wolff SN, Fay JW, et al. Treatment of advanced melanoma with high-dose chemotherapy and autologous marrow transplantation. In: Dicke KA, Spitzer G, Jagannath S, Evinger-Hodges MJ, eds. Autologous Bone Marrow Transplantation. Houston: MD Anderson Cancer Center, 1989:499–508.

27. Williams SF, Bitran JD, Kaminer L, et al. A phase I–II study of bialkylator chemotherapy, high-dose thiotepa and cyclophosphamide with autologous bone marrow reinfusion in patients with advanced cancer. J Clin Oncol 1987;5:260–265.

28. Herzig RH. Unpublished results, 1991.

29. Wolff SN, Herzig RH, Herzig GP, et al. N, N′, N″-triethylene thiophosphoramide (THIO-TEPA) (TT) with autologous bone marrow transplantation for metastatic malignant melanoma (MMM). A phase I–II study of the North American Bone Marrow Transplant Group [Abstract]. Proc ASCO 1988;7:248.

30. Bitran J, Williams S, Robin E, et al. High dose trialkylator chemotherapy (TACT) with thiotepa (TT), cytoxan, and oral melphalan and autologous stem cell rescue (ASCR) in patients with disseminated cancer [Abstract]. Proc ASCO 1988;7:46.

31. Peters WP. Personal communication, 1991.

32. Herzig GP. Personal communication, 1991.

47

HIGH-DOSE THERAPY FOR BRAIN TUMORS: RATIONALE, RESULTS, AND REVELATIONS

Steven N. Wolff

The treatment of patients with high-grade primary tumors of the CNS, especially tumors of brain glial cell origin, is a formidable challenge for the oncologist. Primary treatment exclusively with debulking surgery does not result in prolongation of survival (1). When radiation therapy is added to primary surgery, median survival is increased but is still less than 1 year, and most patients succumb within 18 months (2). Chemotherapy for tumors progressing after initial surgical and radiation therapy is ineffective (3). When all three modalities are combined as an initial approach, modestly improved survival is achieved, with, however, most patients succumbing within the first 2 years. The results of standard therapy are unsatisfactory and offer little curative potential.

The ineffectiveness of standard chemotherapy results partly from the refractoriness of these tumors to cytotoxic drugs together with the difficulty of achieving adequate brain tumor drug levels due to the blood-brain barrier. Additionally, small changes in the size of the tumor and/or surrounding edema can cause profound symptomatology, making the patient's situation quite tenuous. Thus many patients with brain tumors are unable to tolerate the severe side effects of cytotoxic therapy.

Considering the modest gains accomplished with standard chemotherapy, brain tumors were an early focus for the evaluation of high-dose chemotherapy. This chapter will focus on high-grade glial tumors of the brain, which have been the most well studied with high-dose chemotherapy. This review will describe the pharmacology, rationale, results, and future prospects of high-dose therapy for tumors of the CNS.

RATIONALE OF HIGH-DOSE CHEMOTHERAPY

High-dose chemotherapy is based on the observation of a marked dose-response relationship for many cytotoxic agents. When the myelosuppressive toxicity of high-dose therapy is circumvented by bone marrow or peripheral blood stem cell transplantation (rescue), marked cytotoxic dose escalation can be achieved. Dose escalation can be increased only to the level causing severe visceral organ toxicity. For brain tumors, high-dose therapy has two proposed advantages. The first is that drug levels in brain tumors can be increased due to the pharmacologic perturbations caused by high-dose chemotherapy. Secondly, tumor cytotoxic resistance may be relative and overcome by marked dose escalation. These two reasons supported the rationale for high-dose therapy for brain tumors. Contradistinctive to the putative advantages for high-dose therapy are the intense hospital care, the long-term convalescence, and the high patient care expenses. Considering these consequences, high-dose therapy must result in a substantial survival benefit to have widespread utility.

BLOOD-BRAIN BARRIER

The concept of a selective barrier between macromolecular polar (nonlipid) compounds in the blood and the brain was first introduced by Ehrlich in 1885. This selective barrier depends on the molecules' biochemical composition and method of transport through the choroidal epithelium and cerebral capillary endothelium (4). Besides passive diffusion, there are active transport mechanisms in the brain endothelial cells. The existence of the blood-brain barrier is hypothesized as a mechanism to maintain special brain homeostasis by facilitating the entry of needed metabolites and the removal or exclusion of toxic substances. More rapid entry and equilibrium between the blood and the brain occurs with smaller molecular size, higher lipid solubility, lower ionization at physiologic pH, and the absence of binding to plasma proteins. The blood-cerebrospinal fluid (CSF)-barrier and the CSF-brain barrier exist in addition to the blood-brain barrier. The factors that facilitate the passage of substances from the blood to the brain also are operative for these brain barriers. The blood-CSF and the CSF-brain barriers make extrapolation of measured CSF drug levels to brain substance levels fraught with uncertainty.

The blood-brain and blood-CSF barriers undergo modification during certain pathologic conditions. For example, hyperosmolar solutions alter the blood-brain barrier and have been used to therapeutically augment cytotoxic drug levels in brain tumors. Other factors that can influence these barriers include hypoxemia, hypoosmolality, hypertension, carbon dioxide, seizures, chemical toxins, uremia, infections, corticosteroids, kernicterus, and brain tumors. Primary and metastatic tumors have been associated with abnormal endothelial cells, which increase permeability. Tumors may also construct direct neovascularization, which can corrupt the blood-brain barrier. These mechanisms may make the expected blood-brain barrier exclusion of cytotoxic therapy less important for treating brain tumors. The broaching of the blood-brain barrier may be indicated by the response of primary CNS lymphoma and metastases of sensitive tumors (lymphoma and small cell carcinoma) to standard systemic chemotherapy. All regions of the brain may not be identically excluded (5). Tumor response to cytotoxic therapy may also depend on the exact location in the CNS.

CENTRAL NERVOUS SYSTEM PHARMACOLOGY OF CYTOTOXIC DRUGS

The poor ingress of systemically administered cytotoxic therapy to the brain substance is the hallmark of the blood-brain barrier. For most chemotherapeutic agents, the ratio of drug measured in the CSF to its concomitantly measured blood level is less than 10% (6). Like other drugs, chemotherapeutic agents have reasonable penetration into the CNS if they are small nonpolar lipid-soluble molecules or small nonionized compounds that have poor tissue or protein binding characteristics or have affinity for carriers that facilitate transport. For example, the impediment to CNS penetration exerted by protein binding is shown by the differential ingress of corticosteroids. Dexamethasone is less protein bound compared to prednisolone and thus may offer CNS therapeutic advantage. Chemotherapeutic drugs extensively protein bound, such as the vinca alkaloids and the anthracyclines, penetrate the CNS little. The extrapolation of measured levels in normal situations to those achievable in states of CNS pathology, such as the presence of primary or metastatic tumors, is unclear. Considering an intact blood-brain barrier, if a narrow window of blood therapeutic level to cytotoxicity exists, there is a strong likelihood that therapeutic levels may not be achieved in the CNS tumor target tissue.

Chemotherapeutic drugs can be divided into those able to adequately penetrate the CNS when administered at standard dose or those achieving adequate CNS levels only with augmented blood levels (Table 47.1) (7). Chemotherapy for brain tumors has generally relied on those agents achieving adequate CNS penetration. Agents that have been pharmacologically well evaluated for CSF penetration include cytosine arabinoside (ARA-C), methotrexate, etoposide (UP-16), thiotepa, and busulfan. Although useful in the treatment of meningeal leukemia, intrathecal administration does not result in sufficient deep-tissue penetration to justify therapy of brain substance tumors.

Methotrexate and ARA-C are examples of drugs with adequate penetration of the CNS only with high-dose therapy. Methotrexate is a drug that poorly penetrates the CSF at standard dose (3% penetration), resulting in subtherapeutic CSF drug levels. However, when administered at extremely high doses with calcium leucovorin to block systemic toxicity, markedly higher blood levels can be achieved. These high blood levels are associated with a markedly increased CSF level, well into the therapeutic range for cytotoxicity. Systematically administered high-dose methotrexate has been used to treat meningeal leukemia and serve as part of CNS prophylactic therapy.

ARA-C at the standard dose has reasonable ability to penetrate the CNS (10%–25%), which may be influenced by the total amount of systemic drug administered. Similar to methotrexate, ARA-C requires a fixed level and duration of tumor exposure to maximize cytotoxicity. This level is not achieved in the CNS with standard-dose administration. High-dose ARA-C has now become a mainstay in the treatment of acute leukemia. With high-dose ARA-C use, substantial CNS levels are achieved that are equivalent to blood levels obtained with standard-dose ARA-C. A further benefit of adequate ARA-C penetration is the lack of deaminating metabolizing enzymes in the CNS, which prolongs the ARA-C half-life in the CNS. Like high-dose methotrexate, high-dose ARA-C has been used to successfully treat meningeal leukemia. These drugs at normal dose do not cause CNS toxicity. However, both of these drugs when administered at high doses cause novel CNS toxicity, presumably due to the marked increase in brain and CSF drug levels (8). Due to a lack of known activity against glial tumors, these agents have not been well studied for the treatment of brain tumors.

Busulfan, carmustine (BCNU), and thiotepa are highly lipid soluble agents that have substantial ability to penetrate the CNS when administered at normal dose. BCNU has not been adequately pharmacologically studied due to the difficulty in drug measurement. At standard dose, busulfan and thiotepa achieve essentially equivalent CSF and blood levels, with a busulfan CSF-to-plasma ratio from 1.02 to 1.39 (9, 10). In one patient with lymphomatous meningitis, the busulfan CSF-to-plasma ratio was 2.47. At high doses, busulfan causes seizures, more commonly in adults than children. This observed clinical difference is presumably due to enhanced busulfan clearance in children. When busulfan is dosed on body surface area (rather than by weight), the incidence of neurotoxicity and relative drug levels are equivalent between children and adults. This CNS toxicity of busulfan is novel and not recognized at standard dose. BCNU, thiotepa, and other high-dose agents cause another form of CNS toxicity (11, 12)—severe and potentially irreversible cortical abnormalities that appear to be dose depen-

Table 47.1. Drugs with Adequate CNS Penetration

At Normal Dose	Only at High-Dose
Aziridinylbenzoquinone	Cytosine arabinoside
Carmustine (BCNU)	Cyclophosphamide
Busulfan	6-Mercaptopurine
Dexamethasone	Methotrexate
5-Fluorouracil	Etoposide
Procabazine	
Thiotepa	

dent. These novel CNS toxicities have proven to be dose limiting. BCNU is the mainstay of conventional chemotherapy for brain tumors; busulfan has not been adequately studied, and thiotepa has shown modest activity.

CHOICE OF HIGH-DOSE CHEMOTHERAPEUTIC AGENTS FOR CENTRAL NERVOUS SYSTEM TUMORS

Tumors of the CNS are conventionally treated with chemotherapeutic agents that demonstrate adequate CNS penetration. Foremost of these agents are the nitrosoureas and specifically BCNU. Drugs that precipitate CNS toxicity have been evaluated, assuming that CNS toxicity indicates substantial drug penetration (Table 47.2). Considering the special scenario for high-dose therapy, almost any agent could be evaluated, assuming that increased blood level yields increased CNS drug penetration. In this circumstance, drugs that have little activity at standard dose could demonstrate novel utility at high doses. However, assuming a steep dose-response relationship, high-dose therapy would be most effective using agents capable of adequate penetration of the CNS at standard dose, having some degree of effectiveness at standard dose against CNS tumors, and being sufficiently tolerable by ill patients (Table 47.3). However, the lack of effectiveness at standard dose should not discourage the evaluation of a drug at high doses since there are ample examples of drugs that have scant activity at standard dose and demonstrate increased activity only at high doses.

BCNU was the first agent to meet all of the high-dose criteria. This agent was also the first to undergo extensive high-dose phase I and phase II studies encompassing tumors of the CNS (13). Aside from BCNU, cyclophosphamide, nitrogen mustard, busulfan, mitomycin-C, ARA-C, methotrexate, VP-16, carboplatin, and thiotepa have undergone extensive high-dose evaluation.

STANDARD THERAPY FOR HIGH-GRADE GLIAL TUMORS OF THE CENTRAL NERVOUS SYSTEM

The intracranial high-grade astrocytoma developing de nouveau or by progressive anaplasia from a low-grade lesion is rapidly progressive and lethal. Following surgery alone, more than 50% of patients succumb within 6 months and virtually all die within 2 years. When radiation therapy is added to initial surgery, 10%–20% of patients will survive 2 years, and a few patients may survive longer. Younger patients and those with grade-III lesions have the best overall survival. Unfortunately, modifications of dose, schedule, and method of administration of radiation therapy do not substantially improve survival. This bleak outlook is well shown in a recent report of the Brain Tumor Study Group (BTSG) (14). In that study, 571 adult patients were randomized after definitive surgery to

Table 47.2. Drugs Exhibiting CNS Toxicity

5-Azacytidine	Hexamethylmelamine
Cytosine arabinoside	Ifosfamide
Aziridinylbenzoquinone	L-Asparaginase
Carmustine (BCNU)	Methotrexate
Busulfan	Nitrogen mustard
Cisplatin	Procarbazine
Corticosteroids	Thiotepa
2'-Deoxycoformycin	Tiazofurin
5-Fluorouracil	Vindesine
Fludarabine	Etoposide

Table 47.3. High-Dose Drug Requirements for CNS Tumor Therapy

1. Adequate CNS penetration at standard dose
2. Adequate CNS penetration with high-dose administration
3. Demonstrable antitumor activity with standard dose
4. Tolerable CNS toxicity with high-dose administration
5. Tolerable visceral organ tolerance with high-dose administration

one of three chemotherapy regiments; BCNU alone, alternating courses of BCNU and pro-carbazine, and BCNU plus hydroxyurea alter-nating with procarbazine plus teniposide (VM-26). All patients received some form of radiation therapy, either 6020 rads to the whole brain or 4300 rads to the whole brain followed by 1720 rads coned down to the tu-mor volume. The median survival from time of randomization ranged from 11.3 to 13.8 months. Only 29%–37% of the patients sur-vived 18 months, and approximately 20% survived 2 years. Although none of the treat-ment parameters influenced survival, younger age, the diagnosis of anaplastic astrocytoma versus glioblastoma multiforme, and better performance status were all independently related to survival. Aside from the dismal ab-solute survival figures, these curves did not demonstrate any plateau, suggesting few long-term disease survivors. Counter to the adult experience, children may have a better sur-vival, as shown by a study of the Children's Cancer Study Group (15). In that study, pa-tients with glioblastoma had a 20% extended survival, and patients with anaplastic astro-cytoma fared even better, with a 40%–50% long-term survival. Due to their low molec-ular weight and high lipid solubility, the ni-trosoureas were the mainstay of treatment in both of these studies. Unfortunately, no other agent has shown superiority to BCNU, and the studies with combination chemotherapy have not revealed improved survival to BCNU alone.

EVALUATION OF HIGH-DOSE THERAPY

Based on multiple studies of the BTSG for high-grade glial tumors, a median survival of 12 months and an approximate 20% 2-year survival can be anticipated with standard therapy. Considering the many prognostic factors for short-term response and survival, the best determinant for the results of high-dose therapy is long-term survival. Since there are few long-term disease-free survivors, the observation of a large cohort of disease-free

survivors would suggest benefit. Although most rapidly gained, information concerning response rate must be critically evaluated, since at times accurate measurement of CNS tumor mass is difficult and obscured by the edematous normal brain interface (16).

RESULTS OF HIGH-DOSE CHEMOTHERAPY

BCNU was the initial agent to undergo phase I escalation with autologous bone mar-row transplantation (ABMT). These studies demonstrated that myelosuppression was moderated by ABMT, that visceral toxicity (pulmonary and liver) occasionally led to pa-tient death, and that a safe high dose was ap-proximately 3–5 times the standard dose. Of particular interest in these studies was the observation of CNS toxicity and responses in patients with primary and CNS tumors.

Considering that BCNU met all of the criteria for high-dose CNS treatment, high-dose BCNU was studied by multiple investigators for the treatment of high-grade glial tumors (17, 18). These studies initially treated pa-tients with tumors enlarging after standard surgery and radiation therapy. Phillips et al. treated 27 patients with progressive glioma and produced a 44% response rate (19). Al-though a high response rate was observed, most patients again relapsed and succumbed to their tumor. Interestingly, 2 patients re-main alive (presumably tumor-free) 5 and 7 years after treatment. Takvorian et al. treated 20 patients with progressive glioma, includ-ing some who had had prior nitrosourea therapy (20). The percent response of their patients was similar to the prior report's, and some patients were surviving more than 2 years after treatment. Summarizing these two studies, almost one-half of patients re-sponded, although most responses were not durable. Myelosuppression although formi-dable was controlled by ABMT. Occasional visceral (pulmonary and hepatic) toxicity proved fatal. Considering that these patients had progressive disease, the results showed promise as indicated by the high response rate and the observation of a small number of long-term survivors. Based on these studies, additional patients were given high-dose BCNU as part of their initial therapy (21–23). These were crucial phase II studies; patients chosen for their target group were those anticipated to obtain maximal benefit from high-dose treatment. The sequence of therapy varied, with some patients receiving high-dose BCNU prior to radiation and some patients receiving high-dose therapy after completing radiation therapy. A rationale for the sequence of high-dose BCNU prior to radiation was to allow for maximal chemotherapy tumor penetration, with subsequent reduction of the volume of tumor by radiation therapy. At least three series have been published treating patients adjunctively with definitive surgery, radiation therapy, and high-dose BCNU. Early evaluation of these survival curves is interesting, as there is apparently early increased survival. Some of these reports were discussed rather early since they were viewed with optimism. Unfortunately, with more prolonged observation, these series revealed tumor progression in most patients, and overall survival not meaningfully different from that obtained with standard BCNU treatment. When reviewing the results for relatively small numbers of patients with glial tumors, care must be taken to control for the various parameters that influence survival, such as age, histology, performance status, and degree of tumor resection prior to chemotherapy. The influence of prognostic factors was not critically evaluated in these small studies. With this in mind, a recent review of high-dose BCNU compared to a valid historical cohort of patients treated with standard-dose BCNU revealed similar median survival (24). In these series there are anecdotal cases demonstrating extremely long survival. These long-term observations are interesting but not indicative of any major population therapeutic benefit.

Although outright survival was not improved, the studies with high-dose BCNU did demonstrate substantial tumor reduction. However, the degree of cytotoxicity was not adequate for survival benefit. Analogous to other successfully treated tumors, it is unlikely that single-agent therapy would be maximally effective. Therefore, other agents were evaluated to determine synergistic combination chemotherapy. VP-16 and thiotepa were the next agents to be studied for CNS tumors (25–28). High-dose VP-16 in phase I trials was substantially less toxic than BCNU. Unfortunately, high-dose phase II trials for CNS tumors demonstrated marginal activity and were clearly less effective than either standard BCNU or high-dose BCNU. Thiotepa, one of the older alkylating agents, has excellent CNS penetration at standard dose. During high-dose evaluation, CNS toxicity was common and felt to be dose limiting. The knowledge of its excellent brain penetration encouraged thiotepa evaluation. In preliminary trials, antitumor activity has been demonstrated, although more patient accrual and observation are required for definitive evaluation.

Knowing that the best results of chemotherapy are achieved with combinations of active single agents, a few studies have attempted to combine high-dose agents (29). When combining high-dose agents, the possibility of extraordinary visceral organ toxicity may be encountered, as evidenced by an abbreviated trial of high-dose BCNU and high-dose VP-16, which caused severe hepatic toxicity in 50% of patients treated without producing substantial tumor response (30). Additional combination chemotherapy studies are in very preliminary phase I and II evaluation.

SUMMARY OF HIGH-DOSE THERAPY

The basic dilemma in treating unresponsive tumors is chemotherapeutic resistance. Resistance is shown by an overall poor response rate together with the absence of objective complete responses. Nowhere is this problem better demonstrated than in the treatment of primary high-grade glial tumors of the CNS. One of the aspirations of high-dose therapy is the ability to overcome relative drug resistance. Unfortunately, in the completed trials of high-dose therapy for high-grade glial tumors, no substantial improvement in overall survival was noted despite an apparent increase in overall response rate. Although somewhat more effective than standard dose, currently available high-dose regimens still do not eradicate enough tumor mass to affect survival. Since these initial reports, fewer investigators have chosen to study CNS tumors. Future studies in this disease will require the identification of more active single agents that, one hopes, can be combined into effective (ideally synergistic) regimens. High-grade CNS tumors remain a challenge, and patients with these tumors continue to have a very bleak outcome.

REFERENCES

1. Nazzaro JM, Neuwelt EA. The role of surgery in the management of supratentorial intermediate and high-grade astrocytomas in adults. J Neurosurg 1990;73:331–344.
2. Bloom HJG. Intracranial tumors: response and resistance to therapeutic endeavors, 1970–1980. Int J Radiat Oncol Biol Phys 1982;8:1083–1113.
3. Edwards MS, Levin VA, Wilson CB. Brain tumor chemotherapy: an evaluation of agents in current use for phase II and III trials. Cancer Treat Rep 1980;64:1179–1205.
4. Fishman RA. Cerebrospinal fluid in diseases of the nervous system. Philadelphia: WB Saunders, 1980:43–62.
5. Toner GC, Pike J, Schwarz MA. The blood-brain barrier and response of CNS metastases to chemotherapy. J Neurooncol 1989;7:21–24.
6. Balis FM, Poplack DG. Central nervous system pharmacology of antileukemic drugs. Am J Pediatr Hematol Oncol 1989;11:74–86.
7. Chabner BA, Collins JM. Cancer chemotherapy: principles and practice. Grand Rapids, MI: JB Lippincott, 1990.
8. Herzig RH, Hines JD, Herzig GP, et al. Cerebellar toxicity with high-dose cytosine arabinoside. J Clin Oncol 1987;5:927–932.
9. Herzig RH, Herzig GP, Fay JW, et al. Phase I-II studies with high-dose N,N′,N″-triethylene thiophosphoramide and autologous bone marrow transplantation

in patients with refractory malignancies. In: Gale RP, Champlin R, eds. Recent advances in bone marrow transplantation. UCLA symposium of molecular and cellular biology. New York: Alan R. Liss, 1987:889–901.
10. Vassal G, Deroussent A, Hartmann O, et al. Dose-dependent neurotoxicity of high-dose busulfan in children: a clinical and pharmacological study. Cancer Res 1990;50:6203–6207.
11. Leff RS, Thompson JM, Do MB, et al. Acute neurologic dysfunction after high-dose etoposide therapy for malignant glioma. Cancer 1988;62:32–35.
12. Rottenberg DA. Neurologic complications of cancer treatment. Boston: Butterworth-Henneman, 1991.
13. Phillips GL, Fay JW, Herzig GP, et al. Intensive 1,3-bis(2-chloroethyl)-1-nitrosourea (BCNU) and cryopreserved autologous marrow transplantation for refractory cancer. A phase I-II study. Cancer 1983;52:1792–1802.
14. Shapiro WR, Green SB, Burger PC, et al. Randomized trial of three chemotherapy regimens and two radiotherapy regimens in postoperative treatment of malignant glioma. J Neurosurg 1989;71:1–9.
15. Sposto R, Ertel IJ, Jenkin RDT, et al. The effectiveness of chemotherapy for treatment of high grade astrocytoma in children: results of a randomized trial. A report from the childrens cancer study group. J Neurooncol 1989;7:165–177.
16. Grossman Sa, Burch PA. Quantitation of tumor response to anti-neoplastic therapy. Semin Oncol 15:441–454, 1988.
17. Wolff SN, Phillips GL, Fay JW, et al. High-dose chemotherapy with autologous bone marrow transplantation for gliomas of the central nervous system. In: Dicke KA, Spitzer G, Jagannath S, eds. Proceedings of the third international symposium. Houston: University of Texas, 1987:557–563.
18. Phillips GL, Fay JW, Herzig GH, Herzig RH, Lazarus HM, Wolff SN. Intensive monochemotherapy and autologous bone marrow transplantation for malignant glioma. In: Dicke KA, Spitzer G, Jagannath S, eds. Proceedings of the third international symposium. Houston: University of Texas, 1987:543–547.
19. Phillips GL, Wolff SN, Fay JW, et al. Intensive BCNU chemotherapy and autologous bone marrow transplantation for malignant glioma. J Clin Oncol 1986;4:639–645.
20. Takvorian T, Parker LM, Hochberg FH, Canellos GP. Autologous bone-marrow transplantation: host effects of high-dose BCNU. 1983;1:610–620.
21. Wolff SN, Phillips GL, Herzig GP. High-dose BCNU with autologous bone marrow transplantation for the adjuvant treatment of high-grade gliomas of the central nervous system. Cancer Treat Rep 1987;71:183–185.
22. Mbidde EK, Selby PJ, Perren TJ, et al. High dose BCNU chemotherapy with autologous bone marrow trans-

plantation and full dose radiotherapy for grade IV astrocytoma. Br J Cancer 1988;58:779–792.

23. Johnson DB, Thompson JM, Corwin JA, et al. Prolongation of survival for high-grade malignant gliomas with adjuvant high-dose BCNU and autologous bone marrow transplantation. J Clin Oncol 1987;5:783–789.

24. Goodwin W, Crowley J. A retrospective comparison of high-dose BCNU with autologous marrow rescue plus radiotherapy vs. IV BCNU plus radiation therapy in high-grade gliomas: A Southwest Oncology Group review [Abstract]. Proc ASCO 1989;8:90.

25. Ascensao J, Ahmed T, Feldman E, et al. High dose thiotepa with autologous bone marrow transplantation (ABM) and localized radiotherapy (RT) for patients (PTS) with astrocytoma grade III–IV (GLIOMA): a promising approach [Abstract]. Proc ASCO 1989;8:90.

26. Saarinen UM, Pihko H, Mäkipernaa A. High-dose thiotepa with autologous bone marrow rescue in recurrent malignant oligodendroglioma. J Neurooncol 1990;9:57–61.

27. Long J, Leff R, Daly M, et al. Phase II trial of high-dose etoposide (E) and autologous bone marrow transplantation (ABMT) for treatment of progressive glioma [Abstract]. Proc ASCO 1989;8:92.

28. Giannone L, Wolff SN. Phase II treatment of central nervous system gliomas with high-dose etoposide and autologous bone marrow transplantation. Cancer Treat Rep 1987;71:759–761.

29. Finlay JL, August C, Packer R, et al. High-dose multiagent chemotherapy followed by bone marrow "Rescue" for malignant astrocytoma of childhood and adolescence. J Neurooncol 1990;9:239–248.

30. Wolff SN. High-dose BCNU and high-dose VP-16-213: a treatment regimen demonstrating enhanced hepatic toxicity. Cancer Treat Rep 1987;70:1464–1465.

48

Autologous Bone Marrow Transplantation for Miscellaneous Tumors

Bruce D. Cheson

The number of patients treated with high-dose chemotherapy and autologous bone marrow transplantation (ABMT) or peripheral blood stem cell support has been increasing dramatically over the past few years. In an analysis published in 1989 by the International Autologous Bone Marrow Transplant Registry (ABMTR) of ABMT conducted at 112 centers worldwide, the number of transplants had increased from 265 in 1981 to over 1200 in 1987. This figure exceeded 3000 worldwide in 1990, approximately half of which were conducted in the United States (J Armitage, personal communication). Lymphomas and solid tumors have accounted for 94% of the ABMT performed in the United States. This number is divided approximately equally between the two categories of diseases (1). The remaining 6% of ABMT was conducted primarily for leukemia.

The relative frequency with which ABMT has been performed for various solid tumors relates to the overall number of patients with that tumor, the inherent chemosensitivity of the tumor, the availability of effective alternative therapies, the median age of patients with that malignancy (i.e., the number who are young enough to tolerate the procedure),

and the frequency of concurrent comorbid diseases (e.g., pulmonary disease in lung cancer patients, malnutrition in head and neck cancer patients), which would render a patient a poor candidate for ABMT. The majority of 1361 cases described in a recent review of the published literature (2) were performed for lung cancer (214 small cell, 13 non-small-cell, and 30 unspecified diagnoses), melanoma (283), and breast cancer (138). Relatively few cases have been reported for some of the most common, although relatively chemoresistant, tumors (e.g., colorectal cancer, 109 cases) and for some of the less prevalent malignancies (e.g., neuroendocrine tumors, 8 cases); these consist primarily of individual cases accrued to phase I trials, and an occasional phase II trial. These published figures, particularly for breast cancer, substantially underrepresent the number of procedures that have actually been performed.

This chapter will review the available literature on the status of the miscellaneous group of tumors not dealt with elsewhere in this text because they are either rare tumors or less commonly treated with ABMT, and will suggest future directions for research in ABMT for these diseases.

GASTROINTESTINAL MALIGNANCIES

Colorectal Cancer

Colorectal cancer is one of the most common tumors in adults. Approximately 160,000 cases are diagnosed in the United States each year. Recent studies have suggested a survival advantage for patients with Dukes' C colon cancer treated with 5-fluorouracil (5-FU) plus levamisole as an adjuvant following curative surgical resection (3). The addition of leucovorin to 5-FU increases the response rate in patients with metastatic disease compared with 5-FU alone, although not consistently accompanied by a prolongation of survival (4, 5). Unfortunately, no systemic therapy has substantially altered the survival of patients with advanced disease, which primarily reflects a lack of active chemotherapy agents (6).

In spite of the lack of activity of chemotherapy agents at conventional doses to achieve either complete responses or dramatically improve survival, several drugs and combination regimens have been evaluated in the ABMT setting (Tables 48.1, 48.2).

SINGLE AGENTS

Alkylating agents are relatively inactive at standard doses against advanced colorectal cancer. For example, Knight et al. (20) treated 43 patients with 30 mg/m^2 (n = 38) or 40 mg/m^2 (n = 5) of intravenous melphalan and observed only two complete remissions and one partial remission lasting 2 months, 28 months, and 2 months, respectively. Nevertheless, this class of drugs, and melphalan in particular, has been the most extensively evaluated in the ABMT setting. Corringham et al. (7) treated 2 patients with melphalan (1 with 120 mg/m^2, the other with 140 mg/m^2) following cyclophosphamide (CPA) pretreatment in an attempt to accelerate hematologic recovery. One patient achieved a partial response lasting 8 weeks; the other patient progressed. Herzig et al. (8) treated 7 patients at

doses of melphalan more closely approximating the maximum tolerated dose (180–225 mg/m^2) and noted one complete response and three partial responses of 2, 2, 3, and 3 months' duration. Leff et al. (9) treated 20 patients with metastatic colon cancer using melphalan at 180 mg/m^2. They achieved three complete responses and six partial responses for an overall response rate of 45%. Prior therapy with 5-FU did not appear to influence the likelihood of a response. Despite the high response rate, the median survival was only 6½ months. Knight et al. (10) included 20 colon cancer patients in a broad phase II trial in which patients were treated with melphalan at a dose of 180 mg/m^2. There was one complete response and nine partial responses. Although the response duration data were not presented by individual disease, the median duration for their entire series was only 12 weeks.

Spitzer et al. (11) attempted to augment the efficacy of melphalan by combining the drug at a dose of 120–180 mg/m^2 with the radiosensitizer misonidazole. The stated rationale was based on in vitro and animal model data suggesting that misonidazole enhances the tumor cytotoxicity of alkylating agents (21, 22). Of 14 patients, 6 achieved a partial response, with a median duration of response of 4 months (range 3–10 months). Based on this limited experience, the addition of misonidazole to melphalan does not appear to be superior to melphalan alone.

Fay et al. (12) used escalating doses of thiotepa (180–1575 mg/m^2) to treat 22 patients. Three of these patients had received prior radiation therapy and 13 prior 5-FU-based chemotherapy. The investigators noted 1 complete response lasting 96 days and 12 partial responses. The overall median response duration was 5 months. Most of the responses occurred at doses of at least 900 mg/m^2, suggesting a dose-response effect. Thirteen patients died from progression of their colon cancer; in addition there were four treatment-related deaths, three from sepsis and one from hemorrhage into the central ner-

Table 48.1. Response Rates to Single-Agent High-Dose Chemotherapy with Autologous Bone Marrow Transplantation—Miscellaneous Solid Tumors

Tumor	Patients	Complete Remission	Partial Remission	Total Remission	Overall Response (%)	Duration of Response	Reference
High-dose chemotherapy							
Colon	97	7	39	46	47	2 weeks–24 mos.	Corringham (7)
							Herzig (8)
							Leff (9)
							Knight (10)
							Spitzer (11)[a]
							Fay (12)
							Karanes (13)
							Shea (14)
							Lazarus (19)
Gastric	5	0	1	1	20	1 mo.	Herzig (8, 24)
							Karanes (13)
Pancreatic	3	0	0	0	0	—	Herzig (8)
							Karanes (13)
Esophageal	1	0	0	0	0	—	Herzig (8)
Renal cell	5	0	2	2	40	3, 3 mos.	Knight (10)
							Shea (14)
							Lazarus (19)
Unknown primary or undifferentiated	7	1	4	5	71	1, 1+, 2+, 4, 3 mos.	Herzig (8,24) Lazarus (19)
Cervical	2	0	0	0	0	—	Shea (14)
Uterine	1	0	0	0	0	—	Shea (14)
High-dose chemoradiotherapy							
Nasopharyngeal	2	2[b]	0	2	100	8.5, 48.5 mos.	Harada (27)

[a]Misonidazole also administered.
[b]One patient in complete remission, one in partial remission after prior treatment.

Table 48.2. Response Rates to High-Dose Combination Chemotherapy with Autologous Bone Marrow Transplantation—Miscellaneous Solid Tumors

Tumor	Patients	Complete Remission	Partial Remission	Total Remission	Overall Response (%)	Duration of Response	Reference
High-dose chemotherapy							
Colorectal	10	1	5	6	60	2–4 mos.	Williams (15)
							Antman (16)
							Shpall (17)
							Slease (18)
Gastric	3	0	1	1	33	3 mos.	Peters (23)
							Mulder (25)
Cholangiocarcinoma	1	0	0	0	0	—	Elias (26)
Nasopharyngeal	1	0	1	1	100	2 mos.	Antman (16)
Neuroendocrine	8	2	1	3	38	Surv: 2–60 mos.	Stewart (28)
Undifferentiated carcinoma	1	0	0	0	0	NE[a]: ?toxic death	Slease (18)

[a]NE, not evaluable.

vous system as a result of drug-induced thrombocytopenia. Herzig et al. (8) treated 4 patients with carmustine (BCNU) (600–1200 mg/m² doses on 3 consecutive days) and observed 1 complete response and 1 partial response, lasting 24 and 5 months, respectively.

There has been limited evaluation of other classes of chemotherapy drugs. Karanes et al. (13) treated four colon cancer patients with mitomycin-C using a variety of dose schedules, each totaling 60 mg/m². There was one brief partial response. Nonhematologic toxicity, particularly venoocclusive disease of the liver, was felt to be prohibitive. Occasional patients have been treated on phase I studies with other agents, including carboplatin, but the number of cases is insufficient to characterize a response rate (14).

COMBINATION CHEMOTHERAPY

Since most of the single-agent high-dose experience has been with alkylating agents, combination chemotherapy regimens for ABMT to treat colon cancer have most often consisted of multiple alkylating agents. Williams et al. (15) administered a fixed dose of 7.5 g/m² of cyclophosphamide over 3 days, while escalating the dose of thiotepa. One of two patients with colon cancer achieved a partial response. Antman et al. (16) treated two patients with cyclophosphamide, cisplatin, and BCNU in a phase I trial. Neither patient responded. Shpall et al. (17) used cyclophosphamide, cisplatin, and thiotepa, and noted one partial response although it is not clear whether one or two patients with colon cancer were included in the series. The median duration of response in the entire series was 2 months. Slease et al. (18) treated five patients at one of three dose levels of BCNU (600–900 mg/m²) plus cyclophosphamide (160–200 mg/kg). They reported one complete response and three partial responses lasting 3, 4, 2, and 2 months, respectively. Two of the patients experienced a toxic death, including the complete responder. No apparent improvement in response rate or dura-

tion of response or survival with any of these combinations could be detected compared with the similarly disappointing results with single agents.

GASTRIC CANCER

There is considerably less experience with high-dose chemotherapy and ABMT in gastric cancer than with colorectal cancer (Tables 48.1, 48.2). Like colorectal cancer, alkylating agents have been most often used. The few reported patients with gastric cancer have been treated almost exclusively on phase I studies accruing a heterogeneous group of patients with various refractory malignancies. Peters et al. (23) treated two patients with melphalan, cyclophosphamide, and cisplatin, both of whom died; one experienced an early septic death, the other acute cardiac failure. Herzig et al. (24) used high-doses of thiotepa on two patients and reported a single partial response lasting 1 month. Neither of their BCNU-treated patients responded. Mulder et al. (25) treated one patient with the combination of high-dose cyclophosphamide (7 g/m²) and mitoxantrone (45 mg/m²) and observed a partial response that lasted 3 months.

There has been limited experience with other chemotherapy agents in gastric cancer. The single reported patient treated with mitomycin-C failed to respond (13). Similarly poor results have been reported with various regimens in the few cases with esophageal cancer, pancreatic cancer, or cholangiocarcinoma (Tables 48.1, 48.2) (8, 13, 26).

NASOPHARYNGEAL CANCER

Patients with nasopharyngeal cancer are generally poor candidates for ABMT because of the high frequency of associated chronic pulmonary disease and the generally debilitated state of these patients. Antman et al. (16) treated one patient with a combination of cyclophosphamide, cisplatin, and BCNU and achieved a partial response lasting 2 months. Harada et al. (27) used a preparative regimen of cyclophosphamide and TBI to treat two patients, one of whom was already disease-free and the other of whom was in a partial response at the time of high-dose chemotherapy and ABMT. The complete responder remained disease-free at 48.5+ months. However, whether this was the result of the primary therapy or of the ABMT was not clear. The partial responder was converted to a complete response with high-dose chemotherapy; however, the duration of the response was brief, although the patient was alive at 27.5+ months following additional salvage therapy.

NEUROENDOCRINE TUMORS

Stewart et al. (28) treated eight patients with recurrent esthesioneuroblastoma or undifferentiated carcinoma of the nasal or sinus cavity using a variety of high-dose regimens (etoposide/cyclophosphamide, cyclophoshamide/Adriamycin/vinblastine [CAV], BCNU/etoposide/cyclophosphamide, thiotepa). Two complete remissions were achieved in CAV-treated patients, both with an esthesioneuroblastoma. One was disease-free at 18 months; the other relapsed at 60 months and underwent another, unsuccessful, ABMT and died from aspiration pneumonia. Residual tumor was documented at autopsy. One patient with sinonasal carcinoma achieved a 3-month partial response with CAV.

RENAL CANCER

Very few cases of ABMT for renal cancer have been reported in the literature (10, 14, 19). Knight et al. (10) used high doses of melphalan and achieved one partial response of two evaluable patients. Lazarus et al. (19) used high-dose thiotepa in three patients and achieved one partial response that lasted 3 months.

CARCINOMA OF UNKNOWN PRIMARY

Patients have also been treated with ABMT for a tumor that is either too undiffer-

entiated to permit a precise histologic diagnosis or for which the site of the primary cannot be identified (8, 18, 19, 23). The published data have been generated from phase I trials. Herzig et al. (8) achieved a complete response using BCNU in a patient with adenocarcinoma of unknown primary and brain metastases, although the total number of treated cases was not provided. The same investigators (23) used high-dose thiotepa to achieve partial responses in all four patients with an unknown primary. These responses lasted 1, 1+, 2+, and 4 months. Lazarus et al. (19) also used high-dose thiotepa in two cases, neither of whom responded. Slease et al. (18) treated one patient with undifferentiated cancer to a partial response; however, the patient died from treatment-related toxicity at 4 months.

GYNECOLOGIC MALIGNANCIES

Of the gynecologic malignancies treated with ABMT, the majority have been for ovarian cancer (2). Only an occasional patient with cervical or endometrial cancer has been accrued to clinical trials, and responses have been rare (14).

SUMMARY AND CONCLUSIONS

At one time ABMT was conducted exclusively by experienced investigators at established transplant centers with staff who were skilled in supportive care. Now, however, this procedure is being performed at a large, and constantly growing, number of hospitals around the world. Initially, ABMT was an experimental form of clinical research; it is now increasingly being performed as a clinical service, despite the expense and toxicity of this therapy, and the limited number of diseases for which it is effective. ABMT has become a standard approach to a number of disease states, such as relapsed Hodgkin's disease or non-Hodgkin's lymphoma, acute myeloid leukemia and acute lymphocytic leukemia in second or subsequent remission, and neuroblastoma. Several trials are currently attempting to confirm uncontrolled data that suggest that ABMT is superior to standard treatment for women either at high risk for recurrence following mastectomy (e.g., more than 10 positive nodes) or those with metastatic breast disease.

Although responses can be achieved in patients with a variety of other tumor types, survival is not necessarily prolonged. For example, when the data with alkylating agents in advanced colorectal cancer are pooled from Tables 48.1 and 48.2, the complete response rate is 7% and the partial response rate is 41%, for an overall response rate of 49%. Nevertheless, the duration of response ranges from 2 weeks (which does not fulfill the standard time criteria for a response) to 24 months (Tables 48.1 and 48.2), most often 1–3 months. Therefore, it is not appropriate to subject a patient to this treatment as routine therapy outside of a clinical trial setting.

The limited data that are available for ABMT in patients with the miscellaneous refractory tumors included in this chapter are difficult to interpret. Relatively small numbers of patients have been treated with a variety of regimens of different intensities. Complete responses are uncommon, and, in general, the duration of these responses is brief. There are a number of explanations for the disappointing results; patients in these studies have generally failed multiple prior regimens. Although performance status and other important prognostic information are often not provided, it is likely that many of these patients are in relatively poor condition at the time of ABMT. Most of the ABMT data are from phase I trials, which are not designed to assess response but are used to identify a maximum tolerated dose of a drug or regimen. Therefore, a subset of patients in each of these studies is treated at doses that are suboptimal. The disappointing results even in this setting have tempered enthusiasm for further study—a self-fulfilling prophecy in which tumors that are less likely to respond are those least likely to be studied.

There are a number of obstacles to the development of ABMT for patients with advanced, chemoresistant tumors. The first and most critical problem is the lack of effective agents, particularly those with myelosuppression as their dose-limiting toxicity. For example, 5-FU is the most active single agent in advanced colorectal cancer; however, this agent is not useful for ABMT because of its nonhematologic, dose-limiting toxicities such as mucositis and neurotoxicity. Few other drugs have demonstrated activity against this disease (6). To date, most of the data with ABMT are with drugs such as melphalan and thiotepa, which are inactive at conventional doses against colorectal cancer, as well as other gastrointestinal tumors and renal cancer (20). Therefore, there is no justification for continuing to treat patients with currently available agents that are unlikely to induce responses merely because they are the only ones that are amenable for high-dose treatment.

In vitro chemosensitivity studies should make it possible to predict which new agents are most likely to be active at high doses in specific tumor types (30). For example, clinically responsive tumors, such as lymphoma and small cell lung cancer, tend to show the steepest in-vitro dose-response effects, whereas the clinically refractory tumors, such as colon cancer, show the shallowest effects. Unfortunately, these assays are neither readily available nor uniformly predictive.

Once a drug has demonstrated activity at conventional doses, there is a stronger rationale to use that drug at high doses. When dose escalation of certain agents is not possible because of nonhematologic dose-limiting toxicities, analogues may provide a reasonable alternative. For example, cisplatin induces responses in patients with nasopharyngeal cancer; however, the dose of this agent cannot be escalated because of the risk of renal and neurologic toxicity. In contrast, the dose-limiting side effect of carboplatin is myelotoxicity, and therefore, this analogue may be worth evaluating in the ABMT setting (14). A number of other agents are currently in development for high-dose chemotherapy regimens, although few are active against the miscellaneous group of tumors under discussion. When there is a suggestion of activity for a new drug in these tumor types, a careful phase II study should be designed and conducted in an optimal patient population (e.g., those with good performance status and organ function and minimal prior therapy). This approach is particularly relevant for those tumors for which there is no effective conventional treatment.

It is likely that combinations of active drugs will be more effective than single agents. The operating philosophy in the development of combination regimens should be that each of the components must be active against that specific tumor; otherwise the patient will be subjected to additional toxicity from the less active drugs while compromising the potential benefit of the active components because of requisite dose reductions.

To date, simply escalating the dose of currently available chemotherapy drugs has not influenced the survival of patients with refractory tumors. There is a need to identify new drugs and to optimize the delivery of available drugs. Some strategies that are currently being pursued for ABMT in the more sensitive tumors (e.g., multiple transplants, combinations and sequences of agents, and the use of chemoprotectors) are, unfortunately, premature for the chemoresistant tumors until active agents are available. Other alternatives include modulating the activity of available agents; for example, buthionine sulfoxamine is currently being tested for its ability to overcome clinical resistance to alkylating agents.

A second problem compromising the development of ABMT has been the slow accrual to clinical trials. Only a relatively small proportion of patients who receive ABMT are treated on these studies. As a result, the rate at which high-dose chemotherapy programs can be developed for various malignancies is compromised. Clinical trials with ABMT have mostly been phase I studies including a heterogeneous group of patients, conducted primarily at single centers, where accrual and resources are limited. These studies may take years to complete and often do not identify diseases worth pursuing in phase II studies because of the small numbers of patients with each tumor type. Nevertheless, the developmental studies required for the chemoresistant tumors need to be conducted at a restricted number of institutions with expertise in ABMT so that appropriate pharmacokinetic studies and supportive care are available. Patients who are not likely to benefit from conventional therapy should be considered for referral to centers involved in clinical trials of ABMT. A promising result should be rapidly confirmed in a multiinstitutional trial. Currently, the NCI-sponsored cooperative oncology groups are conducting clinical trials with ABMT, although primarily in diseases that have already been demonstrated to be sensitive to high-dose chemotherapy (e.g., breast cancer, leukemia, lymphoma, neuroblastoma). However, for patients with the more refractory malignancies, the cooperative groups could potentially provide a unique resource for testing new ideas, as they become available. Increased participation in clinical trials will permit important clinical questions to be addressed in a timely fashion and will facilitate the availability of improvements in care to the general oncology community.

For most tumors, ABMT has not demonstrated substantial clinical benefit, despite considerable morbidity, mortality, and expense. Therefore, ABMT should be based on a solid scientific foundation and restricted to clinical situations in which a meaningful improvement in survival can be anticipated. Patients with refractory tumors, who are unlikely to experience a clinically meaningful prolongation of survival from ABMT, should only be treated on a clinical trial that is addressing an important scientific question. That is not to say that the indications for ABMT will not change; to the contrary, as new active agents are identified and new strategies are developed, therapeutic advances may broaden the applicability of this modality. Continued study of the biology of these tumors will permit a better understanding of the relevant mechanisms of drug resistance. Future studies should then apply these observations to the treatment of patients with refractory malignancies.

REFERENCES

1. Advisory Committee of the International Autologous Bone Marrow Transplant Registry. Autologous bone marrow transplants: different indications in Europe and North America. Lancet 1989;2:317–318.
2. Cheson BD, Lacerna L, Leyland-Jones B, Sarosy G, Wittes RE. Autologous bone marrow transplantation. Ann Intern Med 1989;110:51–65.
3. Moertel CG, Fleming TR, Macdonald JS, et al. Lavamisole and fluorouracil for adjuvant therapy of resected colon carcinoma. N Engl J Med 1990;322:352–358.
4. Petrelli N, Herrera L, Rustum Y, et al. A prospective randomized trial of 5-fluorouracil versus 5-fluorouracil and high-dose leucovorin versus 5-fluorouracil and methotrexate in previously untreated patients with advanced colorectal carcinoma. J Clin Oncol 1987;5:1559–1565.
5. O'Connell MJ. A phase III trial of 5-flourouracil and leucovorin in the treatment of advanced colorectal cancer. A Mayo Clinic/North Central Cancer Treatment Group study. Cancer 1989;63:1026–1030.
6. Kemeny N. Role of chemotherapy in the treatment of colorectal carcinoma. Semin Surg Oncol 1987; 3:190–214.
7. Corringham R, Gilmore M, Prentice HG, Boesen E. High-dose melphalan with autologous bone marrow transplant. Cancer 1983;52(10):1783–1787.
8. Herzig RH, Phillips GL, Lazarus HM, et al. Intensive chemotherapy and autologous bone marrow transplantation for the treatment of refractory malignancies. In: Dicke KA, Spitzer G, Zander AR, eds. Autologous bone marrow transplantation: proceedings of the first international symposium. Houston: University of Texas MD Anderson Hospital and Tumor Institute, 1985:197–202.
9. Leff RS, Thompson JM, Johnson DB, et al. Phase II trial of high-dose melphalan and autologous bone marrow transplantation for metastatic colon carcinoma. J Clin Oncol 1986;4:1586–1591.
10. Knight WA, Page CP, Kuhn JG, Clark GM, Newcomb TF. High dose L-PAM and autologous marrow infusion for refractory solid tumors [Abstract]. Proc. Am Soc Clin Oncol 1984;3:150.
11. Spitzer TR, Lazarus HM, Creger RJ, Berger NA. High-dose melphalan, misonidazole and autologous bone marrow transplantation for the treatment of metastatic colorectal carcinoma. Am J Clin Oncol 1989; 12:145–151.
12. Fay JW, Herzig RH, Herzig GP, Wolff SN, members of the North American Marrow Transplantation Group. Treatment of metastatic colon carcinoma with intensive thiotepa and autologous marrow transplantation. In: Herzig GP, ed. Advances in cancer chemotherapy: high-dose thiotepa and autologous marrow transplantation. New York: Wiley & Sons, 1987:31–34.
13. Karanes C, Ratanatharathorn V, Schilcher RB, et al. High-dose mitomycin-C with autologous bone marrow transplantation in patients with refractory malignancies. Am J Clin Oncol 1986;9:444–448.
14. Shea TC, Flaherty M, Elias A, et al. A phase I study of high-dose carboplatin. In: Dicke KA, Spitzer G, Jagannath S, Evinger-Hodges MJ, eds. Autologous bone marrow transplantation: proceedings of the fourth international symposium. Houston: University of Texas MD Anderson Hospital and Tumor Institute, 1985:519–523.
15. Williams SF, Bitran JD, Kaminer L, et al. A phase I-II study of bialkylator chemotherapy, high-dose thiotepa, and cyclophosphamide with autologous bone marrow reinfusion in patients with advanced cancer. J Clin Oncol 1987;5:260–265.
16. Antman K, Eder JP, Elias A, et al. High-dose combination alkylating agent preparative regimen with autologous bone marrow support: the Dana-Farber Cancer Institute/Beth Israel Hospital experience. Cancer Treat Rep 1987;71:119–125.
17. Shpall E, Jones R, Egorin M, et al. A phase I trial of high-dose combinatin cyclophosphamide (C), cisplatinum (P) and thiotepa (T) with autologous bone marrow support (ABMS) in the treatment of resistant solid tumors [Abstract]. Proc Am Soc Clin Oncol 1987;6:139.
18. Slease RB, Benear JB, Selby GB, et al. High-dose combination alkylating agent therapy with autologous bone marrow rescue for refractory solid tumors. J Clin Oncol 1988;6:1314–1320.
19. Lazarus HM, Reed MD, Spitzer TR, Rabas MS, Blumer JL. High-dose IV thiotepa and cryopreserved autologous bone marrow transplantation for therapy of refractory cancer. Cancer Treat Rep 1987;71:689–695.
20. Knight WA, Goodman P, Taylor SA, et al. Phase II trial of intravenous melphalan for metastatic colorectal carcinoma. Invest New Drugs 1990;8:S87–S89.
21. Clement JC, Gorman MS, Wodinsky I. Enhancement of antitumor activity of alkylating agents by the radiation sensitizer misonidazole. Cancer Res 1980; 40:4165–4172.
22. Brown JM, Hirst DG. Effect of clinical levels of misonidazole on the response of tumor and normal tissues in the mouse to alkylating agents. Br J Cancer 1982;45:700–708.

23. Peters WP, Stuart A, Klotman M, et al. High-dose combination cyclophosphamide, cisplatin, and melphalan with autologous bone marrow support. Cancer Chemother Pharmacol 1989;23:377–383.

24. Herzig RH, Fay JW, Herzig GP, et al. Phase I-II studies with high-dose thiotepa and autologous marrow transplantation in patients with refractory malignancies. In: Herzig GP, ed. Advances in cancer chemotherapy: high-dose thiotepa and autologous marrow transplantation. New York: Wiley & Sons, 1987:17–23.

25. Mulder POM, Sleijfer, DT, Willemse PHB, de Vries, EGE, Uges DRA, Mulder NH. High-dose cyclophosphamide or melphalan with escalating doses of mitoxantrone and autologous bone marrow transplantation for refractory solid tumors. Cancer Res 1989; 49:4654–4658.

26. Elias AD, Ayash LJ, Eder JP, et al. A phase I study of high-dose ifosfamide and escalating doses of carboplatin with autologous bone marrow support. J Clin Oncol 1991;9(2):320–327.

27. Harada M, Yoshida T, Funada H, Hattori K-I, Kanazawa University Bone Marrow Transplant Team. Clinical trial of intensive therapy and autologous bone marrow transplantation in the treatment of malignant diseases. Jpn J Clin Oncol 1984;14(suppl 1):543–552.

28. Stewart FM, Lazarus HM, Levine PA, Stewart KA, Tabbara IA, Spaulding CA. High-dose chemotherapy and autologous marrow transplantation for esthesioneuroblastoma and sinonasal undifferentiated carcinoma. Am J Clin Oncol 1989;12:217–221.

29. Sarosy G, Leyland-Jones B, Soochan P, Cheson BD. The systemic administration of intravenous melphalan. J Clin Oncol 1988;6:1768–1782.

30. Von Hoff DD, Clark GM, Weiss GR, et al. Use of in vitro dose response effects to select antineoplastics for high-dose or regional administration regimens. J Clin Oncol 1986;4:1827–1834.

INDEX

Page numbers in italic denote figures; those followed by "t" denote tables.